[redacted]

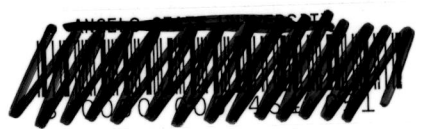

The Best of BYTE

UROLOGIC ONCOLOGY

JOSEPH E. OESTERLING, M.D.
Professor and Urologist-in-Chief
Director, The Michigan Prostate Institute
The University of Michigan
Ann Arbor, Michigan

JEROME P. RICHIE, M.D.
Elliott C. Cutler Professor of Urologic Surgery
Chief of Urology
Brigham and Women's Hospital
Harvard Medical School
Boston, Massachusetts

W.B. SAUNDERS COMPANY
A Division of Harcourt Brace & Company
Philadelphia ▪ London ▪ Toronto ▪ Montreal ▪ Sydney ▪ Tokyo

W.B. SAUNDERS COMPANY
A Division of Harcourt Brace & Company

The Curtis Center
Independence Square West
Philadelphia, Pennsylvania 19106

Library of Congress Cataloging-in-Publication Data

Urologic oncology / [edited by] Joseph E. Oesterling, Jerome Richie.
p. cm.
ISBN 0-7216-6347-8
1. Genitourinary organs—Cancer. I. Oesterling, Joseph E. II. Richie, Jerome P.
[DNLM: 1. Urologic Neoplasms—diagnosis. 2. Urologic Neoplasms—therapy. WJ 160 U7843 1997]
RC280.G4U783 1997
616.99'46—dc20
DNLM/DLC 96-41702

UROLOGIC ONCOLOGY ISBN 0–7216–6347–8

Printed in the United States of America.

Last digit is the print number: 9 8 7 6 5 4 3 2 1

CONTRIBUTORS

RICHARD B. ALEXANDER, M.D.
Associate Professor, Division of Urology, University of Maryland School of Medicine; Chief of Urology, Maryland VA Health Care System, Baltimore, Maryland
Immunotherapy: Basic Principles

ALEX F. ALTHAUSEN, M.D.
Associate Professor of Surgery (Urology), Harvard Medical School; Senior Urologist, Massachusetts General Hospital, Boston, Massachusetts
Transurethral Surgery Plus Chemo-Radiation for Selective Bladder Preservation

ANTONIO PURAS BAEZ, M.D., F.A.C.S.
Associate Professor and Chairman, Urology Section, University of Puerto Rico School of Medicine; University District Hospital, San Juan, Puerto Rico
Invasive Carcinoma of the Penis: Management and Prognosis

GREGORY W. BARAN, M.D.
Assistant Clinical Professor, Department of Radiology, Case Western Reserve University, Cleveland, Ohio
Creative Modalities

MARIO C. BEDUSCHI, M.D.
Fellow in Urologic-Oncology and Research Investigator, The Michigan Prostate Institute, University of Michigan, Ann Arbor, Michigan
Urethral Carcinoma: Diagnosis and Staging

ARIE BELLDEGRUN, M.D., F.A.C.S.
Professor of Urology, Chief, Division of Urologic Oncology, Department of Urology, University of California, Los Angeles; Urologist, UCLA Medical Center, Olive View Medical Center, Los Angeles, California
Tumor Immunity

BRENT A. BLUMENSTEIN, Ph.D.
Affiliate Professor of Urology, Affiliate Professor of Biostatistics, University of Washington; Genitourinary Cancer Biostatistician, Southwest Oncology Group Statistical Center, Fred Hutchinson Cancer Research Center, Seattle, Washington
The Randomized Clinical Trial

BARRY M. BRENNER, M.D.
Samuel A. Levine Professor of Medicine, Harvard Medical School; Director, Renal Division, Brigham and Women's Hospital, Boston, Massachusetts
Acute and Chronic Renal Disease in Urologic Oncology

CHARLES R. BURKE, M.D.
Assistant Clinical Professor—Urology, Tufts University School of Medicine; Formerly Clinical Instructor in Urology, Boston University School of Medicine, Boston, Massachusetts
Surgery of Adrenal Tumors

BRUCE CARLIN, M.D.
Resident in Urology, Case Western Reserve University, Cleveland, Ohio
Creative Modalities

VICTOR L. CARPINIELLO, M.D.
Clinical Associate Professor, University of Pennsylvania; Staff Urologist, Pennsylvania Hospital, Philadelphia, Pennsylvania
Superficial Carcinoma of the Penis: Management and Prognosis

MICHAEL C. CARR, M.D. Ph.D.
Assistant Professor of Urology, University of Washington School of Medicine; Attending Surgeon, Division of Pediatric Urology, Children's Hospital and Medical Center, Seattle, Washington
Neuroblastoma

PETER R. CARROLL, M.D.
Chair, Department of Urology, University of California School of Medicine, San Francisco, California
Noncontinent Urinary Diversion

GLENN M. CHERTOW, M.D.
Instructor in Medicine and Surgery, Harvard Medical School; Assistant Director of Dialysis Services, Brigham and Women's Hospital, Boston, Massachusetts
Acute and Chronic Renal Disease in Urologic Oncology

RALPH V. CLAYMAN, M.D.
Professor of Urology and Radiology, Washington University School of Medicine; Barnes Hospital, St. Louis, Missouri
Laparoscopic Oncology

DONALD S. COFFEY, Ph.D.
Professor of Urology, Oncology, Pharmacology and Molecular Sciences, The Johns Hopkins University School of Medicine; Director, Research Laboratories of the Department of Urology, The Johns Hopkins Hospital, Baltimore, Maryland
The Molecular and Cellular Biology of Urologic Cancers

CHRISTOPHER L. COOGAN, M.D.
Instructor, Department of Urology, Rush Medical College; Attending Urologist, Rush Presbyterian St. Luke's Medical Center, Chicago, Illinois
Testis Tumors: Diagnosis and Staging

MAX J. COPPES, M.D., Ph.D.
Associate Professor of Oncology and Pediatrics, University of Calgary; Director, Pediatric Oncology Program, Tom Baker Cancer Center, Alberta Children's Hospital, Calgary, Alberta, Canada
Wilms' Tumor

E. DAVID CRAWFORD, M.D.
Professor of Urology, Associate Director, University of Colorado Cancer Center, University of Colorado, Denver, Colorado
Metastatic Adenocarcinoma of the Prostate (TxNxM+): Management and Prognosis

JEAN B. deKERNION, M.D.
The Fran and Ray Stark Professor of Urology, Interim Chair, UCLA Department of Urology, UCLA School of Medicine, Los Angeles, California
Diagnosis and Staging of Renal Cell Cancer

S. MACHELE DONAT, M.D.
Assistant Professor of Urology, Memorial Sloan-Kettering Cancer Center, Cornell University Medical College, New York, New York
Transitional Cell Carcinoma of the Renal Pelvis and Ureter: Diagnosis, Staging, Management, and Prognosis

JOHN P. DONOHUE, M.D.
Distinguished Professor Emeritus, Department of Urology, Indiana University Medical School, Indianapolis, Indiana
Radical Orchiectomy and Retroperitoneal Lymph Node Dissection

PEMA DORJE, M.D.
Assistant Professor, Department of Anesthesiology, University of Michigan Health System, Ann Arbor, Michigan
Anesthesia for Major Cancer Surgery

MICHAEL J. DROLLER, M.D.
Chief of Urology, Mt. Sinai Medical Center, New York, New York
Diagnosis and Staging of Bladder Cancer

ROBERT C. FLANIGAN, M.D.
Professor and Chairman, Department of Urology, Stritch School of Medicine, Loyola University Medical Center, Maywood, Illinois; Chief, Urology Service, Hines VA Hospital, Hines, Illinois
Urethrectomy

YVES FRADET, M.D., F.R.C.S.(C)
Professor of Urology, Laval University, Department of Surgery/Urology; Uro-oncologist, Director, Experimental Uro-oncology Laboratory, Laval University Cancer Research Center, Chuq-L'Hotel-Dieu de Quebec, Quebec, Canada
Transurethral Surgery of Bladder Tumors

JENNY J. FRANKE, M.D.
Assistant Professor, Department of Urologic Surgery, Vanderbilt University School of Medicine, Nashville, Tennessee
Surgery for Upper Tract Transitional Cell Carcinoma

JOHN R. FRANKLIN, M.D.
Assistant Clinical Professor, Department of Urology, UCLA School of Medicine; Urologic Oncologist, West Los Angeles Veterans Administration Medical Center, Los Angeles, California
Tumor Immunity

JOHN A. FREEMAN, M.D.
Assistant Professor, Division of Urology, Department of Surgery, University of North Carolina School of Medicine, Chapel Hill, North Carolina
Partial Cystectomy and Radical Cystectomy

J. MIGUEL GARCIA-SCHÜRMANN, M.D.
Resident in Training, Ruhr Universitat-Bochum, Germany
The Molecular and Cellular Biology of Urologic Cancers

INDERBIR S. GILL, M.D.
Associate Professor of Urologic Surgery, University of Nebraska Medical Center, Omaha, Nebraska
Laparoscopic Oncology

MARY K. GOSPODAROWICZ, M.D., F.R.C.P.(C)
Professor, Department of Radiation Oncology, University of Toronto; Director, Clinical Programs, Department of Radiation Oncology, Princess Margaret Hospital, Toronto, Ontario, Canada
Seminoma: Management and Prognosis

MIREILLE GRÉGOIRE, M.D., F.R.C.S.(C)
Assistant Professor, Department of Surgery/Urology, Laval University; Urologist, Chuq-L'Hotel-Dieu de Quebec, Quebec, Canada
Transurethral Surgery of Bladder Tumors

JOSEPH F. HARRYHILL, M.D., F.A.C.S.
Staff Urologist, Pennsylvania Hospital, The University of Pennsylvania, Philadelphia, Pennsylvania
Superficial Carcinoma of the Penis: Management and Prognosis

RICHARD E. HAUTMANN, M.D.
Professor and Chairman, Department of Urology, University of Ulm, Ulm, Germany
Orthotopic Bladder Substitution in the Male and Female

TERRY W. HENSLE, M.D.
Professor of Urology, Columbia University College of Physicians and Surgeons; Director of Pediatric Urology, Babies and Childrens Hospital, Columbia Presbyterian Medical Center, New York, New York
Nutritional Issues for the Cancer Patient

HARRY W. HERR, M.D.
Associate Professor of Urology, Memorial Sloan-Kettering Cancer Center, Cornell University Medical College, New York, New York
Transitional Cell Carcinoma of the Renal Pelvis and Ureter: Diagnosis, Staging, Management, and Prognosis

JORGE RIVERA HERRERA, M.D., F.A.C.S.
Assistant Professor, University of Puerto Rico, School of Medicine; Assistant Professor, University District Hospital, San Juan, Puerto Rico
Invasive Carcinoma of the Penis: Management and Prognosis

REGINA M. HOVEY, M.D.
Chief Resident, Department of Urology, University of California School of Medicine, San Francisco, California
Noncontinent Urinary Diversion

LIAM J. HURLEY, M.D.
Assistant Clinical Professor, Urology, Tufts University School of Medicine; Formerly Clinical Instructor in Urology, Boston University School of Medicine, Boston, Massachusetts
Surgery of Adrenal Tumors

MICHAEL A. S. JEWETT, M.D., F.R.C.S.(C)
Professor and Chairman, Division of Urology, University of Toronto; Head, Division of Urology, Toronto Hospital, Toronto, Ontario, Canada
Seminoma: Management and Prognosis

MARTIN KAEFER, M.D.
Pediatric Urology Fellow, Harvard Medical School; Pediatric Urology Fellow, Children's Hospital, Boston, Massachusetts
Rhabdomyosarcoma of the Pelvis and Paratesticular Structures

DONALD S. KAUFMAN, M.D.
Associate Clinical Professor of Medicine, Harvard Medical School; Physician, Massachusetts General Hospital, Boston, Massachusetts
Transurethral Surgery Plus Chemo-Radiation for Selective Bladder Preservation

GHOLAMREZA KHAKPOUR, M.D.
Urologist and Research Fellow, Division of Urology, University of Toronto; Fellow, Division of Urology, Toronto Hospital, Toronto, Ontario, Canada
Seminoma: Management and Prognosis

ERIC A. KLEIN, M.D.
Head, Section, Urologic Oncology, The Cleveland Clinic Foundation, Cleveland, Ohio
Non–Germ Cell Tumors of the Testis

HOWARD J. KORMAN, M.D.
Urologic Oncology Fellow, Department of Urology, University of Miami, School of Medicine; Urologic Oncology Fellow, Jackson Memorial Hospital, Miami, Florida
Superficial Transitional Cell Carcinoma of the Bladder: Management and Prognosis

JAMES C. KU, M.D.
Chief Resident, Department of Urology, Columbia Presbyterian Medical Center, New York, New York
Nutritional Issues for the Cancer Patient

CHERYL T. LEE, M.D.
Urology Resident-in-Training, University of Michigan, Ann Arbor, Michigan
Cancer of the Prostate: Diagnosis and Staging; Bilateral Pelvic Lymphadenectomy and Anatomical Radical Retropubic Prostatectomy

HOWARD S. LEVIN, M.D.
Staff Pathologist, The Cleveland Clinic Foundation, Cleveland, Ohio
Non–Germ Cell Tumors of the Testis

JOHN A. LIBERTINO, M.D.
Assistant Clinical Professor, Harvard Medical School; Chairman, Department of Urology, Lahey Hitchcock Medical Center, Burlington, Massachusetts
Boston, Massachusetts
Surgery of Adrenal Tumors

BRUCE W. LINDGREN, M.D.
Fellow, Pediatric Urology, Long Island Jewish Medical Center, New Hyde Park, New York; Formerly Chief Resident, Urology, Loyola University Chicago Stritch School of Medicine, Maywood, Illinois
Seminal Vesicles: Diagnosis, Staging, Surgery, Management, and Prognosis

KEVIN R. LOUGHLIN, M.D.
Associate Professor of Surgery (Urology), Harvard Medical School; Brigham and Women's Hospital, Boston, Massachusetts
Squamous Cell Carcinoma of the Penis: Diagnosis and Staging

DONALD F. LYNCH, Jr., M.D.
Associate Professor, Department of Urology, Eastern Virginia Medical School, Norfolk, Virginia
Penectomy and Ilioinguinal Dissection

S. BRUCE MALKOWICZ, M.D.
Associate Professor of Urology, Co-Director, Urologic Oncology, University of Pennsylvania School of Medicine, Philadelphia, Pennsylvania
Retroperitoneal Tumors: Diagnosis, Staging, Surgery, Management, and Prognosis

FRAY F. MARSHALL, M.D.
Professor of Urology and Oncology, The Johns Hopkins University School of Medicine; Director, Division of Adult Urology, The Johns Hopkins Medical Institutions, Baltimore, Maryland
Renal Cell Carcinoma: Management and Prognosis

W. SCOTT McDOUGAL, M.D.
Walter S. Kerr Jr. Professor of Urology, Harvard Medical School; Chief of Urology, Massachusetts General Hospital, Boston, Massachusetts
Continent Urinary Diversion

ELSPETH M. McDOUGALL, M.D., F.R.C.S.(C)
Associate Professor of Urologic Surgery, Washington University School of Medicine, St. Louis, Missouri
Laparoscopic Oncology

RICHARD G. MIDDLETON, M.D.
Professor of Surgery and Chairman, Division of Urology, University of Utah School of Medicine, Salt Lake City, Utah
Clinically Localized Adenocarcinoma of the Prostate (Stage T1a–T2c) Management and Prognosis

GARY J. MILLER, M.D., Ph.D.
Professor of Pathology and Urology, University of Colorado Health Sciences Center, Denver, Colorado
Environmental Carcinogenesis

MICHAEL E. MITCHELL, M.D.
Professor of Urology, University of Washington School of Medicine; Chief, Division of Pediatric Urology, Children's Hospital and Medical Center, Seattle, Washington
Neuroblastoma

JAMES E. MONTIE, M.D.
George F. and Nancy P. Valassis Professor of Urologic Oncology, University of Michigan, Ann Arbor, Michigan
Principles of Surgical Oncology

JOEL B. NELSON, M.D.
Assistant Professor of Urology and Oncology, The Johns Hopkins University School of Medicine; Active, Full-time Staff, Johns Hopkins Bayview Medical Center, The Johns Hopkins Hospital, Baltimore, Maryland
Renal Cell Carcinoma: Management and Prognosis

ANDREW C. NOVICK, M.D.
Chairman, Department of Urology, The Cleveland Clinic Foundation, Cleveland, Ohio
Surgery of Renal Cell Carcinoma

JOSEPH E. OESTERLING, M.D.
Professor and Urologist-in-Chief; Director, The Michigan Prostate Institute, The University of Michigan, Ann Arbor, Michigan
Cancer of the Prostate: Diagnosis and Staging; Bilateral Pelvic Lymphadenectomy and Anatomical Radical Retropubic Prostatectomy; Urethral Carcinoma: Diagnosis and Staging

CARL A. OLSSON, M.D.
John K. Lattimer Professor and Chairman, Department of Urology, Columbia University College of Physicians and Surgeons; Chief, Department of Urology, Chief, Squier Urological Clinic, Columbia Presbyterian Medical Center, New York, New York
Invasive Transitional Cell Carcinoma of the Bladder: Prognosis and Management

ALAN W. PARTIN, M.D., Ph.D.
Associate Professor of Urology, The Johns Hopkins University School of Medicine, Baltimore, Maryland
The Molecular and Cellular Biology of Urologic Cancers

ANUP PATEL, M.S., F.R.C.S. (Urol.)
Urologic Oncology Fellow, Department of Urology, UCLA School of Medicine, Los Angeles, California
Diagnosis and Staging of Renal Cell Cancer

DAVID F. PAULSON, M.D.
Professor of Surgery, Chief of Urology, Duke University Medical Center, Durham, North Carolina
Radical Perineal Prostatectomy

CRAIG A. PETERS, M.D.
Assistant Professor, Harvard Medical School; Assistant in Surgery (Urology), Children's Hospital, Boston, Massachusetts
Pediatric Testicular Tumors

DANIEL P. PETRYLAK, M.D.
Assistant Professor of Medicine, Columbia University College of Physicians and Surgeons; Assistant Attending, Columbia Presbyterian Medical Center, New York, New York
Invasive Transitional Cell Carcinoma of the Bladder: Prognosis and Management

LEE B. PRESSLER, M.D.
Chief Resident, Columbia Presbyterian Medical Center, New York, New York
Invasive Transitional Cell Carcinoma of the Bladder: Prognosis and Management

MARTIN I. RESNICK, M.D.
Professor and Chairman, Department of Urology, Case Western Reserve University, Cleveland, Ohio
Creative Modalities

ALAN B. RETIK, M.D.
Professor of Surgery (Urology), Harvard Medical School; Chief, Department of Urology, Children's Hospital, Boston, Massachusetts
Rhabdomyosarcoma of the Pelvis and Paratesticular Structures

JEROME P. RICHIE, M.D.
Elliott C. Cutler Professor of Urologic Surgery, Chief of Urology, Brigham and Women's Hospital, Harvard Medical School, Boston, Massachusetts
Bilateral Pelvic Lymphadenectomy and Anatomical Radical Retropubic Prostatectomy; Nonseminomatous Germ Cell Tumors: Management and Prognosis

MICHAEL L. RITCHEY, M.D.
Associate Professor, Department of Surgery, University of Texas-Houston Medical School; Chief of Pediatric Urology, Hermann Children's Hospital, Houston, Texas
Wilms' Tumor

RANDALL G. ROWLAND, M.D., Ph.D.
Professor and Acting Chairman, Department of Urology, Indiana University School of Medicine, Indianapolis, Indiana
Testis Tumors: Diagnosis and Staging

THOMAS A. ROZANSKI, M.D.
Chief, Urology Service, Brooke Army Medical Center, San Antonio, Texas
Regionally Advanced Adenocarcinoma of the Prostate (T3a–TNx + M0): Management and Prognosis

PAUL SABBATINI, M.D.
Fellow in Medical Oncology, Genitourinary Oncology Service, Division of Solid Tumor Oncology, Department of Medicine, Memorial Sloan-Kettering Cancer Center, New York, New York
General Principles of Chemotherapy

MARTIN G. SANDA, M.D.
Assistant Professor of Urology and Oncology, University of Michigan Medical School; Chief of Urology, Veterans Administration Medical Center, Ann Arbor, Michigan
Genetic Considerations and Gene Therapy

MICHAEL F. SAROSDY, M.D.
Professor of Surgery, Director, Residency Training, Chief, Division of Urology, University of Texas Health Science Center at San Antonio, San Antonio, Texas
Urethral Carcinoma in the Male and Female: Management and Prognosis

PAUL F. SCHELLHAMMER, M.D.
Professor and Chairman, Department of Urology, Eastern Virginia Medical School; Active Staff, Sentara Health System—Norfolk General Hospital, Leigh Memorial Hospital, and Bayside, Norfolk and Virginia Beach, Norfolk, Virginia
Penectomy and Ilioinguinal Dissection

HOWARD I. SCHER, M.D.
Associate Professor of Medicine, Cornell University Medical College; Chief, Genitourinary Oncology Service; Associate Attending Physician, Division of Solid Tumor Oncology, Department of Medicine, Memorial Sloan-Kettering Cancer Center, New York, New York
General Principles of Chemotherapy

FRANCIS X. SCHNECK, M.D.
Assistant Professor, University of Pittsburgh; Pediatric Urologist, Children's Hospital of Pittsburgh, Pittsburgh, Pennsylvania
Pediatric Testicular Tumors

WILLIAM U. SHIPLEY, M.D.
Professor of Radiation Oncology, Harvard Medical School; Head, Genitourinary Oncology, Department of Radiation Oncology, Boston, Massachusetts
The Rationale for the Use of Radiation Therapy in the Treatment of Urologic Malignancies, Transurethral Surgery Plus Chemo-Radiation for Selective Bladder Preservation

DONALD G. SKINNER, M.D.
Professor and Chairman, Department of Urology, University of Southern California School of Medicine, Los Angeles, California
Partial Cystectomy and Radical Cystectomy

JOSEPH A. SMITH, Jr., M.D.
William L. Bray Professor and Chairman, Department of Urologic Surgery, Vanderbilt University School of Medicine, Nashville, Tennessee
Surgery for Upper Tract Transitional Cell Carcinoma

MARK S. SOLOWAY, M.D.
Professor and Chairman, Department of Urology, University of Miami School of Medicine; Chief, Urology Section, Jackson Memorial Hospital, Miami, Florida
Superficial Transitional Cell Carcinoma of the Bladder: Management and Prognosis

IRA J. SPIRO, M.D., Ph.D.
Assistant Professor, Harvard Medical School; Assistant Radiation Oncologist, Massachusetts General Hospital, Boston, Massachusetts
The Rationale for the Use of Radiation Therapy in the Treatment of Urologic Malignancies

PATRICIA J. TERRY, M.D.
Clinical Instructor, University of Texas Health Science Center at San Antonio, San Antonio, Texas
Urethral Carcinoma in the Male and Female: Management and Prognosis

IAN M. THOMPSON, M.D.
Chairman and Associate Professor, Department of Surgery; Associate Professor, Department of Surgery, Uniformed Services, University of the Health Sciences, Bethesda, Maryland; Chairman, Department of Surgery, Brooke Army Medical Center, San Antonio, Texas
Regionally Advanced Adenocarcinoma of the Prostate (T3a–TNx + M0): Management and Prognosis

KEVIN K. TREMPER, M.D., Ph.D.
Professor and Chair, Department and Anesthesiology, University of Michigan Health System, Ann Arbor, Michigan
Anesthesia for Major Cancer Surgery

E. DARRACOTT VAUGHAN, Jr., M.D.
James J. Colt Professor of Urology, Cornell University Medical College; Urologist-in-Chief, The New York Hospital, New York, New York
Adrenal Tumors

MARK A. WAINSTEIN, M.D.
Chief Resident in Urology, Case Western Reserve University, Cleveland, Ohio
Creative Modalities

W. BEDFORD WATERS, M.D.
Professor of Urology, Loyola University Chicago Stritch School of Medicine, Maywood, Illinois; Associate Director, Department of Urology, Associate Chief, Urology Section, Hines VA Medical Center, Hines, Illinois
Seminal Vesicles: Diagnosis, Staging, Surgery, Management, and Prognosis

ROGER B. WATSON, M.D.
Urologic Oncology Fellow, Department of Urology, University of Miami School of Medicine; Urologic Oncology Fellowship, Department of Urology, Jackson Memorial Hospital, Miami, Florida
Superficial Transitional Cell Carcinoma of the Bladder: Management and Prognosis

STEVE WAXMAN, M.D.
Assistant Clinical Professor of Urology, University of Colorado, Denver, Colorado
Metastatic Adenocarcinoma of the Prostate (TxNxM+): Management and Prognosis

PETER R. WILSON, Ph.D.
Associate Professor, Mayo Medical School, Rochester, Minnesota
Pain Control and Supportive Care of the Terminal Patient

KENNETH I. WISHNOW, M.D.
Associate Professor of Surgery, Harvard Medical School; Active Staff, Beth Israel-Deaconess Medical Center, Boston, Massachusetts
Urethral Carcinoma: Diagnosis and Staging

GILBERT Y. WONG, M.D.
Instructor, Mayo Medical School, Rochester, Minnesota
Pain Control and Supportive Care of the Terminal Patient

PREFACE

The field of urology has undergone significant advances in the past 10 years, with numerous changes occurring in all the domains of urology. Urologic oncology, perhaps more than any other area, has experienced the greatest steps forward. This is particularly true for prostate cancer, where three major developments have altered forever the diagnosis and management of this disease. They are: (1) the discovery of prostate-specific antigen (PSA) as an effective tumor marker for prostate cancer; (2) the development of the anatomic approach to radical prostatectomy in order to enhance cancer removal while reducing associated morbidity; and (3) the bringing together of transrectal ultrasound and the biopsy gun to make prostate biopsy an accurate, pain-free, outpatient procedure. Because of dramatic advances, such as these, that have occurred throughout the entire discipline of urologic oncology, we decided to produce a comprehensive textbook, written predominantly by urologists who are experts in the field, entitled *Urologic Oncology*.

This book is organized into 12 sections, in which the basic principles of medical and surgical urologic oncology are discussed, and each organ of the genitourinary tract (adrenal gland to the penis) is covered in a concise but comprehensive manner. Each section consists of two to seven chapters that review each tumor type for that particular site with regard to (1) incidence, (2) etiology, (3) clinical presentation, (4) diagnosis, (5) staging, (6) nonsurgical and surgical management options, (7) prognosis, and (8) future directions for research.

In addition, the surgical procedures performed for the cancers of the genitourinary tract—conservative and radical, endoscopic and open—are discussed in terms of (1) indications, (2) preoperative preparation, (3) technique, (4) postoperative care, (5) efficacy, and (6) untoward effects.

This textbook reviews all adult malignancies; in addition, pediatric malignancies of the genitourinary tract are discussed in detail, including neuroblastoma, Wilms' tumor, testis tumors of prepubescent boys, and rhabdomyosarcomas of the pelvis and paratesticular structures. The last section of the book addresses clinically important topics that are rarely included in oncology textbooks. The subjects are (1) nutrition and the cancer patient, (2) anesthetic concerns for major cancer surgery, (3) hospital and home care following extirpative and reconstructive surgery, (4) management of renal failure in the setting of genitourinary cancer surgery, and (5) management of pain for the terminally ill patient.

This book concludes with perhaps the most important chapter of all, "The Randomized Clinical Trial." In this treatise, Dr. Brent Blumenstein emphasizes the need for well-designed, prospective, randomized clinical trials to assess the efficacy, side effects, and cost-effectiveness of new treatments. He also stresses the need for proper statistical analysis of data and standardized reporting of results so that findings of different investigations can be compared in a clinically relevant manner. Indeed, it is no longer appropriate to base practice patterns on case reports or retrospective studies when much data are not available for analysis, or investigations with small numbers of patients who have not been followed for a sufficiently long period of time. We, as urologists, must become scientists, astute in the design of clinical trials, and sophisticated with regard to proper statistical techniques for analyzing data. Both the patient and the entire field of urologic oncology will benefit from such endeavors.

This book is written in a clear and concise manner by the leading authorities in the field today. As a result, it is hoped that it will serve as the reference source on urologic oncology for the next several years to come, not only for medical students and residents-in-training but for urologists in private practice, academic urologists, and researchers as well. The text of each chapter is supplemented with appropriate tables and figures. In addition, the bibliography at the conclusion of each chapter is complete and contains the most recent papers published in the urologic and medical literature on that subject. The index to the book is thorough, allowing the reader to identify the topic of interest in a quick and easy manner. Without question, by design, the book is user friendly.

In conclusion, we, the Editors, hope that you, the reader, find this book a valuable addition to your oncology library and that you will refer to it frequently. The world-renowned authors, who contributed the 55 chapters, and we, the Editors, have thoroughly enjoyed the opportunity to bring this book to you. However, if you should have any suggestions as to how this book can be further improved in the second edition, please feel free to contact us at any time.

Joseph E. Oesterling, M.D.
Joseph.Oesterling@umich.edu

Jerome P. Richie, M.D.
jrichie@bics.bwh.harvard.edu

CONTENTS

VI PROSTATE GLAND AND SEMINAL VESICLES

VII TESTIS AND OTHER SCROTAL TUMORS

VIII RETROPERITONEUM

IX URETHRA

X PENIS

NOTICE

I

BASIC SCIENCE ISSUES

1

THE MOLECULAR AND CELLULAR BIOLOGY OF UROLOGIC CANCERS

J. MIGUEL GARCIA-SCHÜRMANN, M.D., ALAN W. PARTIN, M.D., PH.D., *and* DONALD S. COFFEY, PH.D.

The focus of this chapter is to provide an overview of some of the important concepts and discoveries that have recently revolutionized our understanding of cancer. This will be accomplished by giving simple analogies and schematics followed by a more detailed in-depth figure, which shows the complexity and elegance of the control mechanisms involved in controlling life. These processes go astray when cancer develops. This will not be an extensive review with detailed references, but rather an overview of a most important and complex problem.

THE PROBLEM AND IMPACT

Approximately one out of three people living in the United States will develop cancer in their lifetime and about 25% of all will succumb to the ravages of cancer. In the United States, approximately 317,100 new cases of prostate cancer will be diagnosed in 1996, with 41,400 deaths; it is the second leading cause of cancer death in U.S. men. The incidence in blacks is 37% higher than in whites, and their death rate will be almost twice as high. The 5-year survival for all stages is 85.8%, but if there is distant metastasis it is only 29.8%. Prostate cancer is six times more common than bladder cancer, and is the cause of almost four times as many deaths.

Bladder cancer is diagnosed in 52,900 U.S. men per year resulting in 11,700 deaths, and the racial differences are almost opposite to what occurs in prostate cancer. Caucasians in the United States have twice the incidence of bladder cancer as do blacks. Bladder cancer is diagnosed in males two to three times as often as in females. The incidence of bladder cancer is over three times higher if you smoke than if you are a nonsmoker. In contrast to prostate cancer, there does not appear to be a familial tendency to develop bladder cancer. Five-year survival for all stages is 80.7%, with distant metastasis having a 5.9% rate.

Kidney cancer is diagnosed 33,600 times a year in the United States, with an almost twofold higher risk in males as in females. Cigarette smokers have twice the risk of nonsmokers. Five-year survival rate for all stages is 57.9% and with distant metastasis is 9.2%.

In summary, 3 of the top 12 cancers diagnosed in the United States are genitourinary cancers; they afflict 400,600 new cases per year, with 65,100 deaths. Prostate cancer diagnosis has increased at an alarming rate; since 1990 the rate has tripled from less than 100,000 to more than 317,000 per year. This is undoubtedly due to the introduction of serum tests for prostate-specific antigen (PSA) leading to earlier detection of these tumors. Thus, radical prostatectomy has increased sixfold to approximately 160,000 operations per year. Early detection and radical surgery should theoretically result in a dramatic increase in the cure rate, as more localized tumors appear to be detected. The long delay time between diagnosis and death from prostate cancer has resulted in a continuing increase of the mortality rate. Only time and careful analysis will show the results achieved with screening, early detection, and our intervention techniques.

FAMILIAL CANCER

Cancer clusters in some families could be the result of inherited genetic alterations or shared environmental factors. Single or multiple genes could be causing predisposition to cancer. Sporadic occurrence suggests aggravation by the adverse effects of the environment, such as pollutants and carcinogens, as well as socioeconomic differences and cultural habits, such as work, sexual, and dietary factors. It is now possible to apply statistical analysis to these inherited patterns, trying to correlate these with the time of diagnosis in order to determine if there is a genetic predisposition, inherited primarily through genes from either the mother or the father, termed autosomal. In this regard, Patrick C. Walsh and his colleagues have reported that there is a hereditary form of prostate cancer (HPC) with an early onset and a three- to ninefold increased incidence, depending on the number of first-degree relatives involved. Indeed, hereditary prostate cancer appears to be inherited in a mendelian manner and is autosomal dominant, with a penetrance of approximately 85%. The increased incidence is not associated with breast or colon cancer in these families. Intense efforts are underway in many centers to find chromosomal linkage to this hereditary form of cancer and to identify the gene(s) involved in this increased cancer risk. It is hoped that these high-risk genes can be sequenced as they have been in breast cancer. There, BRCA1 and BRCA2 have been identified as hereditary genes. Also, in colon cancer, four genes have been identified, three of which are mismatch DNA repair genes termed MSH2, MLH1, PMS1, 2, as well as the APC tumor suppressor gene. Two kidney cancer genes have been identified to be WT1 in the Wilms' tumor and the VHL gene associated with von Hippel-Lindau syndrome, identified by Marston Lineham and his colleagues.

It is most interesting that there is a familial tendency to prostate and renal cell cancer, without such a tendency yet being identified for bladder cancer. Furthermore, approximately 10% of cancers are inherited through a predisposing gene or genes, but 90% of cancers are acquired through living or by environmental insults; these are termed sporadic cancers. It is believed that if we identify the inherited genes that predispose to familial cancer, these genes will be the same targets that are altered by carcinogens, aging, or biologic damage. This is the basis for Knudson's hypothesis, which has been proven in retinoblastoma.

Since we inherit two genes, one each from our mother and father, we therefore have two alleles for every gene that can be slightly different in sequence (polymorphism) or in methylation (imprinting). If both genes are required to be knocked out to produce cancer, which is the case when a suppressor gene is eliminated, then inheriting the loss of one gene (loss of heterozygosity [LOH]) would increase your chances of getting cancer, because now an environmental insult only needs to eliminate the second allele to inactivate the suppressor gene. This increase in probability results in the early onset of cancer, because one of the two suppressor genes had already been inactivated at birth.

The similarity that approximately 10% of all colon, breast, and prostate cancers are inherited, although the overall frequency of these genes in the population is about 0.3%, is one of the mysteries in cancer research. Is this similarity by chance or does it have a meaning? In addition, in each case when you inherit these predisposing genes you have an approximately 85% chance of getting the cancer, but 15% will not.

One of the difficulties in locating cancer-causing genes is that once you have developed cancer, it is often accompanied by a genetic instability, which produces a series of changes in the genome, which alter the cancerous properties of the cell. This temporal change in the cancer cell clones is called progression and produces the tumor cell heterogeneity. These genetic changes that ensue because of this instability can produce a cell with an increased growth rate, and then this clone will expand and dominate in the tumor. This phenomenon is termed "clonal selection," and since it occurs with time, it is called tumor progression. Ultimately, cells may be selected with not only increased growth rate but also with more aggressive properties, and alterations in many cancer genes such as p53 appear to be related to more aggressive tumors. Therefore, when a tumor is removed from a patient and the karyotype or DNA is examined, it is possible to see tremendous changes in the chromosomes. There are cases of chromosal deletions, amplifications, rearrangements, and duplications, which can result in changes in ploidy and abnormal amounts of DNA in the cancer cell nuclei. This was seen earlier in what we call karyotyping, but this only looked at the shapes and forms of chromosomes and their banding. Later it was possible to differentially stain cancer and normal DNA using either red or green markers as probes to stain and differentially compare the chromosomes. By looking at the presence or absence of the red and green markers on cancer chromosomes, it is possible to visualize changes by their color pattern. This technique has been termed comparative genome hybridization (CGH). For example, it has been possible to find that in certain cancer chromosomes there is a gain in areas on one arm, and a simultaneous loss in areas on the other arm. In prostate cancer, this occurs with loss of material in the short arm (p) and a subsequent gain in the long arm (q) of the eighth chromosome; this is not a simple transposition. Some of these changes may be causal for cancer, but many are just associated with the properties of the tumor as it progresses and are simply epiphenomena. This produces the complex problems that the geneticists face when analyzing tumor cell chromosomes and DNA. Therefore, this requires the meticulous linking of the inherited chromosome changes within the lineages of the families with the tumor types. These linkage studies are most difficult and usually require years of work. New molecular probes and information from the Human Genome Project are speeding this process up and certainly automated and high-throughput systems are accelerating this search, which has been a most difficult problem for cancer research. Certainly, many candidate genes have been identified and are being verified or eliminated by painstaking work. There are more nucleotides (ATGC) in one cell (3×10^9) than there are characters existing in 30 complete sets of the *Encyclopaedia Britannica*. Finding a point mutation in an important cancer gene would be the equivalent of finding a changed character in over 500 volumes of this encyclopedia. It is amazing that this has been accomplished. Within the next several years we will have the entire DNA sequence worked out for the human genome.

The problem then will be linking specific sequences to gene functions, gene control, and disease. There will be much variation and polymorphism within the population, genetic types, and races. Several different types of each inherited cancer may exist. The genome can also change through aging, replication errors, and failures in DNA repair. This is a complex but critical problem in understanding genetic changes associated with cancer.

CANCER GENES

Cancer susceptibility is driven primarily by six types of genes:

1. *Oncogenes*. A series of over 60 genes have been identified that are activated or overexpressed and which have a positive effect in the induction of growth. These constitutive genes have a prefix like c-*myc*. If they are mutated and inserted by viruses this prefix changes to v, like v-*src*.
2. *Suppressor genes*. Loss of the function of a suppressor gene essentially removes a brake on cell growth, thus permitting it to become up-regulated (examples are p53, Rb, and p16).
3. *DNA repair genes*. Normal or induced errors in DNA copying, DNA damage from the environment, or oxidative damage must be corrected or the gene will be mutated or silenced. In colon cancer, a group of mismatch repair genes (MSH2, MLH1, and PMS1,2) have all been shown to be inherited and to induce cancer by accumulation of DNA damage.
4. *DNA defense genes*. These genes protect the DNA from oxidative damage or electrophiles that can form adducts to the bases that are detrimental. There are enzymes that protect the cell against reactive oxygen species that form free radicals and produce oxidative damage to the cell. As the mitochondria carry out their aerobic oxidation, four electrons are required to reduce molecular oxygen to water. In this process, partially reduced intermediates of oxygen produce superoxide, hydrogen peroxide, and hydroxyl radicals that are collectively known as reactive oxygen species (ROS). ROS can also be caused by ionizing radiation, UV light, or certain chemicals in the environment. ROS converts guanine in DNA to 8-oxoguanine, which is highly mutagenic and preferentially mispairs with adenine during replication. There are enzymes such as glutathione-S-transferase (GST), glutathione reductase, quinone reductase, superoxide dismutase, catalase, and other protective enzymes that inactivate electrophiles, carcinogens, and ROS. Carcinogens in our environment often need to be activated by type 1 enzymes or inactivated by type 2 enzymes. For example, procarcinogens like benzpyrene are inactive and must be metabolized by epoxidases to form the active carcinogen that reacts with DNA. This represents a type 1 reaction. Type 2 reactions are represented by the family of glutathione transferases, glucuronosyltransferases, and quinone reductases, all of which can inactivate carcinogens or reactive oxygen species. Type 1 and 2 enzymes can be induced or altered by environment, diet, or inheritance, altering the rate of cancer formation. There are several isoforms and polymorphisms; for example, GST-M is related to bladder and glutathione-S-transferase isoforms (GST-π) methylation to prostate cancer.
5. *Viral genes*. Retroviruses, polyoma, adenoma, and papilloma viruses can also introduce genes into the mammalian cell, which when expressed induce malignant transformation. This includes large T-antigen, E1, E6, and oncogenes.
6. *DNA methylation genes*. DNA methylation is altered in many cancers and for unknown reasons. Hypermethylation of CpG islands in promoter regions can silence genes. DNA methylation can vary in maternal and paternal genes, termed imprinting. Loss of imprinting (LOI) is a common change in cancers.

At present, all of the above six mechanisms are being studied to determine what causes urologic cancers. At the moment, there is only definitive evidence that the VHL gene is associated with von Hippel-Lindau syndrome, and the WT1 gene is associated with Wilms' tumor. The p53 gene is associated with bladder cancer, but it may only be a progression marker, as it is in prostate cancer. No gene has yet been shown to be inherited in prostate cancer, although practically all of these tumors are associated with inactivation of one of the GST-π. This inactivation of expression is accomplished through methylation of the CpG islands in the promoter region, which down-regulates the gene. This genomic change is almost universal in both familial and sporadic prostate cancers, but is not believed to be the inherited gene that causes the cancer.

Since both aging and cancer produce heterogeneity in the stability of various chromosomes, it is hard to eliminate this form of noise in the system, without careful study. In addition, many normal genes have different DNA sequences, which is called polymorphism. These polymorphisms are inherited and can produce different types of isozymes or genetic patterns that may or may not have effects on how these genes function. Some of these polymorphisms are certainly going to increase tendencies towards malignant transformation that would enhance the chances of acquiring cancer, which will add to the complexity. Many suppressor genes not only will be lost through mutation or genetic inactivation but can also be down-regulated and turned off by nongenetic or epigenetic means, such as DNA methylation.

Many traits within the human body, resulting in specific phenotypes, do require many genes operating in concert to produce this specific phenotype. This polygenic phenomenon can be operating in some cancers. Indeed, there are multiple steps involved in the evolution of cancer. It is well known that multiple hits are required, resulting in multiple changes, which occur with time. It has been estimated that three to six changes may be the minimum requirement to produce a clone of cells with the properties to propagate the cancer to a lethal stage. It has been suggested that these hits are cumulative and may not have to occur in a specific order, although this model has not been completely confirmed. Certainly, just inheriting one familial cancer gene seems to guarantee the rest of the hits, since there is an 85% chance of developing cancer when an inherited gene is involved.

How do the aforementioned oncogenes and suppressor genes function within the cell to cause cancer? They appear to regulate cell replication, death, and growth. As is shown in Figure 1–1, oncogenes act as positive signals and function like an accelerator in a car. They are activated and overexpressed in an abnormal manner to speed up growth. There are about 60 oncogenes of primarily four types:

1. Genes for growth factors or their receptors (e.g., platelet-derived growth factor [PDGF], *erb*-B, and RET).
2. Genes affecting cell signaling pathways: such as *ras* and *src*.
3. Genes acting as transcription factors that activate early growth genes, such as the *myc* oncogenes.

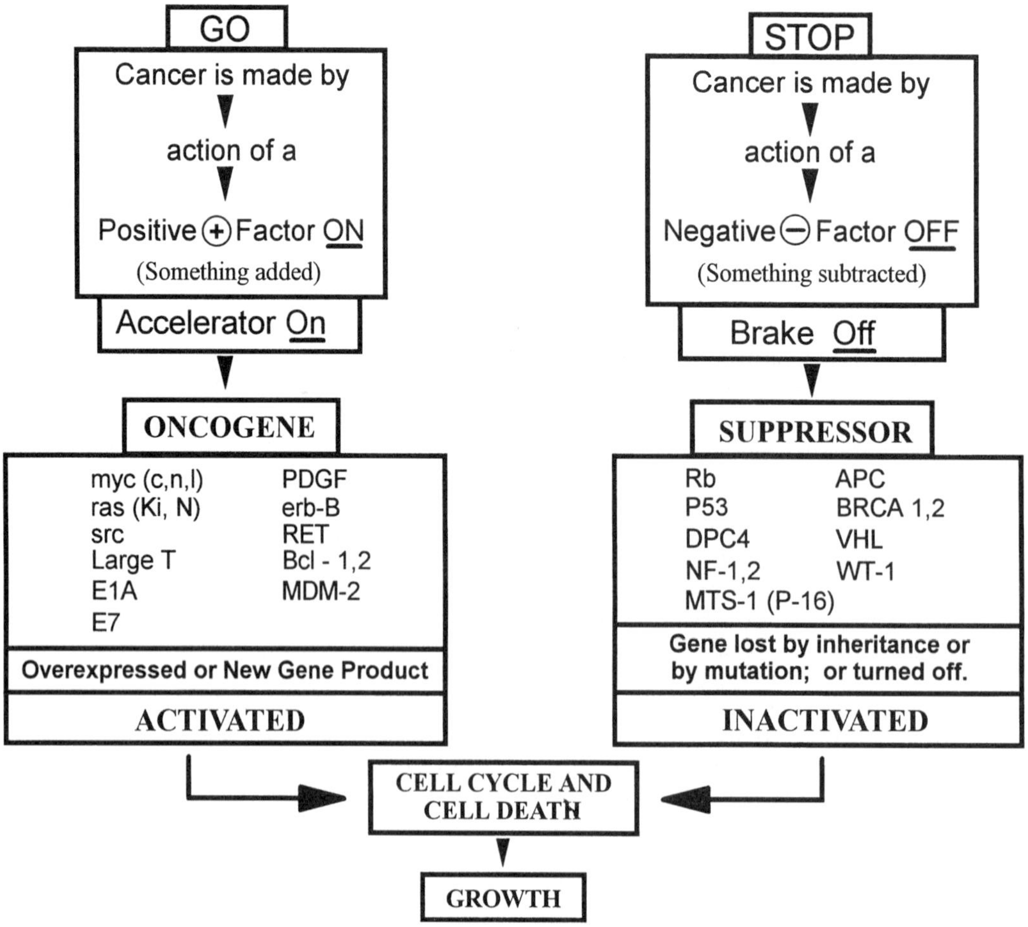
GO
Cancer is made by
action of a
Positive ⊕ Factor ON
(Something added)
Accelerator On
ONCOGENE
myc (c,n,l)
ras (Ki, N)
src
Large T
E1A
E7
PDGF
erb-B
RET
Bcl - 1,2
MDM-2
Overexpressed or New Gene Product
ACTIVATED
STOP
Cancer is made by
action of a
Negative ⊖ Factor OFF
(Something subtracted)
Brake Off
SUPPRESSOR
Rb
P53
DPC4
NF-1,2
MTS-1 (P-16)
APC
BRCA 1,2
VHL
WT-1
Gene lost by inheritance or by mutation; or turned off.
INACTIVATED
CELL CYCLE AND CELL DEATH
GROWTH

FIGURE 1–1. Cancer growth is activated by turning on a class of genes (oncogenes) or by turning off a brake on growth (suppressor). This alters the balance of cell cycle growth over cell death that results in total cell accumulation.

4. Genes affecting the cell cycle: Bcl-1,2 is an inhibitor of cell death which, when overexpressed, blocks apoptosis and allows cells to survive and accumulate. Overexpressing factors that bind to suppressors can remove the brake. For example MDM-2 removes the suppressor brake p53 by binding to it and inactivating it. Many virus proteins are expressed in an infected cell, such as large T, E1A, and E7, and have the ability to complex suppressor molecules such as p53 and Rb. In summary, turning these genes on turns on cell growth.

Suppressors are brake molecules that turn growth off. Removing the brake, of course, turns on the growth. These brakes can be removed either by inheriting the loss of this gene, by mutating the gene and activating it, or by turning off the gene through regulation, which is the case when the DNA in its promoter region is methylated.

How do the suppressor genes function as brakes? Many of these genes are located in the nucleus and affect the cell cycle regulation. The Rb gene is present in all cells and codes for a master brake on the cell cycle that will be discussed in detail in a moment. p53 is one of the best known suppressors and is abnormally regulated in most cancers. It blocks the cell cycle by inducing a series of cell cycle kinase inhibitors (CDKI). This p53 protein is activated when the cell detects damage, such as DNA breakage, and blocks the cell cycle at the G_1/S checkpoint to allow time for DNA repair. If the damage is extensive the p53 induces abnormal cells to undergo a suicide through apoptosis. p53 can also affect the mechanism of mitosis; abnormalities may result in mitotic dysjunction.

MTS-1, also called p16, is another suppressor involved in the braking components of the cell cycle. Other suppressor genes function in the cytoplasm, such as APC, which is involved in colon cancer. APC may affect the cell adhesion molecule mechanisms by interacting with catenin-like molecules. DPC4 is involved in pancreatic cancer and interacts with the cell signaling mechanisms.[1] NF-1, and 2 are suppressor genes involved in cell signaling pathways.

Recently, two genes have been identified to be involved in the inheritance of breast cancer, termed BRCA1, and 2. At the moment it is unknown how they function, although their cellular distribution may change during the cancer state.

Of great interest to the urologist is the WT1 gene, which is involved in the Wilms' tumor of the kidney, and the VHL gene, which is involved in renal cell cancer accompanying von Hippel-Lindau syndrome. VHL can either be lost by inheritance or inactivated by methylation of the cytosine residues of the DNA located in the promotor region of this gene. The VHL gene appears, at the moment, to be involved in the regulation of transcription. Transcription is the conversion of the information of DNA into RNA through the action of RNA polymerase II that forms messenger RNA (mRNA). An important protein binds to the RNA polymerase II and controls the elongation of the mRNA. This transcription and elongation factor is termed elongin or S III. It appears that in normal cells, VHL forms a protein that binds to the elongin and is involved in the control of transcription elongation. When the VHL gene is missing or mutated, it loses its ability to complex to the elongin and, therefore, allows elongin to interact with RNA polymerase II, deregulating the process of mRNA elongation. VHL is the first suppressor gene that has been identified to control the level of transcriptional elongation. This raises the question: Why does the elongation result in cancer? It is believed that this may increase the expression of certain genes involved in growth control, such as *myc* or *fos*.

In summary, the only two genes so far identified for urologic cancers that can be inherited and increase our incidence of cancer are VHL and WT1, which cause renal cell cancers. In urologic cancers, other suppressors have been implicated such as Rb; p53; p16; and the oncogenes PDGF, *myc*, and Bcl-2. However, none of these have been shown to be involved in cancer as inherited factors. Certainly these genes play a major role in urologic cancers in controlling growth and progression, but what is the inherited gene that sets off prostate cancer? This will soon be resolved, as many groups are rapidly mapping in on the target of candidate genes.[2]

THE CONTROL OF THE CELL CYCLE, CELL DEATH, AND TUMOR GROWTH

In normal tissues, the rate of cell replication and the rate of cell death are in a tightly controlled balance. This is shown in Figure 1–2, and it is unknown how this balance is maintained. However, when an imbalance occurs, either through an increase in cell replication or a decrease in cell death, there is an accumulation of cells that forms the tumor. This balance involves growth factors, cell signaling, and control of the cell cycle as well as apoptosis. DNA damage, aging, and senescence activate certain signals, which we believe to be "death" genes that cause the cell to commit suicide. Signaling of the cell cycle for growth and cell death is one of the most active areas of science.

First we will review how the cell cycle functions. The cell is usually quiescent in the nongrowing phase, which is termed G_0. Growth factors, steroids, and hormones can stimulate the cell to grow and undergo an active phase of biochemical events, termed G_1 or the gap period that occurs before DNA synthesis. After the biochemical preparation in G_1, the cell undergoes DNA synthesis, termed the S phase. Following the replication of the complete DNA, there is a second gap called G_2, where the cell prepares itself for mitosis. Then the mitosis (M phase) ensues, in which the mitotic spindle separates the two sets of chromosomes. Then the nu-

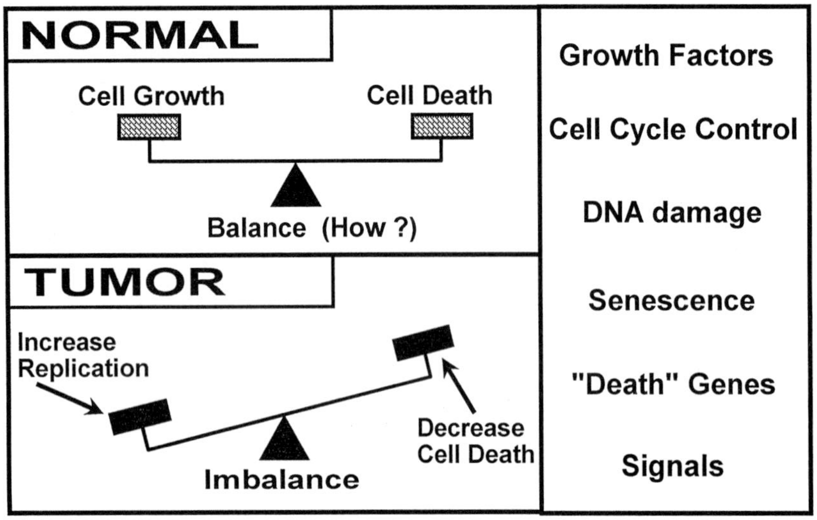
NORMAL
Cell Growth
Cell Death
Balance (How ?)
TUMOR
Increase Replication
Decrease Cell Death
Imbalance
Growth Factors
Cell Cycle Control
DNA damage
Senescence
"Death" Genes
Signals

FIGURE 1–2. In cancer there is a disturbance in the balance of cell replication and cell death that can be accomplished by either increasing replication or decreasing the rate of cell death. The activation (on) of certain genes can induce cell death in specific cell types (TNF, *fas*, bax, etc.). The suppression (off) of survival genes (Bcl-2, etc.) can increase cell death as can alteration in cell contact and structure. These are collectively termed "death" genes.

cleus reorganizes and the cell cycle is completed. Recently, there has been a tremendous amount of research delineating the biochemical controls of the cell cycle. There are specific checkpoints at the interface between each of these phases in which the cell stops to determine its next decision. These decisions in the cycle are primarily controlled by the interaction of regulatory proteins to form heterodimers with kinases that are either active or inactive. This in turn regulates their state of phosphorylation of growth suppressors. A kinase is an enzyme that phosphorylates a protein. In the cell cycle, these kinases are termed cyclin-dependent kinases (CDKs); there are approximately seven of these enzymes (CDK2, CDK4, etc.). They are usually at a constant level and inactive as shown in Figure 1–3. These cyclin-dependent kinases are activated at specific phases of the cell cycle by binding to a second type of molecule, called cyclins (termed cyclin A to H). These are termed cyclins because their concentration varies through the cycle, and it is these transient molecules that regulate the cell cycle. Therefore, you can activate cyclin kinases in a controlled manner by turning on the synthesis and degradation of the cyclins.

Once the CDKs are activated by binding cyclins, they appear to regulate the cell cycle by phosphorylating and turning off the brakes within the nucleus that prevent cell growth. One of the primary brakes or suppressors in the nucleus is Rb, which, when unphosphorylated, is a checkpoint at G_1/S and prevents the cycle from proceeding. When the

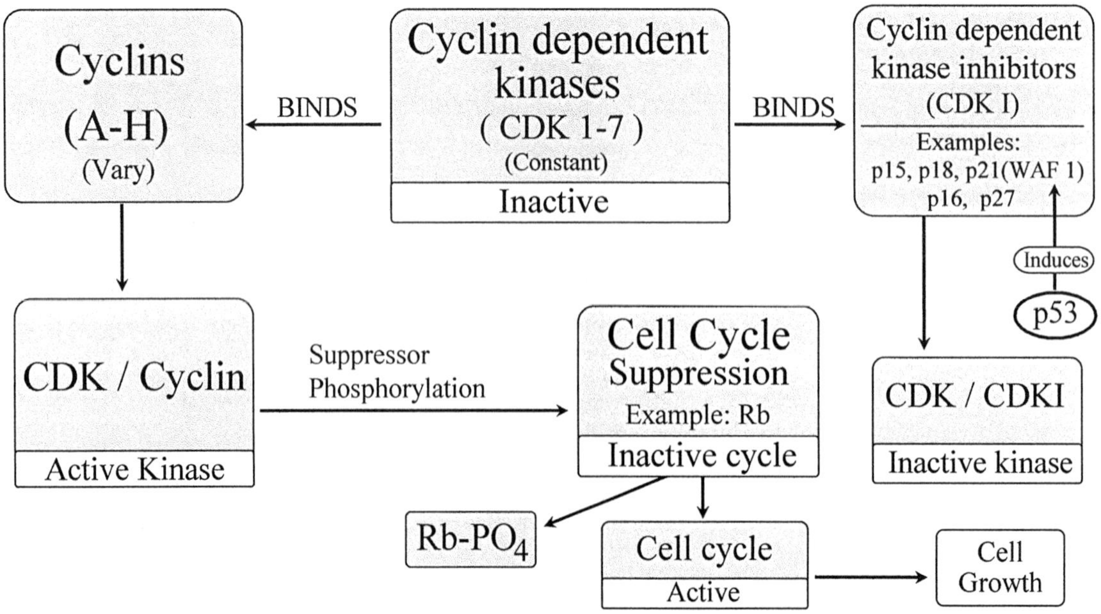
Cyclins
(A-H)
(Vary)
BINDS
Cyclin dependent kinases
(CDK 1-7)
(Constant)
Inactive
BINDS
Cyclin dependent kinase inhibitors
(CDK I)
Examples:
p15, p18, p21(WAF 1)
p16, p27
Induces
p53
CDK / Cyclin
Active Kinase
Suppressor Phosphorylation
Cell Cycle Suppression
Example: Rb
Inactive cycle
CDK / CDKI
Inactive kinase
Rb-PO4
Cell cycle
Active
Cell Growth

FIGURE 1–3. Schematic of how CDKs are activated or inactivated. The active kinases are bound to cyclins and phosphorylate Rb, thus releasing the brake on the cell cycle.

cyclin kinase is activated, it phosphorylates the Rb, thus removing the brake and allowing the cell cycle to initiate DNA synthesis and to continue to complete growth to the daughter cell.

CDKs can also be inactivated by binding to a group of cyclin-dependent kinase inhibitors (CDKIs). Examples of this type of inhibitor are p16 and p21. If these inhibitors are induced, the cell cycle stops, growth is suppressed, and so a checkpoint is formed. How are these inhibitors induced? This occurs through the normal function of p53, which acts like an inducer and can up-regulate these inhibitors. The p53 is usually turned on when cells are damaged. In this case the cell wishes to make the decision not to proceed through cell cycle and to repair itself. In summary, expression of p53 is increased during cell and/or DNA damage and induces a braking system on the cell cycle to prevent defective cells from being made. If the p53 is damaged, lost, or down-regulated, this checkpoint is eliminated. This results in damaged DNA proceeding and accumulating through each cell cycle and may result in the large amount of genetic instability and DNA damage that occur in cancer.

We have just discussed how the cell cycle is regulated, but how does a cell determine to undergo cell death or apoptosis? Damage to the DNA is detected by an unknown mechanism, but appears to involve, in part, poly-ADP ribosylation. Broken ends of the DNA have a special polymer added to them that is made from a breakdown product of nicotinamide-adenine dinucleotide (NAD). NAD is a cofactor in many metabolic energy processes of the cell, and can be metabolized by removing the nicotinic acid. The remaining ribose-phosphate-phosphate-ribose-adenine units can then be involved in a process called poly-ADP ribosylation. These units can be polymerized into long chains, or can be added onto histones and to the ends of damaged DNA molecules. The poly-ADP ribosylation of the ends of damaged DNA appears to set off a signal that can induce cell death.

Other ways to induce cell death are to remove the cell from its extracellular matrix anchorage or to disturb the cytoskeleton. Then, unknown signals from the cell periphery are being sent to the nucleus to induce cell death. In addition, there are large protein molecules like tumor necrosis factor (TNF) and Fas-ligand that act conversely to growth factors and could be termed death factors for some cells. The TNF binds to two types of cell surface receptors and the Fas-ligand binds to its receptor. These complexes move into the cytoplasm and send a signal into the nucleus, which can induce apoptosis.

Sometimes growth factors can induce cell death in certain cells. For example tumor growth factor-β (TGF-β) can activate cell death in epithelial cells. Other growth factors appear to induce cell death when they are absent; these include EGF and FGF2, and 7. Of great importance to the urologist is the fact that the absence of androgen on its receptor can induce cell death in the prostate. Therefore, when the androgen withdrawal occurs following castration, this absence of androgens induces rapid cell death in the prostate epithelial cells. This is, of course, the basis for the hormonal treatment of prostate cancer.

In Figure 1–4 we have a complex figure that shows the balance of cell growth and death with its details. First, let's review the events in cell death. Once the positive signals of TNF, *fas*, or TGF-β are activated through binding to their receptors or, in negative signals, androgen, FGF, or EGF are removed from their receptors, which occurs on the cell surface, a series of biochemical events is induced within the cell that causes death. An early event is the induction of a protease called interleukin-converting enzyme (ICE), which activates a cascade of events. Certain genes appear to be turned on in this period, including the receptor for TGF-β, as well as a nuclease that can degrade DNA and TRPM-2, also known as clusterin. These events occur in the A phase of the D_1 portion of the cell death cascade. John T. Isaacs has proposed that these cascades of events are like the mirror image of the cell cycle, but they only end in the death of the cell. Similar to G_1, he has named these portions D_1 for the events that occur before DNA fragmentation; F stands for the phase that is involved when the DNA is fragmented and degraded in the nucleus. The last phase after fragmentation is termed D_2, when the cell finally undergoes nuclear destruction and phagocytosis.

After the activation of the DNA nuclease by calcium as depicted in phase A, a series of factors is rapidly down-regulated, including ornithine-decarboxylase (ODC). This is followed by the destruction of some of the cyclins as well as some of the CDKs, such as CDK2, and finally the fragmentation of the DNA. A characteristic pattern of DNA fragments can be observed on gel electrophoresis to form the uniform pieces of DNA surrounding the nucleosomes as they are degraded. This produces a stepladder effect on DNA gel analysis. Once the DNA fragmentation occurs, it is irreversible and accompanied by the proteolytic degradation of the nuclear architecture, destroying the lamins around the nuclear periphery and the internal nuclear matrix components. The cell then disintegrates under protease activity, and phagocytosis of the remaining components occurs, destroying the cell. This entire event of cell death has been termed "apoptosis" and is characterized by these morphologic and biochemical events.

As there are brakes or suppressors of growth on the cell cycle, such as p53 and Rb, there are also brakes to stop cell death. One of the leading brakes is Bcl-2. When Bcl-2 is available, it blocks the process of cell death and therefore is termed a survival factor. How is the brake Bcl-2 removed? It can bind to a series of proteins and form a heterodimer. One

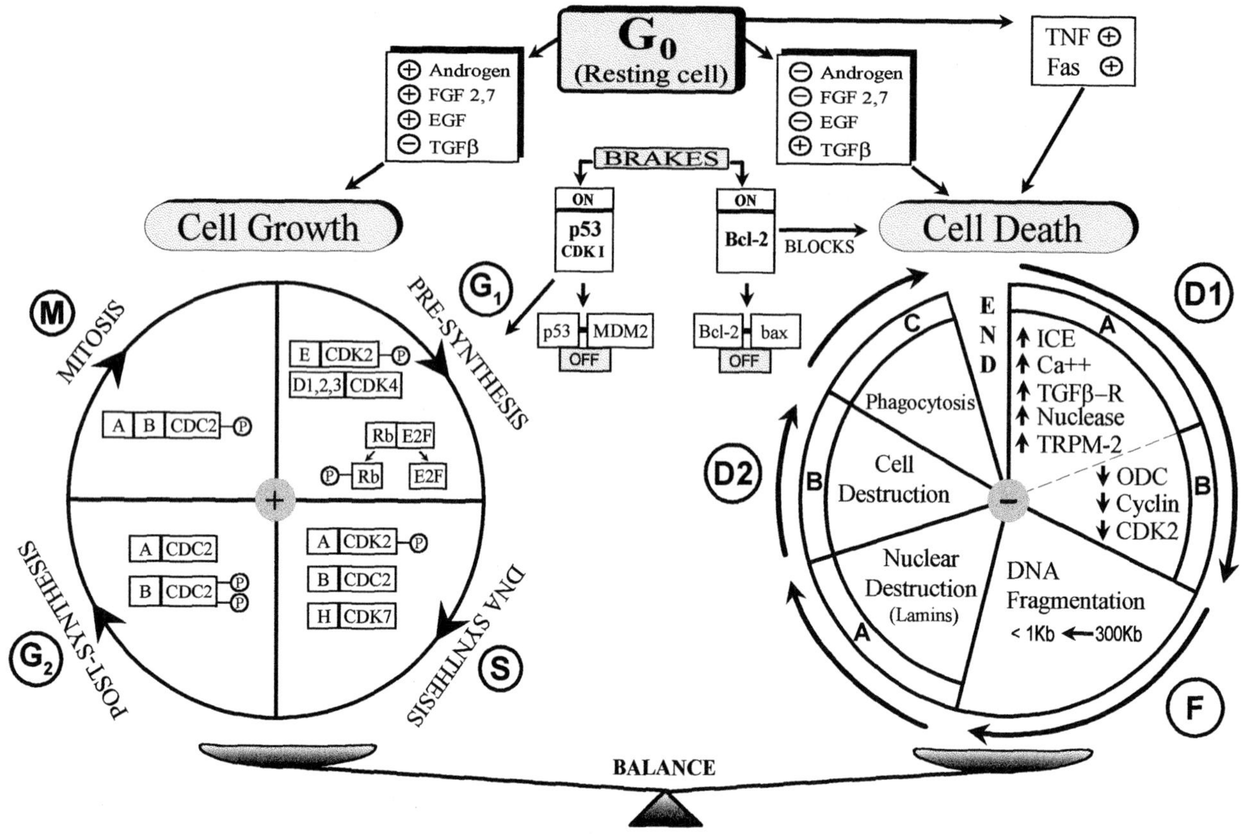

G0
(Resting cell)
⊕ Androgen
⊕ FGF 2,7
⊕ EGF
⊖ TGFβ
⊖ Androgen
⊖ FGF 2,7
⊖ EGF
⊕ TGFβ
TNF ⊕
Fas ⊕
BRAKES
ON
p53
CDK I
ON
Bcl-2
BLOCKS
Cell Growth
Cell Death
p53 MDM2
OFF
Bcl-2 bax
OFF
MITOSIS
PRE-SYNTHESIS
DNA SYNTHESIS
POST-SYNTHESIS
M
G1
G2
S
E CDK2
D1,2,3 CDK4
Rb E2F
Rb
E2F
A B CDC2
A CDC2
B CDC2
A CDK2
B CDC2
H CDK7
D1
D2
F
END
ICE
Ca++
TGFβ–R
Nuclease
TRPM-2
ODC
Cyclin
CDK2
Phagocytosis
Cell Destruction
Nuclear Destruction
(Lamins)
DNA Fragmentation
< 1Kb ← 300Kb
BALANCE

FIGURE 1–4. Detail schematic of the control of the balance between cell cycle growth and cell death. On cell cycle A, B, D, E, and H in boxes are the cyclins. CDK and CDC2 are kinases. See text for discussion.

of these Bcl-2–binding molecules is termed bax, and now a family of these death-inducing molecules is being identified. Combining the Bcl-2 with bax removes the brake and allows cell death to occur.

Now let us turn our attention to the left side of Figure 1–4, where cell replication and cell growth is regulated. Here, a series of growth factors and steroids can either activate or inhibit cell growth, such as the positive factors, like androgens, FGF, EGF, and the inhibitor TGF-β. As shown in the presynthesis G_1 phase, CDK2 and CDK4 can be activated by binding to cyclins, shown here as E, D1, D2, and D3. Rb can be phosphorylated by this active CDK kinase, thus freeing up the transcription factor E2F, which induces the synthesis of some early proteins required for cell growth. Other cyclins, A, B, and H, function in a similar manner in the S period to drive DNA synthesis. The cycle is completed in the G_2 period by a series of interactions of cyclins and kinases and then mitosis ensues in the M phase. The brake on the system can be p53 that induces the CDKI that block the cell cycle by stopping the kinase cascade. In summary, p53 induces CDKI and the cell cycle is checked and cannot proceed. p53 can be taken out of activity and the brake on the cell cycle is removed by forming a heterodimer with MDM2.

While Figure 1–4 may appear complicated, it is truly a simplified version of a very elegant system, which regulates the balance between cell growth and cell death. When this system is out of balance, you have a tumor.[3]

CELL GROWTH FACTORS

There is much direct and indirect signaling that occurs between cells and organs. As shown in Figure 1–5, this signaling can be broken down to various types or categories. Growth factors (GF) are of many types, and they bind to specific transmembrane receptors on the cell surface, setting off kinase cascades and structural information to induce cell growth or death. If the growth factor is made and operates on the cell in which it was manufactured, it is called an autocrine factor. Usually, the autocrine factors are secreted from the cell and then bind to their specific cell surface receptors. If the growth factor operates within the cell, it is called an intracrine mechanism. If the growth factor diffuses to a neighboring cell, it is termed a paracrine stimulation. If the growth factor is transported through the circulation to distant cells, it is termed an endocrine effect. Other special factors can be

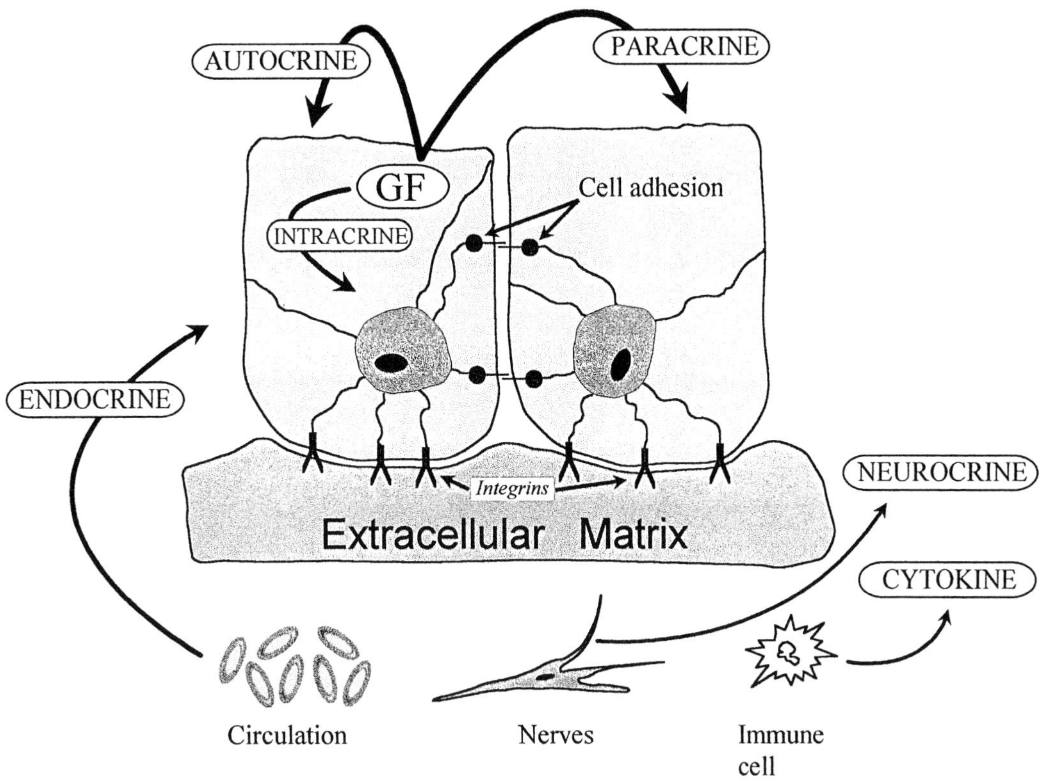
AUTOCRINE
PARACRINE
GF
Cell adhesion
INTRACRINE
ENDOCRINE
Integrins
Extracellular Matrix
NEUROCRINE
CYTOKINE
Circulation
Nerves
Immune cell

FIGURE 1–5. Examples of the types of cell signaling. (Adapted from Partin AW, Coffey DS: *In* Walsh PC, Retik AB, Stamey TA, Vaughan ED Jr [eds]: Campbell's Urology, 7th edition. Philadelphia, WB Saunders Co, 1997, with permission.)

transported by the nerves (neurocrine), or they may come from immunelike cells (cytokine).

Cells can also signal by direct communication through linkages of their structural elements. The extracellular matrix makes direct contact with the cell by binding to integrins, which are molecules that extend through the cellular membrane and link to the cytoskeleton within the cell. Cells can also "hold hands" with their neighbors by direct linkage of the cell adhesion molecules, which form homodimers.

These direct structural linkages, which transfer information in a vectral manner, allow the cell to sense its neighbors. This linkage is like a telephone area code and is one of the most active areas of research in cell biology. These combined units of structural elements form a tissue matrix system, as is shown in Figure 1–6. The cell adhesion molecules (CAMS) form a homopolymer with their neighbors. One of the most prominent of these is E-cadherin, which is a cell surface CAM and extends through the membrane of the cell and organizes cytoskeleton components, such as actin. It does that by interacting with an important molecule called catenin, which appears in several forms called α and β. In cancers, there is aberration in the expression of E-cadherin, whose expression can be regulated by methylation of the DNA in the promoter region for this gene. The linkage to actin can also be disrupted by components that can bind to the catenin, such as the suppressor APC, which has been delineated in colon cancer. The cytoskeleton can also be regulated in its organization by binding to receptors called integrins that detect extracellular matrix components, such as fibronectin. Aberrations in this linking system, which involves vinculin, tailin, and α-actinin, disrupt the organization of the cytoskeleton components such as actin.

The cytoskeleton is made up of microtubules, actin, and keratins, which give the shape to the cell and a different structure to each cell type. The recognition of the cell structure, shape, and organization is the basis of histology. The cytoskeleton links directly to the nuclear matrix, which organizes the DNA into 50,000 loop domains, termed replicons. These loops of about 60,000 base pairs (bp) of DNA are anchored at their base onto the nuclear matrix, where DNA synthesis and DNA methylation can occur. Steroid hormone receptors bind to this nuclear matrix in a tissue-specific manner, and it is this nuclear matrix protein pattern that makes up the tissue specificity. The nuclear matrix protein pattern is altered in cancer. This tissue matrix system is shown in its entirety in Figure 1–6.

In summary, what a cell touches determines what a cell does, and the disturbance in the tissue matrix system causes the variation in shape that we term cancer. Only the pathologist can diagnose cancer, which is done by recognizing aberrations in the nuclear structure in the tissues and cell structure. Cancer is a disease of cell structure.[4]

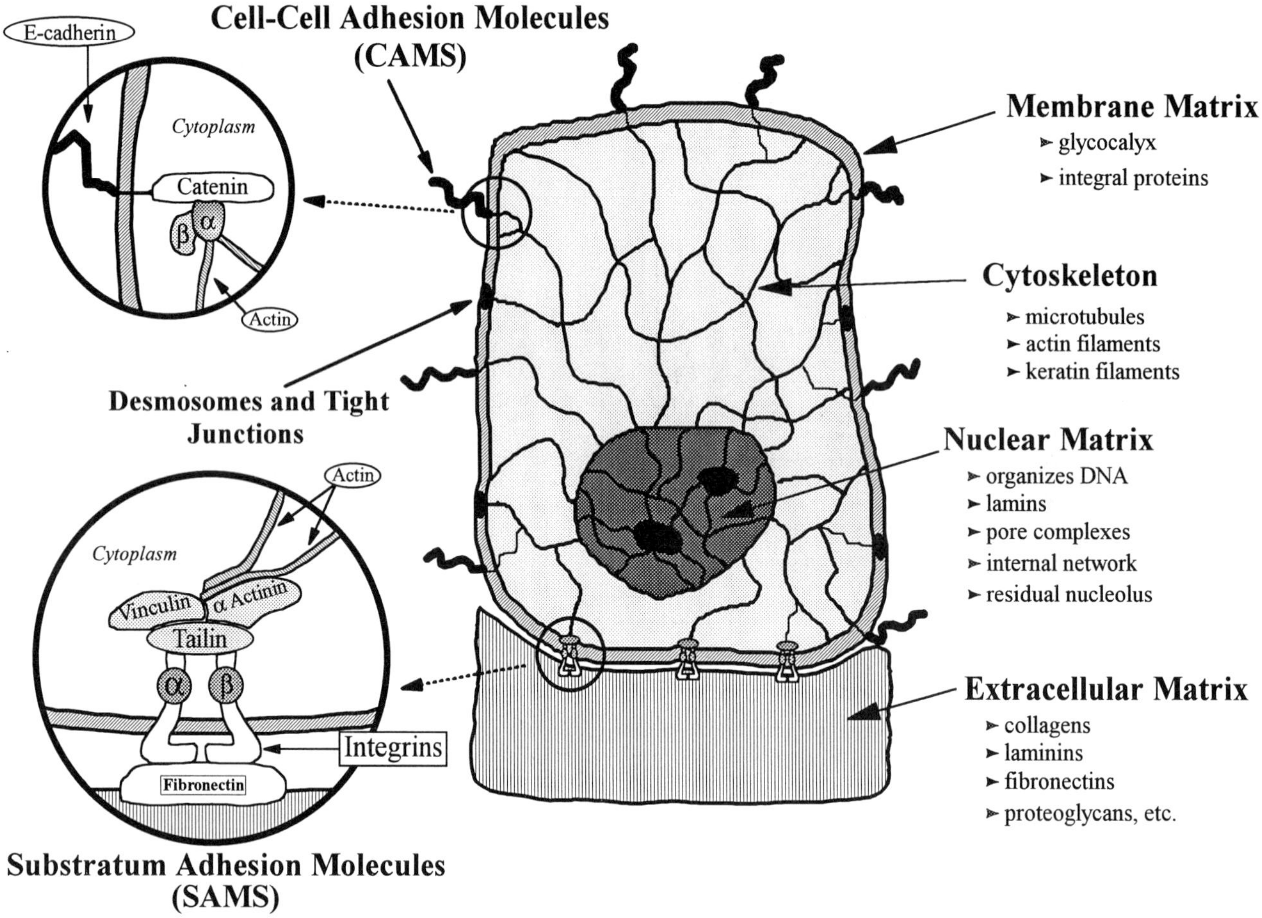
E-cadherin
Cell-Cell Adhesion Molecules
(CAMS)
Cytoplasm
Catenin
α
β
Actin
Membrane Matrix
glycocalyx
integral proteins
Cytoskeleton
microtubules
actin filaments
keratin filaments
Desmosomes and Tight
Junctions
Nuclear Matrix
organizes DNA
lamins
pore complexes
internal network
residual nucleolus
Actin
Cytoplasm
Vinculin
α Actinin
Tailin
α
β
Integrins
Fibronectin
Extracellular Matrix
collagens
laminins
fibronectins
proteoglycans, etc.
Substratum Adhesion Molecules
(SAMS)

FIGURE 1–6. The tissue matrix system composed of interlocking structural components that hardwire the cell to the nucleus and DNA.

CELL SIGNALING

As mentioned, many factors can regulate cell growth and cell death. They do so by interacting with specific transmembrane receptors on the cell surface. Their ligands involve growth factors, cytokines, stress signals, extracellular matrix, and death signals, such as TNF. Once these ligands bind to their cell surface receptors, which span the membrane and activate a series of kinases on the cytoplasmatic portion of the receptor, they set off a cascade of phosphorylation that goes to the nucleus. The kinases can either be tyrosine kinases, which put phosphate groups on tyrosine, or serine kinases, which put phosphate groups on the serine molecules of the target substrate. In Figure 1–7 we demonstrate how these cascades of protein phosphorylations are directed to the nucleus. Each large K indicates a kinase that is activated as the receptor signals down to the nucleus. Three of the major kinase cascades involve a series of phosphorylations of kinase molecules that activate other kinase molecules to phosphorylate, finally reaching phosphorylation of nuclear factors. These three prominent kinases are the jak/stat, MAP kinase, and the jnk/erk pathways. These phosphorylation pathways finally hit the nucleus to activate a series of transcription factors that induce the expression of specific genes of either growth or death. The receptor tyrosine kinase receptor molecule can also link itself to a series of G-protein systems to activate these kinases or can act through another important mechanism that converts the lipids of the membrane into signaling molecules. For example, phospholipase C (PLC) can hydrolyze the lipid molecules of the membrane to become signals by making inositol phosphate (IP-3) or diacylglycerol (DAG). The IP-3 activates calcium release in the cell that is a signal. The DAG activates protein kinase C, which is another major kinase system also signaling to the nucleus.

STROMAL EPITHELIAL INTERACTIONS

All of the aforementioned signaling mechanisms come together and are synchronized in the cell organization forming the tissue that involves the interaction of stromal and epithelial signals. The

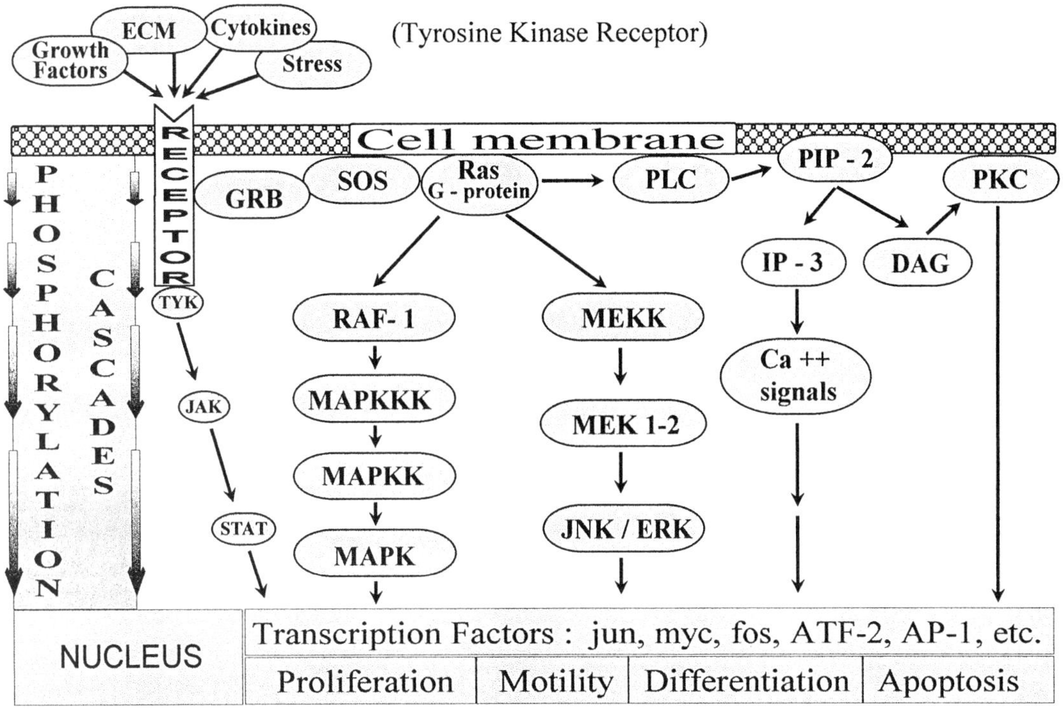
Growth Factors
ECM
Cytokines
Stress
(Tyrosine Kinase Receptor)
RECEPTOR
Cell membrane
PHOSPHORYLATION
CASCADES
TYK
JAK
STAT
GRB
SOS
Ras G - protein
PLC
PIP - 2
PKC
IP - 3
DAG
Ca ++ signals
RAF- 1
MAPKKK
MAPKK
MAPK
MEKK
MEK 1-2
JNK / ERK
NUCLEUS
Transcription Factors : jun, myc, fos, ATF-2, AP-1, etc.
Proliferation
Motility
Differentiation
Apoptosis

FIGURE 1–7. Example of the transmembrane receptor activating the phosphorylation cascade to activate the nucleus. *K*, kinase; *KK*, kinase that phosphorylates a kinase. See text for in-depth discussion.

stroma talks to the epithelium and the epithelial cells talk to the stroma.

The interface between the stromal and epithelial cells is conducted through the formation of the extracellular matrix (ECM), which is formed by secretion from both the stromal and epithelial cells, such as fibronectin, collagen, laminin, and proteoglycans. This structural support system organizes the structure of the cell and polarizes it to receive growth factors and signals that come from the stroma, epithelium, and endocrine hormones.

This action of growth factors and the extracellular matrix making the stromal-epithelial organization and cross-talk is shown in Figure 1–8, which is a diagram of the prostate, where the epithelium is composed of neuroendocrine, secretory, and basal cells. It is believed that the basal cells are the stem cells that differentiate to form both secretory and neuroendocrine cells. The stroma is made up of smooth muscle, fibroblast, and nerve cells. Threading their way through the stroma are the capillaries, lined by endothelial cells, and immune cells, which can move in and out of the prostate. The capillaries bring the steroids, androgens, estrogens, and nutrients to the prostate. Testosterone is converted to dihydrotestosterone (DHT) by 5-α-reductase in the stroma. In the stroma, the DHT stimulates fibroblast growth factor-7 (KGF), which then diffuses up and activates the receptors on the epithelial cells in a paracrine manner. DHT also stimulates fibroblast growth factor 2 (BFGF), which both feeds back in an autocrine effect on the stroma and has a paracrine effect on the epithelial cells. A similar stimulation is induced by DHT on the production of insulin-like growth factor II (IGF-II), which also has an autocrine and paracrine effect. Insulin-like growth factors are bound to insulin-like growth factor binding proteins (IGFBP), which are also made by the stroma. DHT can diffuse from the smooth muscle into the epithelial cells, where it induces the synthesis of epidermal growth factor and TGF-α. In the epithelial cells, the androgen also induces production of IGFBP, which complexes the insulin-like growth factors and keeps it inactive. One of the main secretory proteins made by the prostate is PSA, which hydrolyzes the IGFBP to release active IGF-I and -II, which then can stimulate the growth of the epithelial cells.

This diagram shows the cross-talk between the stroma and epithelial cells via the testosterone and dihydrotestosterone induction of growth factors that can function in an autocrine and paracrine way to these cell components. It is also important to note that many neurotransmitters are made in the prostate, such as nitric oxide (NO). Nitric oxide is produced by the endothelial, immune, and nerve cells and can have a strong stimulatory effect on stromal and epithelial components.

AGING AND TELOMERASE

Although aging is involved in cancer, we know very little about what really brings about this irreversible and deteriorating effect. Certainly, accumulated damage from free radicals from reactive

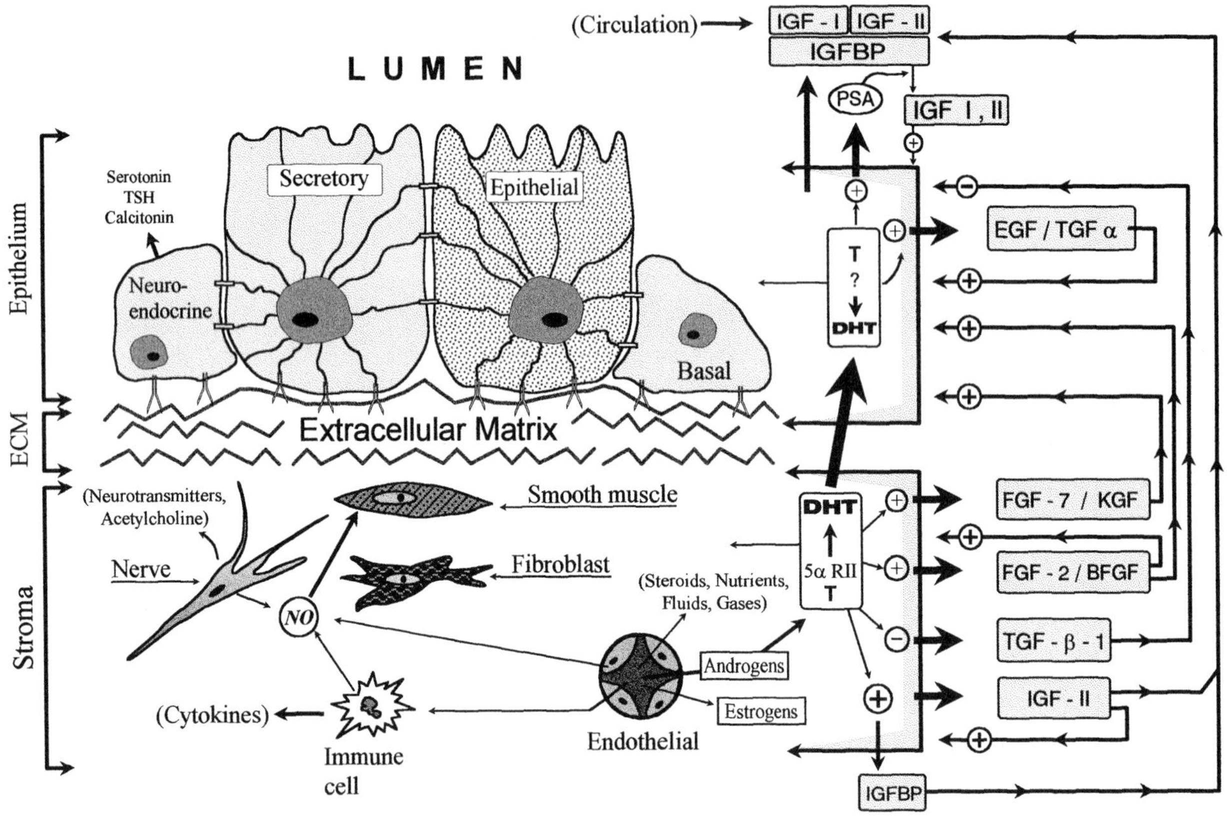
(Circulation)
IGF - I
IGF - II
IGFBP
LUMEN
PSA
IGF I, II
Epithelium
ECM
Stroma
Serotonin
TSH
Calcitonin
Secretory
Epithelial
Neuro-
endocrine
Basal
T
?
DHT
EGF / TGF α
Extracellular Matrix
(Neurotransmitters,
Acetylcholine)
Smooth muscle
Nerve
Fibroblast
NO
(Steroids, Nutrients,
Fluids, Gases)
DHT
5α RII
T
FGF - 7 / KGF
FGF - 2 / BFGF
TGF - β - 1
Androgens
Estrogens
IGF - II
(Cytokines)
Immune
cell
Endothelial
IGFBP

FIGURE 1–8. Stromal-epithelial interactions in the prostate mediated by dihydrotestosterone regulated growth factors; +, stimulation; −, inhibition; NO, nitric oxide. (Adapted from Partin AW, Coffey DS: *In* Walsh PC, Retik AB, Stamey TA, Vaughan ED Jr [eds]: Campbell's Urology, 7th edition. Philadelphia, WB Saunders Co, 1997, with permission.)

oxygen as well as cross-linking and stiffening of collagen are all key components in how we age. Importantly, there is also a biologic clock that counts each cell division; this brings about senescence. At the end of each chromosome are repetitive pieces of DNA called telomeres. Each time the cell divides, it loses a small amount of these telomeres, which is caused by the inability of the DNA synthesis mechanism to fully replicate the last little bit of terminal DNA. The loss of these repetitive pieces of DNA are therefore accumulative and act as a mitotic clock, counting the cell cycles. After approximately 50 doublings, the telomeres of the cell have been reduced to a critical length, resulting in the cell's senescence and death. Every cell is limited by this mitotic clock except cells that have learned how to become immortal. The immortal cells stabilize their telomeres by activating the enzyme called telomerase. Telomerase is an enzyme that carries its own small template made of RNA that is copied into telomere units that allow the cell to replace the telomeres that are lost when the cell divides. In any cell in culture, telomerase has to be activated or the cells would not be immortal. This is also the case only in the stem cells and the germ cells. The other cells do not have telomerase activity and are subject to cell death as the mitotic clock ticks down counting each cell cycle. In cancer cells, telomerase is activated and the cells have become immortal.

We have reported that telomerase is one of the best markers so far in denoting prostate cancer cells from normal and benign prostatic hypertrophy (BPH) cells. This will be a new diagnostic marker when applied in an appropriate manner. Telomerase is one of the most exciting frontiers in understanding senescence, immortality, and how the cancer cell has broken through this aging barrier to become immortal.[5]

OVERCOMING THE TUMOR CELL HETEROGENEITY: APTAMERS AND IN VITRO EVOLUTION

One of the major obstacles in the treatment of urologic cancers is their tremendous heterogeneity. Although clinically appearing as a homogeneous tumor, it actually consists of a heterogeneous pool of cancer cell clones. When we apply any treatment, such as chemotherapy or radiotherapy, we select for subclones in the tumor that are resistant to our treatment. This is not related to the response of the

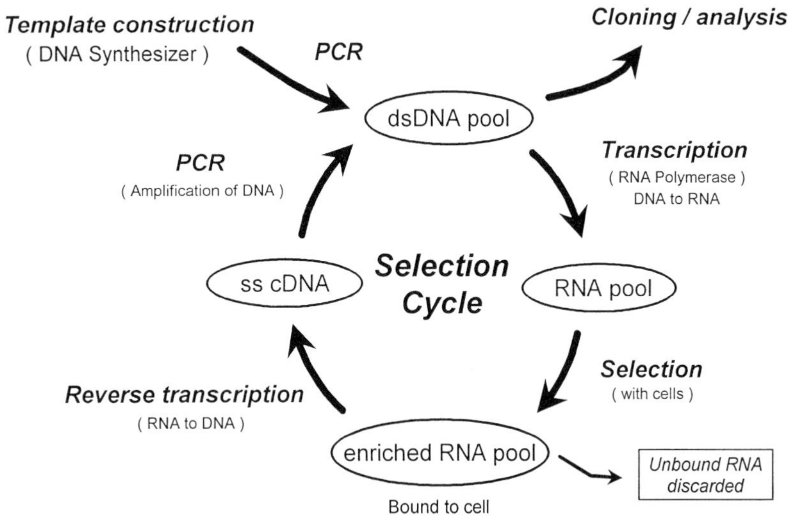
Template construction
(DNA Synthesizer)
PCR
Cloning / analysis
dsDNA pool
Transcription
(RNA Polymerase)
DNA to RNA
PCR
(Amplification of DNA)
ss cDNA
Selection
Cycle
RNA pool
Selection
(with cells)
Reverse transcription
(RNA to DNA)
enriched RNA pool
Bound to cell
Unbound RNA
discarded

FIGURE 1–9. Selection cycle for enriching the binding of a random (10^9) RNA pool to tumor cells. PCR, polymerase chain reaction for amplifying DNA; enriched RNA, aptamer bound to the cells. (Adapted from Garcia-Schürmann JM, Coffey DS: Aptamer adaptability: utilizing tumor cell surface heterogeneity to self-select appropriate diagnostic and therapeutic agents. *In* Getzenberg RH [ed]: Cell Structure 1996 [in press], with permission.)

tumor cells to our treatment but to their ability to use evolutionary techniques to escape any given therapy. There are now new technologies that will allow us to turn therapeutic evolution on the evolution of the tumor and thus beat the cancer at its own game.

Aptamers can be small peptide, DNA, or RNA molecules that will bind in an antibodylike fashion to any given target. Large pools of randomized molecules can be easily made and will provide the molecular diversity to let the tumor cells select the best binding molecules to all the different tumor cell clones. For example, by randomizing the four bases of a 15-nucleotide RNA sequence it is possible to create pools with more than $4^{15} = 10^9$ different molecules. A selection screen is set up in a way allowing us to select the best RNA molecules out of the random pool, that will bind with a high affinity and specificity to our tumor cells. Bound RNA species are then recovered and amplified. This enriched RNA fraction is then subjected to a new round of selection. After 10 to 20 rounds of selection, recovery, and amplification, the pool will contain RNA molecules with high binding specificity. Figure 1–9 gives an overview of a typical selection and amplification cycle that we have involved in in vitro evolution to prostate cancer cells. Those aptamers can then be analyzed and produced in large quantities. They can be used as highly specific cancer probes, to improve diagnosis or, when linked to a cytotoxic "warhead," as a new therapeutic approach to treat cancer.[6]

ACKNOWLEDGMENT

We wish to acknowledge the outstanding effort of Donald Vindivich in designing and creating the figures in this chapter.

REFERENCES

1. Vogelstein B, Kinzler KW: The Multiple Nature of Cancer. Trends Genet 1993; 9:138.
2. Cooper GM: Oncogenes. Boston, Jones & Bartlett, 1995.
3. Bishop JM: Cancer: The Rise of the Genetic Paradigm. Genes Dev 1995; 1309.
4. Rudosalathin E, Reed, JC: Anchorage dependence, integrins and apoptosis. Cell 1994; 77:477.
5. Sommerfeld H-J, Meeker AK, Piatyszek MA, et al: Telomerase activity: a prevalent marker of malignant human prostate tissue. Cancer Res 1996; 56:218.
6. Garcia-Schürmann JM, Coffey DS: Aptamer adaptability: utilizing tumor cell surface heterogeneity to self-select appropriate diagnostic and therapeutic agents. *In* Getzenberg RH (ed): Cell Structure 1996 (in press).
7. Scientific American: What You Need To Know About Cancer. 275, No. 3, September, 1996.

2

GENETIC CONSIDERATIONS AND GENE THERAPY

MARTIN G. SANDA, M.D.

Over 40 years of scientific research following the discovery of DNA[1] have led to recent insights that have set the stage for clinical gene therapy. The enormous volume of scientific research that comprises the foundation for therapeutic use of molecular biology attests to the complexity of linking the most fundamental unit of life, the human genome, to direct clinical intervention.

Preclinical studies have identified several therapeutic strategies based on gene replacement or gene transfer that are under current or planned clinical development. Such gene therapy can correct tumor-specific genetic abnormalities by either inhibiting the function of oncogenes (abnormal tumor genes that promote tumor cell longevity or proliferation) or by restoring functional tumor suppressor genes (such as genes that can regulate DNA repair) that are commonly functionally mutated or absent in cancer. Alternatively, the immune response of patients with cancers harboring any of these abnormalities can be stimulated by gene therapies based on use of recombinant tumor vaccines. Pivotal to all avenues of gene therapy is the gene transfer vector.

GENE TRANSFER VECTORS

As the vehicles for therapeutic gene delivery, gene transfer vectors delegate clinical prospects and limitations. Gene transfer vectors can be generally classified as being of either viral or nonviral origin. Vector design is guided by their desired functions: efficiency of gene transfer, stability of gene expression, and safety of clinical use.

Gene transfer efficiency indicates how well a vector delivers a recombinant gene to a target cell, and how effectively the protein encoded by that gene is subsequently expressed. Highly efficient gene transfer is desirable in almost all clinical strategies using gene transfer. Two critical components determine gene transfer efficiency: gene delivery by the vector and activity of a vector's expression cassette. The first determinant of efficiency, gene delivery, refers to a vector's capacity for cellular attachment, entry, and delivery of the therapeutic gene (within an expression cassette) to a site such as the target cell nucleus at which gene expression can occur. Delivery mechanisms of each vector system are distinct.[2–4] Cell surface density of specific receptors that may be required for vector attachment, as well as stability of the vector itself in the microenvironment surrounding the target cell, affect a vector's capacity for therapeutic gene delivery.[5–7] The second principal determinant of vector efficiency is the vector expression cassette, which contains, in addition to the therapeutic gene, a promoter sequence controlling therapeutic gene transcription. Some vectors (such as poxviruses) encode their own machinery for gene transcription,[4] while others rely entirely on pre-existing polymerases in the target cell[8]; however, all vectors carry a promoter region flanking the therapeutic gene. The promoter profoundly affects therapeutic gene expression and vector efficiency.[9]

The stability of gene expression by a specific vector system depends on the intracellular localization of the therapeutic gene by the vector. Typically, episomal localization (when the therapeutic gene is not integrated in the target cell chromosome) leads to transient expression of the gene because most mammalian cells have efficient mechanisms for extruding episomal foreign DNA. In contrast, vectors that allow the transferred gene to be integrated into the host cell chromosomal DNA, such as retroviral vectors, provide longer duration of stable expression. Although stable, durable expression may be desirable in treating hereditary disorders and chronic disorders, it should be noted that transient gene expression may be equally as desirable if not more so in many strategies of cancer gene therapy.[8]

RETROVIRUS VECTORS

Retroviral vectors were used in the first clinical trials of gene therapy.[10,11] Although retroviral vectors provide distinctly stable long-term expression of therapeutic genes, use of these vectors is limited by complexity of retroviral genetic engineering and vector purification as well as by hypothetical safety obstacles.[6,7] These vectors are currently being used predominantly in ex vivo gene transfer protocols, although in vivo gene transfer applications are emerging.

Vector Production. Production of replication-deficient retroviral vectors is accomplished with vector packaging cell lines (Fig. 2–1). Vector particles secreted into packaging cell supernatant are purified and concentrated in preparation for use for gene transfer.

Gene Delivery. Cells targeted for gene transfer using the purified retroviral vector incorporate the vector by endocytosis via a specific receptor (Fig. 2–2).[12] Reverse transcriptase then converts vector RNA into DNA, which is then integrated into the target cell chromosomal DNA during target cell proliferation. This requirement for target cell proliferation as a prerequisite to transferred gene expression is unique to retroviral vectors; retroviral vectors thus do not readily transfer genes to quiescent cells.[6,7]

Gene Expression. After integration of the retroviral vector expression cassette (the therapeutic gene flanked by sequences that promote gene expression) into the chromosome of the target cell, the therapeutic gene is expressed by the target cell's own polymerases and other mediators of gene expression. Because the therapeutic gene is integrated into the target cell genome, it is stably expressed by the cell long term and is passed on to progeny should the cell continue to proliferate. Further contributing to long-term stability of retroviral transferred gene expression is the immunologically inert phenotype of these vector constructs: immune responses targeting the vector itself have not been an obstacle to retroviral vector use. Although stable genomic integration, as can be achieved with retroviral vectors, may be desirable for some therapeutic strategies (such as tumor suppressor gene replacement), stable and permanent alteration of the target cell genome in vivo also poses potential safety pitfalls such as potentially irreversible untoward genetic effects in vivo.

Attributes and Applications. Due to limitations in the functional concentration (or titer) of retroviral preparations, and also due to rapid inactivation of unbound retrovirus in vivo, direct in vivo gene transfer using retroviral vectors has generally been inefficient, with only a small fraction of target cells expressing the transferred gene. Retrovirus

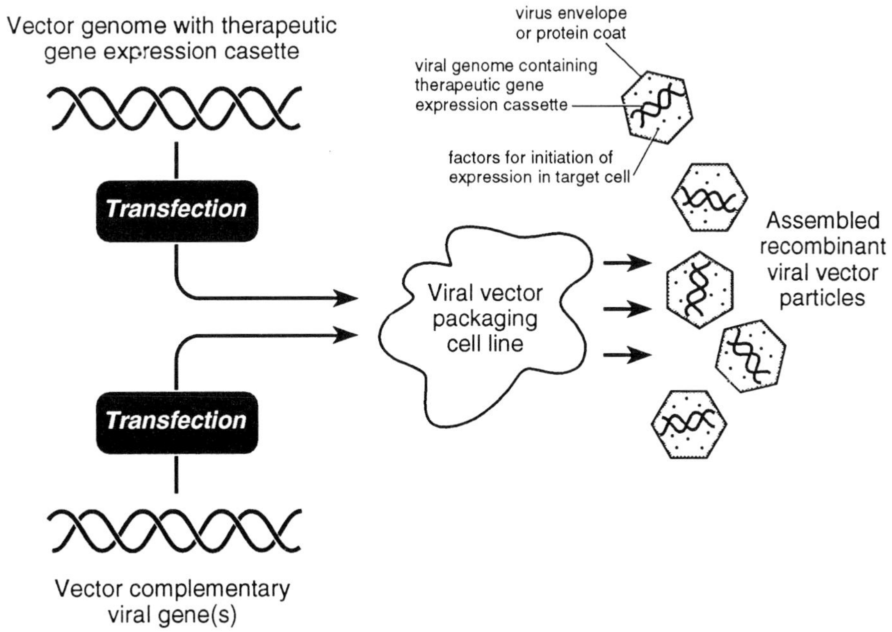
Vector genome with therapeutic gene expression casette
Transfection
Transfection
Vector complementary viral gene(s)
virus envelope or protein coat
viral genome containing therapeutic gene expression cassette
factors for initiation of expression in target cell
Viral vector packaging cell line
Assembled recombinant viral vector particles

FIGURE 2–1. Production of recombinant viral vectors for gene therapy. A schematic representation of retroviral vector production is shown; analogous systems are in use for the production of adenoviral and poxvirus vectors. For retroviral vector production, packaging cell lines in which the therapeutic gene has replaced retroviral *gag*, *pol*, and *env* genes (these genes are normally required for retrovirus particle production and packaging by infected cells). The packaging cell line has been cotransfected with these viral genes *in trans* to complement the replication-defective vector genome, allowing the packaging cell line to produce and package replication-deficient viral vector particles. (Based on references 2, 3, and 6.)

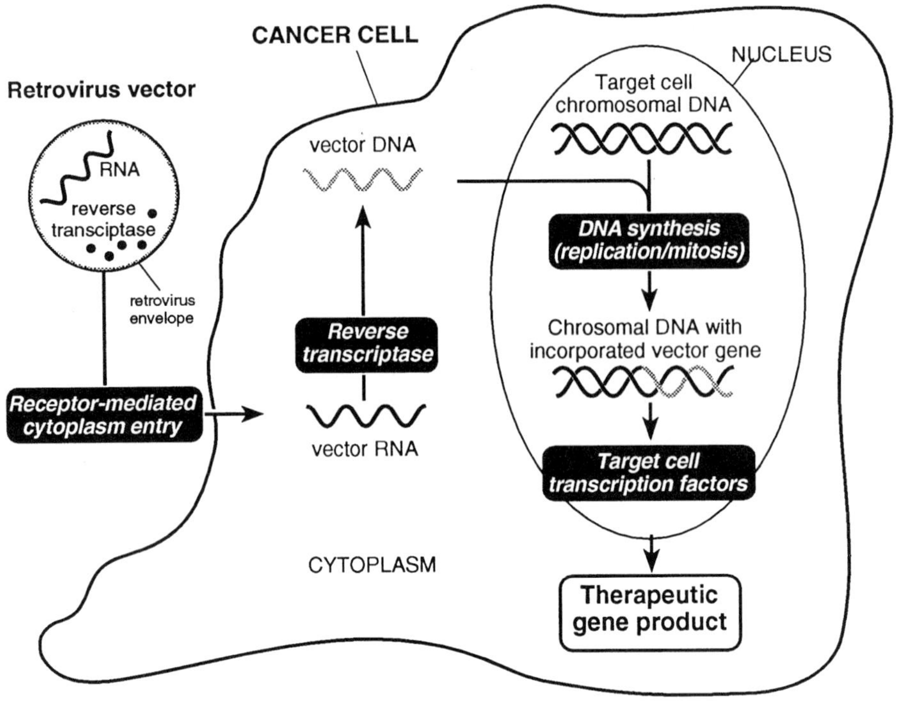
CANCER CELL
Retrovirus vector
RNA
reverse transciptase
retrovirus envelope
Receptor-mediated cytoplasm entry
vector DNA
Reverse transcriptase
vector RNA
CYTOPLASM
NUCLEUS
Target cell chromosomal DNA
DNA synthesis (replication/mitosis)
Chrosomal DNA with incorporated vector gene
Target cell transcription factors
Therapeutic gene product

FIGURE 2–2. Gene transfer by retrovirus vectors. Retroviral gene transfer is mediated by integration of the therapeutic gene into the target cell chromosomal DNA, and therefore requires target cell DNA replication. (Based on references 2, 6, 7, and 9.)

vectors can, however, mediate highly efficient gene transfer ex vivo (Table 2–1).[2] Cancer therapy applications of retroviral vectors have therefore predominantly involved ex vivo gene transfer—for example, to augment the immunogenicity of patient-derived tumor cells (by introducing into such tumor cells an immunostimulatory gene) prior to use of such cells in vivo as a gene-modified tumor cell vaccine or for marker studies.[10,13–15] Because retroviral gene transfer itself neither damages the host cell nor induces undesirable vector-specific immunity, these vectors are ideally suited for gene-modified cancer cell vaccine therapies seeking to elicit tumor-specific immunity.

Two attributes of retroviral vectors may prove advantageous for emerging direct in vivo gene transfer strategies. First, the requirement for target cell proliferation as a prerequisite for integration and expression of the vector hypothetically may provide selective expression of therapeutic genes in rapidly proliferating malignant cells, thereby specifically targeting such cells for functional gene transfer.[9] Second, the durable integration and expression of retroviral vectors may facilitate the long-term efficacy of therapies based on tumor suppressor gene restoration. These two theoretical advantages of retroviral vectors have not yet been realized, as limitations of titer and in vivo instability have hitherto prevailed.

ADENOVIRUS VECTORS

Interest in adenoviral vectors was prompted by their capacity for highly efficient gene transfer in vivo. The propensity of adenovirus vectors to induce nonspecific inflammation and a vector-specific immune response, however, has been a significant limitation of this vector system in clinical trials evaluating adenovirus vectors for gene replacement therapy in, for example, cystic fibrosis.[7,16] Whether the efficacy of antitumor therapies using this vector

TABLE 2–1. ATTRIBUTES OF VECTORS FOR THERAPEUTIC GENE DELIVERY

Vector	Duration of Therapeutic Gene Expression	Efficiency of Gene Transfer	Other
Retrovirus	Stable long-term	Variable	Labile in vivo
Adenovirus	Transient	Highly efficient	Immunogenic
Poxvirus	Transient	Highly efficient	Immunogenic
Nonviral plasmid (liposomal or gene gun)	Transient	Inefficient	Fewer safety concerns

system will be attenuated or augmented by inherent immunogenicity of adenoviral vectors remains to be elucidated.

Vector Production. Recombinant adenoviral vectors are rendered infectious but replication defective (while retaining their capacity to infect cells) by deletions in an early region DNA (E1) required for viral replication.[3] The deleted E1 region and other regions of the adenovirus genome serve as sites for therapeutic genes by using shuttle plasmids and homologous recombination with complementary deletion mutants (Fig. 2–1). A packaging cell line (293 cells, a transformed human embryonic kidney cell line containing the adenovirus E1 DNA) transfected with the E1-deleted adenoviral vector containing a gene of interest is used to produce the replication-deficient adenoviral vectors.[3] High concentrations of adenoviral vector (titer > 10^{11} pfu/ml) can be readily purified.

Gene Delivery. Adenoviruses are taken up by the target cells via binding of the adenoviral vector to target cell integrins ($\alpha_v\beta_5$ or $\alpha_v\beta_3$) and a second cell surface receptor (Fig. 2–3).[7,17,18] The vector is transported from the endosome to the cytoplasm, where the adenoviral protein coat is lost as the adenoviral DNA migrates to the nucleus. In the target cell nucleus, the vector remains epichromosomal and is not integrated into the target cell chromosome. Replication of the target cell is not required for therapeutic gene delivery.

Gene Expression. Nuclear localization of the adenoviral vector allows the target cell's own polymerases and other mediators of gene expression to participate in expression of the therapeutic gene. However, because they remain epichromosomal, expression of adenoviral vector genes is transient, lasting one to several weeks.[7]

Attributes and Applications. Adenovirus vectors are characterized by transient duration of gene expression in target cells, significant induction (by the vector) of inflammation and immunity, and capacity for highly efficient gene transfer in vivo (Table 2–1). The transient gene expression associated with adenoviral vectors is less likely to constrain the utility of these vectors for cancer therapy than for other applications: Gene-targeted immunotherapy, as well as apoptosis-inducing therapies, does not require permanent expression of therapeutic genes, and adenovirus vectors have been effectively applied for such therapeutic strategies in preclinical models.[19,20] Indeed, the transient nature of adenovirus-mediated gene transfer circumvents the safety issue of irreversible undesirable genetic effects such as could be encountered with retroviral gene transfer.

Adenovirus vectors are potent immunogens.[16] Although potentially desirable for gene-targeted immunotherapies, the inherent immunogenicity of adenoviruses may also limit repeated administration of these vectors due to sensitization-induced inflammatory toxicity.[7] Moreover, adenovirus-specific immunity may constrain in vivo gene

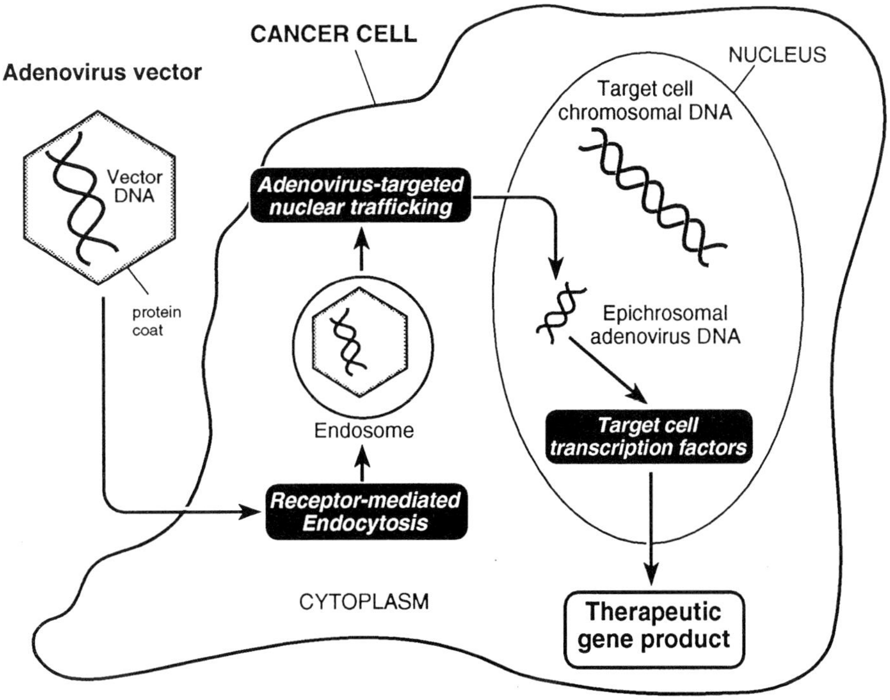
CANCER CELL
Adenovirus vector
Vector DNA
protein coat
NUCLEUS
Target cell chromosomal DNA
Adenovirus-targeted nuclear trafficking
Endosome
Epichrosomal adenovirus DNA
Target cell transcription factors
Receptor-mediated Endocytosis
CYTOPLASM
Therapeutic gene product

FIGURE 2–3. Gene transfer by adenovirus vectors. Adenoviral vectors do not require target cell DNA replication for efficient gene transfer. However, nuclear localization of the vector DNA is required, since target cell nuclear factors are used for gene expression. Because these vectors are epichromosomal, therapeutic gene expression is typically less durable than with retroviral vectors. (Based on references 3, 7, and 9.)

transfer with adenoviral vectors by inducing humoral and cellular responses capable of eliminating the vector and further reducing duration of target gene expression.[16] Despite these limitations, the receptivity of many human cells to adenoviral transfection, coupled with the relative stability and ease of production of adenoviral vectors, has led to significant tumor reduction in several preclinical models of direct in vivo gene transfer.[19–22]

POXVIRUS VECTORS

Vaccinia and other poxvirus vectors are derived from one of the greatest triumphs of postclassical medicine: the smallpox vaccine.[4] Jenner's discovery that a bovine poxvirus was an effective human vaccine against smallpox in 1798 eventually led to implementation of a concerted worldwide vaccination program by the World Health Organization (WHO) implemented in 1967, and Jenner's prediction of "the annihilation of the Small Pox" was finally realized in 1995, nearly 200 years after the introduction of poxvirus vaccines for human use. Current use of poxvirus vectors for experimental cancer therapy relate to the ability of these vectors to induce potent immune responses in vivo.

VECTOR PRODUCTION. Because recombinant poxviruses are used as live, replication-competent viruses (albeit in attenuated or otherwise nonpathogenic forms when administered in vivo), production can be achieved by simply infecting specific host cells that allow productive infection.[4] Genetically engineered packaging cell lines such as those used for retrovirus or adenovirus vector production are not required. Immunostimulatory cytokine, accessory molecule, or tumor antigen genes can be inserted into vaccinia or other poxvirus vectors by flanking these genes with poxvirus sequences in a "shuttle" plasmid, and then introducing this plasmid into a cell that has been infected with whole vaccinia virus. Homologous recombination (as with adenoviral vector systems) in the vaccinia and shuttle plasmid cotransfected cells then leads to insertion of the gene of interest in a small proportion of the viral progeny (Fig. 2–1). Linking the therapeutic gene with an adjacent selectable marker gene allows subsequent purification and production of exclusively recombinant poxvirus containing the gene of interest.[4] Up to 25,000 base pairs (bp) of foreign DNA can be accommodated by vaccinia vectors, representing the greatest size capacity of currently available recombinant viral vectors for transferred genes.[4]

GENE DELIVERY. Infectious poxvirus virions enter the target cell via fusion of the virion lipoprotein envelope with the target cell cytoplasm and intracytoplasmic release of the virion complex core (Fig. 2–4).[4] The virion complex core contains the vector genome as well as RNA polymerases and other enzymes required for expression of the vector genes; the vector remains in the cytoplasm, where gene expression controlled by elements contained in the virion complex core occurs.

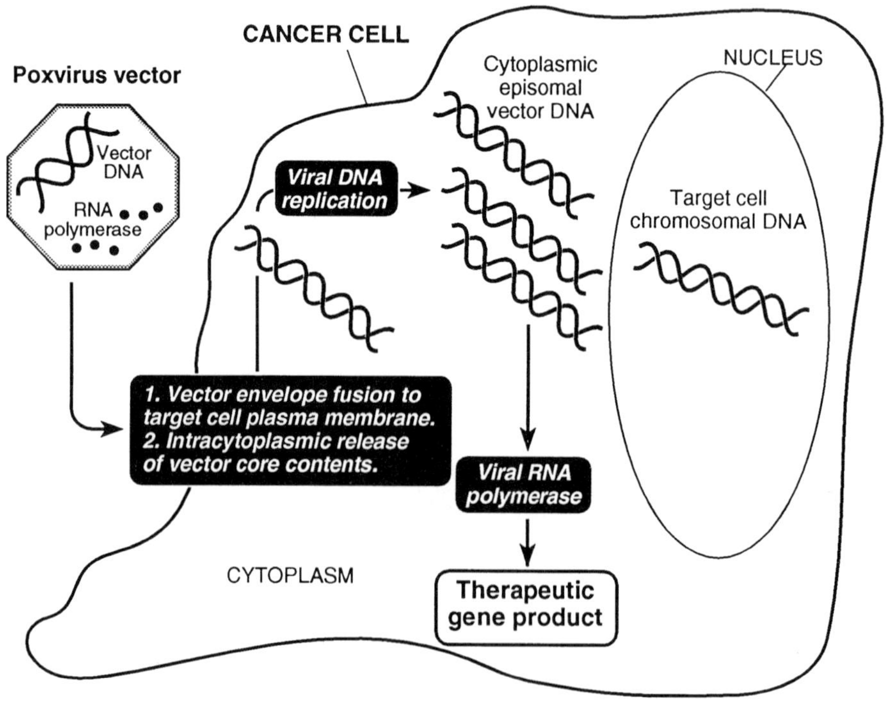
CANCER CELL
Poxvirus vector
Vector DNA
RNA polymerase
Cytoplasmic episomal vector DNA
NUCLEUS
Viral DNA replication
Target cell chromosomal DNA
1. Vector envelope fusion to target cell plasma membrane.
2. Intracytoplasmic release of vector core contents.
Viral RNA polymerase
CYTOPLASM
Therapeutic gene product

FIGURE 2–4. Gene transfer by poxvirus vectors. Poxvirus vector particles contain viral RNA polymerases, obviating any need for nuclear localization or chromosomal integration. Therapeutic gene expression occurs entirely in the target cell cytoplasm. (Based on reference 4.)

Gene Expression. Poxvirus vectors are unique in their ability to express therapeutic genes without requiring transport of the vector to the target cell nucleus. In contrast to other vector systems, which require host cell nuclear factors and enzymes for gene expression, poxviruses carry the apparatus for synthesis of translatable RNA (including virus-encoded RNA polymerases, transcription factors, capping enzymes, and poly[A]polymerases) either prepackaged within the complex virus core or encoded within the viral genome itself.[4] Expression cassettes in poxvirus vectors thus require unique poxvirus-specific promoter regions that can be recognized by viral transcription factors.

Attributes and Applications. Poxvirus transfection is transient and eventually toxic to the target cell (Table 2–1). The successful history of vaccinia use for smallpox eradication and the relative ease of cloning genes into vaccinia vectors has uniquely poised vaccinia and other poxvirus vectors for use as recombinant tumor vaccines. As with adenovirus vectors, use of poxviruses for immunogene therapy is tempered by potentially competitive, antivector, immune response induction.[23]

NONVIRAL VECTORS: LIPOSOMES AND THE GENE GUN

Nonviral approaches to gene therapy avoid disadvantages of viral vectors, such as safety issues related to potential replication-competent virus formation, and limited target cell diversity related to receptor requirements for viral envelope adsorption.[5,7,8,17,18] The most extensively developed nonviral gene delivery systems are liposome-mediated gene transfer and high-velocity particle-mediated gene transfer, also known as the "gene gun."

Vector Production. Plasmid-liposome complexes for gene delivery are comprised of DNA formulated with cationic lipids. The cationic lipid–DNA complexes commonly used for gene delivery in current clinical trials are not true liposomes containing plasmid DNA within a lipid envelope, but rather are particulate complexes in which plasmid DNA is dispersed among the bound lipids.[5,7,24]

Gene Delivery. These complexes promote cellular gene delivery by hydrophobic interaction and fusion of the lipid–DNA complex with the target cell membrane. Unlike viral vectors, however, no signal exists to facilitate transport of the plasmid DNA containing the therapeutic gene to the nucleus (Fig. 2–5).[5] Transfection efficiency is therefore typically relatively inefficient (Table 2–1). In contrast, high-velocity particle-mediated gene transfer, or gene-gun technology, allows the delivery of thousands of copies of DNA into targeted cells. This is achieved by coating 1- to 3-μm gold particles with plasmid DNA or mammalian chromosomal genomic DNA up to 44 kb in size; a gene gun is then used to deliver the particles in vivo by generating a high-pressure gas burst that accelerates the particles to a velocity sufficiently high for penetration of multiple cell layers (Fig. 2–6).[8] As with

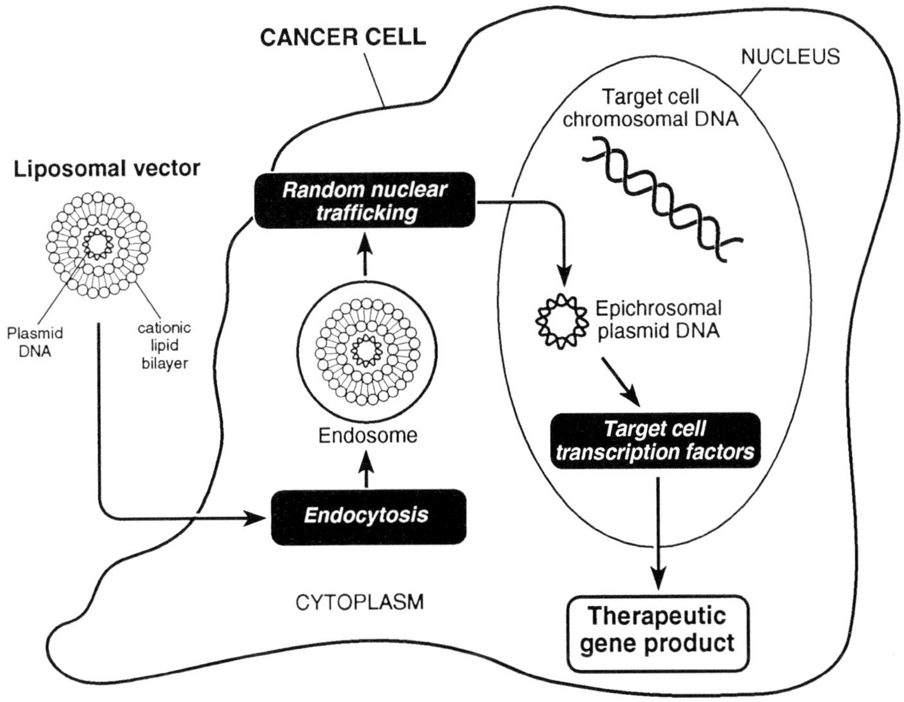
CANCER CELL
NUCLEUS
Target cell chromosomal DNA
Liposomal vector
Random nuclear trafficking
Plasmid DNA
cationic lipid bilayer
Epichrosomal plasmid DNA
Endosome
Target cell transcription factors
Endocytosis
CYTOPLASM
Therapeutic gene product

FIGURE 2–5. Nonviral gene transfer by liposomal vectors. Liposomal vectors in current use are complexes of cationic lipids and plasmid DNA. Although relatively safe and immunologically inert, liposomal vectors require nuclear localization for access to target cell transcription factors. (Based on references 5 and 7.)

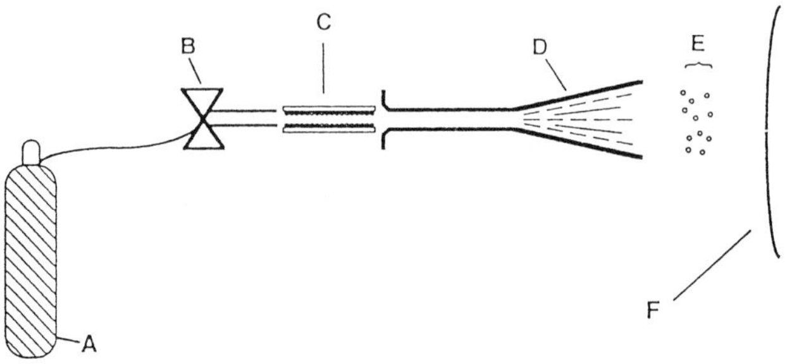
A
B
C
D
E
F

FIGURE 2–6. Nonviral gene transfer via particle bombardment (gene gun). In the helium pulse gene gun, motive force is generated by release of a high-pressure burst of helium gas from a reservoir (*A*) at a preset pressure (150 to 700 psi). A release valve (*B*) discharges helium through a cartridge (*C*) containing DNA-coated gold particles. After being dispersed by an exit nozzle (*D*), the DNA-coated gold particles (*E*) penetrate target cells or tissue (*F*) with sufficient force to penetrate multiple cell layers and deliver plasmid DNA intracellularly. (From Yang NS, Sun WH: Gene gun and other non-viral approaches for cancer gene therapy. Nat Med 1995; 1:481, with permission.)

lipid–DNA complex gene transfer, translocation of plasmid DNA to the nucleus after gene-gun delivery is not a specifically targeted event.

Gene Expression. Plasmid DNA that does manage to translocate to the nucleus usually is not integrated into the target cell genome, and remains epichromosomal (Fig. 2–5).[5] Similar to adenoviral vectors, expression relies on target cell transcription factors and is typically relatively transient.

Attributes and Applications. The principal advantage of nonviral gene delivery systems including cationic lipid–DNA complexes, the gene gun, and other nonviral delivery systems is that these systems circumvent three potentially problematic characteristics of viral vectors: immune reactivity, reliance on viral receptor expression by target cells, and safety issues related to potential pathogenic recombinant contaminants in viral preparations. Enthusiasm and applicability of nonviral vectors is tempered by relatively inefficient gene delivery and transient therapeutic gene expression (Table 2–1). As transient expression systems, nonviral and gene-gun delivery systems have been useful for induction of antitumor immunity. Induction of cytokine secretion using the gene gun has been associated with reduction of renal cell carcinoma progression in a mouse model.[25] Clinical studies using lipid–DNA complexes have shown induction of antitumor immune mediators in melanoma patients, and trials using these vectors for renal cell cancer are underway.[24,26]

EMERGING VECTORS AND OTHER GENE DELIVERY SYSTEMS

The preceding discussion has focused on gene transfer vectors currently being used in clinical trials as investigative agents for urologic cancers. A variety of other, novel viral as well as nonviral vectors are currently under development. Among emerging viral vectors are gene delivery constructs derived from herpesvirus, parvovirus, and adeno-associated viruses.[27–29] Nonviral vectors under development include eukaryote-derived vectors such as *Listeria monocytogenes* and recombinant bacille Calmette-Guérin (BCG), synthetic constructs such as dendrimers, and others.[30] The ideal vector for most gene therapy applications will likely evolve as a hybrid vector merging the desirable properties of viral vectors with advantageous attributes of nonviral delivery systems.[9]

MOLECULAR TARGETS OF GENE THERAPY

Gene therapy for urologic malignancy can be categorized into four distinct strategies based on the molecular target of gene transfer: immunogene therapy, direct tumor cell death induction, anti-oncogene therapy, and tumor suppressor gene restoration (Table 2–2). Immunogene therapy affects tumor growth indirectly by inducing a tumor-

TABLE 2–2. CHARACTERISTICS OF GENE THERAPY STRATEGIES IN CURRENT CLINICAL TRIALS

Therapeutic Gene	Extent of Potential Efficacy In Vivo*	Relative Obstacles
Immunogene: ex vivo transfer	Systemic	Tissue procurement and cell culture required
Immunogene: in vivo transfer	Systemic	Vector-specific immunity may interfere with induction of tumor-specific immunity
Cytotoxicity/apoptosis	Local-regional	Requirement for highly efficient gene delivery in vivo; possibility of cytotoxic injury to normal cells
Anti-oncogene/antisense	Local-regional	Requirement for highly efficient gene delivery in vivo and durable expression of therapeutic gene
Tumor suppressor	Local-regional	Requirement for highly efficient gene delivery in vivo and durable expression of therapeutic gene

*Based on current vector limitations.

TABLE 2–3. NIH-APPROVED CLINICAL TRIALS OF GENE THERAPY FOR UROLOGIC CANCER

Strategy	Principal Investigator	Vector: Therapeutic Gene	Cancer Histology	Status
Immunotherapy: gene transfer ex vivo	Gansbacher	Retrovirus: IL-2	Renal cell	Open
	Simons	Retrovirus: GM-CSF	Renal cell	Completed
	Simons	Retrovirus: GM-CSF	Prostate	Open
	Paulson	Liposome: IL-2	Prostate	Pending
Immunotherapy: gene transfer in vivo	Vogelzang	Liposome: class I MHC	Renal cell	Completed
	Figlin	Liposome: class I MHC	Renal cell	Open
	Lattime	Poxvirus-vaccinia: GM-CSF	Transitional cell	Open
	Chen	Poxvirus-vaccinia: PSA	Prostate	Open
Cytotoxic	Scardino	Adenovirus: HSV-tk	Prostate	Open
Anti-oncogene	Steiner	Retrovirus: *myc* antisense	Prostate	Pending
Tumor suppressor gene restoration	Small	Adenovirus: Rb gene	Transitional cell	Pending

specific immune response either via immunostimulatory gene transfer ex vivo (followed by in vivo administration of genetically altered cells to induce a tumor-specific immune response) or via direct in vivo transfer of immunostimulatory or tumor antigen genes. Direct tumor cell death induction relies on delivery of genes encoding cellular toxins or apoptosis-inducing proteins. Anti-oncogene therapy specifically inhibits or eliminates oncogene activity. Tumor suppressor gene restoration therapy inhibits tumor growth by restoring genes that prevent transformation of the normal cell but which have been functionally disabled during carcinogenesis. The preclinical rationale for these gene therapy strategies and consequent gene therapy clinical trials treating urologic cancers are discussed (Table 2–3).

Immunogene Therapy via Ex Vivo Gene Transfer

Gene therapy via transfer of immunostimulatory genes to induce a tumor-specific immune response is perhaps the most extensively evaluated strategy of gene therapy to date. This is partly because early gene transfer systems limited gene therapy to strategies using ex vivo (rather than in vivo) gene transfer, and this approach is widely applicable as immunogene therapy using, for example, patient-derived cultured tumor cells for a gene-modified tumor cell vaccine.[13,31–38] Generally speaking, clinical applications of these studies used retroviral vectors as the vehicles for gene transfer.[14,15,39] Recently, however, strategies of immunogene therapy have been formulated that rely on gene transfer in vivo.[19,23–26,40–44] It is therefore useful to evaluate immunogene therapy strategies in the context of whether the particular strategy requires ex vivo gene transfer or in vivo gene transfer (Table 2–2).

Therapies using genetically modified, patient-derived cells for a genetically engineered tumor vaccine have comprised the principal use of ex vivo immunogene therapy for urologic malignancies in preclinical studies and clinical trials as well. For these therapies, tumor cells isolated from fresh surgical specimens are genetically transduced during tissue culture with an immunostimulatory gene. The resected genitourinary cancer cells serve principally as vehicles for autologous tumor antigens and are transduced for immunostimulatory gene expression. The gene-modified tumor vaccine is typically irradiated ex vivo prior to being reinjected into the patient as a genetically engineered tumor cell vaccine (Fig. 2–7).

Initial preclinical studies evaluating this strategy of gene therapy showed that a tumor-specific, T-cell–mediated immune response could be augmented by vaccination using tumor cells derived from the same tumor but transduced to secrete interleukin-2 (IL-2); such vaccination protected animals from subsequent tumor challenge.[31,32] Interferon-γ (IFN-γ) gene transfer was shown to promote a similar protective effect.[33] Subsequently, transfer of granulocyte-macrophage colony-stimulating factor (GM-CSF) and other immunostimulatory genes into tumor cells used for vaccination led to elimination of preestablished microscopic tumor cell deposits in animal models. Antitumor immune mediators (such as helper T cells, cytolytic T cells, natural killer [NK] cells, and dendritic cells) are activated by the expression of therapeutic immunostimulatory genes in close proximity to tumor-specific antigens present in the genetically engineered tumor vaccine cells. The immune mediators then circulate and, ideally, eradicate distant micrometastases.[13,34] Preclinical in vivo efficacy of such gene-modified tumor cell vaccines has also been shown in several models of urologic malignancy, including renal cancer, bladder cancer, and prostate cancer (Fig. 2–7).[13,35–38]

Several clinical trials using immunogene therapy with ex vivo gene transfer specifically for urologic cancers are underway or forthcoming (Table 2–3).[14,15,39,45,46] Therapeutic genes encoding IL-2 and GM-CSF targeted prostate cancer or renal cell carcinoma in these studies. In the only study completed at present, no dose-limiting toxicities were

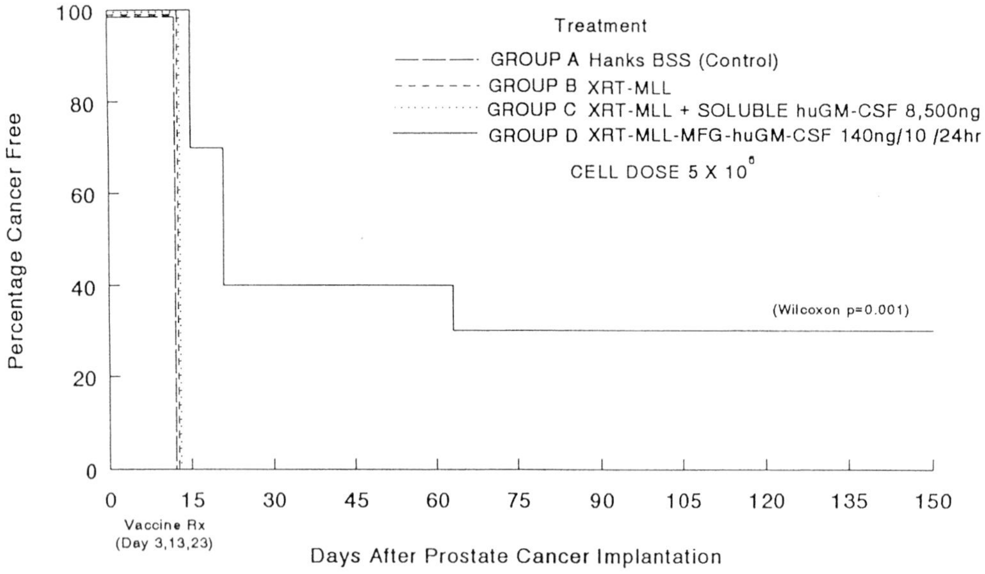
Percentage Cancer Free
100
80
60
40
20
0
Treatment
GROUP A Hanks BSS (Control)
GROUP B XRT-MLL
GROUP C XRT-MLL + SOLUBLE huGM-CSF 8,500ng
GROUP D XRT-MLL-MFG-huGM-CSF 140ng/10 /24hr
CELL DOSE 5 X 10^6
(Wilcoxon p=0.001)
0 15 30 45 60 75 90 105 120 135 150
Vaccine Rx
(Day 3,13,23)
Days After Prostate Cancer Implantation

A

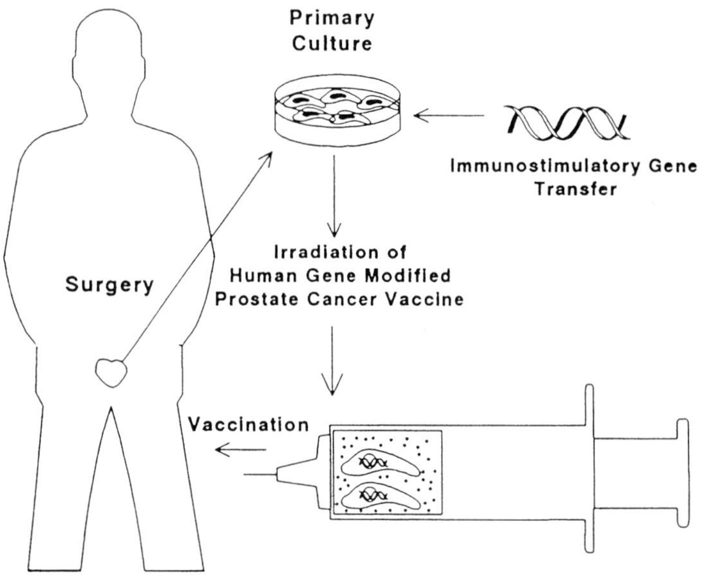
Primary
Culture
Immunostimulatory Gene
Transfer
Surgery
Irradiation of
Human Gene Modified
Prostate Cancer Vaccine
Vaccination

B

FIGURE 2–7. Immunogene therapy via ex vivo gene transfer. *A*, Preclinical models have shown that vaccination of tumor-bearing animals with tumor cells that have been retrovirally transfected ex vivo to produce immunogene products (in this case GM-CSF) can induce complete or partial tumor regression at a distant metastatic site (as shown in the illustrated experiment using hormone-refractory Dunning rat prostate cancer). (From Sanda MG, Ayyagari SR, Jaffee EM, et al: Demonstration of a rational strategy for human prostate cancer gene therapy. J Urol 1994;151:622, with permission.) *B*, Schema of an analogous human gene therapy protocol being evaluated in an ongoing clinical trial based on experiments such as that in *A*. (From Sanda MG, Simons JW: Gene therapy for urological cancer. Urology 1994; 44:617, with permission.)

encountered, and a dose-dependent lymphocyte infiltrate was noted at the vaccine site.[14] The single patient who exhibited a partial response in this phase I study also showed the greatest delayed-type hypersensitivity (DTH) response in the study group, suggesting that GM-CSF–secreting vaccine cells can induce tumor-specific immune responses with minimal toxicity.[14] Evaluation of potential clinical efficacy with this strategy awaits a larger phase II study.

A significant limitation of these ex vivo gene transfer therapies, however, is the need for cell culture of cancer cells that serve as targets for gene transfer (Table 2–2). Problems associated with the need for cell culture include requisite surgery to procure adequate tumor volumes for vaccine cell production; unreliable tumor cell yield with regard to both tumor cell number and tumorigenic genotype; and a requirement for cumbersome, expensive cell culture for each treated subject limiting the widespread applicability of this therapy.[14,36,47] To circumvent these limitations of ex vivo tumor cell culture for gene transfer, the development of nonretroviral gene transfer vectors has led to alternative immunogene therapies using in vivo gene transfer techniques.

Immunogene Therapy via In Vivo Gene Transfer

The advent of vectors capable of efficient and safe direct gene transfer in vivo, such as poxvirus, adenovirus, and liposome vectors, has provided an avenue for overcoming problems unique to ex vivo gene transfer therapies such as the need for tumor cell procurement and culture (Tables 2–1 and 2–2). Two general approaches using in vivo gene transfer for immunogene therapy have been developed through preclinical studies to the arena of clinical trials: one entails in vivo transfer of immunostimulatory genes, and the other entails in vivo delivery of tumor antigen genes by recombinant viral vectors vaccines.

In vivo gene transfer of immunostimulatory genes has been evaluated using poxvirus and liposomal vectors encoding GM-CSF, IL-2, IL-12, and other genes for therapy of renal, bladder, and prostate cancer.[25,26,43,48] Rather than removing tumor cells to achieve genetic modification in vitro, and then using the gene-modified cells as a vaccine, the gene transfer vector is administered directly into tumor in vivo, such as by intravesical instillation or intratumoral injection. The transfected tumor cells essentially function as an in situ vaccine to induce activity both against the transfected primary tumor site and distant metastases, without having undergone ex vivo processing and culture. A potential advantage of this approach is that genuine tumor antigen expression by the in vivo–transfected tumor cells is conserved, while interference by in vitro–artifact antigens is avoided (Table 2–2). This approach has also been extensively evaluated with other vector systems[19,24] in nonurologic tumor models, and clinical trials in urologic and other tumors based on these studies have been undertaken. Two trials have sought to induce antitumor immunity against renal cell carcinoma by direct liposomal gene transfer in vivo of class I major histocompatibility complex (MHC) genes (Table 2–3). This approach is based on studies demonstrating that defective class I MHC expression is a common mechanism of immune evasion in most urologic cancers.[49–52] In addition, intravesical poxvirus vector administration is being evaluated in a clinical trial evaluating potential in situ GM-CSF immunogene transfer for bladder cancer therapy (Table 2–3).[43,53]

Some distinct advantages of bladder cancer and prostate cancer, specifically, support a focus upon these malignancies with in vivo immunostimulatory gene transfer. First, regional targeting of localized bladder and prostate cancer is potentially readily achieved in these sites by either intravesical administration or transrectal prostatic injection. Second, prostate cancer immunogene therapy poses the possibility of using not only tumor antigens, but also potentially of normal prostate antigens (such as prostate-specific antigen [PSA], expressed in normal and malignant prostate cells alike) as targets of immune effector cells.

Use of recombinant vectors encoding specific tumor antigens as agents for recombinant vaccination differs from other immunogene therapy strategies in that the viral vector itself provides the antigen to stimulate a tumor-specific immune response. In this setting, the patient's tumor cells are not relied on as an effective antigen-presenting cell, nor are they a required target of direct immunogene transfer. Instead of targeting tumor cells as the recipients of the therapeutic gene (as shown in Fig. 2–4), systemically administered recombinant vector vaccines target professional antigen-presenting cells as recipients for the therapeutic gene (which in this strategy encodes a tumor antigen). By using antigen-presenting cells, such as dendritic cells, to induce immune mediators which then recognize and eliminate tumor cells, this strategy avoids potential tumor cell mechanisms for actively suppressing immune induction, such as secretion of transforming growth factor-β (TGF-β).[54–56] Initial studies using recombinant vectors as tumor-specific vaccines focused on relatively simple vector constructs encoding a specific tumor antigen alone as the basis for induction of immunity.[23,40] Along these lines, a vaccinia vaccine encoding PSA is soon to enter clinical trials (Table 2–3).[44] The goal of vaccinia-PSA gene therapy is to induce an immune response against any cells expressing PSA under the hypothesis that activated PSA-specific T cells will kill cancer cells that express PSA (as in the setting of recurrence after radical prostatectomy). Innate immune tolerance to PSA as a normal self-antigen, however, will need to be overcome to achieve the desired therapeutic effect.

The efficacy of preclinical immunogene therapy studies should be viewed in context. When evaluated in highly lethal, nonimmunogenic tumor models that most closely mimic human malignancy, the antitumor effect has been modest—in the range of 4-log kill. This would indicate that clinical efficacy of a gene-modified tumor cell vaccine approach may potentially be limited to an adjuvant setting. In addition, characteristics common among urologic cancers, including deficient class I MHC expression, overproduction of immunosuppressive TGF-β, and heterogeneous target tumor antigen expression, all represent potential immune evasion mechanisms that may impede efficacy of immunogene therapies. The immunogene therapy patient conversely may harbor generalized limitations to potential immune stimulation.[57] In addition, immune responses against the vector backbone may interfere with tumor-specific immune effectors.[23,42] A new generation of recombinant vector vaccines seek to address these and other obstacles by combining the advantages of immunostimulatory gene transfer and vector-encoded tumor antigen gene transfer in vectors designed to deliver two therapeutic genes in one vector: an immunostimulatory gene in tandem with a tumor antigen gene.[41] Despite potential obstacles, therapeutic efficacy in the setting of transient gene transfer and durability of tumor-specific immunity comprise advantages of immunogene therapy that fuel continued clinical development.

Gene Transfer for Direct Induction of Target Cell Death

Hypothetical barriers to tumor therapy by transfer of cell death genes traditionally included the potential need for near 100% efficient gene transfer in vivo to achieve remission, and lack of effective strategies for targeting tumor cells specifically without concurrent death induction in normal tissues. The availability of vectors that transfer genes efficiently in vivo, the discovery of bystander effects that allow transmission of cell death signals to nontransduced cells, the characterization of organized cell death (apoptosis) pathway abnormalities in cancer cells, and the development of dominant cell death–inducing genes, however, have all prompted a re-evaluation of these hypothetical barriers (Table 2–2).[3,20,58–63] Three general approaches to targeting cell death (independent of tumor-specific immunity) are in development. First, gene transfer of a drug susceptibility gene (such as herpes simplex virus thymidine kinase [HSV-tk]) renders target cells sensitive to subsequent gancyclovir-mediated cytotoxicity.[64] Second, transfection of cellular toxin genes can induce cell injury, disruption, and necrosis.[65] Third, gene transfer of dominant apoptosis-inducing genes can trigger organized cellular death, or apoptosis.[20]

Gene transfer of HSV-tk, as a means of rendering tumor cells susceptible to subsequent gancyclovir-mediated cytotoxicity, was among the first approaches in efforts to induce tumor cell death via gene transfer.[64,66,67] In this system, gancyclovir acts as a prodrug that becomes cytotoxic only after it is phosphorylated by HSV-tk. Mammalian cells normally lack HSV-tk; hence the requirement for gene transfer. Phosphorylation of gancyclovir by HSV-tk leads to the formation of gancyclovir triphosphate, a potent nucleotide competitor that interferes with DNA synthesis. A bystander effect, whereby nontransduced adjacent malignant cells are killed in part to the transfer of the toxic analogue via gap junctions or apoptotic vesicles, was initially described in HSV-tk gene transfer studies.[58] HSV-tk gene transfer can be accomplished by retroviral or adenoviral vectors in vivo. Due to ease and efficiency of use, adenoviral vectors have been used for HSV-tk gene transfer in animal models of prostate cancer in which in vivo delivery was accomplished by intratumoral injection.[68] Subsequent systemic administration of gancyclovir led to significant reduction of tumor growth. This effect was synergistic with androgen withdrawal in a mouse model of androgen-responsive prostate cancer.[68] A clinical trial based on these findings and using intratumoral injection for delivery is forthcoming (Table 2–3).[69]

A limitation of HSV-tk gene transfer is the need to coordinate and optimize administration of two agents: the sensitizing gene transfer vector and the prodrug gancyclovir. An alternative strategy for direct cytotoxicity is gene transfer of cellular toxin genes, such as ricins, which disrupt plasma membranes or otherwise render lethal cellular injury.[65] Adenovirus vectors encoding ricins have been found to be effective in reducing growth of a variety of tumors in vitro. Direct administration of ricin gene products is cytotoxic to human prostate cancer cells, providing rationale for further development of this strategy.[70]

Third and perhaps most promising of the gene therapy strategies that aim to directly induce cell death is gene transfer of apoptosis-inducing genes. Organized cell death in the form of apoptosis differs from toxic or necrotic cellular disruption (such as ricin-mediated toxicity) in that apoptosis occurs as a normal entity of the eukaryotic life cycle in vivo, without concomitant inflammation or other local toxicity.[63] Prostate biology revealed some of the earliest evidence for apoptosis as a normal component of cellular homeostasis, and prostate cancer was the first among several solid tumors whose growth and progression has been shown to result from defective apoptosis rather than augmented proliferation.[71] Gene products involved in a cascade of intracellular events mediating apoptosis have been successfully targeted for induction of apoptosis in tumor cells. An ideal apoptosis-inducing gene would induce apoptosis in tumor cells without altering homeostasis in normal cells. Candidate genes that may exhibit such selective effects to some degree include Bclx-s and p53; the ability of adenoviral vectors encoding these genes to induce apoptosis in tumor cells in vitro and in vivo has been shown, and effects on normal cells and stem cells are under intensive study.[20,22] Early findings indicate that gene transfer of Bclx-s with adenovirus vectors, for example, has little effect on normal stem cell growth, while tumor cells are profoundly affected.[20]

Anti-oncogene Therapy: Approaches Using Antisense and Ribozyme Constructs

Targeting oncogenes with gene transfer is theoretically advantageous because this strategy can potentially selectively affect tumor cell growth without affecting normal cells, which may lack functional expression of the target oncogene. By exploiting the ability of complementary RNA strands to bind to each other, delivery of genes containing such complementary or "antisense" sequences to specific oncogenes can revert the tumorigenic phenotype by inhibiting expression of specific oncogenes in target tumor cells. Interference with translational machinery due to pairing of antisense RNA constructs with their oncogene-encoding RNA targets is one mechanism of anti-oncogene activity postulated as active in this strategy. By interfering with translation of oncogene RNA, oncogenic proteins are produced at much lower levels, if at all. In addition to interfering with translation, moreover, antisense constructs may activate endogenous ribonucleases, which in turn degrade the bound RNA. Regardless of the mechanism, the net effect of antisense therapy is the reduction of oncogenic protein expression due to binding of oncogene RNA by the antisense gene product (Table 2–2).

Although early antisense strategies focused on direct administration of short antisense oligonucleotides (sometimes modified for improved solubility), more recently the delivery of longer antisense constructs, as well as dominant negative mutation constructs, via recombinant vector systems has emerged.[72–74] Retroviral transfer of a *myc* antisense gene (delivered by direct injection of retroviral vector into small prostate cancer nodules in rodents), for example, was found to impede in vivo prostate cancer growth in a rodent model.[75] Based on these findings, a clinical trial of anti-oncogene therapy using intraprostatic injection of retroviral vector encoding antisense *myc* has been proposed (Table 2–3).[75]

The discovery of ribozymes, or RNA sequences that catalyze RNA cleavage and splicing, opened a promising extension of gene therapy strategies based on oncogene targeting via antisense recognition of oncogene RNA (Fig. 2–8).[76] Ribozymes can be designed to degrade RNA containing a short segment of complementary nucleotides. In theory, almost any RNA containing a unique 15-bp or longer sequence can be specifically degraded by designing a ribozyme containing a complementary binding motif. Adenoviral vectors have been used to deliver oncogene-specific ribozymes (e.g., targeting H-*ras* in a bladder cancer cell line) with consequent repression of in vivo tumorigenesis.[77,78] The efficacy of this strategy in the setting of in vivo gene delivery remains as yet untested. However, the direct target specificity of ribozyme-targeted anti-oncogene therapy, in the setting of a well-characterized effector mechanism, suggests that ribozyme-based strategies may be the most promising antisense-based therapeutic strategy under current development.

Tumor Suppressor Gene Restoration

The recent observation that renal cell cancer tumorigenicity can be reversed by in vitro transfer of the von Hippel-Lindau (VHL) gene, prior to full biochemical and functional characterization of VHL gene product, attests to the potential utility of gene therapy targeting tumor suppressor gene restoration.[79,80] This observation indicates that restoring tu-

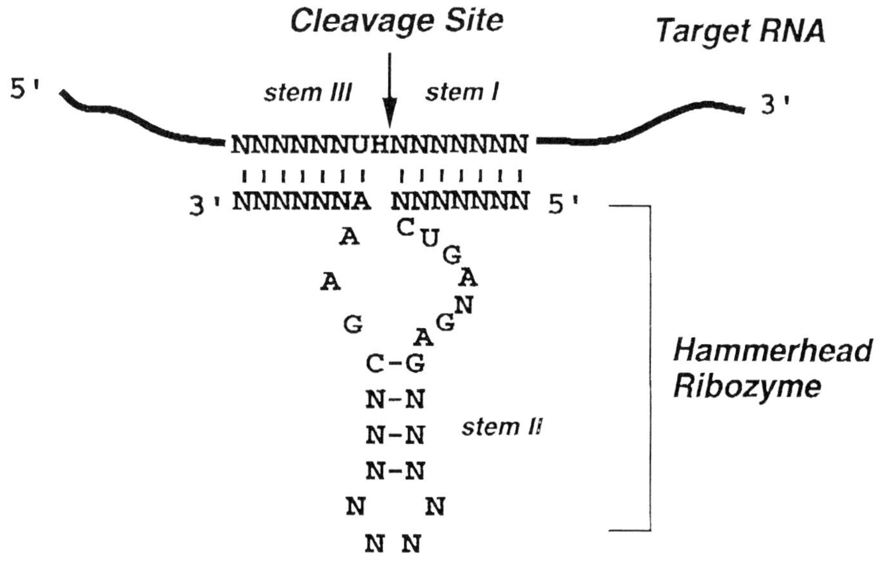
Cleavage Site
Target RNA
5'
stem III
stem I
3'
NNNNNNUHNNNNNNN
3' NNNNNNA NNNNNNN 5'
A
C
U
G
A
A
N
G
G
A
C-G
N-N
N-N
stem II
N-N
N N
N N
Hammerhead
Ribozyme

FIGURE 2–8. Anti-oncogene ribozyme consensus sequence. The hammerhead ribozyme contains three non-conserved helical regions (stems I, II, and III) along with the conserved sequence of the central core. Stems I and III, which determine the specificity of the ribozyme for its target, hybridize to target oncogene RNA. The target RNA is then cleaved at the site indicated by the *arrow*, disabling oncogene expression. Nucleotides designated as "N" can be any nucleotide. (From Thompson JD, Macejak D, Couture L, Stinchcomb DT: Ribozymes in gene therapy. Nat Med 1995; 1:277, with permission.)

mor suppressor genes may reverse tumorigenic potential of individual, in vitro transduced, cells. Tumor suppressor gene transfer in vivo, however, has had less impressive effects than in vitro transfection.[21,22,81] At least two factors may contribute to the discrepancy between in vitro and in vivo effects of tumor suppressor gene restoration. First, intratumoral injection of vectors into solid tumors is not a highly efficient approach for gene delivery—most of the vector is likely cleared before it accesses tumor cells, and the initial vector distribution in injected tissue is unlikely to be uniform. Second, stable long-term integration (as with a retrovirus vector) of the therapeutic suppressor gene, in the setting of 100% efficient in vivo transduction, would be required to arrest tumor growth (Table 2–2).

This strategy could be optimized by using vectors capable of stably integrating the transgene into the target cell genome, such as retroviral vectors, and also capable of highly efficient in vivo transduction, such as adenoviral vectors. In that no vector currently has both of these characteristics (Table 2–1), using any vector system will have limited efficacy at present. For example, one potential tumor suppressor target, c-*cam*, is a cellular attachment molecule that is absent in some prostate cancers, and thereby potentially contributes to the uninhibited and metastatic growth potential of these cells. Intratumoral injection of an adenoviral vector encoding c-*cam*, used to restore expression of this molecule in pre-established prostate cancer xenografts, slowed but did not reverse tumor progression (Fig. 2–9).[81] Similar effects have been seen with adenovirus vector–based therapy targeting restoration of other tumor suppressor genes.[21] Despite these limitations, survival of tumor-bearing animals can be extended with in vivo suppressor gene restoration therapy, and a clinical trial evaluating efficacy of Rb gene delivery via intravesical instillation of adenovirus vector has been proposed (Table 2–3).[82] The association of Rb gene abnormalities in bladder cancer and poor prognosis supports the rationale for intravesical adenovirus-Rb gene therapy.[83]

For many tumor suppressor genes, restoration of suppressor gene function alone may not suffice for cytoreduction of established tumors even in the theoretical setting of totally effective and durable in vivo tumor suppressor gene transfer. Most tumor suppressor genes do not encode signals for direct induction of cell death, but rather affect tumor growth more indirectly, such as by regulating DNA repair, cellular attachment, or cell cycle control.[83] In this setting, restoration of normal suppressor gene via gene transfer may require accompanying cytoreductive systemic or regional therapies (chemotherapy, radiation) to treat established tumors. The

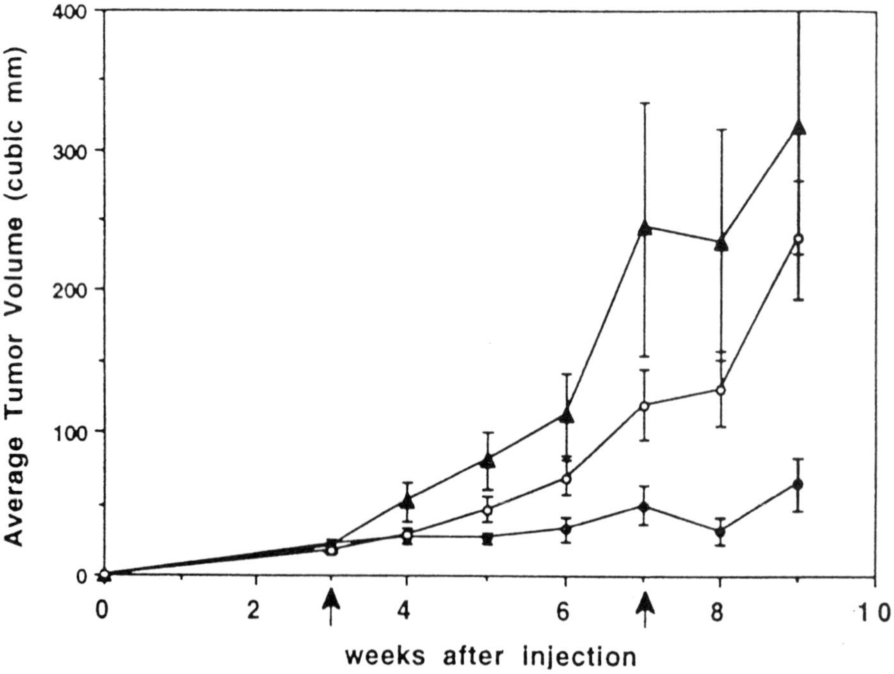
400
300
200
100
0
Average Tumor Volume (cubic mm)
0
2
4
6
8
10
weeks after injection

FIGURE 2–9. Tumor suppressor gene therapy inhibits tumor growth in animal models. Injection of adenovirus encoding c-*cam*1 (*filled circles*) into human prostate cancer nodules grown in nude mice reduced tumor growth compared to saline (*filled triangle*) and vector (*open circle*) controls. Delay of tumor growth without complete tumor remission is typical of strategies relying on local-regional injection of recombinant vectors encoding therapeutic tumor suppressor, anti-oncogene, or cytotoxicity genes. (From Kleinerman DI, Zhang WW, Lin SH, et al: Application of a tumor suppressor [C-CAM1]-expressing recombinant adenovirus in androgen-independent human prostate cancer therapy: a preclinical study. Cancer Res 1995; 55:2831, with permission.)

need for accompanying cytoreductive therapy is further evidenced by the transient expression associated with the most efficient vector systems—once transgene expression fades, the tumorigenic phenotype associated with absence of the suppressor gene will reappear (efficient in vivo vectors are required for this strategy as most, if not all, target cells must directly express, or confer expression via bystander effect, of the transferred gene for effective tumor reduction).

Some tumor suppressor genes may also serve as gatekeepers for intracellular apoptosis-inducing signals.[59] In addition to suppressing the tumorigenic growth potential of individual cells, restoration of these tumor suppressor genes should also be able to reduce established tumors via apoptosis induction. The inability of an adenoviral vector encoding p53 to eliminate pre-established malignancy, however, indicates that near-complete transduction of all tumor cells may be required for optimal therapeutic effect. This level of efficiency is clearly not achieved by direct solid tumor injection with currently available vectors. Improvements in vector and delivery systems will be needed to optimize this, and other, gene therapy strategies that rely on direct effects of gene transfer in the tumor cell target.

FUTURE DIRECTIONS: TARGETING VECTOR SPECIFICITY

Most vectors that, at present, have shown functional efficacy in vivo lack significant specificity in target cell attachment or restriction in transgene expression. The vector envelopes or coats of retroviruses, adenoviruses, and liposomal vectors enter cells via families of receptors that, as a group, are virtually ubiquitous.[12,17] The promoters controlling transgene expression in these vectors are typically potent promoters susceptible to little or no regulation by the host cell. Targeting of gene therapy to specific cells or tissues has therefore been achieved principally via the route of vector administration. The feasibility of conferring specificity via the administration route, in the case of urologic targets, has been demonstrated for renal cancer after renal tubule vector infusion and for bladder epithelium after intravesical instillation of viral vectors.[42,84,85] This approach may be applicable to local-regional therapy of early-stage, organ-confined malignancy (Table 2–2).

Systemic applications of cytotoxic, anti-oncogene, or tumor suppressor, therapeutic gene transfer, however, will require specific targeting based not only on vector administration route: molecular, rather than mechanical, targeting will be needed. Molecular vector targeting can be achieved either by modifying tropism (altering the affinity of the vector coat for attachment and entry to a limited range of human target cells) or by restricting transcription (constructing expression cassettes containing promoters with selective activity in different tissues) (Fig. 2–10).

Modified Vector Tropism

Two approaches have been used for modifying vector tropism. First, vectors can be derived from viruses with inherent tropism for a specific tissue target. Due to the relative paucity of molecular characterization of viruses with natural and specific tropism for the genitourinary tract, this approach has limited utility. Nevertheless, at least one virus (BK virus, which has specific tropism for transitional epithelium) has shown potentially useful tropism specificity for transitional epithelium.[86] Recombinant BK episomal vectors were constructed that led to reporter gene expression specifically in human transitional cell carcinoma (TCC) cell lines relative to absent expression in other tumor cells. Limited characterization of the elements regulating BK specificity, and lack of replication-defective BK vectors, however, has limited further development of this vector system thus far.

Second, molecular engineering and conjugate formation to alter the native vector coats has been used to confer specific tropism. Although attractive in theory, engineering of envelope or vector coat sequences ("pseudotyping") has been limited principally due to the potential of functionally disrupting the ability of engineered envelopes to mediate target cell attachment and entry. Pseudotyping has thus succeeded in producing vectors with extended or altered target cell tropism, without more restricted target specificity per se.[9] Molecular conjugate formation, in contrast, has successfully conferred altered and refined specificity to adenoviral, liposomal, and retroviral vectors alike. This has been achieved via covalent linkage of vectors with ligands such as growth factor receptors or antibody haptens, which confer the desired tropism for cells expressing the specific receptor, and via noncovalent association of hybrid vector components.[87–90]

Restricted Transgene Expression: Transcriptional Targeting

An alternative to vector targeting at the target cell–binding level is to limit expression of therapeutic genes by regulating transcription with a promoter region having either tissue-restricted activity, or preferential activity in malignant cells. Such promoter-regulated specificity has been used to target retroviral and adenoviral vectors alike.[9,91] Tissue-specific promoters are potentially useful for regulating expression of cytotoxic genes in vectors targeting nonvital tissues such as prostate, to widen potential therapeutic windows. To this end, vectors have been constructed with the promoter region

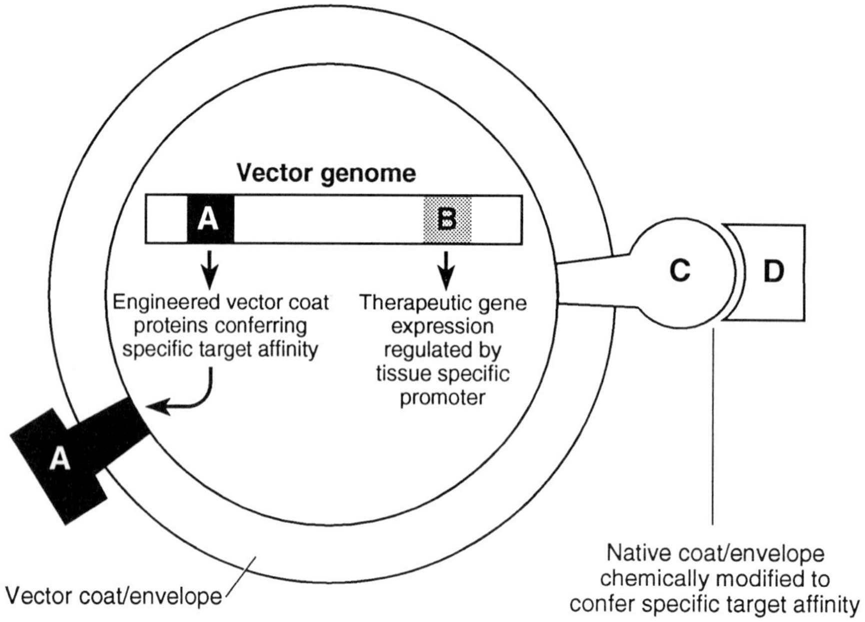
Vector genome
A
B
Engineered vector coat proteins conferring specific target affinity
Therapeutic gene expression regulated by tissue specific promoter
A
C
D
Vector coat/envelope
Native coat/envelope chemically modified to confer specific target affinity

FIGURE 2–10. Restricting target cell specificity of recombinant viral vectors. The ability to specifically target gene delivery can facilitate systemic gene therapy with cytotoxic vectors. Approaches to confer specificity include: *A*, Engineering vector coat specificity. *B*, Restricting promoter-regulated transcription. *C*, Chemically modifying vector-target affinity. (Based on reference 9.)

that normally regulates PSA expression used to control expression of a reporter gene.[92,93] Cloning of therapeutic cytotoxic genes such as HSV-tk into analogous vectors using tyrosinase promoter has been shown to inhibit tumor growth in melanoma animal models[94]; analogous vectors to target prostate cancer are under development.

In contrast to tissue-specific transcriptional targeting, oncogene-associated regulatory sequences may promote selective expression of therapeutic genes in tumor cells that harbor transcriptional overexpression of the oncogene. This has been demonstrated with a vector using ERBB2 promoter sequences to the cytotoxic gene cytosine deaminase; this vector conferred selective sensitivity on ERBB2-overproducing cells.[95] Retroviral vectors requiring target cell replication for integration should also, hypothetically, express therapeutic genes preferentially in highly proliferative tumors such as testicular, renal cell, and transitional cell carcinomas; however, perhaps related to obstacles to effective retroviral gene transfer in vivo, this paradigm remains unproved.

SUMMARY

Based on a growing volume of preclinical data, clinical trials of gene therapy for urologic cancer are underway. Therapeutic genes that are under current or forthcoming clinical study include immunogenes, cell death–inducing genes, anti-oncogenes, and tumor suppressor genes. Although systemic therapy with immunogenes is feasible, other gene therapy strategies, which do not rely on an intervening antitumor immune response, are at present limited to local-regional targeting. This constraint is largely due to limitations of gene transfer vectors as well as in vivo gene delivery systems. Refinement of gene transfer vectors, such as hybrid vector construction, is actively being pursued to broaden the utility and applicability of direct gene therapy strategies.

The early phase of cancer gene therapy clinical trials should be viewed in context. Preclinical models predict modest, if any, therapeutic effects with current forms of human cancer gene therapy. Equally as important as clinical outcome in gene therapy clinical trials, however, are biologic surrogate end-points to guide continued improvement of gene therapy strategies. The earliest clinical trials have indeed shown the ability of clinical gene therapy to alter biology of human urologic cancer.[14] To attain its full potential, gene therapy must be approached with realistic expectations and a recognition of the need for its continued evolution.

REFERENCES

1. Watson JD, Crick FH: Molecular structure of nucleic acids. A structure for deoxyribose nucleic acid. Nature 1953; 171: 737.
2. Danos O, Mulligan RC: Safe and efficient generation of recombinant retrovirus with amphotropic and ecotropic host ranges. Proc Natl Acad Sci U S A 1988; 85:6460.
3. Ghosh-Choudhury G, Haj-Ahmad Y, Brinkley P, et al: Human adenovirus cloning vectors based on infectious bacterial plasmids. Gene 1986; 50:161.

4. Moss B: Vaccinia virus: a tool for research and vaccine development. Science 1991; 2252:1662.
5. Ledley FD: Nonviral gene therapy: the promise of genes as pharmaceutical products. Hum Gene Ther 1995; 6:1129.
6. Mulligan RC: The basic science of gene therapy. Science 1993; 260:926.
7. Crystal RG: Transfer of genes to humans: early lessons and obstacles to success. Science 1995; 270:404.
8. Yang NS, Sun WH: Gene gun and other non-viral approaches for cancer gene therapy. Nat Med 1995; 1:481.
9. Miller N, Vile R: Targeted vectors for gene therapy. FASEB J 1995; 9:190.
10. Rosenberg SA, Aebersold P, Cornetta K, et al: Gene transfer into humans—immunotherapy of patients with advanced melanoma, using tumor-infiltrating lymphocytes modified by retroviral gene transduction. N Engl J Med 1990; 323:570.
11. Blaese M: The ADA human gene therapy clinical protocol. Hum Gene Ther 1990; 1:327.
12. Weiss RA: Cellular receptors and viral glycoproteins involved in retrovirus entry. *In* Levy JA (ed): The Retroviridae, p 1. New York, Plenum Press, 1993.
13. Dranoff G, Jaffee E, Lazenby A, et al: Vaccination with irradiated tumor cells engineered to secrete murine GM-CSF stimulates potent, specific, and long lasting anti-tumor immunity. Proc Natl Acad Sci U S A 1993; 90:3539.
14. Simons JW, Jaffee EM, Weber C, et al: Bioactivity of human GM-CSF gene therapy using autologous irradiated renal cell carcinoma vaccines. (Submitted.)
15. Simons JW: Phase I/II study of autologous human GM-CSF gene transduced prostate cancer vaccines in patients with metastatic prostate carcinoma. RAC Report 1994; 9408–082.
16. Yang Y, Nunes F, Berencsi K, et al: Cellular immunity to viral antigens limits E1-deleted adenoviruses for gene therapy. Proc Natl Acad Sci U S A 1994; 91:4407.
17. Wickham TJ, Mathias P, Cheresh DA, Nemerow GR: Integrins $\alpha_v\beta_5$ and $\alpha_v\beta_3$ promote adenovirus internalization but not virus attachment. Cell 1993; 73:309.
18. Seth P: Adenovirus-dependent release of choline from plasma membrane vesicles at an acidic pH is mediated by the penton base protein. J Virol 1994; 68:1204.
19. Addison CL, Braciak T, Ralston R, et al: Intratumoral injection of an adenovirus expressing IL-2 induces regression and immunity in a murine breast cancer model. Proc Natl Acad Sci U S A 1995; 92:8522.
20. Clarke MF, Apel IJ, Benedict MA, et al: A recombinant bcl-xs adenovirus selectively induces apoptosis in cancer cells but not normal bone marrow cells. Proc Natl Acad Sci U S A 1995; 92:11024.
21. Eastham JA, Hall SJ, Sehgal I, et al: In vivo gene therapy with p53 or p21 adenovirus for prostate cancer. Cancer Res 1995; 55:5151.
22. Yang C, Cirielli C, Capogrossi MC, Passaniti A: Adenovirus-mediated wild-type p53 expression induces apoptosis and suppresses tumorigenesis of prostatic tumor cells. Cancer Res 1995; 55:4210.
23. Wang M, Bronte V, Chen PW, et al: Active immunotherapy of cancer with a non-replicating recombinant fowlpox virus encoding a model tumor-associated antigen. J Immunol 1995; 154:4685.
24. Nabel GJ, Nabel EG, Yang ZY, et al: Direct gene transfer with DNA-liposome complexes in melanoma: expression, biologic activity, and lack of toxicity in humans. Proc Natl Acad Sci U S A 1993; 90:11307.
25. Sun WH, Burkholder JK, Sun J, et al: In vivo cytokine gene transfer by gene gun reduces tumor growth in mice. Proc Natl Acad Sci U S A 1995; 92:2889.
26. Vogelzang NJ, Sudakoff G, McKay S, et al: A phase I study of intralesional (IL) gene therapy in metastatic renal cell cancer (RCC). Proc Annu Meet Am Soc Clin Oncol 1995; 14:A641.
27. Johnson PA, Miyanohara A, Levine F, et al: Cytotoxicity of a replication-defective mutant of herpes simplex virus type I. J Virol 1992; 66:2952.
28. Dupont F, Tenenbaum L, Guo LP, et al: Use of an autonomous parvovirus vector for selective transfer of a foreign gene into transformed human cells of different origin and its expression therein. J Virol 1994; 68:1397.
29. Flotte TR, Afione SA, Conrad C, et al: Stable in vivo expression of the cystic fibrosis transmembrane conductance regulator with an adeno-associated virus vector. Proc Natl Acad Sci U S A 1993; 90:10613.
30. Pan ZK, Ikonomidis G, Lazenby A, et al: A recombinant *Listeria monocytogenes* vaccine expressing a model tumor antigen protects mice against lethal tumour cell challenge and causes regression of established tumours. Nat Med 1995; 1:471.
31. Fearon ER, Pardoll DM, Itaya T, et al: Interleukin-2 production by tumor cells bypasses T helper function in the generation of an antitumor response. Cell 1990; 60:397.
32. Gansbacher B, Gansbacher B, Bannerji R, et al: Retroviral vector-mediated gamma-interferon gene transfer into tumor cells generates potent and long lasting antitumor immunity. Cancer Res 1990; 50:7820.
33. Gansbacher B, Zier K, Daniels B, et al: Interleukin 2 gene transfer into tumor cells abrogates tumorigenicity and induces protective immunity. J Exp Med 1990; 172:1217.
34. Golumbek PT, Lazenby AJ, Levitsky HI, et al: Treatment of established renal cell cancer by tumor cells engineered to secrete interleukin-4. Science 1991; 254:713.
35. Connor J, Bannerji R, Saito S, et al: Regression of bladder tumors in mice treated with interleukin-2 gene modified tumor cells. J Exp Med 1993; 177:1127.
36. Sanda MG, Ayyagari SR, Jaffee EM, et al: Demonstration of a rational strategy for human prostate cancer gene therapy. J Urol 1994; 151:622.
37. Moody DB, Robinson JC, Ewing CM, et al: Interleukin-2 transfected prostate cancer cells generate a local antitumor effect in vivo. Prostate 1994; 24:244.
38. Vieweg J, Rosenthal FM, Bannerji R, et al: Immunotherapy of prostate cancer in the Dunning rat model: use of cytokine gene modified tumor vaccines. Cancer Res 1994; 54: 1760.
39. Gansbacher B, Motzer R, Houghton A, Bander N: Immunization with interleukin-2 secreting allogeneic HLA-A2 matched renal cell carcinoma cells in patients with advanced renal cell carcinoma. RAC Report 1992; 9206–022.
40. Kantor J, Irvine K, Abrams S, et al: Antitumor activity and immune responses induced by a recombinant carcinoembryonic antigen-vaccinia virus vaccine. J Natl Cancer Inst 1992; 84:1084.
41. Bronte V, Tsung K, Rao JB, et al: IL-2 enhances the function of recombinant poxvirus-based vaccines in the treatment of established pulmonary metastases. J Immunol 1995; 154: 5282.
42. Lee SS, Eisenlohr LC, McCue PA, et al: Intravesical gene therapy: in vivo gene transfer using recombinant vaccinia virus vectors. Cancer Res 1994; 54:3325.
43. Lee SS, Eisenlohr LC, McCue PA, et al: In vivo gene therapy of murine tumors using recombinant vaccinia virus encoding GM-CSF. Proc Annu Meet Am Assoc Cancer Res 1995; 36:A1481.
44. Chen AP: A phase I study of recombinant vaccinia that expresses PSA in adult patients with adenocarcinoma of the prostate. RAC Report 1995; 9509–126.
45. Figlin RA: Phase I study of HLA-B7 plasmid DNA/DMRIE/DOPE lipid complex as an immunotherapeutic agent in renal cell carcinoma by direct gene transfer with concurrent low dose bolus IL-2 protein therapy. RAC Report 1995; 9508–121.
46. Paulson D, Lyerly HK: A phase I study of autologous human IL-2 gene modified tumor cells in patients with locally advanced or metastatic prostate cancer. RAC Report 1995; 9510–132.
47. Lahn M, Kohler G, Kulmburg P, et al: Parameters for successful establishment of primary and long-term tumor cell cultures from renal cell carcinoma, melanoma and colon carcinoma for cellular immunotherapy. Gene Ther 1994; 1: S15.

48. Kawakita M, Rao G, Ritchey JK, et al: Canary-pox virus-mediated cytokine gene therapy induces tumor specific and non-specific immunity against mouse prostate tumor. J Urol 1996; 155:516A.
49. Cordon-Cardo C, Fuks Z, Drobnjak M, et al: Expression of HLA-A,B,C antigens on primary and metastatic tumor cell populations of human carcinomas. Cancer Res 1991; 51: 6372.
50. Blades RA, Keating PJ, McWilliam LJ, et al: Loss of HLA class I expression in prostate cancer: implications for immunotherapy. Urology 1995; 46:681.
51. Nouri AM, Hussain RF, Oliver RT: The frequency of major histo-compatibility complex antigen abnormalities in urological tumours and their correction by gene transfection or cytokine stimulation. Cancer Gene Ther 1994; 1:119.
52. Sanda MG, Restifo NP, Walsh JC, et al: Molecular characterization of defective antigen processing in human prostate cancer. J Natl Cancer Inst 1995; 87:280.
53. Lattime EC: Therapy of muscle-invasive bladder carcinoma with intravesical vaccinia. FDA approval, 1996; BB-IND-5002.
54. Torre-Amione G, Beauchamp RD, Koeppen H, et al: A highly immunogenic tumor transfected with a murine transforming growth factor type beta 1 cDNA escapes immune surveillance. Proc Natl Acad Sci U S A 1990; 87:1486.
55. Inge TH, Hoover SK, Susskind BM, et al: Inhibition of tumor-specific cytotoxic T-lymphocyte responses by TGF-beta 1. Cancer Res 1992; 52:1386.
56. Miyamoto H, Kubota Y, Shuin T, et al: Expression of transforming growth factor-beta 1 in human bladder cancer. Cancer 1995; 75:2565.
57. Catalona WJ, Chretien PB, Trahan EE: Abnormalities of cell-mediated immunocompetence in genitourinary cancer. J Urol 1974; 111:229–232.
58. Freeman SM, Abboud CN, Whartenby KA, et al: The bystander effect: tumor regression when a fraction of the tumor mass is genetically modified. Cancer Res 1993; 53: 5274.
59. Symonds H, Krall L, Remington L, et al: p53-dependent apoptosis suppresses tumor growth and progression in vivo. Cell 1994; 78:703.
60. Oltvai ZN, Milliman CL, Korsmeyer SJ: Bcl-2 heterodimerizes in vivo with a conserved homolog, Bax, that accelerates programmed cell death. Cell 1993; 74:609.
61. Boise LH, Gonzalez-Garcia M, Postema CE, et al: Bcl-x, a bcl-2-related gene that functions as a dominant regulator of apoptotic cell death. Cell 1993; 74:597.
62. Raffo AJ, Perlman H, Chen MW, et al: Overexpression of Bcl-2 protects prostate cancer cells from apoptosis in vitro and confers resistance to androgen-depletion in vivo. Cancer Res 1995; 55:4438.
63. Martin S, Green DR: Apoptosis and cancer: failure of controls on cell death and cell survival. Crit Rev Oncol Hematol 1995; 18:137.
64. Furman PA, McGuirt PV, Keller PM, et al: Inhibition by acyclovir of cell growth and DNA synthesis of cells biochemically transformed with herpes virus genetic information. Virology 1980; 102:420.
65. Hoganson DK, Batra RK, Olsen JC, Boucher RC: Comparison of the effects of three different toxin genes and their levels of expression on cell growth and bystander effect in lung adenocarcinoma. Cancer Res 1996; 56:1315.
66. Moolten FL, Wells JM: Curability of tumors bearing herpes thymidine kinase genes transferred by retroviral vectors. J Natl Cancer Inst 1990; 82:297.
67. Culver KW, Ram Z, Wallbridge S, et al: In vivo gene transfer with retroviral vector-producer cells for treatment of experimental brain tumors. Science 1992; 256:1550.
68. Hall SJ, Mutchnik SE, Shaker M, et al: Adenovirus mediated HSV-tk gene transduction and gancyclovir treatment for prostate cancer: suppression of metastasis in an orthotopic model and synergism with androgen ablation. J Urol 1996; 155:528A.
69. Scardino PT, Thompson TC, Woo SLC: Phase I study of adenoviral vector delivery of the HSV-tk gene and the intravenous administration of gancyclovir in men with local recurrence of prostate cancer after radiation therapy. RAC Report 1996; 9601–144.
70. Rodriguez R, Carducci MA, Bartkowski LM, Simons JW: Cytoreductive agents for prostate cancer gene therapy. Proc Am Assoc Cancer Res 1996; 37:346.
71. Kyprianou N, Isaacs JT: Activation of programmed cell death in the rat ventral prostate after castration. Endocrinology 1988; 122:552.
72. McManaway ME, Neckers LM, Loke SL, et al: Tumor-specific inhibition of lymphoma growth by an antisense oligodeoxynucleotide. Lancet 1990; 335:808.
73. Ogiso Y, Sakai N, Watari H, et al: Suppression of various human tumor cell lines by a dominant negative H-ras mutant. Gene Ther 1994; 1:403.
74. Georges RN, Mukhopadhyay T, Zheng Y, et al: Prevention of orthotopic human lung cancer growth by intratracheal instillation of a retroviral antisense k-ras construct. Cancer Res 1993; 53:1743.
75. Steiner MS, Holt JT: Gene therapy for the treatment of advanced prostate cancer by in vivo transduction with prostate-targeted retroviral vectors expressing antisense c-myc RNA. RAC Report 1995; 9509–123.
76. Thompson JD, Macejak D, Couture L, Stinchcomb DT: Ribozymes in gene therapy. Nat Med 1995; 1:277.
77. Kashani-Sabet M, Funato T, Tone T, et al: Reversal of the malignant phenotype by an anti-ras ribozyme. Antisense Res Dev 1992; 2:3.
78. Feng M, Cabrera G, Deshane J, et al: Neoplastic reversion accomplished by high efficiency adenoviral-mediated delivery of an anti-ras ribozyme. Cancer Res 1995; 55:2024.
79. Chen F, Kishida T, Duh FM, et al: Suppression of growth of renal carcinoma cells by the von Hippel-Lindau tumor suppressor gene. Cancer Res 1995; 55:4804.
80. Iliopoulos O, Kibel A, Gray S, Kaelin WG: Tumour suppression by the von Hippel-Lindau gene product. Nat Med 1995; 1:822.
81. Kleinerman DI, Zhang WW, Lin SH, et al: Application of a tumor suppressor (C-CAM1)-expressing recombinant adenovirus in androgen-independent human prostate cancer therapy: a preclinical study. Cancer Res 1995; 55:2831.
82. Small EJ, Carroll PR: Gene therapy of bladder cancer using recombinant adenovirus containing the retinoblastoma gene (ACNRB): a phase I study. RAC Report 1996; 9601–145.
83. Cordon-Cardo C, Dalbagni G, Sarkis AS, Reuter VE: Genetic alterations associated with bladder cancer. Important Adv Oncol 1994; 71.
84. Moullier P, Friedlander G, Calise D, et al: Adenoviral-mediated gene transfer to renal tubular cells in vivo. Kidney Int 1994; 45:1220.
85. Bass C, Cabrera G, Elgavish A, et al: Recombinant adenovirus-mediated gene transfer to genitourinary epithelium in vitro and in vivo. Cancer Gene Ther 1995; 2:97.
86. Cooper MJ, Miron S: Efficient episomal expression vector for human transitional carcinoma cells. Hum Gene Ther 1993; 4:557.
87. Wu GY, Zhan P, Sze LL, et al: Incorporation of adenovirus into a ligand-based DNA carrier system results in retention of original receptor specificity and enhances targeted gene expression. J Biol Chem 1994; 269:11542.
88. Chen J, Gamou S, Takayanagi A, Shimuzu N: A novel gene delivery system using EGF receptor mediated-endocytosis. FEBS Lett 1994; 338:167.
89. Michael SI, Huang CH, Romer MU, et al: Binding-incompetent adenovirus facilitates molecular conjugate-mediated gene transfer by the receptor-mediated endocytosis pathway. J Biol Chem 1993; 268:6866.
90. Vieweg J, Boczkowski D, Roberson KM, et al: Efficient gene transfer with adeno-associated virus-based plasmids complexed to cationic liposomes for gene therapy of human prostate cancer. Cancer Res 1995; 55:2366.
91. Friedman JM, Babiss LE, Clayton DF, Darnell JE: Cellular promoters incorporated into the adenovirus genome: cell

specificity of albumin and immunoglobulin expression. Mol Cell Biol 1986; 6:3791.
92. Taneja SS, Belldegrun A, Dardashti K, et al: In vitro target specific gene therapy for prostate cancer utilizing a prostate specific antigen promoter-driven adenoviral vector. Proc Annu Meet Am Assoc Cancer Res 1994; 35:A2236.
93. Ko SC, Gotoh A, Kao C, et al: Tissue targeted toxic gene therapy for an androgen-independent and metastatic human prostate cancer model. Proc Am Assoc Cancer Res 1996; 37:349.
94. Vile RG, Hart IR: Use of tissue-specific expression of the herpes simplex virus thymidine kinase gene to inhibit growth of established murine melanomas following direct intra-tumoral injection of DNA. Cancer Res 1993; 53: 3860.
95. Harris JD, Gutierrez AA, Hurst HC, et al: Gene therapy for cancer using tumor-specific prodrug activation. Gene Ther 1994; 1:170.
96. Sanda MG, Simons JW: Gene therapy for urological cancer. Urology 1994; 44:617.

3

TUMOR IMMUNITY

JOHN R. FRANKLIN, M.D. *and* ARIE S. BELLDEGRUN, M.D., F.A.C.S.

Malignant tumors or cancers are believed to develop and progress along a common pathway. All tumors have their origin at the genetic level in the form of mutations that affect growth regulation. These mutations either occur spontaneously or are produced by exposure to viral, physical, or chemical carcinogens.[1] The resultant growth pattern of these abnormal cells deviates from the growth of their normal siblings. Consequently, tumor progression culminates in invasive expansion, which may ultimately overwhelm the host. Although it is unclear how tumor development evades the immune system, a growing body of evidence continues to demonstrate tumor responses secondary to manipulation of the host's immune system. Furthermore, modulation of the immune system has been established as the primary modality in the treatment of malignancies such as metastatic renal cell carcinoma and superficial bladder cancer. As a consequence, the relatively new discipline—tumor immunology—has emerged, and is the focus of much basic and clinical research.

The word, *immunis,* meaning "exempting from charges (taxes)" is the Latin origin of the term immune.[2] In Greek, the word also conveys the meaning "memory." Appropriately, the immune system refers to a complex network that protects the host from foreign biologic factors, and accomplishes this task through an ingenious mechanism that relies on the system's ability to recall prior recognition and mount an augmented response. Tumor immunology or tumor immunity defines a phenomenon in which tumor cells are recognized as foreign by the host's immune system, and are attacked by various humoral and cellular factors that combine to promote tumor cell destruction. Because tumor immunity is still a relatively young discipline, and the principles that govern it continue to be unraveled, this chapter will attempt to provide the basic premises upon and through which tumor immunity may be interpreted. A description of the main cellular and humoral components of the immune system will be provided. How these various cellular and humoral factors are integrated in the normal immune response and the proposed mechanisms of action in tumor immunity will be discussed.

COMPONENTS OF THE IMMUNE SYSTEM

The immune system may first be divided into two components (humoral and cellular immunity). Humoral immunity principally includes B lymphocytes and the antibodies they produce, while cellular immunity primarily includes T lymphocytes and other effector cells (Table 3–1).[3] The cells of the immune system are derived from stem cells in the bone marrow through a process called hematopoiesis (Fig. 3–1). The proliferation and maturation of the different types of leukocytes are under the influence of various soluble growth factors such as colony-stimulating factors (CSFs).[3] A very complex network of regulatory factors (cytokines) mediates the cellular responses of the immune system.

Cellular Immunity

Cellular immunity primarily refers to the functions of thymus-derived lymphocytes or T cells.[4] The concept of cellular immunity evolved from an ability to transfer biologic activity to naive hosts utilizing cells only. Delayed-type hypersensitivity (DTH) and rejection of foreign grafts or tumors are some of the functions associated with cellular immunity. T cells originate from bone marrow stem cells, but require the thymus for maturation. The necessity of the thymus to T-cell maturation is evident in conditions of congenital absence of the thymus or following neonatal thymectomy in animal models. In these circumstances, impairment of DTH and certain antibody responses were observed. The development of T cells from their origin in the bone marrow to their maturation in the

TABLE 3–1. LYMPHOCYTE CLASSES*

Class	Functions	Antigen Receptor	Selected Phenotypic Markers	Percentage of Total Lymphocytes: Blood	Lymph Node	Spleen
B Lymphocytes						
	Antibody production (humoral immunity)	Surface antibody (immunoglobulin)	Fc and C3d receptors; class II MHC	10–15	20–25	40–45
T Lymphocytes						
Helper	Stimuli for B-cell growth and differentiation (humoral immunity) Macrophage activation by secreted cytokines (cell-mediated immunity)	αβ heterodimers	CD3+ CD4+, CD8− CD2+†	70–75	70–75	40–45
Cytolytic	Lysis of antigen-bearing (e.g., virally infected) cells, allografts	αβ heterodimers	CD3+ CD4−CD8+ CD2+			
Suppressor	Inhibition of immune response	?	?CD3+ Usually CD4−CD8+			
Natural Killer Cells						
	Lysis of tumor cells, antibody-dependent cellular cytotoxicity	?	Fc receptor for IgG (CD16)	~10	Rare	~10

*From Abbas AK, Litchman AH, Pober JS: Cells and tissues of the immune system. *In* Abbas AK, Litchman AH, Pober JS (eds): Cellular and Molecular Immunology, p 13. Philadelphia, WB Saunders Co, 1991, with permission.

†In most tissues, ratio of CD4+CD8− to CD8+CD4− cells is about 2:1.

thymus is associated with the expression of specialized membrane protein molecules. The antigen-specific T-cell receptor (TCR) exists as either an αβ heterodimer or a γδ heterodimer, and is the hallmark of the mature T lymphocyte.[5,6] The T-cell receptors are similar to the B-cell surface immunoglobulin receptors. Moreover, at the genomic level rearrangements of the α, β, γ, and δ genes take place in a manner much like that of B-cell immunoglobulin genetic rearrangements. Almost exclusively, T cells mediating antigen-specific and major histocompatibility complex (MHC) recognition have been found to express αβ receptors. The α and β molecules are each 40 to 45 kDa in molecular weight and are linked to each other by a disulfide bond. Adjacent to the TCR is a noncovalently associated complex of five additional proteins, which are collectively referred to as the CD3 complex. While the antigen-specificity of the T-cell receptor does not depend on the CD3 complex, the cell surface expression of the TCR clearly does. Additionally, it appears that the transduction of signals from the binding of the TCR to its ligand also depends on CD3 component.[7] The γδ heterodimers represent the second class of T-cell receptors, but are expressed on T cells distinct from those expressing αβ dimers. The γδ heterodimers are similarly associated with the CD3 complex on the T-cell surface. Less is known about T cells expressing the γδ heterodimers; however, evidence suggests that T cells with these receptors may mediate recognition of MHC-encoded antigens or microbial antigens as well as non–MHC-specific recognition.[8,9]

The development of T cells is associated with the expression of a large number of cell surface determinants.[10] Many of these are not unique to T lymphocytes and are, therefore, found on other cells. What is important is that T-cell development may be chronicled by the expression of some of these cell surface determinants. The functional characteristics of T-cell populations can also be defined by the elucidation of these markers. Cells expressing the CD4 and CD8 molecules are among the most frequently studied.[4] CD4+ expression is associated with T-cell helper activity, while CD8+ T cells are commonly associated with T-cell cytotoxic or suppressor activity. MHC class II products are recognized by CD4+ T cells as either foreign antigens in association with self-MHC class II or as foreign class II determinants as alloantigens. CD8+ T cells will predominantly interact with cells presenting foreign antigens in association with self-MHC class I molecules or foreign class I determinants as alloantigens. While the CD4 and CD8 expression corresponds commonly to T-cell helper and cytotoxic activity, respectively, these relationships are not absolute.

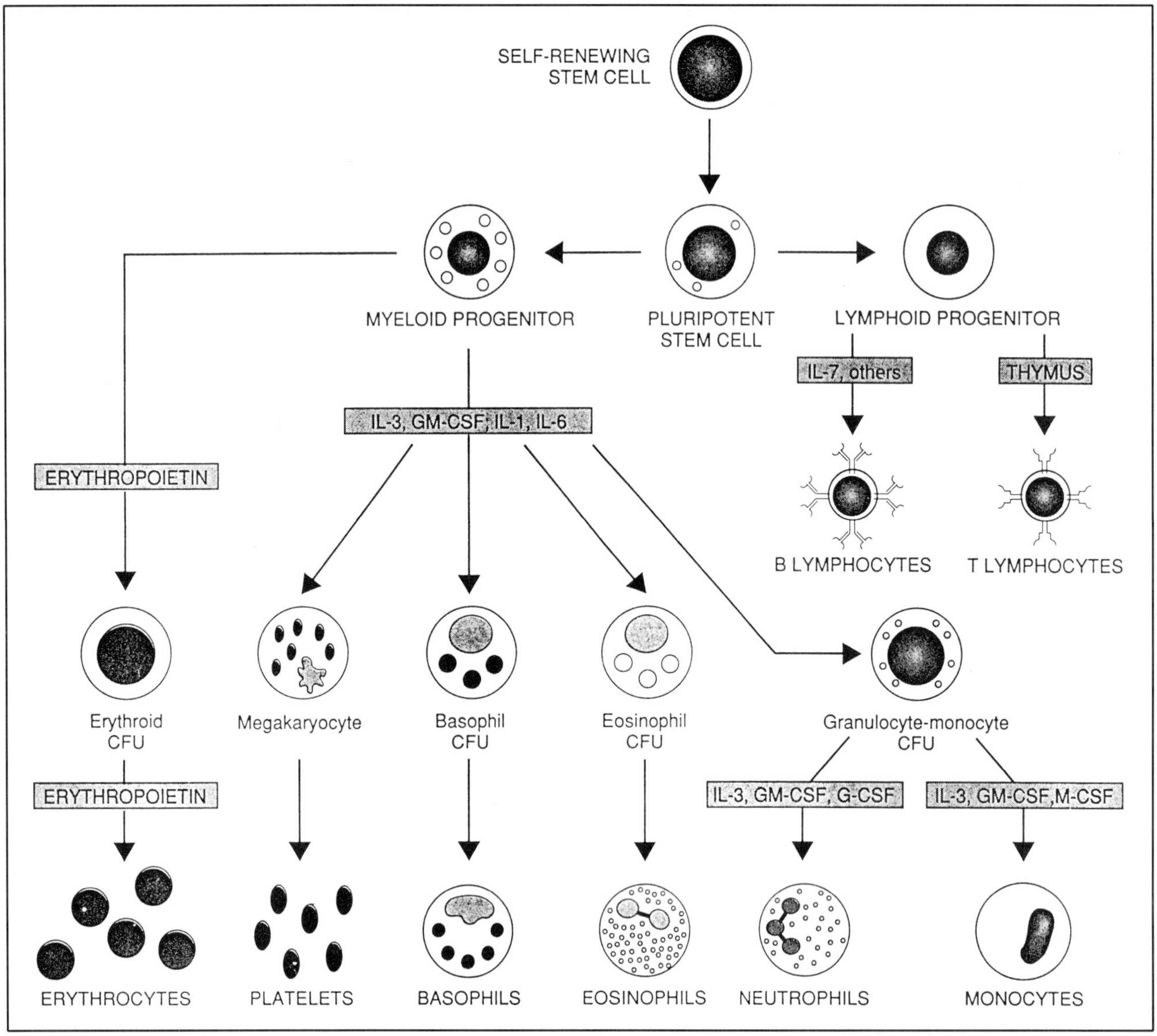
SELF-RENEWING
STEM CELL
MYELOID PROGENITOR
PLURIPOTENT
STEM CELL
LYMPHOID PROGENITOR
IL-7, others
THYMUS
IL-3, GM-CSF, IL-1, IL-6
ERYTHROPOIETIN
B LYMPHOCYTES
T LYMPHOCYTES
Erythroid
CFU
Megakaryocyte
Basophil
CFU
Eosinophil
CFU
Granulocyte-monocyte
CFU
ERYTHROPOIETIN
IL-3, GM-CSF, G-CSF
IL-3, GM-CSF,M-CSF
ERYTHROCYTES
PLATELETS
BASOPHILS
EOSINOPHILS
NEUTROPHILS
MONOCYTES

FIGURE 3–1. Maturation of blood cells: the hematopoietic "tree." The maturation of different lineages of blood cells is regulated by various cytokines. CFU, colony-forming unit; IL, interleukin; GM-CSF, granulocyte-macrophage colony-stimulating factor. (From Abbas AK, Litchman AH, Pober JS: Cells and tissues of the immune system. *In* Abbas AK, Litchman AH, Pober JS [eds]: Cellular and Molecular Immunology, p 13. Philadelphia, WB Saunders Co, 1991, with permission.)

The development of T cells is associated with two important events. The first occurs in the thymus when T cells are subjected to both positive and negative selection. Negative selection culminates in the elimination of T cells that would otherwise be reactive to self-determinants thus preventing autoimmune responses. On the other hand, positive selection allows for the maturation of T cells with specificity for foreign antigens in the context of MHC determinants. Positive selection is mediated by radiation-resistant epithelial thymic cells, whereas negative selection appears to be associated with bone marrow–derived cells.[11] The second phase of T-cell selection occurs when mature and immunocompetent T cells are stimulated by an antigen.[4] This stimulation is specific both for the foreign antigen and the self-MHC determinants with which the foreign antigen is associated. The responding T cells are activated and clonally expanded, resulting in the generation of effector cells and eventually memory cells. These memory cells are now ready to respond to a subsequent antigen challenge with an augmented response.

The T-cell response is triggered when foreign protein antigens are presented on the surfaces of other cells.[12,13] Cells involved in the processing and presenting of antigens are called antigen-presenting cells (APCs), which include dendritic cells, Langerhans cells, B lymphocytes, and cells of the monocyte/macrophage lineage.[14] Tumor cells may play a role in antigen presentation.[15] An APC must encounter an antigen, which is usually in the form of a large soluble protein, or a protein on the surface of a microorganism or foreign cell. The antigen is then cleaved into small soluble peptides, and delivered to the surface of the APC where it is displayed in association with either MHC class I or class II molecules. Exogenous antigens that are taken up and partially lysed in endocytic vesicles of APCs are primarily associated with MHC class II molecules. This association may take place intracellularly or upon release of the antigen on the cell surface. On the other hand, MHC class I molecules appear to be associated principally with endogenously synthesized antigens, such as virally encoded products of infected cells. Here too, the association may occur intracellularly or on the surface of the APC upon delivery of the antigen.

T-cell activation may be divided into two signaling events. The first signal refers to the interaction of antigen-specific TCR with its specific antigen ligand in the context of an MHC molecule. The second signal consists of all other requirements for T-cell activation and includes the interaction of cell surface structures on T cells with complementary structures on accessory cells, as well as signals provided by soluble factors such as cytokines.[13] Both signals are required for a complete T-cell activation (Fig. 3–2). Moreover, T-cell activation with the first signal, in the absence of the second signal, may lead to unresponsiveness of the T cells, which may lead to failure of activation when the cells are challenged on a subsequent occasion.[17] The B7 costimulator factor, expressed on APCs and tumor cells, binds to the CD28 molecule on T cells.[18,19] Tumor cells lacking B7 costimulation (B7−) not only fail to be immunogenic but can be made to acquire immunogenic potential when manipulated to express the B7 antigen. Activation of T cells, therefore, depends on the expression of a complex array of cell surface molecules. Coexpression of B7-1 and intercellular adhesion molecule 1 (ICAM-1) was observed as a requirement for tumor rejection and the establishment of a memory response by T cells against a number of tumor cell lines.[20]

Effector Function of T Cells

HELPER FUNCTION. The ability of CD4+ T cells to enhance the activity of other cells has been characterized as helper function.[1,4] This can be accomplished by direct T-cell interaction with other cells and/or by the production of T-cell lymphokines or cytokines. A notable example is observed in precursors of cytotoxic T lymphocytes (CTLs) requiring T-cell helper activity to generate a full response against its specific antigen. Recognizing not only identical but nonidentical antigens on the same target tumor cell may be sufficient for T-cell helpers to mediate the response of CTL precursors possessing TCRs specific for antigens on the same tumor cell. T cells also participate by promoting help in T-dependent antibody responses of B cells. Differentiation of CD4+ T cells into subsets is dictated by the type of cytokines produced and the potential T-cell function. CD4+ T cells that possess cytotoxic activity and produce the cytokines (interleukin-2 [IL-2], interferon-γ [IFN-γ], tumor necrosis factor-α [TNF-α], and lymphotoxin [LT]) are characterized as Th1 or inflammatory CD4+ T cells. Other CD4+ T cells that produce cytokines (IL-4, IL-5, IL-6, IL-10, IL-13) and exhibit predominantly helper function are designated Th2 cells.[21,22] Differentiation of CD4+ T cells into Th1 is promoted by IL-12 and IFN-γ, as compared to Th2 subsets promoted by IL-4.

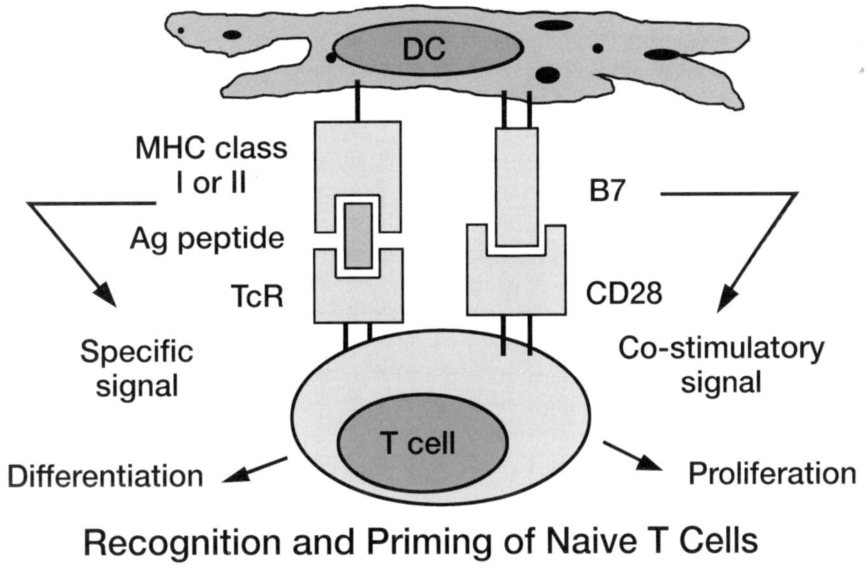
DC
MHC class I or II
Ag peptide
TcR
B7
CD28
Specific signal
Co-stimulatory signal
T cell
Differentiation
Proliferation
Recognition and Priming of Naive T Cells

FIGURE 3–2. Antigens are presented to T cells in a MHC class I– or class II–restricted manner. Costimulatory signals such as B7 are essential for T-cell recognition.

T-cell activity may produce down-regulation of the immune response, a process referred to as immune suppression. Immune suppression may be either antigen specific or antigen nonspecific. Benacerraf et al. described a complex pathway of antigen-specific suppression.[23] They defined three T-suppressor cell populations (TS_1, TS_2, and TS_3), and reported that each population played an essential role in immune suppression either by direct interaction with each other or by production of humoral factors. T cells also play a primary role in the DTH reaction when they produce lymphokines in response to antigenic signals. Some of these lymphokines serve as chemotactic activating agents, which attract a variety of other cells. The vast majority of these cells are not specific for the initiating antigen. Characteristic of the DTH reaction is the alteration of vascular permeability produced by the T-cell lymphokines.[24]

Cytotoxic Cell Functions

Cytotoxic cellular activity is produced predominantly by cytotoxic T lymphocytes, activated macrophages, natural killer (NK) lymphocytes, and activated neutrophils (Table 3–2).[4] The generation of the cytotoxic activity of these cells depends on T-cell responses. These cells are capable of producing and releasing the effector molecules that mediate cytotoxicity, and possess the receptors capable of triggering activation or release of cytotoxic molecules upon binding to a ligand.

Cytotoxic T Lymphocytes. Cytotoxic T lymphocytes have been considered central in tumor immunology. As previously mentioned, CTLs express primarily the CD8+ molecules, which recognize antigens associated with MHC class I determinants. Clones of T cells with CD4+ surface molecules, however, have been identified to release slow-acting cytotoxic products such as lymphotoxins.[22] These cells are referred to as Th1, or inflammatory CD4+ T cells, and may be both helper and cytotoxic. Cytotoxic T-lymphocyte binding to target cells initiates cytotoxic activity. Adhesion molecules on the surface of T cells will facilitate the CTL–target cell binding. Recognized T-cell surface adhesion molecules are leukocyte function–associated antigen 1 (LFA-1), CD2, CD4, and CD8.[4] The LFA-1 (CD11a and CD18) molecule can complex to ICAM-1 (or CD54) as well as to other as yet unidentified ligands on target cells. CD2 binds to LFA-3 (CD58), CD4 binds to class II MHC, and CD8 binds to class I MHC. The functional state of the lymphocytes is reflected by the density of these adhesion molecules on their cell's surface. The higher levels of LFA-1, CD2, and LFA-3 on memory T cells than other T cells may contribute to their enhanced response to restimulation with antigen.

The function of differentiated CTLs is to lyse and

TABLE 3–2. CHARACTERISTICS OF HUMAN CYTOTOXIC CELLS*

Cytotoxic Cell	Partial Phenotype	MHC-Restricted Cytotoxicity	MHC-Nonrestricted Cytotoxicity	ADCC†
CTL‡	CD3Ti+ CD2+ CD4+ (subset) CD8+ (subset) FcR−§ (primarily) CD56‖	Yes	Yes, if precultured with IL-2	No (primarily)
NK†	CD3/Ti− CD2+ CD4− CD8+ (subset) FCr+§ CD56+	No	Yes	Yes
Macrophages	CD3/Ti− CD2+ CD4+ CD8− FcR+§ CD56−	No	Yes	Yes
PMN¶	CD3/Ti− CD2− CD4− CD8− FcR+§ CD56−	No	Yes	Yes

*From Wunderlich JR, Hodes RJ: Principles of tumor immunity: Biology of cellular immune responses. *In* De Vita VT Jr, Hellman S, Rosenberg SA (eds): Biologic Therapy of Cancer, p 3. Philadelphia, JB Lippincott Co, 1991, with permission.

†ADCC, antibody-dependent cellular cytotoxicity.

‡LAK cells represent a combination of activated NK and CTL.

§FcR, cell-surface immunoglobulin receptors, for which there are different molecular forms.

‖CTLs express CD56 if precultured with IL-2.

¶PMN, polymorphonuclear cells.

kill target cells. Mature postthymic CTLs do not possess the machinery to kill target cells. These cells must not only be stimulated by coming into contact with the specific antigen on target cells in association with other accessory molecules but must also be able to receive signals from helper T cells. The development of specific membrane-bound cytoplasmic granules and the capacity to transcribe and secrete cytokines and other proteins mark the differentiation process. The cytoplasmic granules contain pore-forming macromolecules called porforins or cytolysins, serine esterases, protein toxins, and proteoglycans. Among the secreted cytokines, INF-γ, LT, and to a lesser extent IL-2 are observed. The cross-linking of apoptosis-inducing target cell surface molecules, such as APO-1/Fas, by CTL membrane ligands has been described as another mechanism of CTL–target cell killing.[25,26] Cytolytic T-lymphocyte killing is antigen specific. The CTL killing occurs through direct cell contact through the specific antigen receptor and accessory molecules (Fig. 3–3). The lethal agents are, therefore, delivered directly to the target cell, initiating a process of programmed cell death. The activated CTL is spared the cytotoxic effects of the secreted agents, and upon releasing the affected target cell, turns its attention to others. Similar to the observed subdivision of CD4+ T cells, CD8+ T-cell subsets have been determined.[27] Th2 CD8+ T cells that can help B cells at a distance in bystander reactions, but kill them if they are recognized directly, have been described.[4] Much alike the differentiation observed with CD4+ cells, differentiation of naive CD8+ T cells appears to be regulated by the type of cytokines they are exposed to. While IL-12 and IFN-γ promote cytotoxic or Th1 characteristics, IL-4 promotes the helper or Th2 phenotype.[27] CD8+ T cells, therefore, support many regulatory functions such as helper function and immune suppression through the release of various cytokines.

Natural Killer Lymphocytes. Natural killer lymphocytes differ from the classic T lymphocytes in that their cytolytic activity is nonspecific.[4] They recognize target cells in a non–MHC-restricted fashion, and their development is nonthymic dependent. Natural killer lymphocytes do not develop into memory cells with the capability of an augmented response upon restimulation. The NK cells appear to originate and possibly differentiate initially in the bone marrow. They are in a cell lineage separate from that of the CTLs and diverge from the T-cell lineage early in the prethymic phase. No genetic rearrangements occur in these cells as occur in B and T lymphocytes. Natural killer cells, therefore, do not express the TCR, or the closely associated CD3 molecules, on the surface of their cell membrane. The NK lymphocytes are distinguished from CTLs in that they express the CD56+ antigen and a surface receptor for immunoglobulin (FcR), and are efficient mediators of antibody-

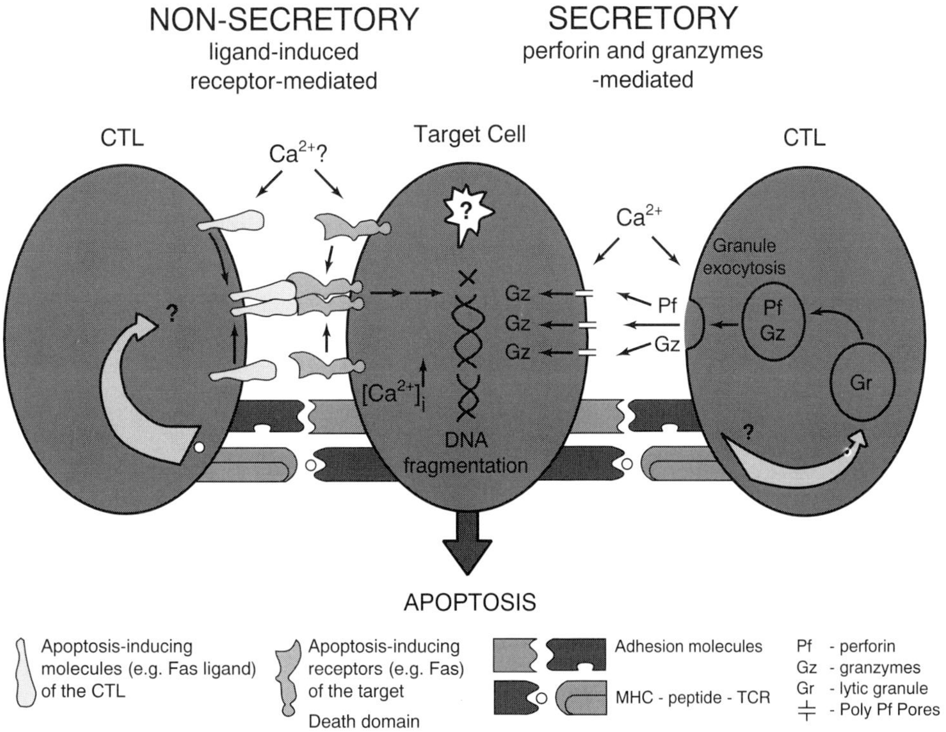
NON-SECRETORY
ligand-induced
receptor-mediated
SECRETORY
perforin and granzymes
-mediated
CTL
Ca2+?
Target Cell
CTL
?
Ca2+
Granule
exocytosis
Gz
Gz
Gz
Pf
Gz
Pf
Gz
Gr
?
[Ca2+]i
DNA
fragmentation
?
APOPTOSIS
Apoptosis-inducing
molecules (e.g. Fas ligand)
of the CTL
Apoptosis-inducing
receptors (e.g. Fas)
of the target
Death domain
Adhesion molecules
MHC - peptide - TCR
Pf - perforin
Gz - granzymes
Gr - lytic granule
- Poly Pf Pores

FIGURE 3–3. Schematic diagram showing the mechanisms of CTL-mediated target cell lysis. (From Berke G: The CTL's kiss of death. Cell 1995; 81:9–12, with permission.)

dependent cellular cytotoxicity. The mechanism of cytotoxicity for NK cells appears to be similar to that of CTLs.[25,28] The NK cells binds to the target cell via adhesion molecules and produce target cell lysis by releasing cytotoxic factors such as cytolysin/perforin and lymphotoxins. Although NK cells are not target specific, they are more toxic for tumor cells, virus-infected, and cultured cells than for normal cells. Different clones of NK cells show different patterns of cytotoxicity with panels of tumor cells from different sources.

Lymphokine-Activated Killer Cells. Lymphokine-activated killer (LAK) cells are produced by exposing lymphocyte culture to high doses of IL-2.[29] The activity of the resultant LAK cells is characteristic for the selective lysis of a broad spectrum of autologous, syngeneic, or allogeneic tumor cells in a non–MHC-dependent fashion. These activated cells are derived from both NK cells and T cells.

Activated Macrophages and Neutrophils. Macrophages activated by high doses of IL-2 are selectively cytotoxic or cytostatic to tumor cells in vitro. Several characteristics of macrophages distinguish them from CTLs and NK cells—macrophages may be phagocytic, express CD68, are commonly adherent, and have a relatively abundant cytoplasm lacking azurophilic granules. Macrophages may express CD4, but they do not express CD2, CD3, or CD8.[30] Macrophages express immunoglobulin Fc receptors, and can mediate antibody-dependent cellular cytotoxicity.[24] The cytotoxicity and cytostatic activity are MHC independent and produced by macrophage target cell binding and/or the secretion of cytotoxic mediators. In addition to tumor-cell contact, macrophages can be activated by IFN-γ, granulocyte-macrophage colony-stimulating factor (GM-CSF), CSF-1, and by bacterial products such as lipopolysaccharides (LPS).[24,31] Mechanisms of macrophage cytotoxicity or inhibition of cell growth mechanisms appear to be dependent on receptor-mediated macrophage–tumor cell binding. Macrophages rarely endocytose tumor cells. Cytotoxic mechanisms include antibody-independent and -dependent cytolysis and separate processes associated with inhibition of DNA synthesis, or cytostasis. Among the cytotoxic factors produced by macrophages, TNF-α appears to be one of the most important.

Humoral Immunity

Humoral immunity essentially refers to the complex system mediated by the production and function of antibodies. Antibody production is unique to B lymphocytes, which are derived from hematopoietic stem cells in the bone marrow.[32] These cells mature in the bone marrow and acquire the ability to synthesize membrane-bound immunoglobulin molecules. The mature B cells then enter the peripheral circulation, where they encounter antigen stimulation and differentiate into activated antibody-secreting cells. Some activated B lymphocytes persist as membrane immunoglobulin-expressing memory cells. Memory B cells can survive for several weeks or months without further antigenic stimulation but respond to antigen restimulation with highly efficient antibody synthesis and secretion. The concept of humoral immunity was advanced by Paul Ehrlich approximately a century ago.[33] It was not until 1959, however, that the basic protein structure and composition of antibodies were defined.[34,35] The basic structure of antibodies is the immunoglobulin molecule (Ig), which consists of four polypeptides (two light chains, two heavy chains). The light chain has a molecular weight of 23 kDa and contains approximately 215 amino acids. The carboxyl-terminal region is largely invariant and is designated the light chain constant region. Two types of light chain constant regions (κ and λ) have been identified. They exist in humans in a κ/λ ratio of 60:40; however, any single immunoglobulin molecule will contain only one light chain type. The NH_2-terminal half of the light chain contains the highly variable antigen-binding site. This site exhibits extensive sequence diversity, which is particularly pronounced at three hypervariable noncontiguous segments. These smaller segments are termed complementary-determining or hypervariable regions, and their three-dimensional relationship with corresponding regions on the heavy chain polypeptide constitutes the antigen-binding site.

Many of the structural features seen in the light chain are present in the heavy chain polypeptide.[33] The NH_2-terminal regions of the heavy chains similarly display marked sequence variability and the three hypervariable regions observed on the light chain. Different heavy chain constant regions varying in length and sequence have been identified and define the various immunoglobulin classes. There are five different classes of immunoglobulins designated as IgG, IgM, IgA, IgD, IgE, which correspond to the heavy chain constant regions γ, μ, α, δ, and ϵ, respectively. The basic structure of the immunoblobulin molecule is depicted in Figure 3–4. Several disulfide bonds maintain the configuration of the variable and constant regions and link the light and heavy polypeptide chains to each other. Antibody synthesis results from a series of genetic rearrangements producing almost unlimited variability in antigen-binding specificity. Papain digestion of the immunoglobulin molecule produces three fragments. Two identical fragments maintaining antigen-binding capacity are designated as fragments Fab. The third fragment was found to crystallize easily, and was termed the Fc fragment.

The role of antibodies in tumor immunology and tumor immunotherapy has been limited. With the development of monoclonal antibodies (MoAbs), some success has been achieved in tumor diagnosis

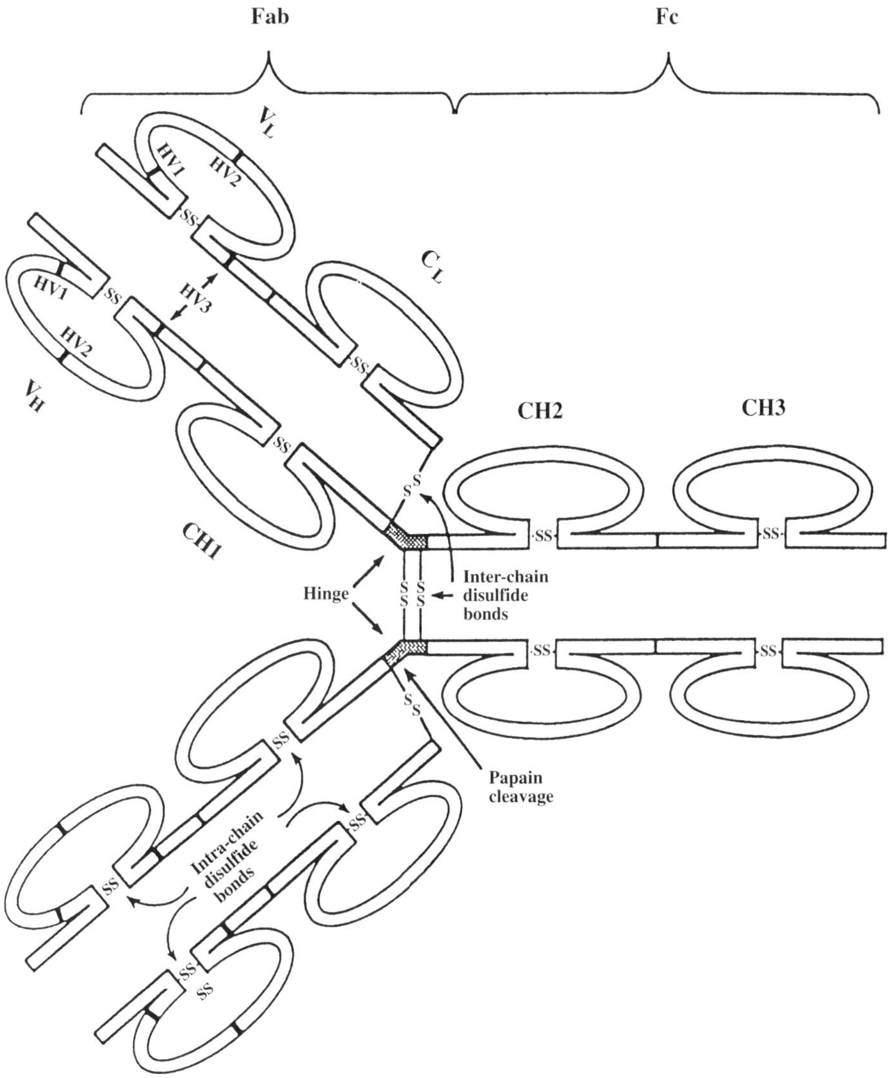
Fab
Fc
VL
HV1
HV2
HV3
CL
HV1
HV2
VH
CH1
CH2
CH3
SS
S S
Hinge
Inter-chain disulfide bonds
Papain cleavage
Intra-chain disulfide bonds

FIGURE 3–4. Schematic representation of an IgG antibody molecule. V_L and V_H, variable domains of the light and heavy chains; CL, constant regions of the light chain; CH1, CH2, and CH3, constant domains of the heavy chain; HV1, HV2, and HV3, hypervariable or complementary-determining regions; SS, disulfide bonds; Fab, papain-derived antigen-binding fragment; Fc, papain-derived crystallizable fragment. (From Rosenberg SA: Principles and applications of biologic therapy. *In* De Vita VT Jr, Hellman S, Rosenberg SA [eds]: Cancer: Principles & Practice of Oncology, 4th edition. Philadelphia, JB Lippincott Co, 1993, with permission.)

and staging. Today, the use of murine MoAbs produced with hybridoma technology is limited by the human antimurine immunoglobulin (HAMA) response. To minimize or eliminate the HAMA response, recombinant/chimeric MoAbs and antibody humanization have been utilized. A wide range of clinical applications for the utilization of MoAbs in tumor diagnosis, monitoring, and therapy has been developed.[36,37] Clinically, antibodies have gained prominence in tumor diagnosis, but progress in the domain of immunotherapy has been slow.[37] Radiolabeled MoAbs are being used to treat some leukemia and lymphomas, but no significant responses have been observed when these agents are used to treat solid tumors. Recently, MoAbs reactive to the G250 renal tumor–associated antigen have been developed. Histologically, these antibodies stain almost all clear cell renal tumors, and approximately 85% of all renal tumors. Using Iodine-133 (^{131}I)–labeled MoAb G250, Oosterwijk et al. were able to detect 90% of primary and metastatic lesions demonstrated on magnetic resonance imaging (MRI) and computed tomography (CT) scans.[38] Only minimal responses were observed when ^{131}I-G250 was utilized as radioimmunotherapy for metastatic renal cell carcinoma.[37] Radiolabeled MoAbs reactive to antigens on prostate cancer cells are also being investigated for imaging and clinical staging.[39] Although the results are encouraging, further studies are needed to determine the role these MoAbs will play in the management of patients with kidney or prostate cancer.

TABLE 3–3. GENERAL PROPERTIES OF CYTOKINES

1. Cytokines are produced during the effector phases of natural and specific immunity and serve to mediate and regulate immune and inflammatory responses.
2. Cytokines secretion is a brief, self-limiting event.
3. Many individual cytokines are produced by multiple diverse cell types.
4. Cytokines not only are produced by different cell types but also act upon many different cell types.
5. Cytokine actions are often redundant.
6. Cytokines often influence the synthesis of other cytokines.
7. Cytokines often influence the action of other cytokines.
8. Cytokines, like other polypeptide hormones, initiate their action by binding to specific receptors on the surfaces of target cells.
9. The expression of many cytokine receptors is regulated by specific signals.
10. Most cellular responses to cytokines are slow, occurring over a period of hours, and require new mRNA and protein synthesis.
11. For many target cells, cytokines act as regulators of cell division (i.e., as growth factors)

Cytokines

Cytokines are biologically active agents produced by cells to promote an effector response in the immune system. The properties of cytokines are outlined in Table 3–3. In general, cytokines are polypeptide proteins that are produced by a variety of cells in response to different stimuli (mononuclear-phagocytes to microbial products such as LPS, T cells secondary to a specific recognition of foreign antigens, or cytokines produced by one cell type may regulate the synthesis of cytokines in other cells).[40] Cytokines are not stored as preformed molecules, but are transiently secreted after brief and self-limiting gene transcription of the cytokine mRNA. These hormones are not only produced by different cell types but also act upon different cell types. Although the actions of cytokines continue to unfold, it has been established that cytokines will influence the synthesis and action of other cytokines and serve as regulatory growth factors for many target cells.[41] Table 3–4 shows the names and functions of several known cytokines.

Interleukin-2

IL-2 is one of the most extensively studied cytokines.[42] Interleukin-2 is produced naturally by T lymphocytes and large granular lymphocytes (LGLs); however, some malignant B-cell lines may produce this cytokine.[43] The major inducer of IL-2 production is recognition of the nominal antigen and MHC by the T-cell receptor. IL-2 exists mainly as the secreted form, although membrane-associated IL-2 epitopes have been identified on the surface of some human T cells. As part of the positive selection of T cells during their development and maturation in the thymus, they acquire IL-2 receptors and a responsiveness to IL-2 stimulation. T cells migrate to peripheral sites such as lymph nodes, where their population is maintained by IL-2 production in a paracrine and endocrine fashion. Persistent T-cell expansion and death in these peripheral pools results in approximately a 50% turnover of the peripheral T cells every 2 to 3 days.[44]

Human IL-2 is a 15-kDa protein, which is dissimilar to murine IL-2 (15 to 31 kDa).[45,46] Although human IL-2 produces some murine cell responses, little murine IL-2 activity on human cells has been noted. The human IL-2 gene is located on chromosome 4, and the final protein product consists of 133 amino acids. Regulation of IL-2 production occurs at the level of DNA transcription. The mRNA of IL-2, like other cytokines, has a short life (2 hours, compared with 10 hours for somatic mRNA). The major inducer of IL-2 production is recognition of the nominal antigen and MHC complex by the T-cell receptor. Only activated T cells (not resting) produce IL-2. Other inducers of IL-2 include cross-linking of the T-cell receptor with antibodies or with mitogens such as phytohemagglutinin (PHA). Although the biochemical pathways leading to IL-2 cellular production are not fully defined, it appears that increased cytosolic calcium and activation of protein kinase C are required.[47,48] The IL-2 molecule is extremely hydrophobic and is stable at pH 2.

There are at least three different types of IL-2 receptors (p55, p70, p55/p70), each composed of α and β chains either singly or in combination.[42] The IL-2 affinity for the receptors varies. The α (p55) receptor molecule binds IL-2 rapidly with a half-life of 1.7 seconds, promoting capture and presentation to the β chain. In contrast to the short half-life of the α chain–IL-2 dissociation, the β (p70) chain–IL-2 dissociation half-life is much longer (46 minutes). IL-2 binding to its receptor complex occurs through a process of rapid high-affinity binding and slow release. Upon binding to the β chain or α-β biomolecular complex, the IL-2 is rapidly internalized.[49] IL-2 binding to the α chain alone fails to trigger receptor-mediated endocytosis. Following IL-2 binding to the β chain, cells rapidly increase their transcription of the α chain receptor, progress through the G_1 phase, and lymphocyte mitogenesis occurs.[50,51] IL-2 protein-receptor binding results in proliferation of T cells, B cells, monocytes, and LGLs. IL-2 promotes chemotaxis of cytotoxic T cells and NK/LAK cells. It stimulates the production and release of various cytokines such as IFN-γ, IL-1, IL-6, and TNF. It has been shown that activation of the JAK-STAT pathway may be a common mechanism through which many cytokines including IL-2 affect cellular responses.[52]

Efforts to unravel the mechanism(s) of action of IL-2 are ongoing. At the same time, IL-2 is utilized in clinical practice as a potent antitumoral agent to treat patients with metastatic renal cell carcinoma and melanoma.[53] Clinical response rates on the order of 15 to 20% have been reported for patients

TABLE 3–4. NAMES AND FUNCTIONS OF SEVERAL KNOWN CYTOKINES*

Cytokines	Biological Effects
INF-α or β	Exerts antiviral activity; enhances the expression of surface (β_2-microglobulin, Fc receptors, tumor-associated antigens, and MHC class I antigens); modulates B-cell function; inhibits suppressor T-cell activity; activates monocytes/macrophages; augments NK cell activity; has fever-inducing and antiproliferative properties; interacts (enhances, inhibits) with growth factors, oncogenes, and other cytokines; activates CTL
INF-γ	Induces MHC class I and class II antigens; activates macrophages and endothelial cells; augments NK cell activity; exerts antiviral activity; augments or inhibits other cytokine activities; induces IL-2 receptors; mediates antimicrobial activity, regulates lipid metabolism; induces B-cell Ig production; suppresses IL-4 activities on B cells; activates CTL; enhances tumor-associated antigen expression; regulates differentiation
IL-1 α or β	Costimulates T cells; induces IL-2 production; increases IL-2 receptor number and binding; growth-factor activation; induction/release of other cytokines; augments IL-2–induced LAK activity; induces CSF production by accessory cells; hemopoietin I activity; activates endothelial cells and macrophages; induces acute-phase responses; mediates catabolic processes, inflammation, and nonspecific resistance to infection; enhances growth of virulent strains of *Escherichia coli*; costimulates proliferation and differentiation of B cells; induces maturation of pre-B cells
IL-2	Costimulates T cells; activates cytotoxic responses in T cells; stimulates monocytes to become tumoricidal; chemotactic for T cells; cofactor for growth and differentiation of B cells; induction/release of cytokines; induces non–MHC-restricted CTL killing; costimulates proliferation and differentiation of B cells
IL-3	Initiates growth of mature inducer T cells (thy-1^+, Lyt-1^+, 2^-) and of Thy-1^+, Lyt-1^-, 2^-, $T3^+$ non–MHC-restricted CTL (in mouse); supports mast cell growth; stimulates early progenitor cell growth (erythrocyte, monocyte, granulocyte, megakaryocyte); supports growth of pre–B-cell lines
IL-4	Costimulates (in proliferation of normal resting T cells); stimulates thymocyte proliferation and differentiation to CTLs (in presence of lectin and phobol myristate acetate); helper factor for CTL generation in primary MLC and induces/amplifies in vitro primed MLC memory cells; promotes growth of TILs cytotoxic for autologous human melanoma; generates LAK activity and augments IL-2–induced LAK activity (in mouse); supports mast cell growth; synergizes with other growth factors to promote colony growth; induces monocyte cytotoxicity (in mouse); induces MHC class II antigens on B cells and monocytes; growth factor for activated B cells; increases expression of Fc receptors; increases IgG1 and IgE secretion by B cells; decreases IgG2a, IgG2b, IgM, and IgG3 secretion by B cells
IL-5	Cofactor for induction of CTL differentiation; induces IL-2 receptor expression on T and B cells; causes release of soluble IL-2 receptor; enhances IL-2–mediated LAK activity (in mouse); induces proliferation and differentiation of eosinophil precursors; increases proliferation of activated normal B cells; increases IgA and IgM secretion of B cells
IL-6	Costimulates T cells; induces IL-2 production; CTL differentiation factor; augments human NK and LAK cytotoxicity; augments human and mouse ADCC; enhances MHC class I expression; enhances tumor-associated antigen (CEA) expression on human colorectal adenocarcinoma cells; induces acute-phase responses; synergizes with other growth factors to promote colony growth; enhances Ig secretion by B cells; induces B-cell differentiation
IL-7	Costimulates purified T cells (in presence of ConA or PMA); induces LAK activity; generates and expands allospecific CTL and antitumor CTL; induces cytokine secretion and tumoricidal activity by human monocytes; supports the growth of B-cell precursors
IL-10	Cytokine synthesis inhibitory factor for T helper-1 cells; inhibits macrophage activity and monocyte-dependent stimulation of NK cell production of IFN-γ; costimulates with IL-2 or IL-4 the proliferation of activated but not resting T cells; increases the number of CTL precursors; augments CTL activity; stimulates B cells; increases viability of resting B cells; costimulates (with IL-3 or IL-4) enhanced growth of mast cell lines and progenitors
IL-12	Stimulates antigen-activated CD4+ and CD8+ T cells (independent or IL-2); synergizes with IL-2 in induction of CTL and additive with IL-2 and CTL proliferation; enhances NK activity; stimulates INF-γ secretion by resting and activated human PBLs
IL-15	Is a cofactor for growth and differentiation of T and B cells; induces T cells to produce IL-5
TNF α or β	Stimulates T-cell proliferation; enhances NK activity; induces macrophage tumoricidal activity; directly cytotoxic to some tumor cells; induces systemic acute-phase responses; activates PMNs; costimulates mitogen-activated B cells; enhances expression of MHC class I and class II molecules; stimulates production of other cytokines; including colony-stimulating factors; affects (reduces or increases) expression of oncogene products; induces cytokine receptor expression; activates endothelial cells (expression of adhesion molecules); mediates catabolic processes, septic shock, and inflammation; induces myeloid differentiation
G-CSF	Stimulates growth of granulocyte colonies and activates mature granulocytes; increases antibody-dependent, neutrophil-mediated cytotoxicity; induces in vitro differentiation of leukemia cell lines; stimulates proliferation of leukemic progenitors
GM-CSF	Stimulates growth of granulocyte, monocyte, and early erythrocyte progenitors, and, less, megakaryocyte progenitors; activates mature granulocytes and monocytes; enhances antibody-dependent, cell-mediated cytotoxoicity; may stimulate proliferation of leukemic progenitors; chemotactic for monocytes and PMNs; up-regulates CR3 receptors on PMNs and monocytes; stimulates production of other cytokines (M-CSF and TNF) by monocytes
M-CSF	Stimulates growth of monocyte colonies; supports in vitro survival of monocytes; activates mature monocytes; enhances antibody-dependent, monocyte-dependent cytotoxicity; stimulates production/secretion of cytokines, plasminogen activator, oxygen reduction products, acidic isoferritins by macrophages; enhances Fc receptor, CR3 receptor, and MHC class II expression on macrophages; stimulates macrophage pinocytosis; chemotactic

*Modified from Rosenberg SA: Principles and applications of biologic therapy. *In* De Vita VT Jr, Hellman S, Rosenberg SA (eds): Cancer: Principles & Practice of Oncology, 4th edition. Philadelphia, JB Lippincott Co, 1993, with permission.

IFN, interferon; IL, interleukin; TNF, tumor necrosis factor; CSF, colony-stimulating factor; G, granulocyte; GM, granulocyte-macrophage; M, macrophage; LAK, lymphokine-activated killer cells; CTL, cytotoxic T lymphocyte; MHC, major histocompatibility complex; MLC, mixed lymphocyte reaction; TIL, tumor-infiltrating lymphocyte; ADCC, antibody-dependent cellular cytotoxicity; CEA, carcinoembryonic antigen; NK, natural killer cell; ConA, concanavalin A; PMA, phobol myristate acetate; PBL, peripheral blood lymphocyte; CR3, complement receptor 3.

with metastatic renal cell carcinoma.[54] Consequently, IL-2 has been approved by the U.S. Food and Drug Administration (FDA) for the treatment of metastatic renal cell carcinoma. In addition to a limited efficacy, IL-2 immunotherapy is tempered by significant dose-related toxicities.[55,56] These toxicities appear to affect major organ systems and may result in single-organ as well as multiorgan failures and death. Among the most noticeable IL-2–associated toxicities is the vascular leak syndrome, which results in pulmonary edema, ascites, oliguria, azotemia, peripheral edema, decreased peripheral resistance, and hypotension secondary to vascular depletion. Cardiorespiratory, renal, and neurologic toxicities are not uncommon and may be quite severe. Hepatic, gastrointestinal, hematologic, and dermatologic toxicities, on the other hand, are typically mild and infrequently affect treatment delivery.

Interferons

Interferons were first discovered by Isaacs and Lindenmann in 1957, and are classified as either IFN-α, IFN-β, or IFN-γ according to their cellular origin and mode of induction.[57] IFN-α can be produced by different cell types, including macrophages; non-B, non-T lymphocytes; and B-cell lines. Fibroblasts and epithelial cells are the main producers of IFN-β. Primary inducers of IFN-α and -β are viral infections and double-stranded RNA. Platelet-derived growth factor (PDGF), TNF, macrophage colony-stimulating factor (M-CSF), and IL-1 have also been shown to induce IFN-α and -β production.[58–60] IFN-γ is produced predominantly by T cells and NK cells, and to a lesser extent by macrophages. IFN-γ production is induced by mitogens and specific antigens.

Interferons-α and -β are proteins, each with 166 amino acids. At least 24 subtypes of IFN-α have been identified and the amino acid sequences have been determined.[61] Only one subtype of IFN-β has been characterized. Another protein formally designated IFN-β2 is now referred to as IL-6. The genes for IFN-α and IFN-β are both located on chromosome 9p21. In general, IFN-α and -β share about 30% homology in amino acid sequence, are both stable at pH 2.0, and bind to the same cellular receptor. The location of the gene responsible for the IFN-α and -β receptor synthesis has been identified at chromosome 21q21. In contrast, IFN-γ is structurally distinct from IFN-β, and has about 12% amino acid homology with IFN-α. Only one species of the IFN-γ protein exists, which is made up of 146 amino acids. The gene for the IFN-γ protein is located on a different chromosome than that of the other interferons (chromosome 12q24). IFN-γ is not acid stable, and binds to a different receptor whose gene is located at chromosome 6q.

Several properties are attributed to interferons.[57] The properties shared by all three groups are immunomodulatory activities such as activation of NK and cytotoxic T cells, and induction of the MHC class I antigens. Interferons are also known for their antiviral and antiproliferative activity, inhibition of angiogenesis, and regulation of differentiation; and for their interaction with growth factors, oncogenes, and other cytokines. Interferons are also capable of enhancing tumor-associated antigens. Properties attributed exclusively to IFN-γ are activation of monocytes/macrophages, stimulation of MHC class II antigens, induction of B-cell immunoglobulin production, and induction of IL-2 receptors. IFN-γ also possesses antimicrobial activity (mediated by monocytes/macrophages), and affects lipid (triglyceride) metabolism.

Many properties of interferon contribute to either a direct or indirect antitumor effect. The antitumor activity of IFNs was further demonstrated when human bladder cancer cells were inhibited by continuous exposure to IFN-α and IFN-β.[63] Additionally, IFN-γ has been shown to stimulate the expression of surface antigens on human bladder cancer cells.[64] In a study by Belldegrun et al., in vitro and in vivo growth of the R11 renal cell carcinoma cell line was abrogated following transfection of the INF-α gene into these cells.[65] Recent developments point to an intracellular mechanism that explains in part the activity of interferon. α- and β-IFN binding to the α/β-receptor leads to the activation of the Janus family of tyrosine kinases (Jak) and subsequently to activation of proteins referred to as signal transducers and activators of transcription (STATs).[66] The STAT proteins, once phosphorylated, migrate from the cytoplasm to the nucleus, where they regulate early response genes. This JAK-STAT pathway is further augmented by additional phosphorylation of the STAT proteins via the mitogen-activated protein (MAP) kinase-Ras pathway. Expanded characterization of these pathways will provide greater insights into the functions of the interferons.

Tumor Necrosis Factor

TNF is a potent cytokine produced by monocytes/macrophages in response endotoxins, phobol esters, and phospholipase-2 activators.[67] Lymphotoxin, also called TNF-β, shares about 30% homology with TNF, and acts on the same receptor.[68,69] The genes for both TNF-α and -β are located on chromosome 6 at 6p23-6p12, near the HLA locus. Regulation of TNF production has been shown to take place at both the transcriptional and translational levels.[70] TNF is synthesized initially as a proprotein of 230 amino acids, which is subsequently cleaved at the amino-terminal end to produce the mature protein of 154–157 amino acids.[71] Following synthesis, the proprotein may exist as a transmembrane molecule. The active TNF protein is released upon cleavage of the hydrophobic signal peptide segment. The membrane-bound proprotein retains cytotoxic activity against TNF-sensitive cells.[72] TNF must bind to receptors on the surface of target cells to induce their activity. Although the TNF receptor number appears to be regulated through several mechanism, the biologic significance of adjusting target cell membrane TNF receptor content remains unclear. Following ligation of TNF to its receptor, the complex is internalized and rapidly degraded.[73] Protein synthesis is, therefore, required to maintain the TNF receptor cell membrane number. Interferons have been shown to upregulate the TNF receptor, while IL-1, lipopolysaccharides, and phobol ester have been observed to down-regulate the TNF receptor.[67] Two major TNF receptor types with molecular weights 55 kDa and 75 kDa have been identified.[74] These receptors may exist in the soluble form in both serum and urine, and may serve as inhibitors of TNF.[75] Not only was increased elaboration of the soluble TNF receptors observed in patients with renal cell carcinoma but an increased secretion of the 55-kDa component was demonstrated following treatment with IL-2 and tumor-infiltrating lymphocytes (TILs).[76]

The actions of TNF emanate from its binding to the TNF receptors on target cells. Although the mechanism(s) of signal transduction is not completely defined, several activities have been observed.[67,77] Secondary intracellular messengers included cyclic adenosine monophosphate (cAMP), inositol phosphates, diacylglycerol, eicosanoids, intracellular calcium, and intracellular pH are known to be associated with TNF activity. Binding of the TNF protein–receptor complex to nucleotide-binding proteins (G proteins) is suspected. The increased enzyme activity observed in phospholipase A_2 and adenyl cyclase is believed to be related to G-protein mechanisms. Another G-protein–associated enzyme (phospholipase C) has not been shown to be altered with TNF activity. TNF activity is also associated with protein kinase C and calcium ionophore activity.

TNF produces both direct and indirect cellular responses. Antiproliferative activity is observed against various tumor cell lines, but not against normal cells. This antiproliferative activity may be either cytolytic or cytostatic, and is limited to approximately one third of the cell lines tested. The variability in TNF cytotoxicity is not yet understood. Cytotoxicity requires TNF binding to the TNF receptor. The receptor–TNF complex is internalized by endocytosis, and then transported to lysosomes. Inhibitors of cytoskeletal action such as cholchicine and cytochalasin B can block TNF killing.[78] Similarly, lysosomal and protease inhibitors can inhibit the cytolytic effects of TNF.[79] Tumor necrosis cell killing is cell cycle specific, dependent on temperature, and involves the elaboration of free radicals.[67] Synergy with TNF cytotoxicity has been shown with a number of other agents, which include the interferons (IFN-α, -β, -γ), inhibitors of mRNA synthesis (actinomycin D, 5-fluorouracil), mitosis inhibitors, alkylating agents (cyclophosphamide, cisplatin, ionizing radiation), and topoisomerase II inhibitors (doxorubicin, etoposide). Another property attributed to the direct action of TNF is the inhibition of cellular differentiation. This property has been observed with mesenchymal cells (adipocytes and muscle cells), and different myeloid cells.

Apart from the direct effects of TNF described above, other activities of TNF are mediated through the induction of other cytokines or growth factors.[67] Both IL-1 and IL-6 are induced by TNF, and these cytokines may contribute to some of the mitogenic properties observed with TNF. In contrast to the antiproliferative characteristics attributed to TNF, TNF may produce proliferation in both normal and malignant cell types. Epidermal growth factor (EGF) and PDGF appear to mediate some of these proliferative effects of TNF. Antitumor effects of TNF have also been demonstrated in vivo. Synergy in TNF's in vivo antitumor effect has been demonstrated with both cytotoxic and other biologic agents. A combination of changes in clotting, endothelial-cell antigen expression, and synthesis of inflammatory mediators results in profound alterations in vascular physiology. These events lead to coagulation and hence necrosis. The activation of neutrophils, lymphocytes, and monocytes by TNF together with the elaboration of other cytokines participate in the antitumor effect. Although TNF is an extremely potent cytokine, its clinical activity has been limited by significant systemic effects including those typical of sepsis (hypotension, metabolic acidosis, hemoconcentration, hypoglycemia, hyperkalemia, and respiratory arrest). Other systemic toxicities are cachexia, hematologic, and hepatic.

Colony-Stimulating Factors

CSFs are a family of glycoproteins that share as their main function the regulation of proliferation of hematopoietic cells. Each CSF is produced by its own gene and binds to a unique receptor on the target cells.[80] The clustering of genes for the GM-CSF, multi-CSF, and M-CSF together with other hematopoietic growth factors (IL-4, IL-5) also suggest a relationship between these genes. The role of CSF in mediating the number and survival of various hematogenous cells appear to be directly related to the normal cellular proliferation of these cellular populations. Infectious and other inflammatory stimuli cause increased production of the CSFs and the attendant enhanced proliferation of the responding cells. CSFs have gained wide clinical applications as adjuncts to standard chemotherapy by reducing myelotoxicity and associated complications. Dose intensification of myelosuppressive agents may be accomplished. Because CSFs are differentiation-inducing agents of hematopoietic cells, this property has been exploited in myelodysplastic syndromes and myloid leukemia.

Antitumor activity has been reported with the CSFs.[81–83] In a number of studies, transduction of

GM-CSF in ex vivo irradiated tumor cells enhanced their tumorigenicity. Moreover, utilization of these transfected cells as tumor vaccines promoted potent, long-lasting, and specific antitumor immunity.[82] The mechanism(s) of this antitumor action remains unclear, but is most likely T-cell mediated. These observations have served as the basis for the initiation of human clinical trials using irradiated tumor cells transduced with GM-CSF as tumor vaccines.[83,84] To date such studies are ongoing in kidney and prostate cancers. Although no dramatic results have been reported, it is still too soon to assess the validity of this approach.

Other Cytokines

The number of recognized cytokines participating in the immune system continues to expand (Table 3–4).[10] Essential to the immune system is the integrated network of these soluble factors, which serve as cell-to-cell signaling agents. Although functional characteristics have been ascribed to individual cytokines, our knowledge of the true activity of these agents in vivo remains incomplete. To date, IL-2 and the IFNs are the most commonly utilized cytokines in clinical practice. Although the CSFs are extensively used as adjuncts to chemotherapy regimens to prevent neutropenia, their role in the treatment of solid malignancies is still being explored. Other cytokines being evaluated for their direct or indirect roles in antitumor therapy are IL-4, IL-6, and IL-7.[85–87] These cytokines were all determined to enhance the cytotoxic activity of TILs against renal tumor cells. The highly potent IL-12 heterodimeric cytokine promotes the maturation and activation of human peripheral blood lymphocytes and NK cells. IL-12 causes the induction of IFN-γ production by both resting and activated CD4+ T cells, CD8+ T cells, and NK cells.[88] Synergy of actions with IL-2 and IL-12 has been observed. Antitumor activity of IL-12 has been demonstrated and presently provides the foundation for existing and future clinical trials.[89]

Nonspecific Stimulants and Immunomodulators

Nonspecific stimulation of the immune system refers to mechanisms that do not directly involve the specific induction or interaction of antibodies or cytoxic T cells with tumor-associated or tumor-specific antigens on the surfaces of tumor cells. Involved in these mechanisms are the nonspecific immunologic defense factors such as macrophage activation, NK cell activation, and the release of cytokines.[90] Microbials such as bacille Calmette-Guérin (BCG) and microbial cell wall and glycoprotein products characterize the nonspecific stimulants (Table 3–5). Purified or synthetic substances such as the peptidoglycans and endotoxins, and interferon inducers (polynucleotides such as poly IC and poly IC-LC, or pyrimidinones such as bropirimine), are also examples of these nonspecific stimulators. Utilizing BCG, the principles of active nonspecific immunotherapy were defined by Bast et al.[91] They described that success of BCG depends upon (1) a small or minimal tumor burden; (2) the immunocompetence of the host and the ability of the host to mount an immune response to the BCG antigens; (3) a high dose of BCG organisms; (4) administration in close proximity to the tumor via intratumoral, intracavitary, or regional lymph node drainage injection; and (5) the ability of the tumor-bearing patient to mount an immune response to the antigens of the tumor.

The concept of immunomodulation refers to up- or down-regulation of specific antitumor cellular or humoral immunity. In cancer immunology, immunomodulation is based on the fact that there is progressive immunodeficiency as cancer progresses.[92] The association between immunocompetence and prognosis is such that immunocompetent patients will respond better to therapies and have a better prognosis than patients who are immunocompromised.[93] Many nonspecific immunomodulatory agents exist (Table 3–6), including thymic hormone extracts (Thymoxin fraction 5), vitamins (retinoids

TABLE 3–5. NONSPECIFIC HOST DEFENSE STIMULANTS*

Category	Example
Intact microorganisms	Viable: BCG
	Viable inactivated: OK-432 (Picibanil)
	Nonviable: *C. parvum*
Microbial cell wall	BCG cell-wall skeleton
	Nocardia cell-wall skeleton
	Methanol extraction residue of BCG
Glucans	Glucan (yeast)
	Lentinan (fungal)
	Pachymaran (fungal)
	Scizophyllan (fungal)
Protein-bound polysaccharide	PSK (Krestin) (fungal)
Microbial glycoproteins	*Klebsiella* glycoprotein (Biostim)
Purified or synthetic components	Peptidoglycans
	Muramyl dipeptide (MDP)
	MDP derivatives
	Trehalose dimycolate (P_3)
	Endotoxins (lipopolysaccharide)
	Modified endotoxins (detoxified)
Interferon induces polynucleotides	Poly IC
	Poly IC-LC
	Poly AU
	Ampligen
Pyan copolymers	MVE-2
Low-molecular-weight inducers	Pyrimidinones (ABPP, AIPP)
Delivery systems	Oil-in-water emulsions: CFA
	Water-in-oil emulsions: Ribi reagents
	Liposomes

*From Hersh EM, Taylor CW: Immunotherapy by active immunization: use of nonspecific stimulants and immunomodulators. *In* De Vita VT Jr, Hellman S, Rosenberg SA (eds): Biologic Therapy of Cancer, p 613. Philadelphia, JB Lippincott Co, 1991, with permission.

BCG, bacille Calmette-Guérin; *C parvum*, *Corynebacterium parvum*; IC, inosinic-cytidylic acid; LC, poly L leucine; AU, adenylic-uridylic acid; CFA, complete Freud's adjuvant; MVE-2, methyl vingl ether fraction 2.

TABLE 3–6. NONSPECIFIC IMMUNOMODULATORY AGENTS*

Category	Example
Natural products and derivatives	
Thymic hormone extracts	Thymosin fraction 5 TP1, thymic humoral factor (THF)
Synthetic thymic hormones	Thymosin-α1, thymopoietin, pentapeptide, THF-α2
Lymphocyte extracts	Transfer factor, immunogenic RNA
Tuftsin	Tuftsin
Enkephalins and endorphins	Methionine enkephalin
Chemical immunomodulators	
Sulfur-containing	Levamisole, diethyldithiocarbamates
Cyanoaziridines	Azimexon, ciamexon, imexon
Tellurium-based	AS101, tellurium chloride
Other	Isoprinosine
Vitamins	Retinoids, vitamin C
Regulators of physiologic mechanisms	PGE_2 synthesis inhibitors: indomethacin H_2-receptor antagonists: cimetidine Suppressor-cell modulation by cytoxic chemotherapy: cyclophosphamide

*From Hersh EM, Taylor CW: Immunotherapy by active immunization: Use of nonspecific stimulants and immunomodulators. *In* De Vita VT Jr, Hellman S, Rosenberg SA (eds): Biologic Therapy of Cancer, p 613. Philadelphia, JB Lippincott Co, 1991, with permission.

and vitamin C), and synthetic chemical agents (levamisole). Active research is ongoing to determine the role of various nonspecific immunomodulators (retinoids in kidney and prostate cancers) and bropirimine (a pyrimidinone derivative) in bladder and prostate cancers.[94–97]

Tumor-Associated Antigens

An essential feature of tumor immunity is the natural or induced stimulation of the immune system to target and eliminate tumor cells. Tumor cells must, therefore, be recognized as foreign to the host's immune system. The concept of tumor cell recognition as foreign by their host was first postulated by Paul Ehrlich at the turn of the century.[98] Early attempts to elucidate this phenomenon led to the definition of tumor-specific transplantation antigens (TSTAs).[1] TSTAs may be induced by chemicals, irradiation, or viruses. In the classic experiment (Fig. 3–5), tumor inoculation followed by excision will confer antitumor immunity to a second challenge by the same tumor.[1,99,100] It was observed that this tumor immunity was specific for the tumor and not for other transplanted tissue of the original mouse. While tumor immunity against TSTAs was strong, these antigens were unique for each individual chemical- or irradiation-induced tumor.[100,101] In contrast to TSTAs induced by chemicals and irradiation, TSTAs associated with the same virus cross-react, while neoplasms caused by different viruses express different TSTAs. Natural tumor occurrences in either animal or human models reveal few examples of tumor-associated TSTAs (Burkitt's lymphoma, mammary tumor virus [MTV]–associated breast carcinoma). Moreover, most tumors induced by low doses of chemical carcinogens are nonimmunogenic.

Some antigens associated with naturally occurring human tumors are referred to as tumor-associated differentiation antigens (TADAs) or tumor-associated antigens (TAAs). These antigens are also expressed on normal cells during some stage of the organism's development.[1] They typically represent molecules that are normally expressed only during fetal development, but are overexpressed by tumors. The TADAs can be subdivided into several subcategories. Embryonic and fetal antigens such as carcinoembryonic antigen (CEA) and alpha-fetoprotein (AFP) are expressed by some malignant cells as a result of retrodifferentiation, amplification, and/or immortalization of stem cells. Other subcategories are the clonal antigens, mutant cellular genes (oncogenes, suppressor genes, and fusion proteins), and antigens encoded by viral proteins.

AFP and CEA are among the most useful TADAs in clinical practice. AFP is an important marker of testicular tumors and hepatic carcinomas, while CEA is significant in colon cancers. Both are useful as diagnostic markers as well as for the monitoring of patient response to therapy. The G250 TAA identified on renal cell carcinoma may also be significant as a diagnostic marker of renal tumors.[38] These TADAs are, for all intents and purposes, nonimmunogenic. More recently, the genes to a family of TADAs associated with melanoma have been defined by Boon and colleagues.[102] This gene family consists of 12 closely related genes (MAGE 1–12) located on chromosome X. Six of these genes (MAGE 1, 2, 3, 4, 6, and 12) were found to be expressed at high levels on a number of histologically different tumors.[103–105] With the exception of testis, none of these genes was expressed in normal tissues.[102] Unlike CEA and AFP, the human melanoma antigens encoded by the MAGE family of genes were discovered as targets of CTLs against melanoma cancer cells.[106,107] The peptide antigens of the MAGE-1 and MAGE-3 gene products, which are recognized by autologous cytotoxic T lymphocytes, have been identified.[108] Synthetic peptide antigens can be expressed by APCs and have been observed to enhance activity of autologous CTLs.[107,109,110]

IMPORTANCE TO UROLOGIC TUMORS

Modulation of the immune system has evolved into effective strategies that are presently incorporated in the management of genitourinary malignancies (Table 3–7). Of particular importance, intravesical administration of the nonspecific im-

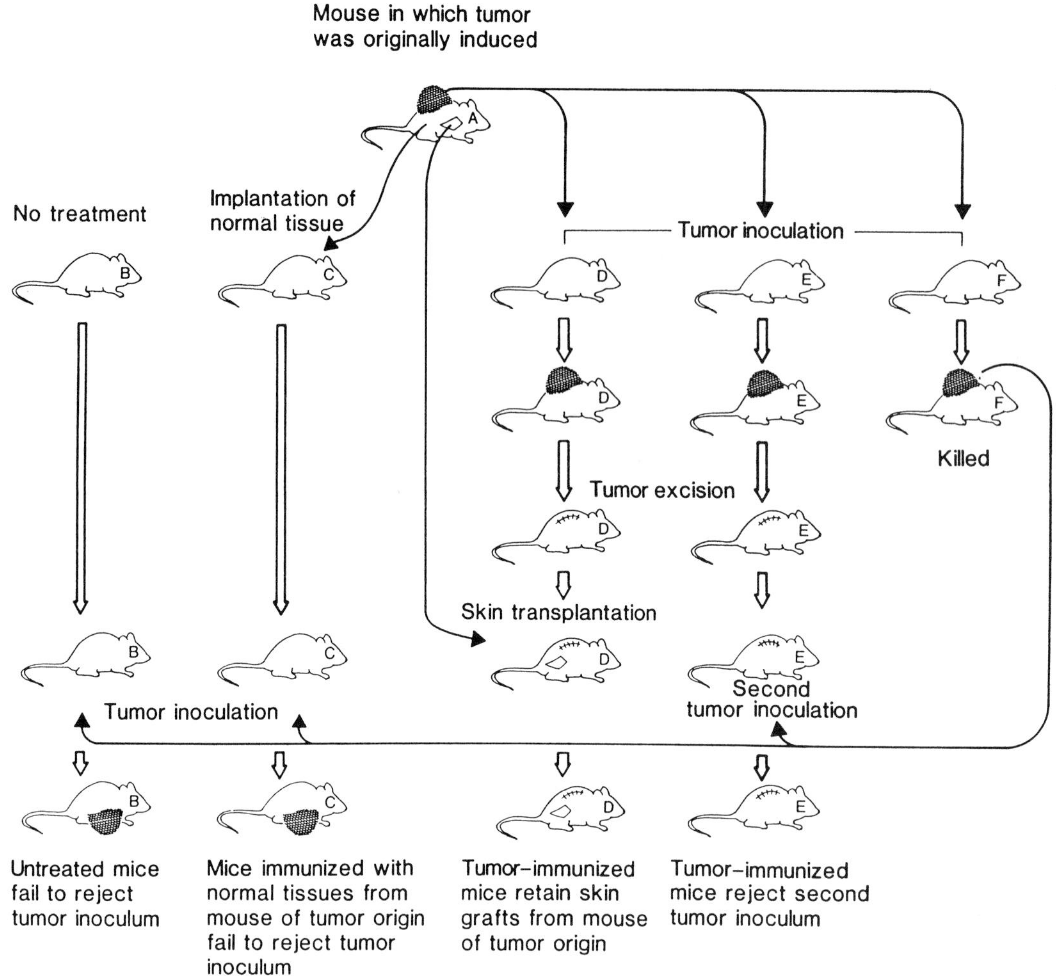
Mouse in which tumor was originally induced
A
No treatment
Implantation of normal tissue
Tumor inoculation
B
C
D
E
F
Killed
Tumor excision
Skin transplantation
Second tumor inoculation
Tumor inoculation
Untreated mice fail to reject tumor inoculum
Mice immunized with normal tissues from mouse of tumor origin fail to reject tumor inoculum
Tumor-immunized mice retain skin grafts from mouse of tumor origin
Tumor-immunized mice reject second tumor inoculum

FIGURE 3–5. Transplantation experiments demonstrating the existence of transplantation antigens on MCA-induced murine sarcomas.[99] Only those mice (*E*) that had been immunized by previous tumor inoculation and removal rejected the tumor upon second inoculation. Tumor-immunized mice (*D*), however, still accepted normal tissue (skin grafts) of the mouse of origin (*A*), and normal tissues of this mouse (*A*) did not protect other mice (C) against tumor challenge. Animal *F* is used simply to "store" the tumor from mouse *A* for the period required to immunize other mice (*C–E*) with normal and malignant tissues. In similar experiments[100] (not shown), the original tumor was removed completely without killing the animal; after an interim period during which the tumor was "stored" in a second mouse, the tumor was reimplanted into the original mouse that now rejected the tumor that once originated from that mouse. This suggested that a mouse can be made immune to its autochthonous tumor after it has been removed completely from the animal. (From Schreiber H: Tumor immunology. *In* Paul WE [ed]: Fundamental Immunology, 3rd edition, p 1143. New York, Raven Press, 1993, with permission.)

mune stimulator (BCG) for superficial transitional cell carcinoma (TCC) of the bladder is recognized as the most potent therapeutic regimen for this disease.[111,112] Although BCG causes the elaboration of various cytokines (e.g., IL-2, IFN-γ, TNF), the exact mechanism(s) of BCG's action remains undetermined.[113,114] Moreover, therapeutic responses with cytokine therapies utilizing IL-2; IFN-α, -β, or -γ; or TNF-α have been lower than those observed with BCG alone.[115–117] A complex immune response including the recruitment of T-helper and cytotoxic lymphocytes is therefore suspected.[118] The effectiveness of BCG therapy has been limited to superficial bladder cancer resulting in complete eradication (61%) of papillary (Ta, T1) tumors, and complete responses (70%) in carcinoma in situ.[111] Furthermore, BCG promotes an increase in the 10-year progression-free rate (62%) and 10-year survival rate (75%), compared with transurethral-resected controls (37% progression-free rate, 55% survival rate).[112]

Spontaneous regression of metastatic lesions following surgical extirpation of the primary renal cell carcinoma has been attributed to effective functioning of the host's immune system. Unfortunately, this occurrence is only too infrequent. A great interest has, ultimately, developed in the utilization of immunotherapeutic regimens for the treatment of metastatic renal cell carcinoma. Manipulation of the immune system in the management of meta-

TABLE 3-7. SUBCATEGORIES OF CLASSIC IMMUNOTHERAPY AND SOME REPRESENTATIVE AGENTS

Subcategories of Immunotherapy	Representative agents
Active immunotherapy	
Specific	Tumor vaccines (e.g., irradiated tumor cells)
Nonspecific	Nonspecific immune stimulators (e.g., bacillus Calmette-Guérin, *Corynebacterium parvum*)
Passive immunotherapy	Monoclonal antibodies
Adoptive immunotherapy	Autologous lymphocytes, lymphokine-acitivated killer cells (LAKs), tumor-infiltrating lymphocytes (TILs)
Restorative immunotherapy	Thymic hormones (Thymosin fraction 5); chemical immunomodulators (levamisole); vitamins (retinoids)

static renal cell carcinoma has proceeded along different paths. Biotherapy with various biologic response modifiers (IL-2, IFN-α), has produced response rates of 15 to 20%.[119-121] There is some indication that higher response rates are observed with combination therapies such as IL-2/IFN.[121,122] Another approach has incorporated cellular or adoptive immunotherapy (LAKs or TILs) to augment the responses of cytokine therapy. A randomized study comparing high-dose IL-2 versus IL-2 plus LAK showed no significant difference in tumor response, duration of response, or overall survival between the two groups.[123] Response rates with IL-2/IFN-α combined with TILs has yielded response rates of approximately 40%.[124] The results of a recently completed randomized trial will shed some light on whether TILs produced an added effect to the cytokine response. The observed responses of metastatic renal cell carcinoma to immunotherapy are encouraging, particularly since metastatic renal cell carcinoma is both chemoresistant and radiation resistant, and is associated with a historical median survival of approximately 10 months.[125] What is becoming clear is that current immunotherapeutic approaches may be altering the natural history of this disease.[126]

A tremendous effort is being made to unravel the mechanisms of the immune system. In parallel with this work are the attempts to devise strategies to manipulate this system for desired clinical outcomes. To this end, innovative efforts are in progress to engineer APCs to stimulate cytotoxic T lymphocytes to specific TAAs.[107-110] It is hoped that these approaches will improve the immunotherapy response rates of malignancies such as renal cell carcinoma and melanoma. Furthermore, cryptic peptides from normally nonimmunogenic antigens may be presented on APCs to induce immunity.[127] This development offers the potential of extending immunotherapeutic approaches to relatively nonimmunogenic malignancies such as advanced prostate cancer and bladder cancer.

REFERENCES

1. Schreiber H: Tumor immunology. *In* Paul WE (ed): Fundamental Immunology, 3rd edition, p 1143. New York, Raven Press, 1993.
2. Narayan P: Immunology of genitourinary tumors. *In* Tanagho EA, McAninch JW (eds): Smith's General Urology, 4th edition, p 334. Norwalk, CT, Appleton & Lange, 1995.
3. Abbas AK, Litchman AH, Pober JS: Cells and tissues of the immune system. *In* Abbas AK, Litchman AH, Pober JS (eds): Cellular and Molecular Immunology, p 13. Philadelphia, WB Saunders Co, 1991.
4. Wunderlich JR, Hodes RJ: Principles of tumor immunity: biology of cellular immune responses. *In* De Vita VT Jr, Hellman S, Rosenberg SA (eds): Biologic Therapy of Cancer, p 3. Philadelphia, JB Lippincott Co, 1991.
5. Allison JP, Lanier LL: Structure, function, and serology of the T-cell antigen receptor complex. Annu Rev Immunol 1987; 5:503.
6. Raulet DH: The structure, function, and molecular genetics of the gamma/delta T-cell receptor. Annu Rev Immunol 1989; 7:175.
7. Clevers H, Alarcon B, Wileman T, et al: The T cell receptor/CD3 complex: a dynamic protein ensemble. Annu Rev Immunol 1988; 6:629.
8. Matis LA, Cron R, Bluestone JA: Major histocompatibility complex-linked specificity of gamma delta receptor-bearing T lymphocytes. Nature 1987; 330:262.
9. O'Brien RL, Happ MP, Dallas A, et al: Stimulation of a major subset of lymphocytes expressing T cell receptor gamma delta by an antigen derived from mycobacterium tuberculosis. Cell 1989; 57:667.
10. Rosenberg SA: Principles and applications of biologic therapy. *In* De Vita VT Jr, Hellman S, Rosenberg SA (eds): Cancer: Principles & Practice of Oncology, 4th edition. Philadelphia, JB Lippincott Co, 1993.
11. Schwartz RH: Acquisition of immunologic self-tolerance. Cell 1989; 57:1073–1081.
12. Braciale TJ, Braciale VL: Antigen presentation: structural themes and functional variations. Immunol Today 1991; 12(4):124–129.
13. Geppert TD, Davis LS, Gur H, et al: Accessory cell signals involved in T-cell activation. Immunol Rev 1990; 117:5–66.
14. Klinkert WEF: Lymphoid dendritic accessory cells of the rat. Immunol Rev 1990; 117:103–120.
15. Runger TM, Klein CE, Becker JC: The role of genetic instability, adhesion, cell motility and immune escape mechanisms in melanoma progression. Curr Opin Oncol 1994; 6:188–196.
16. Denfeld RW, Dietrich A, Wuttig C: In situ expression of B7 and CD28 receptor families in human malignant melanoma: relevance for T-cell-mediated anti-tumor immunity. Int J Cancer 1995; 62:259–265.
17. Lo D, Burkly LC, Flavell RA, et al: Antigen presentation in MHC class II transgenic mice: stimulation versus tolerization. Immunol Rev 1990; 117:121–136.
18. Linsley PS, Ledbetter JA: The role of the CD28 receptor during T cell responses to antigen. Annu Rev Immunol 1993; 11:191.
19. Chen L, McGowan P, Ashe S, et al: Tumor immunogenicity determines the effect of B7 costimulation on T cell-mediated tumor immunity. J Exp Med 1994; 179:523–532.
20. Cavallo F, Martin-Rontecha A, et al: Co-expression of B7.1 and ICAM-1 on tumors is required for rejection and the establishment of a memory response. Eur J Immunol 1995; 25:1154–1162.
21. Mosmann TR, Coffman RL: TH1 and TH2 cells: different patterns of lymphokine secretion lead to different functional properties. Annu Rev Immunol 1989; 7:145–173.

22. Patel SS, Duby AD, Thiele DL, et al: Phenotypic and functional characterization of human T cell clones. J Immunol 1988; 141:3726–3736.
23. Benacerraf B, Germain RN: A single major pathway of T-lymphocyte interactions of antigen-specific immune suppression. Scand J Immunol 1981; 13:1–10.
24. Meltzer MS, Nacy CA: Delayed-typed hypersensitivity and the induction of activated, cytotoxic macrophages. *In* Paul WE (ed): Fundamental Immunology, 2nd edition, p 765. New York, Raven Press, 1989.
25. Berke G: Debate: The mechanism of lymphocyte-mediated killing. Lymphocyte-triggered internal target disintegration. Immunol Today 1991; 12:396–399.
26. Berke G: The CTL's kiss of death. Cell 1995; 81:9–12.
27. Croft M, Carter L, Swain SL, Dutton RW: Generation of polarized antigen-specific CD8 effector population: reciprocal action of interleukin (IL)-4 and IL-12 in promoting type 2 versus type 1 cytokine profiles. J Exp Med 1994; 180:1715–1728.
28. Berke G: Functions and mechanisms of lysis induced by cytotoxic T lymphocytes and natural killer cells. *In* Paul WE (ed): Fundamental Immunology, 2nd edition, p 735. New York, Raven Press, 1989.
29. Rosenberg SA: Immunotherapy of cancer using interleukin-2: current status and future prospects. Immunol Today 1988; 9:58–62.
30. Nathan CF, Cohn ZA: Cellular components of inflammation: monocytes and macrophages. *In* Killey WN, Harris ED Jr, Ruddy S, Sledge CB (eds): Textbook of Rheumatology, pp 144–169. Philadelphia, WB Saunders Co, 1985.
31. Drysdale BE, Agarwal S, Shin HS: Macrophage-mediated tumoricidal activity: mechanisms of activation and cytotoxicity. Prog Allergy 1988; 40:111–161.
32. Abbas AK, Litchman AH, Pober JS: Cells and tissues of the immune system. *In* Abbas AK, Litchman AH, Pober JS (eds): Cellular and Molecular Immunology, p 69. Philadelphia, WB Saunders Co, 1991.
33. Rudikoff S: Principles of tumor immunity: biology of antibody-mediated responses. *In* De Vita VT Jr, Hellman S, Rosenberg SA (eds): Biologic Therapy of Cancer, p 22. Philadelphia, JB Lippincott Co, 1991.
34. Porter RR: The hydrolysis of rabbit γ-globulin and antibodies with crystalline papain. Biochem J 1959; 73:119–126.
35. Edelman GM, Poulik MD: Studies on structural units of the γ-globulins. J Exp Med 1961; 113:861–884.
36. Schlom J: Antibodies in cancer therapy: basic principles of monoclonal antibodies. *In* De Vita VT Jr, Hellman S, Rosenberg SA (eds): Biologic Therapy of Cancer, p 464. Philadelphia, JB Lippincott Co, 1991.
37. Divgi CR: Status of radiolabeled monoclonal antibodies for diagnosis and therapy of cancer [see comments]. Oncology 1996; 10(6):939–958.
38. Oosterwijk E, Debruyne FMJ, Schalken JA: The use of monoclonal antibody G250 in the therapy of renal-cell carcinoma. Semin Oncol 1995; 22:34–41.
39. Burgers JK, Hinkle GH, Haseman MK: Monoclonal antibody imaging of recurrent and metastatic prostate cancer. Semin Urol 1995; 13(2):103–112.
40. Abbas AK, Litchman AH, Pober JS: Cells and tissues of the immune system. *In* Abbas AK, Litchman AH, Pober JS (eds): Cellular and Molecular Immunology, p 225. Philadelphia, WB Saunders Co, 1991.
41. Oettgen HF, Old LJ: The history of cancer immunotherapy. *In* De Vita VT Jr, Hellman S, Rosenberg SA (eds): Biologic Therapy of Cancer, p 87. Philadelphia, JB Lippincott Co, 1991.
42. Lotze MT: Interleukin-2: Basic principles. *In* De Vita VT Jr, Hellman S, Rosenberg SA (eds): Biologic Therapy of Cancer, p 123. Philadelphia, JB Lippincott Co, 1991.
43. Walker E, Leemhuis T, Roeder W: Murine B lymphoma cell lines release functionally active interleukin-2 after stimulation with *Staphylococcus aureus*. J Immunol 1988; 140:859–865.
44. Rocha BB: Population kinetics of precursors of IL-2 producing peripheral T lymphocytes: evidence for short life expectancy, continuous renewal, and post-thymic expansion. J Immunol 1987; 139:365–372.
45. Welte K, Wang CY, Mertelsmann R, et al: Purification of human interleukin-2 to apparent homogeneity and its molecular heterogeneity. J Exp Med 1982; 156:454–464.
46. Robb RJ, Kutny RM, Chowdhry V: Purification and partial sequence analysis of human T-cell growth factor. Proc Natl Acad Sci U S A 1983; 80:5990–5994.
47. June CH, Ledbetter JA, Lindsten T, et al: Evidence for the involvement of three distinct signals in the induction of IL-2 gene expression in human T lymphocytes. J Immunol 1989; 143:153–161.
48. Mills GB, May C, Hill M, et al: Physiologic activation of the protein kinase C limits IL-2 secretion. J Immunol 1989; 142:1995–2003.
49. Fung MR, Ju G, Greene WC: Co-internalization of the p55 and p07 subunits of the high-affinity human interleukin-2 receptor: evidence for a stable ternary receptor complex. J Exp Med 1988; 168:1923–1928.
50. Smith KA, Cantrell DA: Interleukin-2 regulates its own receptors. Proc Natl Acad Sci U S A 1985; 82:864–868.
51. Stern JB, Smith KA: Interleukin-2 induction of T-cell G1 progression and c-myb expression. Science 1986; 233: 203–206.
52. Yoshimura A, Ichihara M, Kinjyo I, et al: Mouse oncostatin M: an immediate early gene induced by multiple cytokines through the JAK-STAT5 pathway. EMBO J 1996; 15(5):1055–1063.
53. Rosenberg SA, Yang JC, Topalain SL, et al: Treatment of 283 consecutive patients with metastatic melanoma or renal cell cancer using high-dose bolus interleukin 2 [see comments]. JAMA 1994; 271:907–913.
54. Fyfe G, Fisher RI, Rosenberg SA: Results of treatment of 255 patients with metastatic renal cell carcinoma who received high-dose recombinant interleukin-2 therapy. J Clin Oncol 1995; 13(3):688–696.
55. Taneja SS, Pierce W, Figlin R, et al: Immunotherapy for renal cell carcinoma: the era of interleukin-2 based treatment. Urology 1995; 45(6):911–924.
56. Lotze MT, Rosenberg SA: Interleukin-2: Clinical applications. *In* De Vita VT Jr, Hellman S, Rosenberg SA (eds): Biologic Therapy of Cancer, p 159, Philadelphia, JB Lippincott Co, 1991.
57. Kurzrock R, Gutterman JU, Talpaz M: Interferon-α,β,γ: basic principles and preclinical studies. *In* De Vita VT Jr, Hellman S, Rosenberg SA (eds): Biologic Therapy of Cancer, p 247. Philadelphia, JB Lippincott Co, 1991.
58. Zullo JN, Cochran BH, Huang AS, et al: Platelet-derived growth factor and double-stranded ribonucleic acids stimulate expression of the same genes in 3T3 cells. Cell 1985; 43:793–800.
59. Moore RN, Larsen HS, Horohov DW, et al: Endogenous regulation of macrophage proliferative expansion by colony-stimulating factor-induced interferon. Science 1984; 223:178–181.
60. Kohase M, May LT, Tamm I, et al: A cytokine network in human diploid fibroblasts: interactions of beta interferons, tumor necrosis factor, platelet-derived growth factor and interleukin-1. Mol Cell Biol 1987; 7:273–280.
61. VanDamme J, DeLey M, Opdenakker G, et al: Homogeneous interferon-inducing 22K factor is related to endogenous pyrogen and interleukin-1. Nature 1985; 314:266–268.
62. Zoon KC: Human interferons: structure and function. *In* Gresser I (ed): Interferon 9, p 1. New York, Academic Press, 1987.
63. Borden E, Groveman D, Nasu T, et al: Antiproliferative activities of interferons against human bladder carcinoma cell lines in vitro. J Urol 1984; 132:800.
64. Hayward S, James K, Prescott S, et al: The effects of recombinant human interferon-gamma on a panel of human bladder cancer cell lines. J Urol 1991; 145:1078.
65. Belldegrun, Tso C-L, Sakata T, et al: Human renal carcinoma line transfected with interleukin-2 and/or inter-

feron-α gene(s): implication for live cancer vaccines. J Natl Cancer Inst 1993; 85:207–216.
66. David M, Petricon E III, Benjamin C, et al: Requirement for MAP kinase (ERK2) activity in interferon α-stimulated gene expression through STAT proteins. Science 1995; 269:1721.
67. Spriggs DR: Tumor necrosis factor: basic principles and preclinical studies. *In* De Vita VT Jr, Hellman S, Rosenberg SA (eds): Biologic Therapy of Cancer, p 354. Philadelphia, JB Lippincott Co, 1991.
68. Nedwin GE, Naylor SL, Sakaguchi AY, et al: Human lymphotoxin and tumor necrosis factor genes: structure, homology and chromosomal localization. Nucl Acids Res 1985; 13:6361–6373.
69. Aggarwal BB, Eessalu TE, Hass PE: Characterization of receptors for human tumour necrosis factor and their regulation by gamma-interferon. Nature 1985; 318:665–667.
70. Sariban E, Imamura D, Luebbers R, et al: Transcriptional and post-transcriptional regulation of tumor necrosis factor gene expression in human monocytes. J Clin Invest 1988; 81:1506–1510.
71. Muller R, Marmenout A, Fiers W: Synthesis and maturation of recombinant human tumor necrosis factor in eukaryotic systems. FEBS Lett 1986; 197:99–104.
72. Kriegler M, Perez C, DeFay K, et al: A novel form of TNF/cachectin is a cell surface cytotoxic transmembrane protein: ramifications for the complex physiology of TNF. Cell 1988; 53:45–53.
73. Watanabe N, Kuriyama H, Sone H, et al: Continuous internalization of tumor necrosis factor receptors in a human myosarcoma cell line. J Biol Chem 1988; 263(21): 10262–10266.
74. Hohmann HP, Remy R, Brockhaus M, Van LAP: Two different cell types have different major receptors for human tumor necrosis factor (TNF alpha). J Biol Chem 1989; 264: 14927–14934.
75. Peete C, Thysell H, Grubb A, et al: A tumor necrosis factor binding protein is present in human biological fluids. Eur J Hematol 1988; 41:414–419.
76. Belldegrun A, Pierce W, Sayah D, et al: Soluble tumor necrosis factor receptor expression in patients with metastatic renal cell carcinoma treated with interleukin-2-based immunotherapy. J Immunol 1993; 13:175–180.
77. Bazzoni F, Beutler B: The tumor necrosis factor ligand and receptor families. N Engl J Med 1996; 334(26):1717–1725.
78. Kull FC, Cuatrecasas P: Possible requirement for internalization in the mechanism of in vitro cytotoxicity in tumor necrosis serum. Cancer Res 1981; 41:4885–4890.
79. Ruggiero V, Johnson SE, Baglioni C: Protection from tumor necrosis factor cytotoxicity by protease inhibitors. Cell Immunol 1987; 107:3317–3325.
80. Metcalf D, Morstyn G: Colony-stimulating factors: general biology. *In* De Vita VT Jr, Hellman S, Rosenberg SA (eds): Biologic Therapy of Cancer, p 417, Philadelphia, JB Lippincott Co, 1991.
81. Dranoff G, Jaffee E, Lazenby A, et al: Vaccination with irradiated tumor cells engineered to secrete murine granulocyte-macrophage colony-stimulating factor stimulates potent, specific, and long-lasting anti-tumor immunity. Proc Natl Acad Sci U S A 1993; 90:3539–3543.
82. Sanda MG, Ayyagari SR, Jaffee EM, et al: Demonstration of a rational strategy for human prostate cancer gene therapy. J Urol 1994; 151:622–628.
83. Cheng L, Sun J, Pretlow TG, et al: CWR22 xenograft as an ex vivo human tumor model for prostate cancer gene therapy. J Natl Cancer Inst 1996; 88(9):607–611.
84. Marshall F, Jaffee E, Wever C, et al: Bioactivity of human GM-CSF gene therapy in metastatic renal carcinoma. J Urol 1996; 155(Suppl):582A.
85. Tso C-L, Duckett T, deKernion JB, et al: Modulation of tumor-infiltrating lymphocytes derived from human renal cell carcinoma by interleukin-4. J Immunother 1992; 12:82–89.
86. Dougherty GJ, Thacker JD, Lavey RS, et al: Inhibitory effect of locally produced and exogenous interleukin-6 on tumor growth in vivo. Cancer Immunol Immunother 1994; 38:339–345.
87. Ditonno P, Tso CL, Sakata T, et al: Regulatory effects of interleukin-7 on renal tumor infiltrating lymphocytes. Urol Res 1992; 20:205–210.
88. Chan SH, Perussia B, Gupta JW, et al: Induction of IFNγ production by NKSTF: characterization of the responder cells and synergy with other inducers. J Exp Med 1991; 173:869.
89. Zitvogel L, Tahara H, Robbins PD: Cancer immunotherapy of established tumors with IL-12: effective delivery by genetically engineered fibroblasts. J Immunol 1995; 155:1393–1403.
90. Hersh EM, Taylor CW: Immunotherapy by active immunization: use of nonspecific stimulants and immunomodulators. *In* De Vita VT Jr, Hellman S, Rosenberg SA (eds): Biologic Therapy of Cancer, p 613. Philadelphia, JB Lippincott Co, 1991.
91. Bast RC, Zbar B, Borsos T, et al: BCG and cancer. N Engl J Med 1973; 290:1413–1420, 1458–1469.
92. Hersh EM, Freireich EJ, McCredie DB, et al: Primary and secondary immune responses in the evaluation of immunocompetence and prognosis in cancer patients. Recent Results Cancer Res 1972; 47:1–11.
93. Eilber FR, Morton DL: Impaired immunologic reactivity and recurrence following cancer surgery. Cancer 1970; 25: 362–367.
94. Moltzer RJ, Schwartz L, Law TM, et al: Interferon alfa-2a and 13-cis-retinoic acid in renal cell carcinoma: antitumor activity in a phase II trial and interactions in vitro. J Clin Oncol 1995; 13(8):1950–1957.
95. Seidmon EJ, Trump DL, Kreis W, et al: Phase I/II dose-escalation study of liarozole in patients with stage D, hormone refractory carcinoma of the prostate. Ann Surg Oncol 1995; 2(6):550–556.
96. Sarosdy MF: Bropirimine in bladder cancer: clinical studies. Ann N Y Acad Sci 1993; 685:301–308.
97. Sarosdy MF, Higdon AL, Demoor CA: In vivo antitumor activity of bropirimine against PAIII and Dunning MAT-lylu rodent prostate cancers. J Urol 1996; 155(6):2085–2089.
98. Himmelweit B (ed): The Collected Papers of Paul Ehrlich. Oxford, England, Pergamon Press, 1975.
99. Prehn RT, Main JM: Immunity to methylocholanthrene-induced sarcomas. J Natl Cancer Inst 1957; 18:769–778.
100. Klein EJ, Sjogren HO, Klein E, et al: Demonstration of resistance against methylcholanthrene-induced sarcomas in the primary autochthonous host. Cancer Res 1960; 20:1561.
101. Old LJ, Boyse EA: Immunology of experimental tumors. Annu Rev Med 1964; 15:167.
102. van der Bruggen P, Traversari C, Chomez P, et al: A gene encoding an antigen recognized by cytolytic T lymphocytes on a human melanoma. Science 1991; 254:1643.
103. Rimoldi D, Romero P, Carrel S: The human melanoma-antigen-encoding gene, MAGE-1, is expressed by other tumor cells of neuroectodermal origin such as glioblastoma and neuroblastomas. Int J Cancer 1993; 54:527–528.
104. Brassuer F, Marchand M, Vanwijck R, et al: Human MAGE-1, which encodes for a tumor rejection antigen, is expressed by some breast tumors. Int J Cancer 1992; 53: 839–841.
105. Weyants P, Lethe B, Brassuer F, et al: Expression of MAGE genes by non-small cell lung carcinomas. Int J Cancer 1994; 56:826–829.
106. Gaugler B, Van den Heynde B, van der Bruggen P, et al: Human gene MAGE-3 codes for an antigen recognized on a melanoma by autologous cytolytic T lymphocytes. J Exp Med 1994; 179:921–930.
107. van der Bruggen P, Bastin J, Gajewski T, et al: A peptide encoded by human gene MAGE-3 and presented by HLA-A2 induces cytolytic T lymphocytes that recognize tumor cells expressing MAGE-3. Eur J Immunol 1994; 24: 3038–3043.
108. Kocher T, Schultz-Thater E, Gudat F, et al: Identification

and intracellular location of MAGE-3 gene product. Cancer Res 1995; 55(11):2236–2239.
109. Yamasaki S, Okino T, Chakraborty NG, et al: Presentation of synthetic peptide antigen encoded by the MAGE-1 gene by granulocyte/macrophage-colony-stimulating-factor-cultured macrophages from HLA-A1 melanoma patients. Cancer Immunol Immunother 1995; 40:268–271.
110. Hu X, Chakraborty NG, Sporn JR, et al: Enhancement of cytolytic T lymphocyte precursor frequency in melanoma patients following immunization with the MAGE-1 peptide loaded antigen presenting cell-based vaccine. Cancer Res 1996; 56:2479–2483.
111. Lamm DL, Torti FM: Bladder cancer, 1996. CA Cancer J Clin 1996; 46(2):93.
112. Herr HW, Schwalb DM, Zhang ZF, et al: Intravesical bacillus Calmette-Guérin therapy prevents tumor progression and death from superficial bladder cancer: ten-year follow-up of a prospective randomized trial. J Clin Oncol 1995; 13(6):1404.
113. Jackson AM, Prescott S, Hawkyard SJ, et al: The immunomodulatory effects of urine from patients with superficial bladder cancer receiving intravesical evans BCG therapy. Cancer Immunol Immunother 1993; 36:25.
114. De Boer EC, De Jong WH, Steerenberg PA, et al: Induction of urinary interleukin-1 (IL-1), IL-2, IL-6, and tumor necrosis factor during intravesical immunotherapy with bacillus Calmette-Guerin in superficial bladder cancer. Cancer Immunol Immunother 1992; 34:306.
115. Glashan R: A randomized controlled study of intravesical α-2b-interferon in carcinoma in situ of the bladder. J Urol 1990; 144:658.
116. Boccardo F, Cannata D, Rubagotti A, et al: Prophylaxis of superficial bladder cancer with mitomycin or interferon alfa-2b: results of a multicentric Italian study. J Clin Oncol 1994; 12:7–13.
117. Sargent ER, Williams RD: Immunotherapeutic alternatives in superficial bladder cancer: interferon, interleukin-2, and keyhole-limpet hemocyanin. Urol Clin North Am 1992; 19(3):581–589.
118. Ratliff TL, Ritchey JK, Yaun JJ, et al: T-cell subsets required for intravesical BCG immunotherapy for bladder cancer. J Urol 1993; 150:1018–1023.
119. Alexander RB, Walther MM, Linehan WM: Immunotherapy of renal cell carcinoma: surgery branch, National Cancer Institute experience. AUA Update Series 1995; Vol XIV (Lesson 40).
120. Graham SD Jr: Interferon. AUA Update Series 1995; Vol XIV (Lesson 39).
121. Taneja SS, Pierce W, Figlin R, et al: Management of disseminated kidney cancer. Urol Clin North Am 1994; 21(4): 625–637.
122. Marincola FM, White DE, Wise AP: Combination therapy with interferon alfa-2a and interleukin-2 for the treatment of metastatic cancer. J Clin Oncol 1995; 13(5):1110–1122.
123. Rosenberg SA, Lotze MT, Yang JC, et al: Prospective, randomized trial of high-dose interleukin-2 alone or in conjunction with lymphokine activated killer cells for the treatment of patients with advanced cancer. J Natl Cancer Inst 1993; 85:622–632.
124. Belldegrun A, Tso C-L, Kaboo R, et al: Natural immune reactivity-associated therapeutic response in patients with metastatic renal cell carcinoma receiving tumor-infiltrating lymphocytes and interleukin-2-based therapy. J Immunother 1996; 21:625.
125. deKernion JB, Ramming KP, Smith RB: Natural history of metastatic renal cell carcinoma: a computer analysis. J Urol 1978; 120:148.
126. Belldegrun A, Franklin J, Dorey F, et al: Long term survival of 181 patients with metastatic renal cell carcinoma (mRCC) treated with IL-2 based immunotherapy with/without tumor infiltrating lymphocytes. J Urol 1996; 155(Suppl):385A.
127. Nanda NK, Sercarz EE: Induction of anti-self-immunity to cure cancer. Cell 1995; 82:13–17.

4

ENVIRONMENTAL CARCINOGENESIS

GARY J. MILLER, M.D., PH.D.

Prostatic cancer incidence continues to increase throughout the United States and the westernized world.[1,2] The major risk factors that are associated with this disease include age, race, diet, and family history.[3,4] The identification of risk factors such as these allows us to formulate general strategies for screening and detection, but they tell us little about the actual etiologic agents that cause prostatic cancer to develop. Although it is obviously desirable to learn how to treat this increasingly common disease, a more effective strategy for influencing overall outcome would be to eliminate its occurrence. To this end, it will be necessary to identify the agents that initiate the malignant transformation of prostatic epithelial cells. Differences in geographic distribution of prostatic cancer have been taken to indicate the potential influence of dietary fat[3] or chemopreventive substances.[5] However, it is also possible that these differences reflect variations in exposure to other causative environmental factors. Ultimately, our environment is largely influenced by human activities such as industry, mining, and other vocational practices. Occupational studies[6,7] point to numerous possibilities that could explain the occurrence of the disease, at least in selected populations. It is the purpose of this review to discuss and summarize specific environmental findings with a view towards understanding the specific agents that lead to prostatic carcinogenesis.

INDUSTRIAL EXPOSURES

The complexity of modern industry provides the opportunity for workers to be exposed to literally thousands of potentially toxic chemicals, many of which may have carcinogenic potential. Regarding the genitourinary tract, it has long been known that there is a direct association between exposure to aniline dyes and transitional cell carcinomas of the urinary bladder.[8] The associations between various chemical agents and prostate cancer are less clear, but distinct possibilities do exist.

Probably the most commonly implicated class of compounds are the heavy metals including nickel, chromium, arsenic, and cadmium.[9] Cadmium exposure has long been considered to be related to cancer risk. It has been estimated, for example, that the cadmium released from burning coal in the United States could account for 20,000 cancer deaths per year.[10] However, the majority of these deaths would result from lung cancer. Cadmium exposure has been related to human prostatic cancer risk in some but not all epidemiologic studies.[11] For example, the incidence of prostate cancer has been found to be elevated among smelter and nickel-cadmium battery workers[12,13] as well as Swedish art glass workers.[14] A high incidence of prostate cancer in the Salamanca province of Spain has also been related to high regional cadmium content of the soil.[15] Other studies on similar populations have failed to reveal such associations.[16,17] These differences may be due to significant methodologic difficulties such as assessment of cadmium exposure, concomitant exposure to other metal carcinogens, or confounding factors such as diet or smoking that could have profound effects on cadmium levels.[18] Support has been given to the association by the finding of a positive correlation between prostate tissue cadmium levels and the presence of prostatic malignancy.[11] Animal models of cadmium carcinogenesis have directly demonstrated the ability of this substance to induce prostatic carcinomas in Wistar rats.[19,20] Cadmium has also been shown to promote prostatic tumorigenesis in a rat ventral prostate model using 3,2′-dimethyl-4-aminobiphenyl as a carcinogen.[21] Susceptibility of the prostate to cadmium is modulated by the ability of epithelial cells to respond to metal toxins by the induction of the cadmium-binding protein metallothionein.[22] Of particular relevance for the population at large, almost 800 National Priorities List waste sites are known to be contaminated with cadmium, which could lead to increased risk of exposure through drinking water, food, or contaminated air.[23] It would appear that although definitive human data do not exist to prove the role of cadmium in prostatic carcinogenesis, this controversial topic merits further investigation.

There are a variety of other studies that suggest a role for chemical exposure in the carcinogenesis of prostatic carcinoma. Workers exposed to formaldehyde had a slight excess of Hodgkin's disease and carcinomas of the lung and prostate.[24] In a case control study of dimethylformamide exposure, there was no statistically significant association between development of prostate cancer and any exposure level.[25] However, prostate carcinoma was significantly elevated at one specific plant using this substance. A nonsignificant association (observed risk 2.66, 90% confidence interval [CI] 0.39 to 18.1) between high exposure to isocyanates used in polyurethane foam manufacture and prostate cancer has also been reported.[26] Nonsignificant excesses of prostate cancer have also been found in textile workers.[27] Specifically, this involved workers in dyeing and finishing businesses as well as those in broad woven fabric mills.

In other specific circumstances, stronger associations between specific exposures and prostate cancer risk have been found. A study of workers in the compounding area of rubber and tire manufacturing found that those involved in batch preparation showed statistically significant ($p < .025$) risk ratios over three different exposure periods.[28] The latent period was estimated to be 29 years and the period of greatest risk occurred during the years 1940 to 1947. Significant risks for blacks were also found in service to batch preparation and the shipping and receiving work areas. In a study of 1345 male employees exposed to acrylonitrile at a fibers-producing plant, a significant excess of prostate cancer (6 cases observed, 1.8 expected) was found.[29] However, death from prostate cancer was not increased among these workers. Eight prostate cancer deaths (4.4 expected, standardized mortality ratio [SMR] 1.82) were found in a 43-year follow-up study on 1008 male oil refinery workers involved in the dewaxing process.[30] This risk increased with increasing duration of employment in the lube oil department, and a latency of at least 20 years was observed. Most recently, a significant excess of prostate cancer mortality was found among 15,818 coke oven workers.[31] Relative risk (RR) values for cancer of the prostate were found to be as high as 1.93, while rates of respiratory tract cancers during the same time period were declining. This suggests a relatively long latent period. It has also been recognized that those individuals exposed to high levels of unspecified carcinogens such as found in fire smoke would be at increased risk for developing this disease. A cohort of 2447 firefighters in Seattle and Tacoma were found to have an elevated risk for prostate cancer (standardized incidence ratio 1.4, 95% CI 1.1 to 1.7) over 16 years of exposure.[32] However, this increase was less than that seen in police officers (incidence density ratio 1.1, 95% CI 0.7 to 1.6) and it was not directly related to the length of exposure. Such studies do justify use of protective equipment in individuals who might be exposed to mixed agents.

FARMING

Studies on the geographic patterns of prostate cancer mortality from 3056 counties in the United States suggest that the increase in mortality associated with high population density results from environmental exposures in the urban setting.[33] However, numerous epidemiologic studies have identified a consistent increase in prostate cancer risk associated with farming. Agricultural workers typically have lower overall and smoking-related (lung and bladder) cancer mortality rates.[34] Deficits of colorectal cancer have also been noted.[35] In spite of this, hematologic malignancies and prostate cancer are often found to be elevated in the same populations. For example, although the proportionate mortality ratio (PMR) for all cancer was found to be lower for Iowa farmers between 1971 and 1978, this was largely due to lower rates of lung, esophageal, and mouth cancers.[36] The mortality rate for prostate cancer was significantly higher (PMR = 1.10). Each of the six types of cancer (including lip, stomach, leukemia, lymphoma, multiple myeloma, and prostate cancers) with significantly elevated mortality in Iowa has also been reported to have elevated mortality in farmers from other states. Some age-standardized PMRs were also calculated for a group of 28,032 male farmers in British Columbia.[37] Elevated risks of cancer mortality were present for prostate (PMR = 1.13, $p < .001$) as well as carcinomas of the lip and stomach, leukemias, and aplastic anemias. The elevated risks were consistent over the 29-year period examined. Again, significant deficits for esophageal, colonic, laryngeal, and lung carcinomas were also found. Cancers in farmers reported to the Illinois State Cancer Registry also indicate that prostate cancer incidence is elevated (odds ratio [OR] 1.15, 95% CI 0.99) in this group.[38] A positive association between cancer of the prostate and hay or beef production was noted. Studies contradicting the elevation of prostate cancer risk associated with farming are relatively rare.[39]

Farmers are recognized to be exposed to a number of chemical agents (pesticides, herbicides, fertilizers, solvents, oils, fuels, and fumes) as well as zoonotic viruses, microbes, and fungi. Among these, the specific etiologic factors associated with prostate cancer risk have begun to be defined. In a cohort study of 1791 pesticide-exposed agricultural technicians, there was no elevation in prostate cancer risk, even though the risk of bronchial carcinoma doubled.[40] A cohort of 2131 male nitrate fertilizer workers were also evaluated for cancer mortality between 1963 and 1986.[41] No significant increase in lung or stomach cancers was found. However, 26 cases of prostate cancer were observed (expected 16), which was statistically significant (SMR 1.61, 95% CI 1.07 to 2.39). The risk was not enhanced by applying a 10-year latency period. The same study found that in a cohort of 1148 male fertilizer workers who had never been exposed to nitrates, there was an increase in lung cancer incidence, but no difference in rates of stomach or prostate cancers. No association between airborne nitrate exposure dose and total cancer, stomach, lung, or prostate cancers could be documented. Recently, a potentially important association with herbicide use has also been documented among the farmers of Manitoba, Saskatchewan, and Alberta, Canada.[42] A total of 1148 prostate cancer deaths among 2,213,478 person-years were investigated. When the analysis was restricted to farmers believed to have the least potential for misclassification, the risk for prostate cancer increased with the number of acres sprayed with herbicides (rate ratio 2.23 for 250 or more acres sprayed, 95% CI 1.3 to 3.84, test for trend $p < .01$). No other farm-related exposures were associated with any detectable pattern of increased or decreased prostate cancer risk. These findings clearly implicate herbicides and nitrate fertilizers in prostatic carcinogenesis; however, experimental confirmation has not yet occurred.

IONIZING RADIATION

In view of the post–World War II emphasis on nuclear contamination and atomic generation of electrical power, surprisingly little information exists regarding the ability of radioactivity to induce prostate cancer. Anecdotal cases have been reported of prostatic carcinoma such as that occurring in a survivor of the Hiroshima bomb.[43] However, a single autopsy series of 1357 individuals from Hiroshima and Nagasaki in which the prostates were step-sectioned at 5-mm intervals indicates that radiation did not raise the risk for prostatic cancer.[44] This was true even for those known to have received 100 rads or more. Experimentally, it is known that pelvic irradiation of male ICR/JCL mice at approximately 7 weeks of age will result in prostatic carcinomas in approximately 4% of those that survive the initial irradiation.[45] The finding that correlations exist between domestic radon exposure and several cancers, including prostate, has led to the hypothesis that α-radiation from natural sources may be an initiator of these diseases.[46] Perhaps the best data supporting a role for ionizing radiation in the initiation of prostatic cancer come from the United Kingdom Atomic Energy Authority. An analysis of 3373 deaths among 39,546 people employed between 1946 and 1979 has revealed that prostatic cancer was the only condition in which mortality clearly increased in relation to exposure.[47] Of the 19 men with a radiation record who died of prostate cancer, 9 had dosimeter readings totalling more than 50 mSv. Later, the same investigators documented that the risk of prostatic cancer was significantly increased in men who were internally contaminated with or worked in an environment potentially contaminated with tritium, chromium-51, iron-59, cobalt-60, or zinc-65 radionuclides.[48] Relative risk increased with increasing duration of exposure and increasing levels of probable contamination. These associations have not, however, been confirmed in international studies of nuclear industry work forces.[49]

SMOKING

Smoking is currently believed to exert a clear carcinogenic effect on the transitional epithelium of the urinary bladder.[50] It is logical, therefore, to expect that a similar effect might be present in the prostate due to their physical proximity and common embryologic origins. As might be expected, conflicting data regarding the association of tobacco smoke with prostatic cancer risk have been presented in the literature. The topic has been extensively reviewed, however, and it has been concluded that "current epidemiologic data link prostate cancer to smoking."[51]

Numerous studies have found an elevated risk for prostatic carcinoma among smokers. Two hundred sixteen case control pairs of middle-aged men were studied for the effects of vasectomy, smoking, and age at first sexual intercourse.[52] Cigarette smoking was associated with an increased risk (RR 1.9, 95% CI 1.2 to 3.0) and there was a significant dose response related to years of smoking ($p = .001$). In a cohort of 17,633 white males 35 and older studied for numerous dietary and behavioral factors, the only factor that did correlate with prostate cancer risk was use of tobacco products.[53] Smoking (RR 1.8, 95% CI 1.1 to 2.9) and use of smokeless tobacco (RR 2.1, 95% CI 1.1 to 1.4) were both found to elevate risk. In a 26-year follow-up of nearly 250,000 U.S. veterans including 4607 who had died from prostate cancer, cigarette smokers were found to have significant increase in risk (RR 1.18, 95% CI 1.09 to 1.28) and a clear dose response, with the relative risk reaching 1.51 for those who smoked 40 or more cigarettes per day.[54] Of potential clinical significance, smokers have been found to be at increased risk for more invasive and high-grade prostate carcinomas compared to control populations.[55] Stage D disease has been independently related to smoking (OR 2.1, 95% CI 1.3 to 4.3, $p = .015$) and again, smokers were found to have higher grade carcinomas.[56] These observations suggest that smoking may contribute to an increased malignant potential for prostatic carcinoma in addition to simply raising its incidence. Contrary to all of these findings, other large case-control studies have failed to show either an elevated risk or dose response associated with tobacco use.[57,58] In general, the largest and best-designed studies indicate an increased risk.

In addition to study design, numerous variables could contribute to the observed differences between groups. Other factors such as detection, hormonal effects, diet, or alcohol use could modulate the incidence and severity of prostatic carcinoma among smokers. For example, cigarette smokers have a lower likelihood of requiring surgery for benign prostatic hyperplasia.[51] It could be expected that this would decrease the number of incidental carcinomas found in smokers at transurethral resection. However, it has been found that more stage A carcinomas are found among smokers,[59] perhaps because their prostates are smaller and a larger portion is examined for pathologic changes. Elevated risk for stage D disease has also been related to lack of obesity, implicating a host of dietary and hormonal factors.[56] Although it might be assumed that smoking risk would be accompanied by risk from alcohol consumption, this has not been found to be the case.[60,61]

CONCLUSIONS

At the present time, it can be concluded that no single substance is likely to cause clinical prostate cancer in westernized societies. There are, however, sufficient data to implicate several classes of substances as being probably carcinogenic for the prostate. These would include heavy metals such as cadmium, and industrial chemicals such as formaldehyde, dimethylformamide, acrylonitrile, lubricating oils, and coke oven fumes. Evidence linking prostate cancer to farming continues to build. At present, the most likely cause is exposure to herbicides and nitrate fertilizers. Only weak links exist for exposure to ionizing radiation. It is interesting to note, however, that some of the radionuclides that are suspect include metal ions such as chromium and zinc that may be concentrated in the prostate by the same protein(s) that can bind cadmium. Finally, the data continue to provide increasing evidence for a link between smoking and prostate cancer incidence. Evidence also exists suggesting that the severity of prostate cancer may be enhanced by tobacco smoke. In view of the complex interactions that could be expected between most of the potential candidates for a "prostate carcinogen" that have been identified to date, it is likely that the final answers to these questions will have to come from experimental studies where exposure to multiple substances can be more carefully controlled.

REFERENCES

1. Parker SL, Tong T, Bolden S, Wingo PA: Cancer statistics, 1996. CA Cancer J Clin 1996; 46(1):5.
2. Boyle P, Maisonneuve P, Napalkov P: Geographical and temporal patterns incidence and mortality from prostate cancer. Urology 1995; 46(3 Suppl A):47.
3. Key T: Risk factors for prostate cancer. Cancer Surv 1995; 23: 63.
4. McLellan DL, Norman RW: Hereditary aspects of prostate cancer. Can Med Assoc J 1995; 153(7):895.
5. Barnes S: Effect of genistein on in vitro and in vivo models of cancer. J Nutr 1995; 125(3 Suppl):777S.
6. Brownson RC, Chang JC, Davis JR, et al: Occupational risk of prostate cancer: a cancer registry-based study. J Occup Med 1988; 30(6):523.
7. van der Gulden JW, Kolk JJ, Verbeek AL: Work environment and prostate cancer risk. Prostate 1995; 27(5):250.
8. Case RA, Hosker ME, McDonald DB, et al: Tumors of the urinary bladder in workmen engaged in the manufacture and use of certain dyestuff intermediates in the British chemical industry. Part I. The role of aniline, benzidine, alpha-naphthylamine, and beta-naphthylamine. Br J Ind Med 1993; 50(5):389.
9. Waalkes MP, Coogan TP, Barter RA: Toxicological principles of metal carcinogenesis with special emphasis on cadmium. Crit Rev Toxicol 1992; 22(3–4):175.
10. Cohen BL: Applications of ICRP 30, ICRP 23, and radioactive waste risk assessment techniques to chemical carcinogens. Health Phys 1982; 42(6):753.
11. Waalkes MP, Rehm S: Cadmium and prostate cancer. J Toxicol Eviron Health 1994; 43(3):251.
12. Elinder CG, Kjellstrom T, Hogstedt C, et al: Cancer mortality of cadmium workers. Br J Ind Med 1985; 42(10):651.
13. Elghany NA, Schumacher MC, Slattery ML, et al: Occupation, cadmium exposure, and prostate cancer. Epidemiology 1990; 1(2):107.
14. Wingren GB: Epidemiologic studies of health hazards related to the Swedish art glass industry. Diss Abstr Int 1992; 53(4):716.
15. Garcia-Sanchez A, Antona JF, Urrutia M: Geochemical prospection of cadmium in a high incidence area of prostate cancer, Sierra de Gatta, Salamanca, Spain. Sci Total Environ 1992; 116(3):243.
16. Kazantzis G, Lam TH, Sullivan KR: Mortality of cadmium-exposed workers. A five-year update. Scand J Work Environ Health 1988; 14(4):220.
17. Sorahan T, Waterhouse JA: Mortality study of nickel-cadmium battery workers by the method of regression models in life tables. Br J Ind Med 1983; 40(3):293.
18. Boffetta P: Methodological aspects of the epidemiologic association between cadmium and cancer in humans. *In* Cadmium in the Human Environment: Toxicity and Carcinogenicity. September 25–27, 1991, Gargnano, Italy, 1991.
19. Waalkes MP, Rehm S, Riggs CW, et al: Cadmium carcinogenesis in male Wistar [Crl:(WI)BR] rats: dose-response analysis of tumor induction in the prostate and testes and at the injection site. Cancer Res 1988; 48(16):4656.
20. Waalkes MP, Rehm S, Riggs CW, et al: Cadmium carcinogenesis in male Wistar [Crl:(WI)BR] rats: dose-response analysis of effects of zinc on tumor induction in the prostate, in the testes, and at the injection site. Cancer Res 1989; 49(15):4282.
21. Shirai T, Iwasaki S, Masui T, et al: Enhancing effect of cadmium on rat ventral prostate carcinogenesis induced by 3,2′-dimethyl-4-aminobiphenyl. Jpn J Cancer Res 1993; 84(10):1023.
22. Coogan TP, Shiraishi N, Waalkes MP: Apparent quiescence of the metallothionein gene in the rat ventral prostate: association with cadmium-induced prostate tumors in rats. Environ Health Perspect 1994; 102(Suppl 3):137.
23. Faroon OM, Williams M, O'Connor R: A review of the carcinogenicity of chemicals most frequently found at National Priorities List sites. Toxicol Ind Health 1994; 10(3): 203.

24. Blair A, Stewart P, O'Berg M, et al: Mortality among industrial workers exposed to formaldehyde. J Natl Cancer Inst 1986; 76(6):1071.
25. Walrath J, Fayerweather WE, Gilby PG, et al: A case-control study of cancer among Du Pont employees with potential for exposure to dimethylformamide. J Occup Med 1989; 31(5):432.
26. Hagmar L, Stromberg U, Welinder H, et al: Incidence of cancer and exposure to toluene diisocyanate and methylene diphenyldiisocyanate: a cohort based case-referent study in the polyurethane foam manufacturing industry. Br J Ind Med 1993; 50(11):1003.
27. Hoar SK, Blair A: Death certificate case-control study of cancers of the prostate and colon and employment in the textile industry. Arch Environ Health 1984; 39(4):280.
28. Goldsmith DF, Smith AH, McMichael AJ: A case-control study of prostate cancer within a cohort of rubber and tire workers. J Occup Med 1980; 22(8):533.
29. O'Berg MT, Chen JL, Burke CA, et al: Epidemiologic study of workers exposed to acrylonitrile: an update. J Occup Med 1985; 27(11):835.
30. Wen CP, Tsai SP, Weiss NS, et al: Long-term mortality study of oil refinery workers. IV. Exposure to the lubricating-dewaxing process. J Natl Cancer Inst 1985; 74(1):11.
31. Costantino JP, Redmond CK, Bearden A: Occupationally related cancer risk among coke oven workers: 30 years of follow-up. J Occup Environ Med 1995; 37(5):597.
32. Demers PA, Checkoway H, Vaughan TL, et al: Cancer incidence among firefighters in Seattle and Tacoma, Washington. Cancer Causes Control 1994; 5(2):129.
33. Blair A, Fraumeni JF: Geographic patterns of prostate cancer in the United States. J Natl Cancer Inst 1978; 61(6):1379.
34. Schenker M, McCurdy S: Pesticides, viruses, and sunlight in the etiology of cancer among agricultural workers. *In* Becker CE, Coye MJ (eds): Cancer Prevention. Strategies in the Workplace, p 29. Washington, DC, Hemisphere Publishing Corporation, 1986.
35. Blair A, Malker H, Cantor KP, et al: Cancer among farmers. A review. Scand J Work Environ Health 1985; 11(6):397.
36. Burmeister LF: Cancer mortality in Iowa farmers, 1971–78. J Natl Cancer Inst 1981; 66(3):461.
37. Gallagher RP, Threlfall WJ, Jeffries E, et al: Cancer and aplastic anemia in British Columbia farmers. J Natl Cancer Inst 1984; 72(6):1311.
38. Keller JE, Howe HL: Case-control studies of cancer in Illinois farmers using data from the Illinois State Cancer Registry and the U.S. Census of Agriculture. Eur J Cancer 1994; 30A(4):469.
39. Pearce NE, Sheppard RA, Fraser J: Case-control study of occupation and cancer of the prostate in New Zealand. J Epidemiol Community Health 1987; 41(2):130.
40. Barthel E: Cancer risk in pesticide exposed agricultural workers. Arch Geschwulstforsch 1981; 51(7):579.
41. Hagmar L, Bellander T, Andersson C, et al: Cancer morbidity in nitrate fertilizer workers. Int Arch Occup Environ Health 1991; 63(1):63.
42. Morrison H, Savitz D, Semenciw R, et al: Farming and prostate cancer mortality. Am J Epidemiol 1993; 137(3):270.
43. Hashimoto M, Akaza H, Shibamoto K, et al: Triple urogenital cancer in a patient with a history of heavy smoking who had been exposed to the Hiroshima atomic bomb explosion. Jpn J Clin Oncol 1988; 18(1):65.
44. Bean MA, Yatani R, Liu PI, et al: Prostatic carcinoma at autopsy in Hiroshima and Nagasaki Japanese. Cancer 1973; 32(2):498.
45. Hirose F, Takizawa S, Watanabe H, et al: Development of adenocarcinoma of the prostate in ICR mice locally irradiated with x-rays. Gann 1976; 67(3):407.
46. Henshaw DL, Eatough JP: Does environmental alpha radioactivity cause cancer in the general population? Br J Radiol 1993; 66(Congress Suppl):28.
47. Beral V, Inskip H, Fraser P, et al: Mortality of employees of the United Kingdom Atomic Energy Authority, 1946–1979. Br Med J 1985; 291(6493):440.
48. Rooney C, Beral V, Maconochie N, et al: Case-control study of prostatic cancer in employees of the United Kingdom Atomic Energy Authority. BMJ 1993; 307(6916):1391.
49. Cardis E, Gilbert ES, Carpenter L, et al: Effects of low doses and low dose rates of external ionizing radiation: cancer mortality among nuclear industry workers in three countries. Radiat Res 1995; 142(2):117.
50. Tobacco Smoking. International Agency for Research on Cancer (IARC): IARC working group on the evolution of the carcinogenic risk of chemicals to humans. Monographs 1986; 38:199.
51. Matzkin H, Soloway MS: Cigarette smoking: a review of possible associations with benign prostatic hyperplasia and prostate cancer. Prostate 1993; 22(4):277.
52. Honda GD, Bernstein L, Ross RK, et al: Vasectomy, cigarette smoking, and age at first sexual intercourse as risk factors for prostate cancer in middle-aged men. Br J Cancer 1988; 57(3):326.
53. Hsing AW, McLaughlin JK, Schuman LM, et al: Diet, tobacco use, and fatal prostate cancer: results from the Lutheran Brotherhood Cohort Study. Cancer Res 1990; 50(21):6836.
54. Hsing AW, McLaughlin JK, Hrubec Z, et al: Tobacco use and prostate cancer: 26-year follow-up of US veterans. Am J Epidemiol 1991; 133(5):437.
55. Hussain F, Aziz H, Macchia R, et al: High grade adenocarcinoma of prostate in smokers of ethnic minority groups and Caribbean Island immigrants. Int J Radiat Oncol Biol Phys 1992; 24(3):451.
56. Danilee HW: A worse prognosis for smokers with prostate cancer. J Urol 1995; 154(1):153.
57. van der Gulden JW, Verbeek AL, Kolk JJ: Smoking and drinking habits in relation to prostate cancer. Br J Urol 1994; 73(4):382.
58. Hayes RB, Pottern LM, Swanson GM, et al: Tobacco use and prostate cancer in blacks and whites in the United States. Cancer Causes Control 1994; 5(3):221.
59. Daniell HW: More stage A prostatic cancers, less surgery for benign hypertrophy in smokers. J Urol 1993; 149(1):68.
60. Hiatt RA, Armstrong MA, Klatsky AL, et al: Alcohol consumption, smoking, and other risk factors and prostate cancer in a large health plan cohort in California. Cancer Causes Control 1994; 5(1):66.
61. Tavani A, Negri E, Franceschi S, et al: Alcohol consumption and risk of prostate cancer. Nutr Cancer 1994; 21(1):24.

II

TREATMENT MODALITIES FOR CANCER: GENERAL PRINCIPLES

5

PRINCIPLES OF SURGICAL ONCOLOGY

JAMES E. MONTIE, M.D.

Cancer surgery comprises a substantial portion of urologic practice. Yet formal training for a urologist in the general principles of surgical oncology is uncommon and few resources are available.[1] It is unfortunate that we do not approach this topic in a more systematic fashion, since it is so central to our specialty. The lack of specific education in surgical urologic oncology rests in the fact that tradition, logic, and intuitive judgment form the basis for many of the principles; there may also be considerable variation among approaches for different cancers at different institutions making it difficult to arrive at widely accepted fundamental principles. For example, can an operation disseminate a cancer by increasing the burden of circulating cancer cells? If so, are strategies or techniques available that may modify the dissemination? The possibility that a surgical procedure could actually increase the risk of metastases may be one of the most fundamental concerns in surgical oncology. Unfortunately, answers to these questions are not available for the operations done by us each day. In addition to reviewing the principles supporting many surgical oncology procedures, this chapter will pose many questions. Table 5–1 lists the issues addressed in the chapter. The reader must realize that a personal philosophy of cancer care and individual experience undoubtedly influences the discussion. The "right" answer is not evident for many topics and disagreement is likely and welcomed. Whenever possible, specific examples in urologic oncology will illustrate a general principle.

PHILOSOPHY ABOUT CANCER OPERATIONS

"Radical" Surgery

The public perception regarding cancer surgery has traditionally focused on the "radical" aspect of an operation, implying a degree of excess. In practical terms, this often only means inclusion of an adequate margin of normal tissue around the cancer to be certain the gross and microscopic cancer is removed entirely. Historically, a radical procedure often caused substantial morbidity and permanent change in the patient's lifestyle. In current vernacular, the surgery adversely affected the patient's "quality of life." Indeed, many operations performed were "mutilating" from a patient's perspective. Radical mastectomy is probably the best known example in general surgery, while in urology, radical cystectomy is perceived as a mutilating procedure because of the need for a stoma and pouch/bag.

A historical view is necessary when discussing these radical operations developed nearly 100 years ago.[2] Radical mastectomy was an operation devised for large, locally advanced cancers, often invading the chest wall. An operation for such an extensive cancer needed to remove the muscles of the chest wall to provide complete removal of the local cancer. However, the standardization of radical mastectomy led to its use in all cases of breast cancer for decades, including small cancers confined to the breast. This rather indiscriminate application of one operation illustrates a concept occasionally overlooked in surgical oncology. The primary goal of an operation is to remove the existing cancer entirely. An operation, possibly combined with other local therapy, must prevent a local recurrence of the cancer. It should not do less but it also cannot do more. If metastases exist at the time of the operation, a bigger operation will not improve survival. Thus, the *smallest* operation that will reliably eliminate the cancer is the procedure of choice because it will likely have the least functional impact.

Let's imagine one operation that removes the tumor, the organ of origin, and surrounding soft tissue with a 5% local recurrence rate and 50% met-

TABLE 5–1. ISSUES ADDRESSED IN DISCUSSION OF SURGICAL ONCOLOGY

1. Philosophy about cancer operations
   a) "Radical" surgery
   b) Patient choice
2. Biopsy
3. Pathology
4. Markers
5. Staging
6. Morbidity from treatment
7. Lymph nodes
8. Combined modalities
9. Inoperable or unresectable cancers
10. Debulking
11. Follow-up
12. Does surgery disseminate cancer?

astatic rate. Simple removal of the tumor with an adequate margin of normal tissue yet preserving function of the organ also has a 5% local recurrence rate and 50% metastatic rate. Is it necessary to do the larger operation? This illustration emphasizes that an operation is local treatment only with success based on the ability to prevent a local recurrence. Local control at the lowest possible price to the patient should be the goal. Sacrificing adjacent tissue not involved with cancer may increase morbidity without improvement in local control. Having stated the above, other factors undeniably complicate the picture. Most critical is the potential for multifocal tumors within the organ, either at the time of detection or in the future. Surgery may need to remove the whole organ for this purpose. Also, technical considerations may make removal of a portion of an organ more difficult than removal of the entire organ with more complications. If there is an increase in risk or complications, there should be corresponding benefit to justify it.

Perhaps a definition of terms will help now to avoid confusion. A local excision means removal of a tumor with a small margin of surrounding apparent normal tissue. A "total" removal of an organ implies removal of just the organ itself with no attempt to include surrounding tissue. A "radical" procedure requires definition specifically for each organ. A radical mastectomy indicates inclusion of adjacent chest wall muscles. A radical nephrectomy means the dissection is outside Gerota's fascia. Radical prostatectomy implies removal of a small amount of soft tissue directly around the organ but no other structures. Radical cystectomy implies removal of the bladder, adjacent soft tissue, and the prostate. Radical orchiectomy means removal of the testicle outside the tunica vaginalis with a wide margin of spermatic cord. For each organ, "radical" has a unique definition. A "radical" operation may be done with or without a regional lymphadenectomy.

Let's examine breast cancer and renal cell carcinoma as illustrations of the previous discussion. At the time radical mastectomy was developed, large cancers were the rule. Early detection provides a preponderance of much smaller cancers. Because a smaller operation may remove the smaller cancer just as well as a larger operation, lumpectomy became possible. Experience taught us that only the smallest tumors were suitable for this approach and there was still a problem with new tumor formation because of the multifocal nature of the cancer.[3] Another modality, external beam radiation therapy, is necessary to prevent new tumors. The outcome of this reasoning is preservation of a cosmetically acceptable breast, providing a substantial benefit to the patient. Cure rates, diminished because of preexisting metastases prior to any therapy, should be the same regardless of the type of local therapy if local recurrence rates are the same. It is noteworthy that the evolution of this approach and the confirmation of its safety took 30 years, thousands of women in well-designed clinical trials, and millions of dollars of clinical research support.

Radical nephrectomy is the standard operation for renal cell carcinoma. The operation became popular when the average diameter of the tumor was approximately 10 cm. Invasion into the surrounding soft tissue or renal vein was common. Earlier detection is now common with widespread use of abdominal ultrasound or computed tomography for a variety of abdominal complaints. Small, asymptomatic, 2- to 3-cm tumors are now visible. Is a radical nephrectomy necessary for all these cases?[4] Since surgery strives for local control, local recurrences either in the renal fossa or in the remaining kidney represent a key outcome. If a recurrence does occur, salvage treatment efficacy is important. Which operation has the fewer complications and what is the ultimate benefit to the patient? The local recurrence rate of a radical nephrectomy for a 3.0-cm renal cell cancer approaches zero. The local recurrence rate in the remaining kidney after a partial nephrectomy for a 3.0-cm incidental lesion approaches 3% or less. Is this too high? How effective is a total nephrectomy after a failed partial nephrectomy? Might some patients develop distant metastases as a consequence of the local recurrence when initial radical nephrectomy might provide a cure? The answers to these questions are currently unavailable. What is the benefit to the patient? Data would suggest that removal of one kidney when the other kidney is entirely normal represents little risk for future compromise of total renal function, although only a 20-year follow-up is available. Bilateral, asynchronous renal cell cancers occur in only 1% of cases. The complication rate after a partial nephrectomy may be slightly higher than that seen for a radical nephrectomy. Thus patients may experience a greater risk from a partial nephrectomy with an uncertain benefit. Currently, there are too many gaps in our data to allow firm conclusions about the ideal approach. We must be cautious because the general idea of organ preservation is attractive to patients when it may not be the right thing to do. The point to be illustrated is that we should strive to do the smallest operation we can to eliminate the cancer while preserving overall benefit to the patient. Sometimes, removal of an entire organ may be a safer operation without sacrificing functional results.

Does this concept apply to other urologic cancers? Prostate cancer is multifocal, and less than a total prostatectomy leaves residual disease. In addition, partial removal of the prostate may carry similar morbidity to a total prostatectomy because of the operative exposure needed. However, an anatomic radical prostatectomy with preservation of the neurovascular bundles next to the prostate depends on the observation that a small cancer confined within the prostate does not need a wide margin of normal tissue excised along with the organ. Preservation of erectile function translates into a significant improvement in quality of life in *selected* prostate cancer patients. Partial cystectomy for bladder cancer preserves important organ function for selected patients but new tumor formation and appropriate patient selection remains problematic. Might a total cystectomy without removal of the prostate provide adequate results in selected cases? What would be the magnitude of the benefit in erectile function or urinary continence? Total orchiectomy through the scrotum instead of a radical orchiectomy would provide no functional benefit and may only increase the risk.

The addition of other modalities to help eliminate the local cancer may allow performance of a smaller operation. Certainly limb-sparing combined-modality treatment using radiation therapy and chemotherapy for extremity sarcomas represents a major advance.[1] The standard treatment for anal carcinoma is a combination of 5-fluorouracil, mitomycin C, and radiation therapy; extensive pelvic surgery is commonly avoided.[5] For urologic cancers, successful combined-modality therapy remains a hope rather than an accepted practice. A combination of systemic chemotherapy followed by partial cystectomy cures some bladder cancer patients, but limited and somewhat discouraging results limit generalized use.[6]

Detection of smaller cancers allows the opportunity to use a smaller operation. We must be cognizant that an operation needed for one type of cancer may be excessive when the pattern of the disease presentation changes. It is necessary to frequently re-examine what we do and to avoid entrapment by tradition when the enemy is no longer the same.

Patient Choice

Surgeons face increasing opportunities to allow the patient to participate in decisions about cancer care. Options are frequently available and the choice of treatment must balance the risks and benefits. For many patients, elimination of the cancer is the primary goal but not at any cost. For example, the loss of erections after urologic cancer surgery may substantially offset a modest survival benefit.[7] The surgeon must provide data on the risk of recurrence and other negative consequences as accurately as possible. Unfortunately, the information available to make a decision is often incomplete, and the physician's judgment becomes an important factor.[8] More information on outcomes of specific operations is essential. These outcomes may even need to be physician specific for some types of surgery. Surgeons should welcome this trend, since it will likely generate a better appreciation of the impact of surgery and lead to better results.

Principle: An operation is local treatment only. The operation is the one that exposes the patient to the smallest risk and least functional impairment and yet reliably eliminates the cancer. Patient choice is an integral part of the decision process.

BIOPSY

Fundamental to any therapy for cancer is an accurate diagnosis. For this, we rely on biopsy of the lesion. Although a clinical presentation may be characteristic of a malignancy, decisions about therapy generally require adequate material for a pathologist to examine. The amount of material needed to establish the diagnosis varies by cancer, and surgeons must be sensitive to the inherent difficulties in making a diagnosis or characterizing a cancer when insufficient tissue is available to the pathologist. In some settings, a cytologic examination of either an aspirate or body fluid may be sufficient. However, in most circumstances, an actual tissue section provides the most information. A currently relevant example in urologic oncology is aspiration biopsy of the prostate. While commonly sufficient to make a diagnosis in expert hands, the information obtained by cytology is inferior to that available with needle biopsy yielding an actual core of tissue.[9]

A general oncologic principle affirms that the method used to obtain the biopsy should not compromise the definitive therapy needed. Methods include needle biopsy, incisional biopsy, and excisional biopsy. Patients may ask if the biopsy can spread the cancer along the biopsy tract. For certain head and neck cancers, an ill-planned biopsy may significantly interfere with later surgery. For most urologic cancers, incisional biopsy does not compromise later therapy, but notable exceptions exist. A transcrotal biopsy of a testis cancer can dramatically alter the risk for local recurrence, lymphatic spread, and ultimate therapy. An "open" biopsy of a bladder cancer can seed the incision and suprapubic space, making subsequent curative treatment impossible. For the common urologic cancers, well-established practice patterns exist for biopsy to make the diagnosis. For prostate cancer, needle biopsy is the standard; for bladder cancer, transurethral biopsy or resection is used; for penile cancer, incisional or excisional biopsy of the lesion is required; for renal and testicular cancers, the involved organ may be removed without prior histologic confirmation based on the characteristic clinical situation, supporting laboratory data, and gross appearance in the operating room. For the latter two cancers, a benign tumor may mimic a cancer on rare occasion and lead to removal of the organ.

Heterogeneity within a cancer sometimes requires sampling of several representative areas. For example, a renal mass may appear to be an oncocytoma in one area and be clearly malignant in other areas. The surgeon must be sure that enough information is available from the biopsy to allow the appropriate clinical decision.

Principle: Biopsy is commonly needed to establish a tissue diagnosis preoperatively, but the method of biopsy should not interfere with possible surgery.

PATHOLOGY

Pathologic examination of biopsy material provides a diagnosis of cancer. Substantial advances are evident in urologic pathology through standardization of interpretation and immunohistochemical staining techniques. It is often not enough just to know the presence or absence of the cancer; grading of a cancer is typically one of the most powerful prognostic factors. The growth pattern or degree of invasion may dictate therapy. For each urologic cancer, specific aspects of the pathology may be extremely helpful in management decisions. For example, Gleason grading of prostate cancer may be the factor that decides if treatment is even necessary.[10] The depth of invasion of bladder cancer may make the difference between a transurethral resection and a cystectomy. The presence of mixed germ cell elements in a testis cancer requires an entirely different treatment algorithm than for a pure seminoma. Experience has shown that the occasionally cryptic diagnosis on the pathology report does not always communicate all the information that may help in treatment decisions. With difficult decisions, reviewing the pathologic material with the pathologist provides an appreciation of the more subtle aspects of the tumor. A bladder cancer may be "invasive" but that distinction could represent a few cells clearly within the resected tissue or a broad front at the base of the specimen. Direct discussion between the surgeon and the pathologist can prevent miscommunication that may have an adverse impact on patient care.

Immunohistochemical staining has become a necessary component of many aspects of pathologic diagnosis and research. The evolution of immunohistochemistry relies on specific differentiation of the organ of origin of the neoplasm or the tumor itself. Polyclonal or monoclonal antibodies directed against enzymes, proteins, or metabolites provide characteristic staining patterns that may be useful in establishing a site of origin, tissue type, or important subtype of a cancer. Automated instruments are now available that simplify the process and bring these techniques further into routine use.

There are three common examples in urologic oncology in which immunohistochemical staining may be extremely valuable.

1. Prostate-specific antigen (PSA) is useful in identifying prostate cancer metastases at remote sites when the presentation or microscopic appearance is unusual. There are also cases in which a tumor at the bladder neck may be either a transitional cell carcinoma of the bladder invading the prostate or a poorly differentiated adenocarcinoma of the prostate invading the bladder neck; PSA staining generally can discriminate between the two, having a profound effect on therapy decisions.
2. The diagnosis of early prostate cancer may be difficult, and use of a basal cell–specific anticytokeratin stain may separate dysplasia or high-grade prostatic intraepithelial neoplasia from cancer.[11]
3. Staining for the tumor markers alpha fetoprotein (AFP) or human chorionic gonadotropin (HCG) may distinguish a metastatic germ cell tumor from other types of cancer.

Oncogene or tumor-suppressor gene products may also become more reliably identified by immunohistochemistry and correlated with tumor prognosis. One example in urology is the identification of the tumor-suppressor gene protein p53 in bladder cancer.[12] Abnormal p53 function is a consequence of mutations on chromosome 17 and is associated with aggressive behavior in superficial and invasive bladder cancer. Although not currently integrated into clinical management strategies, it will not be long before this information will signal the need for more aggressive therapy.[13]

Also in the near future, additional specialized methods of molecular evaluation will become more common.[14] Recombinant DNA technology labels probes to identify DNA in tumor cells. Fluorescent in situ hybridization (FISH) on small tissue samples will identify cellular DNA of specific genes in individual cells while retaining the normal tissue architecture.[15,16] As more specific chromosomal abnormalities and patterns become apparent for cell types or prognostic subgroups, FISH will supplement the microscopic characteristics to define more precisely the actual molecular abnormalities.

Principle: Pathologic confirmation of malignancy is anticipated before organ removal; notable exceptions in urologic oncology may be certain renal or testicular masses.

TABLE 5–2. BIOMARKERS FOR UROLOGIC CANCERS

Tumor	Marker
Prostate	Prostate-specific antigen
	Acid phosphatase
	Prostate-specific membrane antigen
Testes	Alpha fetoprotein
	Beta human chorionic gonadotropin (HCG)
	Placental alkaline phosphatase
Renal	Ferritin
Bladder	HCG
	Carcinoma embryonic antigen (CEA)

MARKERS

Serum biomarkers have long had an important role in urologic oncology. In the 1940s, serum acid phosphatase was a reliable marker for advanced prostate cancer and a reflection of treatment response. Biomarkers from tumor tissue exhibit varying degrees of specificity and sensitivity. They represent enzymes, proteins, metabolites, and more recently oncogenes or tumor-associated antigens. They may be useful for diagnosis, staging, prognosis, monitoring the course of the disease, and potentially as a source for targeting therapy. Urologic oncology is fortunate to have the best marker in oncology, PSA.[17] However, the limitations of this marker are evident. Most men with an elevated PSA do not have prostate cancer; PSA reflects tumor volume but not precisely; the absence of detectable PSA soon after therapy does not preclude return of the disease; earlier detection of residual disease after initial therapy does not reliably translate into an improved outcome. In spite of these limitations, PSA is an example of the enormous value a biomarker can have in the management of a cancer patient. Table 5–2 lists additional markers useful in urologic oncology. Research into biomarkers for the common cancers is extensive in industry; for example, molecular forms of PSA may provide substantially improved performance over total PSA alone.

PRINCIPLE: An ideal tumor marker should provide early detection, improved assessment of prognosis, earlier detection of disease, or earlier discovery of recurrence leading to more effective therapy and a better outcome.

STAGING AND PROGNOSTIC FACTORS

Staging a cancer is such an integral part of cancer patient management that it is easy to take for granted. Prior to treatment decisions, the practitioner must arrive at an assessment of the extent of disease. A clear understanding of the relationship between staging and prognostic factors helps us realize the value and limitations of both. Staging of a cancer defines the anatomic extent of disease. It is certainly not the only prognostic factor but it is usually the best.[18] Prognostic factors predict the natural history of a cancer or the response to a therapy. They help select patients for clinical trials, compare therapies, or define subgroups with particular characteristics.[19–21] Accepted or proposed prognostic factors include stage, grade, sex, age, performance status, comorbidity, serum biomarker level, immunohistochemical marker pattern, and oncogene or suppressor gene function.[22,23] For breast cancer, there are more than 70 putative prognostic factors. The integration of the information obtained from prognostic factors fosters specific statistical methods needed to determine the relative value of the different factors. The American Joint Committee on Cancer (AJCC) recommends that a prognostic factor be (1) independent (i.e., important after controlling other factors), (2) significant (i.e., does not occur by chance), and (3) important (i.e., clinically useful).[20] Criteria for prognostic factors are valuable because of the substantial impact they may have on clinical practice. For example, a new molecular prognostic factor for prostate cancer such as p53 status would have enormous economic implications if performed on each of the 250,000 new prostate cancer patients each year in the United States. Prior to widespread implementation, the value of the marker over existing factors must be clear.[24]

Staging of urologic cancers remains in evolution, a necessary but troublesome feature. Historically, an astute clinician (such as Whitmore, Jewett, or Robson) proposed a cancer staging classification that gradually assumed the name of the author and attained generalized use. In recent years, an effort has been extended to provide a common staging classification for use worldwide and is based on the TNM (tumor, nodes, metastases) system. The goal is a more precise definition of the extent of the disease and easier communication. For urologic cancers, the TNM system was not in common usage in the United States for a variety of reasons; recently, the TNM system reflects clinical practice more precisely and thus it is gaining broader support.[18]

Although the TNM classification system allows more precise definition of the extent of disease in an individual patient, grouping of patients and adding additional prognostic factors becomes problematic.[20,21] For example, the TNM system in prostate cancer allows for 32 "bins" in which to slot a patient based on the extent of disease. Adding one more variable, such as grade with three categories of well, moderate, or poor differentiation, raises the number of "bins" to 96, clearly unworkable. However, the addition of more proven prognostic variables will allow a more precise prediction of outcome for an individual patient and could be of tremendous value in clinical care and research. The incorporation of many prognostic variables will require innovative statistical methods; early research has focused on nomograms, prognostic scores or indices, and neural network analysis. Nomograms are available in prostate cancer to predict the risk of lymph node metastases based on clinical stage, grade, and PSA level.[25] Clearly, important and readily available information such as age and comorbidity provide information to help decide the risk of the disease over time. Such research requires large databases of several thousand patients that are not currently available. Neural network analysis in prostate cancer may yield an improvement in outcome prediction.[26] The future is intriguing when one envisions the use of a hand-held computer containing five, ten, or more variables on an individual patient. The software in the computer could draw on previous experience with thousands of patients using these variables and provide the clinician with a number that describes the relative risk for disease progression with or without a variety of treatments. The required technology is available now but the databases are not. Clinical judgment currently serves this purpose and will persist as the foundation, but the limitations and inherent biases are evident.

Principle: Anatomic extent of disease (staging) is one of many prognostic factors for malignancy. New prognostic factors should be independent, significant, and important.

MORBIDITY FROM TREATMENT

The emphasis on a critical examination of cancer treatment morbidity is increasing. More and more, the patient rather than the treating surgeon is being asked to evaluate and quantify the effect of an operation.[27–30] This is certainly a good trend. Oncologic surgeons tend to view the positive aspects of an operation, focusing largely on the primary goal of cancer elimination. However, the value placed on body function or appearance may vary greatly among cancer patients; some will accept risks about cancer control to preserve an unaltered aspect of their life. In urologic oncology, a prominent example is the choice patients often make about preservation of sexual function. Surgeons must be cognizant that the decisions a patient makes commonly involves relative risks. A slightly increased risk for disease recurrence may be an acceptable trade-off for a better chance of preserving erectile function. Singer and associates documented that many patients will accept a 10% or more increase in risk for treatment failure to improve the potential for maintaining erections.[7] In my experience, if there is not another good option available, almost all patients will accept the negative consequences of the surgery for the opportunity to rid themselves of the cancer. If a treatment option exists that has the potential to cure the cancer while preserving normal function, many patients will opt for this approach. A realization of this should help us as surgeons examine what we do more critically to see if there is a way to modify the surgery and preserve function. An excellent example is the introduction of the anatomic radical prostatectomy by Dr. Patrick Walsh. He modified the traditional operation in selected patients to increase the preservation of a normal function with minimal risk of increasing cancer recurrence.[31] Patient satisfaction should be a compelling force to help us continually scrutinize our procedures to make them better.

The last 10 years have witnessed a remarkable emphasis on quality-of-life (QOL) issues.[32] This research has demonstrated that the ideal person to evaluate the impact on the patient is not the treating physician.[33] Unconsciously, the physician or surgeon will interpret the patient's response from his or her own perspective. This problem is apparent in the evaluation of incontinence after radical prostatectomy or cystectomy and orthotopic neobladder.[28–30] The bother or change in lifestyle induced by incontinence requires the patient's perspective as much as possible. The data acquisition should minimize bias introduced by the treating physician and allow comparison in several settings. Reliable QOL instruments are now becoming available in urology that allow critical assessment and comparison of treatment impacts. This evaluation of results may be a valuable teaching tool to help a surgeon objectively survey results and, if necessary, make adjustments in technique or patient selection. Research into QOL issues after surgery helps patients by making surgeons more aware of areas that need improvement or emphasizing the successful aspects of procedures now used.

Principle: Assessment of the impact of surgery on QOL issues, in addition to the issue of cancer control, should be incorporated into the evaluation of a procedure.

LYMPHADENECTOMY

The discussion up to now has focused on the primary tumor. However, cancer is frequently a regional disease, defined as spread to lymph nodes adjacent to the site of origin. Regional lymph nodes are commonly the first echelon of spread of the cancer. For most epithelial cancers, spread to regional nodes profoundly alters the ability to cure the cancer with only a local therapy.[34] Thus lymphadenectomy is useful in some cancers for staging purposes only, allowing identification of an adverse prognosis.[35] Historically, a "radical" operation often implied the removal of regional nodes with an en bloc dissection if possible. In reality, a wide local excision of an organ is possible with or without removal of the regional nodes. For each cancer, the goal of the lymphadenectomy should be articulated and supported by evidence.

There is uncertainty about the value of quantifying the degree of lymph node metastases. Staging systems rely on either the number of nodes involved or the size of the nodes. Neither system appears ideal for all cancers. The identification of true "micrometastases," visible only with special staining techniques to find epithelial cells in the nodes, is interesting. In breast cancer, step-sectioning of apparently negative nodes increased the yield of positive nodes by 24% and the prognosis of these patients was not substantially different from that of patients with truly negative nodes.[36] In prostate cancer, techniques to identify micrometastases have not greatly increased the yield, and even minuscule volume of spread apparently adversely affects survival.[37,38] Unfortunately, these observations commonly include relatively small numbers of patients because additional sectioning and processing the nodes is labor intensive and expensive.

Urologic cancers demonstrate the spectrum of significance of lymph node involvement. Penile and testis cancers represent two of the most curable cancers in spite of lymph node metastases. Lymphadenectomy for small-volume regional disease may cure up to 50% of patients. Few epithelial cancers behave in this favorable fashion. In bladder cancer, lymphadenectomy and cystectomy cures 20 to 50% of early node-positive cases, dependent somewhat as well on the T stage of the primary.[39] Renal cancer with involved lymph nodes allows cure in only occasional cases. Lastly, prostate cancer, long perceived as a "benign" acting cancer, has few if any long-term cures when any degree of lymph node spread is present. In the Johns Hopkins series, no prostate cancer patient with only microscopic spread had an undetectable PSA greater than 6 years after radical prostatectomy alone.[40] Based on these observations, the extent of surgical removal of the nodes varies greatly among the different cancers. The regional lymphadenectomy for penile and testis cancer aims to remove all first-echelon draining nodes. For renal and bladder cancers, lymphadenectomy removes a majority of the primary nodes but not all potential sites of spread. For prostate cancer, a limited sampling of a common site of spread precludes an attempt at a therapeutic dissection. The reasons for the striking differences among these cancers is not apparent and few data are available.

The function of regional lymph nodes in cancer biology remains perplexing. Few data support early theories that regional nodes function as a "filter" or part of host immunity against cancer. In the 1980s, there was interest in the morphologic patterns in regional nodes that may reflect or correlate with host defenses. That line of research appears to have stalled. Animal studies with chemically or virally induced tumors or transplanted tumors may not be directly relevant to common epithelial tumors. The nagging question of a possible adverse effect of removal of uninvolved lymph nodes remains, although few clinical observations support this. It is perplexing that in spite of substantial progress in understanding cancer, the role of the regional lymph node in the progression of cancer remains a mystery.

Principle: Regional lymphadenectomy is of prognostic value for most cancers and therapeutic for some.

COMBINED MODALITIES

Great expectations surround the use of combined therapies for cancer.[41] Although surgery is by far the most common method to cure cancer, some locally advanced cancers are not amenable to resection. Extension to nearby vital organs or microscopic tentacles approaching surgical margins may preclude an operation from eliminating the local disease entirely. Combining surgery with either radiation therapy or chemotherapy is an attempt to get the most out of all the treatments without excessively increasing side effects or normal-tissue damage.

The desired goal from combining therapies must be clear. If surgery or radiation therapy alone cures the cancer and side effects are low, there is no impetus to combine them. Three goals may be possible: (1) allow organ preservation, (2) improve local control, and (3) prevent distant relapse. Organ preservation is an admirable goal, but one that remains elusive in urologic oncology. The bulk of research of combined treatment for organ preservation has been in invasive bladder cancer using transurethral resection, systemic chemotherapy, and pelvic irradiation. Despite some promising initial results, long-term freedom from cancer recurrence in the remaining bladder is disappointingly low.[42,43] This approach remains investigational but worthwhile because of a potential for improved patient rehabilitation. Pre- or postoperative radiation therapy may decrease local recurrence in selected bladder and prostate cancers. However, improved local control may not translate into improved survival (i.e., necessary but not sufficient). Cancers locally advanced enough to require combined surgery and irradiation to eliminate the cancer may be the ones with pre-existing occult metastases; no amount of further local therapy will have a substantial impact on survival. Lastly, the combination of surgery and chemotherapy, either before surgery (neoadjuvant) or after surgery (adjuvant), may improve survival. Major advances in the future will come primarily in this area.[44] In urologic cancer, combined therapy is clearly beneficial only in testis cancer. The choice of pre- or postoperative timing depends more on patient selection and tolerance. There is no conclusive superiority of one over the other. As a classic rule, systemic therapy for defined metastatic disease should have at least a 50% response rate to justify its use in an adjuvant setting. For bladder cancer, adjuvant chemotherapy is tantalizing but not unequivocally beneficial; for renal cancer, it is nonexistent; for prostate cancer, it is unstudied. In prostate cancer, neither adjuvant nor neoadjuvant hormonal therapy currently provides proven survival benefit.

There is little doubt that combined therapy will be the treatment approach of the future for larger cancers. More effective systemic agents will be forthcoming and integrated into standard care. However, surgery as a discipline to treat cancer will continue. Even in cancers for which very effective chemotherapy is available, surgical resection of the primary and metastatic sites is sometimes valuable.[45]

PRINCIPLE: A combination of radiation therapy and chemotherapy with surgery may increase the local control rate, impact survival, or allow organ preservation. The goal of a combined-modality strategy must be clearly evident.

INOPERABLE OR UNRESECTABLE CANCERS

A most frustrating circumstance for a surgeon is the cancer so locally extensive that it is deemed inoperable prior to surgery or unresectable at the time of surgery. A patient should not be declared inoperable based solely on a blood test or an imaging study known to have false-positive results. In such a situation, the next diagnostic step should confirm or deny a metastasis or local extension to prevent erroneous withholding of a potentially curative procedure. An example is a moderately enlarged regional lymph node identified on computed tomography. Histologic confirmation of metastases is appropriate to avoid overstaging the patient who may have only a benign, reactive node.

A desire to help can overwhelm good judgment to the detriment of the patient. Some patients do have unresectable cancers, and heroic attempts to remove the tumor often leads to more morbidity from the unsuccessful treatment.[1] The patient then suffers the side effects of the surgery without the benefit of removing the disease. Locally advanced prostate or bladder cancer may precipitate this dilemma when the surgeon must decide whether to go on with a planned radical prostatectomy or cystectomy. The ideal management is frequently uncertain, and decisions are based on a balance of the risk from the surgery, the potential for morbidity from unresected local disease, the effectiveness of alternate palliative treatments, and the patient's emotional status. For prostate cancer, other treatments such as radiation therapy or hormonal therapy can provide substantial palliation; locally advanced bladder cancer often responds poorly to attempts to palliate urinary symptoms or ureteral obstruction. These decisions are often difficult for the patient, physician, and family, and are made only after weighing all the options.

PRINCIPLE: Some locally advanced cancers are beyond surgical resection and surgery may actually increase morbidity without a survival benefit.

DEBULKING SURGERY

The term "debulking" occurs in many different settings in surgical oncology. A strict definition greatly limits the use of the term. Let's imagine a scenario of a patient with an abdominal primary cancer with chest metastases. Both sites have not responded to chemotherapy. Does debulking (removal) of the abdominal tumor make the chest metastases any more susceptible to the same or different chemotherapy? Does removal of a portion of a tumor convert the remaining tumor from resistant to sensitive to chemotherapy? There is no firm evidence to support this concept in spite of its application in urologic oncology. A primary renal cell cancer is excised in the hope of rendering the metastases more sensitive to a variety of therapies; data to support such a strategy are negligible.[46] Experience has shown that subtotal removal of a testis cancer metastasis after chemotherapy does not make the remaining mass more sensitive to the previous chemotherapy.[47] Removal of a bulky primary tumor to diminish systemic symptoms such as anorexia or hypercalcemia might be worthwhile, but successful applications are rare.

Applying debulking in a broader sense may expand the justification for surgery. Subtotal removal of a large primary tumor (debulking a primary without metastases) may allow other modalities such as radiation therapy or chemotherapy to focus on a smaller amount of cancer. Occasionally this can be effective but preoperative therapy may work just as well. In gynecologic oncology, debulking is part of established therapy for ovarian cancer.[48] Patients whose tumor can be debulked to less than 1 cm prior to chemotherapy do better than those in whom it is not possible.

The term debulking is not the appropriate description of complete excision of a residual mass after chemotherapy, as is commonly done for testis cancer. The goal of this surgery is to remove *all* residual disease, thereby achieving a complete response with combined therapy; anything less than that is generally of little benefit.

PRINCIPLE: Incomplete resection of a primary tumor in the face of metastases rarely alters sensitivity to systemic treatment using other modalities.

FOLLOW-UP

Patient follow-up is an inherent part of any cancer surgery. Most urologists follow their own cancer patients, and questions about the appropriate studies and timing are common. Surprisingly few firm data exist in urologic cancer about follow-up regimens that have been proven to be of benefit to the patient in ultimate outcome. Philosophically, if no curative treatment is available at the time of relapse as is the case for most solid tumors, why subject the patient to expensive and anxiety-provoking studies? If a bladder cancer patient relapses, systemic chemotherapy as currently available is rarely curative and is associated with substantial morbidity. For this cancer, perhaps we should only focus on potentially treatable recurrence, such as the urethra or upper tract collecting systems.[49] In some situations, it may make as much sense to discharge the patient after the initial postoperative check and say "come back and see us if you have any trouble." The overall survival may be identical to our current practices. However, in this country, follow-up after cancer treatment is ingrained in the public mindset and expected. It is appropriate to scrutinize the type and timing of follow-up tests. The studies should emphasize sites of potentially treatable recurrences such as the lungs over other sites such as bone where palliation only is the rule. A complete scrutiny of this topic is beyond the scope of this chapter, but other reviews are available.[50]

There is a need for follow-up to monitor the impact of our treatment, apart from concerns about a cancer recurrence. For example, after cystectomy and urinary diversion, it is necessary to monitor the upper tracts and renal function for late technical complications. Late functional results must be documented, such as continence and potency. There may also be an increased risk for second malignancies, either inherently or as a consequence of treatment.

Prostate cancer represents a unique dilemma now for follow-up.[51] PSA is such a good marker for disease that patients and physicians alike focus on it tremendously. After radical prostatectomy, some patients obsess over their PSA level and would have it done monthly if we let them. PSA levels may become abnormal years before clinically apparent disease is evident; management of these patients is a difficult issue with no course clearly proven beneficial. Patients are often uncomfortable with observation only in spite of no symptoms and no imaging abnormalities. Earlier initiation of endocrine therapy provides an unquantified survival benefit. In essence, a new "disease" becomes apparent by allowing the patients to know they will relapse years before it may actually take place and yet no potentially curative therapy is available. A serum marker is truly valuable for follow-up only when it allows earlier detection of a recurrence that translates into cure or prolonged disease-free survival. We are not at that point in prostate cancer.

Principle: Follow-up should be tailored to the disease and altered by the risk of recurrence with a goal of detection in the situation that makes salvage therapy possible.

DOES SURGERY DISSEMINATE CANCER?

We have all been confronted with a patient or family member inquiring if "letting air in on the cancer" will make it spread. This cancer myth rests partially on observations that some patients clearly deteriorate rapidly after ineffective surgery. The clinical situation is usually a planned procedure abandoned or the cancer is clearly more advanced than preoperatively anticipated, implying a rapid growth phase starting even before the surgery. Nevertheless, circumstances of worsening nutrition after surgery, an immunosuppressive effect of anesthesia and surgery, or a patient "giving up" after an operation may hasten their demise. From a cancer biology viewpoint, the possibility that surgery may disseminate cancer remains. Metastases developing several years after initial cancer surgery with good local control are generally attributed to micrometastases established at the time of the original operation. However, this is speculative. Studies done 30 to 40 years ago document, albeit crudely, that manipulation of a cancer increases circulating cancer cells.[52] The fate of this potential shower of cells is uncertain, and the cells may not have the right machinery to develop into metastases. Animal studies suggest that manipulation of a tumor can increase spread; classic surgical teaching minimized preoperative examination of the cancer and intraoperative handling through "no-touch" techniques. The improved results associated with no-touch techniques may be secondary to other aspects of the procedure such as wider local excision.

Earlier studies of circulating tumor cells should be repeated with current molecular biology methods that allow identification of a small number of cancer cells more specifically.[53] Either cytokeratin markers for epithelial cells or organ-specific markers, such as PSA, may be useful. Preliminary studies in prostate cancer suggest circulating tumor cells are more common with higher local stage disease, and may increase transiently with surgery.[54,55]

The implications of surgery disseminating cancer cells are noteworthy. If true, then additional tools are necessary in all or selected cases to make the cells less viable or unable to start the metastatic landing process. Preoperative treatment of the tumor with modest doses of chemotherapy or radiation therapy might work; earlier studies with small numbers of heterogeneous patients may not detect small differences in outcome. New agents may be discovered that interfere with metastasis formation without necessarily being cytotoxic. An example of such a compound, modified citrus pectin, has been shown to prevent metastases in animal systems, including prostate cancer models.[56] Perioperative treatment may be valuable to disrupt the metastatic process.

Principle: In spite of suggestive experimental evidence, there is little documentation that commonly performed surgery disseminates cancer. Molecular biologic technology will open new research avenues on this topic.

PERSPECTIVE

Surgery is the dominant component of cancer diagnosis and therapy. In 1993, approximately 90% of the 1,170,000 new patients with cancer had surgery for diagnosis, primary therapy, or complications.[1] Surgery is the preferred modality for cure in 90 to 95% of patients with common solid tumors. The public is constantly seeking a "breakthrough" in the war against cancer, but the battles may not be won or lost that way. More likely, small victories accumulate over time, seemingly imperceptibly. New treatments may not always be necessary; we may only need to apply the currently available ones more safely and earlier in the disease course. Urologic cancers represent excellent examples of such a phenomenon. Bladder cancer surgery is enormously more effective and safer than 20 to 30 years ago. Perioperative mortality rates of cystectomy are 1 to 2% instead of 5 to 10% and orthotopic diversion allows earlier intervention for lethal cancers by improving rehabilitation.[57] Prostate cancer surgery in the 1990s is drastically different from that seen in the 1970s; improved surgery combined with improved detection of earlier cancers has the potential to markedly reduce cancer deaths.[58] The impact of earlier detection of small renal cancers is uncertain. Even for testis cancer, in which effective chemotherapy may be appropriately viewed as a breakthrough, surgery remains an integral part of treatment of all stages of disease.

The changes in surgery in the near future will likely come in the form of smaller operations and minimally invasive surgery. For urologic cancers, minimally invasive surgery has limited current application. However, this will gradually change as technology improves laparoscopic surgery, robotic assisted surgery, and remote site monitoring. Few centers will have the technical or personnel capabilities to undertake this research, but great strides can be taken by those with the vision and the courage to expand our field.

The evolution of surgical oncology will include a stronger emphasis on clinical outcomes. Surgeons have examined complication rates and mortality from operations for decades. The measurements used to evaluate a procedure were often not standardized and applied in a similar fashion among many types of institutions. Changes in health care delivery and funding methods will greatly accelerate the creation of "benchmark" results that hospitals and surgeons will be expected to meet. Table 5–3 lists several outcomes that will be measured by both our own hospitals and payors. Certainly the data will be surgeon-specific and possibly become public knowledge. If obtained and presented in a fair fashion, these activities will help us improve care. Clearly there will be an opportunity for misuse. As long as we all focus on the goal of improved patient care and results and not just cost issues, such scrutiny should be worthwhile. Surgical oncology, including urologists providing urologic cancer care, should provide a leadership role in the process.

Principle: Be prepared to test new ideas and challenge traditional operations for their appropriateness. An appraisal of outcomes of urologic oncology care will provide an opportunity for improved care.

TABLE 5–3. OUTCOME MEASURES FOR UROLOGIC CANCER CARE

Morbidity, mortality
Recurrence and survival rates
Readmits
Preventive care
Malpractice settlements
Complications
Infection rates
Other

REFERENCES

1. Bland KI, Karakousis CP, Amaral JF, et al: Principles of oncologic surgery and assessment of operative risk. *In* Bland KI, Karakousis CP, Copeland EM (eds): Atlas of Surgical Oncology, p 1. Philadelphia, WB Saunders Co, 1995.
2. Rosenberg SA: Principles of surgical oncology. *In* De Vita VT Jr, Hellman S, Rosenberg SA (eds): Cancer: Principles & Practice of Oncology, 4th edition, p 238. Philadelphia, JB Lippincott Co, 1993.
3. Fisher B, Redmond C, Poisson R, et al: Eight-year results of a randomized clinical trial comparing total mastectomy and lumpectomy with or without irradiation in the treatment of breast cancer. N Engl J Med 1989; 320:822.
4. Novick AC: Partial nephrectomy for renal cell carcinoma. Urology 1995; 46(2):149.
5. Martenson JA, Lipsitz SR, Lefkopoulou M, et al: Results of combined modality therapy for patients with anal cancer (E7283). Cancer 1995; 76(10):1731.
6. Sternberg CN: Organ conservation in T2-3 bladder cancer: the role of transurethral resection, partial cystectomy, and primary and adjuvant chemotherapy. World J Urol 1992; 10:2.
7. Singer PA, Tasch ES, Stocking C, et al: Sex or survival: trade-offs between quality and quantity of life. J Clin Oncol 1991; 9:328.
8. Montie JE: Counseling the patient with localized prostate cancer. Suppl Urol 1994; 43(2):36.
9. Miller GJ: New developments in grading prostate cancer. Semin Urol 1990; 8(1):9.
10. Albertsen PC, Fryback DG, Storer BE, et al: Long-term survival among men with conservatively treated localized prostate cancer. JAMA 1995; 274(8):626.
11. Wojno KJ, Epstein JI: The utility of basal cell-specific anti-cytokeratin antibody (34bE12) in the diagnosis of prostate cancer. Am J Surg Pathol 1995; 19(3):251.
12. Sidransky D, von Eschenbach A, Tsai YC, et al: Identification of p53 gene mutations in bladder cancers and urine samples. Science 1991; 251:706.
13. Esrig D, Elmajian D, Groshen S, et al: Accumulation of nuclear p53 and tumor progression in bladder cancer. N Engl J Med 1994; 331:1259.

14. Boyd J: Molecular medicine quietly comes of age. Cancer 1994; 74(8):2215.
15. Macoska JA, Trybus TM, Sakr WA, et al: Fluorescence *in situ* hybridization analysis of 8p allelic loss and chromosome 8 instability in human prostate cancer. Cancer Res 1994; 54:3824.
16. Brown JA, Alcaraz A, Takahashi S, et al: Chromosomal aneusomies detected by fluorescent in situ hybridization analysis in clinically localized prostate carcinoma. J Urol 1994; 152:1157.
17. Partin AW, Oesterling JE: The clinical usefulness of prostate specific antigen: update 1994. J Urol 1994; 152:1358.
18. Montie JE: Staging of prostate cancer current TNM classification and future prospects. Cancer Suppl 1995; 75(7): 1814.
19. Fielding LP, Fenoglio-Preiser CM, Freedman LS: The future of prognostic factors in outcome prediction for patients with cancer. Cancer 1992; 70(9):2367.
20. Burke HB, Henson DE: Criteria for prognostic factors and for an enhanced prognostic system. Cancer 1993; 72(10): 3131.
21. Simon R, Altman DG: Statistical aspects of prognostic factor studies in oncology. Br J Cancer 1994; 69:979.
22. Montie JE: Current prognostic factors for prostate cancer. Cancer 1996; 78:341.
23. Grignon DJ, Hammond EH: College of American pathologist's conference XXVI on clinical relevance of prognostic markers in solid tumors. Arch Pathol Lab Med 1995; 199: 1122–1126.
24. Wolfe HJ: Probing for prognostic markers at the cellular level: potentials and pitfalls. J Natl Cancer Inst 1992; 84(16):1226.
25. Partin AW, Yoo J, Carter HB, et al: The use of prostate specific antigen, clinical stage, and Gleason score to predict pathological stage in men with localized prostate cancer. J Urol 1993; 150:110.
26. Snow PB, Smith DS, Catalona WJ: Artificial neural network in the diagnosis and prognosis of prostate cancer: a pilot study. J Urol 1994; 152:1923.
27. Kornblith AB, Herr HW, Ofman US, et al: Quality of life of patients with prostate cancer and their spouses. Cancer 1994; 73(11):2791.
28. Bjerre BD, Johansen C, Steven K: Health-related quality of life after cystectomy: bladder substitution compared with ileal conduit diversion. A questionnaire survey. Br J Urol 1995; 75:200.
29. Jonler M, Messing EM, Rhodes PR, et al: Sequelae of radical prostatectomy. Br J Urol 1994; 74:352.
30. Litwin MS, Hays RD, Fink A, et al: Quality-of-life outcomes in men treated for localized prostate cancer. JAMA 1995; 273(2):129.
31. Steiner MS, Morton RA, Walsh PC: Impact of anatomical radical prostatectomy on urinary continence. J Urol 1991; 145:512.
32. Gill TM, Feinstein AR: A critical appraisal of the quality of quality-of-life measurements. JAMA 1994; 272(8):619.
33. Osoba D: Lessons learned from measuring health-related quality of life in oncology. J Clin Oncol 1994; 12(3):608.
34. Donahue JP (ed): Lymph Node Surgery in Urology. Oxford, UK, Isis Medical Media, 1995.
35. Donahue JP (ed): Role of lymph node dissection in urological cancer. *In* Lymph Node Surgery in Urology. Oxford, UK, Isis Medical Media, 1995.
36. Fisher ER, Swamidoss S, Lee CH, et al: Detection and significance of occult axillary node metastases in patients with invasive breast cancer. Cancer 1978; 42(4):2025.
37. Gomella LG, White JL, McCue PA, et al: Screening for occult nodal metastasis in localized carcinoma of the prostate. J Urol 1993; 149:776.
38. Moul JW, Lewis DJ, Ross AA, et al: Immunohistologic detection of prostate cancer pelvic lymph node micrometastases: correlation to preoperative serum prostate-specific antigen. Urology 1994; 43(1):68.
39. Lerner SP, Skinner DG, Lieskovsky G, et al: The rationale for en bloc pelvic lymph node dissection for bladder cancer patients with nodal metastases: long-term results. J Urol 1993; 149:758.
40. Partin AW, Pound CR, Clemens JQ, et al: Serum PSA after anatomic radical prostatectomy. Urol Clin North Am 1993; 20(4):713.
41. Shipley WU, Kaufman DS, Heney NM: Can chemo-radiotherapy plus transurethral tumor resection make cystectomy unnecessary for invasive bladder cancer? Oncology 1990; 4(7):25.
42. Kaufman DS, Shipley WU, Griffins PP, et al: Selective bladder preservation by combination treatment of invasive bladder cancer. N Engl J Med 1993; 329(19):1377.
43. Given RW, Parsons JT, McCarley D, et al: Bladder-sparing multimodality treatment of muscle-invasive bladder cancer: a five-year follow-up. Urology 1995; 46(4):499.
44. Fisher B, Mamaunas EP: Preoperative chemotherapy: a model for studying the biology and therapy of primary breast cancer. J Clin Oncol 1995; 13(3):537.
45. Donahue JP, Thornhill JA, Foster RS, et al: The role of retroperitoneal lymphadenectomy in clinical stage B testis cancer: the Indiana University experience (1965 to 1989). J Urol 1995; 153:85.
46. Bennett RT, Lerner SE, Taub HC, et al: Cytoreductive surgery for stage IV renal cell carcinoma. J Urol 1995; 154:32.
47. Fox EP, Weathers TD, Williams SD, et al: Outcome analysis for patients with persistent nonteratomatous germ cell tumor in postchemotherapy retroperitoneal lymph node dissections. J Clin Oncol 1993; 11(7):1294.
48. van der Berg MEL, van Lent M, Buyse M, et al: The effect of debulking surgery after induction chemotherapy on the prognosis in advanced epithelial ovarian cancer. N Engl J Med 1995; 332:629.
49. Montie JE: Follow-up after cystectomy for carcinoma of the bladder. Urol Clin North Am 1994; 21(4):639.
50. Resnick M: Evaluation and management of recurrent malignant disease. Urol Clin North Am 1994; 21(4):xiii.
51. Montie JE: Follow-up after radical prostatectomy or radiation therapy for prostate cancer. Urol Clin North Am 1994; 21(4):673.
52. Cole WH, McDonald GO, Roberts SS, et al: Dissemination of Cancer. New York, Appleton-Century-Crofts, Inc, 1961.
53. Seiden MV, Kantoff PW, Krithivas K, et al: Detection of circulating tumor cells in men with localized prostate cancer. J Clin Oncol 1994; 12(12):2634.
54. Cama C, Olsson CA, Raffo AJ, et al: Molecular staging of prostate cancer. II. A comparison of the application of an enhanced reverse transcriptase polymerase chain reaction assay for prostate specific antigen versus prostate specific membrane antigen. J Urol 1995; 153:1373.
55. Oefelein MG, Kaul K, Herz B, et al: Molecular detection of prostate epithelial cells from the surgical field and peripheral circulation during radical prostatectomy. J Urol 1996; 155:238.
56. Pienta KJ, Naik H, Akhtar A, et al: Inhibition of spontaneous metastasis in a rat prostate cancer model by oral administration of modified citrus pectin. J Natl Cancer Inst 1995; 87(5):348.
57. Montie JE, Pavone-Macaluso M, Tazaki H, et al: What are the risks of cystectomy and the advances in perioperative care? Int J Urol 1995; 2(Suppl 2):89.
58. Zincke H, Bergstrahl EJ, Blute ML, et al: Radical prostatectomy for clinically localized prostate cancer: long-term results of 1,143 patients from a single institution. J Clin Oncol 1994; 12(11):2254.

6

THE RATIONALE FOR THE USE OF RADIATION THERAPY IN THE TREATMENT OF UROLOGIC MALIGNANCIES

IRA J. SPIRO, M.D., PH.D. *and* WILLIAM U. SHIPLEY, M.D.

A successful cancer therapy should render the patient free of local, regional, and distant disease. This therapy should have minimal morbidity and maintain pretreatment functional status. Local therapy alone may be sufficient for patients with very early stage disease. Conversely, patients with advanced but localized cancer are more frequently treated with multiple modalities, often combining surgery, radiation, and chemotherapy. One important advantage of radiation is that it can include major vessels, nerves, connective tissues, and hollow viscera with relatively low risk of producing complications, thus improving functional and cosmetic outcome.

The optimal use of radiation, whether used as a sole treatment modality or as a part of a multimodality program, requires an understanding of the action of radiation from the physical level to the whole-organ level. Generally, there are two strategies to enhance the efficacy of radiation therapy. These include (1) improving the physical dose distribution so as to increase dose in the tumor relative to normal tissues and (2) increase the differential response to radiation between tumors and normal tissues. The former strategy relates to physical parameters, while the latter pertains to biologic considerations.

PHYSICAL ASPECTS OF RADIATION THERAPY

In modern practice, radiation therapy is delivered using linear accelerators. Pelvic tumors are most often treated with equipment capable of delivering beam energies in the range of 10 to 25 MV x-rays. These beams offer the relative advantage of lower surface doses with increased dose at a given depth in tissue, compared to older lower energy equipment. At these high energies, beams also offer sharp lateral field edges with rapid dose fall-off. This characteristic allows for less irradiation of nontarget tissues. Isocentric gantries and patient couches capable of a multitude of movement options allow for an almost infinite choice of beam portals incident on the patient. The ultimate choice of beam energy and treatment technique is based on delivering the highest feasible concentration of dose in the target volume (i.e., the volume judged to contain cancer cells) while minimizing dose to normal tissues. To realize this goal, sophisticated high-speed computers plan treatment in three dimensions, using anatomic information obtained from computed tomography (CT) and/or magnetic resonance imaging (MRI).[1,2] In addition, computer-controlled dynamic treatment systems allow for gantry, collimator (i.e., field borders), and couch movement during the actual treatment. In this manner, the high-dose treatment volume is able to conform more accurately to the target volume. Other modern advances include "on-line" portal imaging systems, which allow for instant verification of the radiation treatment field. Modern radiation oncology is increasingly making use of improved patient immobilization devices.

In addition to conventional external beam irradiation, other specialized modalities are available for the treatment of urologic malignancies. These include the use of brachytherapy (Greek *brachy*, short) implant techniques. This type of treatment has been pursued in prostate cancer therapy[3,4] and more recently has gained a resurgence in interest.[5] In general, temporarily dwelling hollow catheters can be placed at the time of surgery or under ultrasound or CT guidance and remotely loaded with radioactive sources at a later time. These techniques allow for high doses of radiation to be delivered to relatively small volumes of tissue. Brachytherapy became available in the early part of this century, soon after radioactive isotopes were discovered. In addition to brachytherapy, there has also been interest in the use of charged-particle (mostly proton) accelerators, which are available at a small number of institutions.[6,7]

BIOLOGIC AND GENETIC CONSIDERATIONS

The target for radiation-induced lethality in tumor cells is DNA. Unrepaired or misrepaired double-strand breaks or DNA base damage presumably leads to cell killing. In addition, a number of factors alter the response of tumor cells and normal tissues to radiation. These include but are not limited to (1) the inherent radiosensitivity of the cells in question, (2) the capacity of these cells to repair radiation damage, (3) the oxygen and nutrient status of the tumor, (4) the position of an individual cell in the cell cycle, and (5) the capacity for repopulation. In order to improve the therapeutic differential between tumor cells and normal tissues, radiation treatments are given as a series of equal-sized fractions over a number of weeks, in part exploiting these factors.

It is poorly understood why some cells such as seminoma are exquisitely sensitive to radiation while renal carcinoma cells require higher doses for control or why not all patients with a given histology show equal sensitivity. Clearly, genetic factors must play a role in determining the response of cells to radiation, although the molecular basis for these differences is not yet understood. Recently, there has been wider recognition of the process of programmed cell death or apoptosis.[8] This process of cell death is not linked to mitosis and was first appreciated in lymphocytes, although now it is known to occur to varying degrees in normal and tumor tissues. Of interest, the normal p53 gene has been shown to be required for this process.[9] Tumor cells with mutant p53 alleles or lacking a normal p53 allele may therefore be more resistant to cell killing if this process is not functioning.[10]

For the most part, both normal tissues and tumor cells are capable of repair between doses of radiation. Normal tissues may possess greater capacity for repair, although they may require more time to do so. Therefore, spacing radiation fractions by at least 6 hours (usually 24 hours) may provide a greater advantage to normal tissues. Even small therapeutic gains, when exponentially expanded over a course of treatment, can become highly significant. Cells also vary considerably in their radiosensitivity depending on their position in the mitotic cycle. S-phase cells are most radioresistant, while cells in late G_2 and mitosis at the time of irradiation are most sensitive.[11] A dose of 200 cGy (1 cGy = 1 rad) will eradicate tumor cells in the most sensitive phases of the cycle, preferentially leaving cells in resistant phases. If another dose of radiation is given 24 hours later, some of the cells in resistant phases of the cycle will have moved to more sensitive ones. Late-responding normal tissues, which are not actively cycling, will be preferentially spared by this effect.

The absence of molecular oxygen is an effective radioprotector, and tumor cells at low oxygen tensions are relatively resistant to radiation.[12] This phenomenon can occur because tumor cells can outgrow their blood supplies. As well-oxygenated radiosensitive cells within a tumor are killed off, hypoxic cells in the tumor may reoxygenate over time. Fractionated radiotherapy would therefore be more beneficial to normal, well-oxygenated tissues. Repopulation occurs in acutely responding normal tissue, such as the gut epithelium, but also occurs in tumors. Moreover, a therapeutic advantage would occur if the rate of repopulation was more rapid in normal tissues than in tumors. In general, it is best to deliver a course of radiation in the shortest possible period of time that will be tolerated by acutely responding normal tissues. Treatment delays beyond this time, due to radiotherapy toxicity or elective breaks, will favor tumor proliferation.

DOSE-RESPONSE RELATIONSHIPS IN RADIATION THERAPY

The relationship between radiation dose and tumor control probability is shown in Figure 6–1. The

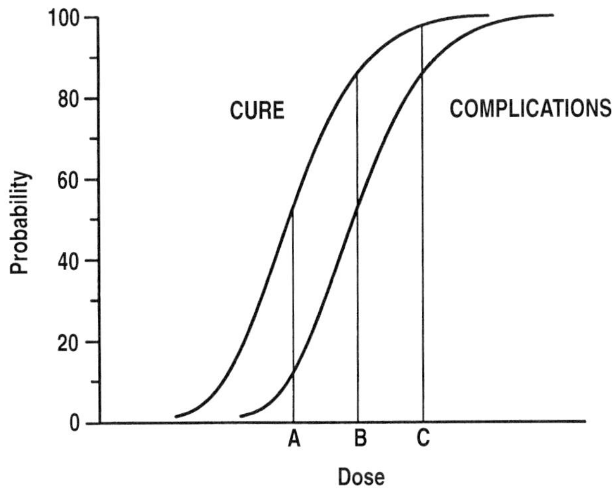
100
80
60
40
20
0
Probability
CURE
COMPLICATIONS
A
B
C
Dose

FIGURE 6–1. The probability of tumor cure or complications versus dose. Doses that produce no complications achieve low cure rates (dose *A*). Doses that achieve high levels of cure produce unacceptably high complication rates (dose *C*).

delivery of the physical dose to the tumor is controlled by the physical factors discussed above, while the shape of the curve is determined by the biologic factors. Normal tissues also display similar sigmoidal dose-response curves, although fractionated therapy generally places this curve to the right of the tumor curve. At doses that produce no level of complications, cure rates are low (e.g., Fig. 6–1, dose *A*) while tumor doses that produce greater than 90% cure rates may produce unacceptable morbidity (e.g., Fig. 6–1, dose C). In general, intermediate doses are chosen so that the benefits and risks of therapy are well balanced (dose B).

The precise number of cells in a tumor that need to be inactivated is also a critical determinant of the probability of tumor cure. For example, if a tumor contains 10^8 clonogenic cells and a dose of 180 cGy (or 1.8 Gy) reduces survival by 50%, then 30 fractions of 2 Gy would reduce survival to 9×10^{-10}. The probability of control would be given by:

$$P_{\text{control}} = \text{e-(cell number* surviving fraction)}$$

$$= \text{e-}(10^8 * 9 \times 10^{-10})$$

$$= 0.91 \text{ or } 91\%$$

Such an analogy could be made to the small burden of bladder tumor cells remaining after a complete transurethral resection of the bladder (TURB). If the cell number were to increase from 10^8 clonogenic cells to 1×10^9, or approximately 1 g, then the probability of cure would decrease to:

$$P_{\text{control}} = \text{e-}(1 \times 10^9 * 9 \times 10^{-10})$$

$$= 0.41 \text{ or } 41\%$$

To achieve the same probability of control, an additional three fractions would have to be delivered.

IMPLICATIONS FOR THE FUTURE

Various strategies for increasing the therapeutic gain of radiation treatment have been recommended. These include judicious use of combined-modality therapy. Surgery is effective in removing bulk disease, but it would be expected to have a lower therapeutic index for subclinical disease. At doses that produce acceptable normal tissue injury, radiotherapy is effective at eliminating small tumors and subclinical disease. Combinations of these local treatments can produce better locoregional control. Similarly, combined chemotherapy and radiation therapy would improve local control rates if chemotherapy against transitional cell cancers[13,14] or androgen suppression of localized prostate cancer[15,16] could kill cells resistant to radiation or further sensitize cells to radiation.

Altered radiation fractionation schemes, which deliver more than one treatment a day with a 4- to 6-hour interfraction interval, are being investigated. Such programs may produce an additional benefit for normal tissues and reduce repopulation of tumor cells during the course of therapy. Strategies that reduce the hypoxic cell burden in a tumor are also being investigated. These include the use of perfluorocarbons and carbogen as oxygen substitutes, and the use of hypoxic cell sensitizers. Normal tissue protection is another means for improving therapeutic gain. Sulfhydryl-containing compounds are able to scavenge the hydroxyl radicals produced by radiation, which are thought to mediate radiation injury. Unfortunately, to date both radioprotectors and hypoxic cell sensitizers have proven to be toxic with limited improvement over conventional treatment. Both areas remain fertile for future research.

Predictive assays, which seek to characterize tumor cells in vitro in terms of radiation response, chemotherapy response, tumor characteristics such as apoptotic fraction, ploidy, genetic polymorphisms, oncogene or suppresser gene expression, oxygen status, growth fraction, and potential doubling time, would allow for therapy selected to the individual patient. Until these factors are studied prospectively, their promise remains unproven. One of the more exciting research developments in cancer therapy is the potential of gene therapy.[17] It will become possible to target genes to cancer cells that would alter their response to chemotherapy, radiotherapy, or ultimately their metastatic potential and cancerous genotype. In addition, such genetic alteration may allow for the restoration of apoptotic death in cells that have lost this capacity. The challenge remains to selectively target genes or antibodies to all clonogenic cancer cells. Recently, it has been shown that a tumor necrosis factor gene, under the control of a promoter/enhancer that is activated by radiation, has efficacy in a human tumor grown in animals.[18] These approaches hold promise for cancer research and therapy over the next 10 years.

REFERENCES

1. Sandler HM, Perez-Tamayo C, Ten Haken RK, Lichter AS: Dose escalation for stage C(T3) prostate cancer: minimal rectal toxicity observed using conformal therapy. Radiother Oncol 1992; 23:53–54.
2. Leibel SA, Heimann R, Kitcher GJ, et al: Three-dimensional conformal radiation therapy in locally advanced carcinoma of the prostate: preliminary results of a phase I dose escalation study. Int J Radiat Oncol Biol Phys 1993; 28: 55–65.
3. Whitmore WF, Hilaris B, Grabstald H: Retropubic implantation of iodine 125 in the treatment of prostatic cancer. J Urol 1972; 108:918.
4. DeLaney TF, Shipley WU, O'Leary MP, et al: Preoperative irradiation, lymphadenectomy and iodine 125 implantation for patients with localized carcinoma of the prostate. Int J Radiat Oncol Biol Phys 1986; 12:1779–1785.

5. Blasko JC, Grimm PD, Radge H: Brachytherapy and organ preservation in the management of carcinoma of the prostate. Semin Radiat Oncol 1993; 3:240–249.
6. Shipley WU, Tepper JE, Prout GR Jr, et al: Proton radiation as boost therapy in patients irradiated for localized prostatic cancer. JAMA 1979; 241:1912–1915.
7. Shipley WU, Verhey LJ, Munzenrider JE, et al: Advanced prostate cancer: the results of randomized comparative trial of high dose irradiation boosting with conformal protons compared with conventional dose irradiation using photons alone. Int J Radiat Oncol Biol Phys 1995; 32:3–12.
8. Lane DP: A death in the life of p53. Nature 1993; 362: 786–787.
9. Clarke AR, Purdie CA, Harrison DJ, et al: Thymocyte apoptosis induced by p53-dependent and independent pathways. Nature 1993; 362:849–852.
10. Lowe SW, Bodis S, McClatchey A, et al: p53 Status and the efficacy of cancer therapy in vivo. Science 1994; 266:807–810.
11. Terasima R, Tolmach LJ: X-ray sensitivity and DNA synthesis in synchronous populations of HeLa cells. Science 1963; 140:490–492.
12. Spiro IJ, Ling CC, Stickler R, Gaskill J: Oxygen radiosensitization at low dose rate. Br J Radiol 1985; 58:357–363.
13. Kaufman DS, Shipley WU, Griffin PP, et al: Selective preservation by combination treatment of invasive bladder cancer. N Engl J Med 1993; 329:1377–1382.
14. Koiso K, Shipley WU, Keuppen S, et al: The status of bladder preserving therapeutic strategies in the management of patients with mucle invasive bladder cancer. Int J Urol 1995; 2(Suppl 2):49–57.
15. Pilepich MV, Krall JM, Al-Sarraf M, et al: Androgen suppression with radiation therapy compared with radiation therapy alone for locally advanced prostatic carcinoma. A randomized comparative trial of the Radiation Therapy Oncology Group. Urology 1995; 45:616–623.
16. Nakfoor BM, Prince EA, Shipley WU, Zietman AL: A randomized trial comparing local tumor control following irradiation alone versus combined androgen withdrawal and irradiation in an androgen sensitive prostate cancer xenograft (Abstract). Int J Radiat Oncol Biol Phys 1995; 32(Suppl 1):189.
17. Blau HM, Springer ML: Gene therapy—a novel form of drug delivery. N Engl J Med 1995; 333(18):1204–1207.
18. Weichselbaum RR, Hallahan DE, Beckett MA, et al: Gene therapy targeted by radiation preferentially radiosensitizes tumor cells. Cancer Res 1994; 54:4266–4269.

7

GENERAL PRINCIPLES OF CHEMOTHERAPY

HOWARD I. SCHER, M.D. *and* PAUL SABBATINI, M.D.

The efficacy of specific chemotherapeutic agents or combinations varies for the tumors that develop in the urogenital tract. These range from highly curable testis cancers to refractory renal cell carcinomas. As such, the aims of ongoing developmental strategies differ. In testis cancer, the aim is to maximize the cure proportion while minimizing long-term toxicity; for renal cell carcinoma, it is to find approaches with efficacy upon which to build. Yet, even for tumors for which effective therapies are available, many patients still die from disease. In these situations, drug development has focused on identifying specific prognostic groups so that patients who are destined to do poorly are offered novel strategies. In many cases, chemotherapy is integrated into a combined-modality approach with the aim of achieving a complete response as initial treatment (neoadjuvant therapy) or as a systemic approach in patients with a high risk of relapse after primary local treatment (adjuvant therapy).

DRUG DEVELOPMENT

A large number of compounds are screened for antitumor activity each year but only a small fraction proceed to clinical testing. One screen performed by the National Cancer Institute and many pharmaceutical houses measured the activity against the P388 and L1210 murine leukemia models. With improvements in cell culture techniques and the availability of robotics, an ever-increasing number of compounds can be rapidly screened against a panel of human tumor cell lines,[1,2] or for their effects on specific genes or gene products. Agents with in vitro activity are then tested in nude mice xenograft systems implanted with human tumor cell lines. Pharmacokinetic data are used to estimate a starting dose for investigation, and toxicity profiles evaluated in at least two animal species prior to human trials.[3]

Clinical testing generally begins with a phase I trial that seeks to assess safety and the determination of a dose for disease-specific phase II investigations. The traditional end-point is the maximally tolerated dose (MTD) based on normal tissue tolerance. However, as the target specificity of compounds improves, and with the extension of trials into the areas of prevention and differentiation, more studies are focusing on the optimal biologic dose to the tumor rather than on toxicity of the host as the end-point. Dose escalation traditionally follows one of several predetermined schemes until the MTD is reached. New methodologies have been proposed that base dose escalation on pharmacokinetic data in the hopes of accelerating the process.[3,4] The decision to proceed to phase II testing is based on the anticipated efficacy from preclinical studies in conjunction with safety profiles and pharmacologic data from phase I trials. Antitumor activity is not formally evaluated in phase I trials and should not affect the decision to proceed. Phase II trials are designed to estimate efficacy in particular tumor types. These trials require measurable disease or an established surrogate to evaluate response. Urogenital tumors vary in the ease with which response may be assessed. Renal cell carcinomas, which frequently present with bidimensionally measurable tumor masses, can be evaluated by serial radiographs or computed tomography (CT) scans. Prostate cancer, where metastasies are typically limited to bone, is difficult to assess in an objective, quantifiable, and reproducible way using serial bone scintigraphy scans.[5] The methods of Fleming or Gehan are commonly used to determine sample size.[6,7] Using the scheme proposed by Gehan, phase II trials are set to accrue and evaluate 14 patients. If no response is observed, the trial is terminated because, based on this sample size, one can conclude that the true response rate does not exceed 20% with 95% confidence.[7] A larger number of patients are needed for more precise estimates of antitumor activity. Agents with activity in single-drug phase II trials that have nonoverlapping toxicity profiles can be given in full doses and be combined in multidrug regimens. The value of combination regimens can only be proven in randomized phase III studies to compare the investigational treatment with a standard (control) arm. These trials must be of sufficient size to detect the often small differences between a standard and novel treatment. The outcomes of phase III testing increasingly include not only efficacy but quality-of-life and cost-effectiveness analysis as end-points.

CLASSIC MODELS AND CHEMOTHERAPY

The development of combination regimens with antineoplastic agents has been based in part on an evolving understanding of tumor kinetics. Nearly 20 years ago, Skipper performed classic experiments with L1210 mouse leukemia cell lines and proposed several principles regarding cancer chemotherapy.[8,9] They observed that L1210 leukemia in BDF_1 or DBA mice grows exponentially from implantation. The doubling time, as well as the fraction of cells killed when treated with a specific chemotherapeutic agent, was constant and independent of initial tumor size. This log-kill model assumed all cells were in cycle and dividing. Furthermore, since tumor cell kill followed first-order kinetics, it was possible to calculate and demonstrate cure probabilities in the cell lines experimentally. Unfortunately, this simple model did not support the clinical observations with most solid tumors.

Rather than the straight-line growth on a semilog plot, solid tumor growth curves typically follow a sigmoid pattern termed "gompertzian."[10,11] This curve takes into account that net tumor growth is a combination of dividing (G_1), quiescent (G_0), and actively dying cells. This concept of a partial proliferative or growth fraction was initially theorized by Mendelsohn in 1960.[12] The importance of gompertzian growth in describing the failure and success of anticancer chemotherapy in a quantitative sense is the focus of the Norton-Simon hypothesis.[13] This model addresses the paradoxical findings of failure to cure small-volume tumors, while rapid regression is seen in larger tumors. It suggests that survival can only be improved by eliminating all cells so that rapid regrowth cannot occur or by preventing the regrowth of resistant cells by inducing differentiation or immunity, or other novel strategies. It also provides a basis for the treatment scheme that uses sequential therapies at high doses to attack the remaining cells after an initially effective therapy has been employed against large-volume disease.[14]

Conceptually, the lower end of the sigmoid gompertzian curve represents the smallest tumors, with the largest growth fraction, presumed to be related to their optimal access to oxygen and nutrients. This next portion of the curve is flat, since the total number of cells are small and despite high proliferation rates, the overall increase in tumor size is small. The upper end of the curve also flattens as the number of necrotic and anoxic cells increases, while the middle portion describes a period of the greatest overall increase in tumor burden. In terms of response, effective chemotherapy applied to a tumor growing in a gompertzian fashion evokes a response that is proportionally related to the growth rate of the tumor prior to treatment.[15,16] The Norton-Simon hypothesis supports the observation of Skipper-Schabel that the rate of response is proportional to the rate of growth, and considers that the regrowth that occurs after treatment is appropriate for a tumor of that size along the growth curve. The greater fractional cell kill in the early period is compensated for by greater fractional growth. The distinction between the Skipper-Schabel model and the Norton-Simon hypothesis is that in gompertzian growth, unlike exponential growth, the growth rate of the tumor is changing. This changing growth rate, which is greatest at the smallest tumor volume, should correlate with changes in overall response rates at different tumor volumes.

TUMOR KINETICS: THE BASIS FOR DOSE INTENSIFICATION

In vitro studies of many chemotherapeutic agents show a steep dose-response curve such that a continued increase in dose parallels an increase in regression or cell kill.[17] The slope of the dose versus cell kill curve varies with the agent used and plateaus in some instances. Figure 7–1 illustrates the hypothetical relationship between administered dose (x axis), response proportion (*X*), and toxicity (*O*) for an agent. As shown, there is a threshold dose of 6 mg/m^2 below which no significant responses are observed. The response proportion reaches a maximum at a dose of 17 mg/m^2 beyond which no further increase in response is noted. Also shown is the relationship between dose and toxicity in which no plateau is observed with increasing doses. Continued increases in dose with this agent beyond the ceiling for response would add toxicity with no increase in efficacy.

Dose intensity is defined as the amount of drug given per unit of time and is generally expressed as milligrams per square meter per week.[18] Dose intensity may be increased either by increasing the total dose of drug, which is termed "dose escalation," or by reducing the time interval between doses, which has been termed "dose density."[19] Dose escalation attempts to exploit the dose-response relationship. If an agent has a plateau in

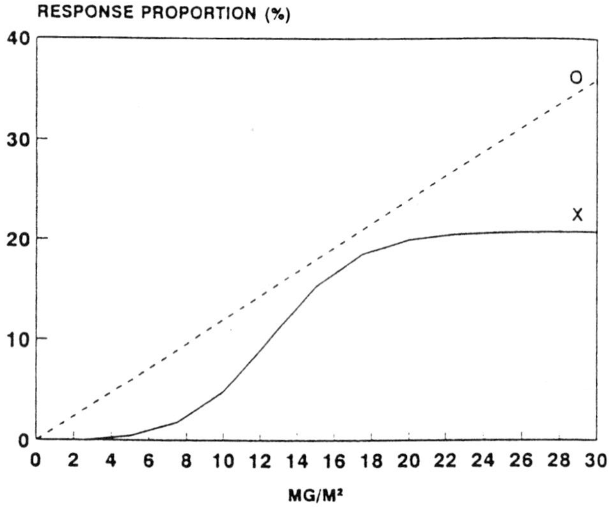
RESPONSE PROPORTION (%)
40
30
20
10
0
O
X
0 2 4 6 8 10 12 14 16 18 20 22 24 26 28 30
MG/M²

FIGURE 7–1. The relationship between dose (x axis), response proportion (*X*), and toxicity (*O*). Note the plateau in response with a linear increase in toxicity. See text for discussion. (Modified from Scher HI, Norton L: Chemotherapy for urothelial tract malignancies: breaking the deadlock. Semin Surg Oncol 1992; 8:316–341. Reprinted by permission of John Wiley & Sons, Inc.)

the dose-response curve, using the gompertzian growth model where the greater fractional cell kill occurs early when the growth rate is most rapid, a dose-dense therapy (more frequent) has the potential to be more advantageous than using simple dose escalation to increase dose intensity. The rapid recycling provides additional fractional cell kill before regrowth occurs. The theoretical impact of a more and less dose-dense therapy is illustrated in Figure 7–2.

The development of recombinant hematopoietic growth factors as well as bone marrow and peripheral blood stem cell support technology have permitted significant increases of dose intensity in vivo.[20] In general, dose intensification is accomplished with combinations of alkylating agents,

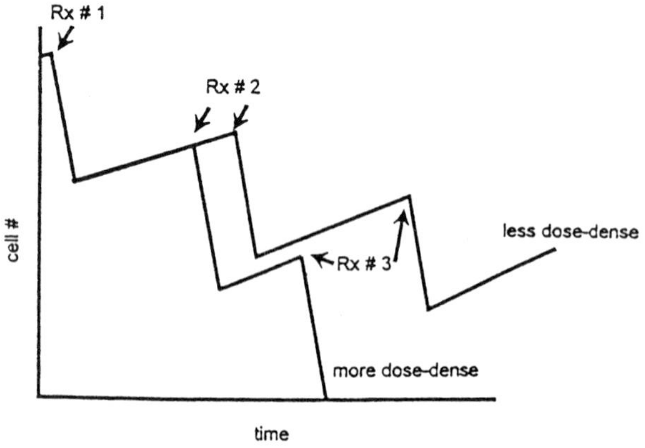
Rx # 1
Rx # 2
Rx # 3
less dose-dense
more dose-dense
cell #
time

FIGURE 7–2. The theoretical advantage in increasing dose density as a means of increasing dose intensity for a tumor with gompertzian growth. See text for discussion. (Modified from Hudis C: New approaches to adjuvant chemotherapy for breast cancer. Pharmacotherapy 1995; 16:88S–93S, with permission.)

since most of their serious nonhematologic side effects do not occur at myeloablative doses and their dose-response curve is steep.[21] High-dose chemotherapy is now widely used in selected patients with acute leukemia, non-Hodgkin's lymphoma, and multiple myeloma.[22,23] The concept of dose escalation has also been tested in several genitourinary tumors.

Dose-intensive therapy with carboplatin, etoposide, and cyclophosphamide followed by peripheral blood stem cell support has been shown to result in long-term survival for 20 to 30% of germ cell tumor patients who are refractory to standard cisplatin therapy and would otherwise die of their disease.[24] The greatest improvement in disease-free survival occurred in patients with poor prognostic features who were transplanted early with a minimal disease burden. This observation has prompted the consideration of applying high-dose chemotherapy as front-line therapy in patients destined to do poorly with standard dose regimens. Randomized phase III studies are ongoing to evaluate this concept.

The success in treating germ cell tumors with high-dose therapy has not been duplicated in other genitourinary malignancies. Several trials explored modest increases in dose intensity in bladder cancer. Seidman et al. reported a study in which drug delivery was increased by 33% over standard methotrexate, vinblastine, doxorubicin, and cisplatin (M-VAC) with granulocyte colony-stimulating factor (G-CSF) support. Further increases in drug doses did not increase dose intensity, as hematologic toxicities and febrile neutropenia necessitated a delay in recycling intervals.[25] Steinberg et al. achieved a dose intensity of 1.95 times that of standard M-VAC with granulocyte-macrophage colony-stimulating factor (GM-CSF) support. The major response rate (70%) and complete response proportion (30%) were similar to standard M-VAC.[26,27] Thus, modest increases in dose intensity in vivo did not appear to improve outcomes.

A previous phase I trial established the maximum tolerated dose of cyclophosphamide that could be administered using GM-CSF without autologous bone marrow transplantation.[28] Phase II testing recently confirmed the feasibility of using dose-escalated cyclophosphamide with doxorubicin and GM-CSF in a cohort of patients with hormone-resistant prostate cancer. This trial showed that patients who showed significant posttherapy declines in prostate-specific antigen (PSA) had a longer median survival than nonresponders (23 versus 7 months). The overall median survival was similar to that of historical controls.[29] Other regimens with conventional dosing, such as estramusine with vinblastine, have shown similar response rates.[29a] A randomized trial is required to draw specific conclusions regarding survival data.

The role of dose-intensive chemotherapy in the treatment of metastatic genitourinary tumors other than germ cell neoplasms remains investigational. The failure to show a benefit in other urogenital tumors demonstrates that it is crucial to have sufficiently effective therapies to dose escalate if a benefit is to be observed.

In addition to kinetic considerations, intrinsic and acquired drug resistance are critical factors that contribute to treatment failure. A mathematical model proposed by Goldie and Coldman related the drug sensitivity of a tumor to its spontaneous mutation rate towards phenotypic drug resistance.[30] It is based on the assumption that all tumors have an intrinsic probability of mutation with each cell division. The model was later expanded to include multiple sublines in a given tumor with varied mutation rates and drug sensitivities.[31] This would suggest that the goal of treatment should be to reduce the total number of cells as rapidly as possible to prevent the development of increasing resistance over time. A strategy to exploit this would be to use all possible effective drugs early in treatment to prevent cells already resistant to one drug from mutating to resistance to others. If drugs have overlapping toxicity, this model suggests using an alternating rather than sequential sequence to provide the broadest early exposure of all cells to sensitive drugs. Translation of the model to clinical use has not been straightforward and alternately therapy has not been shown superior to sequential therapy in terms of overall survival in several diseases including Hodgkin's disease and most recently in the adjuvant treatment of high-risk breast cancer. Advocates of the model point out that alternating regimens have not proven superior because the regimens were not of equal efficacy and not truly cross resistant.[32,33] The notion of very early (within 36 hours of surgery) versus conventional (within 32 days of surgery) adjuvant chemotherapy has also been addressed in breast cancer with no overall difference in survival between the timing of the two treatments.[34]

The kinetic models outlined can explain some biologic observations. Each is dependent, however, on certain assumptions that are not present in all tumor types. These and other theoretical models to date are not subject to simple interpretations when viewed in light of clinical experience.

ANTINEOPLASTIC AGENTS

The standard combination chemotherapy regimens used in genitourinary malignancies encompass a surprisingly limited number of drug classes and agents, which are listed in Table 7–1 with common toxicities.[35,36]

DRUG RESISTANCE

Resistance to the drugs used in the treatment of genitourinary cancers, whether intrinsic or acquired, remains a significant obstacle to improved survival. Clinical drug resistance may occur at the host, tumor, and cellular levels.[37] Examples of potential mechanisms are illustrated in Table 7–2.

The possibility for achieving inadequate tumoricidal doses due to host factors is of obvious importance and may be determined by dose-limiting toxicity of drugs or varied drug metabolism between patients. The contribution of host factors to this type of drug resistance is sometimes modifiable, such as the reduction in hematologic toxicity with growth colony-stimulating factors or by the biochemical modulation of 5-fluorouracil.[38,39] The impact of tumor factors on drug resistance is more difficult to characterize. The aberrant nature of tumor blood vessels and altered flow patterns create physical barriers to therapeutic agent delivery in solid tumors. This microenvironment cannot be duplicated in vitro and animal models that bear smaller tumor burdens do not necessarily reflect the human condition.[40] The interstitium in tumor cells may also have different characteristics. For example, changes in extracellular pH have been shown to increase the cytotoxicity of cisplatin while reducing the activity of doxorubicin and vinca alkaloids.[41]

The most significant increases in our understanding of drug resistance have occurred at the cellular level. Cells may have altered intake or efflux of drugs, abnormal intracellular activation or degradation, or an inability to repair a lethal insult.[42] When exposed to a single agent, many tumors acquire a resistance to a number of unrelated drugs in a simultaneous characteristic fashion. One mechanism for this multiple-drug-resistant phenotype is related to the product of the MDR-1 (multidrug-resistance) gene. This gene encodes a 170-kDa p-glycoprotein that is localized on the cell membrane and functions as an energy-dependent drug efflux pump. Cross-resistance occurs between the plant alkaloids, anthracyclines, actinomycin D, colchicine, mitomycin C, and etoposide in part by this mechanism, which results in reduced intracellular concentrations.[43–46] This p-glycoprotein is normally distributed in areas where detoxification occurs, such as the gastrointestinal tract, kidney, and bile ducts.[47,48] The expression of the MDR-1 gene product on the endothelial cells of the brain and testis is believed to explain why the sites function as pharmacologic sanctuaries; to which drug delivery is poor.[49] MDR-1 mRNA and expression is low in untreated bladder and germ cell tumors, but high in refractory relapsed disease. In contrast, untreated renal cell carcinomas show high expression consistent with the intrinsic resistance to treatment.[49,51] It is important to note that MDR-1 is not the sole mechanism of resistance to agents that are transported by p-glycoprotein. Anthracyclines and other compounds inhibit topoisomerase II, for example, which causes a spectrum of resistance that overlaps with the MDR-1 substrates and is often termed

TABLE 7–1. STANDARD ANTINEOPLASTIC AGENTS, REGIMENS, AND TOXICITIES*

Class	Drug	Major Mechanism	Regimen	Indication	Major Toxicity	Special Comment
Antimetabolite	Methrotrexate	Inhibits dihydrofolate reductase	M-VAC	Bladder tumor	Mucositis, diarrhea, bone marrow	Accumulates in effusions, leucovorin lessens toxicity
	Fluorouracil	Inhibition of thymidylate synthase	Single agent, with leucovorin	Salvage bladder tumor	Bone marrow, diarrhea, mucositis, hand-foot dermatitis	Diarrhea may be profuse and life threatening
Alkylating agent	Ifosfamide	Binds and cross links DNA	VIP, VeIP, single agent, with paclitaxel	Salvage germ cell, salvage bladder tumor	Hemorrhagic cycstitis, CNS depression, N/V, bone marrow	Mesna acts as urothelial protective agent
Antitumor antibiotics	Bleomycin	Single-strand DNA breaks	BEP, PVB	Germ cell tumor	Fever, pulmonary fibrosis, skin reactions	Rare anaphylaxis
Anthracyclines	Doxorubicin	Intercalation and alteration of DNA topology	M-VAC, with ketoconazole, single agent, CAP	Bladder, prostate, germ cell tumor	Alopecia, N/V, bone marrow, mucositis, cardiac	Vessicant, radiation recall dermatitis
Vinca alkaloids	Vinblastine	Binds tubulin, microtubule disruption	PVB, VIP	Germ cell tumor	Bone marrow, neuropathy, ileus, hypertension	Vessicant
Epipodophyllotoxins	Etoposide	Topoisomerase II inhibition	VeIP, EP, single agent	Germ cell tumor, prostate (small cell)	Bone marrow, N/V, mucositis (high doses), alopecia	
Platinum compounds	Cisplatin	DNA cross links	BEP, VIP, VeIP, M-VAC, EP	Germ cell, bladder tumor, prostate	Bone marrow, nephrotoxicity, N/V, neuropathy, hypomagnesemia	Amifostine is under investigation to reduce toxicity
	Carboplatin	DNA cross links	Single agent, with paclitaxel, estramustine	Bladder tumor, prostate	Bone marrow (particularly platelets), N/V, less neuropathy	Inferior to cisplatin in germ cell tumors

*Data from Cancer Chemotherapy and Biotherapy, Principles and Practice (1996)[99]; and The Chemotherapy Sourcebook (1992).[100]

"atypical MDR."[52] Despite the MDR phenotype, this "atypical MDR" pattern of resistance is non–p-glycoprotein mediated and has been consistently shown related to decreased levels of topoiosomerase II and overexpression of a multidrug-resistance–associated protein (MRP).[53] The resistance to alkylating agents such as platinum is believed to be non-MDR mediated. In cisplatin resistance, for example, proposed mechanisms have included decreased cellular uptake,[54] increased cisplatin-induced DNA damage repair abilities,[55] increased metallothionein expression, and increased glutathione (GSH) levels.[56,57] The metallothioneins are protein sulfhydryl compounds that are responsible for heavy metal binding and detoxification. The importance of these compounds in mediating drug resistance has been demonstrated in some tumor types but not consistently in others.[58–60] Multiple mechanisms for glutathione-enhanced resistance have been proposed including drug inactivation by GSH-drug binding, GSH-facilitated DNA repair, and active elimination of biologically functional GSH-drug conjugates.[61,62] Attempts to overcome drug resistance generally involve selecting different classes or formulations of drugs, changing the dose or schedule, or using biochemical modulation of metabolic pathways to potentiate drug effects or reduce dose-limiting toxicity.

BIOCHEMICAL MODULATION TO OVERCOME RESISTANCE

In tumors where a large proportion of cells have high MDR expression, pharmacologic inhibition of the p-glycoprotein efflux pump has been investigated. To effect this agents studied include calcium channel blockers, cyclosporine, tamoxifen, inhibi-

TABLE 7–2. DRUG RESISTANCE (INTRINSIC OR ACQUIRED)

Site of Action	Mechanism	Example(s)
Host	Inadequate drug levels Sanctuary sites Altered metabolism Toxicity preventing dosing	Blood-brain barrier
Tumor (macro)	Inadequate drug delivery Abnormal vasculature Altered interstitial pressures	Postradiation fibrosis
Cellular (micro)	p-Glycoprotein expression MDR associated protein (MRP) Increased DNA repair Metallothionein expression Increased glutathione levels	Multidrug resistance Phenotype Cisplatin resistance Alkylator resistance

tors of protein kinase C, and antibodies to p-glycoprotein have been investigated.[63,64] The use of calcium channel blockers has been particularly limited by the high drug concentrations required for pump inhibition and relative to the untoward cardiovascular side effects. Attempts to ameliorate these effects by using stereoisomers such as dexverapamil have not yielded promising results to date.[65,66]

As the molecular events responsible for neoplastic transformation are elucidated, other novel targets for therapies to overcome resistance are suggested. Apoptosis is the active, energy-dependent process by which cells destroy themselves in a characteristic fashion with shrinkage, chromatin condensation, and the formation of pedunculations.[67] The inhibition of protein kinase C, a family of serine/threonine kinases, is thought to promote apoptosis via a regulatory fashion.[68,69] Several drugs that specifically inhibit protein kinase C such as safingol and UCN-01 (7-OH-staurosporine), for example, are being investigated. Recent investigations have further suggested that protein kinase–induced apoptosis may be independent of p53-mediated growth arrest and could prove to be an additional pathway where modulation may be therapeutically important as in genitourinary malignancies that have a high incidence of p53 mutation as one mechanism for resistance.[70,71] In addition to activating programmed cell death pathways, p53 has been shown to exert an effect at the G_1/S cell cycle checkpoint as well as affecting the cellular response to DNA damage.[71,72] The ability to restore wild-type p53 function in neoplastic cells may also be important to restore drug sensitivity.

CLINICAL APPLICATIONS OF CHEMOTHERAPY

With the exception of gestational trophoblastic disease, germ cell neoplasms, and a proportion of patients with transitional cell carcinoma, chemotherapy alone is rarely curative when used as a single modality in the setting of overt metastatic disease. This has prompted the investigation of chemotherapy in the settings of minimal or microscopic disease (adjuvant) or prior to definitive local therapy (neoadjuvant). These approaches are contrasted in Table 7–3.

Neoadjuvant therapy goals may serve several aims that do not necessarily overlap. These include attempts to reduce the extent of surgical intervention required for local control, to convert unresectable to resectable disease, to improve local control, and most important, to improve overall survival. Neoadjuvant chemotherapy is now the standard of treatment in anal canal neoplasms, Ewing's sarcoma, and osteogenic sarcoma.[73] It has been shown to permit safe organ preservation with equivalent systematic control in patients with laryngeal cancer.[74] In genitourinary neoplasms, neoadjuvant therapy is still investigated and should be administered in the context of clinical trials. Most studied are bladder tumors, but despite a number of randomized comparisons, no definitive survival advantage has been demonstrated. A difficulty in interpreting these trials involves the problems in staging and evaluating the methods used to assess response.[75] Techniques that rely on clinical means, including the transurethral resection and biopsy, have a high risk of understaging, and in particular cannot reliably determine which bladders would be free of tumor if surgically removed. Hall et al. recently reported a 21% pathologic complete response rate of the primary bladder tumor in the preliminary review of a large randomized multicenter trial.[76] This shows the limitations of currently available regimens in rendering the bladder tumor free. The role of neoadjuvant hormonal and antineoplastic chemotherapy in prostate cancer that is locally advanced or has poor prognostic features is also being explored. Pathologic downstaging with hormonal therapy has been reported in patients with clinical T_2 disease as demonstrated by a reduction in positive surgical margins from an average of 47% to an average of 22% in several randomized, prospective, controlled trials.[77] Preliminary results have, however, indicated no difference in the progression rate between treated and untreated patients. This finding demonstrates the caution nec-

TABLE 7–3. COMPARISON OF ADJUVANT AND NEOADJUVANT THERAPY

	Neoadjuvant	Adjuvant
A. Basic principles		
1. Early treatment of micrometastasis	+	+
2. Inverse relationship of tumor volume to cure	+	+
3. Decreased chance of spontaneous resistance	+	+
B. Factors favoring neoadjuvant therapy		
1. Chemosensitivity demonstrated in vivo		
a. Primary response may predict prognosis	+	−
b. Organ preservation possible	+	−
2. Decrease need or extent of additional therapy	+	−
3. Convert inoperable lesion to operable	+	−
4. Drug delivery not compromised by prior surgery	+	−
5. More precise end-point of therapy	+	−
C. Factors favoring adjuvant therapy		
1. Case selection		
a. Uses more accurate pathologic staging	−	+
b. Follows "curative" local procedure	−	+
2. Timing of definitive local therapy		
a. Not delayed with potentially ineffective agents	−	+
b. No refusal of potentially curative surgery	−	+

essary when interpreting early surrogate outcomes such as pathologic downstaging instead of the ultimate end-point, which is improved survival.[78] In settings where improved survival is not demonstrated, therapy should be evaluated in the context of quality-of-life contributions to reducing required radical surgery or extending the time of local and systemic disease control.[79] The need to further identify clinical, laboratory, and pathologic parameters is also essential to define prognosis more precisely.[80] For example, using previously defined prognostic criteria based on clinical stage, digital rectal examination, and PSA, the role of neoadjuvant chemotherapy prior to radiation therapy in patients with poor-risk prostate carcinoma is being investigated (W.K. Kelly, M. Zelefsky, Memorial Sloan-Kettering Cancer Center, personal communication).

The need to identify prognostic features and stratify patients according to risk has prompted ongoing investigations to find a correlation between biologic markers and the degree of response of the primary tumor to neoadjuvant therapy.[81] The ultimate goal is to identify biologic markers that will tailor the need for neoadjuvant therapy as well as predict response and survival. In bladder cancer, for example, disease progression and death from invasive disease has been correlated with alterations in tumor suppressor genes to include altered Rb expression and p53 overexpression.[82,83] A clinical trial investigating a bladder-sparing approach in patients with p53 negative, and a low risk of metastasis, is ongoing at Memorial Sloan-Kettering Cancer Center (D. Bajorin, J. McCaffrey, personal communication).

Adjuvant therapy is presently considered the standard of care for subsets of patients with breast or colon carcinoma, Wilms' tumor, and osteosarcoma. In urogenital cancers, the refinement of an effective adjuvant approach is demonstrated in the treatment of stage II nonseminomatous testicular cancers. Initial studies had shown that standard chemotherapy administered in the adjuvant setting could be of shorter duration and remain highly effective in preventing relapse.[84] Other studies in advanced disease showed that bleomycin could be deleted from a standard platinum-based regimen with a reduction in toxicity with equivalent efficacy.[85] The natural progression of investigation was to evaluate the streamlined chemotherapy regimen in the adjuvant setting. Recent trials have confirmed that two rather than four cycles of etoposide and cisplatin chemotherapy in the adjuvant setting is highly effective in patients with stage II nonseminomatous germ cell tumors, and others have suggested also applying this therapy to high-risk stage I patients.[86,87] The issues surrounding adjuvant chemotherapy for germ cell tumors are unique in that the ultimate ability for cure is the same whether treatment is administered at the minimal disease state or at the time of objective recurrence. Accordingly, the focus of investigation has shifted toward toxicity reduction and an improvement in quality of life without compromising cure. Assessment of the effect of adjuvant chemotherapy on any one patient is difficult, since usual response parameters such as measurable tumor are not present. Its endpoint must ultimately be an increase in overall survival. In bladder cancer, for example, a trial by Skinner reported a 70 versus 46% 3-year disease-free interval in patients receiving adjuvant cisplatin, Cytoxan, Adriamycin (CISCA) combination chemotherapy. The survival at 5 years, however, shows no significant difference.[88] An analysis of the effectiveness of adjuvant chemotherapy in bladder cancer has been hampered by the lack of prospective randomized controlled trials of sufficient sample size. The available data consist largely of phase II trials, with several suggesting a benefit when compared to historical controls.[89] These trials cannot be compared secondary to differences in staging and lack of controls for known prognostic predictors such as p53 overexpression. With the exception of germ cell tumors, the use of adjuvant chemotherapy in genitourinary malignancies remains investigational, with the adjuvant treatment of subsets of patients with bladder cancer holding the most promise based on available data. Adjuvant therapy has been ineffective in all trials to date for renal cell carcinoma.

ADJUNCTS TO CHEMOTHERAPY ADMINISTRATION

Hematopoietic colony-stimulating factors (G-CSF or GM-CSF) have been demonstrated to allow the administration of more dose-intensive chemotherapy regimens.[90] They are also used to mobilize stem cells that are collected in regimens with significant myeloablative potential that require peripheral blood stem cell support.[91] Recent clinical practice guidelines support their routine use following a

TABLE 7–4. SELECTED NEW INDICATIONS, DRUGS, AND REGIMENS UNDER INVESTIGATION FOR GENITOURINARY MALIGNANCIES

Class	Drug	Major Mechanism	Disease Activity	Major Toxicity	Regimens Under Investigation	Comments/ References
Taxanes	Paclitaxel	Binds and stabilizes microtubules	Bladder, germ cell, small cell, prostate	Hypersensitivity, bone marrow, neuropathy, arrhythmias, alopecia	Single agent, with cisplatin, carboplatin, or ifosfamide; with estramustine	McCaffrey et al. (1996)[101] Murphy et al. (1996)[102]
	Docetaxel		Bladder	Hypersensitivity, bone marrow, neuropathy, rash, asthenia, fluid retention		van Oosterom and Schrivers (1995)[103]
Nucleoside analogs	Gemcitabine	Incorporates into DNA, blocks synthesis	Bladder	Bone marrow, nausea, fever, liver function abnormalities	Single agent, with cisplatin; with etoposide	38% response untreated; 28% response in pts with prior treatment TCC Moore et al. (1996)[104] DeLena et al. (1996)[105]
Camptothecins	Irinotecan, topotecan, 9-aminocamptothecin	Inhibits topoisomerase I	No activity as single agent to date in GU tumors	Bone marrow, nausea, diarrhea		No responses in phase II trial with renal cell cancer
Retinoids	13-cis RA, all trans RA	Differentiation	No activity in germ cell, prostate, or bladder cancer	Stomatitis, hand-foot syndrome, generalized rash	Renal cell carcinoma, with interferons	Motzer et al. (1994)[106] Atzpodien et al. (1996)[107]
Antifolates	Edetrexate	Inhibits dihydrofolate reductase	No response in prostate, preliminary response in bladder	Same as fluorouracil		
	Trimetrexate	Inhibits hihydrofolate reductase	No response in prostate	Same as fluorouracil		
Other	Liposomal doxorubicin	Anthracycline, prolonged half-life	No activity in renal cell	Stomatitis, hand-foot syndrome, bone marrow	Prostate trial underway	
	Vinorelbine	Microtubule disruption	? Prostate	Bone marrow, nausea	With estramustine in prostate CA, phase I	Reese et al. (1996)[108]
	Marmistat	Metalloproteinase inhibitor	Unproven	Minimal in initial phase I	Prostate	Boasberg et al. (1996)[109]

documented febrile neutropenia episode in a previous chemotherapy cycle when dose reduction is not appropriate.[92] A recent randomized study suggested that adding G-CSF to antibiotic treatment in established neutropenic fever shortens the duration of neutropenia, the time on intravenous antibiotics, and the duration of hospital stay, and demonstrated a trend towards decreased cost.[93]

Recent investigations have demonstrated that thrombopoietin (TPO) is the factor responsible for regulating platelet production.[94] Recombinant human megakaryocyte growth and development factor (rHuMGDF), with an amino acid sequence identical to the first 163 amino acids of native human TPO, binds to the receptor c-MPL on megakaryocyte progenitors, which induces proliferation and cytoplasmic maturation. Phase I and II testing is underway to define its therapeutic role in the amelioration of chemotherapy-induced thrombocytopenia.[95]

In addition to the application of cytokines to reduce the morbidity of chemotherapy, novel compounds are in several stages of development with specific chemoprotective effects. Amifostine, for example, is shown to lessen the hematopoietic, nephrotoxic, and neurotoxic effects of cisplatin therapy. No interference in cytotoxic activity has been demonstrated in human cell lines or in vivo in palliative combination regimens.[96,97] Carefully conducted studies are required in curative regimens such as those utilized for germ cell tumors before its use can be recommended in this setting. Dexrazoxane has been shown to reduce the incidence of cardiac toxicity in anthracycline-containing regimens, allowing continued use in responding patients. Further investigation is likewise required in regimens with curative potential.[98]

SUMMARY

The selected agents and combinations in Table 7–4 are under investigation either based on preclinical data, indications, efficacy in other tumor types, or as part of a combination regimen.

Most cancers of the genitourinary tract are relatively refractory to current antineoplastic drugs and require innovative strategies to effectively improve outcomes. The need to improve the individual efficacy of current agents is apparent and illustrates the importance of rapidly testing potential compounds. Novel targets for treatment are suggested by the further elucidation of molecular pathways and improvement in our understanding of the process of cellular differentiation and the balance between immunity and cancer. Of equal importance is developing new approaches to identify accurate prognostic models using clinical characteristics, biochemical or genetic markers, or other means to risk-stratify patients so that new agents may be applied in a rational and effective way.

REFERENCES

1. Grever MR, Schepartz SA, Chabner BA: The National Cancer Institute: cancer drug discovery and development program. Semin Oncol 1992; 16:622–638.
2. Driscoll JS: The preclinical new drug research program of the National Cancer Institute. Cancer Treat Rep 1984; 68:63–76.
3. Collins JM, Zaharko DS, Dedrick RL, Chabner BA: Potential roles for preclinical pharmacology in phase I trials. Cancer Treat Rep 1986; 70(1):73–80.
4. Collins JM, Grieshaber CK, Chabner BA: Pharmacologically guided clinical phase I trials based upon preclinical drug development. J Natl Cancer Inst 1990; 82(16): 1321–1326.
5. Yagoda A, Watson RC, Natale RB, et al: A critical analysis of response criteria in patients with prostatic cancer treated with cis-diamminedichloride platinum II. Cancer 1979; 44:1553–1562.
6. Fleming TR: One-sample multiple testing procedure for phase II clinical trials. Biometrics 1982; 38(1):143–151.
7. Gehan EA: The determination of the number of patients required in a preliminary and followup trial of a new chemotherapeutic agent. J Chronic Dis 1961; 13:346–351.
8. Skipper HE: Historic milestones in cancer biology: a few that are important in cancer treatment (revisited). Semin Oncol 1979; 6(4):506–514.
9. Skipper HE: Laboratory models: the historical perspective. Cancer Treat Rep 1986; 70:3–7.
10. Laird AK: Dynamics of growth in tumors and normal organisms. Natl Cancer Inst Monogr 1969; 30:15–28.
11. Norton L: Gompertzian model of human breast cancer growth. Cancer Res 1988; 48:7067–7071.
12. Mendelsohn ML: The growth fraction: a new concept applied to tumors. Science 1960; 132:1496.
13. Norton L, Simon R: Growth curve of an experimental tumor following radiotherapy. J Natl Cancer Inst 1977; 58:1735–1741.
14. Scher HI, Norton L: Chemotherapy for urothelial tract malignancies: breaking the deadlock. Semin Surg Oncol 1992; 8:316–341.
15. Norton L: Implications of kinetics heterogeneity in clinical oncology. Semin Oncol 1985; 12:231–249.
16. Norton L, Simon R: Tumor size, sensitivity to therapy, and the design of treatment schedules. Cancer Treat Rep 1977; 61:1307–1317.
17. Frei EI, Canellos GP: Dose: a critical factor in cancer chemotherapy. Am J Med 1980; 69:585–593.
18. Hryniuk W, Levine MN: Analysis of dose intensity for adjuvant chemotherapy trials. J Clin Oncol 1986; 4:1162–1170.
19. Hudis C: New approaches to adjuvant chemotherapy for breast cancer. Pharmacotherapy 1996; 16(3 Pt 2):88S–93S.
20. Fenelly D, Vahdat L, Schneider J, et al: High intensity chemotherapy with peripheral blood progenitor cell support. Semin Oncol 1994; 21(2)S2:21–25.
21. van der Wall E, Beijnen JH, Rodenhuis S: High dose chemotherapy regimens for solid tumors. Cancer Treat Rev 1995; 21:105–132.
22. Phillip T, Armitage JO, Spitzer G, et al: High dose chemotherapy and autologous bone marrow transplantation after failure of conventional chemotherapy in adults with intermediate grade or high grade non-Hodgkin's lymphoma. N Engl J Med 1987; 316:1493–1498.
23. Harousseau JL, Attal M, Divine M, et al: Autologous stem cell transplantation after first remission induction treatment in multiple myeloma: a report of the French Registry on autologous transplantation in multiple myeloma. Blood 1995; 85(11):3077–3085.
24. Motzer RJ, Mazumdar M, Bosl GJ, et al: High dose carboplatin, etoposide, and cyclophosphamide for patients with refractory germ cell tumors: treatment results and prognostic factors for survival and toxicity. J Clin Oncol 1996; 14(4):1098–1105.

25. Seidman AD, Scher HI, Gabrilove JL, et al: Dose intensification of methotrexate, vinblastine, doxorubicin, and cisplatin with recombinant granulocyte colony stimulating factor as initial therapy in advanced urothelial cancer. J Clin Oncol 1993; 11:408–414.
26. Sternberg C, de Mulder P, van Oosterom AT, et al: Escalated MVAC chemotherapy and recombinant human granulocyte macrophage colony stimulating factor (rhGM-CSF) in patients with advanced urothelial tract tumors. Ann Oncol 1993; 4(5):403–407.
27. Scher HI, Geller NL, Curley T, Tao Y: Effect of relative dose intensity on survival of patients with urothelial cancer treated with MVAC. J Clin Oncol 1993; 11:400–407.
28. Lichtman SM, Ratain MJ, Van Echo DA, et al: Phase I trial of granulocyte macrophage colony stimulating factor plus high dose cyclophosphamide given every two weeks: a Cancer and Leukemia Group B study. J Natl Cancer Inst 1993; 85(16):1319–1326.
29. Small EJ, Srinivas S, Egan B, et al: Doxorubicin and dose-escalated cyclophosphamide with granulocyte colony-stimulating factor for the treatment of hormone-resistant prostate cancer. J Clin Oncol 1996; 14(5):1617–1625.
29a. Scher HI, Logofhetis CJ: Management of androgen independent prostate cancer. *In* Raghavan D, Scher HI, Leibel SA, Lange P (eds): Principles and Practice of Genitourinary Oncology, p 602. Philadelphia, Lippincott-Raven, 1996.
30. Goldie JH, Coldman AJA: A mathematical model for relating the drug sensitivity of tumors to their spontaneous mutation rate. Cancer Treat Rep 1979; 63:1727–1733.
31. Goldie JH: Scientific basis for adjuvant and primary (neoadjuvant) chemotherapy. Semin Oncol 1987; 14:1–7.
32. Canellos GP, Anderson JR, Propert KJ, et al: Chemotherapy of advanced Hodgkin's disease with MOPP, ABVD, or MOPP alternating with ABVD. N Engl J Med 1992; 327(21):1478–1484.
33. Bonadonna G, Zambetti M, Valgussa P: Sequential or alternating doxorubicin and CMF regimens in breast cancer with more than three positive nodes. JAMA 1995; 273(7):542–547.
34. The Ludwig Breast Cancer Study Group: Combination adjuvant chemotherapy for node-positive breast cancer. N Engl J Med 1988; 319:677–683.
35. Clarke NW, McClure J, George NJ: Preferential preservation of bone mineralisation by LHRH agonists in the treatment of metastatic prostate cancer. Eur Urol 1991; 19:114–117.
36. Szepeshazi K, Korkut E, Szende B, et al: Histological changes in Dunning prostate tumors and testes of rats treated with LH-RH antagonist SB-75. Prostate 1991; 18: 255–270.
37. Theyer G, Hamilton G: Role of multidrug resistance of tumors of the genitourinary tract. Urology 1994; 44(6): 942–950.
38. Peters GJ, van Groeningen CJ: Clinical relevance of biochemical modulation of 5-fluorouracil. Ann Oncol 1991; 2:469–480.
39. Hageboutros A, Hudes GR, Brennan J: Phase I trial of fluorouracil modulation by *N*-phosphonacetyl-L-aspartate and 6-methylmercaptopurine ribonucleoside. Cancer Chemother Pharmacol 1996; 37(3):229–234.
40. Curti B: Physical barriers to drug delivery in tumors. Crit Rev Oncol Hematol 1993; 14:29–39.
41. Song CW, Lyons JC, Luo Y: Intra- and extra-cellular pH in solid tumors: influence on therapeutic response. *In* Teicher BA (ed): Drug Resistance in Oncology, pp 25–51. New York, Marcel Dekker, 1993.
42. Vendrik CPJ, Bergers JJ, De Jong WH, Steerenberg PA: Resistance to cytostatic drugs at the cellular level. Cancer Chemother Pharmacol 1992; 29:413–429.
43. Ling V: P-glycoprotein and resistance to anticancer drugs. Cancer 1992; 69:79–89.
44. Cornwell MM: Molecular biology of P-glycoprotein. Cancer Treat Res 191; 57:37–56.
45. Lum BL, Gosland MP: MDR Expression in normal tissues. Pharmacologic implications for the clinical use of p-glycoprotein inhibitors. Hematol Oncol Clin North Am 1995; 9(2):319–336.
46. Roninson IB: The role of the MDR1 (P-glycoprotein) gene in multidrug resistance in vitro and in vivo. Biochem Pharmacol 1992; 43:95–102.
47. Hsing S, Gatmaitan Z, Arias IM: The function of Gp170, the multidrug-resistance gene product, in the brush border of rat intestinal mucosa. Gastroenterology 1992; 102: 879–885.
48. Cordon-Cardo C, O'Brien JP, Boccia J, et al: Expression of the multidrug resistance gene product (p-glycoprotein) in human normal and tumor tissues. J Histochem Cytochem 1990; 38:1277–1287.
49. Cordon-Cardo C, O'Brien JP, Casals D, et al: Multidrug resistance gene (p-glycoprotein) is expressed by endothelial cells at blood-brain barrier sites. Proc Natl Acad Sci U S A 1989; 69:695.
50. Volm M, Kastel M, Mattern J, Efferth T: Expression of resistance factors (p-glycoprotein, glutathione s-transferase-pi, and topoisomerase II) and their inter-relationship to proto-oncogene products in renal cell carcinomas. Cancer 1993; 71(12):3981–3987.
51. Hasegwa S, Abe T, Naito S, et al: Expresion of multidrug resistance associated protein (MRP), MDR1, and DNA topoisomerase II in human multi-drug resistant bladder cancer cell lines. Cancer 1995; 71(5):907–913.
52. Mestadgh N, Pommery N, Saucier JM, et al: Chemoresistance to doxorubicin and cisplatin in a murine cell line. Analysis of p-glycoprotein, topoisomerase II, glutathione, and related enzymes. Anticancer Res 1994; 14(3A):869–874.
53. Naito S, Hasegawa S, Yokomizo A, et al: Non-p-glycoprotein mediated atypical drug resistance in a human bladder cancer cell line. Jpn J Cancer Res 1995; 86(11): 1112–1118.
54. Parker RJ, Eastman A, Bostick-Bruton F, Reed E: Acquired cisplatin resistance in human ovarian cancer cell lines is associated with enhanced repair of cisplatin-DNA lesions and reduced drug accumulation. J Clin Invest 1991; 87:772–777.
55. Masuda H, Ozols RF, Lai GM, Fojo A: Increased DNA repair as a mechanism of acquired resistance to cis-diamminedichloroplatinum (II) in human ovarian cancer cell lines. Cancer Res 1988; 48:5713–5716.
56. Kondo Y, Woo ES, Michalska AE, et al: Metallothionein null cells have increased sensitivity to anticancer drugs. Cancer Res 1995; 55(10):2021–2023.
57. Singh SV, Xu BH, Jani JP, et al: Mechanism of cross resistance to cisplatin in a mitomycin c-resistant human bladder cell line. Int J Cancer 1995; 61(3):431–436.
58. Saika T, Tsushima T, Ochi J, et al: Over-expression of metallothionein and drug resistance in bladder cancer. Int J Urol 1994; 1(2):135–139.
59. Kashahara K, Fujiwara Y, Nishio K, et al: Metallothionein content correlates with the sensitivity of human small cell lung cancer cell lines to cisplatin. Cancer Res 1988; 51:3237–3242.
60. Sark MW, Timmer-Bosscha H, Meijer C, et al: Cellular basis for differential sensitivity to cisplatin in human germ cell tumour and colon carcinoma cell lines. Br J Cancer 1995; 71(4):684–690.
61. Schroeder CP, Godwin AK, O'Dwyer PJ, et al: Glutathione and drug resistance. Cancer Invest 1996; 14(2):158–168.
62. Zaman GJ, Lankelma J, van Tellingen O, et al: Role of glutathione in the export of compounds from cells by the multi-drug-resistance-associated protein. Proc Natl Acad Sci U S A 1995; 92(17):7690–7694.
63. Fisher GA, Sikic BJ: Clinical studies with modulators of drug resistance. Hematol Oncol Clin North Am 1995; 9(2):363–382.
64. Leu BL, Huang JD: Inhibition of intestinal p-glycopro-

tein and effects on etoposide absorption. Cancer Chemother Pharmacol 1995; 35(5):432–436.
65. Motzer RJ, Lyn P, Fischer P, et al: Phase I/II trials of dexverapamil plus vinblastine for patients with advanced renal cell carcinoma. J Clin Oncol 1995; 13(8): 1958–1965.
66. Pereira E, Teodori E, Dei S, et al: Reversal of multidrug resistance by verapamil analogues. Biochem Pharmacol 1995; 50(4):451–457.
67. Wylle AH: The significance of apoptosis. Int Rev Cytol 1980; 68:251–306.
68. Jarvis WD, Turner AJ, Povirk LF, et al: Induction of apoptotic DNA fragmentation and cell death in HL-60 human promyelocytic leukemia cells has been reported for pharmacological inhibitors of protein kinase C. Cancer Res 1994; 54:1707–1714.
69. Sachs CW, Safa AR, Harrison SD, Fine RL: Partial inhibition of multidrug resistance by salfingol is independent of modulation of p-glycoprotein substrate activities and correlated with inhibition of protein kinase C. J Biol Chem 1995; 270(44):26639–26648.
70. Johnson M, Dimitrov D, Vojta PJ, et al: Evidence for a p-53 independent pathway for upregulation of SD11/CIP1/WAF1/p21 RNA in human cells. Mol Carcinog 1994; 11:59–64.
71. Lowe SW, Ruley HE, Jacks T, Housman DE: p53-Dependent apoptosis modulates the cytotoxicity of anticancer agents. Cell 1993; 74:957–967.
72. Prokocimer M, Rotter V: Structure and function of p53 in normal cells and their aberrations in cancer cells: projection on the hematologic cell lineages. Blood 1994; 84: 2391–2411.
73. Trimble EL, Ungerleider RS, Abrams JA, et al: Neoadjuvant therapy in cancer treatment. Cancer 1993; 72: 3315–3324.
74. Pfister DG, Harrison LB, Strong EW, et al: Current status of larynx preservation with multimodality therapy. Oncology 1992; 6(3):33–38.
75. Scher HI, Yagoda A, Herr HW, et al: Neoadjuvant M-VAC (methotrexate, vinblastine, doxorubicin and cisplatin) effect on the primary bladder lesion. J Urol 1988; 139:470–474.
76. Hall RR, for MRC Advanced Bladder Cancer Working Party, EORTC GU Group, et al: Neo-adjuvant CMV chemotherapy and cystectomy or radiotherapy in muscle invasive bladder cancer. First analysis of MRC/EORTC Intercontinental Trial. Proc Am Soc Clin Oncol 1996; 15: 244.
77. Soloway MS, Sharifi R, Wajsman Z, et al: Randomized prospective study comparing radical prostatectomy alone versus radical prostatectomy preceded by androgen blockade in clinical stage B2(T2bNxM0) prostate cancer. J Urol 1995; 154:424–428.
78. Van Poppel H, DeRidder D, Elgamel AA, et al: Neoadjuvant hormonal therapy before radical prostatectomy decreases the number of positive surgical margins in stage T2 prostate cancer: interim results of a prospective randomized trial. J Urol 1995; 154:429–434.
79. Frei E: Randomized clinical trials and other approaches in clinical research. Cancer 1994; 74(9 Suppl):2610–2613.
80. Partin AW, Yoo J, Carter HB, et al: The use of prostate specific antigen, clinical stage and Gleason score to predict pathological stage in men with localized prostate cancer. J Urol 1993; 149:1.
81. Eberlein TJ: Preoperative chemotherapy: where do we go from here? Ann Surg 1995; 222(5):609–611.
82. Sarkis AS, Bajorin DF, Reuter VE, et al: Prognostic value of p53 nuclear overexpression in patients with invasive bladder cancer treated with neoadjuvant MVAC. J Clin Oncol 1995; 13:1384–1390.
83. Logothetis CJ, Xu H, Ro JY, et al: Altered expression of retinoblastoma protein and known prognostic variables in locally advanced bladder cancer. J Natl Cancer Inst 1992; 84:1256–1261.
84. Williams SD, Stablein DM, Einhorn LH, et al: Immediate adjuvant chemotherapy versus observation with treatment at relapse in pathologic stage II testicular cancer. N Engl J Med 1987; 317:1433–1438.
85. Bosl GJ, Geller NL, Bajorin D, et al: A randomized trial of etoposide + cisplatin versus vinblastine + bleomycin + cisplatin + cyclophosphamide + dactinomycin in patients with good prognosis germ cell tumors. J Clin Oncol 1988; 6:1231–1238.
86. Motzer RJ, Sheinfeld J, Mazumdar M, et al: Etoposide and cisplatin adjuvant therapy for patients with pathologic stage II germ cell tumors. J Clin Oncol 1995; 13(11): 2700–2704.
87. Cullen MH, Stenning SP, Parkinson MC, et al: Short course adjuvant chemotherapy in high risk stage I nonseminomatous germ cell tumors of the testis: a medical research council report. J Clin Oncol 1996; 14:1106–1113.
88. Skinner DG, Daniels JR, Russell CA, et al: The role of adjuvant chemotherapy following cystectomy for invasive bladder cancer: a prospective comparative trial. J Urol 1991; 145:459–464.
89. Stockle M, Meyenburg W, Weller S, et al: Adjuvant polychemotherapy of nonorgan-confined bladder cancer after radical cystectomy revisisted: long-term results of controlled prospective study and further clinical experience. J Urol 1995; 153:47–52.
90. Gabrilove JL, Jakubowski A, Scher H, et al: Effect of granulocyte colony-stimulating factor on neutropenia and associated morbidity due to chemotherapy for transitional-cell carcinoma of the urothelium. N Engl J Med 1988; 318:1414–1422.
91. Winter JN, Lazarus HM, Rademaker A, et al: Phase I/II study of combined granulocyte colony stimulating factor and granulocyte-macrophage colony stimulating factor administration for the mobilization of hematopoietic progenitor cells. J Clin Oncol 1996; 14(1):277–286.
92. American Society of Clinical Oncology recommendations for the use of hematopoietic colony-stimulating factors: evidence based, clinical practice guidelines. J Oncol 1994; 12(11):2471–2508.
93. Mayordomo JI, Rivera F, Diaz-Puente MT, et al: Improving treatment of chemotherapy-induced neutropenic fever by administration of colony stimulating factors. J Natl Cancer Inst 1995; 87(11):803–808.
94. Bartley TD, Bolgenberger J, Hunt P, et al: Identification and cloning of a megakaryocyte growth and development factor that is a ligand for the cytokine receptor Mpl. Cell 1994; 77:1117–1124.
95. Kauchansky K, Lok S, Holly RD, et al: Promotion of megakaryocyte progenitor expansion and differentiation by the c-MPL ligand thrombopoietin. Nature 1994; 369: 568.
96. Capizzi RL, Oster W: Protection of normal tissues from the cytotoxic effects of chemotherapy and radiation by amifostine: clinical experiences. Eur J Cancer 1995; 31A(Suppl 1):S8–S13.
97. Dunn TA, Schmoll HJ, Grunewald V, et al: Anti-tumor activity of cisplatin (DDP) in combination with amifostine in DPP-sensitive nude mouse model of human nonseminomatous germ cell tumor (NSGCT). Proc ASCO 1996; 15:687A.
98. Swain S, Whaley FS, Ewer MS: Congestive heart failure after doxorubicin containing therapy in advanced breast cancer patients treated with or without dexrazoxane. Proc ASCO 1996; 15:1739A.
99. Cancer Chemotherapy and Biotherapy, Principles and Practice. Philadelphia, JB Lippincott Co, 1996.
100. The Chemotherapy Sourcebook. Baltimore, Williams & Wilkins, 1992.
101. McCaffrey J, Hilton S, Mazumdar M, et al: A phase II trial of ifosfamide, paclitaxel and cisplatin (ITP) in patients (pts) with advanced urothelial tract tumors (Abstract). Proc Am Soc Clin Oncol 1996; 15:251.
102. Murphy BA, Johnson DR, Smith J, et al: Phase II trial of

paclitaxel (P) and cisplatin (C) for metastatic or locally unresectable urothelial cancer (Abstract). Proc Am Soc Clin Oncol 1996.

103. van Oosterom AT, Schrivers D: Docetaxel, a review of preclinical and clinical experiences (Abstract). Anticancer Drugs 1995; 6(3):356–368.

104. Moore MJ, Tannock S, Ernst S, et al: Gemcitabine demonstrates promising activity as a single agent in the treatment of metastatic transitional cell carcinoma (Abstract). Proc ASCO 1996; 15:637A.

105. DeLena M, Gridelli C, Lorusso V, et al: Gemicitabine activity (objective responses and symptom improvement) in resistant stage IV bladder cancer (Abstract). Proc Am Soc Clin Oncol 1996; 15:622.

106. Motzer RJ, Schwartz L, Law TM, et al: Interferon alfa-2a and 13-cis-retinoic acid in renal cell carcinoma: antitumor activity in a phase II trial and interactions in vitro. J Clin Oncol 1995; 13(8):1950.

107. Atzpodien J, Buer J, Probst M, et al: Clinical and preclinical role of 13 cis-retinoic acid in renal cell carcinoma: Hanover experience (Abstract). Proc Am Soc Clin Oncol 1996; 15:625.

108. Reese D, Burris H, Belledgrun A, et al: A phase I/II study of Navelbine (vinorelbine) and estramustine in the treatment of hormone refractory prostate cancer (HRPC) (Abstract). Proc Am Soc Clin Oncol 1996; 15:673.

109. Boasberg P, Harbaugh B, Roth B, et al: Marimastat, a novel matrix metalloproteinase inhibitor in patients with hormone-refractory prostate cancer. Proc Am Soc Clin Oncol 1996; 15:671.

8

IMMUNOTHERAPY: BASIC PRINCIPLES

RICHARD B. ALEXANDER, M.D.

Immunotherapy is the fourth and newest modality of cancer therapy after surgery, radiation therapy, and chemotherapy. Immunotherapy of cancer is the exploitation of the immune system or its parts as a therapy for neoplastic disease. The principal feature of the immune system that has intrigued investigators searching for cancer therapies is specificity. The immune system can clearly identify and destroy cells it recognizes in some way while sparing cells it does not so recognize. The essential question of cancer immunotherapy is whether this system can recognize and destroy cancer cells while sparing normal cells.

To understand the basic principles of cancer immunotherapy one must understand the nature of antigens and how the immune system recognizes cells. Recent insight into many aspects of this process have been clarified. This chapter will review new information about immune system function including T-cell function, cytokines, major histocompatibility complex (MHC) restriction, and antigen presentation. New insights into the nature of tumor antigens in humans characterized to date will be presented as will a brief review of the use of immunotherapy for patients with cancer.

FUNCTION OF THE IMMUNE SYSTEM

The immune system consists of a family of cell types with many different and overlapping functions as shown in Table 8–1. Because of its ability to rapidly recognize and destroy cells, the immune system has developed a tightly regulated and highly complex series of interactions to control and regulate the immune response. The immune system can be divided into two components with broadly overlapping function: cell-mediated immunity and humoral immunity. The distinction between these two is mostly of historical interest but serves to classify immune responses in a useful way.

Humoral Immunity

The principal mediator of humoral, or soluble, immune function is the antibody or immunoglobulin. Antibodies are multichain glycoproteins containing a framework constant region and a variable region. Through the diversity of the variable region antibodies can manifest a large number of conformations that are complementary to (and can therefore bind to) virtually any potential macromolecular tertiary structure.

Antibodies are made by B lymphocytes. B lymphocytes express the particular antibody they are capable of making (defined by the conformation of the variable region) on their surface. Each B cell expresses a single antibody conformation. The diversity of antibody structure comes from the recombination of regions of the immunoglobulin genes that contain several polymorphic regions that can combine in different ways during the genesis of the B cell in the bone marrow. Even with a relatively small number of different regions and linkers an astonishing diversity of antibody variable regions can be created (estimated at 10^{21} different conformations). The immunoglobulin genes share many similarities with those of the T-cell receptor that defines the specificity of T cells in a similar way. The genes that behave in this way are therefore known as the immunoglobulin gene superfamily.

When a B cell encounters an antigen that binds the antibody it expresses, the cell is activated and undergoes a series of cellular processes resulting in secretion of cytokines, up-regulation of cell surface expression of various functional membrane-bound proteins, and proliferation. Ultimately the B cell becomes a plasma cell and secretes large amounts of

TABLE 8–1. CELLS OF THE IMMUNE SYSTEM AND THEIR BROAD FUNCTION

Cell type	Function
CD4 T lymphocyte	Cytokine secretion, Th1 and Th2 and others B cell help
CD8 T lymphocyte, cytotoxic T cell	Lysis of antigen-bearing target cell in context of MHC class I Cytokine secretion
Natural killer cells (NK cells)	Inherent cytotoxicity to target cells Suppressor cells?
Monocytes and macrophages	Phagocytic function Direct cytotoxicity to infectious organisms Antigen presentation Cytokine secretion
Dendritic cells	Antigen presentation, including primary immune responses Migration to lymph nodes and long-term presentation of antigen to T cells Costimulation to T cells
B lymphocytes	Antibody production Antigen presentation, particularly for specific antigen recognized by surface immunoglobulin
Granulocytes	Phagocytic function Direct cytotoxicity to infectious organisms Proinflammatory cytokine secretion

the antibody it expresses on its surface. In this way the antibodies that are created are in response to the particular antigen to which a humoral immune response is being made.

B cells do not function independently but require help from T cells for maturation and control of the antibody response. This occurs by the secretion of cytokines and by cell-to-cell interactions at the local site of the immune reaction and in lymph nodes. The helper T cell (CD4+) appears to be principally responsible for this function. T cells provide a helper function to B cells resulting in the secretion of higher affinity IgG antibodies against the inciting antigen rather than the lower affinity but more rapidly secreted IgM class of antibody. This is known as immunoglobulin class switching,[1] the control of which is a critical function of helper T cells. It is the pattern of cytokines secreted by CD4 helper T cells that control the creation and maintenance of the particular type of immune response being generated.

Antibodies are ideally suited for attack on an invader that is outside of normal cells and thus available for binding. The binding of antibodies (opsonization) is a critical signal for destruction by the host by means of the complement system as well as phagocytosis by granulocytes and monocytes that contain receptors for the constant region of antibodies.

Cell-Mediated Immunity

Many pathogens do not principally exist outside of host cells but rather within the cells. Viruses are the prototype of this type of pathogen and the immune system generates a different type of response when the invading microorganism is within normal cells. This type of immune response is cell-mediated immunity and is principally controlled and mediated by T lymphocytes. Viruses and other intracellular pathogens take over the synthetic machinery of the cell to create new infectious particles, which then infect other cells. Hence the immune system requires a method to detect the expression of foreign proteins inside normal cells. Antibodies are too large to enter intact cells for this purpose. It is the T lymphocytes that are principally responsible for the detection of cells containing foreign material.

Major Histocompatibility Complex and T-Cell Antigens

T cells do not recognize whole foreign proteins but rather short peptides derived from such proteins presented in the context of self-MHC.[2] The MHC system consists of two major classes of surface markers expressed by cells. Class I MHC consists of a heavy glycoprotein chain noncovalently associated with β_2-microglobulin. Class I antigens include the classic HLA-A, -B, and -C transplantation antigens and are expressed constitutively by all nucleated cells. The class I complex has a groove on its surface in which peptides derived from the cytoplasm of the cell are assembled.[3] It is this peptide–self-MHC complex that is the antigen for T lymphocytes. The phenomenon of the assembly of the peptide–MHC complex is called antigen processing and presentation.

Class II MHC has a different structure and consists of two glycoprotein chains, α and β.[4,5] The structure of class II MHC is very similar to that of class I in that a groove on the extracellular surface of the molecule can bind peptides and serve as the antigen for T cells. Class II MHC is not usually expressed by most cells but is expressed by cells of the immune system with specialized function as antigen-presenting cells such as monocytes, B cells, and dendritic cells.

Antigen Processing and Presentation

The process by which peptides are assembled into the class I and II MHC complexes for display on the cell surface is called antigen processing and presentation.[6] There are two major pathways of antigen processing: the endogenous pathway and the exogenous pathway as shown in Figure 8–1. These correspond to class I and class II MHC in that endogenous pathway antigens are typically found inside the cell in the cytoplasm and are assembled into class I by way of the endoplasmic reticulum. Antigens outside of the cell can also be taken up

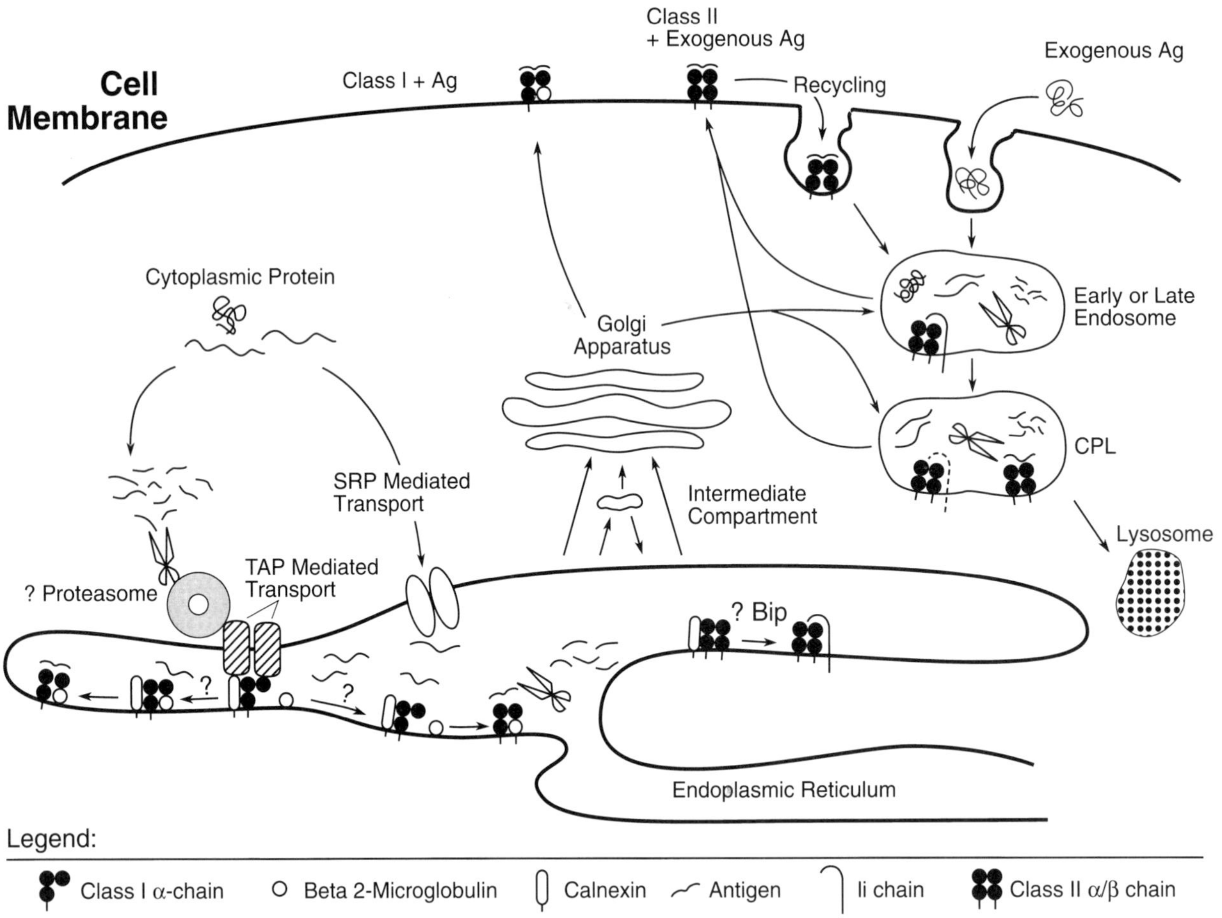
Cell Membrane
Class I + Ag
Class II + Exogenous Ag
Recycling
Exogenous Ag
Cytoplasmic Protein
Golgi Apparatus
Early or Late Endosome
CPL
SRP Mediated Transport
Intermediate Compartment
Lysosome
TAP Mediated Transport
? Proteasome
? Bip
Endoplasmic Reticulum
Legend:
Class I α-chain
Beta 2-Microglobulin
Calnexin
Antigen
Ii chain
Class II α/β chain

FIGURE 8–1. Diagram of antigen processing and presentation. Endogenous antigens in the cytoplasm are digested to peptides, which are transported into the endoplasmic reticulum. They are assembled into complexes with MHC class I and transported to the surface of the cell through the Golgi apparatus. Exogenous antigens are taken up from outside the cell and are broken down into peptides in the endosomal compartment. These peptides are then assembled into complexes with MHC class II and transported to the cell surface. (From Restifo NP, Wunderlich JR: *In* De Vita VT, Hellman S, Rosenberg SA [eds]: Biologic Therapy of Cancer, 2nd edition, pp 3–37. Philadelphia, Lippincott-Raven, 1995, with permission.)

by specialized phagocytic antigen-presenting cells (APC) such as monocytes and dendritic cells. These cells break down the ingested material in the endosomal compartment at low pH and the resultant peptides are assembled into class II MHC and then presented on the surface of the cell. In this way APC are capable of presenting antigens from the surrounding fluid to the immune system.

It is apparent that the reason for the MHC system is the constant monitoring of cells for antigen expressed inside of cells that could be a threat to the host but which might not be the target of an antibody response. Viruses are a good example and are probably the reason the system evolved in the first place. If a virus infected a cell, then the foreign viral proteins expressed inside the cytoplasm would be processed into self–class I MHC through the endogenous pathway, which would generate an immune response against cells infected by virus. Specialized antigen-presenting cells called dendritic cells also exist throughout the host.[7] These cells, so-called professional antigen-presenting cells, exist in high numbers at sites of potential antigen challenge, such as the skin. Dendritic cells are highly efficient at antigen processing through both the endogenous and exogenous pathways and express a variety of costimulatory molecules critical to the development of a T-cell response. Once these cells acquire antigen in the skin, they migrate to lymph nodes where they can present antigen to the T-cell repertoire and engender a specific immune response to antigen.

T Lymphocytes and Antigen Recognition

T lymphocytes recognize antigens through the T-cell receptor (TCR), a surface complex of two glycoprotein chains noncovalently associated with the CD3 complex.[8] The TCR genes are part of the immunoglobulin gene superfamily. As such they undergo somatic rearrangement and reassembly, and through this mechanism the variable region of the TCR genes attains an enormous diversity of differ-

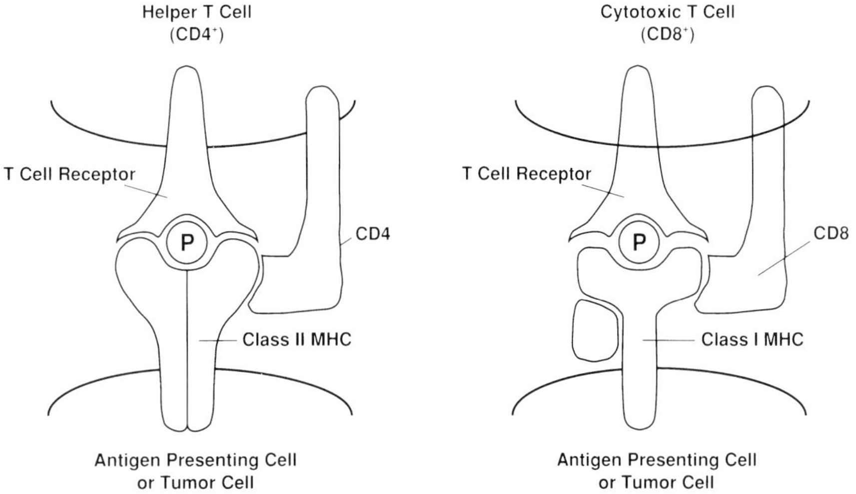
Helper T Cell
(CD4+)
Cytotoxic T Cell
(CD8+)
T Cell Receptor
P
CD4
Class II MHC
Antigen Presenting Cell
or Tumor Cell
T Cell Receptor
P
CD8
Class I MHC
Antigen Presenting Cell
or Tumor Cell

FIGURE 8–2. Schematic structure of the class I and class II complexes along with antigenic peptide (P). CD4 T lymphocytes recognize antigen in the context of self-class II MHC, and CD8 T cells recognize antigen in the context of self-class I MHC. (From Alexander RB, Walther MM, Lineman WM, Rosenberg SA: *In* Lytton B, et al. (eds): Immunotherapy of Renal Cell Carcinoma: Experience of the Surgery Branch, National Cancer Institute. Advances in Urology, pp 101–125. St. Louis, Mosby Year Book, 1993, with permission.)

ent configurations able to bind to a wide variety of antigenic configurations. Each T cell has a single TCR conformation, and it appears that T cells with a TCR configuration with a high affinity for self-antigens are deleted in the thymus. T cells with TCR of low or no binding to self-antigens are able to enter the periphery and participate in immune responses. The diversity of TCR sequences (a potential recombinatorial diversity of 10^{21} combinations) ensures that a TCR able to recognize and bind with high affinity to most potential foreign epitopes will exist in the normal host.

T cells recognize antigen not as intact molecules, as antibodies do, but rather short peptide fragments of antigens complexed with MHC surface molecules. This is schematically shown in Figure 8–2. There are two major classes of T cells defined by the surface markers CD4 and CD8. CD4 T cells, typically called helper T cells because of cytokine secretion, recognize antigen in the context of class II MHC. CD8 T cells, commonly called cytotoxic T cells because of their ability to lyse target cells, recognize antigens in the context of MHC class I. The distinction between helper and cytotoxic functions of T cells is becoming less defined, as CD4 T cells clearly can lyse appropriate class II–bearing cells and CD8 T cells can clearly secrete cytokines in response to appropriate stimulation.

Engagement of antigen by the TCR complex initiates a complex series of events in the T cell known as T-cell activation.[9] Activated T cells up-regulate the expression of certain surface molecules, secrete cytokines, and expand through proliferation. The overall effect is the expansion of specific clones of T cells recognizing the foreign antigen and the development of an immune response at the site of antigen.

After an immune response has been made to a specific antigen and the antigen rejected, T cells remain in the host as memory cells.[10] They are present at a high precursor frequency and recirculate through the vascular and lymphatic systems, retaining the ability to respond quickly to antigenic rechallenge. Strategies for vaccination against infectious diseases, particularly viruses, rely upon this function of T cells.

Helper T-Cell Subsets

The secretion of cytokines that interact with specific surface receptors on other cells of the immune system is a critical function of T cells. The local cytokine environment around a developing immune response is a major determinant of the nature and outcome of the immune response. Helper T cells play a critical role in this process. It has recently been recognized that CD4 T cells secrete cytokines in patterns that can skew the immune response in very different directions.[11] One pattern of cytokine secretion, termed T helper type 1 (Th1), includes the secretion of the cytokines interferon-γ (IFN-γ) and interleukin-2 (IL-2). This pattern of response results in the development of a cell-mediated immune response to antigen. The cytokines IL-4, IL-5, and IL-10 are secreted by T helper type 2 (Th2) cells which engenders principally a humoral or antibody response to antigen.

The distinction between these two types of response is critical. For example, in the human disease leprosy, caused by an infection with *Mycobacterium leprae*, a spectrum of immune responses to the infection can be observed. Patients with lepromatous leprosy have primarily a humoral, Th2 pattern of response to the infection and develop open lesions filled with organisms that cannot be destroyed by the primarily humoral response. Patients with tuberculous leprosy, on the other hand, have principally a Th1 type of response to the infection and mount a cellular immune response to the organism.[12,13] The cell-mediated immune response is quite capable of eliminating the intracellular infection and these patients have healing lesions with few organisms and which are not infectious. Hence, the immune response to the organism can yield very different outcomes that appear to be defined by the local cytokine environment during the developing immune response.

CANCER AND THE IMMUNE SYSTEM

The immune system has long been an attractive potential therapy for malignancy. The reason for this is because of the immune system's specificity (i.e., the ability of the immune system to recognize an organism or cell and bring forth a powerful response to destroy it with little or no injury to normal cells). The question for immunotherapy of cancer, then, is whether the immune system recognizes cancer cells or can be made to recognize cancer cells and whether this recognition can be therapeutic in patients who have established disease. It is important that specificity and efficacy not be confused. In designing a treatment for cancer, specificity without efficacy is of no use; it will do little for patients with cancer if the immune system can recognize tumors but cannot destroy them. It is clear that many therapies with no specificity for cancer can have enormous efficacy as a treatment for the disease, chemotherapy with antiproliferative drugs being the best example. Nevertheless, the prospect of specific recognition of cancer cells and rejection of cancer in the same way that bacteria or virally infected cells are destroyed continues to intrigue immunologists and cancer therapists.

The question of whether tumors contain antigens that can be recognized by the immune system has a long history of debate in immunology. For many years this question was pursued by searching for antibodies that specifically bound tumor cells but not normal cells. A clear demonstration of tumor antigens was never made by this method. Since the part of the immune system principally responsible for the recognition of cells is the T-lymphocyte population, the discovery of IL-2, the first cytokine capable of causing T cells to grow in vitro, and the increased understanding of the nature of antigens recognized by T cells and the clarification of MHC restriction greatly facilitated the study of tumor antigens recognized by T cells.

Human Tumor Antigens

Early studies of lymphocytes in tumor-bearing patients suggested that specific recognition of tumor cells could be observed in lymphocytes derived from the peripheral blood or lymph nodes of patients with melanoma.[14–17] Such cells were also found directly infiltrating the tumor and could be grown by culturing single-cell suspensions of fresh tumors in IL-2.[18] Such proliferating cultures of T cells were called tumor infiltrating lymphocytes (TIL). In murine tumors, TIL were exclusively CD8 T cells and could specifically recognize their syngeneic tumor of origin.[19] Similarly, in human melanoma TIL could readily be produced that specifically recognized the tumor of origin but not other tumors.[20,21] In fact, it became clear following the study of many such TIL derived from melanoma that there were shared melanoma-associated antigens and the specificity of T-cell recognition was due to the MHC restriction element expressed by the tumor cells.[22] For example, TIL were observed that recognized many cultured melanoma tumor cells that were derived from patients who were HLA-A2 and these TIL could also recognize non–HLA-A2 melanoma cells if they were transfected with the gene for HLA-A2.[23,24] Antigen-specific, MHC-restricted recognition of tumor cells by T cells has been demonstrated by a variety of methods including lysis of tumor cells,[21] cytokine secretion by T cells,[25,26] and increases in intracellular calcium concentration[27] demonstrating that the signal transduction and effector functions of these T cells appear to be no different than those observed in allogeneic mixed lymphocyte reactions or viral antigen recognition. Hence, in melanoma, the concept of tumor-associated antigens that could be specifically recognized by lymphocytes within the tumor-bearing host was demonstrated to be valid.

Human Melanoma Antigens

What is the nature of these antigens in melanoma? One expectation would be that because these antigens are derived from tumor cells, mutated or abnormal proteins somehow involved in the genesis of the cancer would result in abnormal peptide expression in the tumor cell and these mutated peptides would be immunogenic and result in an antigen-specific T-cell response. While such mutated antigenic proteins have been detected,[28] most tumor-associated antigens in melanoma that have so far been characterized are components of normal cells as well as cancer cells. The first melanoma-associated antigen to be described was termed melanoma-associated gene (MAGE-1), which is part of a family of proteins expressed by melanomas.[29] A peptide derived from the MAGE-1 gene product, when presented in the context of HLA-A1, was demonstrated to be the antigen recognized by melanoma-specific cytotoxic T lymphocytes (CTL) derived from the same patient.[30] The MAGE-1 gene product is expressed in melanomas but not in normal tissues with the possible exception of testis.

Other melanoma antigens have been described, however, where expression in normal mature tissues is observed. The enzyme tyrosinase, a protein necessary for the synthesis of melanin, is also the target of a T-cell response in melanoma.[31–34] Tyrosinase is expressed in melanocytes, normal skin, and pigmented nevi, all melanin-containing tissues. The melanoma-associated antigen MAGE-3, another of the family of MAGE gene products, contains a peptide sequence that is recognized by autologous CTL in the context of HLA-A1.[35] MAGE-3 is expressed in melanoma cells as well as in melanocytes, normal testis, and in a significant proportion of other cancers.[35] Another peptide derived from melanomas was identified by Cox et al.[36] by tandem mass spectroscopy of peptides eluted from a melanoma cell line DMA. This peptide appears to be derived from the protein Pmel 17, a protein expressed by normal melanocytes and melanoma cells. This peptide, when presented by HLA-A2.1 was recognized by CTL derived from five different melanoma patients. Finally, the melanoma antigen MART-1 is expressed by melanocytes and normal retina tissue and is also an antigen recognized by melanoma TIL in the context of HLA-A2.[37] Thus, the antigens in melanoma that are clearly recognized by T lymphocytes are frequently not abnormal or mutated gene products but are components of normal cells as well as tumor cells.

Self and Altered Self

Antigens expressed in melanomas and recognized by T cells are frequently components of normal cells of the same lineage as the tumor. Peptides derived from these normal cell proteins that bind to self–class I MHC have been synthesized and can be recognized by TIL derived from patients. These peptides, which can bind to MHC on the surface of intact cells,[38] can also be used to detect the precursor frequency of reactive T lymphocytes and to produce cultured T-cell lines from the peripheral blood of patients with melanoma with peptide specificity and specific recognition of the antigen contained in melanoma tumor cells. Interestingly, however, the same cells are present and can be cultured from individuals of the appropriate MHC haplotype who do not have melanoma.[39] For example, the MART-1 tumor antigen contained in the majority of melanoma and melanocyte cell lines contains an immunodominant peptide that binds to HLA-A2 and that can be used to produce CD8 T-lymphocyte cell lines from the peripheral blood of normal HLA-A2 individuals that recognize HLA-A2 melanoma tumor cells.[40]

Thus a growing body of evidence suggests that tumor reactivity in patients with melanoma is self-reactivity. This may help explain the interesting observation that patients with melanoma who develop vitiligo, a depigmenting disease of the skin, have a better prognosis.[41] T cells that recognize normal self-antigens in melanomas are present in normal individuals. These cells are not deleted and are not anergic or nonresponsive. They are present and can respond to appropriate antigenic stimulation. Hence, tumor immunology appears to share much with autoimmunity. Clearly, as we learn more about what controls immune reactivity to self we will learn more about how to use the immune system to treat cancer.

Tumor Antigens in Urologic Malignancies

TIL have been produced from a variety of urologic malignancies.[42] However, just as has been observed in human cancer histologies other than melanoma, specific recognition of tumor cells has been infrequent. For example, in renal cell carcinoma TIL can be readily grown by culturing tumor digests in IL-2 but only rarely has antigen-specific, MHC-restricted recognition of renal cell carcinoma tumor cells been demonstrated.[43,44] Typically, renal cell carcinoma TIL contain heterogeneous populations of T cells and non–T cells with broad reactivity against cultured tumor targets, similar to lymphokine-activated killer (LAK) cells.[45] The reason for the distinction between melanoma TIL, where specific T cells can be detected in 40% of cultures, and renal cell carcinoma TIL is unknown. One potential explanation is the cutaneous origin of melanoma and the presence of dendritic cells in the skin that might result in a primary T-cell response in patients with melanoma more readily than in organ-based malignancies where dendritic cells are less numerous.

It is also very clear that, despite the failure of TIL from renal cell carcinoma to specifically recognize tumor cells, large numbers of T cells are present in renal cell cancers. In fact, the CD4 T cells in renal cell carcinoma primary tumors have the phenotype of activated cells but have not up-regulated IL-2 receptors compared to peripheral blood CD4 T cells.[46] Proliferation defects in T cells infiltrating human renal cell carcinoma have been described[47] as well as aberrations in the signaling pathways of T cells infiltrating human renal cell cancers.[48] Perhaps renal cancer antigen-specific T cells are present in renal cancers but are unable to proliferate, explaining the infrequent finding of specific T cells in cultures from renal cell carcinomas produced with IL-2.

Antigens in Prostatic Cancer

There are few published studies of prostatic TIL, and no reports of specific T cells being produced from prostatic cancers by culture in vitro. Several groups, however, are searching for specific T cells recognizing antigens known to be specific for the prostate based upon the finding that cancer antigens in melanoma are normal self-proteins. Tjoa et al.[49] described an HLA-A2 peptide derived from prostate-specific membrane antigen (PSMA)[50] that was recognized by cultured T cells. We have observed specific recognition of peptides that bind to HLA-A2 derived from the sequence of PSA in HLA-A2 patients with prostatic cancer (R.B. Alexander, submitted for publication). Whether any of these peptide-specific T cells will recognize intact antigen expressed in prostatic cancer cells remains to be determined. Strategies to vaccinate patients with prostatic cancer using a recombinant vaccinia virus expressing prostate-specific antigen (PSA) are in progress.[51] Again the goal of these approaches is to detect or engender an immune response against an antigen known to be expressed only in prostatic epithelial cells.

CLINICAL USE OF IMMUNOTHERAPY

Many strategies for the immunotherapy of cancer have been tested in humans and a few have achieved U.S. Food and Drug Administration (FDA) approval for specific indications. The development of these therapies and the findings about their use in humans can teach important lessons about the basic principles of immunotherapy of cancer.

Adoptive Immunotherapy Versus Vaccination

The immunotherapy of cancer can be divided into two basic approaches. Adoptive immunotherapy is herein defined to mean the administration of components of the normal immune system, either cellular or noncellular, in pharmacologic doses to patients with cancer. Vaccination represents an attempt to engender an immune response within the host against the cancer in order for the host's immune system to bring about the destruction of tumor cells.

Adoptive Immunotherapy

The administration of pharmacologic doses of biologic agents to patients was limited by the small amounts and impure nature of such agents until the development of recombinant DNA technology. This technology allowed for the production of large quantities of very pure materials to be tested as a therapy for cancer in animals and patients. The purity of cytokines and other types of biologic agents is critically important to sort out the desired and adverse effects of these agents. At present there are two cytokines approved by the FDA for the treatment of cancer, IFN-α for the treatment of hairy cell leukemia and IL-2 for the treatment of metastatic renal cell carcinoma.

INTERLEUKIN-2. Interleukin-2 was the first cytokine discovered with the capability to make T lymphocytes proliferate in culture.[52] Given that T cells are principally responsible for the recognition of foreign cells it was this simple fact that stimulated interest in the use of IL-2 as a treatment for cancer. The goal of IL-2 as an anticancer agent was to find or engender specific recognition of cancer by T lymphocytes.

The most readily available source of T cells in patients with cancer is the peripheral blood. It was quickly clear that peripheral blood T cells from patients with cancer, when cultured in IL-2, developed the ability to lyse fresh single-cell suspensions of human cancers in an MHC-independent fashion.[53,54] This activity was called LAK for lymphokine activated killer and was never specific but was always seen in patients with cancer and in normal individuals.

In murine experimental models of cancer it was clear that IL-2 had antitumor effects and caused dose-dependent reductions in experimental metastases of immunogenic and nonimmunogenic tumors in mice. LAK cells could also be produced in mice by culture of murine splenocytes in IL-2 and the addition of LAK cells to IL-2 alone could cure established experimental metastatic tumors in mice.[55] Both LAK and IL-2 were required for cures in animals to be observed. It was these preclinical data that supported the performance of trials of IL-2 and LAK cells in patients with cancer.

Patients with metastatic cancer, the majority of whom had metastatic renal cell carcinoma or melanoma, with evaluable disease were treated with IL-2 and LAK cells. In the initial reports of this therapy in humans dramatic responses were observed in patients with, in some cases, bulky metastatic disease.[56,57] Therapy with the maximum tolerated dose of IL-2 was also toxic, with patients manifesting a capillary leak syndrome with the accumulation of fluid in interstitial spaces, hypotension, and reversible major organ system dysfunction.[58]

A major question when these results were reported was whether the LAK cells contributed to the therapy, as this heterogenous population of cells had no clear counterpart in natural immune responses and were cumbersome to produce and administer. A randomized trial comparing LAK plus IL-2 to IL-2 alone was therefore instituted in patients with advanced cancers. After 5 years of follow-up, there was no difference in response rate, durability of responses, or overall survival in patients with renal cell carcinoma; the difference in survival for patients with melanoma, while favoring LAK plus IL-2, was not statistically significant.[59] The important result of this trial is that, despite compelling preclinical data, the individual components of multiagent regimens must be carefully tested to determine which contributes to desirable effects. This is particularly true of therapies including biologic agents.

Nevertheless, it is clear that IL-2 alone had a significant antitumor effect in patients with metastatic renal cell carcinoma. In the application to the FDA, the overall response rate in patients with metastatic renal cell carcinoma treated on an inpatient, high-dose regimen of 720,000 IU/kg IL-2 intravenously every 8 hours was 15%. A significant portion of these responses, however, were durable complete responses that appear to have extended the survival of patients. Thus, while most patients do not respond to IL-2 and the administration of IL-2 has significant toxicity, the chance to achieve a durable complete response of even bulky metastatic disease resulted in the approval of IL-2 for the treatment of metastatic renal cell carcinoma.

Other schedules of administration of IL-2 have been tested. In the early experience with IL-2 by intravenous bolus given at the maximum tolerated dose, patients tolerated a variable number of doses. The drug was held during cycles of administration depending on toxicity in individual patients and it was observed that patients who received relatively small amounts of IL-2 overall could still be observed to have responses. To address this question, a randomized trial of two arms—standard, high-dose IL-2 at 720,000 IU/kg intravenously every 8 hours, or a dose tenfold lower on the same schedule (72,000 IU/kg intravenously every 8 hours)—was instituted in patients with renal cell carcinoma. An interim analysis of this trial demonstrated no difference in response rates or durability of response but a dramatic decrease in toxicity of the low-dose IL-2 arm compared to the high-dose IL-2 arm, especially in the occurrence of grade 3 or 4 hypotension, which is the dose-limiting toxicity of IL-2 by intravenous administration.[60] This trial demonstrates that the maximum tolerated dose of IL-2 is not necessarily the best dose, an important fact that should be considered in all designs of trials for biologic agents in particular. However, it may still be possible that high-dose IL-2 has a higher complete response rate than lower dose intravenous regimens, hence recruitment into the trial continues.

Following the report of Sleijfer et al.,[61] IL-2 is also being administered by outpatient, subcutaneous regimens to patients with metastatic renal cell carcinoma. This is probably the most frequent way this agent is being used in the United States at present. A variety of regimens, most in combination with interferon-α or chemotherapeutic drugs, is being explored.[62–67] As always, the effect of each part of combination regimens can only be clearly resolved by prospective clinical trials.

Cellular Adoptive Therapies. Since T cells are central to the developing immune response and are the principal means by which foreign cells are recognized, the ability to produce such cells by culture and to administer them as a therapy for cancer has generated great interest. TIL from a variety of malignancies have been administered to patients as a treatment for cancer. The interpretation of these studies is complicated, however, by the different protocols used to produce cultured cells and the variation from patient to patient of the phenotype and function of the cells obtained by culture and administered to patients. TIL from patients with melanoma have been reported to produce a 40% response rate in patients with metastatic melanoma when administered along with IL-2 and cyclophosphamide.[68] As described above, these cultured cells can specifically recognize melanoma cancer cells in an MHC-restricted, antigen-specific fashion, and cultures in which this occurs appear to be more likely to be therapeutic in patients.[69] The response rate to TIL in melanoma also appears to be no different whether or not patients have previously failed IL-2 therapy, which provides indirect evidence that the cellular therapy may be contributing to responses in patients with melanoma.

TIL from other histologies have also been studied in patients with variable results. In renal cell carcinoma TIL can readily be produced by culture in IL-2. The cells resulting from such cultures demonstrate typical heterogeneous mixture of CD4 and CD8 T cells along with other populations similar to LAK cells.[70] Results with the administration of such cells to patients have been variable.[71,72] In combination regimens with other biologic agents the response rates to TIL have been reported in some trials that suggest that the TIL may be contributing in excess of the other cytokines that are concurrently administered to patients.[73] Once again, however, the contribution of each component of multiagent therapies can only be resolved prospectively. Attempts to enrich the CD8 subpopulation of TIL from renal cell carcinoma TIL cultures and to use these as therapy are also underway in a multicenter trial.[74]

Other Cytokine Therapies. The list of human cytokines that have been cloned and expressed as recombinant material continues to grow. Many of these mediators have been and are being tested in pharmacologic doses as a treatment for cancer. Tumor necrosis factor (TNF) was one of the first human cytokines to undergo extensive clinical testing as a treatment for cancer, since it caused necrosis of experimental tumors in mice. However, a large number of trials of systemic TNF in humans demonstrated substantial toxicity and no evidence of significant antitumor effects in patients.[75] IL-4, IL-6,[76] and IL-7 have also entered trials in humans with cancer.

Interleukin-12 is a monocyte-derived cytokine that is central to the developing cell-mediated immune response and the engendering of a Th1 type of response to infectious agents.[77] Since it appears that this is the type of immune response most likely to be effective against cancer, IL-12 has generated substantial interest as a potential therapy for cancer.[78,79]

The major problem with systemic cytokine therapies is toxicity. Cytokines, when secreted by cells of the immune system, generate an effect that is local and do not achieve significant systemic levels for the most part. In addition, cytokines do not act in isolation but provide signals to cells that can be modulated by timing, combinations of different cytokines, and direct cell-to-cell interactions that are complex and highly regulated. Hence, the administration of cytokines systemically is not physiologic, and adverse effects that can be severe and dose-limiting can occur. Targeted delivery of cytokines to tumor deposits is possible in some cases (e.g., the delivery of IL-2 to lung metastases by inhalational therapy[80,81] or the administration of cytokines to tumor-bearing organs by isolated perfusion[82]). These approaches are limited by the ability to target tumors effectively by some technical procedure but may have relevance in some clinical situations.

Vaccination Strategies

The general theme of vaccination strategies for cancer is to induce an immune response to tumor antigens that will bring about the rejection of established disease. The finding of tumor antigens in melanoma that are specifically recognized by T cells has finally demonstrated that it is theoretically possible to do this. However, the finding that most antigens in melanoma are components of normal cells suggests that toxicity from such vaccination is possible and that the tightly controlled means by which the body prevents autoreactivity in most individuals must be understood and circumvented in order to engender a significant immune response to self that will be effective against tumors.

The history of vaccination as a therapy for established cancer is a long one. William Coley observed a patient with an unresectable neck sarcoma who had complete regression of the tumor after he developed a streptococcal infection of the neck. Coley spent his life developing and testing various extracts of bacteria as a therapy for cancer. These came to be known as Coley's toxins.[83] Despite an enormous effort, however, the use of various microbial agents, tumor extracts, and various nonspecific immune stimulants has never resulted in an established therapy for human cancer with the notable exception of bacille Calmette-Guérin (BCG) as a treatment for superficial transitional cell carcinoma of the bladder. The history of this subject is extensively reviewed by Oettgen and Old.[84]

Once tumor antigens recognized by T cells in melanoma were identified, strategies to specifically vaccinate against them became possible. Several approaches to vaccination with known tumor antigens are under consideration. First, one could vaccinate with tumor-associated antigens along with an adjuvant. A fundamental tenet of immunology is that the immune response to proteins that one can induce by vaccination is greatly increased by the inclusion of an adjuvant in the vaccine. The purpose of the adjuvant is to create a local inflammatory response that brings immune cells to the site of antigen. Adjuvants typically contain oils that are difficult for the host to break down and also commonly contain killed bacterial organisms such as BCG or *Corynebacterium parvum.* Adjuvants are essential in the production of monoclonal and polyclonal antibodies to foreign proteins in experimental animals. The type of adjuvant used can profoundly affect the type of immune response.[85] Unfortunately, many adjuvants are not suitable for use in humans because of local toxicity at the site of vaccination.

Peptide Vaccines. It is also possible to use peptides derived from tumor antigens as vaccines to treat cancer. Peptides derived from tumor antigen sequences that bind to intact HLA class I or class II can be chemically synthesized, purified, and administered to patients. Such exogenous peptides can bind to HLA complexes on the surface of cells[38] and engender an immune response to the peptide. The advantage of a peptide approach is that the antigen is highly defined and purified and little toxicity is likely. The problem with the peptide approach is that the immunogenicity of individual peptides is low and patients must have defined MHC haplotypes, which vary greatly in their frequency. Another potential problem with peptide vaccination is the possibility that T cells with reactivity to peptide may be made anergic or unresponsive to antigen because of overstimulation by the peptide vaccine. This effect has clearly been demonstrated in an animal model,[86] and it is well known that overstimulation of T cells with antigen can cause anergy or even deletion of T cells, probably a means of controlling the immune response. Recent evidence that there may be peptide-binding supermotifs among the diverse polymorphism of HLA alleles may simplify the design of peptide vaccines.[87] Clinical trials of peptide-based vaccines using peptides derived from MAGE-3 and MART-1 melanoma antigens are underway in patients.

Another approach to peptide vaccine delivery is to pulse dendritic cells with the peptide and use autologous, pulsed cells as the vaccine. Such experiments have been successful in animal models[88-90] and may serve to make the immune response to the peptide antigen more robust than that occurring from simple peptide vaccination alone. The availability of protocols for the production of dendritic cells from peripheral blood has facilitated these studies.[91]

Another approach to specific vaccination is the use of recombinant vectors that contain tumor antigen sequences and can infect host cells with high efficiency but low toxicity. Viruses are ideally suited for such a purpose. It is essential that the virus not cause disease in humans for such a strategy to be effective. The recombinant virus containing the tumor antigen infects host cells and propagates, and produces the tumor antigen protein within host cells. The immune response directed against the virus would also then be directed against the tumor antigen and the resulting systemic immune response could cause the rejection of tumors at distant sites. The virus acts both as a vector to deliver the tumor antigen to host cells and also as an adjuvant by engendering an immune response against viral proteins.

Several recombinant viral vectors are being explored for this purpose. Vaccinia virus is on orthopox virus widely used throughout the world as a vaccine for smallpox. Recombinant vaccinia viruses expressing foreign genes are readily produced. The virus infects human cells and is cytopathic to cells after 24 to 48 hours of infection. Before lysis of the cell, however, the recombinant gene is expressed in high amounts by the infected cell and can serve as a target for an immune reaction. Recombinant vaccinia virus expressing carcinoembryonic antigen (CEA) is being explored as a therapy for colonic cancer in humans.[92,93] Similarly, vaccinia virus expressing PSA is being explored as a therapy for prostatic cancer.[51] Other viral vectors for delivering tumor antigens to tumor-bearing hosts are being explored as a therapy for cancer including adenovirus[94,95] and fowlpox virus.[96] Finally, vaccination using plain or "naked" DNA vectors may perhaps be the simplest means of creating a specific immune response against a known tumor antigen.[97] The DNA vector is presumably taken up by cells at the site of the injection and an immune response engendered.

Gene Therapy of Cancer. Gene therapy for cancer may be rather broadly defined as any therapy of cancer that involves a recombinant DNA technology. Most approaches to gene therapy are not, in fact, therapies directed against the genetic changes that are increasingly recognized as a major cause of the malignant phenotype, but are rather immunotherapies using genetic manipulation in one form or another.[98]

The most thoroughly studied approach to the gene therapy of cancer is the use of tumor cells transfected with the genes for cytokines. These cytokine-transfected tumor cells have been shown in some cases to be incapable of forming tumors compared to wild-type tumor cells, or in some cases the transfected tumor cells grow and regress.[99] The means by which these cytokine-transfected tumor cells cause the regression of tumors is a paracrine effect in that high local amounts of cytokine along with the tumor cell results in the stimulation of a local immune response that generates an immune response against the tumor (reviewed by Pardoll[100]). The advantage of this approach is that the exact antigen does not need to be known and the vaccine can generate reactivity to any of the many potential antigens simultaneously. Virtually the entire list of cloned cytokines has been explored in murine experiments. In the B16 murine melanoma Dranoff et al. found that granulocyte-monocyte colony-stimulating factor (GM-CSF) was the most active cytokine[101] and produced a CD4 and CD8 T-cell-dependent antitumor response. One problem with the interpretation of these studies is the level of cytokine secretion observed can vary greatly. This probably reflects factors relating to the vector used to transfect the cytokine gene as well as the particular tumor cell line under study. Clinical trials in humans with renal cell carcinoma have demonstrated antitumor effects, and similar trials are ongoing in men with prostatic cancer at high risk for recurrence following radical prostatectomy (J. Simons, unpublished data).

CONCLUSION

The immune system is an enormously complex and highly regulated network our understanding of which continues to increase. It is clear that an immune response to human tumors can and does occur and that, for melanoma, the antigens being recognized in this response are components of normal cells. The factors that keep the immune system from destroying the normal host and the ways in which this self-reactivity might be released to destroy tumors are the critical factors that must be understood for progress in the field of cancer immunotherapy to occur.

REFERENCES

1. Harriman W, Volk H, Defranoux N, Wabl M: Immunoglobulin class switch recombination. Annu Rev Immunol 1993; 11:361–384.
2. Gotch F, Rothbard J, Howland K, et al: Cytotoxic T lymphocytes recognize a fragment of influenza virus matrix protein in association with HLA-A2. Nature 1987; 326: 881–882.
3. Bjorkman PJ, Parham P: Structure, function, and diversity of class I major histocompatibility complex molecules. Annu Rev Biochem 1990; 59:253–288.
4. Jardetzky TS, Brown JH, Gorga JC, et al: Three-dimensional structure of a human class II histocompatibility molecule complexed with superantigen. Nature 1994; 368:711–718.
5. Brown JH, Jardetzky TS, Gorga JC, et al: Three-dimensional structure of the human class II histocompatibility antigen HLA-DR1. Nature 1993; 364:33–39.
6. Restifo NP: Antigen processing and presentation. *In* De Vita VT, Hellman S, Rosenberg SA (eds): Biologic Therapy of Cancer. Philadelphia, JB Lippincott Co, 1995.
7. Steinman RM, Witmer-Pack M, Inaba K: Dendritic cells: antigen presentation, accessory function and clinical relevance. Adv Exp Med Biol 1993; 329:1–9.
8. Clevers H, Alarcon B, Wileman T, Terhorst C: The T cell receptor/CD3 complex: a dynamic protein ensemble. Annu Rev Immunol 1988; 6:629–662.
9. Weiss A, Imboden JB: Cell surface molecules and early events involved in human T lymphocyte activation. Adv Immunol 1987; 41:1–38.
10. Jamieson BD, Ahmed R: T cell memory. Long-term persistence of virus-specific cytotoxic T cells. J Exp Med 1989; 169:1993–2005.
11. Mosmann TR: T lymphocyte subsets, cytokinse, and effector functions. Ann N Y Acad Sci 1992; 664:89–92.
12. Salgame P, Abrams JS, Clayberger C, et al: Differing lymphokine profiles of functional subsets of human CD4 and CD8 T cell clones. Science 1991; 254:279–282.
13. Yamamura M, Uyemura K, Deans RJ, et al: Defining protective responses to pathogens: cytokine profiles in leprosy lesions. Science 1991; 254:277–279.
14. Knuth A, Danowski B, Oettgen HF, Old LJ: T-cell-mediated cytotoxicity against autologous malignant melanoma: analysis with interleukin 2-dependent T-cell cultures. Proc Natl Acad Sci U S A 1984; 81:3511–3515.
15. Anichini A, Fossati G, Parmiani G: Clonal analysis of cytotoxic T-lymphocyte response to autologous human metastatic melanoma. Int J Cancer 1985; 35:683–689.
16. Slingluff CL, Darrow TL, Seigler HF: Human T cells specifically activated against autologous malignant melanoma. Arch Surg 1987; 122:1407–1411.
17. Herin M, Lemoine C, Weynants P, et al: Production of stable cytolytic T-cell clones directed against autologous human melanoma. Int J Cancer 1987; 39:390–396.

18. Rosenberg SA, Spiess PJ, Lafreniere R: A new approach to the adoptive immunotherapy of cancer with tumor infiltrating lymphocytes. Science 1985; 233:1318–1321.
19. Barth RJ, Bock SN, Mule JJ, Rosenberg SA: Unique murine tumor associated antigens identified by tumor infiltrating lymphocytes. J Immunol 1990; 144:1531–1537.
20. Muul LM, Spies PJ, Director EP, Rosenberg SA: Identification of specific cytolytic immune responses against autologous tumor in humans bearing malignant melanoma. J Immunol 1987; 138:989.
21. Topalian SL, Solomon D, Rosenberg SA: Tumor-specific cytolysis by lymphocytes infiltrating human melanomas. J Immunol 1989; 142:3714–3725.
22. Hom SS, Topalian SL, Simonis T, et al: Common expression of melanoma tumor-associated antigens recognized by human tumor infiltrating lymphocytes: analysis by human lympocyte antigen restriction. J Immunother 1991; 10:153–164.
23. O'Neil BH, Kawakami Y, Restifo NP, et al: Detection of shared MHC-restricted human melanoma antigens after vaccinia virus-mediated transduction of genes coding for HLA. J Immunol 1993; 151:1410–1418.
24. Kawakami Y, Zakut R, Topalian SL, et al: Shared human melanoma antigens. Recognition by tumor-infiltrating lymphocytes in HLA-A2.1-transfected melanomas. J Immunol 1992; 148:638–643.
25. Schwartzentruber DJ, Topalian SL, Mancini M, Rosenberg SA: Specific release of granulocyte-macrophage colony-stimulating factor, tumor necrosis factor-alpha, and IFN-gamma by human tumor-infiltrating lymphocytes after autologous tumor stimulation. J Immunol 1991; 146: 3674–3681.
26. Schwartzentruber DJ, Solomon D, Rosenberg SA, Topalian SL: Characterization of lymphocytes infiltrating human breast cancer: specific immune reactivity detected by measuring cytokine secretion. J Immunother 1992; 12:1–12.
27. Alexander RB, Bolton ES, Koenig S, et al: Detection of antigen specific T lymphocytes by determination of intracellular calcium concentration using flow cytometry. J Immunol Methods 1992; 148:131–141.
28. Wolfel T, Hauer M, Schneider J, et al: Ap16^{ink4a}-insensitive CDK4 mutant targeted by cytolytic T lymphocytes in a human melanoma. Science 1995; 269:1281–1284.
29. van der Bruggen P, Traversari C, Chomez P, et al: A gene encoding an antigen recognized by cytolytic T lymphocytes on a human melanoma. Science 1991; 254:1643–1647.
30. Traversari C, Bruggen PV, Luescher IF, et al: A nonapeptide encoded by human gene MAGE-1 is recognized on HLA-A1 by cytolytic T lymphocytes directed against tumor antigen MZ2-E. J Exp Med 1992; 176:1453–1457.
31. Brichard V, Van Pel A, Wolfel T, et al: The tyrosinase gene codes for an antigen recognized by autologus cytolytic T lymphocytes on HLA-A2 melanoma. J Exp Med 1993; 178:489–495.
32. Kang X, Kawakami Y, el-Gamil M, et al: Identification of a tyrosinase epitope recognized by HLA-A24-restricted, tumor-infiltrating lymphocytes. J Immunol 1995; 155: 1343–1348.
33. Topalian SL, Rivoltini L, Mancini M, et al: Human CD4+ T cells specifically recognize a shared melanoma-associated antigen encoded by the tyrosinase gene. Proc Natl Acad Sci U S A 1994; 91:9461–9465.
34. Robbins PF, el-Gamil M, Kawakami Y, et al: Recognition of tyrosinase by tumor-infiltrating lymphocytes from a patient responding to immunotherapy. Cancer Res 1994; 54:3124–3126.
35. Gaugler B, Eynde VE, Bruggen PV, et al: Human gene MAGE-3 codes for an antigen recognized on a melanoma by autologous cytolytic T lymphocytes. J Exp Med 1994; 179:921–930.
36. Cox AL, Skipper J, Chen Y, et al: Identification of peptide recognized by five melanoma-specific human cytotoxic T cell lines. Science 1994; 264:716–719.
37. Kawakami Y, Eliyahu S, Delgado CH, et al: Cloning of the gene coding for a shared human melanoma antigen recognized by autologous T cells infiltrating into tumor. Proc Natl Acad Sci U S A 1994; 91:3515–3519.
38. Christinck ER, Luscher MA, Barber BH, Williams DB: Peptide binding to class I MHC on living cells and quantitation of complexes required for CTL lysis. Nature 1991; 352:67–70.
39. Celis E, Tsai V, Crimi C, et al: Induction of anti-tumor cytotoxic T lymphocytes in normal humans using primary cultures and synthetic peptide epitopes. Proc Natl Acad Sci U S A 1994; 91:2105–2109.
40. Rivoltini L, Kawakami Y, Sakaguchi K, et al: Induction of tumor-reactive CTL from peripheral blood and tumor-infiltrating lymphocytes of melanoma patients by in vitro stimulation with an immunodominant peptide of the human melanoma antigen MART-1. J Immunol 1995; 154: 2257–2265.
41. Rosenberg SA, White DE: Vitiligo in patients with melanoma: normal tissue antigens can be targets for cancer immunotherapy. J Immunother 1996; 19:81–84.
42. Haas GP, Solomon D, Rosenberg SA: Tumor-infiltrating lymphocytes from nonrenal urological malignancies. Cancer Immunol Immunother 1990; 30:342–350.
43. Finke JH, Rayman P, Edinger M, et al: Characterization of a human renal cell carcinoma specific cytotoxic CD8+ T cell line. J Immunother 1992; 11:1–11.
44. Schendel DJ, Gansbacher B, Oberneder R, et al: Tumor-specific lysis of human renal cell carcinomas by tumor-infiltrating lymphocytes. I. HLA-A2-restricted recognition of autologous and allogeneic tumor lines. J Immunol 1993; 151:4209–4220.
45. Kim TY, von Eschenbach AC, Filaccio MLD, et al: Clonal analysis of lymphocytes from tumor, peripheral blood, and nontumorous kidney in primary renal cell carcinoma. Cancer Res 1990; 50:5263–5268.
46. Alexander RB, Fitzgerald EB, Mixon A, et al: Helper T cells infiltrating human renal cell carcinomas have the phenotype of activated memory-like T lymphocytes. J Immunother Emphasis Tumor Immunol 1995; 17:39–46.
47. Alexander JP, Kudoh S, Melsop KA, et al: T-cells infiltrating renal cell carcinoma display a poor proliferative response even though they can produce interleukin 2 and express interleukin 2 receptors. Cancer Res 1993; 53: 1380–1387.
48. Finke JH, Zea AH, Stanley J, et al: Loss of T-cell receptor zeta chain and p56lck in T-cells infiltrating human renal cell carcinoma. Cancer Res 1993; 53:5613–5616.
49. Tjoa B, Boynton A, Kenny G, et al: Presentation of prostate tumor antigens by dendritic cells stimulates T-cell proliferation and cytotoxicity. Prostate 1996; 28:65–69.
50. Israeli RS, Powell T, Fair WR, Heston WDW: Molecular cloning of a complementary DNA encoding a prostate-specific membrane antigen. Cancer Res 1993; 53:227–230.
51. Hodge JW, Schlom J, Donohue SJ, et al: A recombinant vaccinia virus expressing human prostate-specific antigen (PSA): safety and immunogenicity in a non-human primate. Int J Cancer 1995; 63:231–237.
52. Morgan DA, Ruscetti FW, Gallo R: Selective in vitro growth of T lymphocytes from normal human bone marrows. Science 1976; 193:1007–1008.
53. Grimm EA, Mazumder A, Zhang HZ, Rosenberg SA: Lymphokine-activated killer cell phenomenon. Lysis of natural killer-resistant fresh solid tumor cells by interleukin 2-activated autologous human peripheral blood lymphocytes. J Exp Med 1982; 155:1823–1841.
54. Grimm EA, Ramsey KM, Mazumder A, et al: Lymphokine-activated killer cell phenomenon. II. Precursor phenotype is serologically distinct from peripheral T lymphocytes, memory cytotoxic thymus-derived lymphocytes, and natural killer cells. J Exp Med 1983; 157:884–897.
55. Lafreniere R, Rosenberg SA: Adoptive immunotherapy of murine hepatic metastases with lymphokine activated killer (LAK) cells and recombinant interleukin 2 (RIL 2)

can mediate the regression of both immunogenic and nonimmunogenic sarcomas and an adenocarcinoma. J Immunol 1985; 135:4273–4280.

56. Rosenberg SA, Lotze MT, Muul LM, et al: Observations on the systemic administration of autologous lymphokine-activated killer cells and recombinant interleukin-2 to patients with metastatic cancer. N Engl J Med 1985; 313:1485–1492.
57. Rosenberg SA, Lotze MT, Muul LM, et al: A progress report on the treatment of 157 patients with advanced cancer using lymphokine-activated killer cells and interleukin-2 or high-dose interleukin-2 alone. N Eng J Med 1987; 316:889–897.
58. Rosenberg SA, Lotze MT, Yang JC, et al: Experience with the use of high-dose interleukin-2 in the treatment of 652 cancer patients. Ann Surg 1989; 210:474–485.
59. Rosenberg SA, Lotze MT, Yang JC, et al: Prospective randomized trial of high-dose interleukin-2 alone or in conjunction with lymphokine-activated killer cells for the treatment of patients with advanced cancer. J Natl Cancer Inst 1993; 85:622–632.
60. Yang JC, Topalian SL, Parkinson DR, et al: Randomized comparison of high-dose and low-dose intravenous interleukin-2 for the therapy of metastatic renal cell carcinoma: an interim report. J Clin Oncol 1994; 12:1572–1576.
61. Sleijfer DT, Janssen RA, Buter J, et al: Phase II study of subcutaneous interleukin-2 in unselected patients with advanced renal cell cancer on an outpatient basis. J Clin Oncol 1992; 10:1119–1123.
62. Atzpodien J, Kirchner H, Hanninen EL, et al: Interleukin-2 in combination with interferon-alpha and 5-fluorouracil for metastatic renal cell cancer. Eur J Cancer 1993; 29A: S6–S8.
63. Atzpodien J, Kirchner H, Hanninen EL, et al: European studies of interleukin-2 in metastic renal cell carcinoma. Semin Oncol 1993; 20:22–26.
64. Atzpodien J, Hanninen EL, Kirchner H, et al: Multiinstitutional home-therapy trial of recombinant human interleukin-s and interferon alfa-2 in progressive metastatic renal cell carcinoma. J Clin Oncol 1995; 13:497–501.
65. Rosenberg SA, Lotze MT, Yang JC, et al: Combination therapy with interleukin-2 and alpha-interferon for the treatment of patients with advanced cancer. J Clin Oncol 1989; 7:1863–1874.
66. Buter J, Sleijfer DT, van der Graaf TA, et al: A progress report on the outpatient treatment of patients with advanced renal cell carcinoma using subcutaneous recombinant interleukin-2. Semin Oncol 1993; 20:16–21.
67. Angevin E, Valteau-Couanet D, Farace F, et al: Phase I study of prolonged low-dose subcutaneous recombinant interleukin-2 (IL-2) in patients with advanced cancer. J Immunother 1995; 18:188–195.
68. Rosenberg SA, Packard BS, Aebersold PM, et al: Use of tumor-infiltrating lymphocytes and interleukin-2 in the immunotherapy of patients with metastatic melanoma. A preliminary report. N Engl J Med 1988; 319:1676–1680.
69. Schwartzentruber DJ, Hom SS, Dadmarz R, et al: In vitro predictors of therapeutic response in melanoma patients receiving tumor-infiltrating lymphocytes and interleukin-2. J Clin Oncol 1994; 12:1475–1483.
70. Belldegrun A, Muul LM, Rosenberg SA: Interleukin 2 expanded tumor-infiltrating lymphocytes in human renal cell cancer: isolation, characterization, and antitumor activity. Cancer Res 1988; 48:206–214.
71. Bukowski RM, Sharfman W, Murthy S, et al: Clinical results and characterization of tumor-infiltrating lymphocytes with or without recombinant interleukin 2 in human metastatic renal cell carcinoma. Cancer Res 1991; 51: 4199–4205.
72. Finke JH, Murthy S, Alexander J, et al: Tumor infiltrating lymphocytes in human renal cell carcinoma: adoptive immunotherapy and characterization of interleukin-2 expanded tumor-infiltrating lymphocytes. *In* Debruyne FMJ, Bukowski RM, Pontes JE, de Mulder PHM (eds): Immuno-Therapy of Renal Cell Carcinoma, pp 119–130. Berlin Heidelberg, Springer-Verlag, 1991.
73. Belldegrun A, Pierce W, Kaboo R, et al: Interferon-alpha primed tumor-infiltrating lymphocytes combined with interleukin-2 and interferon-alpha as therapy for metastatic renal cell carcinoma. J Urol 1993; 150:1384–1390.
74. Linna TJ, Moody DJ, Feeney LA, et al: Tumor microenvironment and immune effector cells: isolation, large scale propagation and characterization of CD8+ tumor infiltrating lymphocytes from renal cell carcinomas. Immunol Ser 1994; 61:175–178.
75. Alexander RB, Rosenberg SA: Tumor necrosis factor: Clinical applications. *In* De Vita VT, Hellman S, Rosenberg SA (eds): Biologic Therapy of Cancer, pp 378–392. Philadelphia, JB Lippincott Co, 1991.
76. Weber J, Gunn H, Yang JC, et al: A phase I trial of intravenous interleukin-6 in patients with advanced cancer. J Immunother Emphasis Tumor Immunol 1994; 15:292–302.
77. Trinchieri G: Interleukin-12: a proinflammatory cytokine with immunoregulatory functions that bridge innate resistance and antigen-specific adaptive immunity. Annu Rev Immunol 1995; 13:251–276.
78. Zitvogel L, Tahara H, Robbins PD, et al: Cancer immunotherapy of established tumors with IL-12. J Immunol 1995; 155:1393–1403.
79. Zitvogel L, Lotze MT: Role of interleukin-12 (IL12) as an anti-tumour agent: experimental biology and clinical application. Res Immunol 1995; 146:628–635.
80. Huland E, Heinzer H, Huland H: Inhaled interleukin-2 in combination with low-dose systemic interleukin-2 and interferon α in patients with pulmonary metastic renal-cell carcinoma: effectiveness and toxicity of mainly local treatment. Cancer Res Clin Oncol 1995; 120:221–228.
81. Huland E, Huland H, Heinzer H: Interleukin-2 by inhalation: local therapy for metastatic renal cell carcinoma. J Urol 1992; 147:344–348.
82. Lienard D, Ewalenko P, Delmotte JJ, et al: High-dose recombinant tumor necrosis factor alpha in combination with interferon gamma and melphalan in isolation perfusion of the limbs for melanoma and sarcoma. J Clin Oncol 1992; 10:52–60.
83. Coley WB: The therapeutic value of the mixed toxins of the streptococcus of erysipelas and bacillus prodigiosus in the treatment of inoperable malignant tumors. Am J Med Sci 1896; 112:251–281.
84. Oettgen HF, Old LJ: The history of cancer immunotherapy. *In* De Vita VT, Hellman S, Rosenberg SA (eds): Biologic Therapy of Cancer, pp 87–119. Philadelphia, JB Lippincott Co, 1991.
85. Forsthuber T, Yip HC, Lehmann PV: Induction of TH1 and TH2 immunity in neonatal mice. Science 1996; 271: 1728–1730.
86. Toes RE, Blom RJ, Offringa R, et al: Enhanced tumor outgrowth after peptide vaccination. J Immunol 1996; 156: 3911–3918.
87. Sidney J, Grey HM, Kubo RT, Sette A: Practical, biochemical and evolutionary implications of the discovery of HLA class I supermotifs. Immunol Today 1996; 17:261–266.
88. Zitvogel L, Mayordomo JI, Tjandrawan T, et al: Therapy of murine tumors with tumor peptide-pulsed dendritic cells: dependence on T cells, B7 costimulation, and T helper cell 1-associated cytokines. J Exp Med 1996; 183: 87–97.
89. Celluzzi CM, Mayordomo JI, Storkus WJ, et al: Peptide-pulsed dendritic cells induce antigen-specific, CTL-mediated protective tumor immunity. J Exp Med 1996; 183:283–287.
90. Mayordomo JI, Zorina T, Storkus WJ, et al: Bone marrow-derived dendritic cells pulsed with synthetic tumour peptides elicit protective and therapeutic antitumour immunity. Nat Med 1995; 1:1297–1302.

91. Romani N, Gruner S, Brang D, et al: Proliferating dendritic cell progenitors in human blood. J Exp Med 1994; 180:83–93.
92. McLaughlin JP, Schlom J, Kantor JA, Greiner JW: Improved immunotherapy of a recombinant carcinoembryonic antigen vaccinia vaccine when given in combination with interleukin-2. Cancer Res 1996; 56:2361–2367.
93. Tsang KY, Zaremba S, Nieroda CA, et al: Generation of human cytotoxic T cells specific for human carcinoembryonic antigen epitopes from patients immunized with recombinant vaccinia-CEA vaccine. J Natl Cancer Inst 1995; 87:982–990.
94. Chen PW, Wang M, Bronte V, et al: Therapeutic antitumor response after immunization with a recombinant adenovirus encoding a model tumor-associated antigen. J Immunol 1996; 156:224–231.
95. Zhai Y, Yang JC, Kawakami Y, et al: Antigen-specific tumor vaccines. Development and characterization of recombinant adenoviruses encoding MART1 or gp100 for cancer therapy. J Immunol 1996; 156:700–710.
96. Wang M, Bronte V, Chen PW, et al: Active immunotherapy of cancer with a nonreplicating recombinant fowlpox virus encoding a model tumor-associated antigen. J Immunol 1995; 154:4685–4692.
97. Ciernik IF, Berzofsky JA, Carbone DP: Induction of cytotoxic T lymphocytes and antitumor immunity with DNA vaccines expressing single T cell epitopes. J Immunol 1996; 156:2369–2375.
98. Alexander RB: This month in investigative urology. Commentary on immunotherapy, gene therapy and cancer. J Urol 1995; 153:300.
99. Asher AL, Mule JJ, Kasid A, et al: Murine tumor cells transduced with the gene for tumor necrosis factor-alpha. Evidence for paracrine immune effects of tumor necrosis factor against tumors. J Immunol 1991; 146:3227–3234.
100. Pardoll DM: Paracrine cytokine adjuvants in cancer immunotherapy. Annu Rev Immunol 1995; 13:399–415.
101. Dranoff G, Jaffee E, Lazenby A, et al: Vaccination with irradiated tumor cells engineered to secrete murine granulocyte-macrophage colony-stimulating factor stimulates potent, specific, and long-lasting anti-tumor immunity. Proc Natl Acad Sci U S A 1993; 90:3539–3543.

III

ADRENAL GLAND

9

ADRENAL TUMORS

E. DARRACOTT VAUGHAN, JR., M.D.

The major adrenal tumors that will be discussed in this chapter include adrenal cortical adenomas producing primary hyperaldosteronism and Cushing's syndrome, adrenal cortical carcinoma, the incidentally identified adrenal mass, and pheochromocytoma. Actually, since the most common tumors involved in the adrenal gland are metastatic tumors to the adrenal, the management of such lesions generally is dependent upon the treatment of the primary disease entity. It is fortunate that the diagnosis of these adrenal disorders is extremely accurate using the combination of precise analytical methods for the measurement of the abnormal secretion of adrenal hormones and sophisticated radiographic techniques for the localization and characterization of specific adrenal lesions.[1,2]

The management of patients with adrenal tumors requires a clear understanding of the normal physiology of the adrenal, medulla, and cortex; a three-dimensional concept of the adrenal anatomy as well as adjacent structures, and the knowledge of the various pathologic entities that may involve the adrenal. Moreover, the operating surgeon must be well aware of the nuances involved in the diagnosis of the different adrenal entities, be aware of potential intraoperative phenomena that are unique to these patients, and be alert to specific postoperative complications that may occur. This chapter will review the pre-, intra-, and postoperative aspect of each of these specific entities and will outline surgical approaches with operative hints to guide those interested in adrenal surgery.

The adrenal glands are paired retroperitoneal organs that lie within the perinephric fat, at the anterior, superior, and medial aspects of the kidneys. Their location in juxtaposition with other organs as well as the periadrenal fat renders them ideal for sectional imaging by computed tomography (CT). Thin-cut CT scanning allows precise identification of lesions as small as 0.5 cm. The CT scan remains the best imaging device for the identification of small adrenal lesions, whereas magnetic resonance imaging (MRI) gives information concerning cell type and aids in the differentiation of adenomas from medullary tumors or metastatic carcinoma.[3] Other advantages of MRI scanning will be discussed later. The right adrenal lies above the kidney posterior and lateral to the inferior vena cava (IVC) and its solitary venous drainage is via a short stubby vein that enters the IVC in a posterior fashion. Hence, the right adrenal gland is best approached through a posterior or modified posterior incision.[4] The left adrenal is in more intimate contact with the kidney, overlying the upper pole of the kidney with its anterior surface and medial surface behind the pancreas and splenic artery. It is best exposed through a flank approach, or a thoracoabdominal approach if the lesion is large.

The adrenals have a delicate, rich blood supply estimated to be 6 to 7 ml/g/min without a dominant adrenal artery. The inferior phrenic artery is the main blood supply with additional branches from the aorta and renal arteries. The small arteries penetrate the gland in a circumferential stellate fashion leaving both the anterior and posterior surfaces avascular (Fig. 9–1). During adrenalectomy, an important technical goal is to divide the superior and lateral blood supply to the adrenal first, allowing the adrenal to remain attached to the kidney, which can be used to draw the adrenal gland inferiorly and anteriorly during the resection. On the left side, the adrenal vein drains into the left renal vein; however, there is also a medially located phrenic drainage branch which, if not appropriately ligated, can cause troublesome bleeding (Fig. 9–2). The left adrenal vein is also a guide to the left renal artery, which often lies dorsal to the vein; one potential complication of left adrenalectomy is the inadvertent ligation of the apical renal arterial branch to the upper pole, which lies in close contact to the inferior border of an adrenal tumor.

The basic physiology of the adrenal cortex and medulla as well as the various pathologic entities will be discussed under specific disorders.

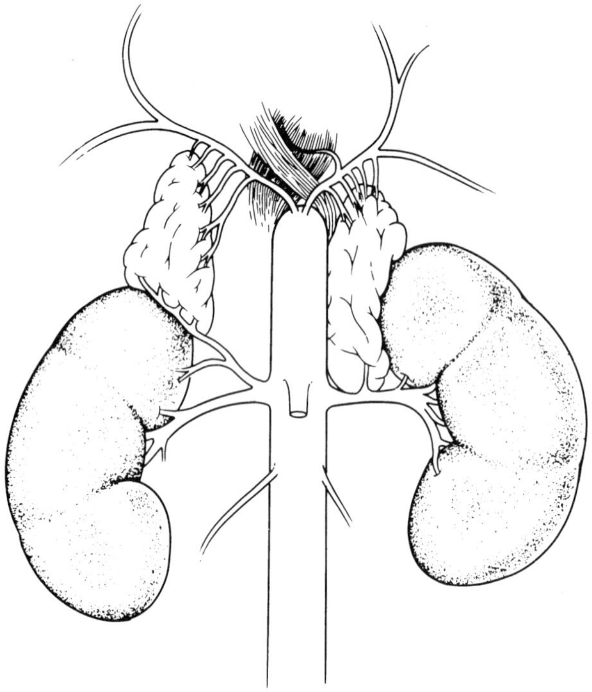

FIGURE 9–1. Arterial supply of left and right adrenal gland. (From Vaughan ED Jr, Carey RM: Adrenal Disorders. New York, Thieme Medical Publishers Inc, 1989, with permission.)

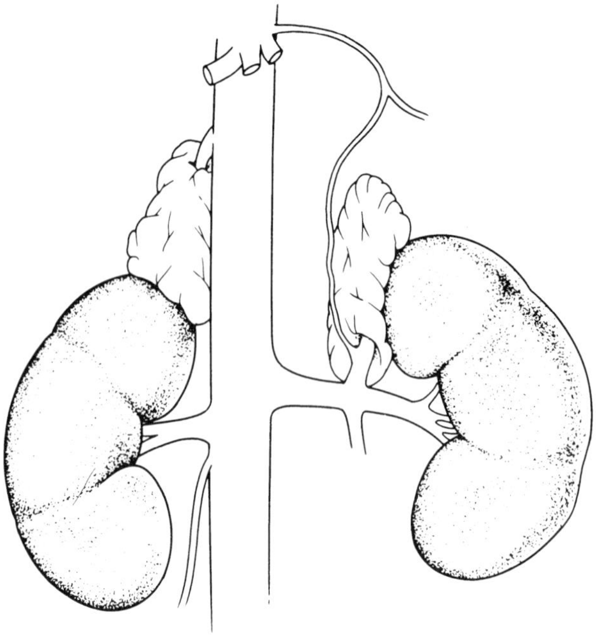

FIGURE 9–2. Venous drainage of left and right adrenal glands with particular attention to the intercommunicating vein on the left. (From Vaughan ED Jr, Carey RM: Adrenal Disorders. New York, Thieme Medical Publishers Inc, 1989, with permission.)

CUSHING'S SYNDROME

Cushing's syndrome is the term utilized to describe the symptom complex caused by excessive circulating glucocorticoids. We must remember that the term is all-encompassing and includes patients with pituitary hypersecretion of ACTH (corticotropin); Cushing's disease, which accounts for 75 to 80% of patients with endogenous Cushing's; patients with adrenal adenomas or carcinomas; and patients with ectopic secretion of ACTH or corticotropin-releasing hormone (CRH) syndrome.[5] Before assuming a patient has one of these pathologic entities there should be a thorough questioning of the patient about the use of steroid-containing preparations. At times patients are unaware that a substance they use, particularly creams or lotions, contains steroids, and if the patient is on any type of medication at all, it should be carefully reviewed for steroid content. There are few diseases in which the clinical appearance of the patient can be as useful in suspecting the diagnosis. Old photographs are helpful in documenting recent changes in appearance that occurred. The more common clinical manifestations of Cushing's syndrome found in different series of patients are shown in Table 9–1. The clinical findings do not distinguish patients with Cushing's disease from those with adrenal adenoma; however, patients with adrenal carcinoma are more likely to show virilization in the female or feminization in the male. Patients with ectopic ACTH may present with manifestations of the primary tumor. It is also important to remember that some nonendocrine disorders mimic the clinical and even the biochemical manifestations of Cushing's syndrome. These patients have been termed to have "pseudo"–Cushing's syndrome; this may

TABLE 9–1. CLINICAL MANIFESTATIONS OF CUSHING'S SYNDROME*

	All† %	Disease‡ %	Adenoma/ Carcinoma§ %
Obesity	90	91	93
Hypertension	80	63	93
Diabetes	80	32	79
Centripetal obesity	80	—	—
Weakness	80	25	82
Muscle atrophy	70	34	—
Hirsutism	70	59	79
Menstrual abnormal/sexual dysfunction	70	46	75
Purple striae	70	46	36
Moon facies	60	—	—
Osteoporosis	50	29	54
Early bruising	50	54	57
Acne/pigmentation	50	32	—
Mental changes	50	47	57
Edema	50	15	—
Headache	40	21	46
Poor healing	40	—	—

*From Scott HW Jr: *In* Scott HW (ed): Surgery of the Adrenal Glands. Philadelphia, JB Lippincott Co, 1990, with permission.
†Hunt and Tyrell, 1978.
‡Wilson, 1984.
§Scott, 1973.

exist in patients with major depression or in patients with chronic alcoholism.[5]

There are a myriad of tests both to diagnose the presence of Cushing's syndrome and then to identify which subentity is present. Fortunately, due to recent development of extremely accurate assays for urinary and plasma cortisol as well as plasma corticotropin this task has become much easier. The approach that has recently been reported by Orth is shown in Figure 9–3.[5]

The clinical diagnosis of Cushing's syndrome is confirmed by the demonstration of cortisol hypersecretion. At the present time the determination of 24-hour urinary excretion of cortisol in the urine is the most direct and reliable index of cortical secretion. Orth recommends that urinary cortisol should be measured in two and preferably three consecutive 24-hour urine specimens, collected on an outpatient basis.

Once the diagnosis has been established, the next chore is to determine whether there is Cushing's disease due to hypersecretion of plasma corticotropin (ACTH) from the pituitary or primary adrenal disease. Herein lies the major change in our ap-

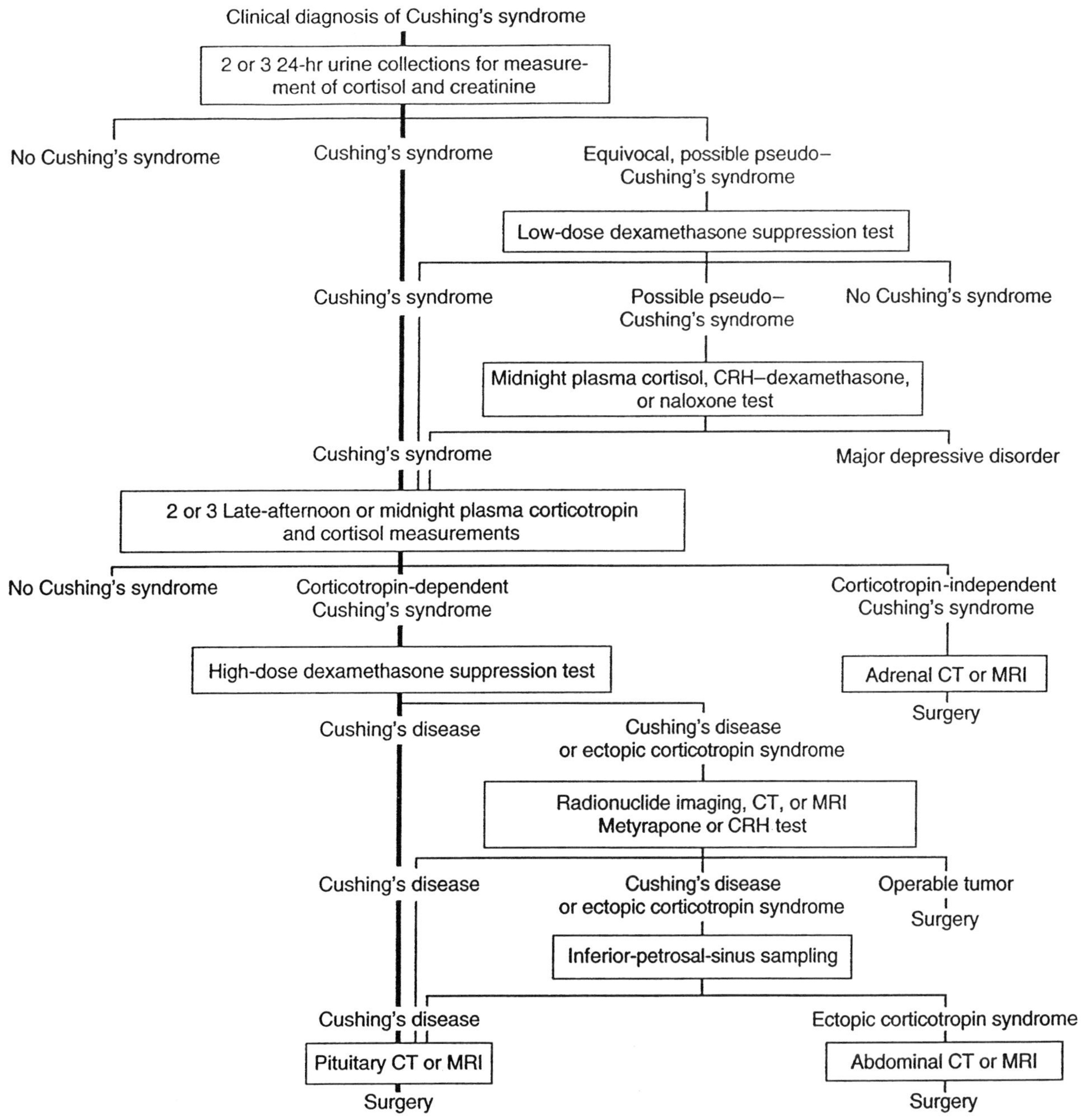
Clinical diagnosis of Cushing's syndrome
2 or 3 24-hr urine collections for measurement of cortisol and creatinine
No Cushing's syndrome
Cushing's syndrome
Equivocal, possible pseudo–Cushing's syndrome
Low-dose dexamethasone suppression test
Cushing's syndrome
Possible pseudo–Cushing's syndrome
No Cushing's syndrome
Midnight plasma cortisol, CRH–dexamethasone, or naloxone test
Cushing's syndrome
Major depressive disorder
2 or 3 Late-afternoon or midnight plasma corticotropin and cortisol measurements
No Cushing's syndrome
Corticotropin-dependent Cushing's syndrome
Corticotropin-independent Cushing's syndrome
High-dose dexamethasone suppression test
Adrenal CT or MRI
Surgery
Cushing's disease
Cushing's disease or ectopic corticotropin syndrome
Radionuclide imaging, CT, or MRI Metyrapone or CRH test
Cushing's disease
Cushing's disease or ectopic corticotropin syndrome
Operable tumor
Surgery
Inferior-petrosal-sinus sampling
Cushing's disease
Ectopic corticotropin syndrome
Pituitary CT or MRI
Abdominal CT or MRI
Surgery
Surgery

FIGURE 9–3. Identifying Cushing's syndrome and its causes. (From: Orth DN: Cushing's syndrome. N Engl J Med 1995; 32:791. Copyright 1995, Massachusetts Medical Society, with permission.)

proach to patients with Cushing's disease. In the past, high- and low-dose dexamethasone suppression tests have been used to accomplish this task. At present the low-dose dexamethasone is generally used to rule out pseudo–Cushing's syndrome. The differentiation of corticotropin-dependent Cushing's versus corticotropin-independent Cushing's syndrome is determined by the concurrent late afternoon or midnight measurement of collection of blood for the simultaneous measurement of plasma corticotropin and cortisol. Thus if the patient's cortisol concentration is above 50 μg/dl and the corticotropin concentration is below 5 pg/ml, then the cortisol secretion is ACTH independent and the patient has a primary adrenal problem. In contrast, if the plasma corticotropin concentration is greater than 50 pg/ml, then the cortisol secretion is ACTH dependent and the patient has Cushing's syndrome or ectopic ACTH or CRH syndrome.[5] In situations where the two-site immunoradiometric assay test is not available, the high-dose dexamethasone suppression test has always been used as the standard test to differentiate between pituitary and adrenal Cushing's syndrome. Patients are given high-dose dexamethasone (2 mg every 6 hours for 2 days), and plasma cortisol and urinary free cortisol levels are measured. In patients with pituitary disease, there should be a 50% or greater suppression in cortisol. Patients with adrenal adenomas or carcinomas fail to suppress cortisol secretion. The high-dose dexamethasone suppression test may also be useful to identify ectopic ACTH syndrome, where there is usually complete resistance to high-dose dexamethasone suppression.

Treatment is obviously dependent on the underlying lesion. Patients with adrenal adenomas or carcinomas are generally treated with surgical extirpation of the lesions. Patients with Cushing's disease have confirmation with pituitary CT or MRI and usually are treated with transsphenoidal pituitary tumor removal, and patients with ectopic ACTH have treatment directed towards the primary tumor. The surgical approach and preparation of patients with adrenal Cushing's disease will be discussed later.

If the patient is identified as having adrenal Cushing's, the next step is radiographic localization with CT scanning.[6] Adrenal adenomas are usually larger than 2 cm, solitary, and associated with atrophy of the opposite gland. The density is low because of the high concentration of lipid (Fig. 9–4). Adrenal carcinomas are often indistinguishable from adenomas except for the larger size, carcinomas usually being greater than 6 cm.[7] Necrosis and calcification are also more common in association with adrenal carcinoma but are not specific. Clearly large irregular adrenal lesions with invasion represent carcinoma; however, metastatic carcinoma to the adrenal has the same appearance.

MRI is not usually necessary in patients with Cushing's syndrome unless the lesion is large; the rationale for MRI is to obtain anatomic information concerning surrounding structures or invasion of the inferior vena cava, a rare but well-recognized entity.[8]

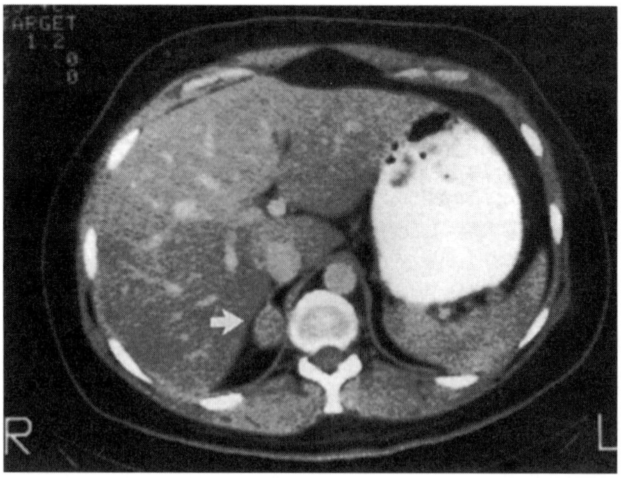
R
L

FIGURE 9–4. Computed tomography scan of a patient with right adrenal adenoma. (From Vaughan ED Jr, Blumenfeld JD: The adrenals. *In* Walsh PC, Retik AB, Stamey TA, Vaughan ED Jr [eds]: Campbell's Urology, 6th edition, p 2373. Philadelphia, WB Saunders Co, 1992, with permission.)

Adrenal cortical scanning with iodinated cholesterol agents is no longer routinely utilized but can be helpful in differentiating functional adrenal tissue from other retroperitoneal lesions.[9]

INCIDENTALLY DISCOVERED ADRENAL MASSES

The increased utilization of abdominal ultrasound and CT scanning has led to a new classification of adrenal lesions termed the "incidentally identified unsuspected adrenal mass" or "incidentaloma."[7] Our approach to the incidentally identified adrenal mass is shown in Figure 9–5. Several points do not warrant controversy. First, there is agreement that all patients with solid adrenal masses should undergo biochemical assessment. If biochemical abnormalities are identified, the lesions should be treated appropriately as described elsewhere in the chapter, usually by removal of the offending lesion. However, the extent of biochemical evaluation has been reviewed and a selective approach has been outlined that markedly limits cost without sacrificing diagnostic accuracy.[10] A very limited evaluation is recommended including tests only to rule out pheochromocytoma, potassium levels in hypertensive cases, and glucocorticoid evaluation only in the presence of clinical stigmata of Cushing's syndrome or virilization. The second point that is noncontroversial is that nonfunctioning solid lesions larger than 5 cm should be removed. This is based on the finding that adrenal

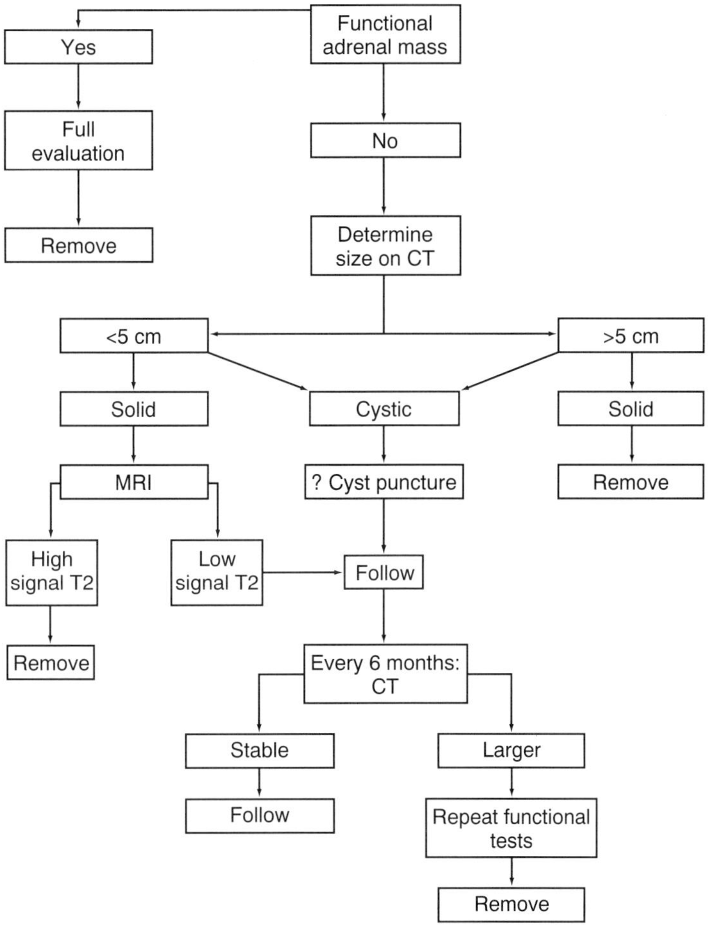
Functional adrenal mass
Yes
Full evaluation
Remove
No
Determine size on CT
<5 cm
>5 cm
Solid
Cystic
Solid
MRI
? Cyst puncture
Remove
High signal T2
Low signal T2
Follow
Remove
Every 6 months: CT
Stable
Larger
Follow
Repeat functional tests
Remove

FIGURE 9–5. Evaluation of incidentally found adrenal mass. (From Vaughan ED Jr, Blumenfeld JD: The adrenals. *In* Walsh PC, Retik AB, Stamey TA, Vaughan ED Jr [eds]: Campbell's Urology, 7th edition. Philadelphia, WB Saunders Co, 1997 [in press] with permission.)

malignancies are almost always larger than 6 cm. However, we feel that CT scanning may underestimate the size of an adrenal and we suggest that exploration be performed when lesions are more than 5 cm on CT or MRI.[11] Furthermore, if lesions are purely cystic by CT or MRI, cyst puncture is often not necessary and these lesions can be followed (Fig. 9–6). The controversy arises in the management strategy for the solid adrenal lesions, smaller than 5 cm in size. The current approach has been to use MRI imaging in this situation. Most adenomas appear slightly hypointense or isointense relative to the liver or spleen on T1-weighted images and slightly hyperintense or isointense relative to hepatic or splenic parenchyma on T2-weighted images. Indeed there is little change in the intensity from T1- to T2-weighted studies. In contrast, the general notion is that adrenal cortical carcinoma is hypointense relative to liver or spleen on T1-weighted images and hyperintense to the liver or spleen on T2-weighted images. Thus if the mean signal intensity ratio between the lesion and the spleen is over 0.8, it is unlikely that the lesion is a benign adenoma. However, it should be remembered that there are a number of entities other than adrenal carcinoma that can cause high intensity including neural tumors, metastatic tumors to the adrenal, adrenal hemorrhage, and other retroperitoneal lesions.[3,12,13] An additional study that has shown accuracy is the fine-needle adrenal biopsy guided by ultrasound or CT. In a large series from Finland, significant cytologic material was obtained in 96.4% and the accuracy to differentiate benign from malignant disease was 85.7%.[14] However, the utilization of aspiration cytology requires an extremely experienced cytologist, and in fact there is often inability to distinguish an adrenal adenoma from a carcinoma even upon pathologic review of the entire specimen.

It is our general approach that if there is either any radiographic evidence that argues against a characteristic benign adenoma or any change in size of an adrenal lesion with repeated studies, then we feel that adrenalectomy is indicated. This fairly aggressive approach is justified in view of the extremely poor prognosis of patients when adrenal carcinoma is diagnosed even when the lesion is localized.

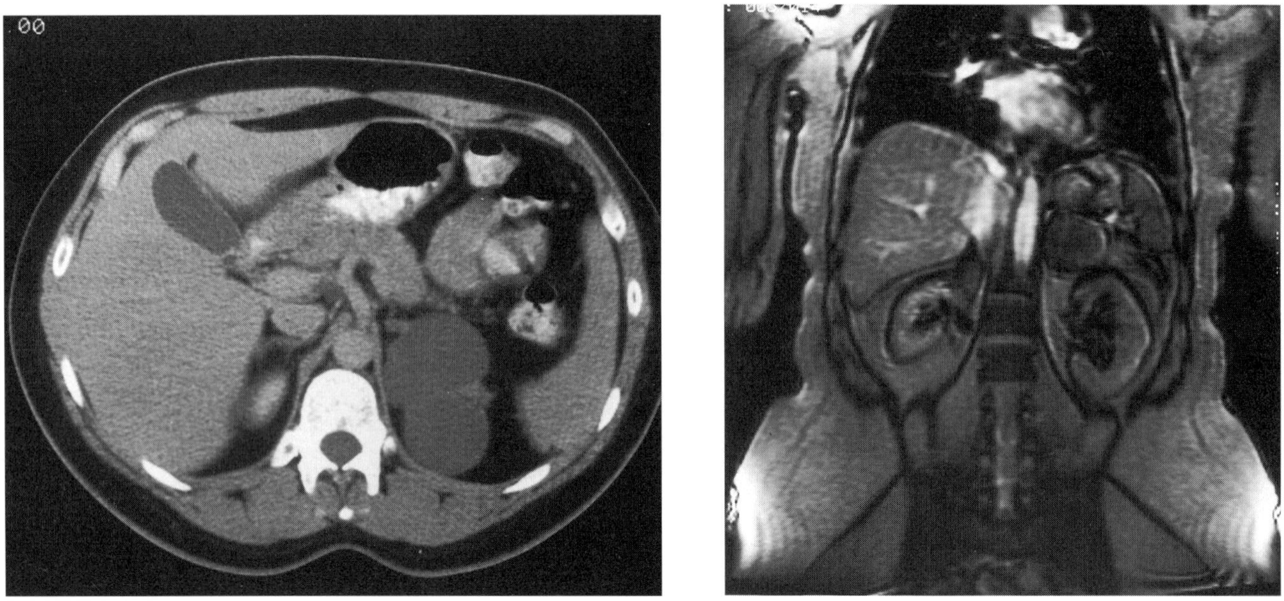

A B

FIGURE 9–6. Multilocular benign renal cyst in an asymptomatic patient that was incidentally identified. *A*, CT scan showing left adrenal cyst. *B*, Coronal MRI showing the lobular suprarenal adrenal cyst. In this case, exploration was carried out because of the multilocular nature. The cyst was benign.

ADRENAL CARCINOMA

Adrenal carcinoma is a rare disease with a poor prognosis. The incidence is estimated as 1 case per 1.7 million, accounting for only 0.02% of cancers. A practical subclassification for adrenal carcinomas is according to their ability to produce adrenal hormones. In a series by Luton et al.,[15] 79% of adrenal tumors were functional, a higher percentage than previously reported due to more sensitive assays. The varieties of functioning tumors are shown in Table 9–2. However, this classification is somewhat contrived, since many of these tumors will produce multiple adrenal hormones and also because of the clear evidence that a tumor may secrete one hormone at one point in its natural history and additional hormones at a later phase when there is increased tumor mass. The most commonly identified functional tumor is one causing Cushing's syndrome. The most common characteristic to delineate Cushing's syndrome due to carcinoma rather than adenoma has been the presence of virilization with elevated 17-ketosteroid levels. More recently the measurement of DHEA has been useful in identifying these patients.

Other rare functional tumors include both testosterone- and estrogen-secreting adrenal cortical tumors. Rarely virilization can occur in the absence of elevated urinary 17-ketosteroids and raises the possibility of pure testosterone-secreting ovarian or adrenal lesions.[16] Of the two sites of origin, adrenal cortical tumors secreting testosterone are exceedingly rare. In contrast to other tumors described in this section, these tumors are usually small, less than 6 cm, and many behave in a benign fashion. In contrast, most feminizing tumors occur in males 25 to 50 years of age, and they are usually larger, often palpable, and highly malignant.[17] Characteristically, the patients present with gynecomastia; in addition they may exhibit testicular atrophy, impotence, or decreased libido. We have also seen a presentation with infertility and oligospermia. These tumors secrete androstenedione, which is converted peripherally to estrogen. Other steroids may also be secreted and the clinical picture may be mixed with associated cushingoid features.

The management of adrenal cortical carcinoma is surgical removal of the primary tumor. The most common sites of metastasis include lung, liver, and lymph nodes.[18] Often these tumors extend directly into adjacent structures, especially the kidney, and surgical removal may require removal of the primary tumor and adjacent organs including the kidney, spleen, as well as local lymph nodes. Unfortunately, despite en bloc resection even in patients without evidence of metastatic disease, the 5-year

TABLE 9–2. CLASSIFICATION OF ADRENAL CARCINOMA

Functional
Cushing's syndrome
Virilization in females
Increased DHEA, 17-ketosteroids
Increased testosterone
Feminizing syndrome in males
Hyperaldosteronism
Mixed combination of above
Nonfunctional

DHEA, dehydroepiandrosterone.

survival rate is only approximately 50% with complete resection and 35% overall.[19] Because of the poor prognosis there has been an intense search for effective adjunctive chemotherapy, but this search has been frustrating and it is generally believed that conventional chemotherapy is not effective, probably because of p-glycoprotein expression.[20] The most success has been reported with the adrenolytic 1,1-dichloro-2-(*o*-chlorophenyl)-2-(*p*-chlorophenyl)-ethane(*o,p*′-DDD) or Mitotane.[21] This DDT derivative has been shown to induce tumor response in 35% in a review of 551 cases reported in the literature.[22] However, despite these response rates, survival time has not been prolonged and there is intense toxicity. Recently it has been suggested that patients even without the presence of metastatic disease be given adjunctive *o,p*′-DDD, and trials are currently in progress to determine if this approach is efficacious.

In general, there is an extremely poor prognosis in patients with adrenal cortical carcinoma and there is obvious need for the development of new treatment strategies.

HYPERALDOSTERONISM

The term "hyperaldosteronism" originally was coined by Dr. Jerome Conn to describe the clinical syndrome characterized by hypertension, hypokalemia, hypernatremia, alkalosis, and periodic paralysis due to an aldosterone-secreting adenoma.[23] We now realize that this metabolic syndrome can be caused by either a solitary adrenal adenoma or by bilateral adrenal zona glomerulosa hyperplasia. One of the clinical chores is to delineate patients with hyperplasia from those with adenoma.[24] The syndrome of primary hyperaldosteronism is now identified by the combined findings of hypokalemia, suppressed plasma renin activity (PRA) despite sodium restriction, and a high urinary and plasma aldosterone level after sodium repletion in hypertensive patients. The current evaluation of patients suspected of having hyperaldosteronism is shown in Figure 9–7. The primary physiologic control of aldosterone secretion is angiotensin II (Fig. 9–8).[25,26] Other control mechanisms are ACTH and potassium. A clear knowledge of the physiology of the renin-angiotensin-aldosterone system (RAAS) is mandatory in order to understand the pathophysiology and evaluate patients with primary hyperaldosteronism. The critical sensor in the RAAS resides in the juxtaglomerular apparatus within the kidney. Thus, in response to a variety of stimuli, but primarily decreased renal perfusion, or a decreased intake of sodium, there is an increased renin release, formation of angiotensin II, and subsequent aldosterone secretion. Therefore, the term "secondary hyperaldosteronism" is utilized when there is increased renin secretion and secondary aldosterone production. The most common examples of secondary hyperaldosteronism would be renovascular hypertension[27] and malignant hypertension.[28] In contrast, with an adrenal adenoma or adrenal hyperplasia there is primary secretion of aldosterone and subsequently the sodium retention that occurs leads to a suppression of plasma renin activity.

Therefore, returning to Figure 9–7, the hallmark of the entity is hypokalemia. However, some patients realize that weakness occurs with increased sodium intake and therefore restrict their sodium, and may have a more normal potassium than that first observed. Therefore, the entity should not be ruled out until the patient has sodium loading with 10 g of sodium a day for several weeks and repeat potassium measurements. A small subset of patients exhibit normokalemic hyperaldosteronism, and if there is a high index of suspicion for the disease, these patients should be studied further. If there is hypokalemia, a 24-hour urine should be collected demonstrating that there is urinary loss of potassium. The critical test is the measurement of plasma renin activity at a time when the patient is either on a low-sodium diet or is challenged with a diuretic. If the patient has hyperaldosteronism, the plasma renin activity remains inappropriately low despite sodium depletion. Because potassium is also a stimulus of aldosterone, the patient should be potassium repleted before measuring 24-hour urine and plasma aldosterone levels. Both of these values should be elevated in hyperaldosteronism.

At this point the question is whether the patient has a unilateral adenoma or bilateral adrenal hyperplasia, and the imaging study of choice is an adrenal CT scan with 3- to 5-mm cuts through both adrenal glands. The next step that is traditionally performed would be adrenal vein sampling. The difficulty with adrenal vein sampling is obtaining adequate collections from the short, stubby, right adrenal vein, and when samples are collected, cortisol levels should always also be collected to ensure proper catheter placement. An appropriate way of analyzing aldosterone levels is with comparative aldosterone/cortisol ratios from each side. It is our general policy to have positive lateralizing information as well as a positive CT scan before recommending exploration and unilateral adrenalectomy. However, more recently in patients who have elevated plasma 18-hydroxy-B levels and elevated urinary 18-hydroxy-F levels at times we have not required sampling when a clear adenoma was demonstrated on CT scan. In contrast, we have demonstrated a subset of patients with radiographic bilateral hyperplasia who will lateralize adrenal vein sampling for aldosterone. In this setting we have performed unilateral adrenalectomy and a significant number of those patients have favorable biochemical and blood pressure responses, although most have required the continuation of some antihypertensive medication.[24]

Finally, in the patients who have normal CT

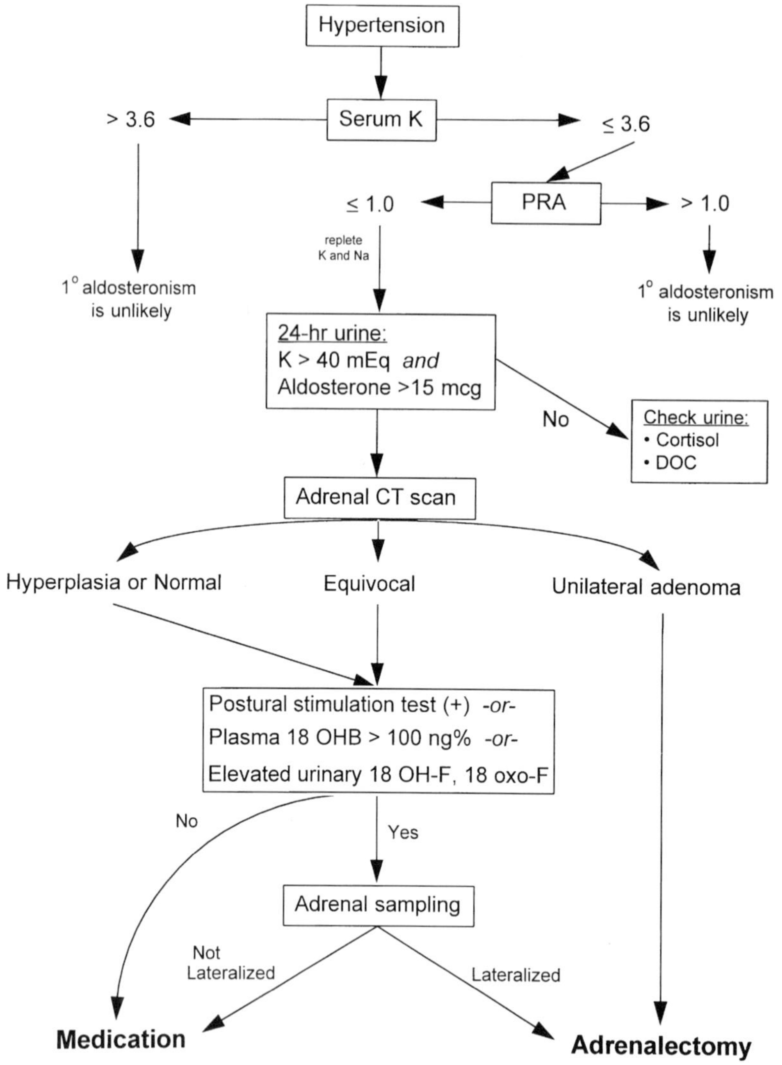
Hypertension
Serum K
> 3.6
≤ 3.6
1° aldosteronism is unlikely
PRA
≤ 1.0
> 1.0
replete K and Na
1° aldosteronism is unlikely
24-hr urine:
K > 40 mEq and
Aldosterone >15 mcg
No
Check urine:
• Cortisol
• DOC
Adrenal CT scan
Hyperplasia or Normal
Equivocal
Unilateral adenoma
Postural stimulation test (+) -or-
Plasma 18 OHB > 100 ng% -or-
Elevated urinary 18 OH-F, 18 oxo-F
No
Yes
Adrenal sampling
Not Lateralized
Lateralized
Medication
Adrenalectomy

FIGURE 9–7. Identifying primary hyperaldosteronism. (From Blumenfeld JD, Schlussel Y, Sealey JE, et al: Diagnosis and treatment of primary hyperaldosteronism. Ann Intern Med 1994; 121:877–885, with permission.)

scans yet lateralize on sampling, if they show elevated 18-hydroxy products we will operate, if not we will follow those patients. The majority of patients with bilateral hyperplasia will not lateralize with adrenal vein sampling for aldosterone. Those patients are treated with spironolactone at an appropriate dose to control blood pressure. Often, they will need other medications such as calcium channel blockers.

PHEOCHROMOCYTOMA

Pheochromocytoma is an uncommon entity but one that has potentially lethal sequelae for the patient if not diagnosed. Therefore, it is generally felt that all patients with sustained hypertension should have the appropriate studies performed to rule out pheochromocytoma (Fig. 9–9).[29]

The clinical manifestations exhibited by patients with a pheochromocytoma are due to the physiologic effects of the catecholamines, dopamine, epinephrine, and norepinephrine. However, other signs and symptom complexes exhibited may be extremely variable, including the asymptomatic patient in whom a lesion is picked up simply on CT scan. In all reported series hypertension is by far the most common sign (Table 9–3). As far as the type of hypertension, the patients may have either sustained hypertension, paroxysmal or dramatic attacks of hypertension, or sustained hypertension with superimposed paroxysms. Most series have shown this latter constellation of findings to be the most common in patients with pheochromocytoma. In addition, the frequency of attacks among patients is quite variable, ranging from a few times a year to multiple daily episodes. In addition, the duration may be minutes or hours and the nature of the attacks can vary dramatically. Most patients will exhibit a paroxysm or an episode once a week,

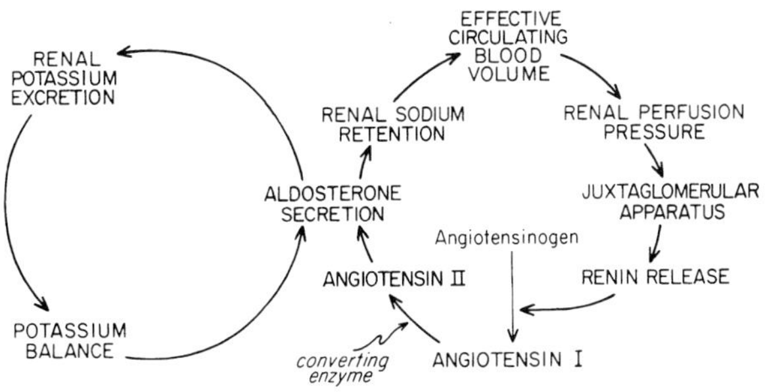
EFFECTIVE CIRCULATING BLOOD VOLUME
RENAL POTASSIUM EXCRETION
RENAL SODIUM RETENTION
RENAL PERFUSION PRESSURE
ALDOSTERONE SECRETION
JUXTAGLOMERULAR APPARATUS
Angiotensinogen
ANGIOTENSIN II
RENIN RELEASE
POTASSIUM BALANCE
converting enzyme
ANGIOTENSIN I

FIGURE 9–8. Control of aldosterone secretion by means of interrelationships between the potassium and renin-angiotensin feedback loops. (From Dluhy RG, Gittes RF: The adrenals. *In* Walsh PC, Gittes RF, Perlmutter AD, Stamey TA [eds]: Campbell's Urology, 5th edition. Philadelphia, WB Saunders Co, 1986, with permission.)

and most of the attacks will last less than an hour. Usually the attacks occur in the absence of recognizable stimuli, but a number of factors—particularly exercise, posture, trauma, or a variety of other situations—may precipitate an attack.

One specific entity is noteworthy: catecholamine-induced myocardiopathy.[30,31] These patients will present with decreased cardiac function and congestive heart failure, and it is mandatory that their cardiac status be stabilized with the use of appropriate α- and β-adrenergic blocking agents as well as α-methylparatyrosine (a tyrosine hydroxylase inhibitor) (Fig. 9–10) to cut down on catecholamine production before surgery is contemplated. Generally the cardiomyopathy is reversible, and the patients can be operated upon within weeks or months after the initial diagnosis and treatment is instituted.

An appreciable number of pheochromocytomas have been found in association with other disease entities and hereditary syndromes. These entities include the association of tumors of the glomus jugulary region, neurofibromatosis, Sturge-Weber syndrome, the von Hippel-Lindau, as well as the familial multiendocrine adenopathy (MEA) syndromes. Pheochromocytomas occur in MEA-2, a triad including pheochromocytoma, medullary carcinoma of the thyroid, and parathyroid adenomas (Sipple's syndrome). Pheochromocytomas may also be a part of MEA-3, which also includes medullary carcinoma of the thyroid, mucosal neuromas, thickened corneal nerves, ganglioneuromatosis, and frequently a marfanoid habitus. It is now believed that the relatives of patients with all of these syndromes should be evaluated for the presence of occult pheochromocytoma. In addition, there is a well-known entity of familial pheochromocytoma whereby multiple members of the kindred will be found to have multiple lesions and all members of such families should be both screened and then followed for the appearance of these tumors. The mechanism of the increased incidence of pheochromocytomas in association with neuroendocrine dysplasias and medullary carcinoma of the thyroid may be explained by the amine precursor uptake and decarboxylation (APUD) cell system of Pierce. The APUD cells derive from the neural crest of the embryo, sharing common ultrastructural and cytochemical features and elaborating amines by precursor uptake and decarboxylation.[32,33]

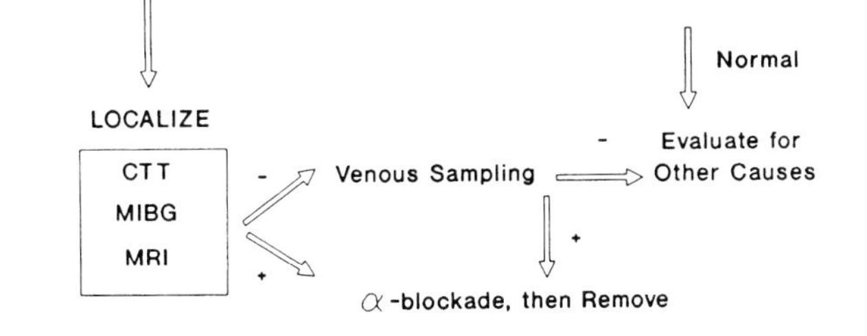
HISTORY
PHYSICAL EXAM
BP X3 › 140/90
BASIC LAB TESTS
SUSPECT
PHEOCHROMOCYTOMA
Plasma Norepinephrine
Epinephrine
Dopamine
Urinary Catechols
Diagnosis
Pheochromocytoma
Elevated
Normal
LOCALIZE
CTT
MIBG
MRI
Venous Sampling
Evaluate for
Other Causes
α -blockade, then Remove

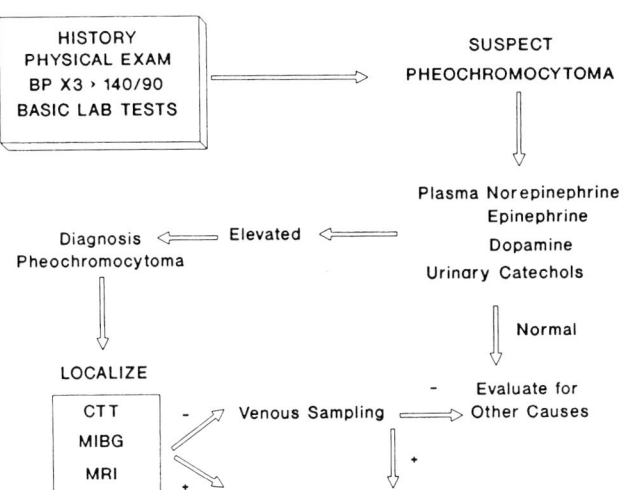

FIGURE 9–9. Identifying pheochromocytoma. (From Vaughan ED Jr: Diagnosis of adrenal disorders in hypertension. World J Urol 1989; 7:111–116, with permission.)

The laboratory diagnosis of pheochromocytoma is now extremely accurate, utilizing the urinary plasma measurements of catecholamines and their by-products (Fig. 9–9). Extremely accurate assays exist for these amines.[34] At the present time it is felt that urinary catecholamines remain the measurement of choice with the measurement of total urinary catecholamines and metanephrines. Approximately 95% of patients will have elevated levels of these substances. In the patient with a severe paroxysmal hypertension who presents in the midst of hypertensive crisis, the plasma catecholamines are almost always elevated and can be utilized.

Stimulation or suppression tests are generally not utilized at the present time. The one situation where they may be useful is in the patient who appears to have essential hypertension but borderline elevated catecholamines, and in this setting a clonidine suppression test may be useful. Follow-

TABLE 9–3. SYMPTOMS REPORTED BY 76 PATIENTS (ALMOST ALL ADULTS) WITH PHEOCHROMOCYTOMA ASSOCIATED WITH PAROXYSMAL OR PERSISTENT HYPERTENSION*

Symptoms	Per Cent Paroxysmal (37 Patients)	Per Cent Persistent (39 Patients)
Symptoms Presumably Due to Excessive Catecholamines or Hypertension		
Headache (severe)	92	72
Excessive sweating (generalized)	65	69
Palpitations ± tachycardia	73	51
Anxiety or nervousness (± fear of impending death, panic)	60	28
Tremulousness	51	26
Pain in chest, abdomen (usually epigastric), lumbar regions, lower abdomen, or groin	48	28
Nausea ± vomiting	43	26
Weakness, fatigue, prostration	38	15
Weight loss (severe)	14	15
Dyspnea	11	18
Warmth ± heat intolerance	13	15
Visual disturbances	3	21
Dizziness or faintness	11	3
Constipation	0	13
Paresthesia or pain in arms	11	0
Bradycardia (noted by patient)	8	3
Grand mal	5	3
Manifestations Due to Complications		
Congestive heart failure ± cardiomyopathy		
Myocardial infarction		
Cerebrovascular accident		
Ischemic enterocolitis ± megacolon		
Azotemia		
Dissecting aneurysm		
Encephalopathy		
Shock		
Hemorrhagic necrosis in a pheochromocytoma		
Manifestations Due to Coexisting Diseases or Syndromes		
Cholelithiasis		
Medullary thyroid carcinoma ± effects of secretions of serotonin, calcitonin, prostaglandin, or ACTH-like substance		
Hyperparathyroidism		
Mucocutaneous neuromas with characteristic facies		
Thickened corneal nerves (seen only with slit lamp)		
Marfanoid habitus		
Alimentary tract ganglioneuromatosis		
Neurofibromatosis and its complications		
Cushing's syndrome (rare)		
Von Hippel-Lindau disease (rare)		
Virilism, Addison's disease, acromegaly (extremely rare)		
Symptoms Caused by Encroachment on Adjacent Structures or by Invasion and Pressure Effects of Metastases		

*From Manger WM, Gifford RW Jr: Pheochromocytoma. *In* Laragh JH, Brenner BM (eds): Hypertension Pathophysiology Diagnosis and Management. New York, Raven Press, 1990, with permission.

ing a single 0.3-mg oral dose of clonidine the patients with neurogenic hypertension at rest show a fall in norepinephrine, whereas patients with pheochromocytomas do not.[34]

The radiographic test that is most useful in both identifying and characterizing neuroendocrine adrenal tumors, and in identifying surrounding structures, is the MRI scan. We've been impressed with the multiple use of MRI scans in patients with pheochromocytoma. Therefore, the test is as accurate as a CT scan in identifying lesions and also has a characteristic bright lightbulb appearance on the T2-weighted study (Fig. 9–10).[3] In addition, sagittal and coronal imaging can provide excellent anatomic information concerning the relationship between the tumor and the surrounding vasculature as well as draining venous channels (Fig. 9–11). Therefore, we feel that the MRI should be the initial scanning procedure in patients with the biochemical findings of pheochromocytoma.

An alternative approach that also is useful at times, particularly for residual or multiple pheochromocytomas, is the metaiodobenzylguanidine (MIBG) scan that images medullary tissue.[35,36] Thus this test may be more sensitive than CT or MRI in picking up small extra-adrenal lesions and has its major use in patients where multiple lesions are suspected.

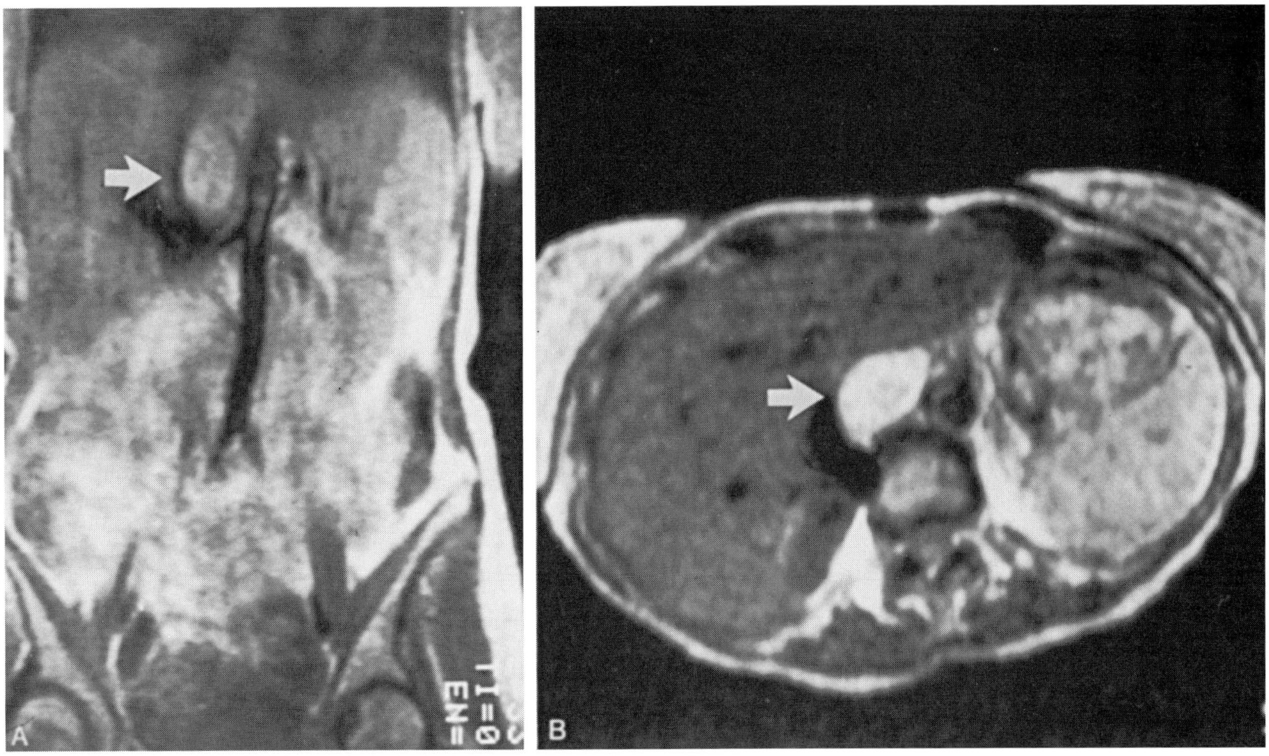
A
B

FIGURE 9–10. Magnetic resonance image of pheochromocytoma. (From Vaughan ED Jr, Blumenfeld JD: The adrenals. *In* Walsh PC, Retik AB, Stamey TA, Vaughan ED Jr [eds]: Campbell's Urology, 6th edition, p 2395. Philadelphia, WB Saunders Co, 1992, with permission.)

ADRENAL SURGERY

Adrenalectomy is the treatment of choice in most patients who have undergone appropriate metabolic evaluation and have been found to have a surgical lesion. However, the surgeon must be aware that there are unique aspects to the care in these patients including specific preoperative management as outlined in Table 9–4. Accordingly, patients with hyperaldosteronism who are generally

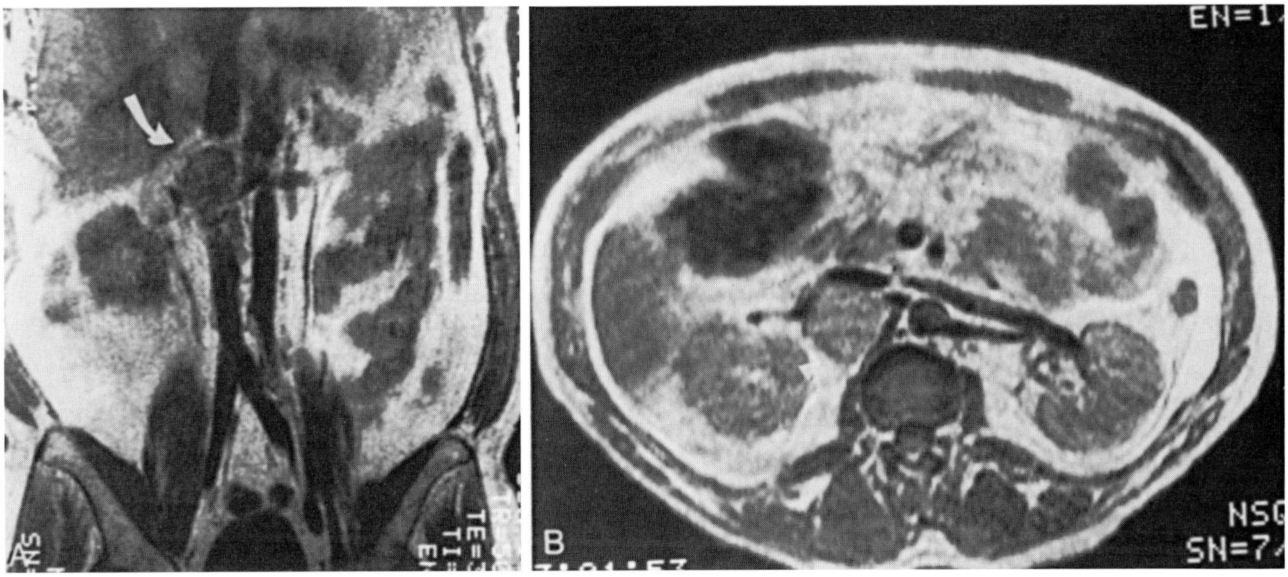
B

FIGURE 9–11. Magnetic resonance image of recurrent pheochromocytoma with an excellent demonstration of anterior crossing right renal vein, feeding lumbar vein, and involvement of right renal artery. (From Vaughan ED Jr, Blumenfeld JD: The adrenals. *In* Walsh PC, Retik AB, Stamey TA, Vaughan ED Jr [eds]: Campbell's Urology, 6th edition, p 2395. Philadelphia, WB Saunders Co, 1992, with permission.)

TABLE 9–4. PREOPERATIVE MANAGEMENT*

	Treatment
Primary hyperaldosteronism	Spironolactone, 100–400 mg/day, 2–3 wk Follow K^+ until normal Blood pressure should fall
Cushing's syndrome	Control of glucose abnormalities Documentation of osteoporosis Glucocorticoid replacement (before, during, and after surgery) Perioperative antibiotics
Pheochromocytoma	Adrenergic blockade Phenoxybenzamine (Dibenzyline), 20–160 mg/day Metyrosine (if needed) Volume expansion Crystalloid β-Blockade if cardiac arrhythmias (only after α-blockade established) Anesthesia consultation

*From Vaughan ED Jr: Adrenal surgery. *In* Marshall FF (ed): Textbook of Operative Urology. Philadelphia, WB Saunders Co, 1996, with permission.

TABLE 9–5. SURGICAL APPROACHES IN ADRENAL DISORDER*

	Approach
Primary hyperaldosteronism	Posterior (left or right) Modified posterior (right) Eleventh rib (left > right) Posterior transthoracic
Cushing's adenoma	Eleventh rib (left or right) Thoracoabdominal (large) Posterior (small)
Cushing's disease Bilateral hyperplasia	Bilateral posterior Bilateral eleventh rib (alternating)
Adrenal carcinoma	Thoracoabdominal Eleventh rib Transabdominal
Bilateral adrenal ablation	Bilateral posterior
Pheochromocytoma	Transabdominal (chevron) Thoracoabdominal (large, usually right) Eleventh rib
Neuroblastoma	Transabdominal Eleventh rib

*From Vaughan ED Jr: Adrenal surgery. *In* Marshall FF (ed): Textbook of Operative Urology. Philadelphia, WB Saunders Co, 1996, with permission.

healthy require spironolactone 100 to 400 mg/day to restore their potassium supply. Patients with Cushing's syndrome have severe systemic effects from the hyperglucocorticoidism. They are often obese, have diabetic tendencies, are poor wound healers, easily sustain bony fractures, and are susceptible to infection. Thus, they are at high risk for complications. In selected patients with markedly elevated cortisol levels the preoperative use of metabolic blockers such as metyrapone is required to reverse some of the clinical findings prior to adrenalectomy. Certainly glucocorticoid replacement is required throughout the surgical procedure and postoperatively until the function of the contralateral adrenal gland occurs. Finally, in patients with a pheochromocytoma, adrenergic blockade generally with Dibenzyline is required, and at times the blockade of catecholamine production with metyrosine is also useful as previously discussed. The additional preoperative evaluation that is mandatory in patients with pheochromocytoma is consultation with the anesthesiologist, who can be well aware of the patient and can plan strategy for management.[37]

Thus the management of patients with an adrenal disorder is approached on a team basis including experienced endocrinologists, radiologists, anesthesiologists, and urologists or general surgeons.

Numerous approaches can be made to the adrenal gland (Table 9–5). The proper approach depends on the underlying cause of adrenal pathology, the size of the adrenal, the side of the lesion, the habitus of the patient, and the experience and preference of the surgeon. In addition to the surgical options, a laparoscopic approach can be utilized, particularly for smaller adrenal tumors. In most cases there are a number of different options available, and a careful review of all the variables is required before a choice is made. Thus each case should be considered individually, although some approaches are preferable for a given disease. For example, in patients with large adrenal tumors a thoracoabdominal approach is often utilized. In contrast, a posterior or modified posterior approach is preferred for small localized lesions. Finally, a patient with multiple lesions, either extra-adrenal or bilateral, will be explored using a transabdominal chevron incision.

Before describing the specific techniques, a number of unifying concepts warrant attention. First, adequate visualization is imperative, as the adrenal glands lie high in the retroperitoneum and quite posterior. Therefore, the use of a headlight by both the surgeon and first assistant is critical, and hemostasis should be rigorously maintained. The operator should bring the adrenal down by initially exposing the cranial attachments and dividing the rich blood supply between either right-angled clips or utilizing a forceps cautery. Thus, it is often simplest to begin the dissection laterally, identifying the vascular supply and working around the cranial edge of the gland. The posterior surface is generally devoid of vasculature and after the gland is freed superiorly with gentle traction on the kidney, the gland can be brought inferiorly for control of the adrenal vein. The only tumor handled in a different fashion would be a pheochromocytoma where intent should be made to obtain control of the adrenal vein early so as to stabilize the patient from a burst of catecholamine release during manipulation. The adrenal gland is extremely friable and fractures easily, which can cause troublesome bleeding. Therefore, tension or traction should be maintained on the kidney or surrounding structures and not on the adrenal itself. The concept has been stated that the "patient should be dissected from the tumor," a view that is particularly true for pheochromocytomas, in which the glands should not be manipulated.

Posterior Approach

The posterior approach can be used for either bilateral adrenal exploration or unilateral removal of small tumors (Fig. 9–12).

The bilateral approach is rarely utilized today because of our excellent localization techniques. It is now utilized primarily for ablative total adrenalectomy. The options for incisions are shown in Figure 9–12; generally rib resection is preferable to gain high exposure. After standard subperiosteal rib resection, care should be taken with the diaphragmatic release, and the pleura should be avoided, and the diaphragm swept cranially.

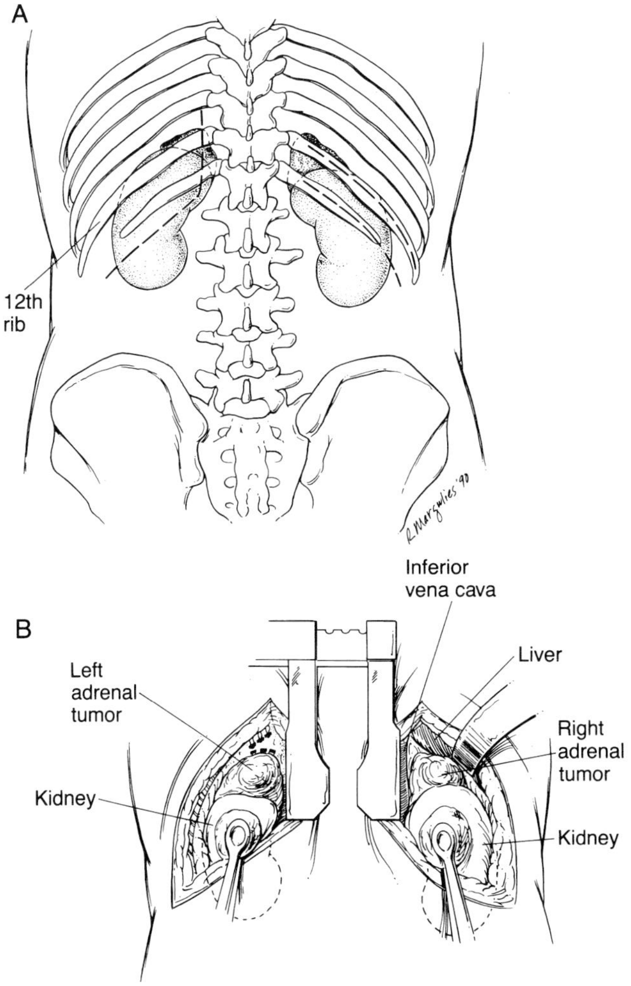
A
12th rib
B
Inferior vena cava
Liver
Left adrenal tumor
Right adrenal tumor
Kidney
Kidney

FIGURE 9–12. Posterior approach to the adrenals. (From Vaughan ED Jr: Adrenal surgery. *In* Marshall FF [ed]: Operative Urology. Philadelphia, WB Saunders Co, 1991, with permission.)

The fibrofatty tissues within Gerota's fascia are swept away from the paraspinal musculature, exposing a subdiaphragmatic "open space" that is at the posterior apex of the resection. The liver within the peritoneum is dissected off the anterior surface of the adrenal and the cranial blood supply is divided. Medially on the right, the IVC is visualized. The short, high adrenal vein entering the cava in a dorsolateral position is identified and can be clipped or ligated. The adrenal can then be drawn caudally by traction on the kidney. The adrenal arteries will issue from behind the inferior vena cava and these must be carefully clipped; otherwise, troublesome bleeding can occur.

Finally, the adrenal is removed from the superior aspect of the kidney and care must be taken to avoid apical branches of the renal artery. On the left, the approach is similar with division of the splenorenal ligament giving initial lateral exposure.

The posterior approach can be modified for a transthoracic adrenal exposure to the diaphragm[38]; however, this more extensive approach is rarely necessary for small adrenal tumors.

Modified Posterior Approach

Although the posterior approach has the advantage of rapid adrenal exposure and low morbidity, there are definite disadvantages. This approach may impair respiration, the abdominal contents are compressed posteriorly, and the visual field is limited. In addition, if bleeding occurs it is difficult to extend the incision to gain a better exposure. Therefore, we have developed a modified posterior approach for right adrenalectomy utilizing the Gil-Vernet position.[39]

The approach is based on the anatomic relationship with the right adrenal, which lies deeply posterior and high in the retroperitoneum behind the liver (Fig. 9–13*A*). In addition, the short, stubby right adrenal vein enters the IVC posteriorly at the apex of the adrenal. Hence, we utilize an approach that is posterior, but the patient is in a modified position, similar to that used for a Gil-Vernet dorsal lumbotomy incision.[40] The patient is first placed in a formal lateral flank position and then allowed to fall forward into the modified posterior position (Fig. 9–13*B*). Subsequently the eleventh or twelfth rib is resected with care to avoid the pleura. The diaphragm then is dissected off the underlying peritoneum and liver in order to gain mobility. Similarly, the inferior surface of the peritoneum, closely associated with the liver, is sharply dissected from Gerota's fascia, which is gently retracted inferiorly. It is of note that the adrenal gland is not identified during the early portion of the dissection, and because of the modified posterior approach, the sur-

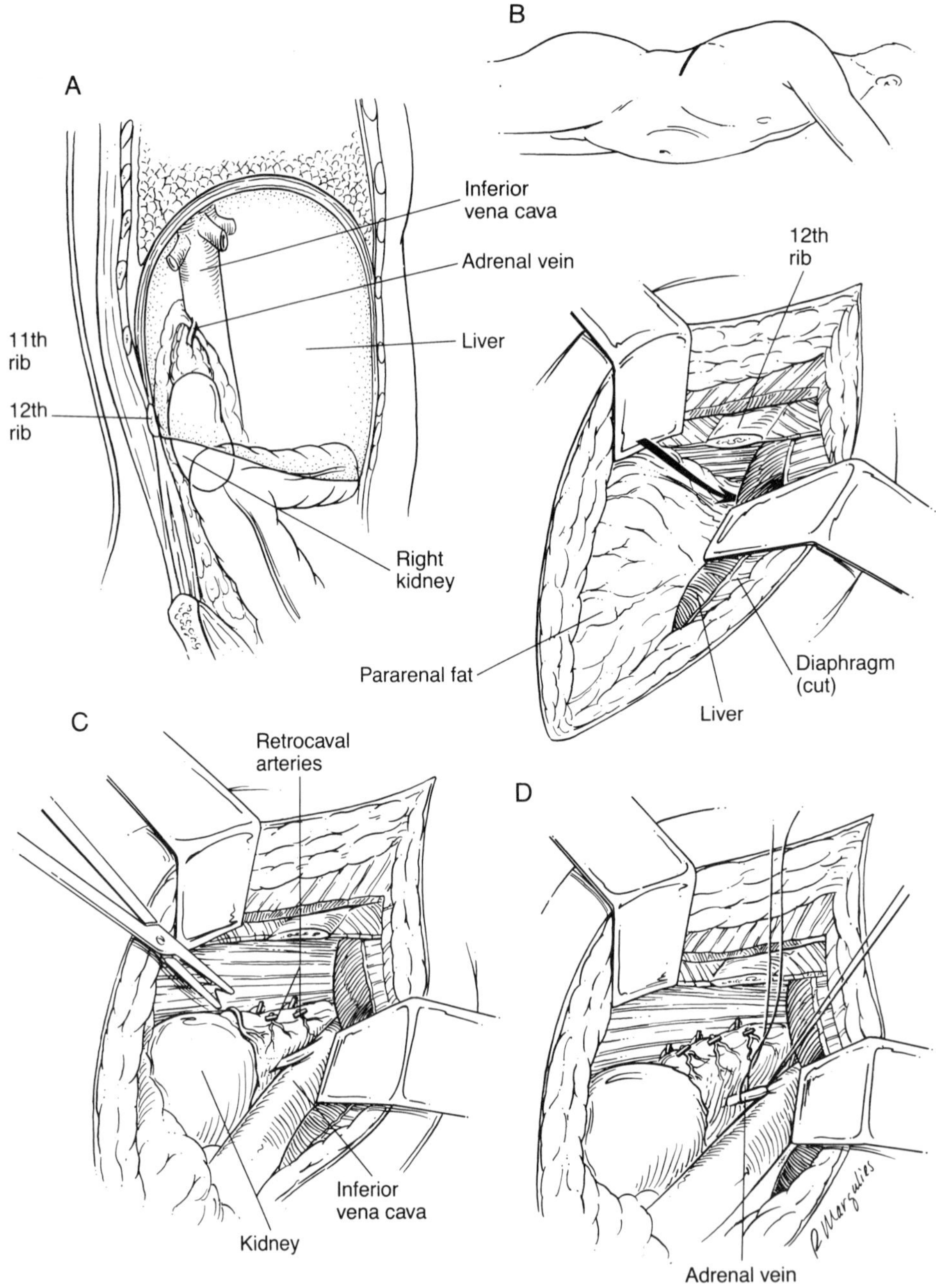
A
B
C
D
Inferior vena cava
Adrenal vein
Liver
11th rib
12th rib
Right kidney
12th rib
Pararenal fat
Diaphragm (cut)
Liver
Retrocaval arteries
Inferior vena cava
Kidney
Adrenal vein

FIGURE 9–13. Modified posterior approach to the right adrenal. (From Vaughan ED Jr: Adrenal surgery. *In* Marshall FF [ed]: Operative Urology. Philadelphia, WB Saunders Co, 1991, with permission.)

geon can become disoriented if not thoroughly familiar with anatomic relationships.

The adrenal will become visible in the depth of the incision as the final hepatic attachments are divided. The lateral, empty space can be found exposing the posterior abdominal musculature and often the inferior vena cava. Multiple small arteries course behind the inferior vena cava and emerge over the paraspinal muscles, and these are clipped and divided.

At this point the adrenal can usually be moved posteriorly against the paraspinal muscles exposing the anterior surface of the inferior vena cava below the adrenal gland.

The major advantage of this approach is that the adrenal vein is easily identified because it emerges from the segment of the IVC exposed and courses up to the adrenal, which now rises toward the surgeon. In other flank or anterior positions the adrenal vein resides in its posterior relationship, requiring caval rotation and the chance of adrenal vein avulsion. After adrenal vein exposure, it is doubly tied and divided or clipped with right-angled clips and divided (Fig. 9–13*D*).

The remaining removal of the adrenal is as was previously described for the posterior approach.

On the left side we do not use this modified approach and use a standard flank approach with a fairly small incision.

We have used the modified posterior approach for all patients with right adrenal aldosterone-secreting tumors and for other patients with benign adenomas of less than 6 cm. We do not recommend the approach for patients with large lesions or malignant adrenal neoplasms. The approach has been used for patients with relatively small pheochromocytomas.

Flank Approach

The standard extrapleural, extraperitoneal eleventh rib resection is excellent for either left or right adrenalectomy. After completion of the incision, the lumbocostal arch is utilized as a landmark showing the point of attachment of the posterior diaphragm to the posterior abdominal musculature. Gerota's fascia, containing the adrenal and kidney, can be swept medially and inferiorly, giving exposure to the splenorenal ligament on the left, which should be divided to avoid splenic injury (Fig. 9–14). Working anteriorly on the left, the spleen and pancreas within the peritoneum can be lifted cranially, exposing the anterior surface of the adrenal gland.

On the right side, a similar maneuver is used to lift the liver within the peritoneum off the anterior surface of the adrenal. Quite often the adrenal gland cannot be identified precisely until these maneuvers are performed. One should not attempt to dissect into the body of the adrenal or to dissect the inferior surface of the adrenal off the kidney. The kidney is useful for retraction. The dissection should continue from lateral to medial along the posterior abdominal and diaphragmatic musculature, with precise ligation or clipping of the small but multiple adrenal arteries. While the operator clips these arteries with one hand, the opposite hand is employed to retract both adrenal and kidney inferiorly. With release of the superior vasculature, the adrenal becomes easily visualized. On the left medially, the phrenic branch of the venous drainage must be carefully clipped or ligated (Fig. 9–15). This vessel is not noted in most atlases but can cause troublesome bleeding if divided. The medial dissection along the crus of the diaphragm and aorta will lead to the renal vein; finally, the adrenal vein is controlled, doubly tied, and divided. The adrenal is then removed from the kidney with care to avoid the apical branches of the renal artery (Fig. 9–15).

On the right side, the dissection is similar. However, after release of the adrenal from the superior vasculature, it is helpful to expose the IVC and divide the medial arterial supply. This maneuver allows mobilization of the cava for better exposure of the high posterior adrenal vein, which is doubly tied or clipped and divided (Fig. 9–16). Patients with large adrenal carcinomas may require en bloc resection of the adrenal and kidney following the principles of radical nephrectomy (Fig. 9–16).

A major deviation from this technique is used for

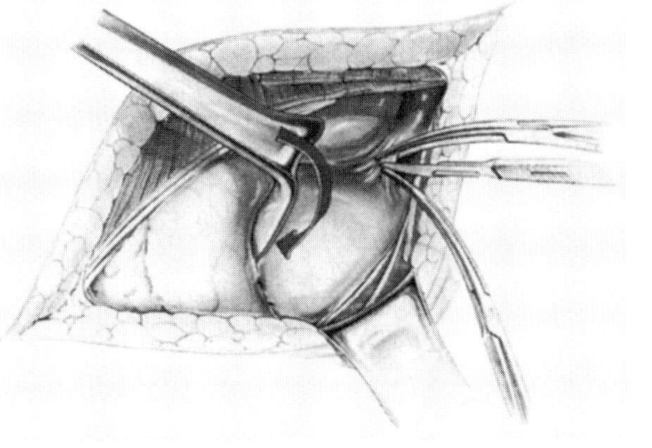

FIGURE 9–14. Release of splenorenal ligament early in exposure of left adrenal. (From Vaughan ED Jr: Adrenal surgery. *In* Marshall FF [ed]: Operative Urology. Philadelphia, WB Saunders Co, 1991, with permission.)

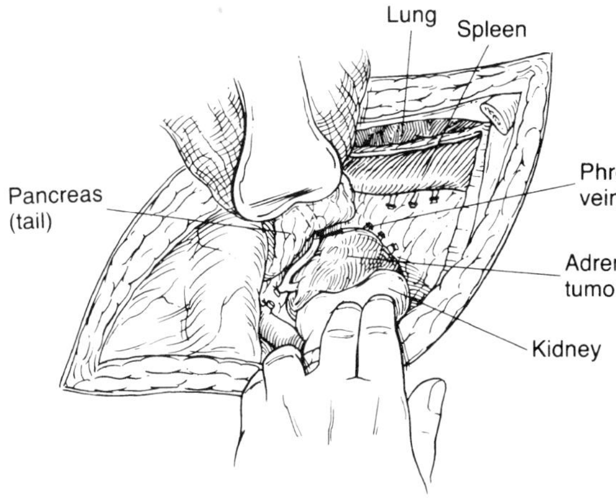
Lung
Spleen
Pancreas (tail)
Phrenic vein
Adrenal tumor
Kidney

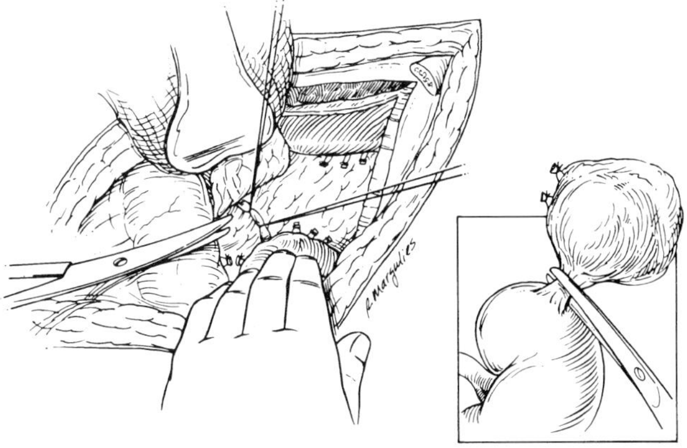

FIGURE 9–15. Further exposure of left adrenal including phrenic vein. (From Vaughan ED Jr: Adrenal surgery. *In* Marshall FF [ed]: Operative Urology. Philadelphia, WB Saunders Co, 1991, with permission.)

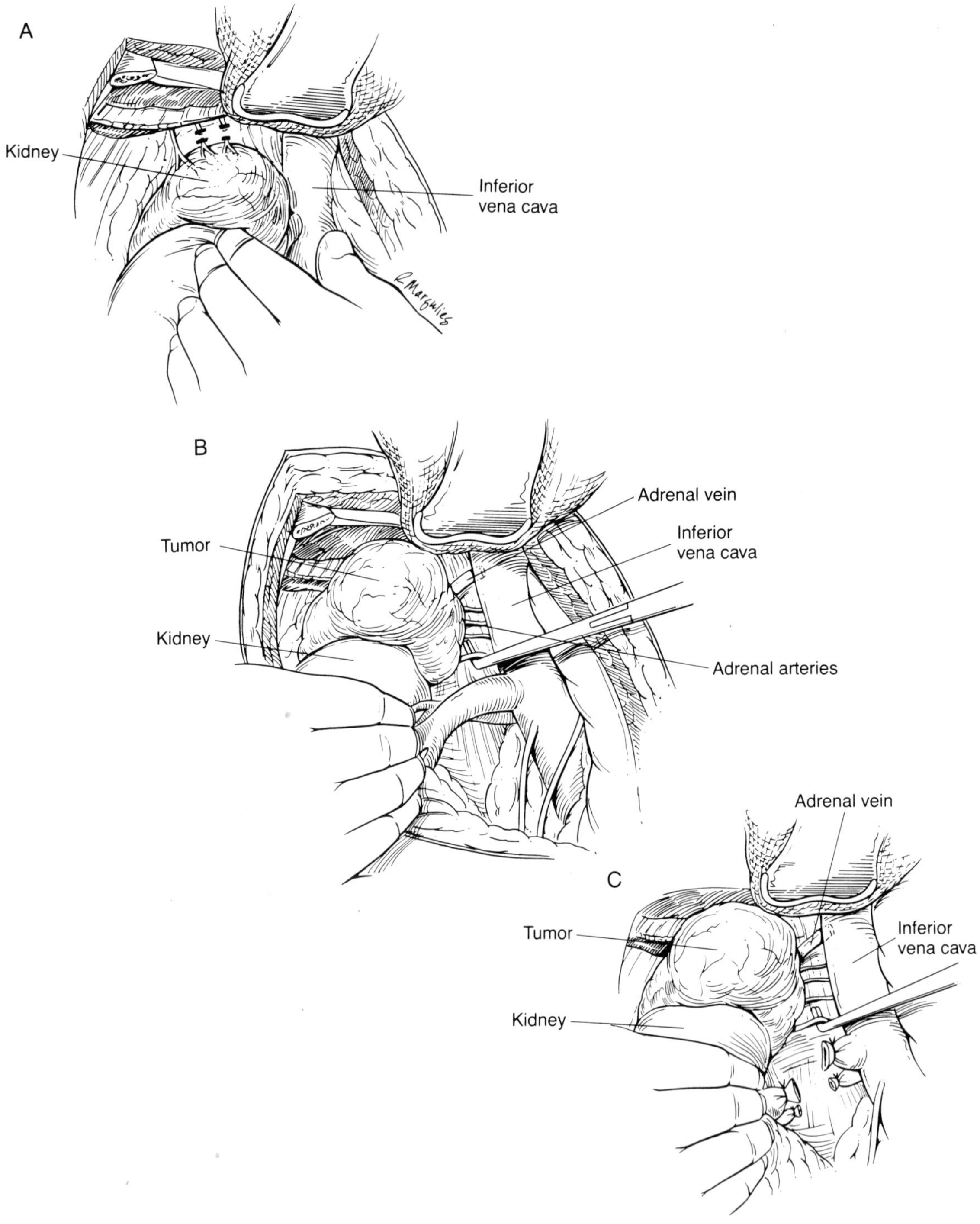
A
Kidney
Inferior
vena cava
B
Adrenal vein
Tumor
Inferior
vena cava
Kidney
Adrenal arteries
Adrenal vein
C
Tumor
Inferior
vena cava
Kidney

FIGURE 9–16. Exposure of right adrenal with and without nephrectomy. (From Vaughan ED Jr: Adrenal surgery. *In* Marshall FF [ed]: Operative Urology. Philadelphia, WB Saunders Co, 1991, with permission.)

the patient with pheochromocytoma, in whom the initial dissection should be aimed toward early control and division of the main adrenal vein on either side. Obviously, in this setting, the anesthesiologist should be notified when the adrenal vein is divided because a marked drop in blood pressure often occurs, even when the patient is adequately hydrated.

After removal of the adrenal, inspection should be made for any bleeding and for pleural tears of the diaphragm. The kidney should also be inspected. The incision is closed without drains with interrupted 0 polydioxanone sutures.

Thoracoabdominal Approach

The thoracoabdominal ninth or tenth rib approach is utilized for large adenomas; for some large adrenal carcinomas; and for well-localized pheochromocytomas. The incision and exposure are standard, with a radial incision through the diaphragm and a generous intraperitoneal extension. The techniques described for adrenalectomy with the eleventh rib approach are used.

Transabdominal Approach

The transabdominal approach is commonly selected for patients with pheochromocytomas, for children, and for some patients with adrenal carcinomas. The concept is to have the ability for complete abdominal exploration to identify either multiple pheochromocytomas or adrenal metastases.

I use the transverse or chevron incision, which I believe gives better exposure of both adrenal glands than a midline incision. The rectus muscles and lateral abdominal muscles are divided, exposing the peritoneum. Upon entering the peritoneal cavity, the surgeon should gently palpate the paraaortic areas and the adrenal areas. Close attention is given to blood pressure changes in an attempt to identify any unsuspected lesions if the patient has a pheochromocytoma. This maneuver is less important today because of the excellent localization techniques previously discussed. In fact, with precise preoperative localization of the offending tumor, the chevron incision does not need to be completely symmetric and may be limited on the contralateral side.

If the patient has a lesion on the right adrenal, the hepatic flexure of the colon is reflected inferiorly. The incision is made in the posterior peritoneum lateral to the kidney and carried superiorly, allowing the liver to be reflected cranially (Fig. 9–17). Incision in the peritoneum is carried downward, exposing the anterior surface of the inferior vena cava to the entrance of the right renal vein. Once the cava is cleared, one or two accessory hepatic veins are often encountered, which should be secured (Fig. 9–18*B*). These veins are easily avulsed from the cava and may cause troublesome bleeding. Ligation of these veins gives 1 to 2 cm of additional caval exposure, which is often useful during the exposure of the short posterior right adrenal vein. Small accessory adrenal veins may also be encountered. The cava is then rolled medially, exposing the adrenal vein, which should be doubly tied or clipped and divided (Fig. 9–18*C*).

After control of the adrenal vein, it is simplest to proceed with the superior dissection, lifting the liver off the adrenal and securing the multiple small adrenal arteries arising from the inferior phrenic ar-

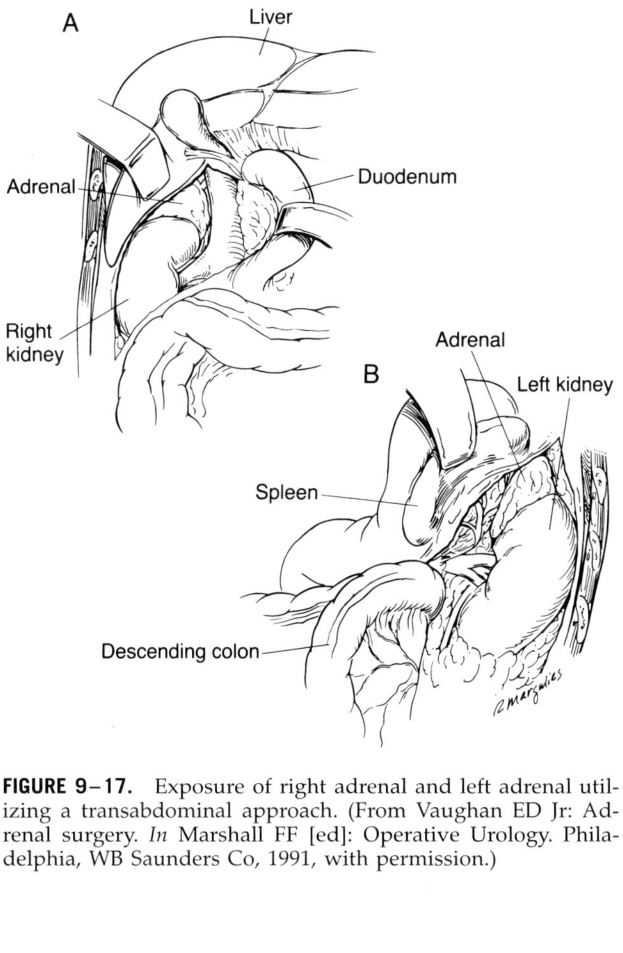
A
Liver
Adrenal
Duodenum
Right kidney
B
Adrenal
Left kidney
Spleen
Descending colon

FIGURE 9–17. Exposure of right adrenal and left adrenal utilizing a transabdominal approach. (From Vaughan ED Jr: Adrenal surgery. *In* Marshall FF [ed]: Operative Urology. Philadelphia, WB Saunders Co, 1991, with permission.)

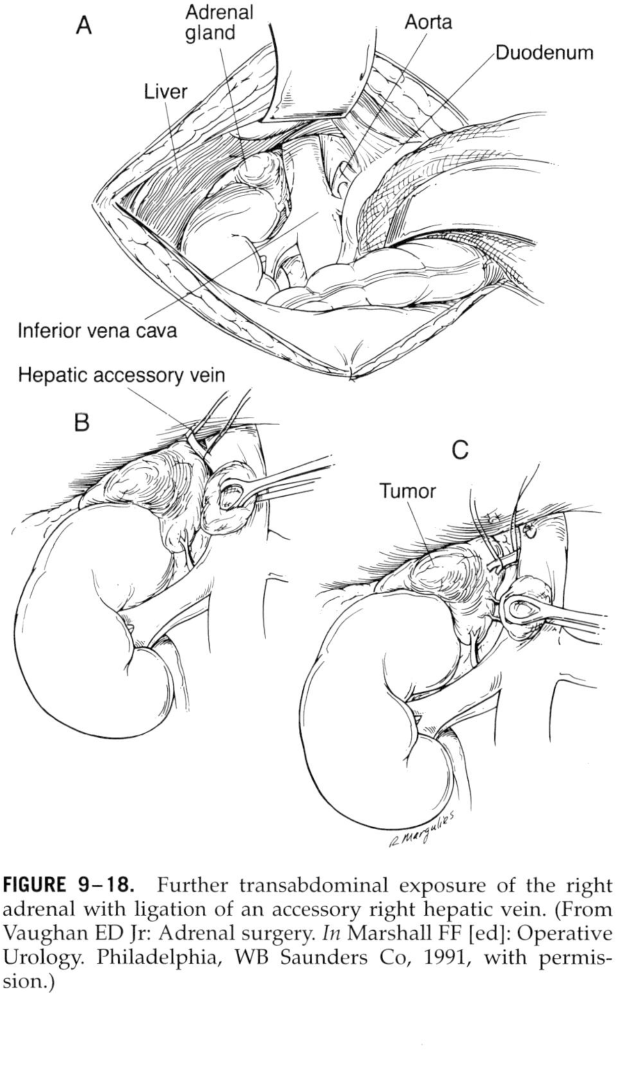
A
Adrenal gland
Aorta
Duodenum
Liver
Inferior vena cava
Hepatic accessory vein
B
C
Tumor

FIGURE 9–18. Further transabdominal exposure of the right adrenal with ligation of an accessory right hepatic vein. (From Vaughan ED Jr: Adrenal surgery. *In* Marshall FF [ed]: Operative Urology. Philadelphia, WB Saunders Co, 1991, with permission.)

tery, which is rarely seen. The adrenal can be drawn inferiorly with retraction on the kidney, and the adrenal arteries traversing to the adrenal from under the cava can be secured with right-angled clips. The final step is removing the adrenal from the kidney.

The left adrenal vein is not as difficult to approach because it lies lower, partially anterior to the upper pole of the kidney, and the adrenal vein empties into the left renal vein. Accordingly, on the left side, the colon is reflected medially, exposing the anterior surface of Gerota's capsule; the initial dissection should involve identification of the renal vein (Fig. 9–17*B*). In essence, the dissection is the same as for a radical nephrectomy for renal carcinoma. Once the renal vein is exposed, the adrenal vein is identified, doubly ligated, and divided. After this maneuver the pancreas and splenic vasculature are lifted off the anterior surface of the adrenal gland. Because of additional drainage from the adrenal into the phrenic system, I generally continue the medial dissection early to control the phrenic vein. I then work cephalad and lateral to release the splenorenal ligament and the superior attachments of the adrenal. The remainder of the dissection is carried out as previously described.

After removal of the tumor, regardless of size, careful inspection is made to ensure hemostasis and the absence of injury to adjacent organs. Careful abdominal exploration is carried out, after which the wound is closed with the suture material of choice. No drains are used.

Patients with multiple endocrine adenopathy or family histories of pheochromocytoma, as well as pediatric patients, should be considered at high risk for multiple lesions. Preoperative evaluation should identify these lesions, but, regardless, a careful abdominal exploration should be carried out.

In patients with suspected malignant pheochromocytomas, en bloc dissections may be necessary to obtain adequate margins, a concept that also applies in patients with adrenal carcinomas. Evaluation with MRI to obtain transverse, coronal, and sagittal images is extremely useful to define clearly the adrenal relationships to the IVC and renal vessels as well as to localize the adrenal vein.

In patients with pheochromocytomas, postoperative management includes maintenance of arterial and venous lines in an intensive care setting until they are stable. Often, 24 to 48 hours is required for the full effect of phenoxybenzamine, the α-blocking agent commonly given, to wear off and for normal α-receptor activity to be restored.

PARTIAL ADRENALECTOMY

The standard treatment for patients with the adrenal lesions described has been total adrenalec-

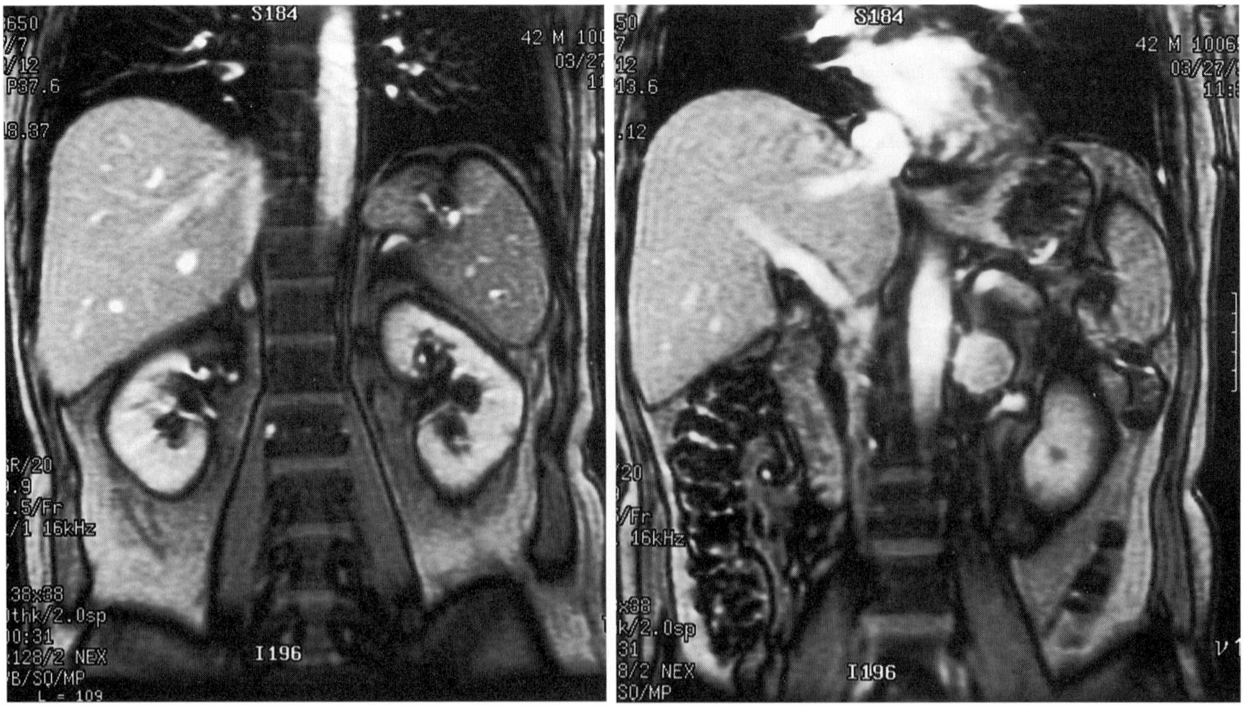
S184
42 M
I196
S184
42 M
I196

A B

FIGURE 9–19. MRI showing bilateral adrenal pheochromocytoma in a patient with bilateral glomus jugulare tumors. *A*, Small right adenoma that was enucleated and which was partially resected. *B*, Large left bright pheochromocytoma that was totally removed. (From Vaughan ED Jr, Blumenfeld JD: The adrenals. *In* Walsh, PC, Retik AB, Stamey TA, Vaughan ED Jr [eds]: Campbell's Urology, 7th edition. Philadelphia, WB Saunders Co, 1997 [in press], with permission.)

tomy. However, there recently has been reported an excellent paper showing the utility of partial adrenalectomy in patients with primary hyperaldosteronism.[41] I have not used partial adrenalectomy in a patient for normal contralateral adrenal, but certainly have used the technique in patients with bilateral disease (Fig. 9–19). Thus, in one patient with a pheochromocytoma on one side and a nonfunctioning adenoma on the other, the adenoma was simply enucleated from the adrenal. In a second patient with bilateral pheochromocytomas, the larger lesion was totally excised and partial adrenalectomy was utilized to remove the contralateral tumor. Care has to be made to obtain thorough hemostasis when performing a partial adrenalectomy because of the vascular nature of the adrenal.

LAPAROSCOPIC ADRENALECTOMY

The techniques of laparoscopic surgery are discussed elsewhere in this text. There is an expanding literature that is now available, describing both the surgical technique and the results of laparoscopic adrenalectomy.[42–44] It is abundantly clear that the technique is feasible, safe, and well tolerated by the patient. One of the major limitations of the widespread usefulness of the procedure is the fact that a coordinated and well-experienced laparoscopic team needs to be available to perform the procedure. In addition, even with an experienced team, the time required to perform a laparoscopic unilateral adrenalectomy far exceeds the time required for an open procedure, and as of yet, there is little cost advantage to performing the procedure other than the fact that the patient can return to work at an earlier time. The specific technical points for the procedure are described elsewhere and are not incorporated into this chapter.

SUMMARY

We are fortunate that our ability to diagnose the specific adrenal entities that mandate a surgical approach is extremely accurate. The combination of analytic methodology to measure the appropriate adrenocortical and medullary hormonal production and the radiologic techniques for localization are superb. The management of these adrenal disorders with surgical precision following localization is highly successful, resulting in a reversal of both metabolic abnormalities and the hypertension that often accompanies these diseases. Indeed, this is a true success story with the evolution of these different techniques over the past 50 years.

REFERENCES

1. Vaughan ED Jr, Blumenfeld JD: The adrenals. *In* Walsh PC, Retik AB, Stamey TA, Vaughan ED Jr (eds): Campbell's Urology, 7th edition. Philadelphia, WB Saunders Co, 1997 (in press).
2. Wilson JD, Foster DW (eds): Williams Textbook of Endocrinology, 8th edition. Philadelphia, WB Saunders Co, 1992.
3. Lee MJ, Mayo-Smith WW, Hahn PF, et al: State-of-the-art MR imaging of the adrenal gland. Radiographics 1994; 14: 1015–1029.
4. Vaughan ED Jr: Adrenal surgery. *In* Marshall FF (ed): Textbook of Operative Urology. Philadelphia, WB Saunders Co, 1996.
5. Orth DN: Cushing's syndrome. N Engl J Med 1995; 32:791.
6. Kazam E, Engel IA, Zirinsky K, et al: Sectional imaging of the adrenal glands, computed tomography and ultrasound. *In* Vaughan ED Jr, Carey RM (eds): Adrenal Disorders. New York, Thieme Medical Publishers Inc, 1989.
7. Belldegrun A, deKernion JB: What to do about the incidentally found adrenal mass. World J Urol 1989; 7:117–120.
8. Hedican SP, Marshall FF: Cardiac bypass and postoperative mitotane in the treatment of adrenocortical carcinoma with caval extension (Abstract 751). Proc Am Urol Assoc 1996; 155:498A.
9. Nakajo M, Nakabeppu Y, Yonekura R, et al: The role of adrenocortical scintigraphy in the evaluation of unilateral incidentally discovered adrenal and juxtaadrenal masses. Ann Nucl Med 1993; 7(3):157–166.
10. Ross NS, Aron DC: Hormonal evaluation of the patient with an incidentally discovered adrenal mass. N Engl J Med 1990; 323:1401.
11. Cerfolio RJ, Vaughan ED Jr, Brennan TG, Hiruela ER: Accuracy of computed tomography in predicting adrenal tumor size. Surg Gynecol Obstet 1993; 176:307.
12. Mayo-Smith WW, Lee MJ, McNicholas MM, et al: Characterization of adrenal masses (<5 cm) by use of chemical shift MR imaging: observer performance vs. quantitative measures. AJR 1995; 165:91–95.
13. Lubat E, Weinreb JC: Magnetic resonance imaging of the kidneys and adrenals. Top Magn Reson Imaging 1990; 2: 17–36.
14. Tikkakoski T, Taavitsainen M, Paivansalo M, et al: Accuracy of adrenal biopsy guided by ultrasound and CT. Acta Radiol 1991; 32:371–374.
15. Luton J-P, Cerdas S, Billaud L, et al: Clinical features of adrenocortical carcinoma, prognostic factors, and the effect of mitotane therapy. N Engl J Med 1990; 322:1195.
16. Imperato-McGinley J, Young IS, Huang T, et al: Testosterone secreting adrenal cortical adenomas. Int J Gynaecol Obstet 1981; 19:421.
17. Gabrilove JL, Sharma DC, Waitz HH, Dorfman R: Feminizing adrenal cortical tumors in the male: a review of 52 cases including a case report. Medicine 44:37, 1965.
18. Richie JP, Gittes RF: Carcinoma of the adrenal cortex. Cancer 1980; 45:1957.
19. Pommier RF, Brennan MF: An eleven-year experience with adrenocortical carcinoma. Surgery 1992; 112:963–971.
20. Haak HR, van Seters AP, Moolenaar AJ, Fleuren GJ: Expression of p-glycoprotein in relation to clinical manifestation, treatment and prognosis of adrenocortical cancer. Eur J Cancer 1993; 29A:1036–1038.
21. Bergenstal DM, Hurtz R, Lipsett MB, Moy RH: Chemotherapy of adrenal cortical cancer with o,p'DDD. Ann Intern Med 1960; 53:672.
22. Wooten MD, King DK: Adrenal cortical carcinoma. Epidemiology and treatment with mitotane and a review of the literature. Cancer 1993; 72:3145–3155.
23. Conn JW: Primary hyperaldosteronism. A new clinical syndrome. J Lab Clin Med 1955; 45:3.
24. Blumenfeld JD, Schlussel Y, Sealey JE, et al: Diagnosis and treatment of primary hyperaldosteronism. Ann Intern Med 1994; 121:877–885.
25. Laragh JH, Angers M, Kelly WG, et al: The effect of epinephrine, norepinephrine, angiotensin II, and others on the secretory rate of aldosterone in man. JAMA 1960; 174:234.
26. Laragh JH, Sealey JE: The renin-angiotensin-aldosterone

system and the renal regulation of sodium, potassium, and blood pressure homeostasis. *In* Windhager EE (ed): Handbook of Physiology. New York, Oxford University Press, 1992.

27. Vaughan ED Jr, Sosa RE: Renovascular hypertension. *In* Walsh PC, Retik AB, Stamey TA, Vaughan ED Jr (eds): Campbell's Urology, 7th edition. Philadelphia, WB Saunders Co, 1997 (in press).
28. Mann SJ, Atlas SA: Hypertensive emergencies. *In* Laragh JH, Brenner BM (eds): Hypertension, Pathophysiology, Diagnosis and Management. New York, Raven Press, 1995.
29. Manger WM, Gifford RW Jr: Pheochromocytoma: a clinical review. *In* Laragh JH, Brenner BM (eds): Hypertension, Pathophysiology, Diagnosis and Management. New York, Raven Press, 1995.
30. Imperato-McGinley J, Gautier T, Ehlers K, et al: Reversibility of catecholamine-induced dilated cardiomyopathy in a child with a pheochromocytoma. N Engl J Med 1987; 316: 793–797.
31. Vaughan ED Jr: Treatment. *In* Manger WM (ed): Pheochromocytoma, 2nd edition, pp 421–422. New York, Blackwell Science Publications, 1996.
32. Bolande RP: The neurocrestopathias: a unifying concept of disease arising in neurocrest maldevelopment. Hum Pathol 1974; 5:409.
33. Pearse AG, Polak JM: Cytochemical evidence for the neural crest origin of mammalian ultimobranchial C cells. Histochemie 1971; 27:96.
34. Bravo EL: Pheochromocytoma: new concepts and future trends. Kidney Int 1991; 40:544–556.
35. Shapiro B, Copp JE, Sisson JC, et al: Iodine-131 metaiodobenzylguanidine for the locating of suspected pheochromocytoma: experience in 400 cases. J Nucl Med. 1985; 26:576.
36. Campeau RJ, Garcia OM, Correa OA, Rege AB: Pheochromocytoma: diagnosis by scintigraphy using iodine-131 metaiodobenzylguanidine. South Med J 1991; 84:1221–1230.
37. Malhotra V (ed): Anesthesia for Renal and Genitourinary Surgery. New York, McGraw Hill, 1995.
38. Novick AC, Straffon RA, Kaylor W: Posterior transthoracic approach for adrenal surgery. J Urol 1989; 141:254.
39. Vaughan ED Jr, Phillips H: Modified posterior approach for right adrenalectomy. Surg Gynecol Obstet 1987; 165: 453–455.
40. Gil-Vernet J: New surgical concepts in removing renal calculi. Urol Int 1965; 20:255–262.
41. Nakada T, Kubota Y, Sasagawa I, et al: Therapeutic outome of primary aldosteronism: adrenalectomy versus enucleation of aldosterone-producing adenoma. J Urol 1995; 153: 1775–1780.
42. Suzuki K, Kageyama S, Ueda D, et al: Laparoscopic adrenalectomy: clinical experience with 12 cases. J Urol 1993; 150:1099–1102.
43. Naito S, Uozumi J, Shimura H, et al: Laparoscopic adrenalectomy: review of 14 cases and comparison with open adrenalectomy. J Endourol 1995; 9:491–495.
44. MacGillivray DC, Shichman SJ, Ferrer FA, Malchoff CD: A comparison of open versus laparoscopic adrenalectomy. J Surg Endosc (in press).

10

SURGERY OF ADRENAL TUMORS

LIAM J. HURLEY, M.D., CHARLES R. BURKE, M.D., *and* JOHN A. LIBERTINO, M.D.

Surgery of the adrenal gland involves the infradiaphragmatic great vessels and associated viscera, including the pancreas, liver, and spleen. These structures increase the technical challenge of adrenal surgery. Historically, urologists, such as Cahill,[1,2] Flint,[3–5] and Glenn et al.[6–9] have contributed greatly to the understanding of adrenal disease and adrenal surgery. They have fostered a generation of adrenal surgeons who maintain an interest in and have developed centers of excellence for the management of patients with adrenal endocrinopathies and neoplasia.

The diagnostic dilemmas that confronted our predecessors have been lessened by advances in computed tomography (CT), magnetic resonance imaging (MRI), and radioisotopic scanning. The surgical management of patients with adrenal disease requires understanding of the functional nature of the endocrinopathy as well as a thorough knowledge of adrenal anatomy and the various surgical approaches to the adrenal gland.

SURGICAL ANATOMY OF THE ADRENAL GLANDS

The location of the adrenal glands in the retroperitoneum adjacent to the upper pole of the kidney is constant. They are paired retroperitoneal organs within perinephric fat, anterosuperior and medial to the kidney. The average size is 5 × 3 × 1 cm and each weighs 5 g. The right adrenal gland is posterolateral to the inferior vena cava and contacts the inferior surface of the liver and diaphragm. It lies higher than the left adrenal gland. The left adrenal gland lies in more intimate contact with the kidney and requires special care on removal to avoid injury to left renal vessels. The arterial supply arises from the inferior phrenic artery above, the aorta laterally, and the renal artery inferiorly and is more variable than the venous drainage (Fig. 10–1). The variable arterial supply rarely causes problems surgically. The adrenal venous supply, although more constant, presents more surgical problems. The right adrenal vein is short and enters the vena cava on its posterolateral aspect. Visualization of this vein may be obscured at its entrance into the vena cava by enlargement of the gland. Failure to ligate this vein securely results in considerable blood loss, which may be difficult to control. On the left, the adrenal vein is prominent and exits from the anteroinferior aspect of the adrenal gland and drains into the left renal vein.

Congenital anomalies of the adrenal gland, such as agenesis, presence of accessory adrenal tissue, and heterotopia, have been reported. Heterotopic adrenal tissue may be intrahepatic, and, rarely, the adrenal gland has been found beneath the renal capsule. If the kidney is absent, the adrenal gland is still usually found in its normal position. It is rare to have unilateral absence of an adrenal gland.

The adrenal cortex is divided into three anatomically and functionally important zones: the zona glomerulosa, the zona fasciculata, and the zona reticularis. The adrenal cortex develops from mesoderm, which invades the mesenchyme between the root of the mesentery and the developing gonad before proliferating. This intimate relationship between the developing gonad, kidney, and adrenal explains the ectopic and aberrant adrenal tissue as mentioned earlier. In the adult, the adrenal cortex constitutes 90% of the gland volume. The zona glomerulosa produces aldosterone; the zona fasciculata, cortisol; and the sex hormones are provided in the zona reticularis. The adrenal medulla, which produces catecholamines, is centrally located and develops from neuroectoderm.

SYNOPSIS OF ADRENAL PHYSIOLOGY

The adrenal cortex produces steroid hormones, which include corticoids, androgens, aldosterone,

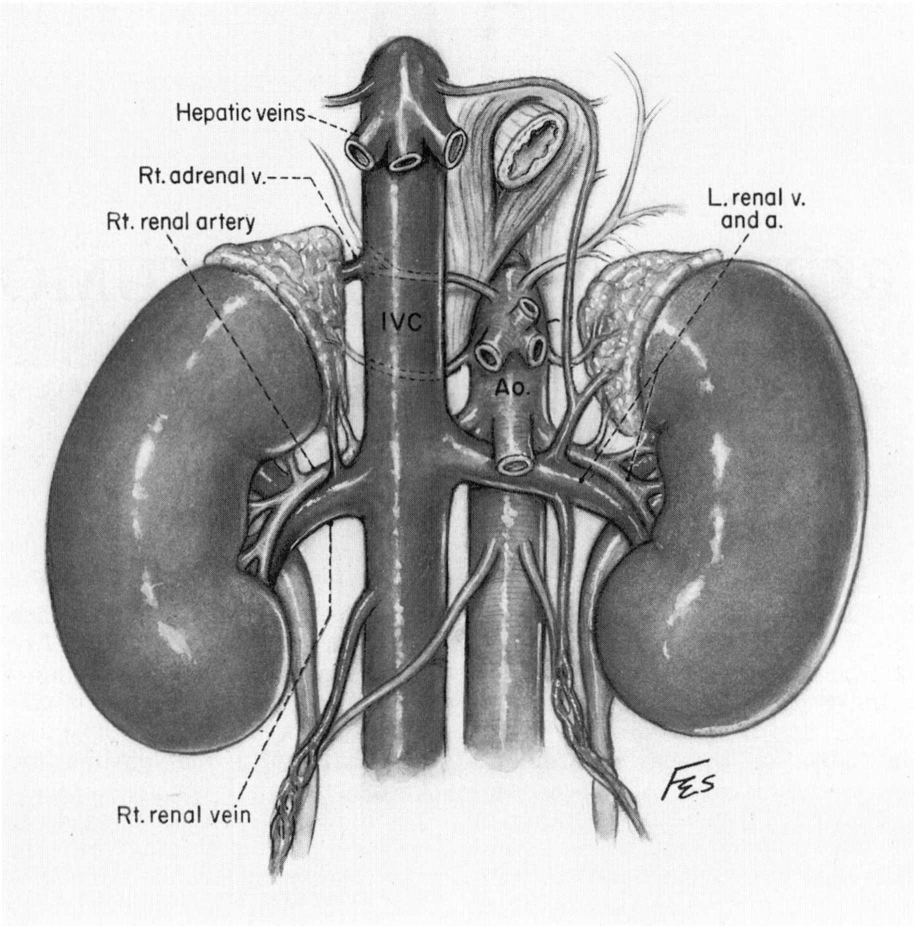
Hepatic veins
Rt. adrenal v.
Rt. renal artery
L. renal v.
and a.
IVC
Ao.
Rt. renal vein
FES

FIGURE 10–1. Normal adrenal anatomy. (By permission of Lahey Clinic.)

and progesterone. The activity of the adrenal cortex is regulated by hormonal mechanisms, whereas the adrenal medulla is stimulated by the sympathetic nervous system. The structure, growth, and secretory activity of the adrenal cortex are controlled primarily by adrenocorticotropic hormone (ACTH) from the anterior pituitary gland, whereas aldosterone, which is produced by the zona glomerulosa, is regulated by angiotensin. Corticotropin-releasing factor (CRF) from the hypothalamus modulates release of ACTH from the pituitary gland. Of the hormones produced by the adrenal cortex, only cortisol (hydrocortisone) has an important inhibitory feedback mechanism. The higher the cortisol level, the lower the ACTH level, and vice versa.

This homeostatic mechanism maintains the level of circulating plasma cortisol within narrow limits unless a stress induces an increase in secretion of ACTH, which can occur regardless of the level of circulating cortisol.

All adrenal steroids are derived from cholesterol (Fig. 10–2). The rate-limiting step in steroid synthesis is the production of pregnenolone from cholesterol. Glucocorticoids are distinguished by the 11-deoxycortisol and 17α-hydroxyprogesterone groups, ultimately resulting in production of cortisol. Under basal conditions, the normal adult produces 10 to 24 mg of cortisol a day. Mineralocorticoids include aldosterone, which is produced at a rate of 30 to 150 mg/day. Weak androgens, the 17-ketosteroids, include dehydroepiandrosterone (DHEA), dehydroepiandrosterone sulfate (DHEAS), and androstanedione. These constitute the remainder of the hormones produced by the adrenal cortex and are secreted in quantities of 25 to 30 mg/day.[10] The adrenal androgens, estrogens, and aldosterone are not involved in the feedback mechanism that exists between the pituitary gland and the adrenal gland. The effects of corticoid excess, as is well known, leads to the classic stigmata of Cushing's syndrome. In addition, excess steroid products can be produced by Conn's syndrome or adrenal carcinoma.

The renin-angiotensin-aldosterone relationship is an important one. Production of aldosterone is increased by an elevated circulating angiotensin level and, to a lesser extent, by ACTH (Fig. 10–3). The mineralocorticoid function of aldosterone controls retention of sodium as well as excretion of potassium and hydrogen by the kidney. Deficiency of mineralocorticoid secretion can lead to water loss, hyponatremia, hyperkalemic acidosis, and a con-

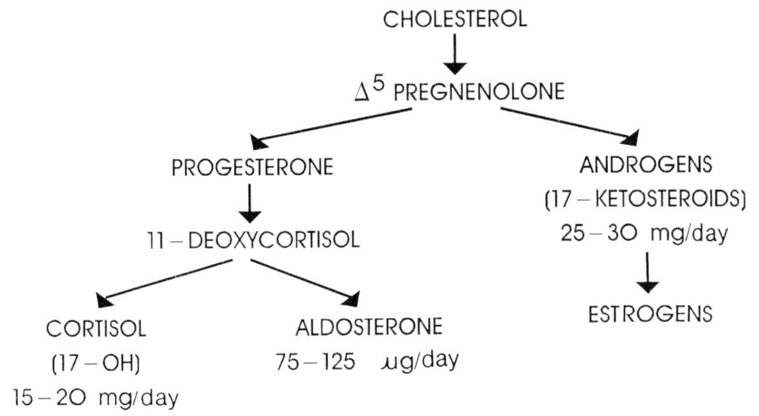
CHOLESTEROL
Δ5 PREGNENOLONE
PROGESTERONE
ANDROGENS
(17 – KETOSTEROIDS)
25 – 30 mg/day
11 – DEOXYCORTISOL
ESTROGENS
CORTISOL
(17 – OH)
15 – 20 mg/day
ALDOSTERONE
75 – 125 μg/day

FIGURE 10–2. Adrenal physiology.

tracted blood volume. Excess aldosterone causes the opposite effects, with volume-dependent hypertension and severe hypokalemic alkalosis secondary to potassium wasting. Thus, primary hyperaldosteronism, such as is seen with an adrenal aldosteronoma, will cause retention of sodium, increased blood volume, and suppression of renin. Conversely, in secondary hyperaldosteronism, such as is seen in renal artery stenosis, an elevation in renin results in chronic stimulation and overproduction of aldosterone.[11]

Metabolisms of the adrenocortical steroids vary. Cortisol has a half-life of 70 minutes, and most is metabolized by the liver; 80% of cortisol is bound to transcortin, a binding globulin. The remainder is found either bound to globulin (10 to 15%) or free (7 to 10%).[12] Variations in these binding proteins will change the total cortisol measured but not the free cortisol value, which represents the active component. Cortisol is released in a diurnal rhythm, with the highest concentration in the morning.

Aldosterone has a half-life of 20 to 30 minutes and is poorly bound by proteins. When plasma values are measured, the sodium and peripheral renin activity of the patient must be noted in relation to aldosterone.[13]

The adrenal medulla functions as a separate unit in the adrenal gland, as would be expected from its distinct embryologic origin. The production of epinephrine and norepinephrine is controlled by sympathetic nerves that innervate the medulla. The physiology of catecholamine secretion and their action are complex. Norepinephrine is synthesized in the tyrosine-dopa-dopamine pathway and is secreted at postganglionic sympathetic nerve fibers, including those in the adrenal medulla. In the adrenal gland, chromaffin cells convert norepinephrine to epinephrine using phenylethanolamine-*N*-methyl transferase. This event occurs only in the adrenal medulla, and information so gained is sometimes helpful in determining whether a pheochromocytoma is located in an adrenal gland or in an ectopic location.

Hypovolemia, upright posture, pain, heat, and cold can activate release of norepinephrine from the adrenal gland, whereas hypoglycemia stimulates production of epinephrine. Because of specific cellular receptor sites, catecholamines have a direct effect on target organs. β-Adrenergic receptors respond more to epinephrine than to norepinephrines and are responsible for arterial dilation, venous constriction, bronchodilation, and increased cardiac rate and contractility. α-Adrenergic receptors are primarily responsive to norepinephrine and result in arterial constriction, increased contraction of the gastrointestinal musculature, diaphoresis, and secretion of insulin.

In summary, norepinephrine stimulates α-adrenergic receptors primarily, whereas epinephrine stimulates both α-adrenergic and β-adrenergic receptor sites.

Catecholamine physiology is complex and is detailed in other texts. The half-life of these substances is 20 seconds.[14] Their primary metabolite is vanillylmandelic acid (VMA) by means of degradation by monamine oxidase (MAO) and catechol-

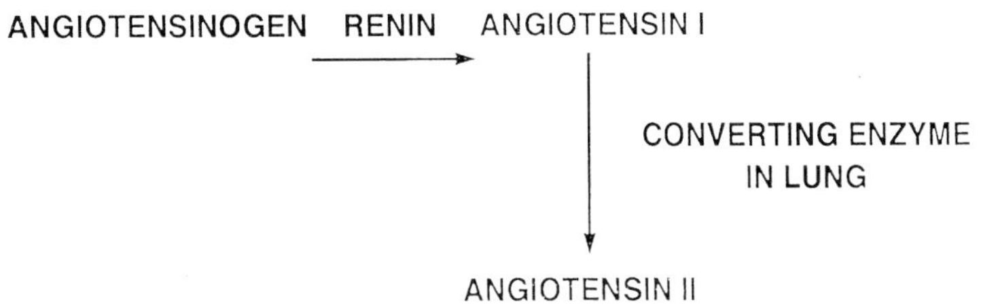
ANGIOTENSINOGEN
RENIN
ANGIOTENSIN I
CONVERTING ENZYME
IN LUNG
ANGIOTENSIN II

FIGURE 10–3. Renin-angiotensin-aldosterone relationship.

O-methyltransferase (COMT). Secondary metabolites include metanephrine from epinephrine and normetanephrine from norepinephrine, which can also be degraded to VMA.

Less than 5% of circulatory epinephrine and norepinephrine is excreted intact in the urine, with the vast majority of urinary products being VMA, metanephrine, and normetanephrine.[15]

CUSHING'S SYNDROME

Cushing's syndrome is not a single disease entity. The clinical picture is secondary to chronic hypersecretion of cortisol by the adrenal cortex. Adrenocortical hypersecretion is classified into Cushing's disease (pituitary dependent) and Cushing's syndrome (pituitary independent). During this discussion, Cushing's syndrome will be used to cover both conditions.

The underlying pathologic findings include pituitary tumor (70%), adrenal adenoma (10 to 15%), adrenal carcinoma (5 to 10%), adrenal hyperplasia (5%), and ectopic ACTH production (5%).[16] In the series reported by Orth and Liddle,[17] 75% of patients had an elevated level of ACTH and 25% did not. Of those with elevated ACTH, 79% will have a pituitary adenoma, either a microadenoma in the anterior lobe (Cushing's disease) or a macroadenoma (Nelson's syndrome), whereas 21% will have an ectopic source outside the pituitary. When electron microscopy and immunohistochemistry techniques are used, cortitroph adenoma cells can be demonstrated in more than 90% of Cushing's disease tumors. Most of these tumors will show basophilic hematoxylin and eosin staining. In patients with an adrenal cause of Cushing's syndrome (an adrenal adenoma or carcinoma), the circulating ACTH will be low or not measurable.

Cushing's syndrome can affect the patient's hematologic system, cardiovascular system, gastrointestinal system, and central nervous system as well as altering metabolism and protein catabolism. Clinical features include stria, truncal obesity, buffalo hump, hypertension, proximal muscle weakness, round face, easy bruisability, and psychiatric symptoms and can resemble those of iatrogenic steroid excess. It is difficult to distinguish patients with Cushing's disease from patients with adrenal adenomas or carcinoma. Ectopic ACTH tumor, however, may produce severe cachexia and hypertension, which may be distinguishable features.[18]

The diagnosis of Cushing's syndrome is best made by measuring cortisol levels. Obtaining morning and afternoon plasma cortisol levels will identify patients with Cushing's syndrome because of the loss of their diurnal variation. Confirmatory evidence is a 24-hour urinary free cortisol determination, with an excess of 125 mg/day being diagnostic.[10]

Further testing includes the overnight dexamethasone suppression test. Failure of urine and plasma steroids to suppress normally with dexamethasone is essential to the diagnosis. Dexamethasone, 1 mg, is given at midnight, and a cortisol level is measured at 8 AM. Failure to suppress indicates Cushing's syndrome. False-positive values occur 20% of the time, whereas false-negative values are rare.[16]

When Cushing's syndrome is suspected, a high-dose dexamethasone suppression test can be administered in an attempt to determine the site of disease. Dexamethasone, 2 mg every 6 hours for 2 or 3 days, is given, and the cortisol level is measured. If cortisol is suppressed by 50%, a pituitary source (Cushing's disease) is likely. In patients with adrenal adenomas, carcinomas, or ectopic ACTH sources, cortisol usually fails to suppress.[19]

Cushing's syndrome can be divided into two major groups: those with an elevated or normal level of circulatory ACTH and those with a low or unmeasurable level of ACTH. If ACTH is low, an adrenal tumor with autonomous function resulting in suppression of ACTH production should be suspected. If ACTH is normal or less than twice normal (<200 pg/dl), a pituitary source of ACTH is suspected. If ACTH is more than twice normal (>200 pg/dl), an ectopic ACTH syndrome is most likely present.[11]

Ectopic ACTH tumors are most commonly oat cell carcinomas of the lung (52%), followed in frequency by bronchial adenoma, carcinomas of the thymus and pancreas, and carcinoid and neural crest tumors.[20]

The metyrapone test also distinguishes between Cushing's disease and adrenal or ectopic sources. Metyrapone inhibits the 11β-hydroxylase enzyme in cortisol production, resulting in a decrease in cortisol and a resultant increase in ACTH by feedback augmentation. If Cushing's disease is present, an exaggerated response is seen, whereas no effect is present with adrenal tumors or ectopic ACTH secretion.

Radiologic studies may be appropriate, depending on the level of ACTH. If ACTH is low, CT of the abdomen is the best initial test because a pituitary lesion is unlikely. Adrenal hyperplasia will produce bilateral diffuse cortical thickening, whereas a functioning adenoma greater than 2 cm will produce contralateral adrenal atrophy. Adrenal carcinoma is usually larger than 6 cm and usually shows calcification and necrosis.[10]

Magnetic resonance imaging can alternatively be used to diagnose adrenal disease. An adenoma is isointense on T2-weighted images, whereas an adrenal carcinoma is hyperintense on T2-weighted images although less so than a pheochromocytoma.[16] Adrenal vein sampling for suspected adrenal sources of Cushing's syndrome can be performed and is precise although invasive.[15]

Adrenal arteriography is not useful for diagnostic purposes, although it may aid in distinguishing a renal from adrenal mass and can identify all vessels before operation on a complex large mass.[16]

Adrenal scanning with 19-norcholesterol iodine-133 (^{131}I) or NP-59 may help to identify hypersecreting adrenal tumors, especially with Conn's syndrome, but it is expensive and not readily accessible.[15]

When neither CT nor MRI suggests adrenal disease, other sources, such as the pituitary or ectopic sources, should be suspected.

When the diagnosis of Cushing's syndrome associated with an elevated level of ACTH is made, it is necessary to investigate the pituitary gland. High-resolution CT is vital in demonstrating tumors greater than 6 mm in diameter.[21] Magnetic resonance imaging with gadolinium-diethylene-triamine-pentaacetic acid (Gd-DTPA) can improve diagnostic accuracy to 80%.[22] Should the tumor not be visualized on CT or MRI, which can occur in 50% of patients with Cushing's disease, selective sampling of ACTH levels in the inferior petrosal sinuses with comparison to peripheral blood ACTH levels will point to a pituitary source of the ACTH and will indicate the correct site of the microadenoma.[23]

The treatment of Cushing's syndrome depends on the site of the tumor. When a pituitary adenoma is the source of the hormonal hypersecretion, the treatment is transsphenoidal removal of the tumor. In patients with a microadenoma (<1 cm), the cure rate for patients with Cushing's disease approaches 90%.[19,24,25] Cure can be obtained with preservation of normal anterior pituitary function in most patients, although return of normal ACTH-adrenal function may take 6 to 9 months. The cure for patients with suprasellar or invasive tumors is significantly lower, 48% in the series of Boggan et al.[24] It has been demonstrated that recurrence is related to regrowth of the tumor and not to hyperplasia of corticotroph cells in the pituitary.[5] In patients in whom a discrete tumor cannot be found or in whom it is not possible to excise the tumor completely, it is reasonable to perform total hypophysectomy in adults past reproductive age.[24,25] It is preferable to perform hypophysectomy than to risk leaving a residual lesion, resulting in persistence of Cushing's disease. In patients in whom it is not possible to effect cure by transsphenoidal surgery, radiotherapy should be administered with 5000 rads. Cure rates are 50 to 80%, with higher rates in children.[26]

Bilateral adrenalectomy for Cushing's disease is no longer the treatment of choice because it results in adrenal insufficiency and the 8% chance of the development of Nelson's syndrome, which is a macroadenoma of the pituitary resulting from lack of feedback.[27] The tumor associated with Nelson's syndrome tends to be more aggressive and is less responsive to surgery or radiotherapy.[28] Bilateral adrenalectomy, however, may still be required if pituitary surgery fails to cure the disease, and the addition of cortisol enzyme inhibitors, such as cyproheptadine, ketoconazole, and aminoglutethimide, may be required to lessen agonizing signs and symptoms.[10]

The treatment of unilateral adrenal tumors is adrenalectomy. The surgical approach is determined by tumor size. Small tumors may be approached extraperitoneally or intraperitoneally (Fig. 10–4). Large tumors can be approached through an anterior transperitoneal or thoracoabdominal incision. Advantages of the anterior approach include direct access to the liver, to the retroperitoneal lymph nodes, and to the tumor and the opposite adrenal gland. Vascular access may also be easier with this approach. A half chevron incision (unilateral subcostal) is usually used. A thoracoabdominal incision provides excellent exposure to the suprarenal area without the morbidity of a transabdominal approach. Disadvantages include longer operative time, pulmonary complications, and less access to intraperitoneal organs and the contralateral adrenal gland.

Supplementation with mineralocorticoids and glucocorticoids is usually required in the postoperative period because the function of the contralateral adrenal gland is usually suppressed by the lowered level of ACTH. After initial high-dose cov-

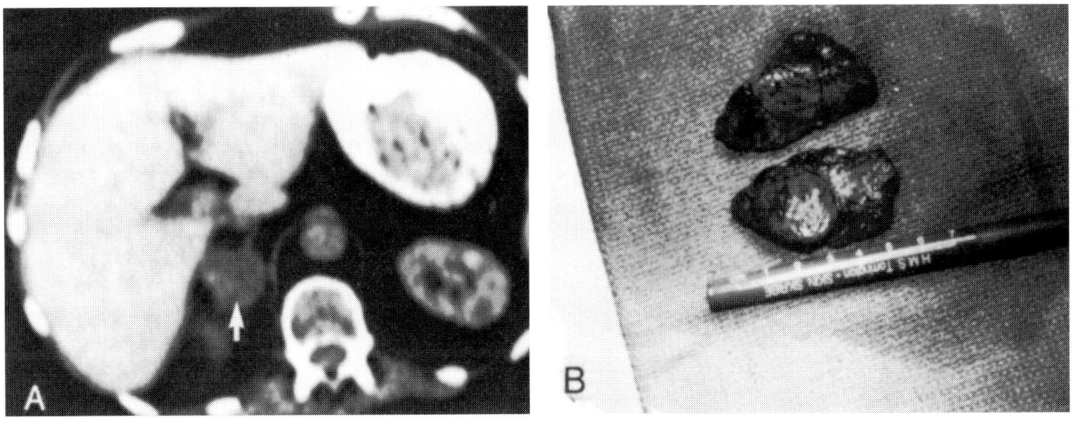
A
B

FIGURE 10–4. *A*, Computed tomogram showing a small adrenal adenoma (*arrow*). *B*, Surgical specimen. (From Libertino JA: Surgery of adrenal disorders. Surg Clin North Am 1988; 68:1027–1056, with permission.)

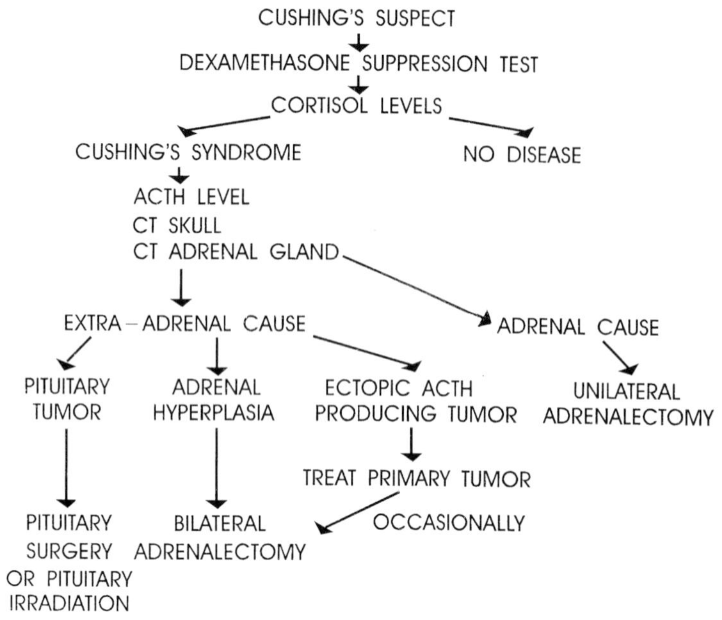
CUSHING'S SUSPECT
DEXAMETHASONE SUPPRESSION TEST
CORTISOL LEVELS
CUSHING'S SYNDROME
NO DISEASE
ACTH LEVEL
CT SKULL
CT ADRENAL GLAND
EXTRA-ADRENAL CAUSE
ADRENAL CAUSE
PITUITARY TUMOR
ADRENAL HYPERPLASIA
ECTOPIC ACTH PRODUCING TUMOR
UNILATERAL ADRENALECTOMY
TREAT PRIMARY TUMOR
OCCASIONALLY
PITUITARY SURGERY OR PITUITARY IRRADIATION
BILATERAL ADRENALECTOMY

FIGURE 10–5. Flow chart for evaluating patients suspected of having Cushing's syndrome.

erage with corticosteroids for the stress of the operative procedure, the dose is slowly tapered to a maintenance level, which should be continued for several months after the operation.[11]

Ectopic production of ACTH is treated by resection of the primary tumor if possible. If this is not possible, cortisol production must be inhibited by the administration of metyrapone, aminoglutethimide, or ketoconazole.[10] Adrenal insufficiency can result with some of these drugs, and supplemental cortisol and mineralocorticoid may be required. Bilateral adrenalectomy is a treatment of last resort because of the 20% incidence of Nelson's syndrome.[29] Preoperative radiation of the pituitary in low doses may prevent this complication should bilateral adrenalectomy be necessary[12] (Fig. 10–5).

ADRENOCORTICAL CARCINOMAS

Adrenocortical carcinoma is a rare tumor, representing 0.02% of all cancers, and is seen with a variety of clinical pictures. Approximately 50% of these tumors are hormonally active, but the remainder may produce no early symptoms.[16] Because of this, nonfunctioning tumors often attain a large size before being detected on physical examination or before symptoms of abdominal pain, fatigue, or weight loss occur. The mean age of patients with adrenal carcinoma is in the fourth decade, although adrenal carcinoma occurs in patients of all ages.

Clinical features include abdominal pain, fatigue, and symptoms of hormonal aberrations. Cushing's syndrome (50% of patients) and virilization (10 to 20% of patients) are commonly associated with these malignant tumors. Aldosterone-producing adrenal tumors are rare (2% of patients), although aldosterone production is usually seen with concomitant glucocorticoid or sex hormone excess.[30] Hormone aberrations in the male are much less obvious because steroids commonly produced with carcinoma are androgens. Males can undergo feminization, but this occurs much less commonly than does virilization in the female. Adrenal carcinoma is the most common cause of Cushing's syndrome in children and any combination of Cushing's syndrome with virilization is strongly suggestive of adrenal carcinoma.[31] Virilization associated with an adrenal tumor portends a poor prognosis.

Males present with feminization secondary to an adrenal tumor as a result of conversion of androgen to estrogen. These male patients have gynecomastia, testicular atrophy, impotence, and a decreased libido on presentation and invariably die of their disease within a few years.

Female patients with virilization have hirsutism, acne, amenorrhea, clitoral hypertrophy, and increased muscle mass on presentation. The differential diagnosis in these patients should include adrenal adenoma and ovarian tumor as well as the more commonly found adrenal carcinoma.

The diagnosis of adrenal carcinoma relies on endocrine studies and radiologic procedures. Patients who have apparent cortisol excess on presentation can be screened with a simple overnight dexamethasone suppression test. Unlike adenomas, adrenal carcinoma often elaborates high levels of 17-ketosteroids, in the range of 50 to 200 mg per 24 hours. A marked increase in the DHEA fraction of the 17-ketosteroid determination is also highly suggestive of malignant tumor.[32,33]

A 24-hour urine collection can be obtained to measure 17-ketosteroids, 17-hydroxycorticosteroids (precursor to cortisol), and 18-hydroxycorticosteroids (precursor to aldosterone). The addition of serum tests for testosterone can be made in female patients with virilization, and estrogen levels can be determined by means of serum and urine in feminizing adrenal tumors in male patients.

A low ACTH level with high cortisol production is indicative of adrenal carcinoma or adenoma because, as we stated, these tumors are autonomous and suppress ACTH.

Radiologic procedures for diagnosis include CT, MRI, and arteriography. Computed tomography has the advantages of revealing the characteristics of adrenal carcinoma, such as inhomogeneity, calcification, and areas of tumor necrosis or local invasion, and also helps to assess the resectability of the tumor. Tumors are usually 5 or 6 cm or larger.[34,35]

Magnetic resonance imaging, with its increased signal on T2-weighted image, may become the preferred procedure if adrenal carcinoma is suspected and cannot be confirmed by CT.[30]

Arteriography is occasionally required in a patient with an adrenal carcinoma and characteristically demonstrates neovascularity and inferior renal displacement (Fig. 10–6). Adrenal carcinomas can invade renal veins and vena cava, as is seen with renal cell carcinoma (Fig. 10–7).[11]

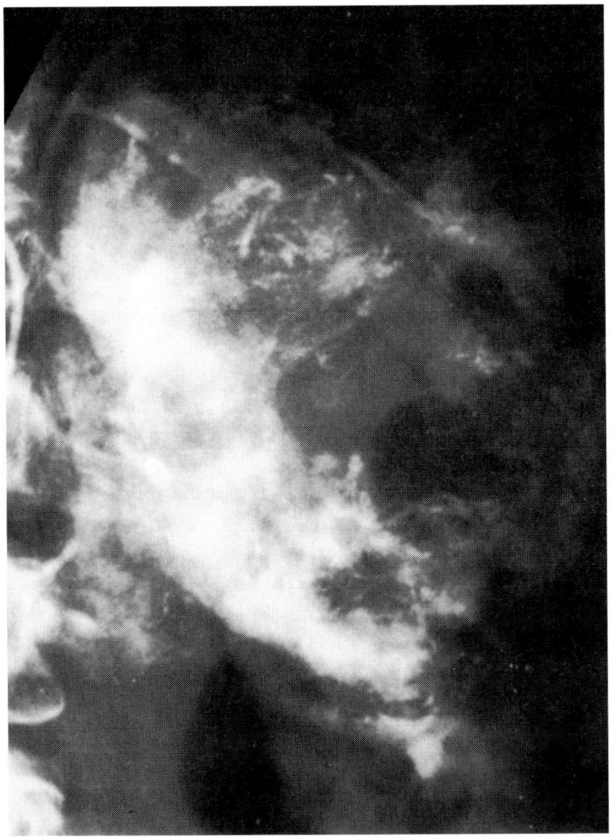

FIGURE 10–6. Adrenal angiogram demonstrating neovascularity and downward renal displacement secondary to a left adrenocortical carcinoma. (From Libertino JA: Surgery of adrenal disorders. Surg Clin North Am 1988; 68:1027–1056, with permission.)

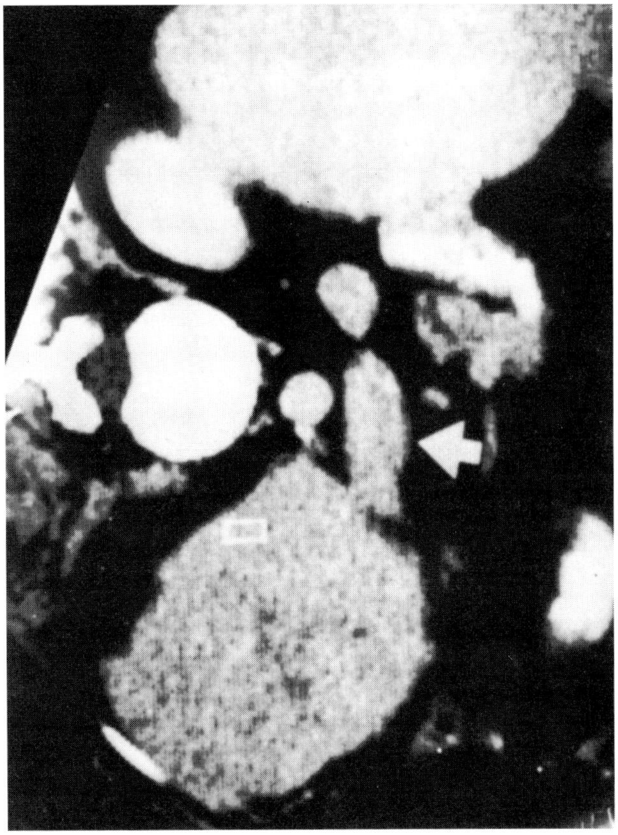

FIGURE 10–7. Computed tomogram showing adrenocortical carcinoma with involvement of left renal vein (*arrow*). (From Libertino JA: Surgery of adrenal disorders. Surg Clin North Am 1988; 68:1027–1056, with permission.)

Surgical extirpation remains the primary treatment and only chance for cure. An anterior or thoracoabdominal approach is required to achieve good surgical margins. Histologically, it is difficult to distinguish between benign and malignant tumors on the basis of their cellular characteristics alone, although ploidy studies may help predict metastatic potential in the future.[30] At present, a tumor can clearly be labeled malignant only when distant metastasis or local invasion is present at operation.

Prognosis depends on the stage of the tumor. Stage I indicates tumor is confined to the adrenal gland, stage II indicates extra-adrenal local spread, and stage III denotes metastatic disease, usually to the lung, liver, or lymph nodes. One can expect a 50% 5-year survival rate with stage I disease and a 10% 5-year survival rate with stage II or III disease.[16]

Postoperative steroid coverage for the contralateral adrenal gland is required for hypercortisol-producing tumors. However, with virilizing tumors, supplemental steroids are not needed because there is no negative feedback of ketosteroids on ACTH production.

Adrenal carcinoma is radioresistant, and therefore radiotherapy is of little value in increasing survival. In patients with metastatic disease, removal of the tumor followed by chemotherapy is now the treatment of choice, although adjuvant chemotherapy has shown no survival advantage. Chemotherapy using *o,p′*-DDD (mitotane) as a primary adrenolytic agent in patients with adrenal carcinoma is associated with a 60 to 70% response rate as evidenced by a reduction in steroid production and excretion. Results are not seen for a minimum of 6 weeks, and the side effects are largely dose related.[11,36] Adrenal insufficiency usually results from this agent, and cortisol and mineralocorticoids must be replaced.

Other chemotherapeutic agents include alkylating agents and doxorubicin, which have been shown to be effective. The antifungal drug, ketoconazole, will inhibit adrenal steroidogenesis as will aminoglutethimide, which blocks the conversion of cholesterol to pregnenolone.[37] With both of these agents, glucocorticoid replacement is necessary.

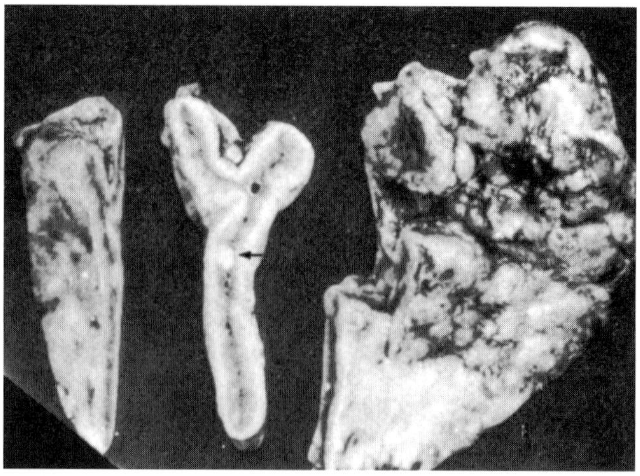

FIGURE 10–9. Adrenal microadenoma (*arrow*) causing primary hyperaldosteronism. (From Libertino JA: Surgery of adrenal disorders. Surg Clin North Am 1988; 68:1027–1056, with permission.)

PRIMARY ALDOSTERONISM

Primary aldosteronism is a syndrome caused by increased production of aldosterone by the zona glomerulosa, first described by Conn in 1955.[38]

Primary aldosteronism is an uncommon condition occurring in less than 1% of patients with hypertension.[11] Manifestations include sodium retention, leading to hypertension, and metabolic alkalosis secondary to potassium wasting. As a result of this potassium wasting, symptoms, such as muscle weakness, headache, nocturia, tetany, and nephropathy, may occur.

The cause of primary hyperaldosteronism is unilateral adenoma in 60 to 80% of patients; bilateral adrenal hyperplasia produces the other 20 to 40% of cases (Figs. 10–8 and 10–9).[11,16] Adrenal carcinoma rarely can produce Conn's syndrome but is usually associated with Cushing's syndrome or virilism or both. Micronodular adrenal hyperplasia is more common in children than in adults.[16]

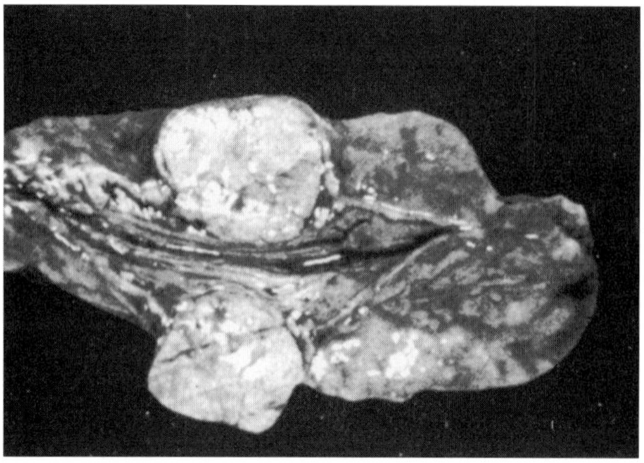

FIGURE 10–8. Adrenal aldosteronoma. (From Libertino JA: Surgery of adrenal disorders. Surg Clin North Am 1988; 68: 1027–1056, with permission.)

Unilateral aldosterone-producing adenomas are small tumors, averaging 1 or 2 cm in size. Diagnosis is made by identifying the above-mentioned clinical manifestations and carrying out screening tests. At presentation, hypokalemia (<3.5 mEq/L) is usually seen associated with diastolic hypertension. This hypokalemia is worse (<3.0 mEq/L) when the patient is taking diuretics and potassium supplementation. However, 7 to 38% of patients with primary aldosterone may be normokalemic. The presence of greater than 30 mEq/L of potassium in a 24-hour urine specimen in a hypokalemic patient suggests hyperaldosteronism. Plasma renin activity (PRA) value is usually low because of increased blood volume.[16] In 25% of these patients, however, the PRA values may be normal or elevated. A plasma aldosterone (PA)/plasma renin activity (PRA) ratio of greater than 20 suggests the presence of disease. When results of any of these screening tests are positive, more definitive testing should be carried out.[16]

Confirmatory tests include failure of aldosterone suppression with instillation of 2 L of saline solution over a 4-hour period as well as demonstration of PRA to increase after volume contraction using diuretics.[10] Perhaps the best test is a 24-hour urinary aldosterone excretion level obtained after prolonged sodium repletion because PA measurements can be highly variable and are less accurate.[16]

In secondary hyperaldosteronism caused by renal artery stenosis or renin-secreting tumors, increased release of renin leads to increased production of angiotensin, which in turn results in increased serum aldosterone levels. Thus, secondary hyperaldosteronism is characterized by an increased aldosterone level along with an increase in the renin level in contradistinction to primary hyperaldosteronism, which is characterized by an increase in aldosterone level and a suppression in renin level.[11]

When the diagnosis of primary aldosteronism is biochemically confirmed, radiographic evaluation with CT usually localizes the adenoma. Computed tomography has a resolution of approximately 1 cm, so that even small adenomas are usually detected. With MRI, resolution is a potential problem. Left-sided lesions are two to three times more common than right-sided lesions. Attempts must be made to identify the site of the lesion before operation. If CT or MRI fails to localize the tumor, adrenal venous sampling is an accurate means of localizing an adenoma (Fig. 10–10). However, adrenal venous sampling and adrenal venography can lead to adrenal infarction (Fig. 10–11).[11] Arteriography and NP-59 scanning are rarely useful.

Occasionally, the surgeon must approach the patient without preoperative knowledge of the location of the lesion. In such instances, bilateral adrenal exploration may be warranted. The left side is usually explored first: when the adenoma is not found in this gland, the right side is explored. Before blind exploration, however, granulosa hyperplasia must be ruled out. Simple tests include documenting severe spontaneous hypokalemia (<3.0 mEq/L), an anomalous postural decrease in plasma aldosterone, and an increased 18-OH-corticosteroid (>100 mg/dl), a precursor to aldosterone, all usually indicative of an adenoma versus hyperplasia.[16] A more invasive technique to distinguish these two entities is to sample aldosterone levels from both adrenal veins. If both adrenal veins display high aldosterone levels, granulosa hyperplasia is likely.[11] Renin levels are not as suppressed in this entity as they are in patients with an adenoma. The hypertension fails to respond to bilateral adrenalectomy,

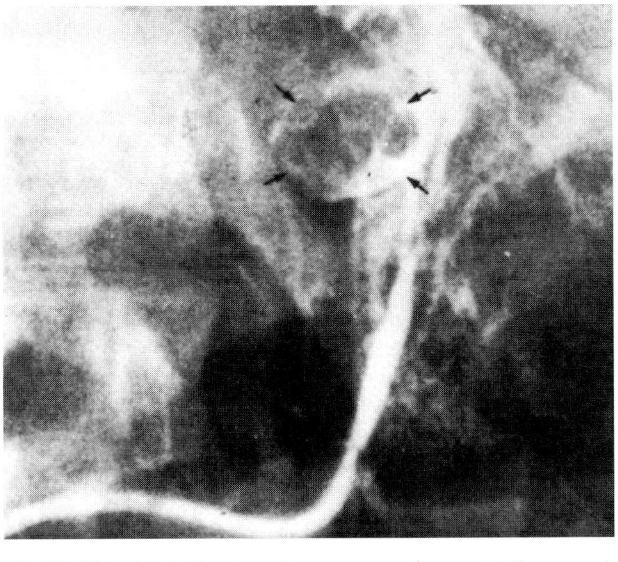

FIGURE 10–10. Left adrenal venogram demonstrating a primary aldosterone-producing adenoma (*arrows*). (From Libertino JA: Surgery of adrenal disorders. Surg Clin North Am 1988; 68: 1027–1056, with permission.)

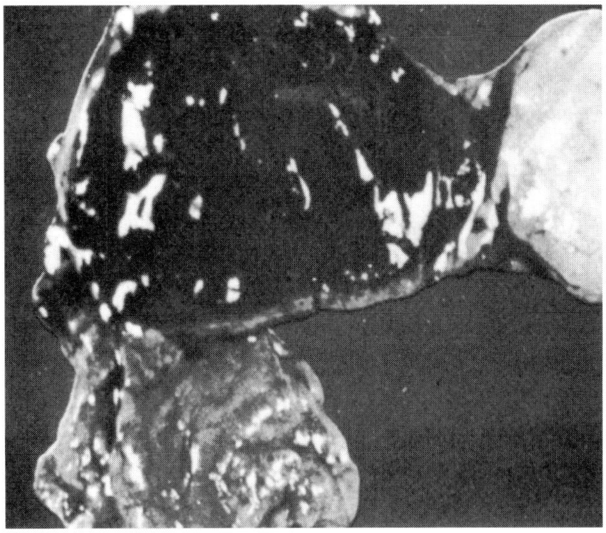

FIGURE 10–11. Adrenal hemorrhage secondary to adrenal venography. (From Libertino JA: Surgery of adrenal disorders. Surg Clin North Am 1988; 68:1027–1056, with permission.)

making medical treatment preferable. Medical treatment in the form of aldosterone antagonists include spironolactone, triamterene, and amiloride.

Primary aldosteronism from an adenoma must be surgically corrected. Preoperatively, spironolactone is given to correct hypokalemia, and if normotensive parameters are maintained, this is a good prognostic sign that the patient will be cured or improved by surgical removal of the adenoma.

Because of the small size of the tumor and its unilaterality, an extraperitoneal approach is best. This may include a posterior approach, which provides the most direct approach to the adrenal gland without transecting major muscles, or a standard flank incision.[16] A flow chart (Fig. 10–12) has been devised for evaluating patients suspected of having primary aldosteronoma.

PHEOCHROMOCYTOMA

Tumors arising in cells of neural crest origin in the adrenal medulla or sympathetic ganglia are called pheochromocytomas. Pathologically, these are chromaffin tumors with excess excretion of catecholamines. Because these tumors derive from neural crest tissue, they may be found in various locations in the body.

Pheochromocytoma is often associated with other endocrinopathies and can cause life-threatening hypertension. Of these tumors, 95% are located in the abdomen or retroperitoneum; the remainder are found in the mediastinum or the skull. Most (90%) are located in the adrenal gland and the remainder in the periaortic sympathetic chain or in the organ of Zuckerkandl just below the aortic bifurcation. Ectopic tumors have also been found in the bladder, vagina, ovaries, testes, spleen, and ca-

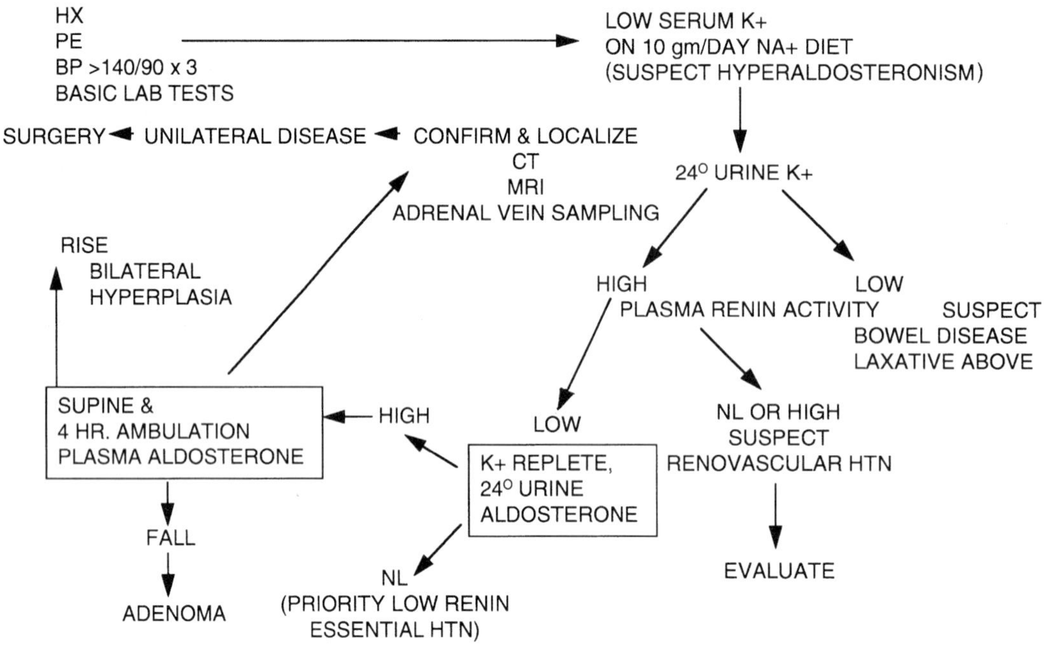
HX
PE
BP >140/90 x 3
BASIC LAB TESTS
LOW SERUM K+
ON 10 gm/DAY NA+ DIET
(SUSPECT HYPERALDOSTERONISM)
SURGERY
UNILATERAL DISEASE
CONFIRM & LOCALIZE
CT
MRI
ADRENAL VEIN SAMPLING
24° URINE K+
RISE
BILATERAL
HYPERPLASIA
HIGH
LOW
PLASMA RENIN ACTIVITY
SUSPECT
BOWEL DISEASE
LAXATIVE ABOVE
SUPINE &
4 HR. AMBULATION
PLASMA ALDOSTERONE
HIGH
LOW
NL OR HIGH
SUSPECT
RENOVASCULAR HTN
K+ REPLETE,
24° URINE
ALDOSTERONE
FALL
EVALUATE
NL
ADENOMA
(PRIORITY LOW RENIN
ESSENTIAL HTN)

FIGURE 10–12. Evaluation of patients suspected of having primary aldosteronism.

rotid bodies.[11] These tumors may be familial and associated with multiple endocrine neoplasia (MEN) syndromes. In adults, the "rule of 10" of pheochromocytoma states that 10% are bilateral, malignant, extra-adrenal, multiple, or associated with MEN syndrome. In children, 40% have extra-adrenal tumors and 25% are bilateral.[10,16]

The clinical presentation of pheochromocytoma is hypertension, with 50% being paroxysmal and 50% being sustained. The most common presenting symptoms include the triad of headache, sweating, and palpitations. Other symptoms include chronic weakness, tiredness, and apprehension. In children, nausea, weight loss, headache, and visual complaints are more common than in adults. In older patients, one may see cardiomyopathy, strokes, retinopathy, congestive heart failure, renal failure, a dissecting aneurysm, myocardial infarction, or arrhythmia. A sudden elevation of blood pressure during initiations of anesthesia or during pregnancy is suggestive of pheochromocytoma.

The diagnosis of a pheochromocytoma is made biochemically. Urinary catecholamines and catecholamine metabolites should be measured. Urinary VMA, normetanephrine, and metanephrine levels are elevated by pheochromocytoma.

The most sensitive test for pheochromocytoma is by measuring the serum catecholamine level. Of patients with pheochromocytoma, 98% will have an elevated serum or urinary level of catecholamines. A serum level greater than 2000 pg/ml is definitely abnormal, whereas a level less than 500 pg/ml is normal. A level between 500 and 2000 pg/ml is equivocal; overlapping values are seen in essential hypertension.[16,39]

Urinary measurement of metanephrines is probably the best initial screening test because these metabolites are chemically more stable and less affected by stress.[40] If more than 1 μg metanephrines per mg creatinine is present in a random urine sample, a pheochromocytoma may be present.[10] Urinary vanillylmandelic levels will produce the largest numbers of false-positive and false-negative studies.[16] Samples showing significantly elevated dopamine indicate a malignant pheochromocytoma because these tumors are deficient in enzymes needed to produce epinephrine.

Patients who are suspected of having a pheochromocytoma but whose catecholamine levels are normal may be candidates for a glucagon stimulation test. In the glucagon stimulation test, intravenous administration of a 0.5- to 1-mg dose of glucagon will stimulate a substantial rise in blood pressure in a patient with pheochromocytoma, whereas no change occurs in normal individuals. Care with this test is essential because a hypertensive crisis may occur in some patients with a pheochromocytoma.[39]

The clonidine suppression test uses a 300-mg dose of clonidine that will inhibit centrally mediated adrenergic influences and will lower blood pressure in essential hypertension but will not suppress the function of a pheochromocytoma. Severe hypotension may occur in patients with essential hypertension.[10,15]

Other provocative tests include the use of naloxone and metoclopramide, which will cause an elevation of blood pressure in patients with pheochromocytomas.[39]

Other neuroectodermal diseases associated with pheochromocytoma are von Recklinghausen's disease (neurofibromatosis), Sturge-Weber disease, and von Hippel-Lindau disease. As mentioned before, MEN II or Sipple's syndrome, consisting of medullary thyroid carcinoma and hyperparathyroidism, is also associated with pheochromocytoma.[11]

The location of a pheochromocytoma varies according to whether the tumor is sporadic or familial and whether it occurs in children or in adults. Bilateral adrenal pheochromocytomas occur in 50% of familial cases and in 25% of children. In addition, 25% of children have extra-adrenal tumors.[39]

Computed tomography of the abdomen and pelvis is the best initial test because 97% of tumors are below the diaphragm. This test has excellent resolution, is 98% sensitive, and is cost effective (Fig. 10–13).[16]

Magnetic resonance imaging has 100% sensitivity and the advantage of not exposing the patient to radiation. Sagittal and coronal images give excellent anatomic information concerning the tumor and its vascularity. In addition, the increased signal intensity on a T2-weighted image is a classic finding.[12,41]

Arteriography is infrequently used but may be required when CT or MRI does not visualize a pheochromocytoma. When angiography is required, patients should be given phenoxybenzamine before the study because of the likelihood of hypertensive crisis in an unprotected patient. Even when the patient has been prepared, it is necessary to have phentolamine or propranolol (Inderal) ready for administration in the angiography suite. Aortic angiography with digital subtraction marks most pheochromocytoma with a neovascular blush. Subtraction also eliminates confusing bony shadows (Fig. 10–14).[42]

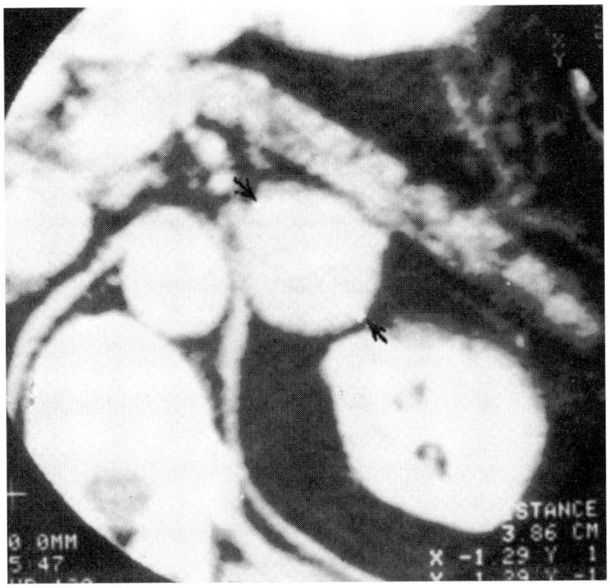

FIGURE 10–13. Computed tomogram showing left adrenal pheochromocytoma (*arrows*). (From Libertino JA: Surgery of adrenal disorders. Surg Clin North Am 1988; 68:1027–1056, with permission.)

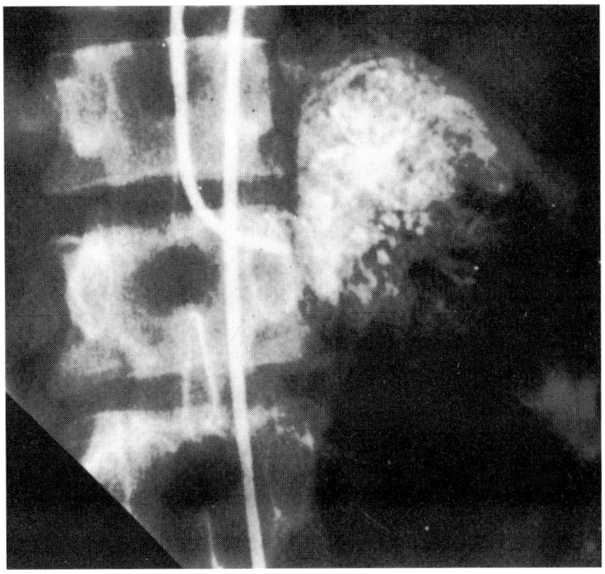

FIGURE 10–14. Adrenal angiogram showing left adrenal pheochromocytoma. (From Libertino JA: Surgery of adrenal disorders. Surg Clin North Am 1988; 68:1027–1056, with permission.)

When angiography, CT, or MRI does not localize an ectopic pheochromocytoma, other tests are required. Computed tomography of the chest and skull may be required to locate an ectopic tumor. Tumors of the bladder and vagina may be discovered at the time of cystoscopy or bimanual pelvic examinations.[13,43,44]

Multiple venous sampling at sites along the superior and inferior vena cava for catecholamines is often helpful. Pheochromocytomas that secrete epinephrine predominantly with only small amounts of norepinephrine are almost always adrenal in origin.[44]

Metaiodobenzylguanidine (MIBG) is useful in seeking occult, multiple, metastatic, or recurrent pheochromocytomas. It is an analogue of guanethidine and is taken up by adrenergic granules and the adrenal medulla. It has a 78% sensitivity, with a 10% false-negative rate. Disadvantages are its expense and limited availability. It may be useful to rule out metastatic disease on a yearly basis after primary treatment.[16,44,45]

Removal of a pheochromocytoma presents a surgical challenge. Preoperative pharmacologic manipulation is necessary to prevent cardiovascular complications. Most pheochromocytomas secrete norepinephrine, and α-blockers, such as phentolamine and phenoxybenzamine, are used to control its hypertensive effects. α-Blockade must be performed first to avoid rebound hypertension or angina from unopposed α-receptor stimulation, which occurs if β-blockade is accomplished first. Theoretically, one can carry out a β-blockade first if the pheochromocytoma secretes only epinephrine, but usually α-blockade is still believed necessary. β-Blockade is added when tachycardia or arrhythmias are still present despite α-blockade. Some drugs, such as labetalol, combine α- and β-blockade. Angiotensin-converting enzyme inhibitors and calcium channel blockers may be used in addition to the above-mentioned medications.[10,16] All medications should be administered 2 weeks before operation and continued to the day of operation.

For malignant pheochromocytomas, α-methyltyrosine inhibits tyrosine hydroxylation, the rate-limiting enzyme for catecholamine biosynthesis. This reduces the catecholamine excess and its resulting symptoms in inoperable tumors but has severe side effects, including extrapyramidal signs, crystalluria, diarrhea, sedation, and anxiety.[12,39,44]

The usual dose of preoperative α- and β-blockade is phenoxybenzamine, 10 mg every 6 hours as a starting dose, increasing to 30 to 40 mg every 6 hours as needed, and propranolol, 5 to 10 mg every 4 to 6 hours.

Some controversy exists regarding the degree of pharmacologic blockade desired in the preoperative patient. Some physicians prefer complete α- and β-blockade, whereas other physicians prefer no blockade so that intraoperative palpation of the contralateral adrenal gland, celiac ganglia, sympathetic chain, preaortic tissue, and organ of Zuckerkandl will result in increased catecholamine activity that is not pharmacologically blunted. Intraoperative palpation is helpful in localizing ectopic pheochromocytomas; however, with no preoperative blockade, the immediate use of intravenous phentolamine or sodium nitroprusside is needed to control the hypertension caused by palpation.[11]

Another important consideration preoperatively is intravascular volume status. Many patients are severely volume depleted secondary to chronic α-stimulation. Transfusion of whole blood preoperatively was once used; now, vigorous intravenous hydration the day before operation with 0.9% saline solution is usual. Hydration also prevents intraoperative and postoperative hypotension.

Induction and maintenance of anesthesia during operation are difficult and require special precautions. The anesthesia team must be experienced with the management of patients with pheochromocytoma. Intensive monitoring is required and includes a central venous catheter, Swan-Ganz catheter, and an arterial line. Anesthetic agents that can be used safely are enflurane and isoflurane. Halothane is unsafe because it causes a high incidence of ventricular arrhythmias.[12]

The intraoperative exploration must be carried out methodically, especially along the sympathetic chain, and resulting hypertensive crisis must be managed appropriately and calmly. When a pheochromocytoma is removed, a wide margin of adjacent tissue should be included because 10% of these lesions are malignant.[11]

Tumors that invade adjacent structures are considered malignant despite the fact that they are difficult to differentiate histologically and require further adjuvant treatment if unresectable. This includes further α-blockade as well as α-methyltyrosine, an inhibitor of catecholamine synthesis. Some studies have advocated multiple chemotherapeutic agents, including cyclophosphamide, vincristine, and dacarbazine, as possibly being effective. Other treatments may include MIBG or tumor embolization and radiation.[10,46]

Postoperatively, hypotension as a result of removed α-blockade is treated with volume replacement. If hypotension does not improve with volume, monitor for hypoglycemia, which may also be present.

Long-term follow-up studies after operation are required for surveillance for metastatic disease and to monitor blood pressure.

Pheochromocytoma during pregnancy is a difficult problem. If diagnosed in the first trimester, the pheochromocytoma may be removed surgically after preoperative medical α- and β-blockade. In the second and third trimesters, α- and β-blockade is continued to near term when a cesarean section can be performed before the tumor is localized and resected.[47]

INCIDENTAL ADRENAL MASS

With the increase of modern imaging modalities, incidental adrenal masses are being found more commonly. These are adrenal masses discovered during evaluation of an unrelated disease in the absence of malignancy or signs suggesting adrenal disease. These masses are seen in 0.4 to 1.3% of all

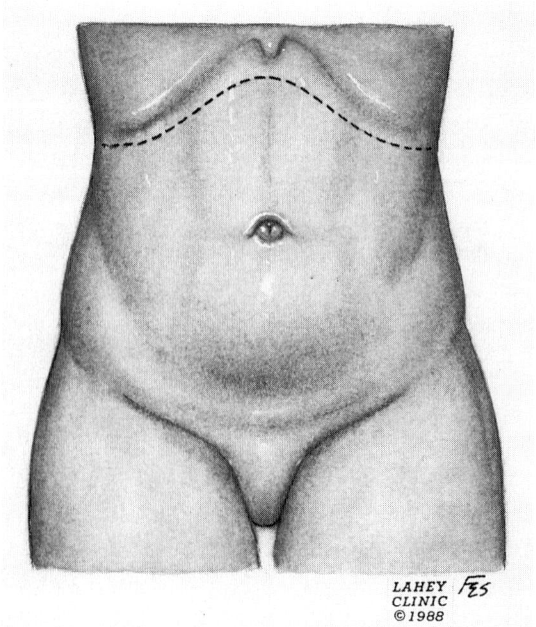
LAHEY CLINIC ©1988

FIGURE 10–15. Chevron incision. (By permission of Lahey Clinic.)

CT scans of the abdomen and produce no symptoms.[16] These incidental masses represent many entities, with benign cortical adenomas constituting 50% of these masses. Benign cortical adenomas are found in 1 to 9% of all autopsy studies,[10] and only a small percentage are functional, with Cushing's syndrome and hyperaldosteronism comprising 3% of these adenomas. Adrenocortical carcinoma accounts for 3 to 8%, and pheochromocytoma, 10 to 20%, whereas the remaining 20 to 30% of adrenal masses are adrenal cysts, myelolipoma, pseudocysts, focal hyperplasia, ganglioneuroma, abscess, and metastatic carcinoma (especially lung).[16] These masses require clinical, endocrinologic, and radiologic evaluation.[48,49]

If the adrenal mass is functional as described previously, the patients may show signs of Cushing's syndrome, hirsutism, feminization, obesity, myopathy, and stria.

Endocrine work-up includes a 24-hour urinary cortisol and metanephrines as well as serum catecholamines, potassium, testosterone, estrogen, aldosterone, cortisol, ACTH, DHEAS, and pregnenolone. An overnight dexamethasone suppression test may also be helpful.[10]

Radiologic evaluation includes CT or MRI. Magnetic resonance imaging on T2-weighted images can differentiate an adrenal adenoma, which is isointense with the liver, from a cortical carcinoma or metastatic lesion, which shows an increased intensity.[16] Pheochromocytomas produce a high T2-weighted image, which some consider pathognomonic for this disease.[41,50]

NP-59 or ^{131}I-iodomethyl-norcholesterol scintiscan may be used in patients with adrenal masses with normal results on biochemical evaluation. When the mass shows uptake, the diagnosis is probably a benign adenoma. When the mass shows no uptake, the differential diagnosis includes primary carcinoma, metastatic lesion, or cyst.[10]

Management of these adrenal masses depends on their size and endocrine activity. All hormonally active masses must be resected. If the size is greater than 6 cm, the mass should be resected. A mass less than 5 cm and hormonally inactive can be watched safely with repeat CT at 2, 6, and 18 months. Also, a 3- to 6-cm mass can be assessed with MRI. With these criteria of MRI, a diagnosis can usually be made.[10]

Fine-needle aspiration is useful when concurrent malignancy is present or when the adrenal mass is larger than 6 cm and is cystic. It is not useful to differentiate an adrenal adenoma from an adrenocortical carcinoma because of their similar histology.[15,16] Again, the patient should be protected from a hypertensive crisis by administering blockers should a pheochromocytoma be suspected.[44]

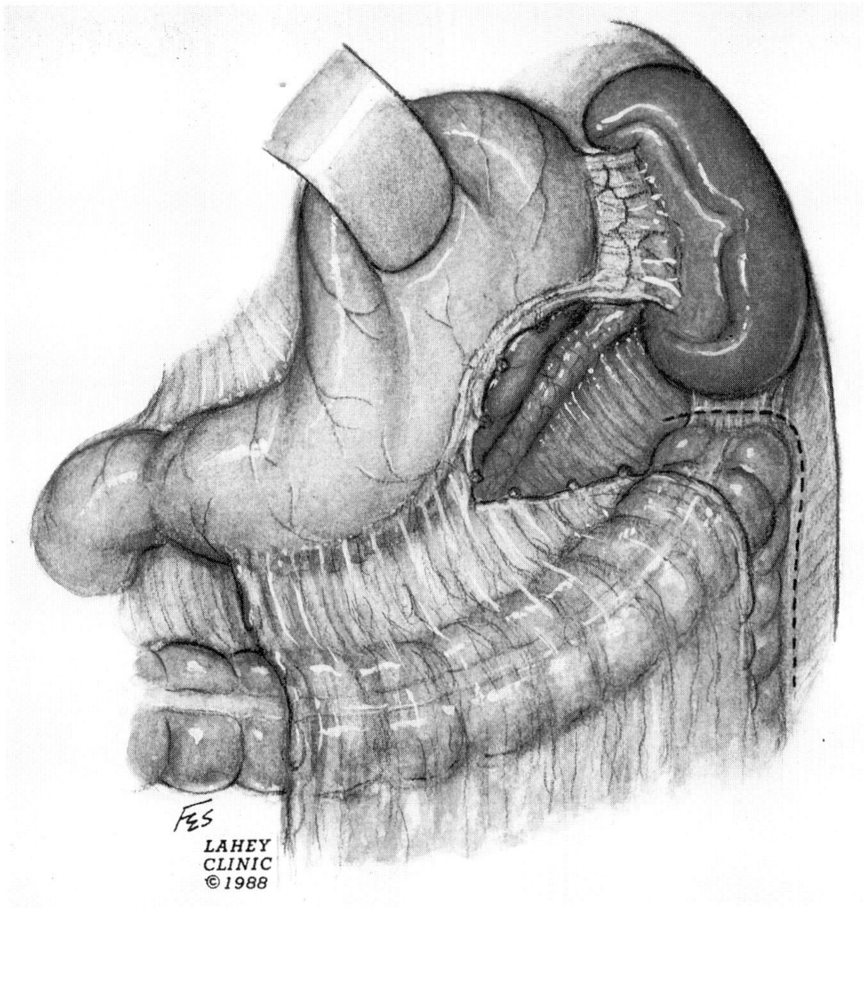
FES
LAHEY
CLINIC
©1988

FIGURE 10–16. Anterior approach to left adrenal gland. (By permission of Lahey Clinic.)

SURGICAL APPROACHES FOR ADRENAL SURGERY

The three major routes to the adrenal gland are the anterior transabdominal approach, the flank or thoracoabdominal approach, and the posterior approach.

Anterior Approach

The anterior approach is preferred in most patients with bilateral hyperplasia when pituitary surgery is not appropriate and in patients with pheochromocytoma or adrenal neoplasm when exploration of the extra-adrenal organs is necessary. In obese patients or whenever bilateral exposure of the adrenal glands is required, a chevron incision is preferred (Fig. 10–15).

The anterior exposure of the left adrenal gland is shown in Figure 10–16. After the peritoneal cavity has been entered and explored, the posterior peritoneum lateral to the left colon is incised along the white line of Toldt and carried upward to divide the splenocolic ligament. Care must be taken to protect the delicate capsule of the spleen. The plane between the pancreas and the spleen anteriorly and the kidney and the adrenal gland posteriorly is developed by sharp dissection (Fig. 10–17). The pancreas and duodenum are mobilized and reflected medially, and the spleen is mobilized cephalad. The anterior surface of the adrenal gland is exposed. The dissection is started laterally and carried up toward the apex of the adrenal gland (Fig. 10–18). Downward traction of the kidney is maintained; this maneuver will aid in gaining exposure of the adrenal gland. The apex of the adrenal gland is brought into view, and the inferior phrenic vessels are clipped with hemostatic clips (Fig. 10–19). The gland can now be rotated medially, and the posterior surface of the gland is completely mobilized (Fig. 10–20). Dissection is carried medially, and the arteries and veins supplying the adrenal gland are ligated with small clips. The adrenal vein is ligated in continuity with 2-0 silk sutures and divided. The adrenal gland is then removed (Fig. 10–21). When the left adrenal gland is being removed for pheochromocytoma (Fig. 10–22), the approach differs in that the initial steps should be ligation and division of the left adrenal vein. This will decrease release of catecholamine from the left adrenal gland during operative manipulation.

Anterior Exposure of Right Adrenal Gland

The posterior peritoneum lateral to the right colon is incised vertically, and the incision is carried

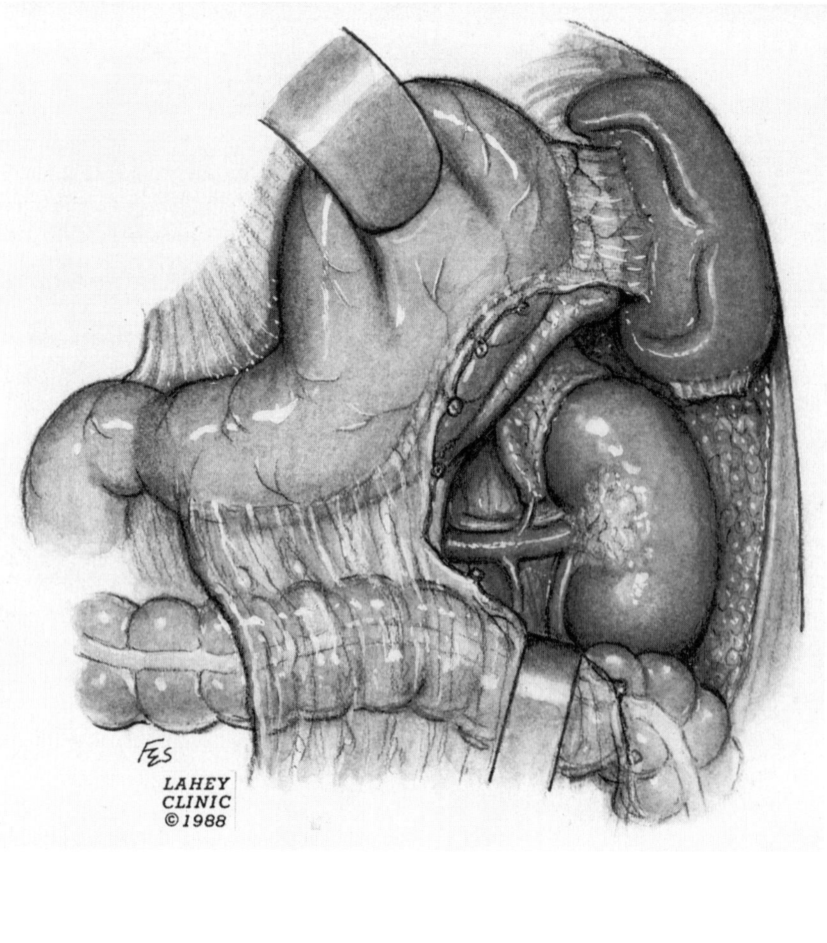
LAHEY
CLINIC
©1988

FIGURE 10–17. Plane is developed between pancreas and spleen and kidney and adrenal gland. (By permission of Lahey Clinic.)

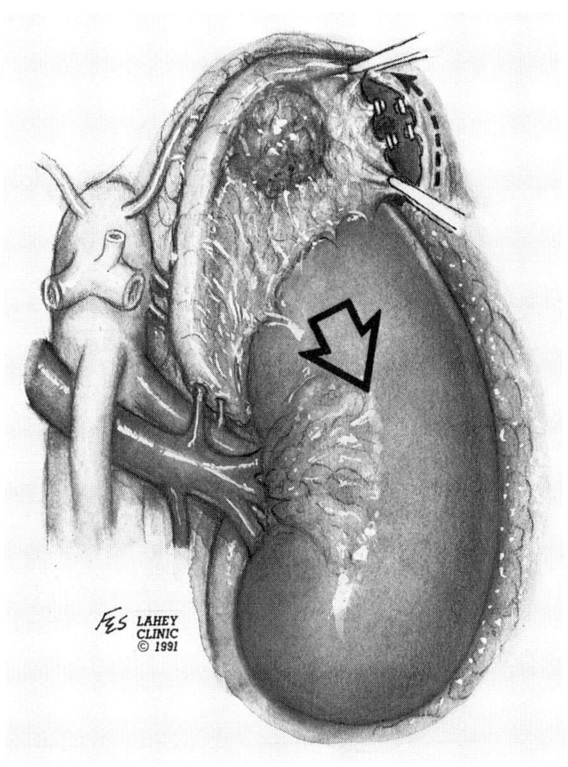
LAHEY
CLINIC
© 1991

FIGURE 10–18. Mobilization of left adrenal gland. (By permission of Lahey Clinic.)

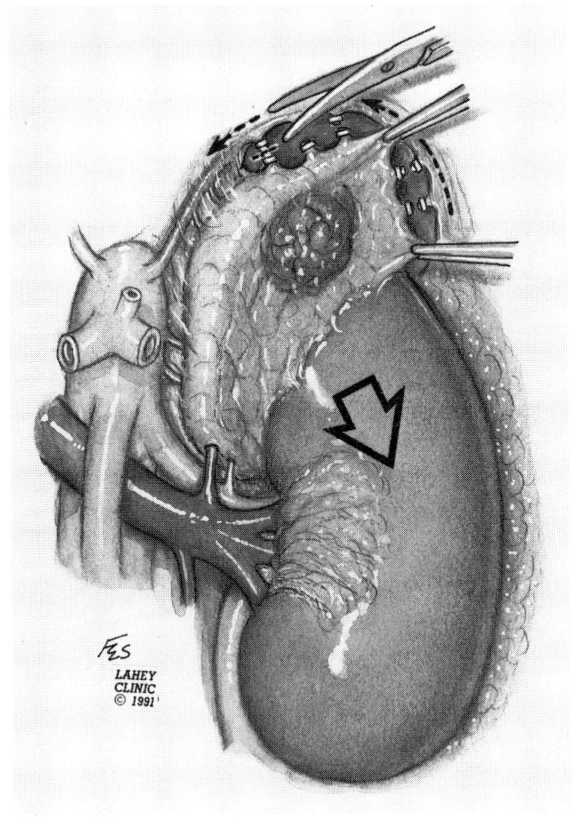
LAHEY
CLINIC
© 1991

FIGURE 10–19. Division of left inferior phrenic artery and vein. (By permission of Lahey Clinic.)

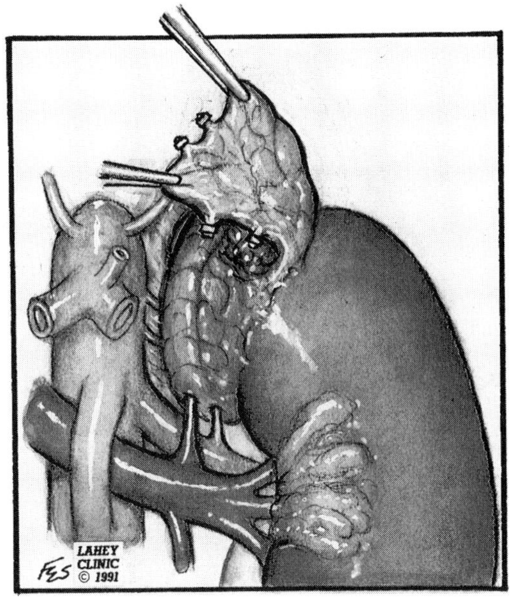
LAHEY
CLINIC
© 1991

FIGURE 10–20. Mobilization of posterior aspect of left adrenal gland. (By permission of Lahey Clinic.)

up around the hepatic flexure. The colon is reflected medially, the liver and gallbladder are retracted upward, and the kidney is gently retracted inferiorly to bring the anterior surface of the right adrenal gland into view (Fig. 10–23). Several of the small hepatic veins may be noted at this point and should be ligated and divided. After the fatty and areolar tissue is dissected off the anterior surface, the adrenal gland is mobilized laterally and posteriorly, meticulously dividing the small vessels between clips and avoiding any direct handling of the adrenal gland itself (Fig. 10–24). The apex of the gland is mobilized, and the inferior phrenic vessels are divided and ligated. The medial aspect of the adrenal gland is approached. The central vein is ligated with 2-0 silk sutures and divided. The remainder of the medial blood supply is ligated with clips (Fig. 10–25). The adrenal gland is freed from the upper pole of the right kidney and removed.

When the anterior approach is used to remove the adrenal gland and its contained pheochromocytoma, control of the major venous outflow of the adrenal gland is the first maneuver in the operative procedure. After the pheochromocytoma has been removed, the entire retroperitoneum is palpated carefully. Any suspicious masses are exposed and samples taken for biopsy. Any area that on palpation produces an elevation in blood pressure should be exposed widely; if a second pheochromocytoma is found, it should also be excised. A wide variety of adjacent structures, including the bladder, ureter, bowel or its mesentery, and the great vessels, may be involved. In general,

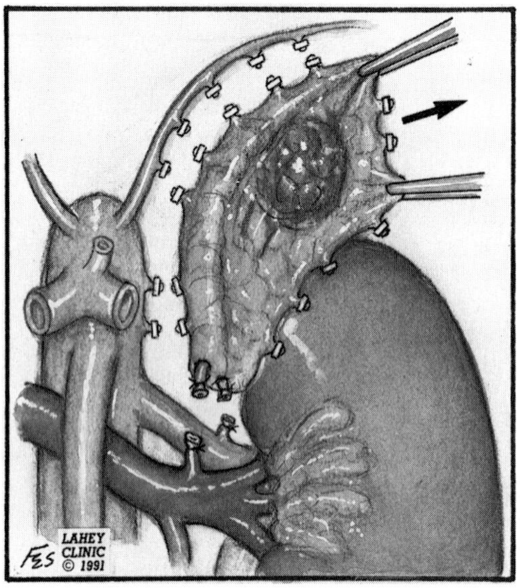
FES
LAHEY
CLINIC
© 1991

FIGURE 10–21. Ligation of major left adrenal artery and vein. (By permission of Lahey Clinic.)

the principles of cancer surgery should apply in such instances, with specific operative techniques varying according to local anatomy. In addition, the anterior approach is usually required in patients undergoing secondary or tertiary operative procedures for recurrent pheochromocytoma.

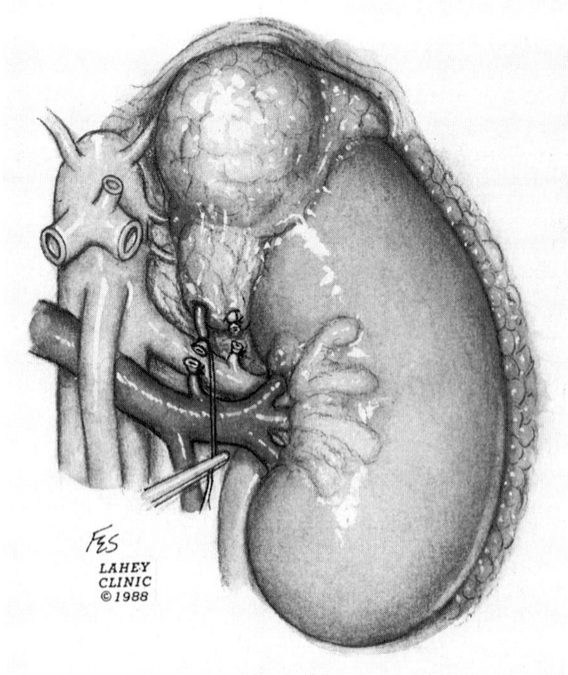
FES
LAHEY
CLINIC
©1988

FIGURE 10–22. Approach for left pheochromocytoma. (By permission of Lahey Clinic.)

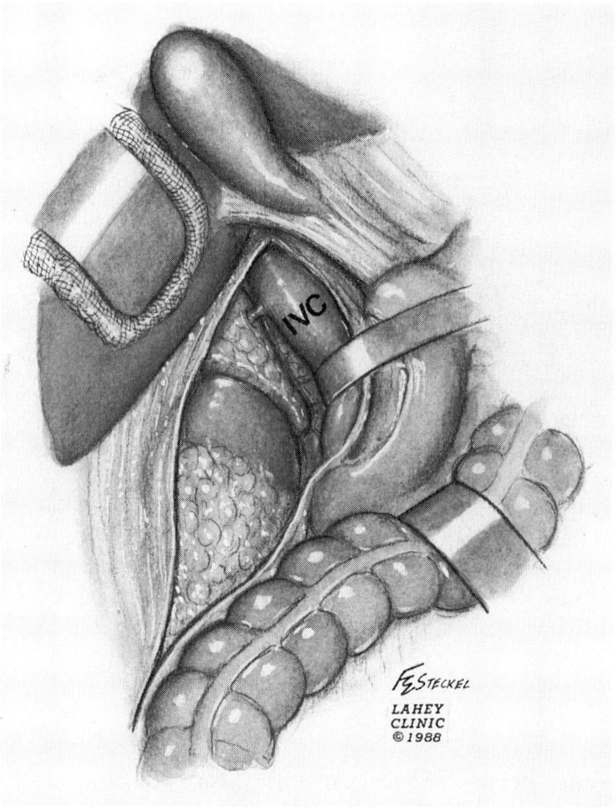
IVC
FESTECKEL
LAHEY
CLINIC
©1988

FIGURE 10–23. Anterior approach to right adrenal gland. (By permission of Lahey Clinic.)

Flank or Supracostal Approach

In patients with unilateral adrenal endocrinopathy, a supracostal eleventh or twelfth rib approach to the adrenal gland is used, depending on the site

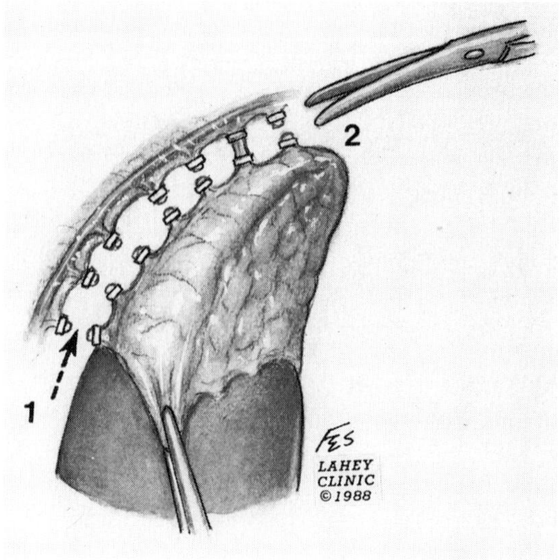
2
1
FES
LAHEY
CLINIC
©1988

FIGURE 10–24. Posterolateral (*1*) and superior (*2*) mobilization of the right adrenal gland. (By permission of Lahey Clinic.)

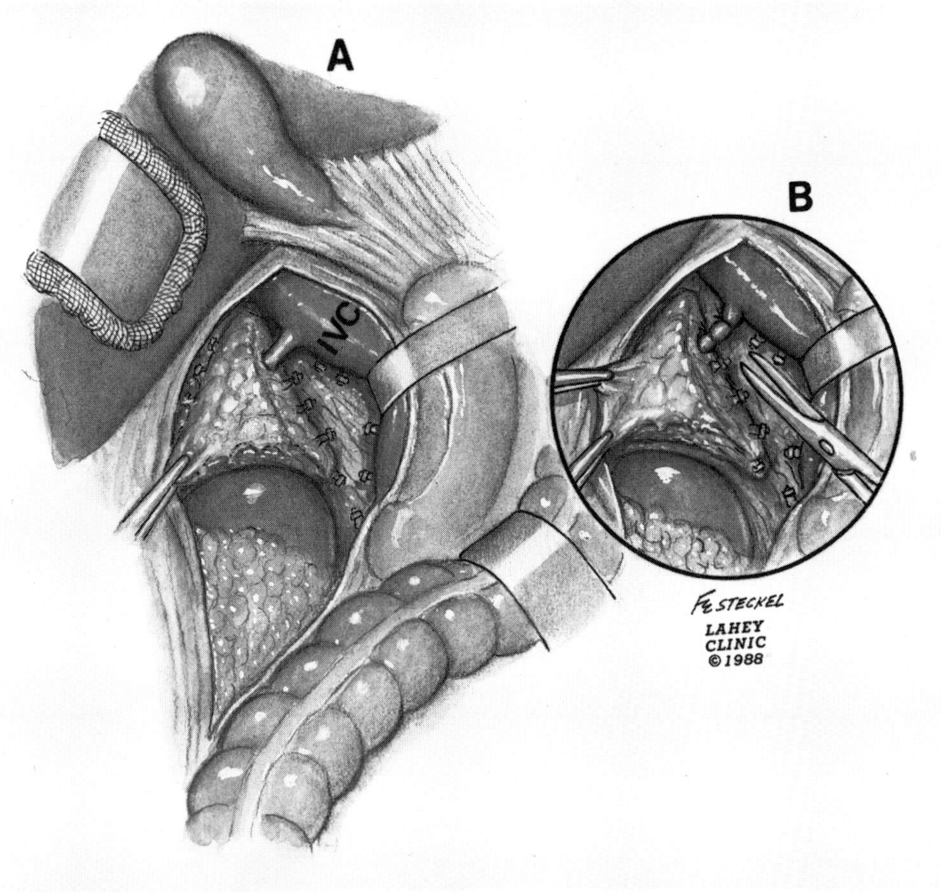
A
B
IVC
F.E. STECKEL
LAHEY
CLINIC
©1988

FIGURE 10–25. Ligation of right central vein. (By permission of Lahey Clinic.)

of the lesion. A flank approach is usually appropriate for a patient with an aldosteronoma, small adrenal adenoma, or small adrenal carcinoma. The advantage of this approach, its familiarity to urologic surgeons, is, however, outweighed by two disadvantages. First, only one adrenal gland can be seen at one time, and a decision for total removal, subtotal adrenalectomy, or no surgical intervention must be made without the knowledge of the condition of the contralateral adrenal gland. Second, the standard subcostal incision may result in low access to a high adrenal gland. Therefore, our preference is the supracostal approach in patients undergoing unilateral adrenalectomy.

The patient is positioned for a flank approach supracostal incision (Fig. 10–26). The incision is made at the tip of either the eleventh or twelfth rib and carried posteriorly along the border of the

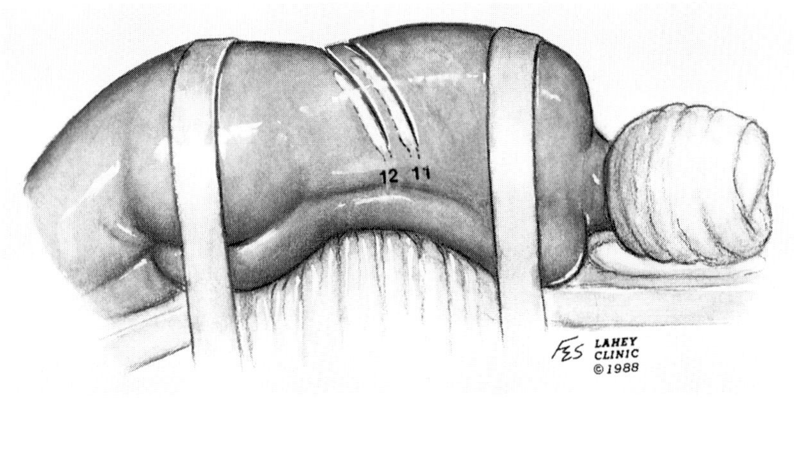
12
11
FES
LAHEY
CLINIC
©1988

FIGURE 10–26. Supracostal eleventh or twelfth rib approach. (By permission of Lahey Clinic.)

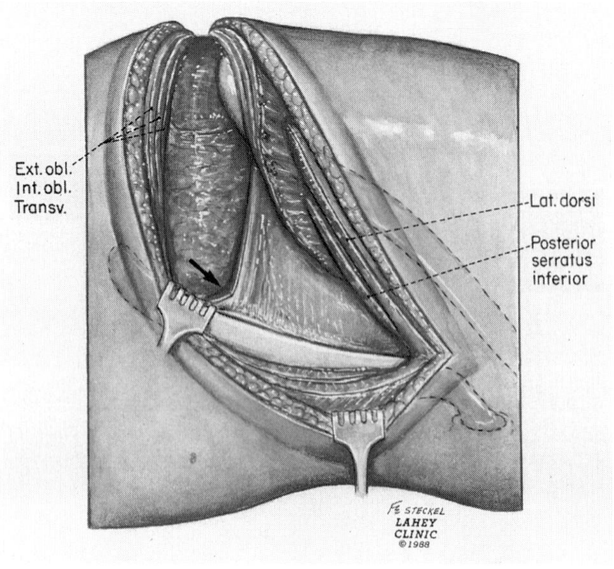
Ext. obl.
Int. obl.
Transv.
Lat. dorsi
Posterior serratus inferior
FE STECKEL LAHEY CLINIC ©1988

FIGURE 10–27. Division of muscles. (By permission of Lahey Clinic.)

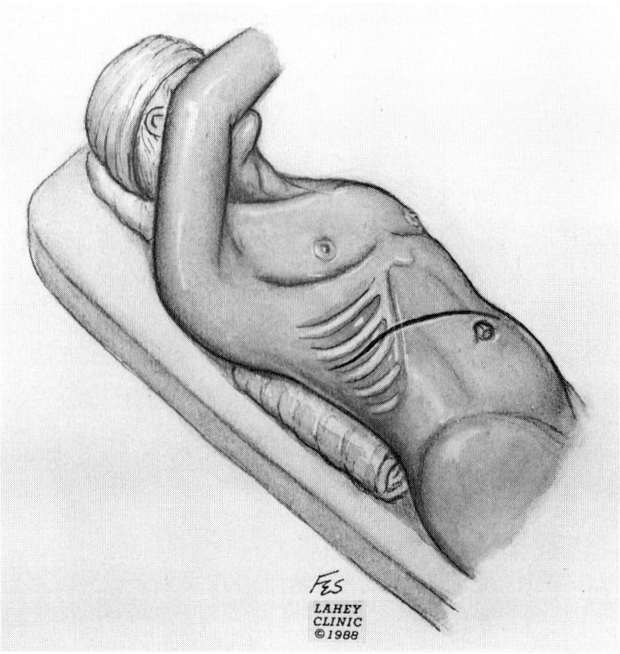
FES LAHEY CLINIC ©1988

FIGURE 10–29. Thoracoabdominal incision. (By permission of Lahey Clinic.)

rib. The latissimus dorsi, external oblique, internal oblique, transversus abdominis, and intercostal muscles are divided along the upper border of the rib (Fig. 10–27). The course of the intercostal nerve is followed to dissect the pleura from the inner aspect of the rib (Fig. 10–28). The cleavage plane between the diaphragm and the retroperitoneal space is mobilized, and the retroperitoneal space is entered.

Thoracoabdominal Approach

The thoracoabdominal approach is useful in patients with a large adrenal carcinoma who might also require concomitant splenectomy, distal pancreatectomy, or radical nephrectomy. In addition,

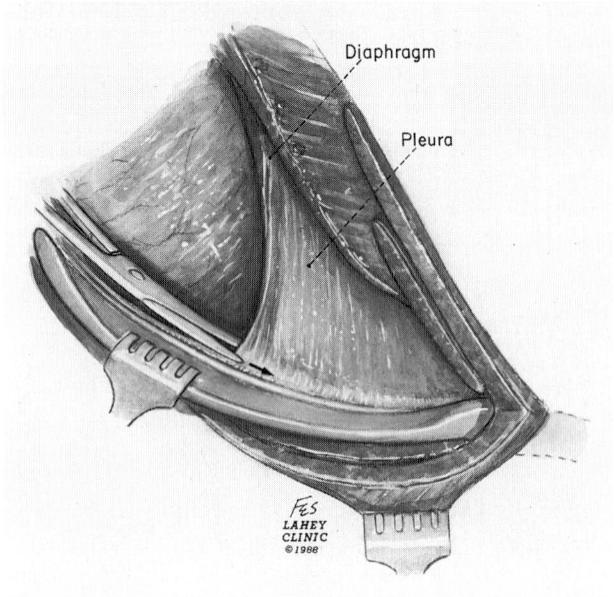
Diaphragm
Pleura
FES LAHEY CLINIC ©1988

FIGURE 10–28. Pleura dissected. (By permission of Lahey Clinic.)

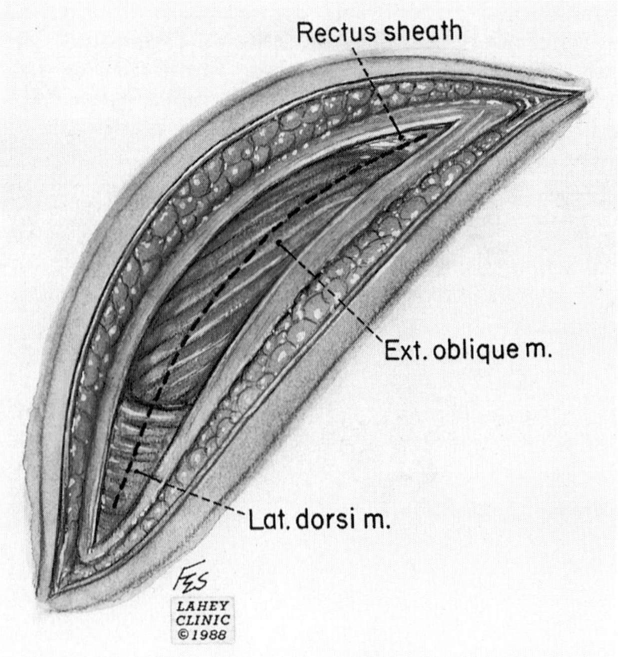
Rectus sheath
Ext. oblique m.
Lat. dorsi m.
FES LAHEY CLINIC ©1988

FIGURE 10–30. Incision carried through muscles. (By permission of Lahey Clinic.)

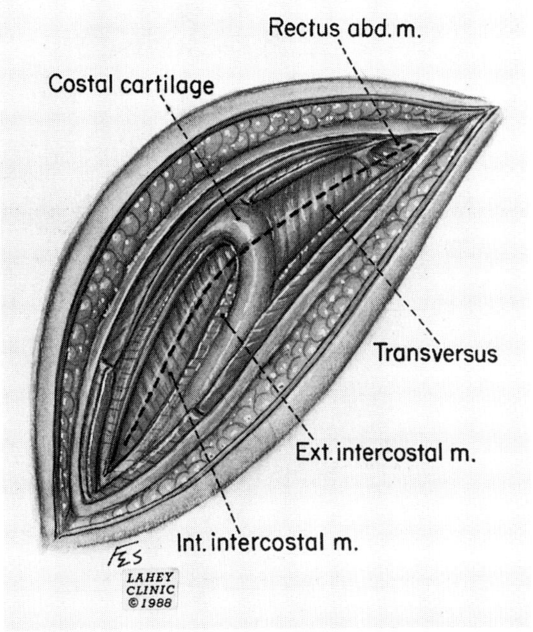
Rectus abd. m.
Costal cartilage
Transversus
Ext. intercostal m.
Int. intercostal m.
FES
LAHEY CLINIC ©1988

FIGURE 10–31. Division of costal cartilage. (By permission of Lahey Clinic.)

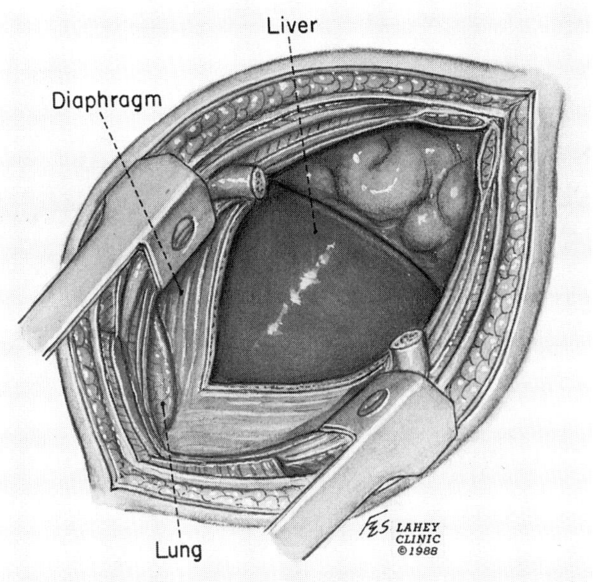
Liver
Diaphragm
Lung
FES LAHEY CLINIC ©1988

FIGURE 10–32. Complete thoracoabdominal incision. (By permission of Lahey Clinic.)

this is a reasonable approach for patients with a large pheochromocytoma because it affords exposure and palpation of the entire retroperitoneum and abdominal viscera through a single incision. It is also appropriate for patients having secondary or tertiary procedures, such as for recurrent pheochromocytoma or an adrenal carcinoma, which is large and locally infiltrating. The patient is placed in a semioblique position (45-degree angle) with a rolled sheet placed longitudinally beneath the flank. The incision is begun in the ninth intercostal space near the angle of the rib and carried across the costal margin at the midpoint of the contralateral rectus muscle just above the umbilicus (Fig. 10–29). As an alternative, this incision can be made either in the bed of the ninth or tenth rib. The incision is carried down through the latissimus dorsi, external oblique, internal oblique, transversus abdominis, and the rectus muscles (Fig. 10–30). After the latissimus dorsi, external oblique, and rectus muscles have been divided, the intercostal muscles are divided in the direction of the incision. The costal cartilage between the ninth and tenth rib is divided (Fig. 10–31). The peritoneal and pleural cavities are entered. The diaphragm is divided, taking care to avoid injury to the phrenic nerve. The lungs are protected with Mikulicz pads, and a large Finochietto retractor is placed in the incision (Fig. 10–32).

Bilateral Posterior Approach

This is an older approach for removal of both normal adrenal glands as well as for aldosteronoma. The patient is placed in the prone position on the operating table with rolls beneath the hips and rib cages (Fig. 10–33). Two incisions are made over either the eleventh or twelfth rib and extended medially to paraspinal muscles (Fig. 10–34). If necessary, the kidney bar can be elevated to give further

FIGURE 10–33. Position for posterior approach. (By permission of Lahey Clinic.)

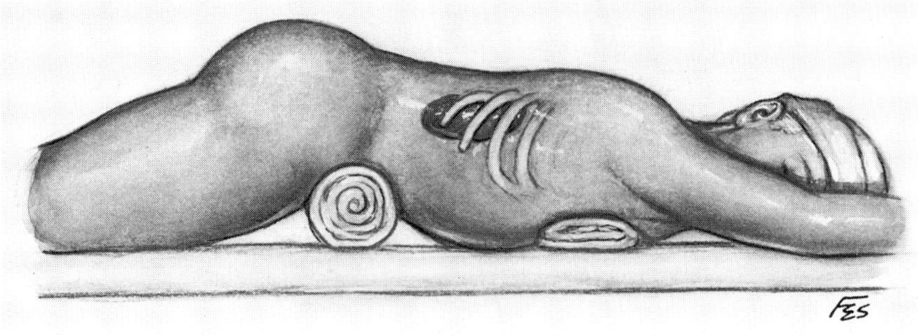
FES

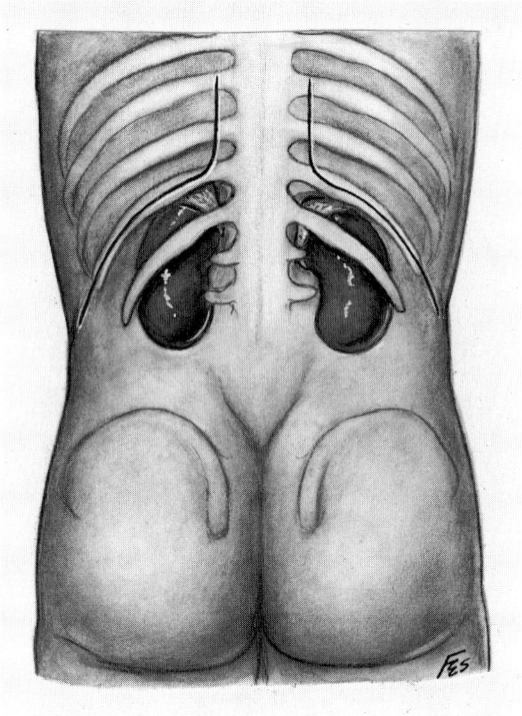

FIGURE 10–34. Posterior approach. (By permission of Lahey Clinic.)

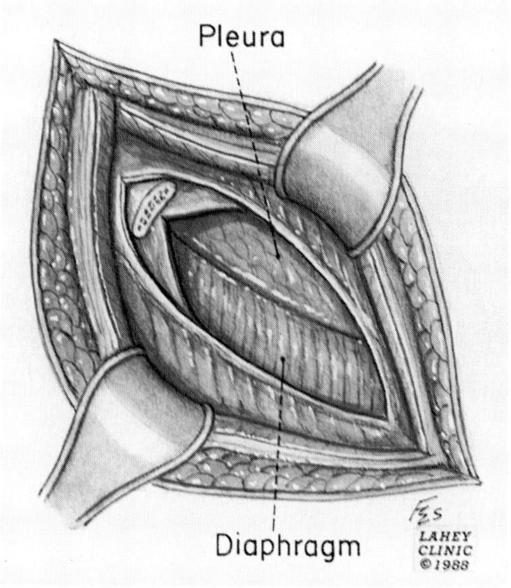
Pleura
Diaphragm
LAHEY CLINIC ©1988

FIGURE 10–36. Incision extended through periosteum. (By permission of Lahey Clinic.)

flexion. The incision can be made over the eleventh and twelfth ribs, depending on the level of each adrenal gland. The ribs are excised subperiosteally (Fig. 10–35), and the incision is carried down through the periosteum of the rib (Fig. 10–36). After the periosteum has been divided, the pleura is mobilized superiorly. The diaphragm and pleura are retracted superiorly, and the paraspinal muscles are retracted medially, exposing the adrenal gland and the upper pole of the kidney (Fig. 10–37).

The major difficulty with this operative approach is controlling the right adrenal vein where it enters the inferior vena cava. When it is difficult to secure this vessel or if the ligature slips off, life-threatening hemorrhage from the inferior vena cava will ensue. It is essential, then, to gain control of the inferior vena cava through an anterior approach in an urgent fashion. For this reason, we are reluctant to use the posterior approach for adrenal surgery and prefer the other approaches described.[11]

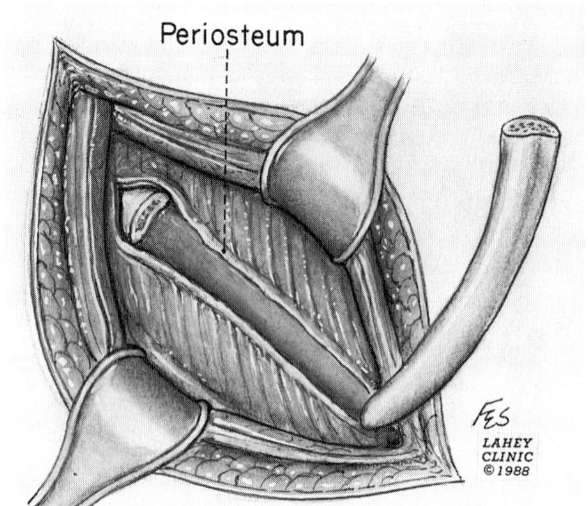
Periosteum
LAHEY CLINIC ©1988

FIGURE 10–35. Excision of ribs. (By permission of Lahey Clinic.)

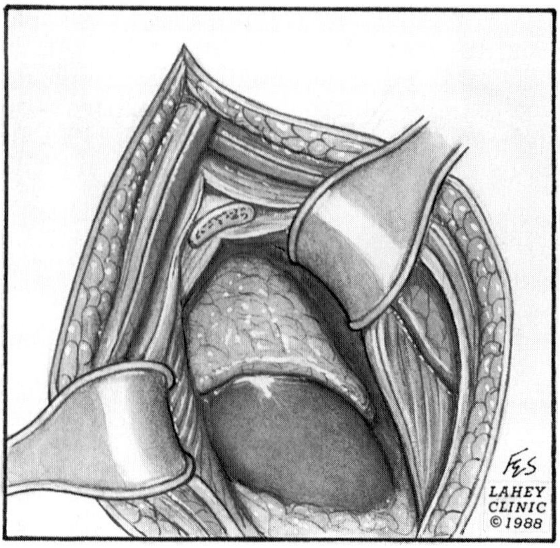
LAHEY CLINIC ©1988

FIGURE 10–37. Exposure of adrenal gland. (By permission of Lahey Clinic.)

REFERENCES

1. Cahill GF: Hormonal tumors of the adrenal. Surgery 1944; 16:233–265.
2. Cahill GF: Adrenalectomy for adrenal tumors. J Urol 1954; 71:123–133.
3. Flint LD: Complications of adrenal surgery from the surgeon's viewpoint. Surg Clin North Am 1957; 37:699–714.
4. Flint LD: A urologist's experience with 17 cases of pheochromocytoma. J Urol 1963; 90:491–499.
5. Flint LD: Surgical exposures for adrenal endocrinopathies. Surg Clin North Am 1973; 53:445–454.
6. Glenn JF: Surgical treatment of chromaffin tumors. Am Surg 1971; 37:6–11.
7. Glenn JF: Nonfunctioning adrenal tumors and aldosteronism. *In* Glenn JF, Boyce WH (eds): Urologic Surgery, 3rd edition, pp 1–25. Philadelphia, JB Lippincott Co, 1983.
8. Glenn JF: Surgery of the adrenal glands. *In* Glenn JF, Boyce WH (eds): Urologic Surgery, pp 1–36. New York, Harper & Row, 1969.
9. Glenn JF, Karl RL, Horwith M: Surgical treatment of Cushing's syndrome. Am Surg 1958; 148:365–374.
10. Waldstein SS: Diseases of the adrenal in the National Center for Advanced Medical Education. Urology Review, 1993, pp 1–29.
11. Libertino JA: Surgery of adrenal disorders. Surg Clin North Am 1988; 68:1027–1056.
12. Vaughan ED Jr, Blumenfeld JD: The adrenals. *In* Walsh PC, Retik AB, Stamey TA, Vaughan ED Jr (eds): Campbell's Urology, 6th edition, pp 2360–2412. Philadelphia, WB Saunders Co, 1992.
13. Laragh JH, Sealey JE: The renin-angiotensin-aldosterone system and the renal regulation of sodium, postassium, and blood pressure homeostasis. *In* Windhager EE (ed): Handbook of Physiology. New York, Oxford University Press, 1991.
14. Ferreira SH, Vane JR: Half-lives of peptides and amines in the circulation. Nature 1967; 215:1237–1240.
15. Howards SS, Carey R: The adrenals. *In* Gillenwater JY, Grayhack JT, Howards SS, Duckett JW (eds): Adult and Pediatric Urology, 2nd edition, pp 523–543. St. Louis, Mosby-Year Book, 1991.
16. Goldfarb DA: Surgical adrenal disease in the National Center for Advanced Medical Education. Urology Review, pp 1–13. Cook County Hospital, Chicago, 1993.
17. Orth DN, Liddle GW: Results of treatment in 108 patients with Cushing's syndrome. N Engl J Med 1971; 285:243–247.
18. Bagshawe KD: Hypokalaemia, carcinoma and Cushing's syndrome. Lancet 1960; 2:284–287.
19. Chandler WF, Schteingart DE, Lloyd RV, et al: Surgical treatment of Cushing's disease. J Neurosurg 1987; 66:204–212.
20. Martin JB, Reichlin S, Brown GM: Clinical Neuroendocrinology, p 192. Philadelphia, FA Davis Co, 1977.
21. Teasdale E, Teasdale G, Mohsen F, Macpherson P: High-resolution computed tomography in pituitary microadenoma: is seeing believing? Clin Radiol 1986; 37:227–232.
22. Dwyer AJ, Frank JA, Doppman JL, et al: Pituitary adenomas in patients with Cushing disease: initial experience with Gd-DTPA-enhanced MR imaging. Radiology 1987; 163:421–426.
23. Zovichian J, Oldfield EH, Doppman JL, et al: Usefulness of inferior petrosal sinus venous endocrine markers in Cushing's disease. J Neurosurg 1988; 68:205–210.
24. Boggan JE, Tyrrell JB, Wilson CB: Transsphenoidal microsurgical management of Cushing's disease: a report of 100 cases. J Neurosurg 1983; 59:195–200.
25. Nakane T, Kuwayama A, Watanabe M, et al: Long term results of transsphenoidal adenomectomy in patients with Cushing's disease. Neurosurgery 1987; 21:218–222.
26. Halberg FE, Sheline GE: Radiotherapy of pituitary tumors. Endocrinol Metab Clin North Am 1987; 16:667–684.
27. Moore TJ, Dluhy RG, Williams GH, et al: Nelson's syndrome: frequency, prognosis and effect of prior pituitary irradiation. Ann Intern Med 1976; 85:731–734.
28. Wilson CB, Tyrrell JB, Fitzgerald PA, Pitts LH: Cushing's disease and Nelson's syndrome. Clin Neurosurg 1980; 27: 19–30.
29. Cohen KL, Noth RH, Pechinski T: Incidence of pituitary tumors following adrenalectomy: a long-term follow-up study of patients treated for Cushing's disease. Arch Intern Med 1978; 138:575–579.
30. Barzilay JI, Pazianos AG: Adrenocortical carcinoma. Urol Clin North Am 1989; 16:457–468.
31. Richie JP, Gites RF: Carcinoma of the adrenal cortex. Cancer 1980; 45(7 Suppl):1957–1964.
32. Bloom LS, Libertino JA: Surgical management of Cushing's syndrome. Urol Clin North Am 1989; 16:547–565.
33. Lipsett MB, Hertz R, Ross GT: Clinical and pathophysiologic aspects of adrenocortical carcinoma. Am J Med 1963; 35:374–383.
34. Dunnick NR, Heaston D, Halvorsen R, et al: CT appearance of adrenal cortical carcinoma. J Comput Assist Tomogr 1982; 6:978–982.
35. Hussian S, Belldegrun A, Seltzer SE, et al: Differentiation of malignant from benign adrenal masses: predictive indices on computed tomography. AJR 1985; 144:61–65.
36. Gutierrez ML, Crooke ST: Mitotane (o,p′-DDD). Cancer Treat Rev 1980; 7:49–55.
37. Fishman LM, Liddle GW, Island DP, et al: Effects of aminoglutethimide on adrenal function in man. J Clin Endocrinol Metab 1967; 27:481–490.
38. Conn JW: Presidential address: part I: painting background. Part II: primary aldosteronism, a new clinical syndrome. J Lab Clin Med 1955; 45:3–17.
39. Greene JP, Guay AT: New perspectives in pheochromocytoma. Urol Clin North Am 1989; 16:487–503.
40. Hengstmann JH: Evaluation of screening tests for pheochromocytoma. Cardiology 1985; 72(Suppl 1):153–156.
41. Glazer GM, Woolsey EJ, Borrello J, et al: Adrenal tissue characterization using MR imaging. Radiology 1986; 158: 73–79.
42. Mendoza EA, Lueg MC, Puyau FA, Sutherland CM: Pheochromocytoma: localization with CT scan and selective angiogram. J LA State Med Soc 1986; 18:45–47.
43. Cariem AK, Green JAS, Fraser AG, Smith LR: Phaeochromocytoma of the bladder: a case report. S Afr Med J 1987; 71:178–179.
44. Malone MJ, Libertino JA, Tsapatsaris NP, Woods BO: Preoperative and surgical management of pheochromocytoma. Urol Clin North Am 1989; 16:567–582.
45. Shapiro B, Sisson JC, Eyre P, et al: 131I-MIBG—new agent in diagnosis and treatment of pheochromocytoma. Cardiology 1985; 72(Suppl 1):137–142.
46. Averbuch SD, Steakley CS, Young RC, et al: Malignant pheochromocytoma: effective treatment with a combination of cyclophosphamide, vincristine, and decarbazine. Ann Intern Med 1988; 109:267–273.
47. Fudge TL, McKinnon WM, Geary WL: Current surgical management of pheochromocytoma during pregnancy. Arch Surg 1980; 115:1124–1125.
48. Copeland PM: The incidentally discovered adrenal mass. Ann Intern Med 1983; 98:940–945.
49. Gross MD, Shapiro B, Bouffard JA, et al: Distinguishing benign from malignant euadrenal masses. Ann Intern Med 1988; 109:613–618.
50. Reinig JW, Doppman JL, Dwyer AJ, et al: Adrenal masses differentiated by MR. Radiology 1986; 158:81–84.

IV

KIDNEY AND URETER

11

DIAGNOSIS AND STAGING OF RENAL CELL CANCER

ANUP PATEL, M.S., F.R.C.S. (UROL.) *and* JEAN B. deKERNION, M.D.

Cancers of the kidney represent only 2 to 3% of all human neoplasms. The evolution of knowledge of renal tumors began in earnest with pathologic examinations, initially by Konig's accurate gross descriptions of kidney tumors in 1826[1] and subsequently by histologic studies published by Robin (1855)[2] and Waldeyer (1867),[3] which culminated in the opinion that these cancers arose from proliferation of renal tubular epithelium, with the aftermath of invasion through the membrana propria and cancerous nodulation. Grawitz, whose name has been eponymously linked to renal cell cancer, noted that these tumors were frequently located beneath the renal capsule near to the adrenal gland, often had a gross appearance suggesting fat content, and were composed of clear cells and amyloid material that resembled adrenal tissue rather than uriniferous tubules. In retrospect, he therefore mistakenly surmised these findings to suggest an origin from adrenal rests within the kidney and coined the descriptive narrative of "struma lipomatodes aberrata renis."[4] In the late nineteenth century, the phrase "hypernephroid tumor" was introduced by Doederlein and Birch-Hirschfeld[5] and this in turn culminated in the misconceived but popular descriptive term "hypernephroma," which for many years encompassed parenchymal tumors of primary renal origin. In modern practice, the concept that both renal adenomas and renal cell carcinomas arise from cells of the proximal convoluted tubule has been undisputed.[6] However, recent immunohistologic findings have shown that they may also develop from the distal convoluted tubule and collecting ducts, with a few tumors exhibiting all three types. Gu and coworkers found that distal convoluted tubule and collecting duct determinants were present in 39% of tumor specimens; clear cell tumors were most consistently linked with proximal convoluted tubular origin (89%), and granular cell tumors reacted in 88% with distal convoluted tubule or collecting duct markers.[7] Origin of renal cell cancer from the duct of Bellini is extremely unusual but has also been described.[8] The reader is referred to Chapter 12 for a comprehensive description of the various histologic types of renal cell cancer and their prognostic significance.

Renal cell carcinoma (RCC) accounts for up to 90% of all kidney tumors, has a projected incidence in excess of 28,000 new cases per year,[9] and has an estimated annual mortality of 11,700 in the United States. It is the third most common site of urinary tract malignancy after the prostate and the bladder. Although it can occur at any age, there is a propensity for most cases to be discovered in the fifth to seventh decades of life. Occurrence in males was twice as common as in females, but current statistics suggest that the male/female ratio both for incidence and disease-related death has changed and now stands at 1.5:1. Furthermore, recent trends have highlighted an increased frequency of renal cell cancer in urban dwellers and in younger adults, particularly in females and adolescents.[10] Overall, there appears to be little evidence to support the influence of race or geographic variations as independent variables that affect the incidence of renal cell cancer, while socioeconomic factors may contribute through different smoking patterns within different groups.

A higher incidence of this tumor has been reported in those with a known familial predilection (hereditary papillary renal cell carcinoma), those with von Hippel-Lindau disease, and those with acquired polycystic kidneys. The hereditary cancers do not show a male preponderance and generally arise two decades earlier than sporadic cancers. Acquired cystic renal disease (ACRD) was reported by Dunnill and colleagues in 1977 in patients treated by long-term hemodialysis.[11] Cystic change and hyperplasia of the tubular epithelium in this group seem to correlate well with the duration of uremia and are not particular to a specific type of dialysis. The risk of these changes occurring in the native kidneys is higher in black patients and those with nephrosclerosis. Renal cell carcinoma occurs as a complication of ACRD with a four times increased incidence over the general population and in a younger age group. Male gender, large renal size, and black race escalate the chance of a malignant complication.[12]

Occurrence of renal cell tumor in the pediatric and adolescent age group (below an upper age limit of 20 years) accounts for 3 to 5% of all reported cases and less than 7% of all solid neoplasms of childhood.[13] Although over 100 cases have been reported, Wilms' tumor is far more common in this age group and presents on average at the age of 2 years, compared to renal cell cancer, which presents around 9 years of age. The youngest reported case of renal cell carcinoma was at an age of 10 months.[14] Childhood RCC has an equal sex distribution and no racial predilection. Children are more likely to present with an abdominal mass than their adult counterparts. Up to 50% have hematuria, 24% exhibit renal calcification on plain abdominal radiographs, and 10% have bilateral tumors. In contrast, both hypertension and a palpable mass are more common in Wilms' tumor cases. Vascular invasion is particularly ominous in the child and mortality is high for disseminated tumors (80 to 100%). Almost all recurrences of RCC in this age group occur within 2 years. The overall survival is only 50 to 60%, a difference that can be explained by the greatest single difference between childhood RCC and Wilms' tumor, which is its inherent lack of chemosensitivity. Raney and associates suggested from a series of 20 patients that a better outcome was observed in patients below the age of 11 years than in older patients.[15]

Although the exact cause of renal cell carcinoma is unknown, a multifactorial etiology is likely. Sporadic reports implicating various substances have appeared in the literature over the years. Renal tumors have been produced in animal models through long-term administration of diethylstilbestrol,[16] but no human parallels have been reported. In another study, administration of the radiographic contrast agent colloidal thorium dioxide was causally linked to a high incidence of renal cell carcinoma.[17] More recently, tumors have been reported in young patients with the acquired immunodeficiency syndrome (AIDS)[18] and others have detected human papilloma virus DNA in both renal tubular cells and in renal cell tumors, but not in glomeruli.[19] Observations such as these have tenuously implicated a possible viral etiology.

Circumstantial epidemiologic evidence has strongly implicated smoking as an important risk factor.[20] Although a specific carcinogen has not been described, a statistically significant dose-dependent relative risk, ranging from 1.1 in moderate smokers to 2.3 for heavy smokers, was reported by these workers. The risk was time related and greatest in those with a long smoking history from young age. This may in part explain the rising incidence in younger patients, where the prevalence of cigarette smoking is ominously increasing. Conversely, cessation of smoking can inversely reduce the risk with time.

Advances in cytogenetics, molecular biology, and immunology in the past decade have unveiled a plethora of possible mechanisms of oncogenesis in renal cell cancer and have also played a significant part in the management and prognosis of those with advanced disseminated disease. Consistent chromosomal deletions and translocations have been localized to regions on the short arm of chromosome 3 (3p), with break points at 3p13-14.2 in familial tumors, at 3p21-24 in the sporadic variety, and at 3p25-26 in the von Hippel-Lindau (VHL). In the last group (VHL), the high prevalence of clear cell renal carcinoma with a compact growth pattern has been linked to the predisposition of somatic or germ line mutations characterized by chromosome 3:8 balanced translocation. In hereditary papillary renal cell carcinoma, 41 affected individuals have been reported from ten families.[21] In this select group, bilateral and multiple tumors have pervaded two to three generations of family members. Father-to-son transmission in three of the families was thought to be traced by linkage analysis to a possible chromosome-1 oncogene, which may have been responsible for a translocation to the X chromosome: t(X;1)(p11.2;q210). Others have observed a high occurrence of allele deletion at locus 3(ph3H2) in sporadic renal cell cancers, suggesting that the loss of a tumor suppressor gene at this site may facilitate oncogenesis. Although no single oncogenetic abnormality has been characterized, c-*myc* and (c-*erb* B-1) mRNA for epidermal growth factor are consistently overexpressed and HER-2 (*erb* B-2) mRNA is underexpressed in many patients with renal cell carcinoma. The significance of these and other altered oncogenetic expression patterns and their possible interplay with autocrine growth control mechanisms (overexpression of growth factors such as tumor growth factor-alpha (TGF-α), epidermal growth factor, and truncated fibronectin) continues to stimulate avid research interest.

Tuberous sclerosis is yet another disease complex associated with renal manifestations. Although the association with renal angiomyolipoma is well recognized in these patients, there have been no systematic studies of renal cell carcinoma in tuberous sclerosis patients. At least 22 case reports have been published citing the coexistence of RCC and angiomyolipomas, and of these 10 were bilateral. It seems likely that the two tuberous sclerosis complex (TSC) genes may predispose to renal cell carcinoma through a two-hit mechanism as first proposed by Knudsen for retinoblastoma.[22] Although the human TSC2 gene has been recently isolated from chromosome 16 and seems to have tumor suppressor gene properties, the TSC1 gene has not yet been mapped from chromosome 9. The Eker rat strain, which has an insertional mutation affecting the homologue of the human TSC gene[23] and develops multifocal RCC as a dominant trait, is the first animal model that has implicated the TSC2 gene in renal cell carcinogenesis. The recent report by Sampson and colleagues[24] of multifocal RCC in siblings from a chromosome 9–linked (TSC1) multigenerational tuberous sclerosis family has for the first time suggested a similar role for the TSC1 gene. Further studies of the exact mechanisms whereby TSC1 and TSC2 gene mutations cause RCC are sure to follow.

PRESENTATION OF RENAL CELL CARCINOMA: SYMPTOMS AND SIGNS

There have been many large studies that sought to address the dilemma of diagnosis in the hope that early diagnosis would in turn lead to curative surgery. Since nature has protected the human kidney from external harm by virtue of location high under the diaphragm and costal flange, the palpation of a mass at physical examination rarely contributes to an early diagnosis of surgically curable disease. The majority of renal diseased states are expressed through the production of abnormal urine. In a recent retrospective analysis of 314 patients, hematuria was still the most common presenting symptom, with flank pain and paraneoplastic syndromes as the next most common modes of presentation in rank order.[25] Pain usually signifies invasion or compression of surrounding tissues and organs but can also occur when bleeding leads to clot formation and clot colic, or obstruction of the collecting system. Acute flank pain can in fact be the mode of presentation after spontaneous intratumoral hemorrhage, or as blood is released into the subcapsular space resulting in a hematoma that expands the renal capsule. Renal cancers are found to be an underlying cause of spontaneous perinephric hemorrhage in up to 60% of cases.[26,27] The classic clinical triad of flank pain, an abdominal mass, and hematuria, which accounted for 5 to 15% of diagnoses before the early 1970s,[28–31] is now exceptional[32] and is usually associated with a tumor that may no longer be organ confined.

In the early 1970s, Skinner and coworkers[29] retrospectively reviewed their experience of patients with renal cell cancer treated by nephrectomy in a general hospital between 1935 and 1965. They reported that 7% of the patients studied had tumors that were incidentally discovered at laparotomy or during the course of other surgery. The quality of current diagnostic imaging has banished this diagnostic entity to one of historical significance only. The majority of renal tumors in the modern era are discovered by serendipity during imaging studies performed either for vague abdominal and flank pain, or for musculoskeletal symptoms, or during the course of targeted investigation of other abdominal organ systems (e.g., barium enema, hepatobiliary sonography, abdominoperipheral anteriography, abdominal or spinal computed tomography [CT] or magnetic resonance imaging [MRI]).

Unfortunately, signs of advanced metastatic disease such as malaise, unexplained weight loss, fever, or anemia are still not uncommon diagnostic clues, particularly when supported by marked elevation of the erythrocyte sedimentation rate. An occasional cause of concern and specialist referral is the so-called newly discovered left varicocele in the young adult male. Skinner and colleagues[29] reported that 3.3% of males in their series were referred with an acute-onset varicocele. The incidence of varicocele in patients with renal cell cancer was 0.6% in another large series of 2314 renal tumors.[33] Of the 14 positive patients in this series, only 2 had a right-sided varicocele. In one of these two, the varicocele disappeared after right nephrectomy, while the other had a left-sided tumor! Rarely, then, does this sign correspond to the presence of an advanced venoinvasive renal cell tumor and it is therefore of no practical significance. In the majority of such patients, a subclinical varicocele may have been present for several years and gone unnoticed. Manifestations of inferior vena caval occlusion by tumor, such as varicocele, leg edema, deep venous thrombosis, recurrent pulmonary emboli, engorged abdominal veins leading to caput medusae, and proteinuria, are only found in 36 to 50% due to compensatory collateral venous drainage through the lumbar and azygos systems.[34,35] Hypertension is not a prominent feature, but may occur if the tumor secretes renin or renin-like substances,[36] secretes erythropoietin which results in polycythemia, compresses a segmental renal artery, obstructs the ureter, metastasizes to the brain, or produces arteriovenous fistulae. When a large renal mass is present and has parasitized an abundance of new vessels leading to significant arteriovenous shunting, auscultation over the mass may reveal an audible bruit.

Renal cell tumors are renowned for an incidence of systemic syndromes. This may account for a high index of suspicion of the presence of an occult renal cell cancer when inexplicable paraneoplastic clinical manifestations are encountered. An important aspect of normal renal function is the production of a diverse range of hormones (renin and erythropoietin), and prostanoid modulators of smooth muscle function (prostaglandins, prostacyclins, and thromboxanes). It is also responsible for the conversion of the vitamin D precursor 25-hydroxycholecalciferol to the active form 1α,25-dihydroxycholecalciferol. The tumor may either elaborate greater amounts of these substances or secrete new hormones such as parathormone-like factors, insulin, glucagon, and human chorionic gonadotropin.

These tumor markers are often useful to follow disease progression after therapeutic intervention. Hypercalcemia, a typical example, has been reported in 6 to 10% of patients with renal cell cancer and can be used as a marker of early or occult disease recurrence after nephrectomy, if skeletal metastases have been excluded by baseline bone scintigraphy. Although the exact mechanism relating to hypercalcemia is still obscure, it is likely that a tumor peptide analogous to N-terminal region of a parathyroid-like hormone is the causative agent.[37] Erythropoietin, a renal cortical glycoprotein secreted in response to hypoxia,[38] has also been detected at elevated levels in up to 47% of patients with metastatic renal cell tumors and up to 37% of those with localized disease[39] but is not always accompanied by erythrocytosis. It is not clear whether this occurs de novo within the tumor, or as a homeostatic response of normal cortical tissue to relative local renal hypoxia from tumor compression of the adjacent parenchyma.[40] Ljungberg and associates[41] observed a lack of correlation between tumor size and erythropoietin production, casting doubt on the concept of tumor-induced renal hypoxia. Since elevations of serum erythropoietin levels are also described in a variety of other renal disease states (e.g., hydronephrosis, renal cyst) as well as in other conditions,[42] by no means is this finding pathognomonic of renal cell cancer. A significant survival difference ($p < .01$) has been noted in one series between those with normal and those with elevated serum erythropoietin levels.[41] This study also reported an increased sensitivity in those with high-grade tumors and, although they suggested that raised serum eythropoietin may have prognostic value, the data were not stratified for stage and grade in a multivariate analysis.

A curious though often dramatic occurrence of nonmetastatic hepatocellular dysfunction manifested by abnormal liver function tests, leukopenia, fever, and areas of hepatic necrosis can occur in association with renal cell carcinoma and is called Stauffer's syndrome. Here, liver function can be normalized by nephrectomy and represents a relatively good prognostic sign with 88% surviving 1 year or more. Persistence or recurrence of the syndrome indicates residual or recurrent tumor.

TABLE 11–1. DIAGNOSTIC POSSIBILITIES FOR A PARENCHYMAL RENAL MASS

Simple cyst (Bosniak I—benign)
Minimally complicated cyst (Bosniak II—does not require follow-up)
Minimally complicated cyst (Bosniak IIF—requires follow-up)
Moderately complex cyst (Bosniak III—indeterminate)
Cystic carcinoma (Bosniak IV—malignant)
Solid tumor with fatty tissue (angiomyolipoma)
Solid tumor with calcification (renal cell cancer)
Renal medullary carcinoma
Pseudotumor
Junctional parenchyma (hypertrophied column of Bertin—cortical septum between fused embryonic upper and lower calyceal groups)
Lobar dysmorphism
Renal abscess
Acute renal infarct
Focal acute pyelonephritis
Hypertrophied parenchyma adjacent to renal scar of chronic reflex
Hematoma
Renal artery aneurysm
Renal arteriovenous malformation
Lipomatosis circumscripta or peripelvic fibrolipomatosis
Dromedary hump
Reninoma
Lymphoma
Oncocytoma
Hemangioma
Sarcomas
Leiomyosarcoma
Liposarcoma
Fibrosarcoma
Rhabdomyosarcoma
Primary osteosarcoma
Chondrosarcoma
Angiosarcoma
Clear cell sarcoma
Sarcomatoid carcinoma
Hemangiopericytoma
Malignant neurilemmoma
Neurofibrosarcoma
Malignant fibrous histiocytoma
Renal metastases
Carcinoma of bronchus
Carcinoma of breast
Carcinoma of the colon
Tumors of the head and neck
Melanoma
Endometrial carcinoma
Appendiceal carcinoma
Leukemia
Seminoma
Benign mesenchymal tumors (fibroma and leiomyoma)
Transitional cell carcinoma
Adult Wilms' tumor

THE ROLE OF DIAGNOSTIC IMAGING OF A RENAL MASS

Hematuria unquestionably raises the specter of renal parenchymal or urothelial neoplasia, but it can be absent in up to 40% of patients with renal cell tumor at diagnosis. The presence of microscopic hematuria cannot be ignored and demands further evaluation of the upper tracts. Urine cytology seldom alludes to the correct diagnosis of RCC, in contrast to transitional cell cancer. Traditionally, intravenous urography is still the first choice but may ultimately be superseded by CT urography (Z.L. Barbaric, personal communication, 1995). In general, using all available imaging criteria, a parenchymal renal mass can be characterized as shown in Table 11–1.

INTRAVENOUS EXCRETORY UROGRAPHY

Intravenous excretory urography (IVU) with nephrotomography as needed, has withstood the test of time as the most popular radiologic screening examination for patients with hematuria or clinical suspicion of a renal cancer. In order for this investigation to detect the presence of a renal mass, several criteria must be fulfilled. The patient must have adequate venous access and no history of allergic reaction to intravenous iodinated contrast medium; the mass must have a location and/or size sufficient to cause distortion of the normal renal architecture (capsule and intrarenal collecting system or ureter), or appear as a filling defect because of diminished or absent function within the tumor tissue. Dogma dictates that any renal mass that enhances with intravenous contrast should be considered a renal cell carcinoma until proven otherwise, but unfortunately, not all enhancing renal masses are tumors or need surgery. Other diagnostic possibilities include complex benign cysts, abscess, hematoma, infarct, inflammatory pseudotumors, angiomyolipomas, lymphoma, and renal metastases.

Detected tumor often appears as an exophytic contour bulge, or through splayed dilated calyces from expansive growth. Occasionally tumors grow in an explosive manner outwards into Gerota's space leaving little detectable distortion of the collecting system. When the predominant growth of tumor is anterior or posterior, the diagnosis may be missed on urography (Fig. 11–1) through the limitations of two-dimensional imaging, compounded by the superimposed shadow of the normal kidney. Size of the lesion must also be factored into the equation, and in a recent report, one third of renal cell tumors 3 cm or less in size were undetectable on urography.[43] Radiographically visible calcifications are present in 13% of renal cell carcinomas.[44] Conversely, 58% of all renal masses with foci of calcification are RCCs. Central dense or amorphous calcifications represent RCC in 87% of cases, while pure rim-like calcification is caused by benign renal cysts in 80%.[45] Other subtle features such as notching of the renal pelvis or upper ureter result from enlarged ureteral vessels recruited into the hypervascular tumor circulation. Active bleeding with clot formation may be represented by long filling defects in the ureter or renal pelvis. Occasionally, these or an infiltrative growth pattern with invasion of the collecting system may be difficult to distinguish from transitional cell cancer (Fig. 11–2) and require further elaboration by retrograde ureteropyelography. Absent renal function is rare but may result from long-standing tumor-induced hydronephrosis or renal vein occlusion. Despite all of these features, the overall diagnostic sensitivity and specificity of urography is low, and invariably additional imaging is required both in those with an apparent parenchymal abnormality and in those where upper and lower tracts appear to be normal but microscopic hematuria persists, if small adenomas and renal cancers are not to be missed.

ULTRASOUND

Most curable renal cancers are asymptomatic and are found serendipitously on CT or ultrasound. Widespread use of these modalities probably explains the apparent rising trend in the incidence of renal cell cancer. In the past two decades, ultrasound and CT imaging have revolutionized the diagnosis and staging of renal neoplasms, and yet there remain areas of uncertainty with each modality. Unfortunately, there are few prospective comparisons of ultrasound and CT in this situation, but both of these investigations have been recommended with regularity as second-line tests in patients with an abnormal IVU.

Sonography with 3.5- and 5-MHz sector scan and linear array probes not only has a place in detecting parenchymal lesions but also, more importantly, distinguishes simple cysts from complex cystic and solid neoplasms. Although its sensitivity in detecting solid renal masses is operator dependent and influenced by other factors such as patient build and co-operation (controlled respiratory excursion), overlying bowel gas, a small acoustic window for lesions at the left upper pole, and echogenic pattern variations in the tumor contrasted to the normal adjacent parenchyma, high-resolution real-time ultrasound has played an emerging role in the detection of renal cell cancer. The argument in favor of implementation of abdominal sonography as a low-cost diagnostic tool in large-scale screening programs for renal cancer is still unproven, as the detection rate was only 1.02% in one large series.[46] The positive yield in this series was significantly better in those with microscopic hematuria or symptoms compared to asymptomatic subjects. This finding reaffirms the view that, ultimately, it may have greatest value in the surveillance of groups at high risk of developing renal tumors.

Simple cysts are round or ovoid in shape; have a thin, smooth, well-defined wall; are devoid of internal echoes; and exhibit good through-transmission of sound. The typical sonographic appearance of renal cell cancer, on the other hand, is that of an exophytic isoechoic inhomogeneous irregular mass with varying hypoechoic areas of cystic degeneration and echo foci with contiguous distal shadowing at sites of tumor calcification. In between these two extremes are lesions that are difficult to characterize on sonography alone and require further imaging. Small renal cancers 3 cm or less in maximum dimension are typically hyperechoic on ultrasound[47] but can be isoechoic to the renal parenchyma and difficult to localize when centrally placed. Larger tumors are less likely to exhibit increased echogenicity. When an isoechoic small renal mass is discovered, absence of through-transmission may be a useful feature in distinguishing tumor from normal parenchyma. Detection rates for small renal tumors have been reported to be as high as 79% for ultrasound (compared to 67% for urography)

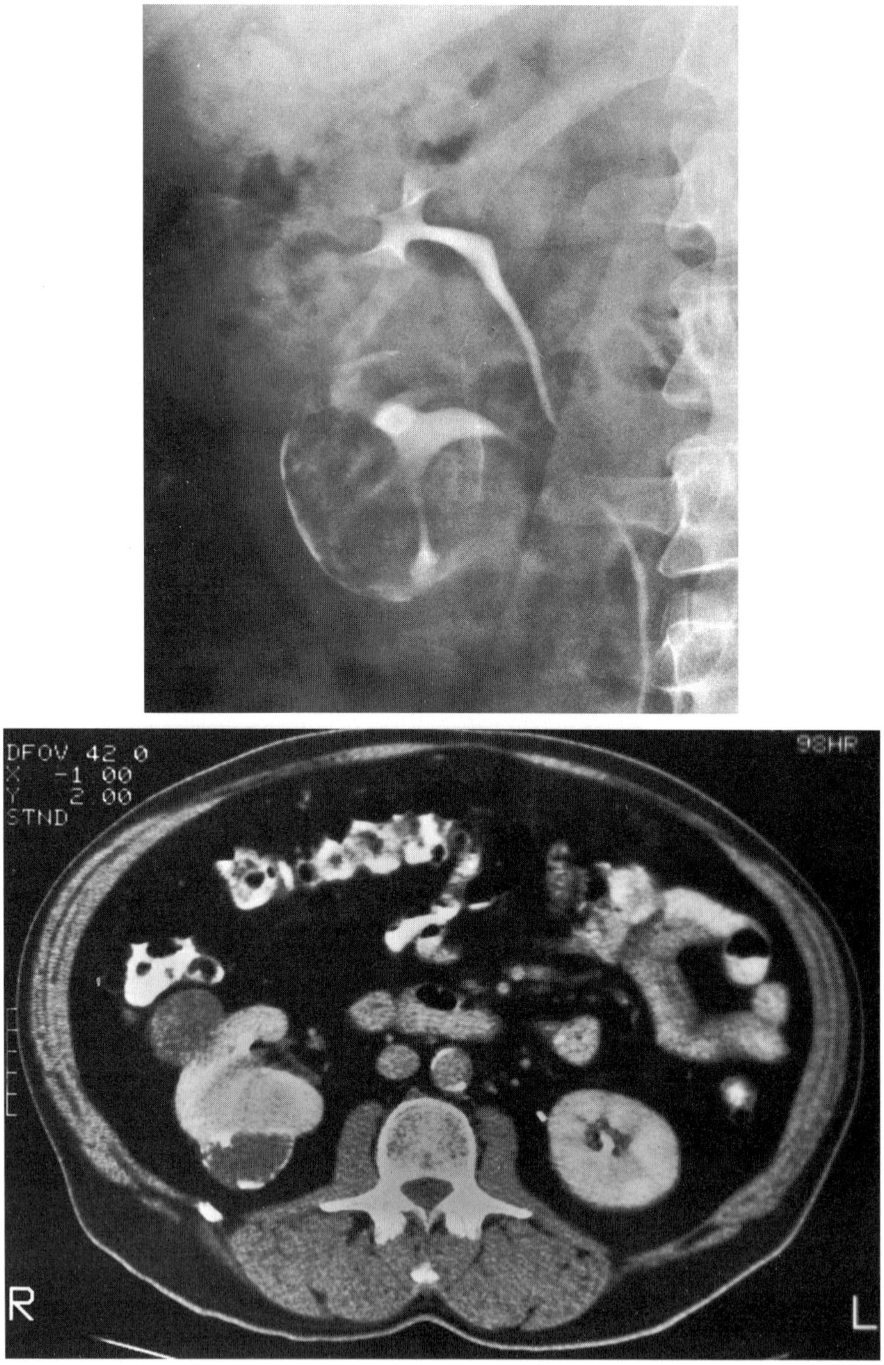
DFOV 42.0
STND
R
L

FIGURE 11–1. Renal tumor of the upper pole in anterior position (with coexistent lower pole calcified cyst) missed on intravenous urography and only seen on CT. (Courtesy of Dr. S.T. Cochran, M.D., Department of Radiology, UCLA School of Medicine.)

and have not substantially improved despite ongoing improvements in transducer technology and hardware. Tumors in this size range (≤3 cm) cannot always be reliably distinguished from angiomyolipomas in up to 32% of cases, purely on the basis of their echo texture.[48] Other diagnostic possibilities for lesions of this size range include pseudotumors, some reninomas, and metastatic renal deposits. In a global era of medical cost containment, it has been suggested that sonography is less time consuming and more cost effective than CT for the work-up of a renal mass detected at urography.[49] The additional cost of CT incurred in this study, where 18% of the sonographic findings were indeterminate, did not economically justify preliminary use of CT even for small lesions less than 3 cm in size.

The addition of Doppler and color duplex Doppler-enhanced sonographic imaging in the ultrasonographer's armamentarium has occasionally been

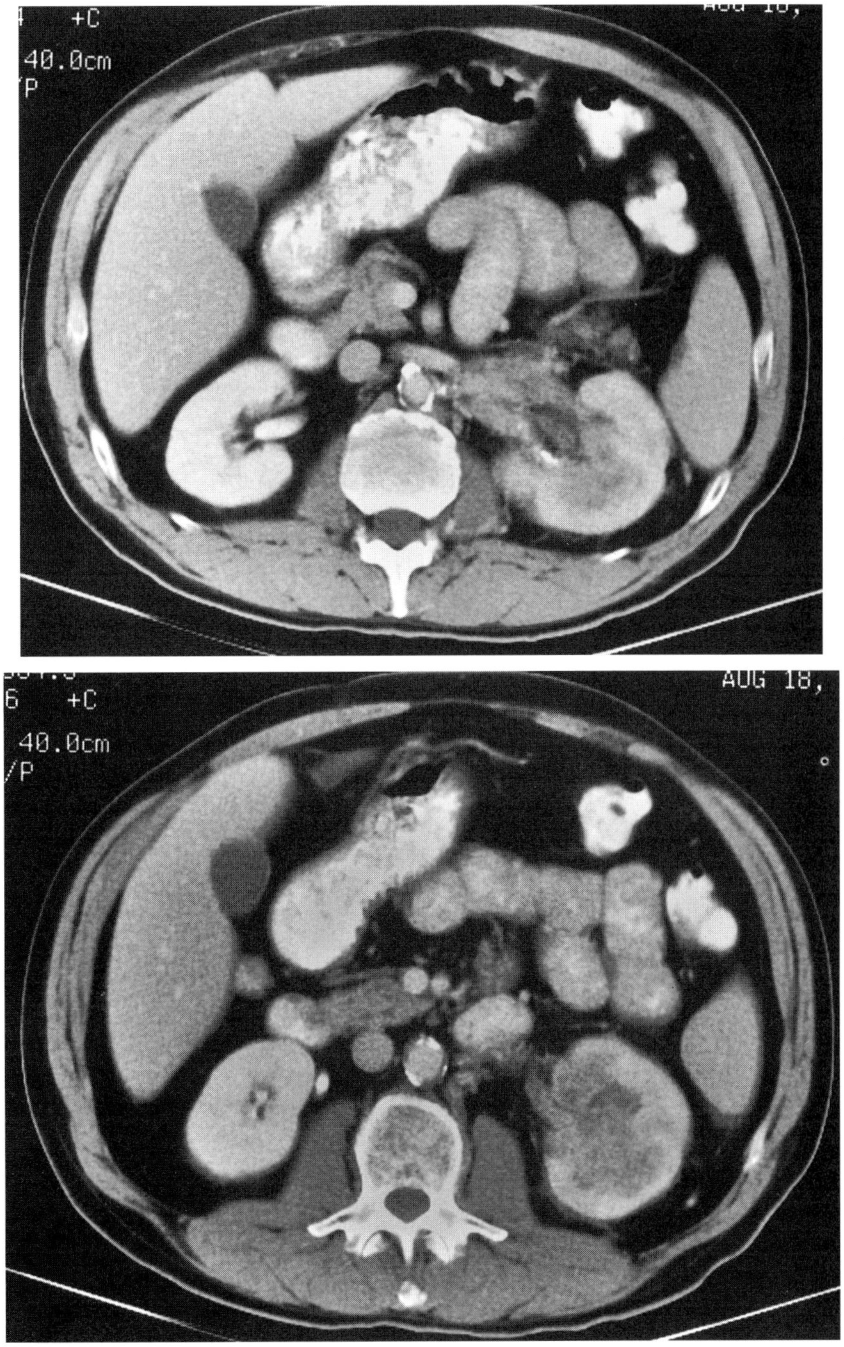
+C
40.0cm
P
+C
AUG 18,
40.0cm
P

FIGURE 11–2. Infiltrative renal cell carcinoma resembling a transitional cell carcinoma. (Courtesy of Dr. S.T. Cochran, M.D., Department of Radiology, UCLA School of Medicine.)

useful to highlight tumor neovascularity or demonstrate parasitized vessels around an indeterminate renal mass in order to sway the diagnosis towards malignancy,[50] but as 20% of renal cell cancers are not hypervascular, the diagnostic limitations of this innovation are self-evident.

Complicated cystic lesions, pseudotumors, lymphoma, and renal lesions 2 cm or less, account for the vast majority of diagnostic "gray areas." Differentiation of cystic lesions that are benign from those that require surgical exploration and excision, is the most vexing task for both the sonographer and the urologist. When the thickness of a cyst wall and its internal architecture cannot be demonstrated, or the cyst contains old degenerated or coagulated blood (50% of hyperdense cysts do not show cystic characteristics on ultrasound), additional imaging by CT scan will be required to characterize the lesion through its ability to enhance with contrast. Renal cell carcinoma coexistent with adult cystic renal disease is also difficult to diagnose on sonography alone and requires MRI imaging without and with gadolinium-diethylenetriamine-pentaacetic acid (Gd-DTPA) to demonstrate enhancement. If a tumor greater than 2 cm is found, bilateral nephrectomy should be undertaken, for the risk of multifocal and bilateral renal cell cancer is high in these patients.

INTRAOPERATIVE ULTRASOUND

Initially performed for stone disease in the early 1960s, a number of authors have recently reported experience with the intraoperative application of ultrasound,[51] both to determine the appropriateness of parenchymal sparing surgery in those with sporadic renal cancer and in defining the cephalad level of a caval tongue of tumor. Used to complement other preoperative imaging, the potential attraction to its use in parenchymal sparing procedures is twofold. First, it may allow the accurate targeting of nephrotomy to ensure adequate margins, thus lowering the risk of tumor bed recurrences while at the same time optimizing parenchymal preservation. Moreover, a 5- or 7.5-MHz linear array probe used to sequentially image the renal cortex from pole to pole may indicate the presence of multifocal and small satellite tumors (e.g., in patients with VHL or familial renal cell cancer), while a 10-MHz probe is better in defining capsular invasion. Both of these intraoperative findings should militate against partial nephrectomy or enucleation. In the publication by Walther and associates,[52] it was found to be most useful in characterizing lesions deep to the capsule in the area of the renal hilum. The addition of color Doppler imaging technology in this study also appeared to help in displaying the vascular architecture adjacent to the tumor.

To place this technology in its proper perspective, although it extends the range of renal imaging, the specific indications guiding its broader application are ultimately quite small due to the high quality of modern CT scans. The limitations of intraoperative ultrasound are self-evident. Benign solid lesions that coexist in the same kidney cannot be reliably distinguished from cancers, while small tumors can be missed.[53] The adrenal gland is also hard to visualize. It is also not clear whether this form of imaging at open surgery should be the domain of the urologist (who may be inexperienced in sonographic renal imaging) or the subspecialist radiologist.

COMPUTERIZED TOMOGRAPHY

Sectional imaging is without doubt the most useful and sensitive means of characterizing an indeterminate lesion of the kidney, provided that the equipment available can produce images of high quality. This requires communication of pertinent clinical information to the radiologist before the sequence of images is planned, and exclusion of previous contrast allergy. An optimal scan consists of thin-section (5-mm) renal imaging with a 2-second scan time in fast sequence, before and after rapid mechanical intravenous injection of an adequate amount of iodinated contrast. If Hounsfield units are measured, regular calibration of the equipment is essential, technical factors should not be varied on the pre- and postcontrast scans, and multiple cursor measurements from small regions of interest in all portions of the lesions are the rule. Provided these criteria are fulfilled, CT alone can enable a diagnostic accuracy of better than 95% for renal cell carcinoma.[54] Classic features typical of renal cell carcinoma on CT include a solid or predominantly exophytic complex cystic soft tissue mass, devoid of fat, that may be lobulated with irregular margins, is isodense to the remainder of the renal parenchyma, but appears hypodense in comparison to the normal parenchyma after contrast enhancement, and has inhomogeneity of internal density with central and/or peripheral calcification. The interface with the normal parenchyma (pseudocapsule) is generally indistinct. Unfortunately, there is great variation in the CT appearance of renal cell carcinoma. Many of the characteristics described above are dependent on the size of the tumor and may be absent in smaller tumors. In one pathologically validated study of 78 tumors imaged preoperatively by CT,[27] precontrast enhancement was evenly distributed between three groups (hyperdense, isodense, and hypodense) and consequently this feature was not pathognomonic for malignancy. Less than 6% of tumors demonstrated a pattern of diffuse local infiltration in this series, while 22% were predominantly cystic. Hyperdensity can be a feature common to both renal cell tumors that contain an area of focal hemorrhage and benign cystic lesions containing old, clotted, or degenerated blood. The differentiation of these lesions therefore relies on the evaluation of enhancement with contrast and extremely high-quality thin-section scans are essential to allow multiple measurements of Hounsfield units. Those indeterminate small lesions that do show enhancement should be surgically explored and treated as cancers.

In 1986, Morton Bosniak described features that distinguished different types of renal cysts and encompassed these within a classification system useful to clinicians in the management of these lesions.[55] The essential aspects of this classification system were centered on an evaluation of the contour and thickness of the wall of the lesion; the number, thickness, and contour of any septae; the amount, location, and character of any calcifications; the fluid density within cystic spaces; the presence of solid components; and margination of the lesion. Bosniak category II lesions are septated, minimally calcified, and may contain infected fluid but have a very low malignant potential. Of more concern are the slightly more complex cysts which are hyperdense and have more wall calcification, for these require interval follow-up imaging over a

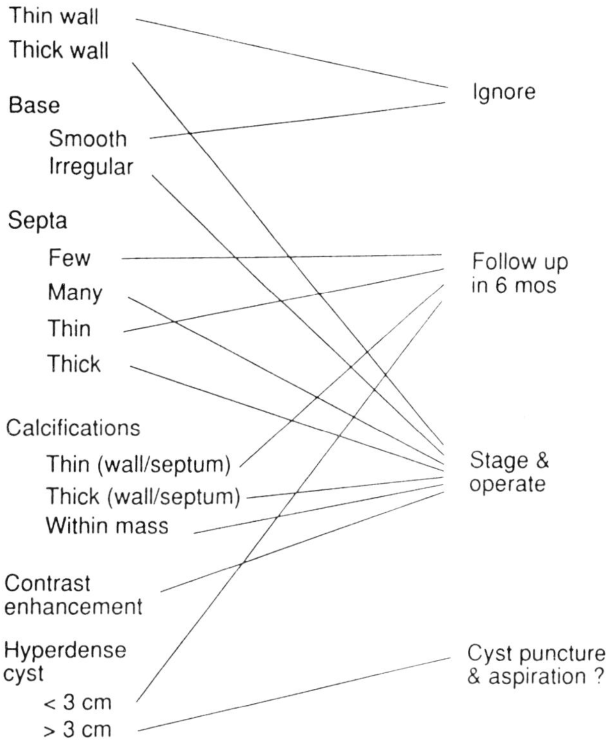
Thin wall
Thick wall
Base
Smooth
Irregular
Septa
Few
Many
Thin
Thick
Calcifications
Thin (wall/septum)
Thick (wall/septum)
Within mass
Contrast enhancement
Hyperdense cyst
< 3 cm
> 3 cm
Ignore
Follow up in 6 mos
Stage & operate
Cyst puncture & aspiration ?

FIGURE 11–3. Algorithm for management of a complex renal cyst. (From Barbaric ZL: Principles of Genitourinary Radiology, 2nd edition. New York, Thieme Medical Publishers, Inc, 1994. Copyright Thieme Medical Publishers, 1994, with permission.)

period of a year or more. Growth and change in character from baseline are indications for surgical intervention where such management is clinically appropriate in the fit patient with a normal contralateral kidney. Complicated Bosniak category III cysts cannot be clinically distinguished from renal cancers and should be excised by enucleation, partial nephrectomy, or total radical nephrectomy, but ultimately, some of these will turn out to be benign lesions (hemorrhagic multiloculated cysts and nephromas). The surgical approach is usually determined by the size and location of the lesion. Lesions that are cystic with a solid nodular base, demonstrate numerous focally thick septa, some of which enhance with contrast, have irregular margins and large amounts of calcification, are Bosniak grade IV lesions. They either represent cystic or necrotic renal carcinoma, with few exceptions.[56]

Lesions in Bosniak category I are undoubtedly benign and may be adequately imaged by sonography, but those in higher categories or associated with poor-quality gray-scale scans should be evaluated by high quality pre- and postcontrast CT scans. A practical schematic depicting management recommendations based on CT findings of indeterminate lesions is shown in Figure 11–3.

Acquired cystic renal change in native and retained nonfunctioning transplant kidneys occurs in those with end-stage renal disease after long-term dialysis (80 to 90% in patients dialyzed for 5 years or more). Here, the incidence of renal cell cancer (Fig. 11–4) is estimated to be 1%. A positive diagnosis on ultrasound, CT, or MRI may be impossible, particularly when the original cause of renal failure was polycystic kidney disease, and is reliant on the demonstration of a solid enhancing lesion. Consequently, routine CT surveillance is not recommended for these patients.[58]

Adenomas of the kidney are semantically distinguished from carcinomas purely by virtue of size, but clearly, many similarities exist between the two lesions. Both have a higher propensity to occur in tobacco users, exhibit cellular differentiation akin to

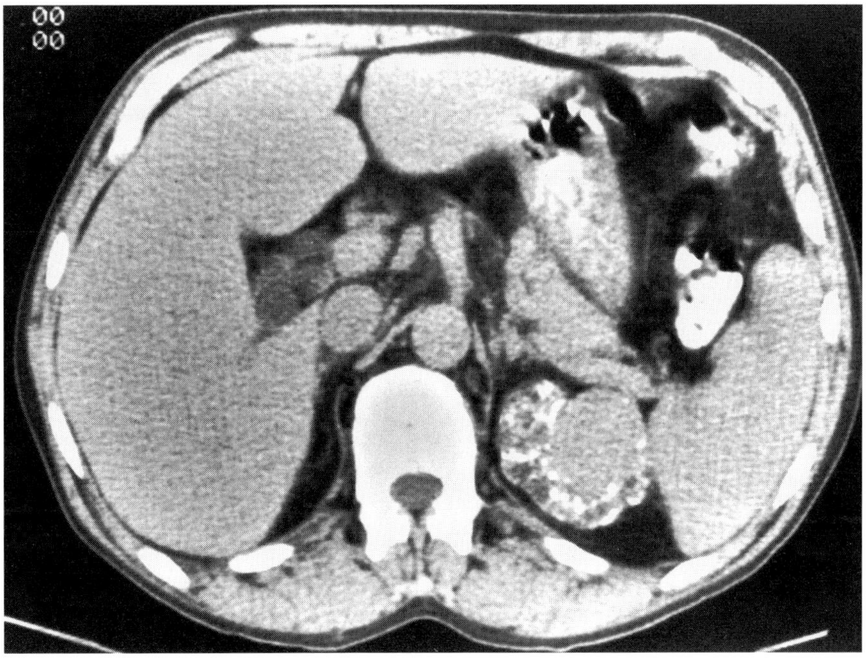
00
00

FIGURE 11–4. Renal cell cancer in acquired cystic renal disease after dialysis. (Courtesy of Dr. S.T. Cochran, M.D., Department of Radiology, UCLA School of Medicine.)

those of the proximal convoluted tuble, may coexist synchronously, occur in the same age group, and show the same male preponderance. The term "adenoma" is therefore a misnomer and these small tumors are more appropriately redesignated as renal carcinoma of low malignant potential.[58,59]

The incidence of incidental solid renal tumors less than 3 cm is as high as 22% in autopsy studies. Bell[60] reported in 1950 that cortical renal tumors smaller than 3 cm rarely metastasized (4.6% in 65 cases), and yet one such tumor in his original publication[61] had already metastasized at the time of diagnosis. Misinterpretation of this article has falsely popularized the distinction between adenomas and adenocarcinomas based on a size threshold of 3 cm. In the intervening 45 years, no reliable biochemical markers for metastatic potential have been identified. Even though the potential for precocious dissemination of a "youthful tumor" based on size alone is still accepted to be low, it cannot be guaranteed. Surgical excision is appropriate if growth can be confidently discerned, for a small percentage of these lesions may have advanced in local stage and possess a propensity to disseminate through early aggressive behavior. Whether such lesions could have been surgically cured through early detection at a lower stage is a matter for debate. Partial nephrectomy is an appropriate option for confined singular tumors, for the risk of ipsilateral local recurrence and asynchronous contralateral tumor is as low as 1% for incidentally discovered renal cell cancers[62,63] as opposed to a 6.6% local recurrence rate for suspected or symptomatic tumors.

Small size is undoubtedly a confounding factor in the radiologic diagnosis of renal cell cancer. Since the advent and wider application of ultrasound and CT, the detection of incidental solid renal masses less than 3 cm is an increasingly common contemporary occurrence. The difficult question as to need for surgical "cure" and the degree of urgency for such a cure is frequently posed. The mere fact that the lesion is small, asymptomatic, and incidentally discovered does not ensure future indolent behavior. Other factors to be weighed in the balance of risk versus benefit of excisional surgery include age at diagnosis, comorbidity, and patterns of familial longevity.

Information provided by high-quality CT scans from a third- or fourth-generation machine is essential to assist in the decision-making process, particularly when the lesion in question is 1.5 cm or smaller. Rapid (3-minute) bolus injection of 40 g of iodinated contrast (in patients with normal renal function) ensures an adequate blood level of the contrast material and must be coordinated with rapid scanning using thin sections (3 to 5 mm) just before the peak of the vasculotubular phase of contrast excretion. Enhancement suggests relative vascularity of the tumor indicating that the lesion in question is likely to be a cancer, an adenoma, or an oncocytoma. Comparative control measurements of enhancement must be made to ensure quality control and rule out blush artifacts caused by a drift in settings between pre- and postcontrast scans. These should include sampling from an attenuated gallbladder and any adjacent renal cysts on both sequences in order to minimize unreliability. Use of a maximum milliampere setting increases the number of photons and reduces "noise." These and other aspects of high-quality CT imaging are comprehensively discussed elsewhere.[64,65] Bosniak has recommended that a lesion that registered more than 25 Hounsfield units and was greater than 1.5 cm in a young healthy individual should be treated as a potential neoplasm amenable to partial nephrectomy (as governed by anatomic location in the kidney). Approximately 10% of these will turn out to be oncocytomas, but the majority will be small renal cancers. On the other hand, follow-up imaging in patients with lesions smaller than 1.5 cm, and in those with significant comorbidity, relative renal insufficiency, or a life expectancy shorter than 10 years is economically unsound, for these lesions are unlikely to impact on the patient's life expectancy. In between these two extremes, patients should be reimaged at 6-month intervals in the first year and annually thereafter. Provided there is no demonstrable growth, an expectant policy may be continued. Appropriate reproducible and comparable settings are crucial and must be carefully selected at the outset for both baseline and follow-up scans. This will optimize the evaluation of change. Interval growth—be it slow (<1 cm per annum) or fast (≥1 cm per annum)—is ominous. Furthermore, it is important to remember that growth patterns differ, are not always linear, and may be exponential or occur in unpredictable spurts with periods of apparent remission. Lesion margination can also be better demonstrated on thin-cut CT. Well-marginated lesions in general are likely to be of low grade, while irregular ones are of higher grade and more likely to disseminate.

The clinical history is usually reliable, but one must be aware that patients who present with symptoms, signs, and scans that suggest a diagnosis of a small renal abscess may occasionally be found to harbor a tumor with a necrotic center. If such a lesion is not to be missed, follow-up scans are prudent after symptomatic resolution with an appropriate course of antibiotic treatment. Persistence of a complex cystic lesion at this time is an indication for needle biopsy.

When the presence of fat is suggested by the sonographic finding of an echogenic focus within a renal mass lesion, confirmation by CT must be sought. Fat, which is registered as a hypodense area within a renal mass on an unenhanced scan, usually excludes a diagnosis of renal cell cancer and is virtually pathognomonic of angiomyolipoma,[66] a hamartomatous lesion of the kidney composed of abundant thick-walled vessels devoid of an internal elastic lamina, variable amounts of spindle-shaped smooth muscle–like cells, and fat. The incidence of angiomyolipoma at routine autopsy is 0.3 to 2.1%. This diagnosis is even more certain in young adult females, and in those with a family history of phacomatoses or stigmata of tuberous sclerosis. Angiomyolipomas in women with the tuberous sclerosis complex are often multifocal, bilateral, and develop during late childhood. On occasion, patients with tuberous sclerosis may have coexistent cystic renal lesions that have the potential to harbor renal cell cancers.[67] The majority of patients with angiomyolipoma are female, have asymptomatic single lesions that are found during middle age, and do not have the tuberous sclerosis complex.

Symptoms most frequently attributed to angiomyolipomas include urinary, intralesional, or retroperitoneal hemorrhage; pain; a mass effect; and fever of unknown origin. Many studies have shown that tumor size correlates well with symptoms. CT is the diagnostic modality of choice and ultrasound can be used to follow small asymptomatic lesions after diagnosis. Occasionally, pitfalls can arise in the CT diagnosis of angiomyolipoma. Such is the case when the fat content is small but there is an abundance of smooth muscle and blood vessels. Here, the demonstration of small fatty areas requires focused thin-sectional imaging and careful measurement of Hounsfield units. If any dystrophic calcification is present in a fat-containing tumor, it is likely to be imaged adequately only by CT and may be missed by both ultrasound and MRI. This unusual finding is indicative that the tumor is most likely a carcinoma, and should not be dismissed as an angiomyolipoma.[68]

Uncertainty after such an examination requires surgical excision for pathologic examination. Rarely, renal cell carcinoma may produce peritumoral edema or hemorrhage, or encompass a small area of perirenal fat, but it must be remembered that CT is reliable only when fat is located within the tumor rather than at its periphery. Furthermore, these features are uncommon for small renal cell tumors, and consequently, the decision to advocate surgical excision and pathologic examination of large lesions is ensured when one considers the propensity for catastrophic hemorrhage for large angiomyolipomas.[69] The accurate preoperative characterization of an angiomyolipoma in this instance may, however, favor renal parenchymal sparing surgery. Conversely, when hemorrhage is the primary mode of presentation, as is often the case for both large renal cell cancers and angiomyolipomas, the characteristic features of the original tumor may be obscured by the hematoma contained within Gerota's space (Fig. 11–5) and nephrectomy is virtually always indicated. Other adult tumors that demonstrate fat content are liposarcomas, but these clearly have a perirenal location and the diagnosis is seldom in doubt. In children, the recent case report of a teratoid Wilms' tumor containing fat[70] is daunting though exceptional. It is well known that angiomyolipomas can be multifocal in origin and may involve not only one or both kidneys but also the regional lymph nodes, renal vein, and inferior vena cava, thereby mimicking an advanced renal cell cancer.[71,72] Cognizance of such a possibility in conjunction with CT scan information may raise suspicion to a point where intraoperative partial nephrectomy and frozen section may be electively undertaken as a planned procedure.

A tumor that is sharply marginated, bears no calcification, is isodense with a homogeneous pattern of enhancement, and demonstrates an area of central stellate scarring on CT, with lesser attenuation on both pre- and postcontrast scans, is most likely an oncocytoma, but even this appearance can be mimicked by a renal cell tumor. Furthermore, the two lesions may also coexist.[73] For the most part, hemorrhage, cystic degeneration, and necrosis are rare in an oncocytoma[73,74] and yet the assured distinction between these two entities by CT scan continues to be elusive.[75] The importance of such distinction between these lesions preoperatively is important in the asymptomatic patient with a small lesion to determine if surgical intervention is indicated at all and, if so, the urgency of the procedure. In the symptomatic patient and in those with diminished renal reserve with a single lesion, the choice once again lies between a renal parenchymal sparing approach and radical nephrectomy.

Lymphoma is another disease entity with a propensity for renal involvement (5% at initial staging and 33% at autopsy). Almost without exception, renal lymphoma does not occur in the absence of systemic lymphadenopathy, may have an invasive interstitial pattern, and may have distinctive CT enhancement characteristics (isodense on precontrast scans with reduced enhancement compared to renal parenchyma on postcontrast scans (see Table 11–2). Diffuse renal enlargement and expansion into the perinephric space are uncommon. If present, neovascularity is sparse and characterized by palisading vessels of small diameter. Non-Hodgkin's lymphoma is more common than Hodgkin's disease and renal involvement is usually discovered during a staging CT examination. The collecting system and ureter can either be encompassed by the retroperitoneal node mass (resulting in uni- or bilateral hydronephrosis), or displaced by it. Multiple renal masses are the rule,[76] and one or both kidneys can be synchronously involved, leaving little doubt of the diagnosis. However, renal cell carcinoma can occur, albeit infrequently in patients with lymphoma. A solitary solid renal mass in a patient with an established diagnosis of lymphoma is most likely to be a lymphoma, but doubt is cast by the presence of areas of cystic degeneration and necrosis. This is one of the few scenarios where CT-guided needle biopsy is indicated to determine the need for surgical excision. The other main indica-

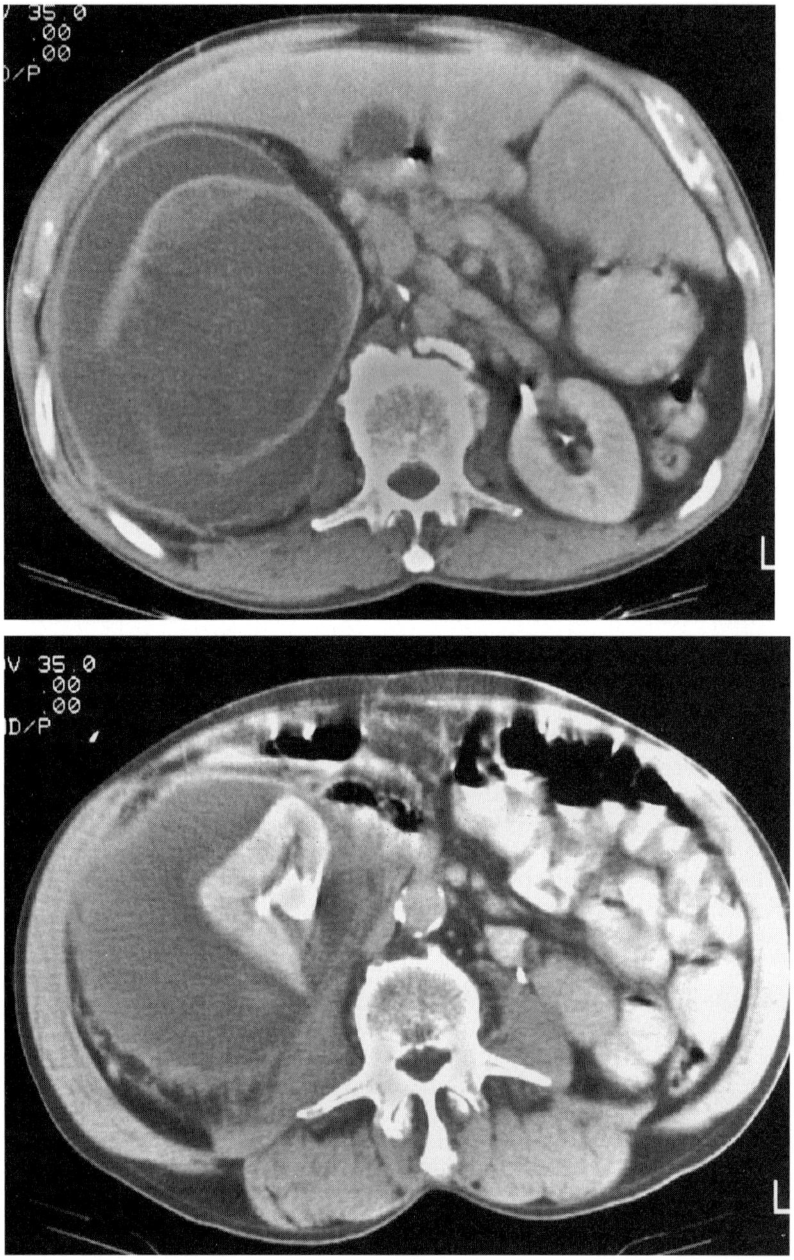
V 35.0
.00
.00
D/P
L

FIGURE 11–5. Tumor obscured by large retroperitoneal hematoma contained within Gerota's space.

tion for needle biopsy in this setting applies when lymphadenopathy regresses with chemotherapy, but the renal lesion persists. Some may justifiably recommend proceeding directly to nephrectomy for a large residual renal mass in this instance.

Renal sarcomata are uncommon in the overall spectrum of renal cancers and account for 1.1% of all malignant renal tumors. In the majority, the diagnosis can only be made from the microscopic examination of the nephrectomy specimen but might be suspected preoperatively if there is CT evidence in favor of an origin from the renal capsule or renal sinus, or if the tumor is large but hypovascular.

Adult Wilms' tumors are extremely rare as evidenced by the sporadic case reports in the literature.[77] They have no clinical or radiologic distinguishing features that are of practical significance and, once again, the diagnosis is one of unexpected surprise when the pathologist's report appears. Equally rare, fortunately, are the cancers that arise in adjacent structures or organs and extend with a contiguous growth pattern to invade the renal parenchyma, leaving doubt of the true organ of origin. Such can be the case for tumors of the pancreas, stomach, colonic flexures, adrenal, and retroperitoneum. Biopsy may be justified in the hope of discovering diagnostic information that may usefully contribute to a multimodal treatment strategy.

Finally, the possibility of renal involvement as a host site for metastatic cancer should not be forgotten, particularly when faced with multiple small parenchymal masses.[78] Metastases may also infil-

TABLE 11–2. TYPICAL CT VALUES FOR HOUNSFIELD UNITS FOR RENAL IMAGING

	Hounsfield Units	
Tissue	Unenhanced	Enhanced
Fat	0 to −100	No change
Fluid	0 to 20	No change
Fresh hematoma	30 to 70	No change
Old blood	10 to 20	No change
High attenuation cyst	50 to 90	No change
Muscle	30 to 35	40 to 45
Lymphoma	10 to 25	No change
Renal parenchyma	20 to 25	200 to 300
Renal cancer	20 to 35	40 to 90

trate the perinephric space. Even after excluding high-risk groups, sporadic renal cell cancer itself can be multifocal (16% incidence in one prospective analysis).[79] Secondary deposits from nonlymphomatous primary tumors (Table 11–1) must be excluded in the presence of such a finding in those with a prior history of other advanced malignancy. Indeed, in this selected group, metastases outnumbered renal cell carcinoma by a ratio of 4:1. Moreover, it is highly unlikely that a renal cell cancer in this situation is likely to impact on the patient's expected survival. Carcinomas of the bronchus (both squamous and adenocarcinoma) and breast can cause large solitary renal deposits, while colon cancer has the propensity to produce an exophytic renal lesion.[78] The indications for radical nephrectomy or diagnostic biopsy are tenuous and only apply to those with an occult primary or those with a prior history of locoregional cancer that has been successfully treated or is in remission, and in whom there is no other evidence of metastatic disease at the time that the solitary renal lesion is discovered.

SPIRAL CT

This technique utilizes rapid continuous volume data acquisition by combining continuous patient transport and scanner rotation during a single-breath-hold, in a bid to eliminate respiratory misregistration (imaging gaps between individual CT sections resulting from variations in the subject's tidal volumes).[80] In this way, three-dimensional surface topography of renal tumors and surrounds can be reconstructed through the use of software algorithms. Postcontrast enhancement is essential as is the selection of the phase of enhancement (vascular, nephrographic, and pyelographic) if small renal cell cancers are to be discovered; therefore, the limitations previously discussed in this chapter pertaining to the use of contrast agents in CT scanning apply. Furthermore, partial voluming is minimized only when slice thickness is at least one half that of the lesion in question. Manual editing of the segmented data even when performed by a skilled radiologist can take up to 2 hours and this in itself limits more than occasional use. At first glance, it would appear that the three-dimensional image did not improve on the diagnostic information provided by the two-dimensional images and may even be deficient with regard to spatial resolution and attenuation. Silverman and associates[81] reported that of the 35 lesions in their study where pathologic correlation was available, 17% of the masses surgically excised were benign, and certainly there was no advantage in characterizing lesions with borderline enhancement or multiple septations. On the other hand, enthusiasts of the technique have suggested that ease of perception of hilar vasculature and its relationship to the tumor, by the surgeon, may facilitate adequate tumor clearance and optimize nephron-sparing surgery where this is appropriate.[82] Comparative data between this variation and conventional high-quality CT is not available at this time, and until such time as these studies are performed, it is hard to justify wider diagnostic application of this new technique for renal cell cancer.

MAGNETIC RESONANCE IMAGING

Magnetic resonance imaging, the youngest of the noninvasive imaging technologies, has been available for over a decade. Although it has become an invaluable tool in the diagnosis and staging of many human cancers, the early promise of this modality in imaging the abdomen and its contents has not been fulfilled, particularly for organs that are mobile with respiration. CT is undoubtedly still the most popular diagnostic modality, for it is less expensive (although the cost differential has steadily declined), widely available, and has standardized imaging parameters for better spatial resolution. Nevertheless, MRI does have a definite place in the diagnostic armamentarium, primarily when there is renal impairment, a strong history of iodinated contrast reaction, and when CT has been indeterminate or there is a contraindication to the use of ionizing radiation. The disadvantage of claustrophobia has been overcome by modern open magnet machines, and yet long acquisition times require considerable patient cooperation if motion artifacts are not to spoil the quality of the acquired images. The sensitivity of MRI was refined with the contribution of special pulse sequences and has been further improved by the use of the intravenous contrast agent gadopentetate dimeglumine. The safety and tolerance of this agent in patients with chronic renal insufficiency has also been firmly established.[83,84] The multiplanar capacity of imaging in sagittal, coronal, or angled radial planes may be useful in determining the organ of origin if this is in doubt after CT. Unfortunately, despite high-resolution, multiplanar imaging capability and the ability to detect vascularity without contrast enhancement, MRI is plagued by similarities in signal intensity from cancerous and normal parenchyma on both T1- and T2-weighted unenhanced spin-echo sequenced images, limiting its usefulness in both detection and diagnosis of small renal cell tumors.

The hardware specifications desired of state-of-the-art MRI imaging for indeterminate renal tumors are incorporation of a 1.5-T (tesla)-unit electromagnet for high signal-to-noise ratio from increased chemical shift and software versatility that enables variations in imaging parameters. This combination of features can reduce the shortcomings of conventional spin-echo sequences. New fast sequences with respiratory gating (single breath-hold), such as enhanced gradient-echo fast low-angle shot (FLASH), spoiled gradient-recalled acquisition in steady state (spoiled-GRASS), and those that enable fat suppression (FS) or water suppression (WS) but require a longer acquisition time, are currently being tested. Corticomedullary differentiation, if desired to distinguish between masses of extrarenal or intrarenal origin (e.g., adrenal or renal), is most apparent on the immediate postcontrast FLASH image after rapid whole-organ coverage. A wider bandwidth for gradient techniques reduces chemical shift artifact and minimizes edge misregistration that can mask small cortical lesions. The main drawback of the breath-hold imaging method is that signal-to-noise ratios and spatial resolution are reduced.

The FS technique reduces chemical shift and respiratory artifact from high-signal-intensity fat in the abdominal wall. Contrast-to-noise ratio between renal parenchyma and surrounding fat is thereby reduced on T2-weighted and gadolinium-enhanced sequences. Consequently, better definition of tumor margins and cyst homogeneity can be attained. In reality, however, artifactual inconsistencies may still occur because of field inhomogeneities, shimming errors, etc., and it is therefore important to remember that the measurement of ipsilateral control values from adjacent tissues (liver, which enhances with Gd-DTPA, and psoas muscle, which does not enhance) other than the organ of interest is an essential part of the examination for the purpose of quality control.

Gadopentetate dimeglumine is excreted exclusively by the kidney and thereby allows enhancement of both the renal parenchyma and vascular tumors through equilibration in the extracellular fluid space. It persists in the nephrons longer and with greater uniformity than it does in the interstitial spaces of renal cell tumors. Consequently, the detection of smaller tumors may be improved, but does not exceed that of CT. Conversely, a uniformly high-signal-intensity cortical blush on dynamic images may hide a small renal cancer. As with CT, no single MRI sequence is error-free in the accurate diagnosis of small renal lesions. Identical imaging parameters must be judiciously selected and reproduced before and after contrast enhancement. Thin sections appropriate to the size of the lesion in

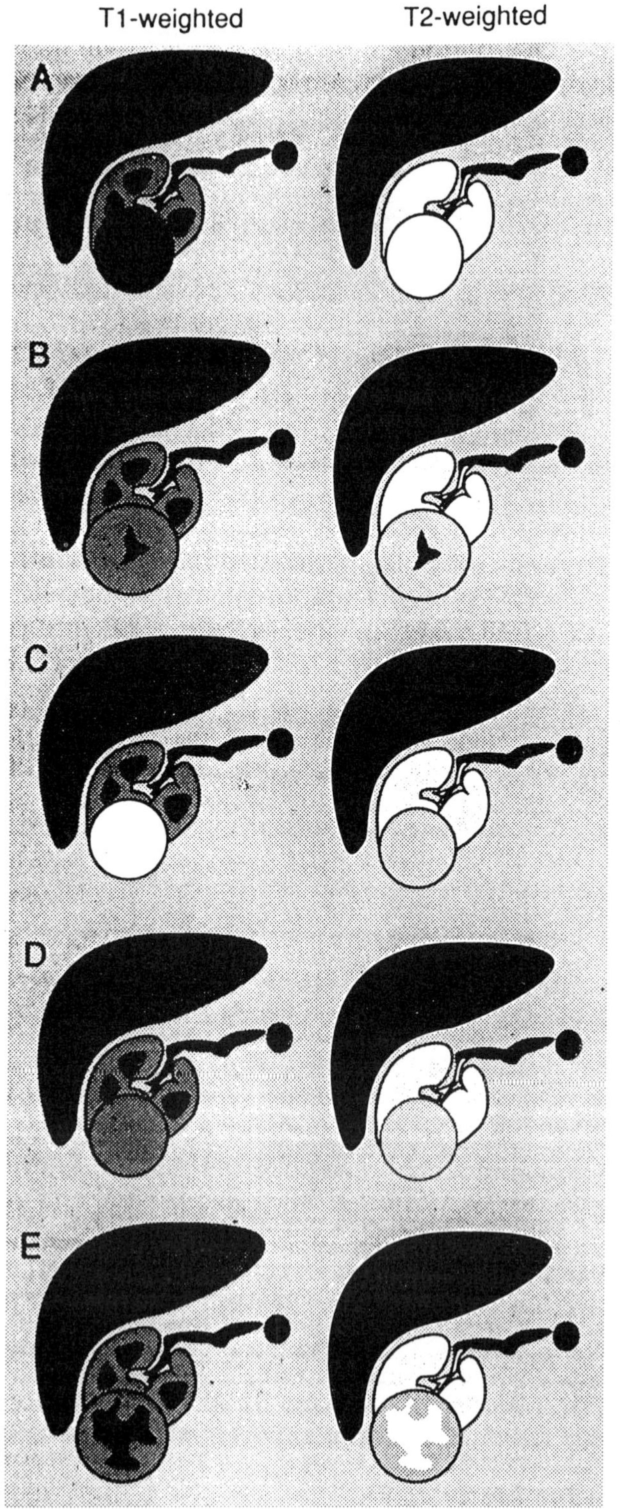
T1-weighted
T2-weighted
A
B
C
D
E

FIGURE 11–6. MRI findings in different renal masses. *A*, Simple cyst. *B*, Oncocytoma. *C*, Angiomyolipoma. *D*, Renal carcinoma. *E*, Necrotic renal carcinoma or metastasis. (From Barbaric ZL: Principles of Genitourinary Radiology, 2nd edition. New York, Thieme Medical Publishers, Inc, 1994. Copyright Thieme Medical Publishers, 1994, with permission.)

question must be judiciously selected and reproduced before and after contrast enhancement in order to minimize loss of definition from partial voluming effects. These features may be useful both when attempting to distinguish between cystic renal cancers and benign complex cysts by the demonstration of absence of contrast enhancement in the benign lesions, and when distinguishing a renal cell carcinoma with hemorrhagic cystic areas from a hemorrhagic cyst. In the study of patients selected because of contraindications to CT imaging, Rominger and associates[85] found that of the nine patients with cystic lesions that did not enhance after gadolinium, none went on to develop malignant features on subsequent imaging, but the follow-up in their study was short (2 to 20 months) and their findings are yet to be corroborated in a larger series of patients. The presence of an enhancing thick irregular wall in a lesion with cystic appearance is always an ominous sign. In a complicated cyst, protein or hemorrhage often alters signal intensity (Table 11–2), but this cannot always be appreciated on CT alone. Since oxyhemoglobin is diamagnetic and consequently has little effect on signal intensity, the appearance of hemorrhage (high intensity on T1-weighted images and low intensity on T2-weighted images) can be related to para- or superparamagnetic properties of hemoglobin breakdown products. Signal intensity can be seen to evolve and change over time as the hematoma ages. Calcification, on the other hand, requires CT and cannot be readily demonstrated with MRI, an important limitation of the technique. A prospectively evaluated contrast-enhanced comparison of CT and MRI (T1, FS, and FLASH) showed no difference in detection rates for renal tumors.[86] Unfortunately, the majority of such studies have not utilized thin-sectional (3 mm) imaging during CT scanning for the purposes of comparison. Typical T1- and T2-weighted MRI appearances of kidney lesions commonly encountered are depicted in Figure 11–6.

TABLE 11–3. ANGIOGRAPHIC CHARACTERISTICS OF KIDNEY TUMORS

Renal Cell Cancer
Hypervascularity (88%)
Neovascularity
Random distribution of vessels
Perivascular cuffing
Irregularity of vessel caliber and branching pattern
Arteriovenous shunting with early filling of the renal vein (causes high-output cardiac failure in 5% of patients with large tumors)
Parasitization of extrarenal vasculature
Accentuation of capsular vessels
Feeding vessels that have diminished vascoconstrictive response to intra-arterial epinephrine
Hypovascularity (17%)
Avascularity (5%)
Multilocular Cystic Nephroma
Septal neovascularity in wall
Oncocytoma
Spoke wheel pattern
Angiomyolipoma
Hypervascular without perivascular cuffing
Small aneurysms
Venous lakes with swirled appearance
Lymphoma
Hypovascular—sparse neovascularity
Palisading vessels around intralobular arteries
Irregular renal outline
Adult Wilms' Tumor
Hypovascular
Neovascularity
Fine zig-zag ("spaghetti") pattern
Creeping vine pattern
No arteriovenous shunting
Liposarcoma
As for angiomyolipoma but with arterial encasement
Reninoma
Hypovascular lesion
Absent renal artery stenosis in the presence of hypertension and secondary aldosteronism
Metastases
Angiographic characteristics mimic that of primary tumor

ANGIOGRAPHY

The place of angiography, once an important diagnostic technique for renal cell cancer, has dwindled in the face of competition from the new noninvasive imaging modalities. Comparisons of the cost versus benefits of this investigation are limited at the present time. The Seldinger technique with aortic flush is still used, followed by selective and subselective catheterization of main and branch segmental renal arteries as indicated in the individual case. Both kidneys are thus imaged. Tumor characteristics that assist in the correct identification of renal cell cancer by angiography are listed in Table 11–3.

Some have deemed CT to be more sensitive to the flow of contrast material than arteriography, on the basis that a negative arteriogram can be discounted in the face of a lesion that enhances by 10 to 25 Hounsfield units on CT scan. On the other hand, it can be superior to CT on those rare occasions when renal failure precludes adequate excretion of intravenous contrast. Nowadays angiography is mainly used to plan parenchymal sparing surgery ("road-mapping") in patients with small tumors and those with a low functional renal reserve (e.g., solitary kidney). Diagnosis can be combined with therapeutic occlusion of arterial tumor feeding vessels as a pre-emptive maneuver to limit intraoperative blood loss when faced with a large hypervascular tumor. In patients unsuitable for surgical treatment, angiography also permits palliative embolization and reduces life-threatening hematuria or perinephric hemorrhage (a technique useful both for renal cell cancer and angiomyolipomas <4 cm). It has been surpassed by nuclear scintigraphy and CT when distinguishing true tumors from pseudotumors in a scarred kidney.

RADIOISOTOPIC IMAGING

Renal imaging with radionuclide tracers has been popular because it can provide quantifiable physiologic information complementary to the anatomic information provided by other imaging tests. The sensitivity of imaging space-occupying lesions of the renal parenchyma with technetium-99m (^{99m}Tc) dimercaptosuccinic acid (DMSA) and ^{99m}Tc-glucoheptonate is improved by the single photon emission CT (SPECT) technique, which can incorporate single-, double-, and triple-headed machines. Dynamic studies can be used to demonstrate intralesional blood pooling. Gallium (Ga) -67 citrate is considered to be an important tumor-seeking radiopharmaceutical for lymphomas and may be a useful adjunct in the characterization of a sonolucent or hypodense renal lesion. The AIDS epidemic has had a significant impact on this disease, for the incidence of non-Hodgkin's lymphoma in these patients has increased 60-fold over that in the general population and Burkitt's lymphoma is 1000 times more common. Unfortunately, gallium scans in this select group may be confounded by renal parenchymal infection or inflammation; by the use of nephrotoxic, recreational, antibiotic, and chemotherapeutic agents; and by collecting system obstruction, any of which can cause gallium uptake,[87,88] limiting its usefulness in the diagnosis of renal cell carcinoma. However, patients with high gallium uptakes in renal tumors were found to have higher grade lesions with a poor prognosis, often from advanced disease.[89]

The tagging of radionuclides onto specific monoclonal antitumor antibodies has sought to open new horizons in diagnostic nuclear oncology by overcoming the lack of sensitivity and specificity of many popular renal radiopharmaceuticals. A variety of antibodies raised against tubular glycoprotein antigens from human renal cell cancers have been tested (Table 11–4), with the hope that not only will they improve upon diagnostic imaging but also will enable tissue-specific targeted therapy. Unfortunately, encouraging results from animal models have not been realized in phase I human trials.[90,91]

TABLE 11–4. RENAL CELL CANCER ANTIGEN–ANTIBODY COMPLEXES TESTED IN AUTORADIOGRAPHIC IMAGING

120-kDa adenosine deaminase binding glycoprotein expressed in 90% proximal tubules and loops of Henle–S23 (IgG1 murine antibody)
115-kDa glycoprotein expressed only in RCC–^{131}I–S22 (IgG2 murine antibody)
Renal cell tumor line G250–IgG1 murine antibody

POSITRON EMISSION TOMOGRAPHY (PET) SCANNING

In the last few years, after initial studies in the murine xenograft model, autoradiographic imaging has evolved to take advantage of differences in regional glucose metabolism between a variety of tumors and host tissue. Malignant cells are recognized to have increased glycolytic metabolism in comparison to their normal or benign counterparts. After uptake of the D-glucose analog 2-deoxy-2[18F]fluoro-D-glucose (FDG) and 6-phosphorylation by intracellular hexokinase, the substrate is metabolically trapped within the tumor cell. This substrate accumulation is accentuated in cancer cells that are deficient in glucose-6-phosphatase activity, enabling both high uptake and retention of the tracer, which translates into a better separation of tumor and normal parenchyma. The most cost-effective use of this exciting new modality for the urologic imaging of renal cell cancer is in the detection of occult primary lesions and the localization of metastatic sites.[93] Renal vein involvement and lymphatic metastases have also been accurately demonstrated by Wahl and colleagues in a small series of five patients.[93] More recently, the urologic indications for PET scanning in patients with an established diagnosis of renal cell cancer have increased to include the confirmation of tumor recurrence in the renal bed (when fibrosis is a possibility) or in local nodes after radical nephrectomy (Fig. 11–7), and to localize metastases in normal sized nodes. It may even enable evaluation of responses to systemic treatment of local recurrences or advanced disseminated disease in the future. Other applications of PET scanning may lie in selecting out patients unsuitable for partial nephrectomy by identifying multifocal disease in the affected kidney. Clearly the early promise of this new modality must be confirmed in a larger series of patients and prospectively tested in the murky waters of upper tract obstruction (particularly as FDG is excreted into the urine and would accumulate in a baggy renal pelvis to confound the interpretation of PET images), the differentiation of complex cysts from cystic cancers, and the distinction between scarring and local recurrence. Whether lesions such as oncocytomas can be discerned from renal cell cancer by this technique is as yet unknown.

THE ROLE OF PERCUTANEOUS NEEDLE ASPIRATION AND BIOPSY IN THE DIAGNOSIS OF RENAL CELL CANCER

In situations where indeterminate renal lesions are identified by conventional imaging, invasive percutaneous sampling has been abandoned as a routine procedure for a variety of extremely good reasons other than the obvious concern of breaching natural tumor barriers with the risk of seeding cancer cells in the needle track. The risk of such a mishap occurring is reportedly small, but it is likely that the true incidence is underestimated.[94] Should

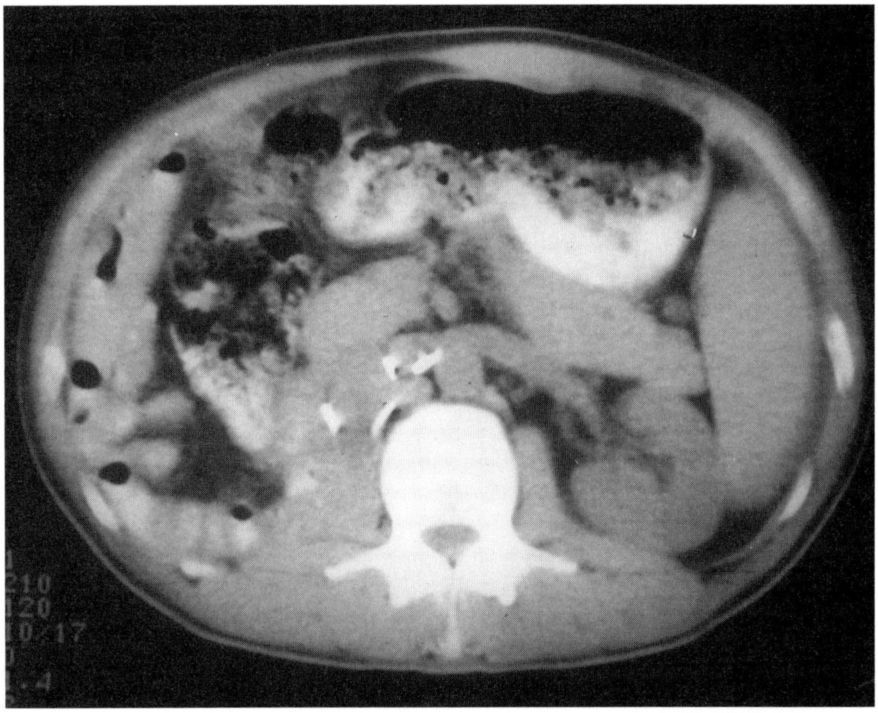

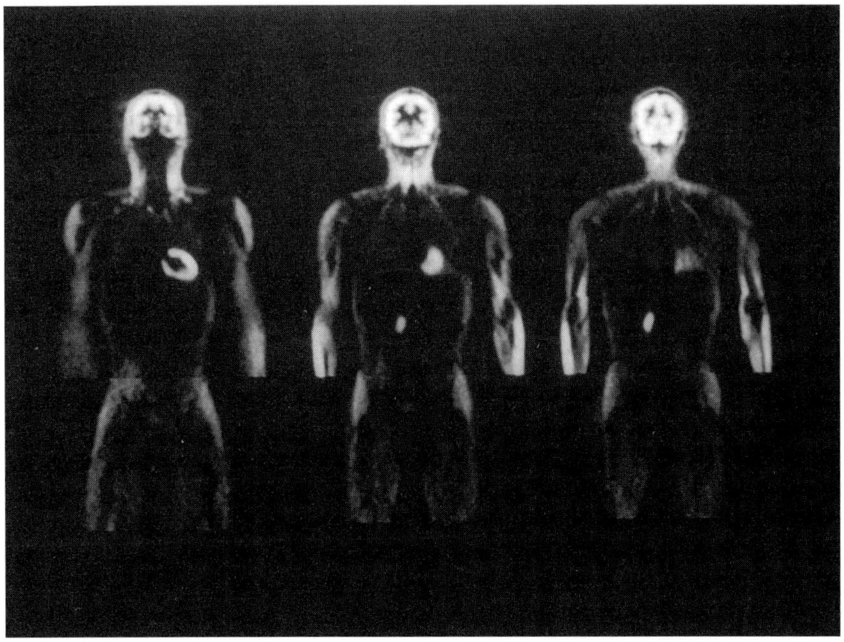

FIGURE 11–7. PET scan showing tumor recurrence in local nodes after right nephrectomy when abdominal CT scan has been indeterminate. (PET scan courtesy of Dr. Carl Hoh, Department of Nuclear Medicine, UCLA School of Medicine.)

this calamity happen, the opportunity of surgically curing a potentially organ-confined renal cancer will have been squandered irretrievably. Although fine-needle aspiration or biopsy of the kidney under ultrasound or CT guidance is regarded as a relatively safe and quick procedure, it is not entirely without risk (bleeding and arteriovenous fistulation). The main argument against the routine biopsy of a solid renal mass, however, lies in the twin possibilities of equivocal or false-negative results from a sampling error. Furthermore, if the imaging modalities previously discussed in this chapter cannot distinguish between a renal cell cancer and an oncocytoma, the mere presence of oncocytes in a core biopsy should not be greeted with relief, for it is well known that oncocytic features may be contained within the more ominous of these two solid renal tumors (Fig. 11–8). Unfortunately, the addition of DNA ploidy studies has not proved useful either.[95]

The indications for percutaneous biopsy of a renal mass that are listed in Table 11–5 have been refined over the years and are specific to those situations where a positive discrimination between a renal cell cancer and an indolent renal tumor is likely to spare the patient who is a high surgical

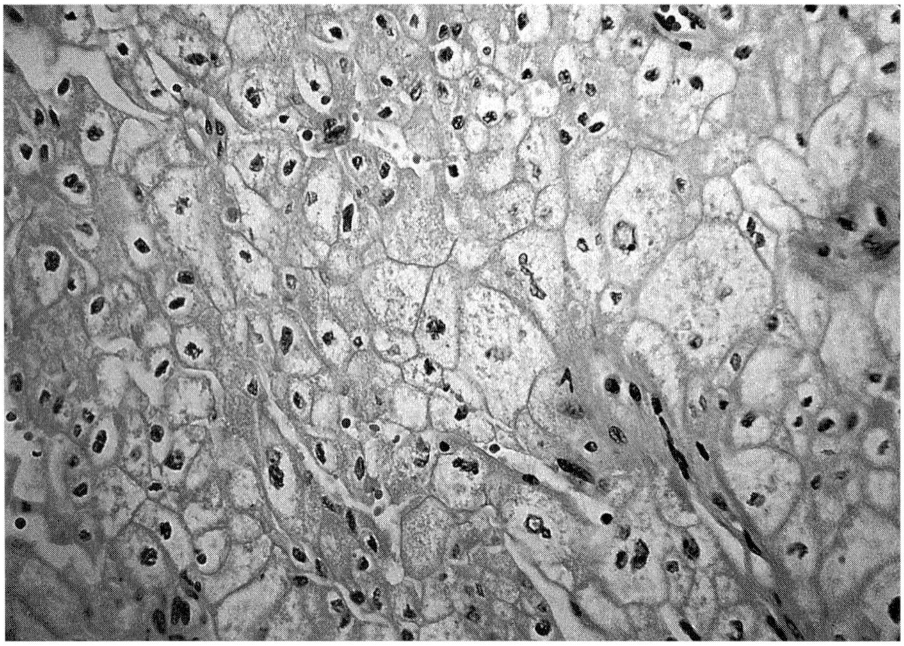

FIGURE 11–8. Oncocytic cells in a renal cell tumor. (Hematoxylin and eosin stain, magnification ×78.)

risk from the rigors of an unnecessary operation or allow the elective preservation of precious functioning parenchyma in the face of a limited functional reserve.

Many malignant cysts can contain small foci of well-differentiated cancer and would not be expected to shed a sufficient number of malignant cells to confirm the diagnosis at needle aspiration. It must be noted that a bloody fluid aspirate from an indeterminate cystic lesion increases suspicion of cancer but clear fluid with a negative Papanicolaou smear does not exclude it. Several aspirations are inevitably needed if multiple loculations are present. It is unknown whether visually targeted laparoscopic excision biopsy of a complex cyst wall and frozen section will reliably improve diagnostic accuracy in difficult cases. Although this procedure is undoubtedly feasible and can be combined with electrosurgical or laser fulguration of the cyst wall should it prove to harbor low-grade superficial malignancy, the risk of tumor spillage and local recurrence has not made it attractive other than in exceptional circumstances.

The diagnostic pathways recommended for an indeterminate solid renal mass are summarized in Figure 11–9.

RENAL CELL CANCER—STAGING

Once the diagnosis of renal cell cancer has been reached, attention is turned to staging the disease. In this way, appropriate steps in management can be orchestrated to optimize treatment outcome and prognostic information can be related to the individual patient. Historically, two staging systems, the Robson classification, which was introduced in 1968 as a modification of the system of Flocks and Kadesky (Fig. 11–10), and more recently, the TNM (tumor, node, and metastases) classification advocated by the International Union Against Cancer (UICC) (Table 11–6), have proved to be popular in this regard. The latter, which is predominantly used in modern practice, has compensated for deficiencies in older systems by accounting for primary tumor size and different degrees of lymphatic and venous extension, but is still by no means perfect in the prediction of outcomes. As with many other cancers, there is a discrepancy between the accuracy of clinical and pathologic staging, which remains difficult to overcome.

TABLE 11–5. INDICATIONS FOR PERCUTANEOUS BIOPSY OF AN INDETERMINATE RENAL MASS

When a renal lesion is present in a patient with a lymphoma or persists after the remainder of the disease bulk regresses with systemic chemotherapy
When trying to distinguish between a primary and a secondary lesion of the kidney in a patient with other malignancy
When trying to differentiate between an infected cyst or chronic abscess and a cystic or infected solid renal cancer (n.b., several aspirations will be required)
When a discernible solid parenchymal abnormality persists after appropriate antibiotic therapy of a renal abscess

ACCURACY OF STAGING FOR LOCAL AND REGIONAL DISEASE

The extent of the preoperative evaluation in surgical candidates as far as blood work and imaging

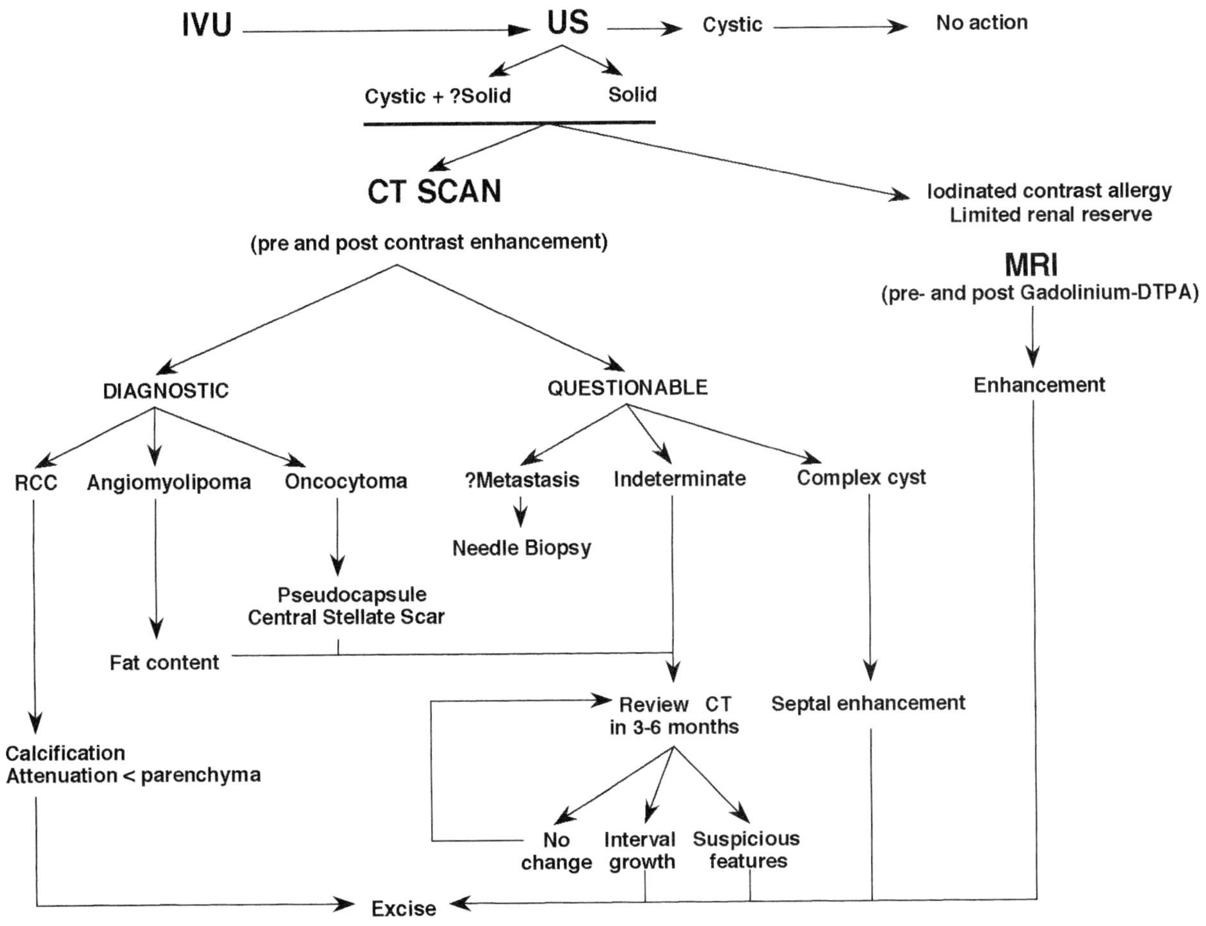
IVU
US
Cystic
No action
Cystic + ?Solid
Solid
CT SCAN
(pre and post contrast enhancement)
Iodinated contrast allergy
Limited renal reserve
MRI
(pre- and post Gadolinium-DTPA)
DIAGNOSTIC
QUESTIONABLE
Enhancement
RCC
Angiomyolipoma
Oncocytoma
?Metastasis
Indeterminate
Complex cyst
Needle Biopsy
Pseudocapsule
Central Stellate Scar
Fat content
Review CT
in 3-6 months
Septal enhancement
Calcification
Attenuation < parenchyma
No change
Interval growth
Suspicious features
Excise

FIGURE 11–9. Algorithm for diagnosis of a renal mass.

are concerned must be tempered by an awareness of the positive or negative yield of each test as well as its cost effectiveness. Tests should be selected only if they are likely to alter the management of the patient (Fig. 11–11).

If the diagnosis of renal cell cancer was made incidentally by ultrasound or CT, excretory urography adds little further useful staging information. Rarely can sonography be used as the sole staging modality. It has long been superseded by contrast-enhanced CT scanning techniques. Towards the end of the last decade, the accuracy of ultrasound had been compared favorably to that of CT with regard to T-stage.[96] However, this was prior to the advent of dynamic CT[97] and contrast-enhanced MRI. Sonography has certainly been utilized as an adjunct when CT findings were suboptimal or ambivalent. Problems arise with the identification of regional lymphatic disease due to overlying bowel gas if transperitoneal imaging is attempted, and intervening echogenic tumor and/or renal sinus fat if retroperitoneal imaging is desired.

The meticulous use of CT for staging renal cell cancer yields an accuracy of 90% or more.[98] To a great extent, errors in locoregional clinical staging can be correlated to tumor size (being greater for large tumors), but occasionally, a small peripherally located high-grade lesion that has poor margination and a propensity for micrometastases may also be understaged. Preoperative differentiation of stage T1 and T2 lesions is probably not critical for practical purposes, since the surgical management is the same for both. The exception to this rule is when a renal-sparing procedure is being considered. The only CT sign that correlates well with extracapsular tumor spread is the presence of discrete soft tissue masses at least 1 cm in diameter in Gerota's space. The sensitivity of this finding is low in T2 lesions (46%) but the specificity is 98%. Other findings such as stranding or cob-webbing, obliteration of perinephric fat, and visualization of collateral vessels in this location are less reliable, as indicated by the finding of demonstrable perinephric stranding in 50% of stage I patients in the study group of Johnson and coworkers. Fascial thickening is often due to direct tumor spread but can also occur from remote inflammation, reactive edema, and hyperemia, particularly when a large primary is present. Another difficult issue for CT in local staging is the problem of abuttal with adjacent organs such as the liver and second part of the duodenum and the question of contiguous invasion,

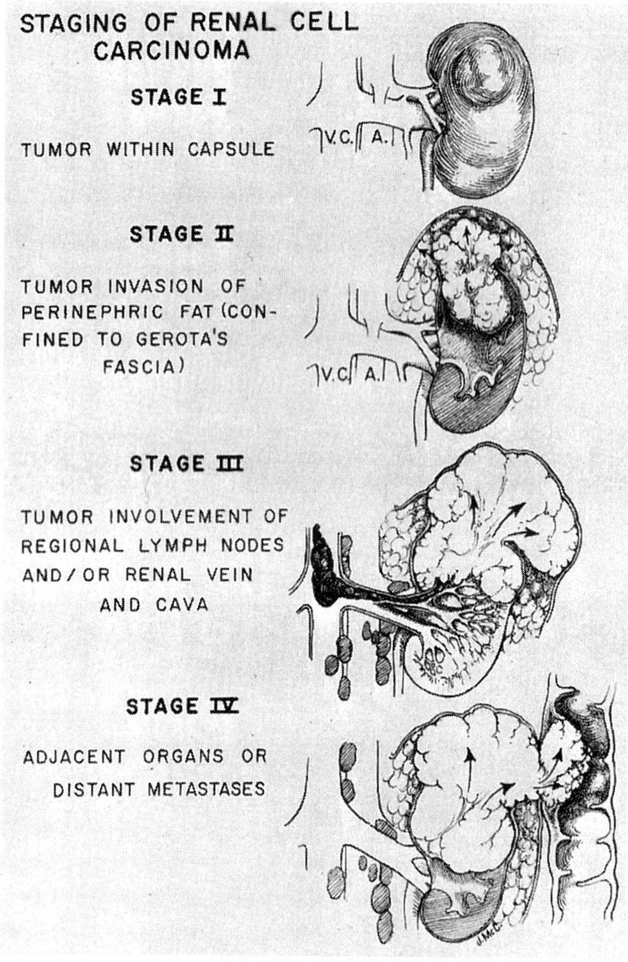
STAGING OF RENAL CELL CARCINOMA
STAGE I
TUMOR WITHIN CAPSULE
V.C.
A.
STAGE II
TUMOR INVASION OF PERINEPHRIC FAT (CONFINED TO GEROTA'S FASCIA)
V.C.
A.
STAGE III
TUMOR INVOLVEMENT OF REGIONAL LYMPH NODES AND / OR RENAL VEIN AND CAVA
STAGE IV
ADJACENT ORGANS OR DISTANT METASTASES

FIGURE 11–10. Robson classification for the staging of renal cell cancer. (From deKernion JB, Belldegrun A: Surgery of the kidney. *In* Walsh PC, Retik AB, Stamey TA, Vaughan ED Jr [eds.]: Campbell's Urology, 6th edition, p 1073. Philadelphia, WB Saunders Co, 1992, with permission.)

TABLE 11–6. COMPARISON OF STAGING SYSTEMS*,†

TNM Clinical Classification

T	Primary tumor
TX	Primary tumor cannot be assessed
TO	No evidence of primary tumor
T1	Tumor 2.5 cm or less in greatest dimension, limited to the kidney
T2	Tumor more than 2.5 cm in greatest dimension, limited to the kidney
T3	Tumor extends into major veins or invades adrenal gland or perinephric tissues but not beyond Gerota's fascia
T3a	Tumor invades adrenal gland or perinephric tissues but not beyond Gerota's fascia
T3b	Tumor grossly extends into renal vein(s) or vena cava
T4	Tumor invades beyond Gerota's fascia
N	Regional lymph nodes
NO	No identifiable nodes in a specified clinical assessment
N1	Metastasis in single lymph node, 2 cm or less in greatest dimension
N2	Metastasis in single lymph node, 2 cm but not more than 5 cm in greatest dimension; in multiple lymph nodes, none more than 5 cm in greatest dimension
N3	Metastasis in a lymph node more than 5 cm in greatest dimension
M	Distant metastasis
MO	Tumors without distant metastasis
M1	Tumors with distant metastasis
G	Histopathologic grading
G1	Well differentiated
G2	Moderately differentiated
G3–G4	Undifferentiated, anaplastic

Stage Grouping

Stage I	T1	NO	MO
Stage II	T2	NO	MO
Stage III	T1	N1	MO
	T2	N1	MO
	T3a	NO, N1	MO
	T3b	NO, N1	MO
Stage IV	T4	Any N	MO
	Any T	N2, N3	MO
	Any T	Any N	M1

*Adapted from International Union Against Cancer: Hermanek P, Sobin LH (eds): TNM Classification of Malignant Tumors, 4th edition. Berlin, Springer-Verlag, 1987.

†The regional lymph nodes are the hilar, abdominal para-aortic, and paracaval nodes. Laterality does not affect the N categories.

particularly for bulky right-sided upper pole tumors. Whether multiplanar tangential imaging with MRI will enable better separation of thinned, stretched but intact tissue planes remains to be seen, for although fat planes can be visualized on T2-weighted sequences, compressed congested liver segments may cause enough signal changes to mimic direct invasion. Spontaneous perinephric hemorrhage from a renal cell cancer adds yet another confounding element to the accuracy of local clinical staging regardless of modality. Local staging accuracy improves, however, with locally advanced disease.

LYMPH NODE METASTASES

The correct identification of lymph node metastases on CT scan or MRI cannot be based on demonstrable abnormalities of internal architecture and therefore relies upon an arbitrary size threshold of 1 cm. Using this criterion for CT scans, the false-negative rate from microscopic metastases is low (4%),[99] while the positive rate has varied from 3 to 43%,[98,100,101] and was higher in patients with demonstrable tumor necrosis and venous extension as a consequence of reactive hyperplasia.[99] Nodal asymmetry is also unreliable, for the left and middle periaortic channels are often fused, resulting in a larger nodal group than that on the right. Thus isolated enlargement in the right pararenal region might be of significance, but too often, this is obscured by ventral tumoral overhang and partial volume effect. MRI is only superior to CT when attempting to distinguish lymphadenopathy from a cluster of small vessels.[100] The unenhanced MRI appearance of lymph nodes on T1-weighted images

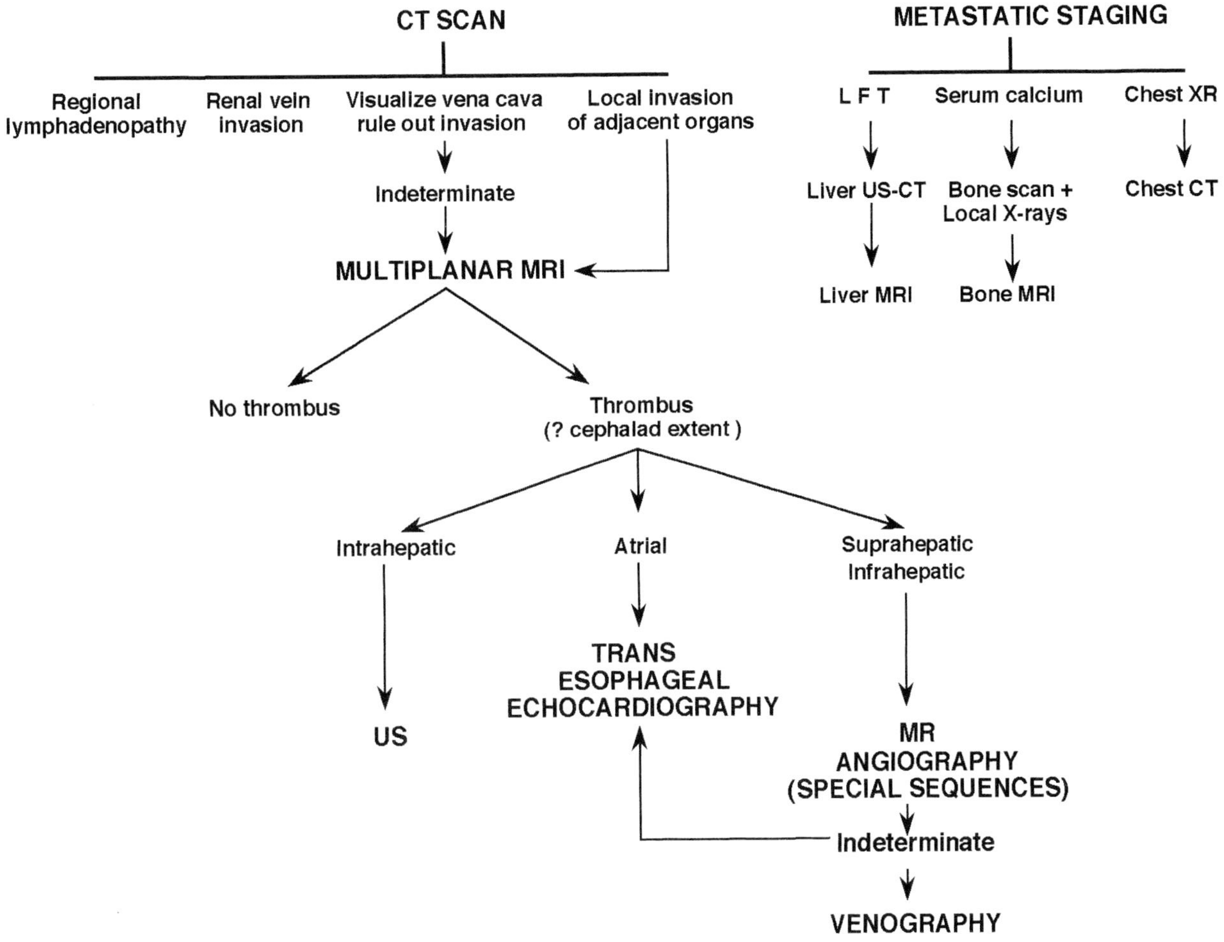
CT SCAN
Regional lymphadenopathy
Renal vein invasion
Visualize vena cava rule out invasion
Local invasion of adjacent organs
Indeterminate
MULTIPLANAR MRI
No thrombus
Thrombus (? cephalad extent)
Intrahepatic
Atrial
Suprahepatic Infrahepatic
US
TRANS ESOPHAGEAL ECHOCARDIOGRAPHY
MR ANGIOGRAPHY (SPECIAL SEQUENCES)
Indeterminate
VENOGRAPHY
METASTATIC STAGING
L F T
Serum calcium
Chest XR
Liver US-CT
Bone scan + Local X-rays
Chest CT
Liver MRI
Bone MRI

FIGURE 11–11. Algorithm for staging of renal cell cancer.

of low to medium signal intensity surrounded by high-intensity fat is optimal. An increase in signal intensity after gadolinium contrast enhancement on T1 sequences is counterproductive, for there is less contrast-to-noise ratio, making a nodal cluster less easily recognized. On T2-weighted images, nodes have a high signal intensity.

Lastly, it must be remembered that angiomyolipoma can be multifocal and occur in regional lymph nodes as well as the renal parenchyma and the vena cava. Gadolinium enhancement may be of value to demonstrate lympathic pooling of contrast in the rare instances when CT is indeterminate and this possibility is entertained.

DETECTION OF VENOUS INVASION

Renal cell carcinoma has a unique propensity for extension into the renal vein and beyond into the inferior vena and even, on occasion, into the right atrium. Although this finding has been associated with a higher incidence of recurrences and metastatic disease, the same sinister prognosis does not apply to those in whom only microscopic venous invasion is seen at pathologic examination of the surgical specimen. Unfortunately, this distinction is seldom accounted for in the majority of staging systems currently in use. In a recent report from the National Institutes of Health, Horan and colleagues[102] cited an incidence of 39% for renal vein involvement at operation and 25% for caval extension. Larger historical series have reported lower rates of between 4 and 10%.[103,104] Success with inferior vena cavotomy and tumor thrombectomy have been reported as long ago as the beginning of this century.[105] The relatively better outcomes after complete surgical clearance in patients with venous invasion alone, as opposed to those with lymphatic invasion only, serve to reinforce the importance of accurate venous staging. Hence, a thorough knowledge of the extent of venous involvement is imperative if adequate preoperative preparations are to be undertaken and the optimal surgical approach for safe en bloc tumor thrombectomy can then be carefully planned. In this respect, the relationship of the cephalad extent of the tumor thrombus to the hepatic veins and the right atrium is critical. Imaging techniques have been tried in abundance to clarify the presence and upper limit of tumor thrombus, and yet each has been found to be wanting in one respect or another, especially when diaphragmatic and cardiac movement causes blurring during image acquisition.

In a bid to avoid doubly invasive superior and inferior venacavography and the small but definite potential morbidity of femoral or jugular catheter venipuncture, modern imaging techniques have been tested and compared prospectively to this time-honored standard. Ultrasound is usually the first choice, is cheap to perform, but can be limited by the skills of the operator and build of the patient. It can produce excellent visualization of the intrahepatic inferior vena cava (100% sensitivity) and the right atrium, but is less good at imaging the renal vein and the infrahepatic vena cava (68 to 96% sensitivity and 97 to 100% specificity). Unfortunately, it can be technically inadequate in up to 26% of cases, particularly for left-sided tumors where the renal vein is harder to visualize. MRI, on the other hand, has sensitivity ranging from 82 to 100% and a specificity of 85 to 97%, but is hampered by its expense. Although it can be used theoretically without limitation in patients with contrast allergy or renal failure, long acquisition sequences are the rule rather than the exception. It is unsuitable for the claustrophobic patient, a drawback that has not yet been compensated for by the quality of venous imaging from open magnet systems and phased surface array coils. Each of the remaining imaging modalities require the use of iodinated contrast medium, and this is certainly contraindicated in a small minority of patients with a history of contrast allergy or impaired renal function (either from intrinsic pre-existing parenchymal disease or renal vein invasion). In bygone days when selective high-dose renal arteriography was popular, failure to visualize the renal vein on late films was presumptive evidence for tumor thrombus in the renal vein.

In the present era, there is little to choose between good-quality sonography and CT when it comes to the accuracy of staging renal vein involvement provided there is no gross hilar lymphadenopathy, but the additional bonus of capturing other staging information on CT images undoubtedly makes it the test of first choice. The sensitivity and specificity of detecting vascular extension by CT has been quoted at approximately 78% and 96%, respectively.[106] Accuracy is greatest for the vena cava (86%) and less good for the renal vein (50%).[107] Once the level of the renal vein has been identified on unenhanced scans, 5-mm-thick contiguous sections can be chosen at this level before dynamic scanning is undertaken. This should coincide with the venous phase of circulation after a contrast bolus is rapidly injected. If necessary, images thus acquired can be further improved by manipulations such as sagittal, helical, or three-dimensional reconstruction where rapid imaging sequences and techniques previously discussed in this chapter minimize both motion and partial volume-based artifacts. Further improvements in image quality are possible with respiratory gating. A final repeat study performed almost without delay on a machine with a high tube heat capacity should complete the image acquisition. The most reliable sign indicating renal vein invasion on images obtained in this way is a persistent low-attenuation filling defect in an otherwise opacified vein, in combination with thrombosis of collateral venous tributaries (e.g., adrenal and gonadal veins). Renal vein enlargement alone can suggest thrombosis, but this can be misleading, for the alteration in vein size can also result from tumor hypervascularity and a hyperdynamic circulation (78%), or from the "nutcracker syndrome" in the case of the left renal vein.[108] Consequently, on its own, this finding had a 90% false-negative rate and a 65% false-positive rate.[109] Rarely, the paradox of a tumor thrombus that conformed to the venous lumen without causing gross enlargement can be encountered. The renal vein can also be displaced from its normal course by a bulky tumor mass, enlarged lymph nodes, or other extrinsic disease, and this finding is also unreliable. CT has been limited in its capacity to differentiate bland organized venous thrombosis from true venous tumor thrombus. This subtle distinction has been possible only when a solid mass can be seen to emanate directly from the kidney into the vein, has intrinsic enhancing neovascularity, and invades beyond the wall of the inferior vena cava. Unfortunately, the true accuracy of CT in staging venous invasion may be underestimated, for by including scans performed at a variety of outside institutions, variances such as the inclusion of unenhanced scans only (patients with poor renal function or contrast allergy), imaging on different units, and the adoption of different protocols must be factored into the final analysis.

Although MRI does not have advantages over CT for clarification of nodal status due partly to the absence of an efficacious oral contrast agent, its capacity to discern between the flow of venous blood and an intraluminal soft tissue mass without the use of iodinated contrast increases its attraction for staging venous extension. Sequences in the sagittal and coronal planes are most useful; the latter clearly shows the juncture of the hepatic veins draining into the inferior vena cava. Blood appears black on standard T1-weighted scans and is enhanced either by a low-flip-angle shot or a GRASS sequence with flow compensation. These techniques are preferred for the clarity with which the extent of tumor thrombus is depicted. The addition of Gd-DTPA should enhance a tumor thrombus and separate it from bland thrombus. Such a distinction undoubtedly adds to the expense of MRI, but has no practical purpose, for all thrombus in a patient with renal cell carcinoma should be surgically treated as tumor thrombus. A large vein that is patent and contains flowing blood should not register an MRI signal when the spin-echo technique is used. This is known as the "flow-void" phenomenon. The presence of an intermediate signal within such a vessel is indicative of either slow flow or tumor thrombus.

MR angiography (MRA) is a supplementary technique that has continued to evolve through the combination of two-dimensional time-of-flight acquisition and phase-contrast angiography. Parameters that were used to control spin-echo sequences and variations of the flip angle to 45 degrees can also be manipulated at the same time to improve vascular evaluation. Unfortunately, in the abdomen, respiratory motion confounds the accurate evaluation of low venous flow. MR venography, which has combined parameters of MRA with short TR and TE values (33/7 msec), may go a long way to solving some of these inherent problems.[110] Cardiac gating enhances the resolution of tumor thrombi in the heart and the suprahepatic portion of the inferior vena cava. Other advantages of MR include the detection of venous transmural invasion (sagittal and coronal gradient-recalled echo images) with greater than 60% accuracy.[111]

Horan and associates prospectively studied the staging of venous invasion by MRI and inferior venacavography.[102] They concluded that MR was superior at localizing thrombus in the renal vein, while the sensitivity and specificity for detecting inferior vena caval thrombus at 82% and 97%, respectively, was equivalent for the two tests. Since the magnet used in this study was only 0.5 T, it is a reasonable assumption that modern machines that have incorporated higher field strength (1.5 T) magnets have improved accuracy. This was confirmed by the study of Amendola and coworkers.[112] However, numerous investigators have rightly pointed out the shortcomings of both invasive and noninvasive imaging studies when the veins in question have been deformed or compressed by a bulky soft tissue mass (primary tumor or regional adenopathy), probably as a consequence of slower blood flow. A possible solution is to combine both tests, since this is virtually infallible. In considering the high cost of each, one might rightly argue that this is unlikely to prove cost effective in the current health care climate of judicial fiscal restraint.

Venography itself is not error free[113] as a consequence of slow flow and suboptimal contrast filling, and may also risk detachment of tumor thrombus. In many institutions, venacavography has become almost obsolete in the staging of venous invasion, in favor of less invasive tests such as external echocardiography and intraoperative transesophageal echocardiography. Both of these tests can accurately exclude right atrial tumor extension and delineate the cephalad level of tumor thrombus, but the hazards of venography are undoubtedly greater by virtue of the need for two punctures and catheters (superior and inferior) when the vena cava is completely occluded. If intracardiac tumor is detected, the surgical approach can be amended, and at the same time the elective participation of cardiac surgeons and a bypass team can be ensured at an early stage of the proceedings.

Intraoperative transesophageal echocardiography was evaluated in five patients with a right-sided renal cell tumor after the induction of anesthesia, by Treiger and associates.[114] A gastroscope was used to guide the attached 5-MHz transducer safely through the esophagus, and the heart and liver were imaged in turn as the endoscope was advanced and rotated appropriately. Accurate delineation of the upper extent of tumor thrombus was confirmed at open surgery in all cases, with the additional bonus of assessing valvular function and enumerating ventricular ejection fraction before and after cardiopulmonary bypass, hypothermia, exsanguination, and temporary cardiac arrest. The issue of preventing intraoperative tumor embolus leading to potentially fatal outcome by such an evaluation must be addressed prospectively in a larger series of patients. These authors, however, rightly pointed out the possibility of tumor growth during an extended interval between preoperative imaging with CT or MRI as a possible source of staging error for these modalities in selected patients.

METASTATIC DISEASE

The incidence of first presentation with metastatic renal cancer has remained virtually undiminished despite improvements in imaging technology. Rates as high as 50 to 60% have been cited at the time of diagnosis in the literature.[115,116] Common sites of distant metastatic disease are the adrenal gland (ipsilateral and contralateral), the lung, the liver, the bones, subcutaneous tissues, and the brain. In general, larger tumors are associated with a higher stage of disease and poorer survival. In a recent large retrospective review of 2473 cases of renal cell carcinoma, Guinan and coworkers found a direct correlation between solid tumor size and metastatic potential.[117]

Numerous special investigations have been used to screen patients for metastatic disease both before and after nephrectomy. An appropriately directed history and physical examination can be excellent indicators of systemic disease. Pain, fever, night sweats, and abnormal serum liver function tests (alkaline phosphatase, γ-glutamyltransferase, glutamic-oxaloacetic transaminase, and glutamate pyruvate transaminase) have a reported sensitivity of 92% in distinguishing metastases or abdominal recurrence[118] from renal cell cancer. It is uncommon for a patient to harbor skeletal metastasis in the absence of either bone pain or elevations of serum alkaline phosphatase and calcium when other pathology that might cause erroneous results have been excluded. A history of cough, dyspnea, pleuritic pain, and hemoptysis has a 74% yield for detecting pulmonary metastases and is improved to

100% by the addition of a chest x-ray. Indeed, we would argue that there is sparse evidence to suggest that the routine addition of a bone scan or chest CT is of any value whatsoever. Others hold the conflicting view that CT is more sensitive than plain radiography in excluding pulmonary and mediastinal metastases[119] in patients who are candidates for curative surgery. In our practice, isotope scans have been discarded as part of the preliminary metastatic work-up.[120] Liver function tests, serum calcium, and good-quality bidirectional (posteroanterior and lateral) chest radiographs are the only tests that are routinely performed preoperatively in all patients with a diagnosis of renal cell carcinoma after history and physical examination. Chest CT and bone scan are selectively used in the staging of patients where coexistent disease confounds the results of the first-line investigations, or when these tests are abnormal and further clarification is indicated. Isolated hot spots on a bone scan often need further confirmation by local radiographs, while exceptionally, additional characterization is indicated in the asymptomatic patient by the exquisite bone marrow imaging capability of unenhanced MRI. On T1-weighted images, a bone metastasis appears as an area of low signal intensity surrounded by high-signal-intensity marrow fat. This contrast between the tissues is rendered inconspicuous by gadolinium enhancement or fat suppression sequences, and hence, both are unnecessary.

Liver metastases are associated with an ominous prognosis, far worse than when the lung is the sole site of metastatic disease. Fortunately for the clinician, intrahepatic metastasis rarely represents the sole site of systemic disease.[121] On the rare occasion where this situation arises, questionable liver lesions must be accurately characterized if such patients are to be honestly counseled about the prospects for response to immunotherapy treatment. This may not always be possible with CT, particularly when focal hepatic lesions fail to enhance after contrast administration, or are too small for the diagnosis to be certain. In a specific situation of this nature, MRI may once again prove useful, for true metastases have a lower signal intensity than the normal liver parenchyma on T1-weighted scans. Furthermore, these foci do not enhance as strongly as benign hemangiomas or simple cysts on T2-weighted sequences.[122]

ADRENAL METASTASIS

When all cancers are considered, only 3% of adrenal metastases have a renal origin. Involvement of the ipsilateral adrenal gland by renal cell cancer has been found in up to 10% of radical nephrectomy specimens[123] but is more common in subjects with established metastatic disease at postmortem.[124] In an autopsy study of 1828 patients with metastatic renal cell cancer, Saitoh and associates found ipsilateral adrenal involvement in 19.1%, while the contralateral gland was affected in 11.5%.[125] Location within the envelope of Gerota's fascia and intimacy with the renal capsule favor direct invasion of the ipsilateral adrenal by contiguous growth, or local vascular or lymphatic permeation, while shared venous drainage on the left side presumably facilitates direct retrograde vascular extension. Unfortunately, the mechanism of these events is by no means clear. Certain groups of patients are felt to be at particularly high risk of this eventuality, namely those with a large tumor in an upper pole location, when the tumor has replaced virtually the entire kidney and those with capsular invasion.[126]

As far as imaging is concerned, a recent retrospective study of the usefulness of CT scans reported by Gill and associates[127] suggested detectable abnormality in 38 of 157 patients, a negative predictive value of 100%, and a positive predictive value of 26%. It is not clear from this study whether all the scans that were evaluated were performed in a standardized fashion at a single institution, for together with section thickness, this could have influenced the detection rate. Certainly, microscopic disease continues to evade detection by any imaging modality, and this fact coupled with the occurrence of adrenal metastasis in occasional patients with small mid or lower pole tumors has until recently fueled the argument for the time-honored surgical ritual of en bloc excision of the gland at radical nephrectomy or upper pole partial nephrectomy. It is unlikely that the positive contribution to cure of such practice outweighs the potential morbidity. Since the risk of leaving behind tumor in the adrenal in this particular group is recognized to be low (1.9%),[126] routine excision is not justified except perhaps in patients prone to multifocal sites of intraparenchymal renal cancer.

Much has been made of the recent discovery by radiologists that the use of chemical shift MRI (which uses in-phase and out-of-phase gradient-echo pulse sequences) can distinguish between benign adrenocortical masses, which have a high lipid (triglyceride) content, and metastases or pheochromocytomas, which do not,[128,129] with an accuracy of 96 to 100%. As a general rule, metastases to the adrenal glands generally mirror the histologic features of the primary tumor. Metastases of tumors such as renal cell carcinoma may occasionally continue to be a source of difficulty in this respect, for a variable cytoplasmic lipid content is seen not infrequently,[130] even when there is none in the primary. The observation that patients with renal cell cancer have 4 to 12 times as many benign adrenal adenomas as the general population[131] can further confuse the evaluation of these masses.

It is not yet certain that the allure of newer imaging techniques such as PET scanning will be able to reliably bridge the gaps in diagnostic imaging of the adrenal that remain after conventional scans have been completed and are indeterminate. Initial experience in 14 patients has shown promise in discriminating between metastatic lesions from a variety of tissue primaries and nonmalignant adrenal masses,[132] but in this study only one of the patients had renal cell cancer. Clearly these findings are interesting and further prospective work is required in this new diagnostic arena in many insitutions. Whether the promise of improved diagnostic accuracy of an adrenal mass in a patient with renal cell cancer is necessary (except perhaps in the patient who is being considered for partial nephrectomy or where the adrenal mass in question is contralateral to the tumor-bearing kidney), or can be realistically translated to reduce unnecessary adrenal sacrifice at the time of nephrectomy, to the ultimate benefit of our patients, is unknown, but cost is certain to play an important part in the selection of the best diagnostic strategy.

REFERENCES

1. Koenig G: Praktische Abhandlungen ueber die Krankheiten der Nieren durch Krankheitsfaelle erlaeutert, pp 307, 21, VII, 8°, Leipzig, C. Cnobloch, 1826.
2. Robin CP: Memoire sur l'epithelioma du rein et sur les minces filaments granuleux des tubes urinares expulses avec les urines. Gaz. d. hop. 1855, 28, 186–187, 194–195, 202–203.
3. Waldeyer W: Die entwickelung der carcinome. Arch Pathol Anat Physiol Klin Med 1867; 41:470–523.
4. Grawitz P: Die sogenannten lipome der niere. Virchows Arch Pathol Anat Klin Med 1883; 93:39–63.
5. Doederlein A: Birch-Hirschfeld FV: Embryonale Druesengeschwulst der Nierengegend im Kindesalter. Centralbl Krankh Harn Sex Org 1894; 3, 88:1pl.
6. Tannenbaum M: Ultrastructural pathology of human renal cell tumors. Pathol Ann 1971; 6:249–277.
7. Gu FFL, Cai SL, Cai BJ, Wu CP: Cellular origin of renal cell carcinoma: an immunohistochemical study on monoclonal antibodies. Scand J Nephrol 1991; 138(Suppl): 203–206.
8. Rumpelt HJ, Storkel S, Moll R, et al: Bellini duct carcinoma: further evidence for this rare variant of renal cell carcinoma. Histopathology 1991; 18(2):115–122.
9. Wingo PA, Tong T, Bolden S: Cancer statistics, 1995. CA Cancer J Clin 1995; 45(1):8–30.
10. Lieber MM, Tomera FM, Taylor WF, Farrow GM: Renal adenocarcinoma in young adults, survival and variables affecting prognosis. J Urol 1981; 125(2):164–168.
11. Dunnill MS, Millard PR, Oliver D: Acquired cystic disease of the kidneys: a hazard of long term intermittent maintenance hemodialysis. J Clin Pathol 1977; 30(9):868–877.
12. MacDougall ML, Welling LW, Wiegmann TB: Prediction of carcinoma in acquired cystic disease as a function of kidney weight. J Am Soc Nephrol 1990; 1(5):828–831.
13. Broecker B: Renal cell carcinoma in children. Urology 1991; 38(1):54–56.
14. Pochedly C, Suwansirikul S, Penzer P: Renal call carcinoma with extrarenal manifestations in a 10 month old child. Am J Dis Child 1971; 121(6):528–530.
15. Raney RB Jr, Palmer N, Sutow WW, et al: Renal cell carcinoma in children. Med Pediatr Oncol 1983; 11(2):91–98.
16. Kirkman H, Bacon RL: Renal adenomas and carcinomas in diethylstilbestrol-treated male golden hamsters (Abstract 77). Anat Rec 1949; 103:475–476.
17. Wenz W: Tumors of the kidney following retrograde pyelography with colloidal thorium dioxide. Ann NY Acad Sci 1967; 145(3):806–810.
18. Bleiweiss IJ, Pervez NK, Hammer GS, Dickman SH: Cytomegalovirus induced adrenal insufficiency and associated renal cell carcinoma in AIDS. Mt Sinai J Med 1986; 53(8):676–679.
19. Kamel D, Turpeenniemi-Hujanen T, Vahakangas K, et al: Proliferating cell nuclear antigen but not p53 or human papillomavirus DNA correlates with advanced clinical stage in renal cell carcinoma. Histopathology 1994; 25(4): 339–347.
20. La Vecchia C, Negri E, D'Avanzo B, Francheschi S: Smoking and renal cell carcinoma. Cancer Res 1990; 50(17): 5231–5233.
21. Zbar B, Glenn G, Lubensky I, et al: Hereditary papillary renal cell carcinoma: clinical studies in 10 families. J Urol 1995; 153(3 pt 2):907–912.
22. Knudsen AG: Mutation and cancer: statistical study of retinoblastoma. Proc Natl Acad Sci U S A 1971; 68(4): 820–823.
23. Yeung RS, Xiao GH, Jin F, et al: Predisposition to renal cell carcinoma in the Eker rat is determined by germ-line mutation of the tuberous sclerosis 2 (TSC2) gene. Proc Natl Acad Sci U S A 1994; 91(24):11413–11416.
24. Sampson JR, Patel A, Mee AD: Multifocal renal cell carcinoma in sibs from a chromosome 9 linked (TSC1) tuberous sclerosis family. J Med Genet 1995; 32:848–850.
25. Dinney CPN, Awad SA, Gajewski JB, et al: Analysis of imaging modalities, staging systems and prognostic indicators for renal cell carcinoma. Urology 1992; 39(2): 122–129.
26. McClennan BL: Oncologic imaging. Staging and follow-up of renal and adrenal carcinoma. Cancer 1991; 67(4 Suppl):1199–1208.
27. Zagoria RJ, Wolfman NT, Karstaedt N, et al: CT features of renal cell carcinoma with emphasis on relation to tumor size. Invest Radiol 1990; 25(3):261–266.
28. Warren MM, Kelalis PP, Utz DC: The changing concept of hypernephroma. J Urol 1970; 104(3):376–379.
29. Skinner DG, Colvin RB, Vermillion CD, et al: Diagnosis and management of renal cell carcinoma. Cancer 1971; 28(5):1165–1177.
30. Ochsner MG, Brannan W, Pond HS III, Goodier EH: Renal cell carcinoma: review of 26 years of experience at the Ochsner clinic. J Urol 1973; 110(6):643–646.
31. Kaufman JJ, Mimms MM: Tumors of the kidney. *In* Current Problems in Surgery, pp 1–44. Chicago, Year Book Medical Publishers, 1966.
32. Sigalow DA, Waldbaum RS, Lowe FC: Identification of asymptomatic renal cell carcinomas utilizing modern radiographic techniques. NY State J Med 1991; 91(5):200–202.
33. Riches EW, Griffiths IH, Thackeray AC: New growths of kidney and ureter. Br J Urol 1951; 23(4):297–356.
34. Pritchett TR, Lieskovsky G, Skinner DG: Extension of renal cell carcinoma into the vena cava, clinical review and surgical approach. J Urol 1986; 135(3):460–464.
35. Clayman RV, Gonzalez R, Fraley EE: Renal cell cancer invading the inferior vena cava, clinical review and anatomical approach. J Urol 1980; 123(2):157–163.
36. Sufrin G, Chasan S, Golio A, Murphy GP: Paraneoplastic and serologic syndromes of renal adenocarcinoma. Semin Urol 1989; 7(3):158–171.
37. Kemp BE, Moseley JM, Rodda CP, et al: Parathyroid hormone-related protein of malignancy: active synthetic fragments. Science 1987; 238(4833):1568–1570.
38. Erslev AJ: Renal biogenesis of erythropoietin. Am J Med 1975; 58(1):25–30.
39. Murphy GP, Kenny GM, Mirand EA: Erythropoietin levels in patients with renal tumors or cysts. Cancer 1970; 26(1):191–194.
40. Erslev AJ, Caro J: Physiologic and molecular biology of erythropoietin. Med Oncol Tumor Pharmacother 1986; 3(3–4):159–164.
41. Ljungberg B, Rasmuson T, Grankvist K: Erythropoietin in

renal cell carcinoma: evaluation of its usefulness as a tumor marker. Eur Urol 1992; 21(2):160–163.

42. Murphy GP, Mirand EA, Johnston GS, et al: Erythropoietin alterations in human genitourinary disease states: correlation with experimental observations. J Urol 1968; 99(6):802–810.
43. Amendola MA, Bree RL, Pollack HM, et al: Small renal cell carcinomas: resolving a diagnostic dilemma. Radiology 1988; 166(3):637–641.
44. Levine E: Renal cell carcinoma. Radiological diagnosis and staging. Semin Roentgenol 1987; 22(4):248–259.
45. Daniel WW Jr, Hartman GW, Witten DM, et al: Calcified renal masses: a review of ten years experience at the Mayo Clinic. Radiology 1972; 103(3):503–508.
46. Tosaka A, Ohya K, Yamada K, et al: Incidence and properties of renal masses and asymptomatic renal cell carcinoma detected by abdominal ultrasonography. J Urol 1990; 144(5):1097–1099.
47. Yamashita Y, Takahashi M, Watanabe O, et al: Small renal cell carcinoma: pathologic and radiologic correlation. Radiology 1992; 184(2):493–498.
48. McClennan BL, Deyoe LA: The imaging evaluation of renal cell carcinoma, diagnosis and staging. Radiol Clin North Am 1994; 32(1):55–69.
49. Einstein DM, Herts BR, Weaver R, et al: Evaluation of renal masses detected by excretory urography: cost effectiveness of sonography versus CT. AJR 1995; 164(2): 371–375.
50. Kuijpers D, Jaspers R: Renal masses: differential diagnosis with pulsed Doppler ultrasound. Radiology 1989; 170(1): 59–60.
51. Gilbert BR, Russo P, Zirinsky K, et al: Intra-operative sonography: application in renal cell carcinoma. J Urol 1988; 139(3):582–584.
52. Walther MM, Choyke PL, Hayes W, et al: Evaluation of color Doppler intraoperative ultrasound in parenchymal sparing surgery. J Urol 1994; 152(6 pt 1):1984–1987.
53. Assimos DG, Boyce H, Woodruff RD, et al: Intraoperative renal ultrasonography: a useful adjunct to partial nephrectomy. J Urol 1991; 146(5):1218–1220.
54. Weyman PJ, McClennan BL, Stanley RJ, et al: Comparison of CT and angiography in the evaluation of renal cell carcinoma. Radiology 1980; 137(2):417–424.
55. Bosniak MA: The current radiologic approach to renal cysts. Radiology 1986; 158(1):1–10.
56. Selzman AA, Hampel N, Hassan MO: Renal oncocytoma arising from a renal cyst: a case report and review of the literature. J Urol 1994; 151(6):1610–1611.
57. Levine E: Renal cell carcinoma in uremic acquired renal cystic disease: incidence, detection and management. Urol Radiol 1992; 13(4):203–210.
58. Peterson RO: Urologic Pathology, pp 85–110. Philadelphia, JB Lippincott Co, 1986.
59. Talamo TS, Shonnard JW: Small renal adenocarcinoma with metastases. J Urol 1980; 124(1):132–134.
60. Bell ET: Renal Diseases, 2nd edition, p 435. Philadelphia, Lea & Febiger, 1950.
61. Bell ET: A classification of renal tumors with observations on the frequencies of various types. J Urol 1938; 39(3): 238–243.
62. Licht MR, Novick AC, Goormastic M: Nephron sparing surgery in incidental versus suspected renal cell carcinoma. J Urol 1994; 152(1):39–42.
63. Montie JE, Novick AC: Partial nephrectomy for renal cell carcinoma (Editorial). J Urol 1988; 140(1):129–130.
64. Bosniak MA: The small (≤3 cm) renal parenchymal tumor: detection, diagnosis and controversies. Radiology 1991; 179(2):307–317.
65. Warshauer DM, McCarthy SM, Street L, et al: Detection of renal masses: sensitivities and specificities of excretory urography, linear tomography, US and CT. Radiology 1988; 169(2):363–365.
66. Sherman JL, Hartman DS, Friedman AC, et al: Angiomyolipoma: computed tomographic-pathologic correlation of 17 cases. AJR 1981; 137(6):1221–1226.
67. Bernstein J: Hereditary renal disease. *In* Churg J, Spargo BH, Mostofi FK, Abell MR (eds): Kidney Diseases, Present Status, Int Acad Pathol Monogr 20, pp 295–326. Baltimore, MD, Williams & Wilkins, 1979.
68. Strotzer M, Lehner KB, Becker K: Detection of fat in a renal cell carcinoma mimicking angiomyolipoma. Radiology 1993; 188(2):427–428.
69. Van Baal JG, Smits NJ, Keeman JN, et al: The evolution of renal angiomyolipomas in patients with tuberous sclerosis. J Urol 1994; 152(1):35–38.
70. Williams MA, Schropp KP, Noe HN: Fat containing renal mass in childhood: a case report of teratoid Wilms' tumor. J Urol 1994; 151(6):1662–1663.
71. Tallarigo C, Baldassare R, Bianchi G, et al: Diagnostic and therapeutic problems in multicentric renal angiomyolipoma. J Urol 1992; 148(6):1880–1884.
72. Umeyama T, Saitoh Y, Tomaru Y, Kitaura K: Bilateral renal angiomyolipoma associated with bilateral renal vein and inferior vena caval thrombi. J Urol 1992; 148(6): 1885–1887.
73. Maatman TJ, Novick AC, Tancinco BF, et al: Renal oncocytoma: a diagnostic and therapeutic dilemma. J Urol 1984; 132(5):878–881.
74. Defossez SM, Yoder IC, Papanicolaou N, et al: Non-specific magnetic appearance of renal oncocytomas, report of three cases and review of the literature. J Urol 1991; 145(3):552–554.
75. Davidson AJ, Hayes WS, Hartman DS, et al: Renal oncocytoma and carcinoma: failure of differentiation with CT. Radiology 1993; 186(3):693–696.
76. Cohan RH, Dunnick NR, Leder RA, et al: Computed tomography of renal lymphoma. Comput Assist Tomogr 1990; 14(6):933–938.
77. Kioumehr F, Cochran ST, Layfield L, et al: Wilms tumor (nephroblastoma) in the adult patient: clinical and radiologic manifestations. AJR 1989; 152(2):299–302.
78. Choyke PL, White EM, Zeman RK, et al: Renal metastases: clincopathologic and radiologic correlation. Radiology 1987; 162(2):359–363.
79. Kletscher BA, Qian J, Bostwick DG, et al: Prospective analysis of multifocality in renal cell carcinoma: influence of histological pattern, grade, number, size, volume and deoxyribonucleic acid ploidy. J Urol 1995; 153(3 pt 2): 904–906.
80. Kalender WA, Seissler W, Lotz E, Vock P: Spiral volumetric CT with single breath-hold technique, continuous transport and continuous scanner rotation. Radiology 1990; 176(1):181–183.
81. Silverman SG, Lee B, Seltzer SE, et al: Small (≤3 cm) renal masses: correlation of spiral CT features and pathologic findings. AJR 1994; 163(3):597–605.
82. Chernoff DM, Silverman SG, Kikinis R, et al: Three-dimensional imaging and display of renal tumors using spiral CT: a potential aid to partial nephrectomy. Urology 1994; 43(1):125–129.
83. Rofsky NM, Weinreb JC, Bosniak MA, et al: Renal lesion characterization with gadolinium-enhanced MR imaging: efficacy and safety in patients with renal insufficiency. Radiology 1991; 180(1):85–89.
84. Haustein J, Niendorf HP, Krestin G, et al: Renal tolerance of gadolinium-DTPA/dimeglumine in patients with chronic renal failure. Invest Radiol 1992; 27(2):153–156.
85. Rominger MB, Kenney PJ, Morgan DE, et al: Gadolinium-enhanced MR imaging of renal masses. Radiographics 1992; 12(6):1097–1116.
86. Semelka RC, Shoenut JP, Kroeker MA, et al: Renal lesions: controlled comparison between CT and 1.5-T MR imaging with non-enhanced and gadolinium-enhanced fat-suppressed spin-echo and breath-hold FLASH techniques. Radiology 1992; 182(2):425–430.
87. McLaughlin AF, Magee MA, Greenough R, et al: Current role of gallium scanning in the management of lymphoma. Eur J Nucl Med 1990; 16(8–10):755–771.
88. Maderazo EG, Hickingbotham NB, Woronick CL, Sziklas JJ: The influence of various factors on the accuracy of gal-

lium-67 imaging for occult infection. J Nucl Med 1988; 29(5):608–615.
89. Kawamura J, Itoh H, Hida S, et al: Significance of Ga-67 citrate tomographic scan in renal cell carcinoma. Kaku Igaku 1985; 22(4):491–499.
90. Bander NH, Welt S, Houghton AN, et al: Radio-nuclide imaging of human renal cancer with labeled monoclonal antibodies. Surg Forum 1984; 35:652–655.
91. Real FX, Bander NH, Yeh SDJ, et al: Monoclonal antibody F23. Radiolocalization and phase 1 study in patients with renal cell carcinoma (Abstract 946). Proc Am Soc Clin Oncol 1987; 6:240.
92. Kawamura J, Hida S, Yoshida O, et al: Validity of positron emission tomography (PET) using 2-deoxy-2[18F]fluoro-D-glucose (FDG) in patients with renal cell carcinoma (preliminary report). Kaku Igaku 1988; 25(11):1143–1148.
93. Wahl RL, Harney J, Hutchins G, Grossman HB: Imaging of renal cancer using positron emission tomography with 2-deoxy-2[18F]fluoro-D-glucose: pilot animal and human studies. J Urol 1991; 146(6):1470–1474.
94. Shenoy PD, Lakhkar BN, Ghosh MK, et al: Cutaneous seeding of renal oncocytoma by Chiba needle aspiration biopsy. Case report. Acta Radiol 1991; 32(1):50–52.
95. Rainwater LM, Farrow GM, Lieber MM: Flow cytometry of renal oncocytoma: common occurrence of deoxyribonucleic acid polyploidy and aneuploidy. J Urol 1986; 135(6):1167–1171.
96. Frohmuller HGW, Grups JW, Heller V: Comparative value of ultrasonography, computerized tomography, angiography and excretory urography in the staging of renal cell carcinoma. J Urol 1987; 138(3):482–484.
97. London NJM, Messios N, Kinder RB, et al: A prospective study of the value of conventional CT, dynamic CT, ultrasonography and arteriography for staging renal cell carcinoma. Br J Urol 1989; 64(3):209–217.
98. Johnson CD, Dunnick NR, Cohan RH, Illescas FF: Renal adenocarcinoma: CT staging of 100 tumors. AJR 1987; 148(1):59–63.
99. Studer UE, Scherz S, Scheidegger J, et al: Enlargement of regional lymph nodes in renal cell carcinoma is often not due to metastases. J Urol 1990; 144(2 pt 1):243–245.
100. Fein AB, Lee JKT, Balfe DM, et al: Diagnosis and staging of renal cell carcinoma: a comparison of MR imaging and CT. AJR 1987; 148(4):749–753.
101. Hatcher PA, Paulson DF, Anderson EE: Accuracy in staging of renal cell carcinoma involving vena cava. Urology 1992; 39(1):27–30.
102. Horan JJ, Robertson CN, Choyke PL, et al: The detection of renal carcinoma extension into the renal vein and inferior vena cava: a prospective comparison of venacavography and magnetic resonance imaging. J Urol 1989; 142(4):943–948.
103. Ney C: Thrombosis of the inferior vena cava associated with malignant renal tumors. J Urol 1946; 55(6):583–590.
104. Arkless R: Renal carcinoma: how it metastasizes. Radiology 1965; 84(3):496–501.
105. Berg AA: Malignant hypernephroma of the kidney, its clinical course and diagnosis, with a description of the author's method of radical operative cure. Surg Gynecol Obstet 1913; 17(4):463–471.
106. Hricak H, Thoeni RF, Carroll PR, et al: Detection and staging of renal neoplasms: a reassessment of MR imaging. Radiology 1988; 166(3):643–649.
107. Hietala S, Ekelund L, Ljungberg B: Venous invasion in renal cell carcinoma: a correlative clinical and radiologic study. Urol Radiol 1988; 9(4):210–216.
108. de Schepper A: "Nutcracker" phenomenon of the renal vein and venous pathology of the left kidney. J Belge Radiol 1972; 55(5):507–511.
109. Zeman RK, Cronan JJ, Rosenfield AT, et al: Renal cell carcinoma: dynamic thin-section CT assessment of vascular invasion and tumor vascularity. Radiology 1988; 167(2): 393–396.
110. Finn JP, Goldman A, Hartnell GG: Venography in the abdomen and pelvis. *In* Potchen EJ, Haacke EM, Siebert JE, Gottschalk A (eds): Magnetic Resonance Angiography, pp 607–624. St. Louis, Mosby-Year Book, 1993.
111. Myneni L, Hricak H, Carroll PR: Magnetic resonance imaging of renal carcinoma with extension into the vena cava: staging accuracy and recent advances. Br J Urol 1991; 68(6):571–578.
112. Amendola MA, King LR, Pollack HM, et al: Staging of renal carcinoma using magnetic resonance imaging at 1.5 tesla. Cancer 1990; 66(1):40–44.
113. Selby JB Jr, Pryor JL, Tegtmeyer CJ, Gillenwater JY: Inferior vena caval invasion by renal cell carcinoma: false positive diagnosis by venacavography. J Urol 1990; 143(3): 464–467.
114. Treiger BF, Jumphrey LS, Peterson CV Jr, et al: Transesophageal echocardiography in renal cell carcinoma: an accurate diagnostic technique for intracaval neoplastic extension. J Urol 1991; 145(6):1138–1140.
115. Buzaid AC, Todd MB: Therapeutic options in renal cell carcinoma. Semin Oncol 1989; 16(Suppl):12–19.
116. Patel NP, Lavengood RW: Renal cell carcinoma: natural history and results of treatment. J Urol 1978; 119(6): 722–726.
117. Guinan PD, Vozelgang NJ, Fremgen AM, et al: Renal cell carcinoma: tumor size, stage and survival. J Urol 1995; 153(3 pt 2):901–903.
118. Sandock DS, Seftel AD, Resnick MI: A new protocol for the follow-up of renal cell carcinoma based on pathological stage. J Urol 1995; 154(1):28–31.
119. Coppage L, Shaw C, Curtis AM: Metastatic disease to the chest in patients with extra-thoracic malignancy. J Thorac Imaging 1987; 2(4):24–37.
120. Lindner A, Goldman DG, deKernion JB: Cost effective analysis of prenephrectomy radio-isotope scans in renal cell carcinoma. Urology 1983; 22(2):127–129.
121. Saitoh H: Distant metastasis of renal adenocarcinoma. Cancer 1981; 48(6):1487–1491.
122. Kressel HY: Strategies for magnetic resonance imaging of focal liver disease. Radiol Clin North Am 1988; 26(3): 607–615.
123. Angervall L, Wahlqvist L: Follow-up and prognosis of renal carcinoma in a series operated by peri-fascial nephrectomy combined with adrenalectomy and retroperitoneal lymphadenectomy. Eur Urol 1978; 4(1):13–17.
124. Hellsten S, Berge T, Linell F: Clinically unrecognized renal carcinoma: aspects of tumor morphology, lymphatic and hematogeneous metastatic spread. Br J Urol 1983; 55(2): 166–170.
125. Saitoh H, Nakayama M, Nakamura K, Satoh T: Distant metastasis of renal adenocarcinoma in nephrectomized cases. J Urol 1982; 127(6):1092–1095.
126. Sagalowsky AI, Kadesky KT, Ewalt DM, Kennedy TJ: Factors influencing adrenal metastasis in renal cell carcinoma. J Urol 1994; 151(5):1181–1184.
127. Gill IS, McClennan BL, Kerbl K, et al: Adrenal involvement from renal cell carcinoma: predictive value of computerized tomography. J Urol 1994; 152(4):1082–1085.
128. Mitchell DG, Crovello M, Matteucci T, et al: Benign adrenocortical masses: diagnosis with chemical shift MR imaging. Radiology 1992; 185(2):345–351.
129. Tsushima Y, Ishizaka H, Matsumoto M: Adrenal masses: differentiation with chemical shift, fast low-angle shot MR imaging. Radiology 1993; 186(3):705–709.
130. Someren A, Zaatari GS, Campbell WG, et al: The kidneys. *In* Someren A (ed): Urologic Pathology with Clinical and Radiologic Correlations, pp 1–243. New York, MacMillan, 1989.
131. Ambos MA, Bosniak MA, Lefleur RS, Mitty HA: Adrenal adenoma associated with renal cell carcinoma. AJR 1981; 136(1):81–84.
132. Boland GW, Goldberg MA, Lee MJ, et al: Indeterminate adrenal mass in patients with cancer: evaluation at PET with 2-[F-18]-fluoro-2-deoxy-D-glucose. Radiology 1995; 194(1):131–134.

12

RENAL CELL CARCINOMA: MANAGEMENT AND PROGNOSIS

JOEL B. NELSON, M.D. *and* FRAY F. MARSHALL, M.D.

Approximately 30,000 people will be diagnosed with renal cell carcinoma and 12,000 will die from it in 1996.[1] This malignancy is noted for its bizarre manifestations and unusual clinical courses. Consider, for example, the case of an 81-year-old woman who died of renal cell carcinoma after 50 years of metastatic, untreated disease.[2] Or the rare but well-documented cases of spontaneous remission.[3–7] Renal cell carcinoma metastasizes to both usual (lymph node, liver, lung, bone, and brain) and unusual (thyroid, skin, heart, penis) locations.[8–10] In fact, renal cell carcinoma is the most common metastatic tumor to the nose and perinasal sinuses.[11–13] Even in the absence of metastases, paraneoplastic syndromes are frequent.[14] Nephrogenic hepatic dysfunction, Stauffer's syndrome, occurs in the absence of metastases, is mediated by cytokines, and can resolve following nephrectomy.[15,16] Late local recurrences and a unique sensitivity to immunotherapy yet stubborn radio- and chemoresistance make renal cell carcinoma both intriguing and frustrating to treat. The goal of this chapter is to discuss the management and prognosis of renal cell carcinoma.

DIFFERENTIAL DIAGNOSIS

The classic triad of hematuria, flank mass, and pain is becoming rare in the age of axial imaging.[17,18] A solid renal mass found on computed tomography (CT) scan must be considered renal cell carcinoma until that diagnosis is ruled out.[19–21] In this increasingly common clinical scenario, several clues may aid in the differential diagnosis of an indeterminate renal mass. Other malignancies can metastasize to kidney, with lymphoproliferative and lung carcinomas the most common causes of secondary renal masses.[22] Of those tumors metastasizing to the genitourinary (GU) tract besides lymphomas (33%) and lung carcinoma (13%), gastric (11%) and breast (8%) carcinomas can metastasize to the kidney.[23] In the age of acquired immunodeficiency syndrome (AIDS)–related malignancies, a solid renal mass in an at-risk individual must be considered lymphoma and, after tissue diagnosis, managed with appropriate systemic therapy. Classically, oncocytoma and chromophobe tumors are correctly diagnosed only following resection, but a characteristic central stellate scar in both lesions and a spoke-wheel vascular appearance on angiography with oncocytoma may provide preoperative clues.[24,25] The association of renal cell carcinoma with oncocytoma and the malignant potential of an otherwise very favorable prognosis with chromophobe tumor dictate prudent resection of both of these lesions. Finally, a history of tuberous sclerosis and the presence of fat on imaging studies makes the diagnosis of angiomyolipoma very likely. These benign tumors can be managed expectantly when small and asymptomatic.[26] See Chapter 11 for further discussion of the differential diagnosis of a renal mass.

SURGICAL MANAGEMENT AND PROGNOSIS OF RENAL CELL CARCINOMA

Nephron-Sparing Surgery

The indications, operative techniques, complications, and results from nephron-sparing surgery are discussed elsewhere. The long-term prognosis of nephron-sparing surgery depends upon correct patient selection and operative technique.[27] Table 12–1 lists cumulative data from several recent series, with a predicted 87% 5-year survival rate in 314 reported patients.

TABLE 12–1. PROGNOSIS FOLLOWING NEPHRON-SPARING SURGERY FOR RENAL CELL CARCINOMA

Reference	Year	No. of Patients	5-Year Survival
Jacobs et al.[28]	1980	51	84.4%
Palmer[29]	1983	7	57%
Novick et al.[30]	1989	100	84%
Petritsch et al.[31]	1990	52	96%
Morgan and Zincke[32]	1990	104	88.9%
Total		314	86.8%*

*Weighed for the number of patients per study.

Radical Nephrectomy

The indications, operative techniques, complications, and results of radical nephrectomy are discussed elsewhere. The prognosis following radical nephrectomy for renal cell carcinoma pathologic stage I, defined as tumor confined to the kidney, is presented in Table 12–2. In 256 reported patients, the 5-year survival rate is 75%; in 65 reported patients followed for 10 years the survival rate is 59%.

The prognosis following radical nephrectomy for renal cell carcinoma pathologic stage II, defined as tumor involving the perinephric fat but confined within Gerota's fascia, is presented in Table 12–3. In 65 reported patients the 5-year survival rate was 66%; in 34 patients, the 10-year survival was approximately 40%. It is interesting that in most larger studies patients defined in pathologic stage II make up the smallest subset of the four pathologic stages. This may indicate the long, relatively indolent nature of a stage I tumor followed by accelerated pathogenesis into stage III and IV disease.

Much of the confusion about the prognosis of renal cell carcinoma comes from a historic staging system that included patients with tumor metastatic to the regional lymph nodes and patients with tumor extending into the inferior vena cava in the same stage.[38] It is clear that the prognosis from these two manifestations of renal cell carcinoma are different. For example, the prognosis following radical nephrectomy for renal cell carcinoma pathologic stage III, defined as renal vein invasion, both gross and microscopic, is similar to patients who have inferior vena cava tumor extension and very different from those patients who have renal cell carcinoma metastatic to regional lymph nodes. Table 12–4 indicates the prognosis following radical nephrectomy for renal cell carcinoma, stage III with renal vein invasion and shows a 5-year survival rate of approximately 56% in 112 patients and a 10-year survival rate of 33% in 84 patients.

These data are similar to the prognosis following radical nephrectomy for renal cell carcinoma stage III with extension into the inferior vena cava. In seven studies, independent of the cephalad extension of the tumor thrombus, a 5-year survival of 53% was observed in 156 reported patients (Table 12–5). In a recent study from the Cleveland Clinic, long-term survival after surgical resection for patients with otherwise localized renal cell carcinoma with extension into the right atrium was achieved.[45] That study found that the cephalad extent of the inferior vena caval tumor thrombus did not appear to be prognostically important, confirming several other previous reports.

The prognosis of renal cell carcinoma metastatic to the regional lymph nodes is summarized on Table 12–6. In 13 studies, including 220 patients, the 5-year survival rate was 25%. It is interesting that the 92 patients followed for 10 years had a survival rate of 16.5%, supporting the observation that some patients with tumor metastatic to lymph nodes are cured by the removal of those lymph nodes.

The issue whether or not the ipsilateral adrenal gland should be removed at the time of radical nephrectomy for renal cell carcinoma is being revisited in the age of laparoscopic and nephron-sparing surgical techniques. An early series reported by Angervall found 10% of patients with renal cell carcinoma to have ipsilateral adrenal metastases.[53] Subsequent series uniformly report a much lower rate of adrenal metastases: notably, the series by Hohenfellner, including 429 patients, revealed only five patients with ipsilateral adrenal metastases or a rate of 1.2%.[55] Table 12–7 summarizes the findings in nearly 2000 patients in whom adrenal metastases were noted. The 4.2% incidence in this pooled series should be considered from the following perspectives: (1) larger tumors and tumors involving the upper pole are more frequently associated with ipsilateral adrenal metastases; (2) in those series in which the information was provided, three quarters of the patients with ipsilateral adrenal metastases also had metastatic disease to

TABLE 12–2. PROGNOSIS FOLLOWING RADICAL NEPHRECTOMY FOR RENAL CELL CARCINOMA: STAGE I: TUMOR CONFINED TO KIDNEY

Reference	Year	No. of Patients	5-Year Survival	No. of Patients	10-Year Survival
Robson et al.[33]	1969	32	66%	15	60%
Skinner et al.[34]	1972	59	65%	34	56%
Siminovitch et al.[35]	1983	80	82%		
Golimbu et al.[36]	1986	52	88%	16	66%
Best[37]	1987	33	64%		
Total		256	75%*	65	59.4%*

*Weighed for the number of patients per study.

TABLE 12–3. PROGNOSIS FOLLOWING RADICAL NEPHRECTOMY FOR RENAL CELL CARCINOMA: STAGE II: TUMOR INVOLVING PERINEPHRIC FAT, BUT CONFINED TO GEROTA'S FASCIA

Reference	Year	No. of Patients	5-Year Survival	No. of Patients	10-Year Survival
Robson et al.[33]	1969	14	64%	6	67%
Skinner et al.[34]	1972	8	47%	2	20%
Golimbu et al.[36]	1986	39	67%	26	35%
Best[37]	1987	4	100%		
Total		65	65.9%	34*	39.7%*

*Weighed for the number of patients per study.

TABLE 12–4. PROGNOSIS FOLLOWING RADICAL NEPHRECTOMY FOR RENAL CELL CARCINOMA: STAGE III WITH RENAL VEIN INVASION (GROSS AND MICROSCOPIC)

Reference	Year	No. of Patients	5-Year Survival	No. of Patients	10-Year Survival
Skinner et al.[34]	1972	48	66%	35	49%
Siminovitch et al.[35]	1983	15	40%		
Golimbu et al.[36]	1986	49	51%	36	20%
Total		112	56%*	84	33%*

*Weighed for the number of patients per study.

TABLE 12–5. PROGNOSIS FOLLOWING RADICAL NEPHRECTOMY FOR RENAL CELL CARCINOMA: STAGE III WITH IVC INVASION (INDEPENDENT OF LEVEL OF THROMBUS)

Reference	Year	No. of Patients	5-Year Survival	No. of Patients	10-Year Survival
Skinner et al.[39]	1972	11	55%	11	43%
Heney and Nocks[40]	1982	9	67%		
Cherrie et al.[41]	1982	18	53%		
Neves and Zincke[42]	1987	29	68%		
Libertino et al.[43]	1987	44	44%		
Hatcher et al.[44]	1991	27	42%		
Glazer and Novick[45]	1996	18	60%		
Total		156	53%*	11	43%

*Weighed for the number of patients per study.

TABLE 12–6. PROGNOSIS FOR RENAL CELL CARCINOMA METASTATIC TO REGIONAL LYMPH NODES

Reference	Year	No. of Patients	5-Year Survival	No. of Patients	10-Year Survival
Flocks and Kadesky[38]	1958	21	14%	12	16%
Petkovic[46]	1959	22	5%		
Robson[47]	1963	10	40%		
Robson et al.[33]	1969	20	38%	13	38%
Rafla[48]	1970	14	21%	14	8%
Skinner et al.[34]	1972	19	16%	12	8%
Middleton and Preston[49]	1973	7	43%		
Peters and Brown[50]	1980	13	44%		
Cherrie et al.[41]	1982	13	0%		
Siminovitch et al.[35]	1983	9	11%		
Golimbu et al.[36]	1986	24	17%	21	5%
Hermanek and Schrott[51]	1990	28	34%		
Giuliani et al.[52]	1990	20	52%	20	26%
Total		220	25%*	92	16.5%*

*Weighed for the number of patients per study.

TABLE 12–7. ADRENAL INVOLVEMENT BY RENAL CELL CARCINOMA

Reference	Year	No. of Patients	Total No. with Adrenal Metastases	% with Adrenal Metastases and Stage III–IV Disease
Angervall and Wahlquist[53]	1978	58	6	
Robson[54]	1982	88	4	
Hohenfellner and Zingg[55]	1982	429	5	
Jaeger and Vahlensieck[56]	1985	161	9	
Robey and Schelhammer[57]	1986	82	2	
O'Brien and Lynch[58]	1987	72	4	
Winter et al.[59]	1990	138	8	50%
Haab et al.[60]	1993	119	6	100%
Sagalowsky et al.[61]	1993	695	30	87%
Gill et al.[62]	1994	157	10	30%
Total		1999	84 (4.2%)	75%*

*Weighed for the number of patients per study.

either regional lymph nodes or distant metastatic disease. Therefore, if an ipsilateral adrenalectomy is being performed with curative intent, and there is disease in that adrenal gland, there is a high likelihood that the patient will have other metastatic disease. While there is no apparent controversy about the surgical management of the ipsilateral adrenal gland in patients with a large and/or upper pole tumor, the long-term morbidity from total adrenal steroid replacement therapy for a patient who has no contralateral adrenal gland should be weighed against the relatively low incidence of adrenal metastases in those patients with lower pole and/or smaller tumors. It is startling to realize how relatively infrequently the adrenal gland is involved at the time of radical nephrectomy.

SURGICAL MANAGEMENT OF METASTATIC RENAL CELL CARCINOMA

The management of metastatic renal cell carcinoma should be viewed from the perspective provided by Table 12–8. The 1- and 5-year survival rates of 28.6 and 4.5%, respectively, in these large pooled series are dismal. On the other hand, there are patients who will survive with metastatic renal cell carcinoma much longer than 5 years, independent of the treatment employed.[2] The aggressive surgical management of a primary renal tumor and solitary metastasis stems, in least at part, from the lack of other effective therapies.

The prognosis following this treatment, radical nephrectomy and simultaneous excision of a solitary metastasis, is summarized on Table 12–9. Five-year survivals range from 7 to 50% in these collected series, with an overall weighted 5-year survival of 22%. If the primary tumor and the metastasis were discovered simultaneously, the prognosis is worse than if the metastasis appeared later. Evidence for this observation is shown in Table 12–10: the 5-year prognosis following excision of a solitary metastasis at some time remote from the radical nephrectomy is better than the synchronous group. Furthermore, in this small subset, a longer interval between nephrectomy and the appearance of the metastasis was associated with a better survival. In most series, the only long-term disease-

TABLE 12–8. PROGNOSIS OF DISTANT METASTATIC RENAL CELL CARCINOMA

Reference	Year	No. of Patients	1-Year Survival	No. of Patients	5-Year Survival
Flocks and Kadesky[38]	1958			116	3.5%
Robson[47]	1963	7	14%	7	0%
Middleton[63]	1967	105	6.6%	105	0%
Robson et al.[33]	1969			9	11%
Böttinger[64]	1970			32	5%
Skinner et al.[65]	1972			77	8%
Thompson et al.[66]	1975	65	21.5%	65	0%
Montie et al.[67]	1977	77	18%		
Siminovitch et al.[35]	1983			71	0%
Selli et al.[68]	1983			20	13%
Maldazys and deKernion[69]	1986	181	48%	181	9%
Golimbu et al.[36]	1986	88	31%	88	2%
Best[37]	1987	21	30%	21	0%
Neves and Zincke[42]	1987			18	12.5%
Giuliani et al.[52]	1990			29	7%
Total		544	28.6%*	839	4.5%*

*Weighed for the number of patients per study.

TABLE 12–9. PROGNOSIS FOLLOWING RADICAL NEPHRECTOMY AND SIMULTANEOUS EXCISION OF A SOLITARY METASTASIS

Reference	Year	No. of Patients	5-Year Survival	No. of Patients	10-Year Survival
Middleton[63]	1967	8	12.5%		
Skinner et al.[65]	1972	76	7%	55	5%
Tolia and Whitmore[70]	1975	19	32%		
Montie et al.[67]	1977	5	20%		
Klugo et al.[71]	1977	10	50%		
O'Dea et al.[72]	1978	18	5.5%		
Golimbu et al.[36]	1986	8	50%		
Total		144	22%*	55	5%*

*Weighed for the number of patients per study.

free survivors had soft tissue metastases. This led to the belief that patients with osseous metastases had a worse prognosis. In fact, about 30% of patients with a surgically resected solitary osseous metastasis from renal cell carcinoma can survive for 5 years.[74] It should be noted, however, that a solitary osseous metastasis, while most common to renal cell carcinoma and neuroblastoma, is still rather unusual.

RADICAL NEPHRECTOMY AND LYMPHADENECTOMY

As indicated by the data presented above, the prognosis is worse if renal cell carcinoma has spread to regional lymph nodes than if the lymph nodes are not involved with tumor. Of patients undergoing radical nephrectomy, approximately 25% will have positive lymph nodes at the time of surgery, a figure that increases if the lymphadenectomy is extended: Robson, who routinely performed mediastinoscopy prior to radical nephrectomy, noted 31% of his patients had positive lymph nodes.[33] Lymph node involvement is microscopic in three quarters of patients.[50] Although CT scanning can detect lymphadenopathy with 95% sensitivity, in one series more than half of the lymphadenopathy was caused by reactive changes and not metastatic disease. This was particularly true when tumor necrosis was present in the primary lesion.[75] Therefore, given microscopic involvement and false-positive imaging studies, certain diagnosis requires microscopic examination of resected tissue.

The benefits of an extended lymph node dissection are: (1) better staging of the tumor; (2) if disease is limited to the primary tumor and lymph nodes, removing all disease is potentially curative; and (3) by removing microscopic residual disease there is a decreased incidence of fossa recurrences. As newer adjuvant therapy is brought to clinical trial, careful systematic staging of patients will be necessary to determine the real impact of such therapy. In both retrospective and nonrandomized prospective studies, patients who underwent an extended retroperitoneal lymph node dissection had improved long-term survival when compared to patients who either did not have a retroperitoneal lymph node dissection or in whom that dissection was limited.[52,76–78] It should be clear, however, that such studies in no way prove that an extended lymph node dissection should be done in each case as a curative maneuver. The potential for skewed results secondary to selection bias is obvious. Theoretically, if 25% of patients undergoing a radical nephrectomy have lymph nodes as the only site of metastatic disease and the 5-year survival is otherwise 30 to 40%, then 5 to 10% of the patients would have been cured by having their diseased lymph nodes removed. To our knowledge, no good prospective randomized study has been done to determine whether lymphadenectomy has any real therapeutic benefit.

There are several problems with performing a lymph node dissection for renal cell carcinoma.

TABLE 12–10. PROGNOSIS FOLLOWING EXCISION OF A SOLITARY METASTASIS FOLLOWING RADICAL NEPHRECTOMY

Reference	Year	No. of Patients	5-Year Survival	No. of Patients	10-Year Survival
Skinner et al.[65]	1972	41	29%	41	22%
O'Dea et al.[72]	1978	26	50%		
McNichols et al.[73]	1981	13	69%	13	54%
Golimbu et al.[36]	1986	13	25%		
Total		93	40%*	54	30%*

*Weighed for the number of patients per study.

1. Renal cell carcinoma metastasizes by both a lymphatic and hematogenous route. Therefore, removing diseased lymph nodes does nothing for circulating malignant cells.[79]
2. The lymphatic drainage from the kidney is quite predictable at the level of the hilum, but beyond the immediate confines of the kidney is quite unpredictable.[80–82] The rationale of simply expanding the margins of resection must, therefore, be questioned.
3. There is no effective adjuvant therapy for patients with node-positive disease. While several proponents would argue this is precisely the reason why an extended lymph node dissection should be performed, this information provides little comfort to the patient.
4. An extended retroperitoneal lymph node dissection increases the operative risks of the procedure.

There are merits to performing a lymphadenectomy, and it does not represent simple surgical desperation. It is sensible to remove residual readily accessible tissue that would otherwise harbor malignant cells. While the collected series do not prove efficacy, there is a clear trend toward survival benefit in those patients treated with a lymphadenectomy. The controversial role of lymphadenectomy in the surgical management of renal cell carcinoma persists in the absence of well-conducted prospective randomized studies. It remains, however, part of the surgical management of renal cell carcinoma.

RENAL CELL CARCINOMA INVADING OTHER ORGANS

The ominous finding of renal cell carcinoma invading adjacent organs is supported by a relatively dismal overall survival. In Robson's series, 9% of his patients had adjacent organ invasion, with a 3-year survival of approximately 20%.[33] This is in agreement with the report from Gittes, in which long-term survival with invasion of the liver or bowel was negligible.[83] It should be noted, however, that patients with recurrences from local extension or incomplete resection at the time of initial nephrectomy tend to do much worse than those with distant metastases and no local disease.[84] If the goal is palliation, then the surgeon should be prepared to carry out the resection of additional structures such as liver or bowel when these are found to be invaded at the time of surgery. Bahnson and colleagues reported on three patients who underwent en bloc liver and kidney resections for direct hepatic extension from renal cell cancer and noted that these were not only technically feasible but were associated with good local control.[85]

Locally extensive disease reported at autopsy has been associated with diffuse metastases. In fact, it is much more common for renal cell carcinoma to involve the liver from metastatic disease than from direct invasion. We have personally resected the liver, the pancreas, the colon, and the psoas to achieve negative margins. Pain has been associated with extensive invasion and one should be prepared to resect these structures as a palliative maneuver. Debulking or partial resection should be avoided. In the age of new adjuvant immunotherapy or gene therapy protocols an increasing number of these locally advanced tumors will be encountered and require surgical management.

Solitary Renal Fossa Recurrence

Following radical nephrectomy, patients are at risk to develop fossa recurrence. There are two relatively distinct patterns of recurrence: either within 24 months following radical nephrectomy or remote late recurrences, which have been reported between 10 and 31 years following the presumed successful resection of the kidney.[73,86,87] These late recurrences underscore the slow doubling time and tenacious quality of renal cell carcinoma.

A solitary recurrence of renal cell carcinoma in the renal fossa is distinctly unusual. Most often patients have evidence of metastatic disease. In the age of CT imaging, however, small fossa recurrence may be diagnosed and successfully surgically removed.[88] CT scanning following radical nephrectomy has been successfully employed to identify patients who have benefited from surgical resection of these recurrences.[89,90] A new mass in the renal fossa, irregularity of the psoas muscle, or alteration in the great vessels may indicate recurrent disease. Unopacified bowel has produced both false-positive and false-negative results using CT scanning.[91] Serial studies or angiography have been proposed to better define subtle abnormalities. Finally, needle aspiration and tissue diagnosis may be necessary.

We recommend a thoracoabdominal approach using an incision above the previous nephrectomy scar in the surgical management of these recurrences.[92] The only reasonable goal of a surgical approach to fossa recurrences is the complete resection. This may require the resection of adjacent organs and/or structures. For example, we have resected psoas and quadratus muscles, ribs, the tail of the pancreas, spleen, and diaphragm to obtain negative margins. An understanding that complete resection with curative intent may require deep and extensive resection of the lateral parietes with Marlex or Gore-Tex reconstruction should be discussed preoperatively.

The prognosis from resection of a solitary renal fossa recurrence is unknown given the lack of reported, well-documented cases. The largest series reported by Skinner and associates included 11 patients, 10 of whom had no metastatic disease. The operative mortality was 20%, but 40% of patients had no evidence of disease with a 60% 1-year and 30% 4-year survival.[91] The subset of patients with a long interval free of obvious disease probably have a more indolent tumor, and aggressive surgical approaches should be strongly considered.[93] We have successfully managed a late, 11-year postoperative, massive scar recurrence with aggressive surgery.[94]

Embolization

Embolic occlusion of feeding vessels, either the renal artery or other parasitic vessels, has been used in the treatment of renal cell carcinoma for a variety of indications:

1. Prenephrectomy renal artery embolic occlusion for large, hypervascular primary tumors with no evidence of metastatic disease.
2. Preoperative embolic renal artery occlusion for patients with demonstrable metastatic disease who subsequently undergo nephrectomy followed by hormonal therapy.
3. For palliation in patients with life-threatening AV fistulas, recurrent gross hematuria, or other severe symptoms, such as flank pain, from advanced renal cell carcinoma.
4. Palliation for metastatic lesions. Embolization of feeding vessels to hypervascular metastases is prudent prior to attempted resection: catastrophic bleeding can occur from the aggressive injudicious use of surgery for metastatic lesions in which no effort has been made to control feeding vessels.

Prenephrectomy Renal Artery Embolization for Nonmetastatic Disease

Several surgeons continue to routinely use preoperative renal artery embolization to shrink large hypervascular tumors. A variety of techniques have been used to occlude the renal artery and its branches. The procedure is performed angiographically with advancement of a catheter through a transfemoral approach. A variety of agents including Silastic spheres, silicone rubber, glass beads, stainless steel pellets, barium, Gianturco stainless steel coils, Gelfoam, detachable silicone balloons, 95% ethyl alcohol, absolute alcohol, autologous blood clot, autologous muscle, polyvinyl alcohol, and ferromagnetic silicone microspheres, and mixtures of compounds such as ducrylate, iophendylate, gangalum, and cyanoacrylate are injected through the catheter for embolization.[95–99] The procedure should be done under fluoroscopic control with and without contrast media with interval films to ensure that embolization has occurred.

The postinfarction syndrome could be considered a complication of this procedure, but because it occurs so frequently and, in fact, has been directly related to the effectiveness of the treatment, should be considered a natural outcome of the procedure. In general, successful embolization of the renal artery is immediately followed by pain, fever, nausea, and vomiting. Although these symptoms are generally of a short duration, less than 72 hours, patients are so debilitated as to require hospitalization and close monitoring. The severity of symptoms following renal artery embolization has been linked to the supposed effectiveness of the procedure. Patients who retain a blood supply to the kidney by way of parasitic arterial vessels do not tend to have severe postinfarction symptoms. Narcotics, often parenteral, are usually required to control the pain. Hiccups from diaphragmatic irritation can occur in as many as 10% of patients.[100]

The major complication associated with renal artery embolization is the inadvertent embolization of other parts of the body as the embolic material is seeded into the peripheral circulation. The reported complications are the direct result of ischemia following inadvertent embolization, and include renal failure following embolization of the contralateral kidney or the administration of too much contrast media, renal abscesses, aneurysm formation, hypertension, paraplegia, colonic infarction, and Ogilve's syndrome.[101–105] We do not use embolization preoperatively primarily because of postinfarction syndrome and the potential consequence of inadvertent and potentially catastrophic embolic material migration. In general, the risks of the procedure almost always outweigh the benefits that may be achieved. Furthermore, the presence of a foreign body in the renal artery may complicate intraoperative vascular control of the pedicle.

Prenephrectomy Renal Artery Embolization for Metastatic Disease

In the early 1970s Almgard reported the use of renal artery occlusion followed by nephrectomy for patients with metastatic renal cell carcinoma.[106–108] He reported that several of their patients' tumors remained dormant. Mindful of the unpredictable nature of metastatic renal cell carcinoma progression, investigators at M.D. Anderson Hospital undertook a prospective study that included 50 patients with metastatic renal cell carcinoma and subjected them to renal artery occlusion, transabdominal radical nephrectomy, followed by parenteral progestins.[100] The proposed mechanism of therapeutic effect came from the shower of tumor antigens into the circulation and subsequent antitumor immune response. Following nephrectomy, such a response would be focused on the residual metastatic disease. In the initial group of 50 patients, there were 7 complete responders, 5 partial responders, and 6 with "stable" disease. This 36% overall response rate was greeted with great enthusiasm and propelled a subsequent multi-institutional trial by the Southwest Oncology Group.[109] Unfortunately, of the 30 patients with metastatic re-

TABLE 12–11. RESPONSE TO ANGIOINFARCTION, NEPHRECTOMY ± PROGESTATIONAL AGENTS IN PATIENTS WITH METASTATIC RENAL CELL CARCINOMA

Reference	Year	No. of Patients	Complete Response	Partial Response	Tumor Stabilization
Swanson et al.[100]	1980	50	7 (14%)	5 (10%)	6 (12%)
Swanson et al.[110]	1983	50	0	3 (6%)	7 (14%)
Gottesman et al. (SWOG)[109]	1985	30	0	1 (3%)	3 (10%)
Kurth et al. (EORTC)[111]	1987	34	1 (3%)	0	3 (9%)
Total		164	8 (4.8%)	9 (5.5%)	19 (11.6%)

nal cell carcinoma treated with renal infarction followed by delayed nephrectomy, there were no complete responses, only 1 partial response, and the 3 patients who had stable disease enjoyed this status for only 6 months. All patients enrolled eventually showed progression. The resulting 21% 1-year survival rate in a 7-month medium survival were very similar to series in which no therapy had been given. The early indication that patients with metastases limited to the lungs enjoyed a unique sensitivity to the expected antitumor immune response that followed infarction and nephrectomy was not substantiated by the multi-institutional studies[112] (Table 12–11).

Embolization of symptomatic, inoperative, primary renal cell carcinoma has been used successfully to control bleeding and pain. Indeed, repeat selective embolization of a solitary kidney with renal cell carcinoma has successfully palliated a patient for 18 months who suffered from massive bleeding from this lesion.[113] Furthermore, advances in angiographic techniques allow selective therapeutic embolization of renal cell carcinoma. In several patients with solitary kidneys who are not considered candidates for nephron-sparing surgery, repetitive therapeutic embolization can be performed. This has been successfully employed by Kozac and colleagues in a series of elderly patients.[114] Finally, patients who have large arterial venous communications in association with renal cell carcinoma may present with high-output congestive heart failure.[115] These AV fistulas can be successfully treated with selective embolization.

Renal Cell Carcinoma in von Hippel-Lindau Disease

Von Hippel-Lindau disease is a genetic disorder characterized by tumors at multiple sites in the body, including multifocal renal cysts and renal cell carcinoma, hemangioblastomas of the central nervous system, retinal angiomas, pheochromocytomas, pancreatic cysts, and epididymal cyst adenomas. The gene responsible for von Hippel-Lindau disease has been localized to the 3p26 region of chromosome 3.[116]

In a review of 267 selected cases of von Hippel-Lindau disease with renal lesions, 47% of the reported deaths were attributed to renal cell carcinoma, but historically, about one third of patients with von Hippel-Lindau disease died of renal cell carcinoma.[117] This percentage should increase with the improved detection and treatment of central nervous system tumors, the other major source of mortality. While a major advancement has been made in the understanding of this disease following the identification of the von Hippel-Lindau tumor suppressor gene,[116] the diverse nature of the renal lesions, high local recurrence rates following nephron-sparing surgery, and a desire to preserve native renal function have made optimal surgical management controversial. It is well known that tumors presenting in the kidney are multifocal, often cystic, with low-grade, clear-cell renal cell carcinoma.[118]

Two recent reviews of renal tumors in von Hippel-Lindau disease provide useful guidelines in the surgical management of these lesions.[117,119] There is no correlation between the size of a lesion and the presence of renal cell carcinoma. In both studies, the overwhelming majority of benign lesions were cystic but, unfortunately, between 25 and 35% of the malignant lesions were also cystic. Solid lesions were almost invariably malignant. With these three observations it is clear that neither size nor appearance of a lesion will determine whether or not it is malignant. Therefore all lesions, whether cystic or solid, should be resected at the time of nephron-sparing surgery, if feasible. Some intrarenal small cysts may be difficult to treat.

It was also observed that the cystic lesions, including renal cell carcinoma, were well encapsulated. Solid lesions, while tending to be well encapsulated, could be invasive. The technical strategy of enucleation of cystic lesions is sound. A wider margin of resection is indicated for solid lesions.

At what point is nephron-sparing surgery no longer indicated? Patients with a diffuse distribution are readily identifiable: the removal of all lesions would also remove the entire cortical surface. Such kidneys should be removed. Large or deeply seeded lesions are probably also best treated with radical nephrectomy. If lesions can be removed safely and allow a reasonable balance of functioning renal parenchyma, then nephron-sparing surgery should be considered. The status of the contralateral kidney obviously needs to be considered.

TABLE 12–12. PROGNOSIS FOLLOWING RADICAL NEPHRECTOMY: CELL TYPE

		Clear Cell Alone		Any Granular Cell		Spindle, Sarcomatoid, Anaplastic	
Reference	Year	No. of Patients	5-Year Survival	No. of Patients	5-Year Survival	No. of Patients	5-Year Survival
Skinner et al.[34]	1972	67	58%	169	46%	36	23%
Selli et al.[68]	1983	70	88%	40	85%	1	0%
Golimbu et al.[36]	1986	201	57%	56	50%	53	25%
Total		338	63.6%*	265	52.7%*	90	24%*

*Weighed for the number of patients per study.

For patients with bilateral diffuse disease it is recommended that they undergo bilateral nephrectomies and subsequent transplantation. Because this is a systemic field change, patients should be expected to recur and lifetime surveillance is mandatory.

The long-term outcome following nephron-sparing surgery is one of recurrence.[120] In series from both the Mayo Clinic and the Cleveland Clinic local recurrence rates and secondary operations were common.[121,122] Nephron-sparing surgery, while technically feasible in many cases,[123] should be reserved for patients with cystic and low-volume nondiffuse solid lesions. Patients should be informed of the risk of recurrence following nephron-sparing surgery.

PROGNOSIS

Grade

Although it is well known that the overall prognosis of renal cell carcinoma is best determined by the stage of the tumor, one third of patients who undergo presumably curative surgery will recur at metastatic sites. While these metastases may be the result of clinically undetected microscopic disease present at the time of surgery, it would be useful to identify those patients provided effective adjuvant therapy becomes available. Histologic evaluation does not, alone, reliably identify those patients. The presence of spindle, sarcomatoid, or anaplastic cell types in a primary tumor portends a poor prognosis. Table 12–12 indicates the 5-year survivals from three different cellular histologies. Fortunately, the spindle cell type is also the most rare.

Tumor grading can provide some prognostic information. Not surprisingly, higher grade tumors have a worse prognosis as summarized on Table 12–13. Fuhrman studied 103 patients with renal cell carcinoma and applied four nuclear grades in analyzing these tumors.[125] She found that nuclear grade was more effective than other parameters in predicting the development of distant metastases following nephrectomy. Unfortunately this technique has been criticized because of its subjective nature. Using more objective measurements, such as nuclear morphometry, may accurately predict those patients destined to recur who have clinically localized renal cell carcinoma.[126]

Nuclear morphometric techniques have been used to predict those patients destined to recur.[126] Multivariate analysis of the four best individual shape descriptor-statistical test pairs predicted the prognosis in 23 of 26 patients analyzed in a blinded retrospective study. No patient predicted to recur remained disease free for a period longer than 65 months and over half of the patients predicted to recur by morphometric analysis relapsed in under 2 years. This stratification is particularly useful in trying to identify high-risk patients who have presumably low stage disease.

TABLE 12–13. PROGNOSIS FOLLOWING RADICAL NEPHRECTOMY: TUMOR GRADE

		Grade I		Grade II		Grade III	
Reference	Year	No. of Patients	5-Year Survival	No. of Patients	5-Year Survival	No. of Patients	5-Year Survival
Riches[124]	1958	24	71%	18	39%	12	25%
Robson[47]	1963	21	87%	24	64%	12	40%
Robson et al.[33]	1968	49	57%	15	47%	15	40%
Bottinger[64]	1970	4	100%	78	46%	8	0%
Guiliani et al.[52]	1990	36	70%	64	30%	11	16%
Total		134	69%*	199	42%	58	27%*

*Weighed for the number of patients per study.

Novel Biomarkers

Despite the current lack of effective therapies for advanced metastatic renal cell carcinoma, there is hope that the developing immunologic and gene therapeutic approaches will be efficacious. Since between 25 and 50% of patients who undergo radical nephrectomies with presumed localized renal cell carcinoma will ultimately develop demonstrable metastatic disease, it is important to identify those patients and enroll them in adjuvant treatment. None of the current prognostic factors, including pathologic tumor stage, size, histologic and/or architectural patterns, and nuclear grade, provide clear independent reliable prognostic information.[127–137] For example, when DNA flow cytometry was applied to stage I renal cell carcinoma lesions, the presence of nondiploid cells indicated a worse prognosis than diploid tumors, but it did not provide an independent prognostic indicator.[138]

An evaluation of tumor cell kinetics using in vivo labeling with iododeoxyuridine was used to determine potential tumor doubling time.[139] In a study of 29 patients who received 100 mg of iododeoxyuridine (used to label dividing cells) immediately prior to nephrectomy, no statistical difference in labeling was identified between the various clinical stages and there was frequent intratumor heterogeneity of potential tumor doubling times. Diploid and aneuploid tumors did have significantly different potential tumor doubling times, which had a significant impact on survival. Whether in vivo labeling and determination of cell kinetics will provide an independent reliable prognostic indicator will require a larger data set than was performed in this preliminary study.

Evaluation of nucleolar organization regions (NORs) has been performed to determine whether a measurement of these regions was of prognostic significance.[140] Malignant tissue is known to contain greater numbers of visible silver-binding NOR-associated proteins than benign tumors or normal tissue of an equivalent histologic type. It appears that NORs are indicative of the proliferative activities of the tissues being examined. Applying this staining technique to renal cell carcinoma may provide new prognostic information but, again, will require larger prospective evaluation. A variety of other markers associated with proliferation, such as proliferation cell nuclear antigen, using monoclonal antibodies Ki-67 or PC 10, may provide another useful prognostic parameter in renal cell carcinoma.

Serum ferritin is another potential marker for renal cell carcinoma. In one study of 30 patients, serum ferritin did correlate with tumor volume. The tumor did appear to be the source of the ferritin. Histologic sections of tumor stained intensely for iron and normal tissue did not. Higher ferritin levels were measured in the renal vein.[141]

Perhaps the most promising new biomarkers will come from evaluation of molecular changes in renal cell carcinoma. Some chromosomal changes, such as 3p loss which has commonly been described in renal cell carcinoma, will probably not provide prognostic information. Furthermore, in a study by Brooks et al., interactivation of p53 RB and DCC genes by allelic loss appear to be uncommon events in the early stages of renal cell carcinogenesis and these markers will probably not be useful prognostic indicators.[142] In a recent study using comparative genomic hybridization techniques, the number of DNA losses per tumor were associated with recurrence-free survival with statistical significance; DNA gains were not associated with clinical outcome.[143] Interestingly, loss of chromosomal arm 9p was the only individual locus associated with recurrence, suggesting that a yet-unidentified tumor suppressor gene may play a role in renal cell carcinoma progression.

Paraneoplastic Syndromes

Renal cell carcinoma has been called the "internist's disease" because of the many unusual presentations of this malignancy. The nonspecific, systemic manifestations of renal cell carcinoma are common: fever, weight loss, fatigue, and cachexia occur in approximately one third of patients. Otherwise unexplained anemia and hypertension are also common (20%).[14]

The paraneoplastic syndromes associated more specifically with a factor or factors produced by the tumor are less common (3 to 10%), but will often resolve following nephrectomy. These syndromes include hypercalcemia, amyloidosis, erthrocytosis, and nephrogenic hepatic dysfunction syndrome (Stauffer's syndrome).[14]

Among the unusual manifestations of renal cell carcinoma, the nephrogenic hepatic dysfunction syndrome is, perhaps, the most curious. This paraneoplastic process occurs in the absence of hepatic metastases and often resolves following resection of the primary tumor. Some degree of hepatic dysfunction is common, although the characteristic manifestations of this syndrome are variable.[144–151] The syndrome has been associated with a poor prognosis.[150] Kozlowski and associates isolated a renal cell carcinoma line from a patient who died of fulminant hepatic failure as a result of this syndrome. This cell line, BA1119, produced a syndrome of hepatic necrosis, splenomegaly, neutrophilia, and cachexia in nude mice bearing BA1119 tumors.[152] Analysis of this cell line in vitro and in vivo revealed the production of massive amounts of cytokines, interleukin-6 (IL-6), and granulocyte colony-stimulating factor (G-CSF). Recapitulation of the syndrome following administration of these cytokines in the absence of the tumor appears to confirm an etiologic role of IL-6 and G-CSF in this syndrome. Interestingly, an elevated IL-6 level is associated with a worse prognosis in renal cell carcinoma.[153]

RADIATION THERAPY

Surgery is the most effective treatment of renal cell carcinoma. It is reasonable to ask, therefore, why one would consider radiation therapy in the management of renal cell carcinoma. It has been proposed that preoperative radiation therapy has several benefits[48]: (1) it may lessen the risk of tumor dissemination at the time of nephrectomy; (2) it can reduce the size of the tumor; (3) it can render a "fixed" lesion resectable; and (4) it can decrease the vascularity. Postoperatively, radiation therapy has the theoretical benefit of providing local control of an incompletely resected primary tumor or grossly positive lymph nodes.[154] The problem with radiation therapy is that primary renal cell carcinoma is a relatively radioresistant lesion, given its frequent necrotic, cystic or otherwise anaerobic qualities. Futhermore, the natural history of tumors with invasion is for early and extensive metastatic disease. The large volume of normal tissue that can be included in a radiation treatment field carries with it potential and real morbidity. The surrounding bowel will not tolerate a very large dose of radiation.

In a large retrospective review of 248 cases over a 25-year period, Peeling found that postoperative radiation therapy did not improve prognosis of renal cell carcinoma over nephrectomy alone.[155] Van Der Werf-Messing performed a randomized prospective study in 141 patients and showed that for each stage preoperative radiation therapy did not improve prognosis.[156] The investigators noted, however, that for each stage metastases occurred more frequently in the surgery-only arm. Also, with higher stage tumors, there was an increase in the residual growth (i.e., fossa recurrence) in the nephrectomy-only group. Finney performed a randomized prospective study of 100 patients who received postnephrectomy radiation.[157] He did not find any influence on local recurrence or distant metastases but he did note an increase in death rate from coincidental causes including radiation-induced liver damage. Considering crude survival data, patients with surgery only did better than those receiving surgery and postoperative radiation therapy. Lang performed embolization of tumors with iodine-125 (^{125}I) for palliation in 14 patients with metastatic disease and 8 patients with greatly locally advanced disease.[158] He was able to achieve an 80% pain control when pain was the major symptom. In patients in whom hemorrhage was a significant problem, this therapy resulted in a 90% response rate. Tumor size decreased in all patients in which this was evaluated.

In a small recent series from the Mayo Clinic, selected patients with a solitary local recurrence or persistence following a radical nephrectomy for renal cell carcinoma benefited from aggressive local treatment including maximal surgery debulking and both pre- and intraoperative radiation.[159] This study was limited to patients who had either local persistent or local regional recurrence and no evidence of metastatic disease. Once again, considering the rare solitary fossa recurrence, it is unclear whether surgery alone would have achieved similar results to those in which surgery was combined with pre- and intraoperative radiation therapy. Clinical trials in favor of radiation therapy have been nonrandomized and retrospective. In randomized prospective studies, matching stage for stage, there has been no change in the prognosis with preoperative radiation therapy; however, it was noted that there was decrease in subsequent metastatic disease and a decrease in local recurrences in patients treated with preoperative therapy.

The current role of radiation in the management of renal cell carcinoma is for palliation, most often in bone metastases. It has been well documented that symptomatic response rates are excellent for painful or bleeding metastases. The role of radiation therapy in the management of metastatic renal cell carcinoma was studied by Halpeirn et al.[160] Thirty-five patients with metastatic disease received palliative radiation therapy to the metastatic site. Seventy-seven per cent of those with bone pain responded at the treated site but he noted only a 30% response for central nervous system lesions. High-dose radiation was not necessary to achieve the desired effect. In conclusion, the well-documented radioresistance of renal cell carcinoma has blunted its widespread use for primary renal cell carcinoma.[161] Radiation clearly has a role, however, for palliation of metastatic lesions.

HORMONE THERAPY

Progestational therapy was based on the following observations: (1) the estrogen diethylstilbestrol (DES) -induced tumors in the Syrian golden hamster model responded to progestational agents[162,163]; (2) the male predominance of both renal cell carcinoma and spontaneous regressions supported a sex-hormonal sensitivity of renal cell carcinoma.[164] In the initial reports by Bloom in the early 1970s, the overall "objective" response rate to hormonal manipulation was 15% with, interestingly, a reported male predominance. This report, however, represented a summary of nonrandomized studies with varying response criteria and unclear subjective and objective response measurements. In a review of therapeutic trials using progestins and/or androgens before 1971, a response rate of 17%, or 40 of 228 so-treated individuals, was reported.[165] Following 1971, with well-defined objective response criteria employed, less than 2% response rate was observed in 416 patients from five separate large trials. Enthusiasm for this form of therapy has, therefore, waned considerably. In the absence, however, of other effective treatment, patients with advanced renal cell carcinoma are still treated with progestational agents.

A variety of agents have been employed including testosterone, tamoxifen, nafoxidine and estramustine phosphate, and medroxyprogesterone acetate. Progesterone is the only agent that has been shown to have an antitumor effect. Compared to systemic cytotoxic chemotherapeutic agents, there are almost no side effects from hormonal therapy. An occasional patient will suffer from nausea, vomiting, painful gynecomastia, and/or uterine bleeding. However, these are usually not limiting toxicities. Given the mild side effects from the hormonal agents, this form of therapy can be considered in the advanced renal cell carcinoma patient who is not a candidate for investigational trials.

CHEMOTHERAPY

Despite the remarkable response of some solid tumors to single and combination chemotherapy, renal cell carcinoma remains doggedly chemoresistant. Such a conclusion is based on multiple studies using single and combination chemotherapy for renal cell carcinoma with generally dismal results. Alkylating agents (cyclophosphamide, chlorambucil); antimetabolites (hydroxyurea, 5-FUDR, methotrexate, 6-mercaptopurine, ARA-C); antimitotic agents (vincristine, vinblastine); and other agents including Adriamycin, atenomycin, mithramycin, and mitomycin C have been employed as single agents.[166] Initial enthusiasm for vinblastine, as a single agent, has been tempered by other studies showing partial responses in the range of approximately 5%.[167] In general, there have been no complete responders to chemotherapy and most partial responses are short-lived. Employing strict criteria in both single and combination chemotherapy, response ranges between 4 and 6%. The agent floxuridine (5-FUDR) employed in a continuous-infusion schedule utilizing circadian rhythms and, potentially, less toxicity, have shown some encouraging results with combined and partial responses in the range of 15%.[168–175]

The multidrug-resistance (MDR) gene and its protein product P-glycoprotein actively pump chemotherapeutic and toxic agents out of cells in which MDR is expressed.[176,177] Agents such as cyclosporine, a potent inhibitor of P-glycoprotein, have been employed in combination with vinblastine.[178] This strategy attempts to disable the biologic basis for renal cell carcinomas' chemoresistance, and while initial results are discouraging, this is a rational and strategic approach to the chemoresistant phenotype. In phase I and phase II trials there does not appear to be improved efficacy. The exhaustive application of single and combination chemotherapeutic regimens to advanced renal cell carcinoma clearly indicates that other strategies need to be employed to provide treatment for this disease. Such an impetus has encouraged us to explore an immunotherapeutic approach using ex vivo gene transfer techniques.

IMMUNOTHERAPY

Interleukin-2 (IL-2) was identified in 1976 by its selective growth effect on T lymphocytes.[179] It was found that incubation of T cells in IL-2 produced cytotoxic immune cells that could selectively lyse tumor cells, the so-called lymphokine-activated killer (LAK) cells.[180,181] The activity of these killer cells was not restricted by major histocompatibility class (MHC) expression. In animal models, IL-2 alone or LAK cells and IL-2 could mediate the regression of established lung and liver metastases.[182–186] This antitumor effect was dose related and, in animals, combined IL-2 and LAK were better than IL-2 alone. In animals, the best antitumor effects were observed at the maximum tolerated dose of both IL-2 and LAK. Based on these observations, high-dose IL-2 was brought to human clinical trials. Currently, IL-2 is the only agent approved by the U.S. Food and Drug Administration (FDA) for the treatment of advanced renal cell carcinoma.

High-Dose IL-2

In the initial trials with high-dose IL-2, including 255 patients, there were 12 (5%) complete responders and 24 (9%) partial responders.[187] Those complete responses were often quite durable, with some 5- to 6-year long-term patients with no evidence of disease. Table 12–14 summarizes the results of several trials using high-dose IL-2 by bolus infusion. The major drawback of high-dose IL-2 therapy is profound cardiovascular toxicity, primarily hypotension. To circumvent this problem, trials using continuous infusion IL-2 have been performed. Table 12–15 summarizes those results. Al-

TABLE 12–14. RESPONSE TO HIGH-DOSE IL-2 BY BOLUS INFUSION IN PATIENTS WITH METASTATIC RENAL CELL CARCINOMA

Reference	Year	No. of Patients	Complete Response	Partial Response
Abrams et al.[188]	1990	16	0	0
Poo et al.[189]	1991	15	0	4 (27%)
Atkins et al.[190]	1993	71	4 (6%)	8 (11%)
Rosenberg et al.[191]	1994	149	10 (7%)	20 (13%)
Yang et al.[192]	1994	65	3 (5%)	17 (26%)
McCabe et al.[193]	1991	37	1 (3%)	3 (8%)
Total		353	18 (5%)	52 (15%)

TABLE 12–15. RESPONSE TO HIGH-DOSE IL-2 BY CONTINUOUS IV INFUSION IN PATIENTS WITH METASTATIC RENAL CELL CARCINOMA

Reference	Year	No. of Patients	Complete Response	Partial Response
Bajorin et al.[194]	1990	24	1 (4%)	2 (8%)
Geertsen et al.[195]	1992	30	1 (3%)	4 (13%)
Negrier et al.[196]	1992	25	2 (8%)	1 (4%)
Palmer et al.[197]	1992	225	8 (4%)	20 (9%)
Escudier et al.[198]	1992	88	0	16 (18%)
Lopez et al.[199]	1993	30	1 (3%)	3 (10%)
Total		422	13 (3%)	46 (11%)

though there is generally less toxicity with continuous infusion and response rates are similar, durable, long-term responses are rare.

The clinical trials with the highest rates of durable response use IL-2 at maximum tolerable doses. Because of the toxicity and resulting intensive and expensive supportive care required in these patients, trials using lower doses of IL-2 have been performed.

Low-Dose IL-2

Trials using low-dose IL-2 by intravenous or subcutaneous administration consistently report less toxicity with similar antitumor responses. In the absence of a consensus definition for low-dose IL-2, IL-2 given on an outpatient basis is considered low dose.[200] Unlike high-dose IL-2, low-dose regimens tend to be protracted. Furthermore, because of the toxicity associated with high-dose IL-2, patients often do not complete therapy. While the cumulative dose is severalfold greater with high-dose IL-2, the tolerability of low-dose therapy allows patients to get IL-2 over a longer period of time.[200]

In an interim report of a randomized phase III trial, Yang reported similar response rates with much less toxicity.[201] For example, hypotension requiring pressors occurred in 52% of those receiving the high-dose IL-2 and in only 3% of those receiving low-dose IL-2. It should be recognized that this is an interim report with short follow-up. The durability of responses from low-dose therapy is currently unknown. Table 12–16 summarizes the response to low-dose IL-2 by either continuous infusion or subcutaneous administration. Because of the brief half-life of IL-2 when given intravenously, it has been combined with polyethylene glycol (PEG) to increase the half-life of the drug. These trials were associated with severe systemic toxicities without a marked improvement in response.[208,212]

IL-2 Toxicity

The major toxicity from IL-2 stems from the induction of increased vascular permeability leading to hypotension, fluid retention, and respiratory distress. Clinically, the patients exhibit a septic, low-systemic-vascular-resistance picture. The mediation of this response is myriad and includes LAK-induced endothelial damage, induction of secondary cytokines including interferon, IL-1, IL-5, IL-8, as well as the potent vasodilator nitric oxide (NO).[213] The relative contributions of the host and the tumor to this response are unknown. We have shown that following IL-2 administration to RCCa in vitro, there is a marked enhancement of the production of several inflammatory cytokines.

Bolus administration of high-dose IL-2 often results in profound hypotension 1 to 2 hours later. Like sepsis, management requires fluids and pressors with α-agonistic activity. Infectious complications, stemming from a reversible defect in neutrophil activity, are associated with an increased risk of gram-positive bacteremia.[214] Cutaneous toxicities include edema, skin lichenization, and desquamation.[213] This pruritic erythematous rash resolves af-

TABLE 12–16. RESPONSE TO LOW-DOSE IL-2 BY CONTINUOUS INFUSION OR SUBCUTANEOUSLY IN PATIENTS WITH METASTATIC RENAL CELL CARCINOMA

Reference	Year	No. of Patients	Intravenous (IV) or Subcutaneous (SQ)	Complete Response	Partial Response
Richards et al.[202]	1988	12	IV	0	0
Whitehead et al.[203]	1990	15	SQ	0	0
Atzpodien et al.[204]	1990	17	SQ	0	0
Bukowski et al.[205]	1990	23	IV	1 (4%)	4 (17%)
Stein et al.[206]	1991	9	SQ	0	2 (22%)
Perez et al.[207]	1991	12	IV	1 (8%)	1 (8%)
Meyers et al.[208]	1991	16	IV (PEG)	0	2 (13%)
Sleijfler et al.[209]	1992	47	SQ	2 (4%)	7 (15%)
Buter et al.[210]	1993				
Vlasveld et al.[211]	1992	9	IV	0	0
Bukowski et al.[212]	1993	35	IV (PEG)	0	2 (6%)
Yang et al.[201]	1994	60	IV	4 (7%)	5 (8%)
Total		255		8 (3%)	23 (9%)

TABLE 12–17. RESPONSE TO INTERFERON THERAPY FOR METASTATIC RENAL CELL CARCINOMA

Reference	Year	No. of Patients	INF-α (α) or INF-γ (γ)	Complete Response	Partial Response
Neidhart et al.[215]	1984	23	α	1 (4%)	4 (17%)
Quesada et al.[216]	1985	50	α	3 (6%)	10 (20%)
Quesada et al.[217]	1985	56	α	1 (2%)	11 (20%)
Kirkwood et al.[218]	1985	30	α	1 (3%)	2 (7%)
Vugrin et al.[219]	1985	21	α	0	1 (5%)
Umeda et al.[220]	1986	108	α	2 (2%)	13 (12%)
Rinehart et al.[221]	1986	13	γ	0	0
Eisenhauer et al.[222]	1987	37	α	0	4 (11%)
Buzaid et al.[223]	1987	22	α	0	5 (23%)
Trump et al.[224]	1987	39	α	0	5 (13%)
Muse et al.[225]	1987	97	α	2 (2%)	6 (6%)
Quesada et al.[226]	1987	16	γ	0	1 (1%)
Figlin et al.[227]	1988	19	α	1 (5%)	4 (21%)
Garnick et al.[228]	1988	41	γ	1 (2%)	3 (7%)
Grups and Frohmuller[229]	1989	9	γ	0	3 (33%)
Auliktzky et al.[230]	1989	16	γ	2 (13%)	4 (25%)
Ellerhorst et al.[231]	1994	34	γ	1 (3%)	4 (12%)
Total		631		15 (2%)	80 (13%)

ter discontinuation of IL-2. Gastrointestinal toxicity, including nausea and vomiting, occurs in nearly all patients treated with IL-2.[213]

Low-dose, outpatient, IL-2 administration is generally not associated with the dramatic systemic responses to high-dose IL-2. The most common toxicity from subcutaneous or low-dose intravenous IL-2 regimens are fatigue and an increase in serum creatinine. We have also noted troublesome, often profound, central nervous system effects manifest by nightmares and frank night terrors.

Interferon Therapy

Interferons were first described as naturally occurring proteins produced by cells to blunt viral reproduction. There are now identified many interferons that exert pleiotrophic actions. The role of interferon in tumor biology is discussed elsewhere.

Clinical trials employing interferons from a variety of crude and purified sources are listed in Table 12–17. Responses are most frequent in patients with low tumor burden, pulmonary metastases as the only site of disease, and in those patients with better performance status. The optimal route, frequency, and dose of administration are not known and probably do not greatly impact the antitumor response. Malaise, low-grade fever, and flulike symptoms are the major side effects.

Low-Dose IL-2 Plus Interferon-α

Preclinical data from the National Cancer Institute (NCI) indicated a synergistic antitumor effect by combining IL-2 and interferon in a mouse model.[232] This has led to a series of trials combining these two agents in the treatment of metastatic renal cell carcinoma. Table 12–18 summarizes these studies, which appear to have activities in combination similar to, and perhaps greater than, either agent alone. Toxicities included constitutional symptoms and weight loss. In a small series, Hu-

TABLE 12–18. RESPONSE TO LOW-DOSE IL-2 PLUS INF-α IN PATIENTS WITH METASTATIC RENAL CELL CARCINOMA

Reference	Year	No. of Patients	IL-2: IV or SQ	Complete Response	Partial Response
Hirsch et al.[233]	1990	15	IV	3 (20%)	3 (20%)
Ilson et al.[234]	1992	35	IV	1 (3%)	3 (9%)
Lipton et al.[235]	1993	39	IV	6 (15%)	7 (18%)
Figlin et al.[236]	1993	52	IV	3 (6%)	10 (19%)
Atzpodien et al.[237]	1993	51	SQ	4 (8%)	10 (20%)
Dutcher et al.[238]	1993	31	SQ	1 (3%)	4 (13%)
Ratain et al.[239]	1993	21	SQ	0	4 (19%)
Vogelzang et al.[240]	1993	42	SQ	2 (5%)	4 (10%)
Huland et al.[241]	1994	15	SQ	1 (7%)	6 (40%)
Thiounn et al.[242]	1995	15	SQ	0	0
Total		316		21 (7%)	51 (16%)

land used inhalation IL-2 administration in combination with systemic IL-2 and interferon-α and noted an overall response rate of 47%.[241]

LAK/IL-2 Therapy

The discovery and preclinical studies showing activity and rationale for LAK cells are discussed elsewhere. The startling in vitro efficacy of LAK cells to lyse tumor tissue did not translate to the clinic. Table 12–19 summarizes the response to IL-2/LAK in patients with metastatic renal cell carcinoma. The goal of combined therapy—to improve responses over IL-2 alone—was prospectively tested in three randomized studies.[254] Collectively, they showed that the combination of LAK/IL-2 is not superior to IL-2 alone.

TIL/IL-2 Therapy

Tumor-infiltrating lymphocytes (TIL) have been shown to be 50 to 100 times more potent on a per-cell basis than LAK cells in lysing target tumor cells.[255] Clinical trials using TIL/IL-2 therapies are summarized in Table 12–20. Again, the exciting in vitro and preclinical data are not reflected in the clinical responses. It should be noted, however, that TIL/IL-2 is still being developed and strategies using cytokine priming, specific CD8+ TIL cells may enhance response rates.

Immunotherapy and Surgery

The role of surgery in patients with widely metastatic renal cell carcinoma is clear. There is no benefit to perform palliative nephrectomy for patients who are otherwise asymptomatic. On the other hand, the effectiveness of an immunologic therapy is dependent on the tumor burden. Some investigators have proposed that patients undergo a "debulking" radical nephrectomy prior to the initiation of any immunotherapy. Following this strategy at the NCI, more than one third of the patients who underwent a nephrectomy in anticipation of subsequent IL-2 treatment failed to ever receive that IL-2 treatment because of progressive disease or other medical issues. More recently, several investigators have shown that patients responding to up-front immunotherapy can be rendered complete responders with the subsequent resection of their primary tumor.[261–264] This strategy has been shown for both IL-2 immunotherapy and interferon-α therapy. Clearly, this is not the case in TIL therapy where lymphocytes are harvested from resected tumors. Outside of these indications, however, the well-established axiom that there is no role for nephrectomy in a patient with widely metastatic renal cell carcinoma holds.

TABLE 12–19. RESPONSE TO IL-2 AND LYMPHOKINE-ACTIVATED KILLER (LAK) CELLS IN PATIENTS WITH METASTATIC RENAL CELL CARCINOMA

Reference	Year	No. of Patients	Complete Response	Partial Response
Fisher et al.[243]	1988	32	2 (6%)	3 (9%)
Parkinson et al.[244]	1990	47	2 (4%)	2 (4%)
Palmer et al.[245]	1992	95	5 (5%)	12 (13%)
Rosenberg[246]	1992	72	8 (11%)	17 (24%)
Foon et al.[247]	1992	23	2 (9%)	4 (17%)
Weiss et al.[248]	1992	94	5 (5%)	11 (12%)
Thompson et al.[249]	1992	42	4 (10%)	10 (24%)
Sznol et al.[250]	1992	40	0	8 (20%)
Dillman et al.[251]	1992	46	0	7 (15%)
Total		491	28 (6%)	71 (14%)

TABLE 12–20. RESPONSE TO IL-2 AND TUMOR-INFILTRATING LYMPHOCYTES (TIL) IN PATIENTS WITH METASTATIC RENAL CELL CARCINOMA

Reference	Year	No. of Patients	Complete Response	Partial Response
Topalian et al.[256]	1988	4	0	1 (25%)
Kradin et al.[257]	1989	7	0	2 (29%)
Bukowski et al.[258]	1991	18	0	0
Dillman et al.[251]	1993	6	0	0
Pierce et al.[259]	1994	40	7 (18%)	6 (15%)
Olencki et al.[260]	1994	16	1 (6%)	3 (19%)
Total		91	8 (9%)	12 (13%)

Gene Therapy

A new form of immunotherapy involves tumor vaccines and gene therapy. This experimental approach utilizes a paracrine (local) immune response to irradiated autologous tumor that then becomes systemic.[265] A cytolytic immune response then results in the destruction of distant metastatic disease.[266] This novel approach has recently been applied to a group of metastatic renal cell carcinoma patients in our institution. The gene for granulocyte-macrophage colony-stimulating factor (GM-CSF) was inserted into autologous tumor cell grown in vitro by a retroviral vector after radical nephrectomy in patients with metastatic disease. This phase I study was recently completed. Ultimately, high-risk patients with low tumor burdens will probably be the best candidates for this new treatment or some variation of it.

REFERENCES

1. Parker SL, Tong T, Bolden S, Wingo PA: Cancer statistics, 1996. CA Cancer J Clin 1996; 46:5.
2. Walter CW, Gillespie DR: Metastatic hypernephroma of fifty years' duration. Minn Med 1960; 43:123.
3. Everson TC, Cole WH: Spontaneous Regression of Cancer. Philadelphia, WB Saunders Co, 1966.

4. Freed SZ, Halperin JP, Gordon M: Idiopathic regression of metastases from renal cell carcinoma. J Urol 1977; 118: 538.
5. Snow RM, Schellhammer PF: Spontaneous regression of metastatic renal cell carcinoma. Urology 1982; 20:177.
6. Vogelzang NJ, Priest ER, Borden L: Spontaneous regression of histologically proven pulmonary metastases from renal cell carcinoma: a case with five-year follow-up. J Urol 1992; 148:1247.
7. Oliver RT, Nethersell AB, Bottomley JM: Unexplained spontaneous regression and alpha-interferon as treatment for metastatic renal carcinoma. Br J Urol 1989; 63:128.
8. Saitoh H: Distant metastasis of renal adenocarcinoma in patients with a tumor thrombus in the renal vein and/or vena cava. J Urol 1982; 127:652.
9. Saitoh H, Nakayama M, Nakamura K, et al: Distant metastasis of renal adenocarcinoma in nephrectomized cases. J Urol 1982; 127:1092.
10. Saitoh H, Hida M, Nakamura K, et al: Metastatic processes and a potential indication of treatment for metastatic lesions of renal adenocarcinoma. J Urol 1982; 128: 916.
11. Cinberg JZ, Solomon MP, Ozbardacki G: Thyroid carcinoma and secondary malignancy of the sinonasal tract. Arch Otolaryngol 1980; 106:239.
12. Matsumoto Y, Yanagihara N: Renal clear cell carcinoma metastatic to the nose and paranasal sinuses. Laryngoscope 1982; 92:1190.
13. Kent SE, Majumdar B: Metastatic tumors in the maxillary sinus: a report of two cases and the review of the literature. J Laryngol Otol 1989; 99:459.
14. McDougal WS, Garnick MB: Clinical signs and symptoms of renal cell carcinoma. *In* Vogelzang NJ, Scardino PT, Shipley WU, et al (eds): Comprehensive Textbook of Genitourinary Oncology, p 154. Baltimore, Williams & Wilkins, 1996.
15. Chang S-Y, Yu D-S, Sherwood ER, et al: Inhibitory effects of suramin on a human renal cell carcinoma line causing nephrogenic hepatic dysfunction. J Urol 1992; 146:1147.
16. Utz DC, Warren MM, Gregg JA, et al: Reversible hepatic dysfunction associated with hypernephroma. Mayo Clin Proc 1970; 45:161.
17. Weyman PJ, McClennan BL, Stanley RJ, et al: Comparison of computed tomography and angiography in the evaluation of renal cell carcinoma. Radiology 1980; 137:417.
18. Lang EK: Comparison of dynamic and conventional computed tomography, angiography, and ultrasonography in the staging of renal cell carcinoma. Cancer 1984; 54:2205.
19. Fein AB, Lee JKT, Balfe DM, et al: Diagnosis and staging of renal cell carcinoma: a comparison of MR imaging and CT. AJR 1987; 148:749.
20. Frohmüller HGW, Grups JW, Heller V: Comparative value of ultrasonography, computerized tomography, angiography and excretory urography in the staging of renal cell carcinoma. J Urol 1987; 138:482.
21. Zeman RK, Cronan JJ, Rosenfield AT, et al: Renal cell carcinoma: dynamic thin-section CT assessment of vascular invasion and tumor vascularity. Radiology 1988; 167:393.
22. Sampaio CA, McLain D, Klein E, et al: Renal masses simulating primary renal cell carcinoma in patients with advanced malignancies. J Urol 1994; 151:1505.
23. Klinger ME: Secondary tumors of the genito-urinary tract. J Urol 1951; 65:144.
24. Crotty TB, Farrow GM, Lieber MM: Chromophobe cell renal carcinoma: clinicopathological features of 50 cases. J Urol 1995; 154:964.
25. Morra MN, Das S: Renal oncocytoma: a review of histogenesis, histopathology, diagnosis and treatment. J Urol 1993; 150:295.
26. Steiner MS, Goldman SM, Fishman EK, et al: The natural history of renal angiomyolipoma. J Urol 1993; 150:1782.
27. Licht MR, Novick AC: Nephron sparing surgery for renal cell carcinoma. J Urol 1993; 149:1.
28. Jacobs SC, Berg SI, Lawson RK: Synchronous bilateral renal cell carcinoma: total surgical excision. Cancer 1980; 46:2341.
29. Palmer JM: Role of partial nephrectomy in solitary or bilateral renal tumors. JAMA 1983; 249:2357.
30. Novick AC, Streem SB, Montie JE, et al: Conservative surgery for renal cell carcinoma: a single-center experience with 100 patients. J Urol 1989; 141:835.
31. Petritsch PH, Rauchenwald M, Zechner O, et al: Results after organ-preserving surge for renal cell carcinoma. Eur Urol 1990; 18:84.
32. Morgan WR, Zincke H: Progression and survival after renal-conserving surgery for renal cell carcinoma: experience in 104 patients and extended followup. J Urol 1990; 144:852.
33. Robson CJ, Churchill BM, Anderson W: The results of radical nephrectomy for renal cell carcinoma. J Urol 1969; 101:207.
34. Skinner DG, Vermillion CD, Colvin RB: The surgical management of renal cell carcinoma. J Urol 1972; 107:705.
35. Siminovitch JMP, Montie JE, Straffon RA: Prognostic indicators in renal adenocarcinoma. J Urol 1982; 130:20.
36. Golimbu M, Tessler A, Joshi P, et al: Renal cell carcinoma: survival and prognostic factors. Urology 1986; 25:291.
37. Best BG: Renal carcinoma: a ten-year review 1971–1980. Br J Urol 1987; 60:100.
38. Flocks RG, Kadesky MC: Malignant neoplasms of the kidney: an analysis of 353 patients followed five years or more. J Urol 1958; 79:196.
39. Skinner DG, Pfister RF, Colvin R: Extension of renal cell carcinoma into the vena cava: the rationale for aggressive surgical management. J Urol 1972; 107:711.
40. Heney NM, Nocks BN: The influence of perinephric fat involvement on survival in patients with renal cell carcinoma extending into the inferior vena cava. J Urol 1982; 128:18.
41. Cherrie RJ, Goldman DG, Lindner A, et al: Prognostic implications of vena caval extension of renal cell carcinoma. J Urol 1982; 128:910.
42. Neves RJ, Zincke H: Surgical treatment of renal cancer with vena cava extension. Br J Urol 1987; 59:390.
43. Libertino JA, Zinman L, Watkins E Jr: Long-term results of resection of renal cell cancer with extension into inferior vena cava. J Urol 1987; 137:21.
44. Hatcher PA, Anderwon EE, Paulson DF, et al: Surgical management and prognosis of renal cell carcinoma invading the vena cava. J Urol 1991; 145:20.
45. Glazer AA, Novick AC: Long-term followup after surgical treatment for renal cell carcinoma extending into the right atrium. J Urol 1996; 155:448.
46. Petkovic SD: An anatomical classification of renal tumors in the adult as a basis for prognosis. J Urol 1959; 81:618.
47. Robson CJ: Radical nephrectomy for renal cell carcinoma. J Urol 1963; 89:37.
48. Rafla S: Renal cell carcinoma—national history and results of treatment. Cancer 1970; 25:26.
49. Middleton RG, Presto AJ III: Radical thoracoabdominal nephrectomy for renal cell carcinoma. J Urol 1973; 110:36.
50. Peters PC, Brown GL: The role of lymphadenectomy in the management of renal cell carcinoma. Urol Clin North Am 1980; 7:705.
51. Hermanek P, Schrott KM: Evaluation of the new tumor, nodes and metastases classification of renal cell carcinoma. J Urol 1990; 144:238.
52. Giuliani L, Giberti C, Martorana G, et al: Radical extensive surgery for renal cell carcinoma: long-term results and prognostic factors. J Urol 1990; 143:468.
53. Angervall L, Wahlqvist L: Follow-up and prognosis of renal carcinoma in a series operated by perifascial nephrectomy combined with adrenalectomy and retroperitoneal lymphadenectomy. Eur Urol 1978; 4:13.
54. Robson CJ: Results of radical thoraco-abdominal nephrectomy in the treatment of renal cell carcinoma. *In* Küss R, Murphy GP, Khoury S, Karr JP (eds): Renal Tumors: Proceedings of the First International Symposium on Kidney Tumors, p 481. New York, Alan R Liss, Inc, 1982.

55. Hohenfellner R, Zingg EJ: Urologie in Klinik and Praxis, Vol I, p 504. New York, Georg Thieme Verlag, 1982.
56. Jaeger N, Vahlensieck W: Prognose bein Mierenkarzinom. Lebensversicherungsmedizin 1985; 37:75.
57. Robey EL, Schelhammer PF: The adrenal gland and renal cell carcinoma: is ipsilateral adrenalectomy a necessary component of radical nephrectomy. J Urol 1986; 135:453.
58. O'Brien WM, Lynch JH: Adrenal metastases by renal cell carcinoma. Urology 1987; 29:605.
59. Winter P, Miersch WD, Vogel J, Jaefer N: On the necessity of adrenal extirpation combined with radical nephrectomy. J Urol 1990; 144:842.
60. Haab F, Gattengo B, Duclos JM, et al: Should adrenalectomy be performed systematically as part of radical nephrectomy for renal cancer? Review of 119 cases. Prog Urol 1993; 3:41.
61. Sagalowsky AI, Kadesky KT, Ewalt DM, et al: Factors influencing adrenal metastasis in renal cell carcinoma. J Urol 1994; 151:1181.
62. Gill IS, McClennan BL, Kerbl K, et al: Adrenal involvement from renal cell carcinoma: predictive value of computerized tomography. J Urol 1994; 152:1082.
63. Middleton RG: Surgery for metastatic renal cell carcinoma. J Urol 1987; 97:973.
64. Böttinger LE: Prognosis in renal carcinoma. Cancer 1970; 26:780.
65. Skinner DG, Colvin RB, Vermillion CD, et al: Diagnosis and management of renal cell carcinoma: a clinical and pathologic study of 309 cases. Cancer 1971; 28:1165.
66. Thompson IM, Shannon H, Ross G Jr, et al: An analysis of factors affecting survival in 150 patients with renal carcinoma. J Urol 1975; 114:836.
67. Montie JE, Stewart BH, Straffon RA, et al: The role of adjunctive nephrectomy in patients with metastatic renal cell carcinoma. J Urol 1977; 117:272.
68. Selli C, Hinshaw WM, Woodard BH, et al: Stratification of risk factors in renal cell carcinoma. Cancer 1983; 52: 899.
69. Maldazys JD, deKernion JB: Prognostic factors in metastatic renal carcinoma. J Urol 1986; 136:376.
70. Tolia BM, Whitmore WF Jr: Solitary metastasis from renal cell carcinoma. J Urol 1975; 114:836.
71. Klugo RC, Detmres M, Stiles RE, et al: Aggressive versus conservative management of stage 4 renal cell carcinoma. J Urol 1977; 118:244.
72. O'Dea MF, Zincke H, Utz DC, et al: The treatment of renal cell carcinoma with solitary metastasis. J Urol 1978; 120: 540.
73. McNichols DW, Segura JW, DeWeerd JH: Renal cell carcinoma: long-term survival and late recurrence. J Urol 1981; 126:17.
74. Swanson DA, Orovan WL, Johnson DE, et al: Osseous metastases secondary to renal cell carcinoma. Urology 1981; 18:556.
75. Studer UE, Scherz S, Scheidegger J, et al: Enlargement of regional lymph nodes in renal cell carcinoma is often not due to metastases. J Urol 1990; 144:243.
76. Giuliani L, Martorana G, Giberti C, et al: Results of radical nephrectomy with extensive lymphadenectomy for renal cell carcinoma. J Urol 1983; 130:664.
77. Herrlinger A, Schrott KM, Schott G, et al: What are the benefits of extended dissection of the regional renal lymph nodes in the therapy of renal cell carcinoma? J Urol 1991; 146:1224.
78. Pizzocaro G, Piva L: Pros and cons of retroperitoneal lymphadenectomy in operable renal cell carcinoma. Eur Urol 1990; 18:22.
79. deKernion JB: Lymphadenectomy for renal cell carcinoma. Urol Clin North Am 1980; 7:697.
80. Tsukamoto T, Kumamoto Y, Miyao N, et al: Regional lymph node metastasis in renal cell carcinoma: incidence, distribution and its relation to other pathological findings. Eur Urol 1990; 18:88.
81. Wood DP Jr: Role of lymphadenectomy in renal cell carcinoma. Urol Oncol 1991; 18:421.
82. Marshall FF, Powell KC: Lymphadenectomy for renal cell carcinoma: anatomical and therapeutic considerations. J Urol 1982; 128:677.
83. Gittes RF: Locally extensive renal cell carcinoma—current surgical management of invasion of vena cava, liver, or bowel. Prog Clin Biol Res 1982; 100:497.
84. deKernion JB, Berry D: The diagnosis and treatment of renal cell carcinoma. Cancer 1980; 45:1947.
85. Bennett BC, Selby R, Bahnson RR: Surgical resection for management of renal cancer with hepatic involvement. J Urol 1995; 154:972.
86. Takatera H, Maeda O, Oka T, et al: Solitary late recurrence of renal cell carcinoma. J Urol 1986; 136:799.
87. Kradjian RM, Bennington JL: Renal carcinoma recurrent 31 years after nephrectomy. Arch Surg 1965; 90:192.
88. Sease WC, Belis JA: Computerized tomography in the early postoperative management of renal cell carcinoma. J Urol 1986; 136:792.
89. Montie JE: Follow-up after partial or total nephrectomy for renal cell carcinoma. Urol Clin North Am 1994; 21: 589.
90. Campbell SC, Novick AC: Management of local recurrence following radical nephrectomy or partial nephrectomy. Urol Clin North Am 1994; 21:593.
91. Esrig D, Ahlering TE, Lieskovsky G, et al: Experience with fossa recurrence of renal cell carcinoma. J Urol 1992; 147:1491.
92. Chute R, Soutter L, Kerr WS Jr: The value of the thoracoabdominal incision in the removal of kidney tumors. N Engl J Med 1949; 241:951.
93. Newmark JR, Newmark GM, Epstein JI, et al: Solitary late recurrence of renal cell carcinoma. Urology 1994; 43:725.
94. Tanguay S, Pisters LL, Lawrence DD, et al: Therapy of locally recurrent renal cell carcinoma after nephrectomy. J Urol 1996; 155:26.
95. Wallace S, Schwarten DE, Smith DC, et al: Intrarenal arteriovenous fistulas: transcatheter steel coil occlusion. J Urol 1978; 120:282.
96. Mazer MM, Baltaxe HA, Wolff GL: Therapeutic embolization of the renal artery with Gianturco coils: limitations and technical pitfalls. Radiology 1981; 138:37.
97. Grinnell VS, Hieshima GB, Mehringer CM, et al: Therapeutic renal artery occlusion with a detachable balloon. J Urol 1981; 126:233.
98. Kadir S, Marshall FF, White RI, et al: Therapeutic embolization of the kidney with detachable silicone balloons. J Urol 1982; 129:11.
99. Crotty KL, Orihuela E, Warren MM: Recent advances in the diagnosis and treatment of renal arteriovenous malformations and fistulas. J Urol 1993; 150:1355.
100. Swanson DA, Wallace S, Johnson DE: The role of embolization and nephrectomy in the treatment of metastatic renal carcinoma. Urol Clin North Am 1980; 7:719.
101. Bergreen PW, Woodside J, Paster SB: Therapeutic renal infarction. J Urol 1977; 118:372.
102. Withlin LS, Gross WS, James TP, et al: Renal artery occlusion with migration of stainless steel coils. JAMA 1980; 243:2064.
103. Cox GG, Lee KR, Price HI, et al: Colonic infarction following ethanol embolization of renal-cell carcinoma. Radiology 1982; 145:343.
104. Teertstra HJ, Winter WA, Frensdorf EL: Ethanol embolization of a renal tumor, complicated by colonic infarction. Diagn Imaging Clin Med 1984; 53:250.
105. Terhune DW, Petrochko N, Jordan GH, et al: Ogilvies syndrome developing after ethanol ablation of renal cell carcinoma. J Urol 1985; 133:838.
106. Almgard LE, Ljundgqvist A: Experimental occlusion of the renal circulation in the dog. Scand J Urol Nephrol 1971; 5:268.
107. Almgard LE, Fernstrom I, Haverling M, et al: Occlusion of the renal circulation facilitating later nephrectomy for carcinoma of the kidney. J Urol Nephrol (Paris) 1971; 77: S521.
108. Almgard LE, Fernstrom I, Haverling M, et al: Treatment

of renal adenocarcinoma by embolic occlusion of the renal circulation. Br J Urol 1973; 45:474.
109. Gottesman JE, Scardino P, Crawford ED, et al: Infarction-nephrectomy for metastatic renal carcinoma. Urology 1985; 25:248.
110. Swanson DA, Johnson DE, von Eschenbach AC, et al: Angioinfarction plus nephrectomy for metastatic renal cell carcinoma—an update. J Urol 1983; 130:449.
111. Kurth KH, Debruyne FMJ, Hall RR, et al: Embolization and postinfarction nephrectomy in patients with primary metastatic renal adenocarcinoma. Eur Urol 1978; 13:251.
112. Flanigan RC: The failure of infarction and/or nephrectomy in stage IV renal cell cancer to influence survival or metastatic regression. Urol Clin North Am 1987; 14:757.
113. Cos LR, Gutierrez O: Repeat selective embolization of solitary kidney with renal cell carcinoma: case report. J Urol 1989; 141:115.
114. Kozac BE, Keller FS, Rosch J, et al: Selective therapeutic embolization of renal cell carcinoma in solitary kidneys. J Urol 1987; 137:1223.
115. Barth KH, White RI, Marshall FF: Quantification of arteriovenous shunting in renal cell carcinoma. J Urol 1981; 125:161.
116. Latif F, Tory K, Gnarra J, et al: Identification of the von Hippel-Lindau disease tumor suppressor gene. Science 1993; 260:1317.
117. Nelson JB, Oyasu R, Dalton DP: The clinical and pathological manifestations of renal tumors in von Hippel-Lindau disease. J Urol 1994; 152:2221.
118. Walther MM, Lubensky IA, Venzon D, et al: Prevalence of microscopic lesions in grossly normal renal parenchyma from patients with von Hippel-Lindau disease, sporadic renal cell carcinoma and no renal disease: clinical implications. J Urol 1995; 154:2010.
119. Poston CD, Jaffe GS, Lubensky IA, et al: Characterization of the renal pathology of a familial form of renal cell carcinoma associated with von Hippel-Lindau disease: clinical and molecular genetic implications. J Urol 1995; 153: 22.
120. Steinbach F, Novick AC, Zincke H, et al: Treatment of renal cell carcinoma in von Hippel-Lindau disease: a multicenter study. J Urol 1995; 153:1812.
121. Frydenberg M, Malek RS, Zincke H: Conservative renal surgery for renal cell carcinoma in von Hippel-Lindau's disease. J Urol 1993; 149:461.
122. Novick AC, Streem SB: Long-term followup after nephron sparing surgery for renal cell carcinoma in von Hippel-Lindau disease. J Urol 1992; 147:1488.
123. Shinohara N, Nonomura K, Harabayashi T, et al: Nephron sparing surgery for renal cell carcinoma in von Hippel-Lindau disease. J Urol 1995; 154:2016.
124. Riches EW: Factors in the prognosis of carcinoma of the kidney. J Urol 1958; 79:190.
125. Fuhrman SA, Lasky LC, Limas C: Prognostic significance of morphologic parameters in renal cell carcinoma. Am J Surg Pathol 1982; 6:655.
126. Pound CR, Partin AW, Epstein JI, et al: Nuclear morphometry accurately predicts recurrence in clinically localized renal cell carcinoma. Urology 1993; 42:243.
127. Myers GH, Fehrenbaker LG, Kelalis PP: Prognostic significance of renal vein invasion by hypernephroma. J Urol 1968; 100:420.
128. Holland JM: Cancer of the kidney—natural history and staging. Nat History Staging (Holland) 1973; 32:1030.
129. deKernion JB, Ramming KP, Smith RB: The natural history of metastatic renal cell carcinoma: a computer analysis. J Urol 1978; 120:148.
130. Patel NP, Lavengood RW: Renal cell carcinoma: natural history and results of treatment. J Urol 1978; 120:722.
131. McDonald MW: Current therapy for renal cell carcinoma. J Urol 1982; 127:211.
132. deKernion JB: Treatment of advanced renal cell carcinoma—traditional methods and innovative approaches. J Urol 1983; 130:2.
133. Hoehn W, Hermanek P: Invasion of veins in renal cell carcinoma—frequency, correlation and prognosis. Eur Urol 1983; 9:276.
134. Elson PJ, Witte RS, Trump DL: Prognostic factors for survival in patients with recurrent or metastatic renal cell carcinoma. Cancer Res 1988; 48:7310.
135. Marroncle M, Irani J, Dore B, et al: Prognostic value of histological grade and nuclear grade in renal adenocarcinoma. J Urol 1994; 151:1174.
136. Targonski PV, Frank W, Stuhldreher D, et al: Value of tumor size in predicting survival from renal cell carcinoma among tumors, nodes and metastases stage 1 and stage 2 patients. J Urol 1994; 152:1389.
137. Ljungberg B, Stenling R, Österdahl B, et al: Vein invasion in renal cell carcinoma: impact on metastatic behavior and survival. J Urol 1995; 154:1681.
138. Grignon DJ, el-Naggar A, Green LK, et al: DNA flow cytometry as a predictor of outcome of stage I renal cell carcinoma. Cancer 1989; 63:1161.
139. Ljungberg B, Larsson P, Roos G, et al: Cell kinetics of renal cell carcinoma studied with in vivo iododeoxyuridine incorporation and flow cytometry. J Urol 1994; 151: 1509.
140. Shimazui T, Tomobe M, Hattori K, et al: A prognostic significance of nucleolar organizer region (AgNOR) in renal cell carcinoma. J Urol 1995; 154:1522.
141. Partin AW, Steiner MS, Hsieh K, et al: Serum ferritin as a clinical marker for renal cell carcinoma: influence of tumor volume. Urology 1995; 45:211.
142. Brooks JD, Bova SG, Marshall FF, et al: Tumor suppressor gene allelic loss in human renal cancers. J Urol 1993; 150: 1278.
143. Moch H, Presti JC, Sauter G, et al: Genetic aberrations detected by comparative genomic hybridization are associated with clinical outcome in renal cell carcinoma. Cancer Res 1996; 56:27.
144. Stauffer MH: Nephrogenic hepatosplenomegaly (Abstract). Gastroenterology 1961; 40:694.
145. Walsh PN, Kissane JM: Nonmetastatic hypernephroma with reversible hepatic dysfunction. Arch Intern Med 1968; 122:214.
146. Pochedly C, Suwansirikul S, Penzer P: Renal-cell carcinoma with extrarenal manifestations in a 10-month-old child. Am J Dis Child 1971; 121:528.
147. Ramos CV, Taylor HB: Hepatic dysfunction associated with renal carcinoma. Cancer 1972; 29:1287.
148. Hanash KA, Utz DC, Ludwig J, et al: Syndrome of reversible hepatic dysfunction associated with hypernephroma: an experimental study. Invest Urol 1971; 8:399.
149. Strickland RC, Schenker S: The nephrogenic dysfunction syndrome: a review. Am J Dig Dis 1977; 22:49.
150. Boxer RJ, Waisman J, Lieber MM, et al. Non-metastatic hepatic dysfunction associated with renal carcinoma. J Urol 1978; 119:468.
151. Hanash KA: The nonmetastatic hepatic dysfunction syndrome associated with renal cell carcinoma (hypernephroma): Stauffer's syndrome. Prog Clin Biol Res 1982; 100:301.
152. Sherwood ER, Kee HN, Fike W, et al: The role of colony stimulating factors in the pathogenesis of nephrogenic hepatic dysfunction (Stauffer's) syndrome. J Urol 1988; 139: 175a.
153. Nelson JB, Sutkowski DM, Kozlowski JM: Association of interleukin 6 (IL-6) and granulocyte colony simulating factor (G-CSF) to nephrogenic hepatic dysfunction (Stauffer's) syndrome. J Urol 1994; 151:484a.
154. Riches E: The place of radiotherapy in the management of parenchymal carcinoma of the kidney. J Urol 1966; 95: 313.
155. Peeling WB, Mantell BS, Shepheard BGF: Post-operative radiation in the treatment of renal cell carcinoma. Br J Urol 1968; 23.
156. van der Werf-Messing B: Carcinoma of the kidney. Cancer 1973; 32:1056.
157. Finney R: The value of radiotherapy in the treatment of hypernephroma—a clinical trial. Br J Urol 1973; 45:258.

158. Lang EK, deKernion J: Transcatheter embolization of advanced renal cell carcinoma with radioactive seeds. J Urol 1981; 120:581.
159. Frydenberg M, Gunderson L, Hahn G, et al: Preoperative external beam radiotherapy followed by cytoreductive surgery and intraoperative radiotherapy for locally advanced primary or recurrent renal malignancies. J Urol 1994; 152:15.
160. Halperin EC, Harisiadis L: The role of radiation therapy in the management of metastatic renal cell carcinoma. Cancer 1983; 51:614.
161. Cox CE, Lacy SS, Montgomery WG, et al: Renal adenocarcinoma: 28-year review, with emphasis on rationale and feasibility of preoperative radiotherapy. J Urol 1970; 104:53.
162. Kirkman H, Bacon RL: Estrogen-induced tumors of the kidney. 1. Incidence of renal tumors in intact and gonadectomized male Golden hamsters treated with diethylstilbestrol. J Natl Cancer Inst 1952; 13:745.
163. Soloway MS, Myers GH Jr: The effects of hormonal therapy on a transplantable renal cortical adenocarcinoma in syngeneic. J Urol 1973; 109:356.
164. Bloom HJG: Hormone induced and spontaneous regression of metastatic renal cancer. Cancer 1973; 32:1066.
165. Hrushesky WJ, Murphy GP: Current status of the therapy of advanced renal carcinoma. J Surg Oncol 1977; 9:277.
166. Talley RW: Chemotherapy of adenocarcinoma of the kidney. Cancer 1973; 32:1062.
167. Fossa SD, Droz JP, Pavone-Macaluso MM, et al: Vinblastine in metastatic renal cell carcinoma: EORTC phase II trial 30882. The EORTC Genitourinary Group. Eur J Cancer 1992; 28A:878.
168. von Roemeling R, et al: Progressive metastatic renal cell carcinoma controlled by continuous 5-fluoro-2-deoxyuridine infusion. J Urol 1988; 139:259.
169. Conroy T, Geoffois L, Guillemin F, et al: Simplified chronomodulated continuous infusion of floxuridine in patients with metastatic renal cell carcinoma. Cancer 1993; 72:2190.
170. Stadler WM, Vogelzang NJ, Vokes EE, et al: Continuous-infusion fluorodeoxyurodine with leucovorin and high-dose interferon: a phase II study in metastatic renal cell cancer. Cancer Chemother Pharmacol 1992; 31:213.
171. Damascelli B, Marchiano A, Frigerio LF, et al: Flexibility and efficacy of automatic continuous fluorodeoxyuridine infusion in metastases from a renal cell carcinoma. Cancer 1991; 68:995.
172. Hrushesky WJ, von Roemeling R, Lanning RM, et al: Circadian-shaped infusion of floxuridine for progressive metastatic renal cell carcinoma. J Clin Oncol 1990; 8:1504.
173. Damascelli B, Marchiano A, Spreafico C, et al: Circadian continuous chemotherapy of renal cell carcinoma with an implantable, programmable infusion pump. Cancer 1990; 66:237.
174. von Roemeling R, Hurshesky WJ: Circadian patterning of continuous floxuridine infusion reduces toxicity and allows higher dose intensity in patients with widespread cancer. J Clin Oncol 1989; 7:1710.
175. Falcone A, Cianei C, Ricci S, et al: Alpha-2B interferon plus floxuridine in metastatic renal cell carcinoma. A phase I-II study. Cancer 1993; 72:564.
176. Nishiyama K, Shirahama T, Yoshimura A, et al: Expression of the multidrug transporter, P-glycoprotein, in renal transitional cell carcinoma. Cancer 1993; 71:3511.
177. Naito S, Sakamoto N, Kotoh S, et al: Expression of P-glycoprotein and multidrug resistance in renal cell carcinoma. Eur Urol 1993; 24:156.
178. Samuels BL, Mick R, Vogelzang NJ, et al: Modulation of vinblastine resistance with cyclosporine: a phase I study. Clin Pharmacol Ther 1993; 54:421.
179. Morgan DA, Ruscetti FW, Gallo RG: Selective in vitro growth of T-lymphocytes from normal bone marrow. Science 1976; 193:1007.
180. Yron I, Wood TA, Spiess PJ, et al: In vitro growth of murine T cells. V. The isolation and growth of lymphoid cells infiltrating syngeneic solid tumors. J Immunol 1980; 125:238.
181. Lotze MT, Line BR, Mathisen DJ, et al: The in vivo distribution of autologous human and murine lymphoid cells grown in T cell growth factor (TCGF): implications for the adoptive immunotherapy of tumors. J Immunol 1980; 125:1487.
182. Grimm EA, Mazumder A, Zhang HZ, et al: Lymphokine-activated killer cell phenomenon: lysis of natural killer-resistant fresh solid tumor cells by interleukin-2 activated autologous human peripheral blood lymphocytes. J Exp Med 1982; 155:1823.
183. Grimm EA, Ramsey KM, Mazumder A, et al: Lymphokine-activated killer cell carcinoma. II. Precursor phenotype is serologically distinct from peripheral T lymphocytes, memory cytoxic thymus-derived lymphocytes, and natural killer cells. J Exp Med 1983; 157:884.
184. Grimm EA, Robb RJ, Roth JA, et al: Lymphokine-activated killer cell phenomenon. III. Evidence that IL-2 is sufficient for direct activation of peripheral blood lymphocytes into lymphokine-activated killer cells. J Exp Med 1983; 158:1356.
185. Rosenstein M, Yron J, Kaufmann Y, et al: Lymphokine-activated killer cells: lysis of fresh syngeneic natural killer-resistant murine tumor cells by lymphocytes cultured in interleukin-2. Cancer Res 1984; 44:1946.
186. Rayner AA, Grimm EA, Lotze MT, et al: Lymphokine-activated killer (LAK) cells: analysis of factors relevant to the immunotherapy of human cancer. Cancer 1985; 55:1327.
187. Hawkins MJ: Management of metastatic disease. 15A. Immunotherapy with high-dose interleukin 2. *In* Vogelzang NJ, Scardino PT, Shipley WU, Coffey DS (eds): Comprehensive Textbook of Genitourinary Oncology, p 242. Baltimore, Williams & Wilkins, 1996.
188. Abrams JS, Rayner AA, Wierni PH, et al: High-dose recombinant interleukin 2 alone: a regimen with limited activity in the treatment of advanced renal cell carcinoma. J Natl Cancer Inst 1990; 82:1202.
189. Poo WJ, Fynan T, Davis C, et al: High-dose recombinant interleukin 2 alone in patients with metastatic renal cell carcinoma (Abstract). Proc Annu Meet Am Soc Clin Oncol 1991; 10:A557.
190. Atkins MB, Rayner Sparano J, Fisher RI, et al: Randomized phase II trial of high-dose interleukin 2 either alone or in combination with interferon alfa-2b in advanced renal cell carcinoma. J Clin Oncol 1993; 11:661.
191. Rosenberg SA, Yang JC, Topalian SL, et al. Treatment of 283 consecutive patients with metastatic melanoma or renal cell cancer using high-dose bolus interleukin 2. JAMA 1994; 271:907.
192. Yang JC, Topalian SL, Parkinson D, et al: Randomized comparison of high-dose and low-dose intravenous interleukin 2 for the therapy of metastatic renal cell carcinoma: an interim report. J Clin Oncol 1994; 12:1572.
193. McCabe MS, Stabliem D, Hawkins MJ: The modified group C experience-phase III randomized trials of IL-2 vs IL-2/LAK in advanced renal cell carcinoma and advanced melanomia. (Abstract 714). Proc Am Soc Oncol 1991; 10:213.
194. Bajorin DF, Sell KW, Richards JM, et al: A randomized trial of interleukin 2 plus lymphokine-activated killer cells versus interleukin 2 alone in renal cell carcinoma. Proc Am Assoc Cancer Res 1990; 31:A1106.
195. Geertsen PF, Hermann GG, von der Maase H, et al: Treatment of metastatic renal cell carcinoma by continuous intravenous infusion of recombinant interleukin 2: a single-center phase II study. J Clin Oncol 1992; 10:753.
196. Negrier S, Mercatello A, Bret M, et al: Intravenous interleukin 2 in patients over 65 with metastatic renal carcinoma. Br J Cancer 1992; 65:723.
197. Palmer PA, Vinke J, Evers P, et al: Continuous infusion of recombinant interleukin 2 with or without autologous lymphokine-activated killer cells for the treatment of advanced renal cell carcinoma. Eur J Cancer 1992; 28A:1038.

198. Escudier B, Rossi JF, Tancini G, et al: French experience of high-dose IL-2 on a two-days-a-week schedule in metastatic renal cell carcinoma: a multicentric study (Abstract). Proc Annu Meet Am Soc Clin Oncol 1992; 11: A651.
199. Lopez M, Carpano S, Cancrini A, et al: Phase II study of continuous intravenous infusion of recombinant interleukin 2 in patients with advanced renal cell carcinoma. Ann Oncol 1993; 4:689.
200. Sparano JA, Dutcher JP, Wiernik PH: Adrenal and kidney cancer. 15B. Low-dose interleukin 2 for advanced renal cell carcinoma. *In* Vogelzang NJ, Scardino PT, Shipley WU, Coffey DS (eds): Comprehensive Textbook of Genitourinary Oncology, p 242. Baltimore, Williams & Wilkins, 1996.
201. Stein RC, Malvoska V, Morgan S, et al: The clinical effects of prolonged treatment of patients with advanced cancer with low-dose subcutaneous interleukin 2. Br J Cancer 1991; 63:275.
202. Richards JM, Barker E, Latta J, et al: Phase I study of weekly 24-hour infusions of recombinant human interleukin 2. J Natl Cancer Inst 1988; 80:1325.
203. Whitehead RP, Ward D, Heminway L, et al: Subcutaneous recombinant interleukin 2 in a dose-escalating regimen in patients with metastatic renal cell adenocarcinoma. Cancer Res 1990; 50:6708.
204. Atzpodien J, Korfer A, Evers P, et al: Lose-dose subcutaneous recombinant interleukin 2 in advanced human malignancy: a phase II outpatient study. Mol Biother 1990; 2:18.
205. Bukowski RM, Goodman P, Crawford ED, et al: Phase II trial of high-dose intermittent interleukin 2 in metastatic renal cell carcinoma: a Southwest Oncology Group study. J Natl Cancer Inst 1990; 82:143.
206. Stein RC, Malvoska V, Morgan S, et al: The clinical effects of prolonged treatment of patients with advanced cancer with low-dose subcutaneous interleukin 2. Br J Cancer 1991; 63:275.
207. Perez EA, Scudder SA, Meyers FA, et al: Short communication: weekly 24-hour continuous infusion interleukin 2 for metastatic melanoma and renal cell carcinoma: a phase I study. J Immunol 1991; 10:57.
208. Meyers FJ, Paradise C, Scudder SA, et al: A phase I study including pharmacokinetics of polyethylene glycol conjugated interleukin 2. Clin Pharmacol Ther 1991; 49:307.
209. Sleijfer DTh, Janssen RAJ, Buter J, et al: Phase II study of subcutaneous interleukin 2 in unselected patients with advanced renal cell cancer on an outpatient basis. J Clin Oncol 1992; 10:1119.
210. Buter J, Sleijfer DTh, van der Graaf WTZ, et al: A progress report on the outpatient treatment of patients with advanced renal cell carcinoma using subcutaneously recombinant interleukin 2. Semin Oncol 1993; 20 (Suppl 9):16.
211. Vlasveld LT, Rankin EM, Hekman A, et al: A phase I study of prolonged continuous infusion of low-dose recombinant interleukin 2 in melanoma and renal cell cancer. Part I: clinical aspects. Br J Cancer 1992; 65:744.
212. Bukowski RM, Young J, Goodman G, et al: Polyethylene glycol conjugated interleukin 2: clinical and immunologic effects in patients with advanced renal cell carcinoma. Invest New Drugs 1993; 11:211.
213. Lestingi TM, Thompson JA: Management of Metastatic Disease. 15C. Management of interleukin 2 toxicity. *In* Vogelzang NJ, Scardino PT, Shipley WU, Coffey DS (eds): Comprehensive Textbook of Genitourinary Oncology, p 242. Baltimore, Williams & Wilkins, 1996.
214. Klempner MS, Noring R, Mier JW. An acquired chemotactic defect in neutrophils from patients receiving interleukin 2 immunotherapy. N Engl J Med 1990; 322:959.
215. Neidhart JA, Gagan MM, Young D, et al: Interferon-alpha therapy of renal cancer. Cancer Res 1984; 44:4140.
216. Quesada JR, Swanson D, Gutterman JU: Phase II study of interferon alpha in metastatic renal cell carcinoma: a progress report. J Clin Oncol 1985; 3:1086.
217. Quesada JR, Rios A, Swanson DEA: Antitumor activity of recombinant-derived interferon alpha in metastatic renal cell carcinoma. J Clin Oncol 1985; 3:1522.
218. Kirkwood JM, Harris JE, Vera R, et al: A randomized study of low dose and high doses of leukocyte alpha-interferon in metastatic renal cell carcinoma: The American Cancer Society Collaborative Trial. Cancer Res 1985; 45:863.
219. Vugrin D, Hood L, Laslo J, et al: Phase II study of human lymphoblastoid alpha interferon in patients with advanced renal carcinoma. Cancer Treat Rep 1985; 69:817.
220. Umeda T, Niijima T: Phase II study of alpha interferon on renal cell carcinoma. Cancer 1986; 58:1231.
221. Rinehart JJ, Malspeis L, Young D, et al: Phase I/II trial of human recombinant interferon gamma in renal cell carcinoma. J Biol Response Mod 1986; 5:300.
222. Eisenhauer EA, Silver HK, Venner PM, et al: Phase II study of high dose weekly intravenous human lymphoblastoid interferon in renal cell carcinoma. Br J Cancer 1987; 55:541.
223. Buzaid AC, et al: Phase II study of interferon alfa-2a, recombinant (Roferon-A) in metastatic renal cell carcinoma. J Clin Oncol 1987; 5:1083.
224. Trump DL, Elson PJ, Borden EC: High-dose lymphoblastoid interferon in advanced renal cell carcinoma: an Eastern Cooperative Oncology Group study. Cancer Treat Rep 1987; 71:165.
225. Muse HB, Costanzi JJ, Leavitt R, et al: Recombinant alfa interferon in renal cell carcinoma: a randomized trial of two routes of administration. J Clin Oncol 1987; 5:286.
226. Quesada JR, Kuzrock R, Sherwin SA, et al: Phase II studies of recombinant human interferon gamma in metastatic renal cell carcinoma. J Biol Response Mod 1987; 6:20.
227. Figlin RA, deKernion JB, Mukamel E, et al: Recombinant interferon alfa-2a in metastatic renal cell carcinoma: assessment of antitumor activity and anti-interferon antibody formation. J Clin Oncol 1988; 6:1604.
228. Garnick MB, Reich SD, Maxwell BEA: Phase I/II study of recombinant interferon gamma in advanced renal cell carcinoma. J Urol 1988; 139:251.
229. Grups JW, Frohmuller HG: Cyclic interferon gamma treatment of patients with metastatic renal carcinoma. Br J Urol 1989; 64:218.
230. Auliktzky W, Gasti G, Aulitzky ME, et al: Successful treatment of metastatic renal cell carcinoma with a biologically active dose of recombinant interferon gamma. J Clin Oncol 1989; 7:1875.
231. Ellerhorst JA, Kilbourn RG, Amato RJ, et al: Phase II trial of low-dose γ-interferon in metastatic renal cell carcinoma. J Urol 1994; 152:841.
232. Cameron RB, McIntosh JK, Rosenberg SA: Synergistic antitumor effects of combination immunotherapy with recombinant interleukin 2 and a recombinant hybrid interferon in the treatment of established murine hepatic metastases. Cancer Res 1988; 48:5810.
233. Hirsh M, Lipton A, Harvey H, et al: Phase I study of interleukin-2 and interferon alfa-2a as outpatient therapy for patients with advanced malignancy. J Clin Oncol 1990; 10:1657.
234. Ilson DH, Motzer RJ, Kradin RL, et al: A phase II trial of interleukin 2 and interferon alfa-2a in patients with advanced renal cell carcinoma. J Clin Oncol 1992; 10:114.
235. Lipton A, Harvey H, Givant E, et al: Interleukin 2 and interferon α-2a outpatient therapy for metastatic renal cell carcinoma. J Immunother 1993; 13:122.
236. Figlin RA, Pierce WC, Belldegrun A: Combination biologic therapy with interleukin 2 and interferon alfa in the outpatient treatment of metastatic renal cell carcinoma. Semin Oncol 1993; 20 (Suppl 9):11.
237. Atzpodien J, Kirchner H, Hanninen EL, et al: Interleukin 2 in combination with interferon alpha and 5-fluorouracil for metastatic renal cell cancer. Eur J Cancer 1993; 29 (Suppl 5):6.
238. Dutcher JP, Fisher RI, Weiss G, et al: An outpatient (OPT) regimen of subcutaneous SC) interleukin 2 (IL-2) plus al-

pha-interferon (IFN) in metastatic renal cell carcinoma (RCC). Proc Am Soc Clin Oncol 1993; 12:248.
239. Ratain MJ, Priest ER, Janisch L, et al: A phase I study of subcutaneous recombinant interleukin 2 and interferon alfa-2a. Cancer 1993; 71:2371.
240. Vogelzang NJ, Lipton A, Figlin RA: Subcutaneous interleukin 2 plus interferon alfa-2a in metastatic renal cell cancer: an outpatient multicenter trial. J Clin Oncol 1993; 11:1809.
241. Huland E, Heinzer H, Huland H, et al: Inhaled interleukin 2 in combination with low-dose systemic interleukin 2 and interferon alpha in patients with pulmonary metastatic renal-cell carcinoma: effectiveness and toxicity of mainly local treatment. J Cancer Res Clin Oncol 1994; 120: 221.
242. Thiounn N, Mathiot C, Dorval T, et al: Lack of efficacy of low-dose subcutaneous recombinant interleukin-2 and interferon-alpha in the treatment of metastatic renal cell carcinoma. Br J Urol 1995; 75:586.
243. Fisher RI, Coltman CA Jr, Doroshow JH, et al: Metastatic renal cancer treated with interleukin-2 and lymphokine-activated killer cells. A phase II clinical trial. Ann Intern Med 1988; 108:518.
244. Parkinson DR, Fisher RI, Rayer AA, et al: Therapy of renal cell carcinoma with interleukin 2 and lymphokine-activated killer cells: phase II experience with a hybrid bolus and continuous infusion interleukin 2 regimen. J Clin Oncol 1990; 8:1630.
245. Palmer PA, Vinke J, Evers P, et al: Continuous infusion of recombinant interleukin 2 with or without autologous lymphokine-activated killer cells for the treatment of advanced renal cell carcinoma. Eur J Cancer 1992; 28A:1038.
246. Rosenberg SA: Karnofsky Memorial Lecture: the immunotherapy and gene therapy of cancer. J Clin Oncol 1992; 10:180.
247. Foon KA, Walther PJ, Bernstein ZP, et al: Renal cell carcinoma treated with continuous-infusion interleukin 2 with ex vivo-activated killer cells. J Immunother 1992; 11: 184.
248. Weiss GR, Margolin KA, Aronson FR, et al: A randomized phase II trial of continuous infusion interleukin 2 or bolus injection interleukin 2 plus lymphokine-activated killer cells for advanced renal cell carcinoma. J Clin Oncol 1992; 10:275.
249. Thompson JA, Shulman KL, Benyunes MC, et al: Prolonged continuous intravenous infusion interleukin 2 and lymphokine-activated killer cell therapy for metastatic renal cell carcinoma. J Clin Oncol 1992; 10:960.
250. Sznol M, Clark JW, Smith JW, et al: Pilot study of interleukin 2 and lymphokine-activated killer cells combined with immunomodulatory doses of chemotherapy and sequenced with interferon alpha-2A in patients with metastatic melanoma and renal cell carcinoma. J Natl Cancer Inst 1992; 84:929.
251. Dillman RO, Church C, Oldham RK, et al: A randomized phase II trial of continuous infusion interleukin 2 in 788 patients with cancer. The National Biotherapy Study Group Experience. Cancer 1993; 71:2358.
252. McCabe M, Stablein D, Hawkins MJ: The modified group C experience—phase III randomized trials of IL-2 versus IL-2/LAK in advanced renal cell cancer and advanced melanoma (Abstract 714). Proc Am Soc Oncol 1991; 10: 213.
253. Rosenberg SA, Lotze MT, Yang JC, et al: Prospective randomized trial of high-dose interleukin-2 alone or in conjunction with lymphokine-activated killer cells for the treatment of patients with advanced cancers. J Natl Cancer Inst 1993; 85:622.
254. Bajorin D, Sell KW, Richards JM, et al: A randomized trial of interleukin 2 plus lymphokine-activated killer cells versus interleukin 2 alone in renal cell carcinoma (Abstract 1106). Proc Am Assoc Cancer Res 1990; 31:A1106.
255. Rosenberg SA, Speiss PJ, Lafreniere R: A new approach to the adaptive immunotherapy of cancer with tumor-infiltrating lymphocytes. Science 1986; 233:1318.
256. Topalian SL, Solomon D, Frederick P, et al: Immunotherapy of patients with advanced cancer using tumor-infiltrating lymphocytes and recombinant interleukin 2: a pilot study. J Clin Oncol 1988; 6:839.
257. Kradin RL, Lazarus DS, Dubinett SM, et al: Tumour-infiltrating lymphocytes and interleukin 2 in treatment of advanced cancer. Lancet 1989; 1:577.
258. Bukowski RM, Sharfman W, Murthy S, et al: Clinical results and characterization of tumor-infiltrating lymphocytes with or without recombinant interleukin 2 in human metastatic renal cell carcinoma. Cancer Res 1991; 51: 4199.
259. Pierce WC, Belldegrun A, deKernion JB, et al: Immunotherapy of patients with metastatic renal cell carcinoma (RCCa) using tumor-infiltrating lymphocytes (TIL) in combination with an outpatient regimen of interleukin 2 (IL-2) with or without interferon alpha (IFN-alpha): UCLA Kidney Cancer Program (Abstract 736). Proc Am Soc Clin Oncol 1994; 13:238.
260. Olencki T, Finke J, Lorenzi V, et al: Adoptive immunotherapy (AIT), for renal cell carcinoma (RCC) tumor infiltrating lymphocytes (TILs) cultured in vitro with rIL-2, rhIL-4, and autologous tumor: a phase II trial (Abstract 762). Proc Am Soc Clin Oncol 1994; 13:244.
261. Fleischmann JD, Kim B: Interleukin-2 immunotherapy followed by resection of residual renal cell carcinoma. J Urol 1991; 145(5):938.
262. Sella A, Swanson DA, Ro JY, et al: Surgery following response to interferon-α-based therapy for residual renal cell carcinoma. J Urol 1993; 149:19.
263. Long JP, Walther MM, Linehan WM, et al: The management of isolated renal recurrence of renal cell carcinoma following complete response to interleukin-2 based immunotherapy. J Urol 1993; 150(1):176.
264. Rackley R, Novick A, Klein E, et al: The impact of adjuvant nephrectomy on multimodality treatment of metastatic renal cell carcinoma. J Urol 1994; 152:1399.
265. Mulligan RC: The basic science of gene therapy. Science 1993; 260:926.
266. Dranoff G, Jaffee EM, Lozenby A, et al: Vaccination with irradiated tumor cells engineered to secrete murine GM-CSF stimulates potent, specific and long-lasting anti-tumor immunity. Proc Natl Acad Sci U S A 1993; 90:3539.

13

SURGERY OF RENAL CELL CARCINOMA

ANDREW C. NOVICK, M.D.

Notwithstanding recent advances in our understanding of the genetics and biology of renal cell carcinoma (RCC), surgery remains the mainstay of curative treatment for this disease. Nevertheless, the role of surgery is changing with respect to both localized RCC and patients with metastatic disease. Nephron-sparing surgery has assumed an increasing role in the management of localized tumors. The advent of promising immunotherapy regimens and their adjunctive use with surgery offers new hope for patients with disseminated malignancy. This chapter will review the contemporary role of surgery and specific operative techniques in the management of patients with RCC.

RADICAL NEPHRECTOMY

Indications and Evaluation

Radical nephrectomy is the treatment of choice for patients with localized renal cell carcinoma.[1,2] The preoperative evaluation of patients with renal cell carcinoma has changed considerably in recent years due to the advent of new imaging modalities such as ultrasonography, computed tomography (CT) scanning, and magnetic resonance imaging (MRI). In many patients, a complete preliminary evaluation can be performed using these noninvasive modalities. Renal arteriography is no longer routinely necessary prior to performing radical nephrectomy. All patients should undergo a metastatic evaluation including a chest x-ray, abdominal CT scan and, occasionally, a bone scan; the latter is only necessary in patients with bone pain or an elevated serum alkaline phosphatase. Radical nephrectomy is occasionally done in patients with metastatic disease to palliate severe associated local symptoms, to allow entry into a biologic response modifier protocol, or concomitant with resection of a solitary metastatic lesion.

Involvement of the inferior vena cava (IVC) with renal cell carcinoma occurs in 3 to 7% of cases and renders the task of complete surgical excision more complicated.[3] Yet, operative removal offers the only hope for cure and, when there are no metastases, an aggressive approach is justified. Five-year survival rates of 40 to 68% have been reported after complete surgical excision.[4–7] The best results have been achieved when the tumor does not involve the perinephric fat and regional lymph nodes.[8] The cephalad extent of vena caval involvement is not prognostically important and, even with intra-atrial tumor thrombi, extended cancer-free survival is possible following surgical treatment when there is no nodal or distant metastasis.[9] In planning the appropriate operative approach for tumor removal, it is essential for preoperative radiographic studies to define accurately the cephalad limits of a vena caval tumor thrombus.

Renal cell carcinoma involving the IVC should be suspected in patients who have lower extremity edema, a varicocele, dilated superficial abdominal veins, proteinuria, pulmonary embolism, a right atrial mass, or nonfunction of the involved kidney. Currently, MRI is the preferred diagnostic study for demonstrating both the presence and distal extent of IVC involvement.[10,11] Transesophageal echocardiography[12] and transabdominal color flow Doppler ultrasonography[13] have also proven to be useful diagnostic studies in this regard. Inferior vena cavography is reserved for patients in whom an MRI or ultrasound study is either nondiagnostic or contraindicated. Renal arteriography is particularly helpful in patients with renal cell carcinoma involving the IVC since, in 35 to 40% of cases, distinct arterialization of a tumor thrombus is observed. When this finding is present, preoperative embolization of the kidney often causes shrinkage of the thrombus that facilitates its intraoperative removal. When adjunctive cardiopulmonary bypass with deep hypothermic circulatory arrest is considered, coronary angiography is also performed preoperatively.[5,14] If significant obstructing coronary lesions are found, these can be repaired simultaneously during cardiopulmonary bypass.

Radical nephrectomy encompasses the basic principles of early ligation of the renal artery and vein, removal of the kidney outside Gerota's fascia, removal of the ipsilateral adrenal gland, and performance of a complete lymphadenectomy from the crus of the diaphragm to the aortic bifurcation.[1] Perhaps the most important aspect of radical nephrectomy is removal of the kidney outside Gerota's fascia, because capsular invasion with perinephric fat involvement occurs in 25% of patients. Recent studies suggest that removal of the ipsilateral adrenal gland is not routinely necessary unless the malignancy either extensively involves the kidney or is located in the upper portion of the kidney.[15] Although lymphadenectomy allows for more accurate pathologic staging, the therapeutic value remains controversial.[16] A recent study from Giuliani and associates suggests that a subset of patients with micrometastatic lymph node involvement may benefit from performance of a lymphadenectomy.[17] At the present time, the need for routine performance of a complete lymphadenectomy in all cases is unresolved, and there remains a divergence of clinical practice among urologists with respect to this aspect of radical nephrectomy.

Surgical Anatomy

The anatomic relationship of the kidneys to surrounding structures is illustrated in Figure 13–1. The kidneys are located on either side of the vertebral column in the lumbar fossa of the retroperitoneal space. Each kidney is surrounded by a layer of perinephric fat that is in turn covered by a distinct fascial layer termed Gerota's fascia. Posteriorly, both kidneys lie on the psoas major and quadratus lumborum muscles. Posteriorly and superiorly, the upper pole of each kidney is in contact with the diaphragm.

A small segment of the anterior medial surface of the right kidney is in contact with the right adrenal gland. However, the major anterior relationships of the right kidney are the liver, which overlies the upper two thirds of the anterior surface, and the hepatic flexure of the colon, which overlies the lower one third. The second portion of the duodenum covers the right renal hilum.

A small segment of the anterior medial surface of the left kidney is also covered by the left adrenal gland. The major anterior relationships of the left kidney are the spleen, body of the pancreas, stomach, and splenic flexure of the colon.

Surgical Incisions

The surgical approach for radical nephrectomy is determined by the size and location of the tumor

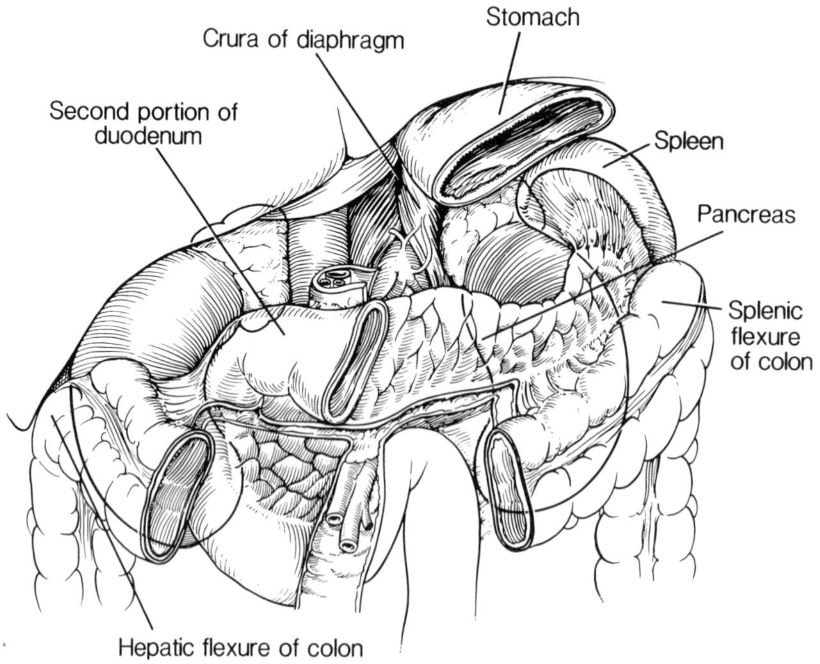
Stomach
Crura of diaphragm
Second portion of duodenum
Spleen
Pancreas
Splenic flexure of colon
Hepatic flexure of colon

FIGURE 13–1. The anatomic relationship of the kidneys to the surrounding structures. The liver is retracted superiorly in this illustration. (From Novick AC, Streem SB: Surgery of the kidney. *In* Walsh PC, Retik AB, Stamey TA, Vaughan ED Jr [eds]: Campbell's Urology, 6th edition. Philadelphia, WB Saunders Co, 1992, with permission.)

as well as by the habitus of the patient.[18] The operation is usually performed through a transperitoneal incision to allow abdominal exploration for metastatic disease and early access to the renal vessels with minimal manipulation of the tumor. Occasionally, an extraperitoneal flank incision is employed in elderly patients or in patients with small tumors who are also classified as poor risks.

The author prefers an extended subcostal or a bilateral subcostal incision for most patients undergoing radical nephrectomy (Fig. 13–2). This incision provides better access to the lateral and superior portion of the kidney than a midline abdominal incision. When employing an anterior subcostal incision, the patient is in the supine position with a rolled sheet beneath the upper lumbar spine. The incision begins approximately one to two fingerbreadths below the costal margin in the anterior axillary line and then extends with a gentle curve across the midline, ending at the midportion of the opposite rectus muscle. The incision is carried through the subcutaneous tissues to the anterior fascia, which is divided in the direction of the incision. In the lateral aspect of the incision, a portion of the latissimus dorsi muscle is divided. The external oblique muscle is divided, exposing the fibers of the internal oblique muscle (Fig. 13–3*A*). The rectus, internal oblique, and transversus abdominis muscles are divided along with the posterior rectus sheath (Fig. 13–3*B*, *C*). The peritoneal cavity is entered in the midline, and the ligamentum teres is divided (Fig. 13–3*D*).

The thoracoabdominal approach is preferable for performing radical nephrectomy in patients with large tumors involving the upper portion of the kidney (Fig. 13–4). It is particularly advantageous on the right side, where the liver and its venous drainage into the upper vena cava can limit exposure and impair vascular control as the tumor mass is being removed. Less need exists for a thoracoabdominal incision on the left side because the spleen and pancreas can usually be readily elevated away from the tumor mass. The patient is placed in a semioblique position, with a rolled sheet placed longitudinally beneath the flank. The incision is begun in the eighth intercostal space, near the angle of the rib, and is carried across the costal margin to the midpoint of the opposite rectus muscle, above the umbilicus. The latissimus dorsi, external oblique, rectus, and intercostal muscles are divided in the direction of the incision (Fig. 13–5*A*). The costal cartilage between the tips of the adjacent ribs is divided (Fig. 13–5*B*). The pleura is then opened to obtain complete exposure of the diaphragm (Fig. 13–5*C*).

The diaphragmatic incision is made at the periphery about 2 cm inside its attachment at the chest wall with the incision then being carried around circumferentially to the posterior aspect of the diaphragm (Fig. 13–5*D*). Circumferential incision of the diaphragm obviates damage to the phrenic nerve and also creates a diaphragmatic flap, which can be pushed into the chest to provide complete exposure of the liver, which is then retracted upward (Fig. 13–5*E*). If further mobilization of the liver is needed, the right triangular ligament and coronary ligament can be incised to mobilize the entire right lobe of the liver upward. This maneuver provides excellent additional exposure of the suprarenal vena cava. Medial to the ribs, the internal oblique and transversus abdominis muscles are divided and the peritoneal cavity is entered. The kidney and great vessels may then be exposed by upward retraction of the liver and medial visceral mobilization (Fig. 13–5*F*).

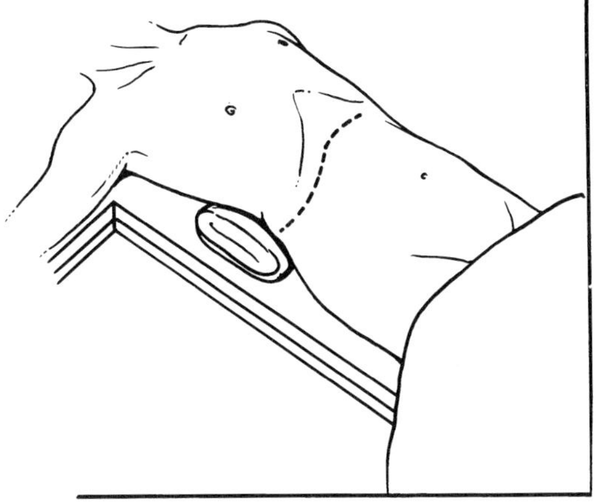

FIGURE 13–2. Patient positioning for anterior subcostal transperitoneal incision. (From Novick AC, Streem SB: Surgery of the kidney. *In* Walsh PC, Retik AB, Stamey TA, Vaughan ED Jr [eds]: Campbell's Urology, 6th edition. Philadelphia, WB Saunders Co, 1992, with permission.)

Left Radical Nephrectomy

After the peritoneal cavity is entered, a thorough exploration is done to rule out metastatic disease. The posterior peritoneum lateral to the left colon is incised vertically and the incision is carried upward to divide the lienorenal ligament. Care must be taken to avoid tearing the delicate capsule of the spleen. The plane between the kidney and adrenal gland posteriorly, and the pancreas and spleen anteriorly, is developed by blunt dissection. The left colon and duodenum are reflected medially, and the pancreas and spleen are reflected cephalad, with care taken not to injure the spleen or the pancreas (Fig. 13–6). When adequate exposure of the kidney and great vessels has been obtained, a self-retaining ring retractor is inserted to maintain the operative field (Fig. 13–7).

The operation is initiated with dissection of the renal pedicle. The left renal vein is quite long as it passes over the aorta. The vein is mobilized completely by ligating and dividing gonadal, adrenal, and lumbar tributaries. The vein can be retracted

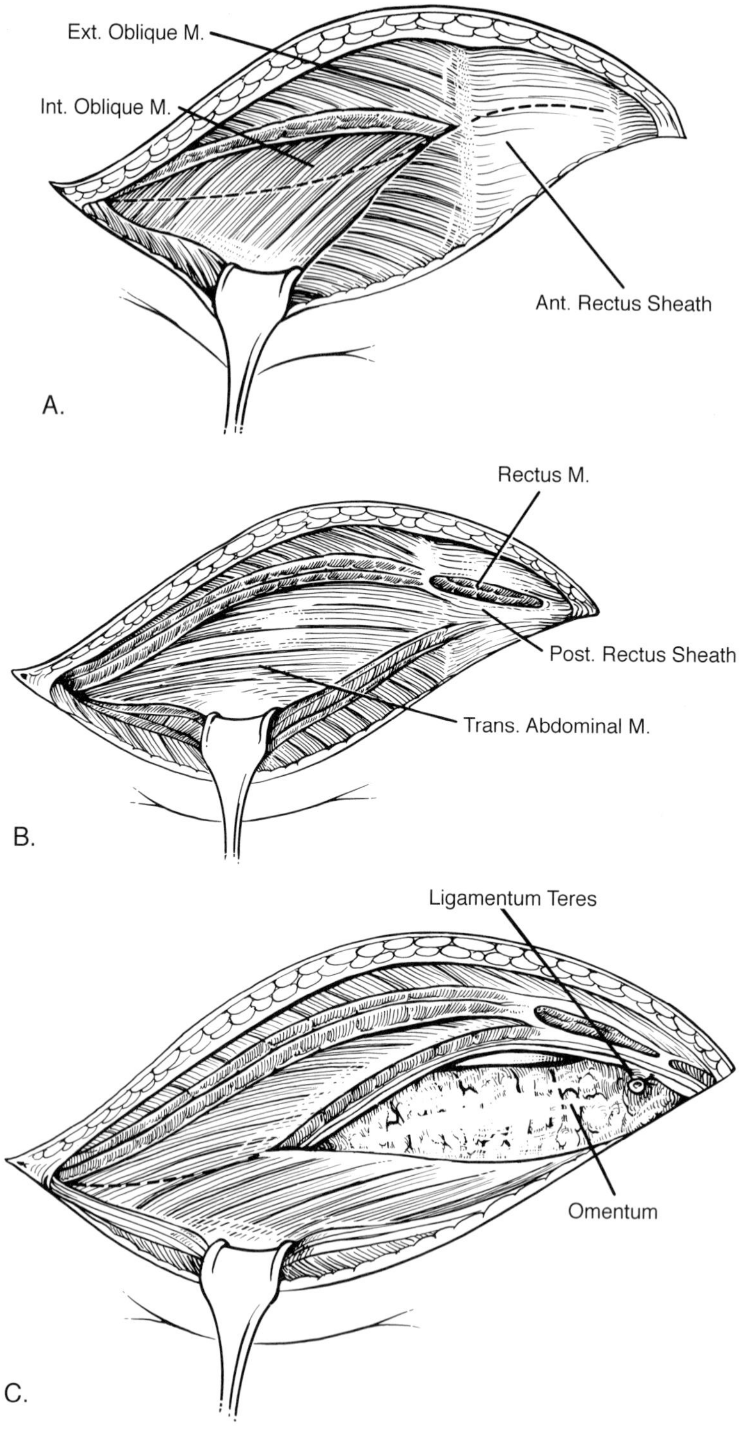
Ext. Oblique M.
Int. Oblique M.
Ant. Rectus Sheath
A.
Rectus M.
Post. Rectus Sheath
Trans. Abdominal M.
B.
Ligamentum Teres
Omentum
C.

FIGURE 13–3. The various steps in performing an anterior subcostal transperitoneal incision are illustrated (see accompanying text). (From Novick AC, Streem SB: Surgery of the kidney. *In* Walsh PC, Retik AB, Stamey TA, Vaughan ED Jr [eds]: Campbell's Urology, 6th edition. Philadelphia, WB Saunders Co, 1992, with permission.) *Illustration continued on opposite page*

to expose the artery posteriorly, which is then mobilized toward the aorta (Fig. 13–8). The renal artery is ligated with 2.0 silk ligatures and divided, and the renal vein is then similarly managed.

The kidney is mobilized outside Gerota's fascia with blunt and sharp dissection as needed (Fig. 13–9). Remaining vascular attachments are secured with nonabsorbable sutures or metal clips. Visualization of the upper vascular attachments is facilitated by downward retraction of the kidney. The ureter is then ligated and divided to complete the removal of the kidney and adrenal gland (Fig. 13–10).

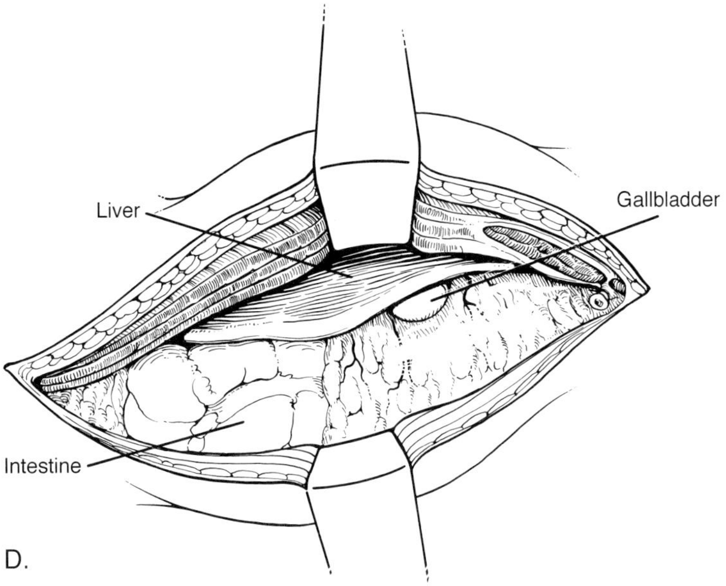
Liver
Gallbladder
Intestine
D.

FIGURE 13–3. *Continued*

The classic description of radical nephrectomy includes the performance of a complete regional lymphadenectomy. The lymph nodes can be removed en bloc with the kidney and adrenal gland or separately, following the nephrectomy. The lymph node dissection is begun at the crura of the diaphragm just below the origin of the superior mesenteric artery. A readily definable periadventitial plane is seen close to the aorta that can be entered. The dissection may then be carried along the aorta and onto the origin of the major vessels, to remove all the periaortic lymphatic tissue. Care must be taken to avoid injury to the origins of the celiac and superior mesenteric arteries superiorly, as they arise from the anterior surface of the aorta. The dissection of the periaortic and pericaval lymph nodes is then carried downward en block to the origin of the inferior mesenteric artery. The sympathetic ganglia and nerves are removed together with the lymphatic tissue. The cisterna chyli is identified medial at the right crus. Entering lymphatic vessels are secured to prevent the development of chylous ascites.

Right Radical Nephrectomy

On the right side, after entering the peritoneal cavity, the posterior peritoneum lateral to the right colon is incised vertically and the incision is carried high up along the vena cava to the level of the hepatic veins. The right colon and duodenum are reflected medially, and the liver and gallbladder are retracted upward (Fig. 13–11). Care is taken to avoid trauma to the delicate hepatic veins, which may enter the vena cava at this level. When adequate exposure of the kidney and adrenal gland is obtained, a self-retaining ring retractor is inserted to maintain the operative field.

The vena cava and renal vein are retracted medially and downward to expose the right renal artery. Alternatively, with a large medial tumor, the renal artery may be exposed between the vena cava and the aorta (Fig. 13–12). Ligation of the renal artery and vein is performed as described on the left side with 2.0 silk ligatures. Since the right renal vein is usually short, ligation should take place at the level of its entrance to the vena cava. The remainder of the radical nephrectomy is performed as described for left-sided tumors.

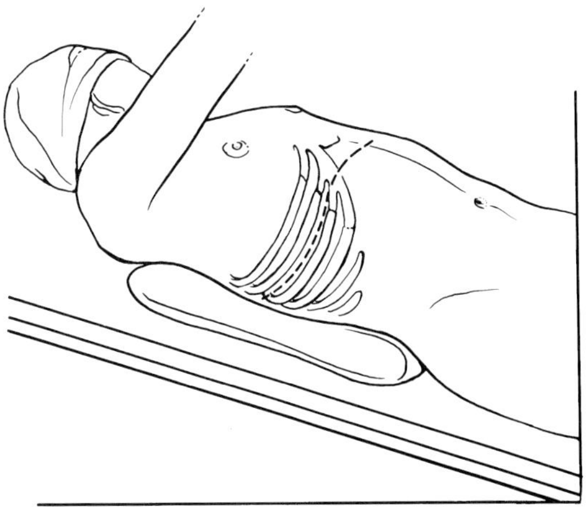

FIGURE 13–4. Patient positioning for a right thoracoabdominal incision. (From Novick AC, Streem SB: Surgery of the kidney. *In* Walsh PC, Retik AB, Stamey TA, Vaughan ED Jr [eds]: Campbell's Urology, 6th edition. Philadelphia, WB Saunders Co, 1992, with permission.)

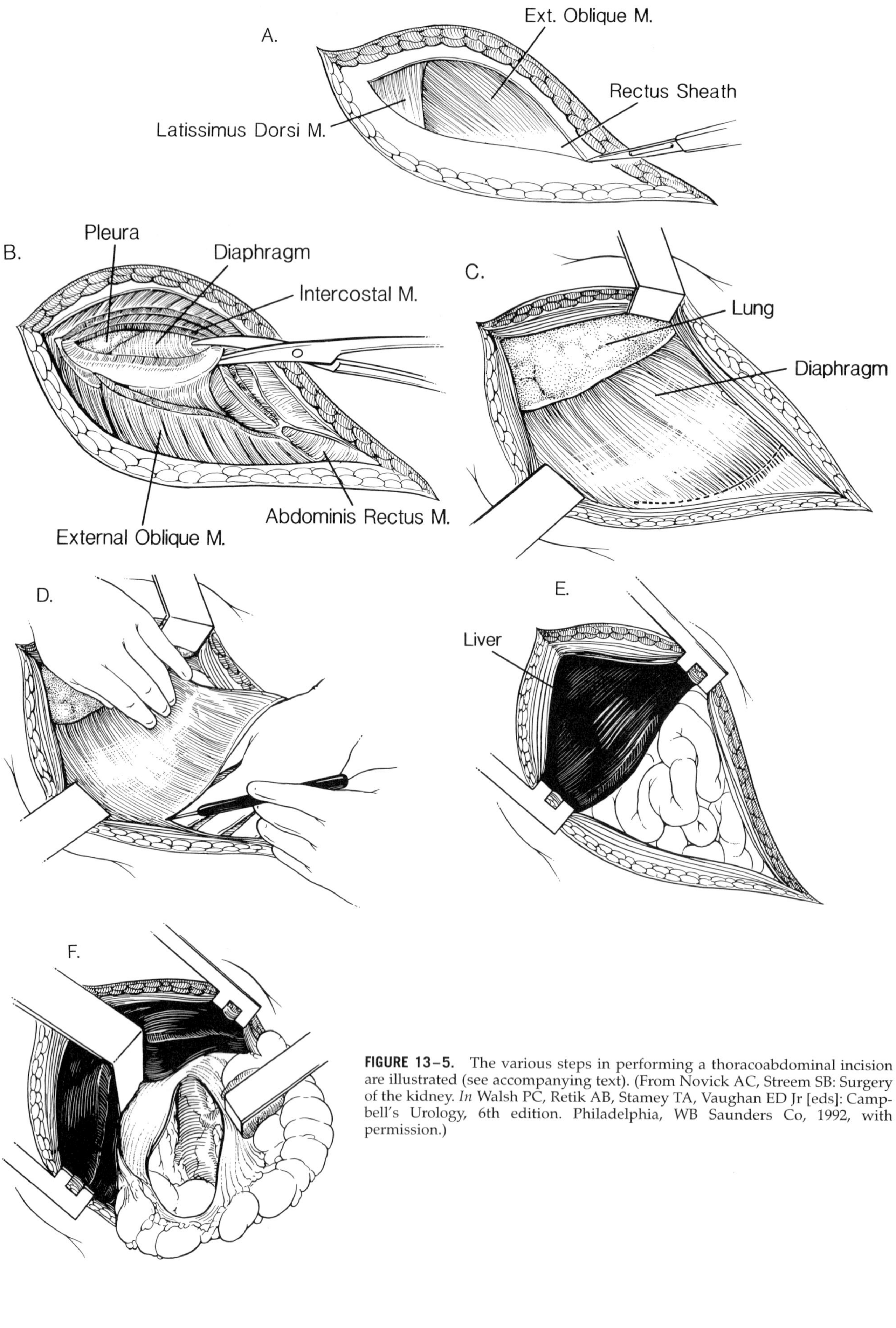
A.
Ext. Oblique M.
Rectus Sheath
Latissimus Dorsi M.
B.
Pleura
Diaphragm
Intercostal M.
Abdominis Rectus M.
External Oblique M.
C.
Lung
Diaphragm
D.
E.
Liver
F.

FIGURE 13–5. The various steps in performing a thoracoabdominal incision are illustrated (see accompanying text). (From Novick AC, Streem SB: Surgery of the kidney. *In* Walsh PC, Retik AB, Stamey TA, Vaughan ED Jr [eds]: Campbell's Urology, 6th edition. Philadelphia, WB Saunders Co, 1992, with permission.)

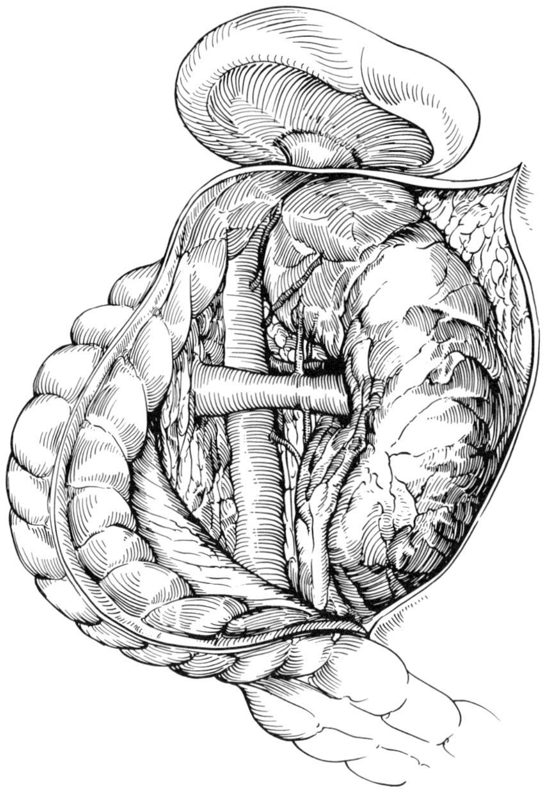

FIGURE 13–6. After entering the peritoneal cavity, the colon is reflected medially to expose the left kidney and great vessels. (From Novick AC: Stewart AC [ed]: Stewart's Operative Urology. Baltimore, Williams & Wilkins, 1989, with permission.)

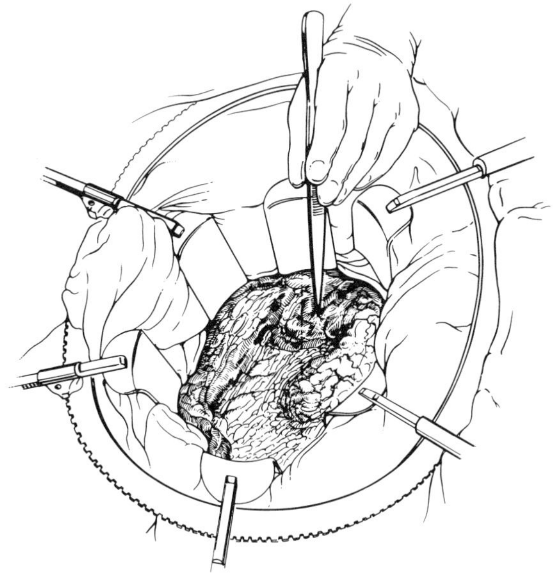

FIGURE 13–7. A self-retaining ring retractor is inserted to maintain exposure of the operative field. (From Novick AC: Stewart AC [ed]: Stewart's Operative Urology. Baltimore, Williams & Wilkins, 1989, with permission.)

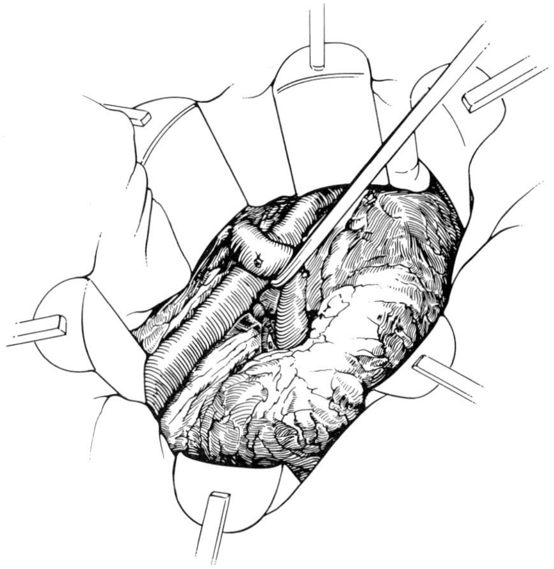

FIGURE 13–8. The left renal vein is mobilized by ligating its major branches to expose the artery posteriorly. (From Novick AC: Stewart AC [ed]: Stewart's Operative Urology. Baltimore, Williams & Wilkins, 1989, with permission.)

Radical Nephrectomy with Infrahepatic Vena Caval Involvement

There are four levels of vena caval involvement in renal cell carcinoma that are characterized according to the distal extent of the tumor thrombus (Fig. 13–13). A bilateral subcostal transperitoneal incision usually provides excellent exposure for performing radical nephrectomy and removal of a perirenal or infrahepatic IVC thrombus. For extremely large tumors involving the upper pole of the kidney, a thoracoabdominal incision may alter-

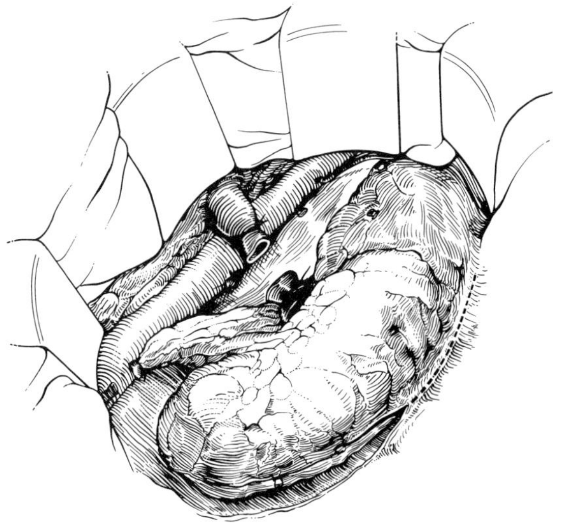

FIGURE 13–9. After securing the pedicle and dividing the ureter, the kidney is mobilized outside Gerota's fascia. (From Novick AC: Stewart AC [ed]: Stewart's Operative Urology. Baltimore, Williams & Wilkins, 1989, with permission.)

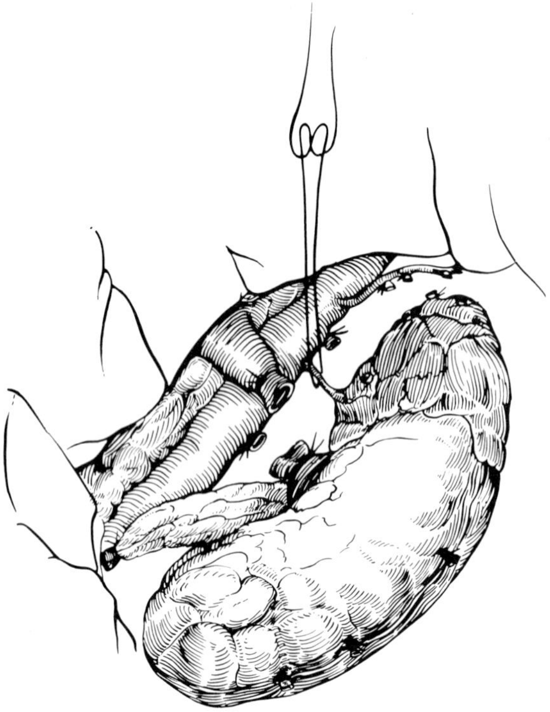

FIGURE 13–10. Remaining medial vascular attachments are secured and divided to complete the nephrectomy. (From Novick AC: Stewart AC [ed]: Stewart's Operative Urology. Baltimore, Williams & Wilkins, 1989, with permission.)

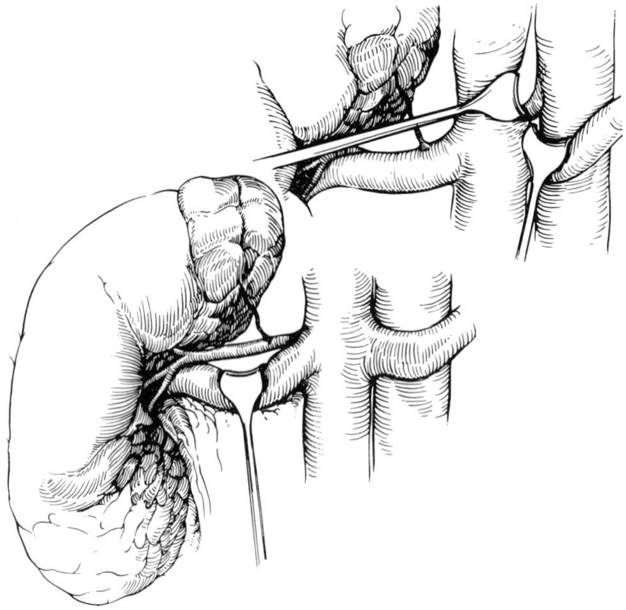

FIGURE 13–12. The right renal artery may be mobilized either lateral to the vena cava (below) or between the vena cava and the aorta (above). (From Novick AC: Stewart AC [ed]: Stewart's Operative Urology. Baltimore, Williams & Wilkins, 1989, with permission.)

natively be used. After the abdomen is entered, the colon is reflected medially and a self-retaining ring retractor is inserted to maintain exposure of the retroperitoneum (Fig. 13–14*A*). The renal artery and the ureter are ligated and divided, and the entire kidney is mobilized outside Gerota's fascia leaving the kidney attached only by the renal vein (Fig. 13–14*B*, *C*). During the initial dissection, care is taken to avoid unnecessary manipulation of the renal vein and vena cava.

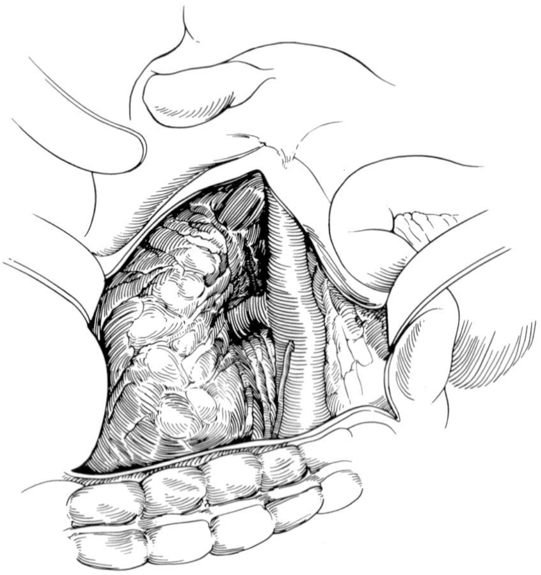

FIGURE 13–11. After entering the peritoneal cavity, the right colon and duodenum are reflected medially to expose the right kidney and great vessels. (From Novick AC: Stewart AC [ed]: Stewart's Operative Urology. Baltimore, Williams & Wilkins, 1989, with permission.)

The vena cava is then completely dissected from surrounding structures above and below the renal vein, and the opposite renal vein is also mobilized. It is essential to obtain exposure and control of the suprarenal vena cava above the level of the tumor thrombus. If necessary, perforating veins to the caudate lobe of the liver are secured and divided to allow separation of the caudate lobe from the vena cava. This maneuver can allow an additional 2- to 3-cm length of vena cava to be exposed superiorly. The infrarenal vena cava is then occluded below the thrombus with a Satinsky venous clamp, and the opposite renal vein is gently secured with a small bulldog vascular clamp. Finally, in preparation for tumor thrombectomy, a curved Satinsky clamp is placed around the suprarenal vena cava above the level of the thrombus (Fig. 13–14*D*).

The anterior surface of the renal vein is then incised over the tumor thrombus and the incision is continued posteriorly with scissors, passing just beneath the thrombus (Fig. 13–14*E*). In most cases, there is no attachment of the thrombus to the wall of the vena cava. After the renal vein has been circumscribed, gentle downward traction is exerted on the kidney to extract the tumor thrombus from the vena cava (Fig. 13–14*F*). After removal of the gross specimen, the suprarenal vena caval clamp may be released temporarily as the anesthetist applies positive pulmonary pressure; this maneuver

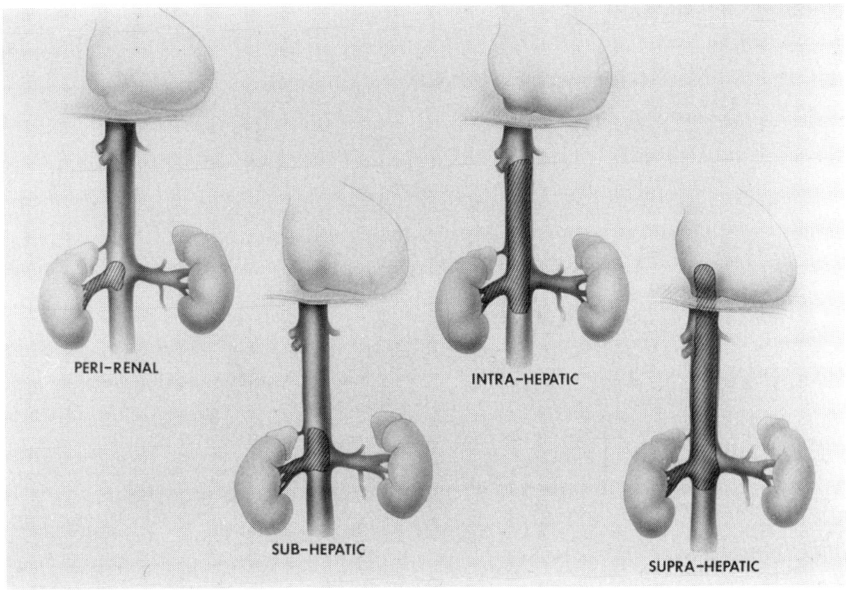
PERI-RENAL
SUB-HEPATIC
INTRA-HEPATIC
SUPRA-HEPATIC

FIGURE 13–13. Classification of inferior vena caval thrombi according to the distal extent of the thrombus as perirenal, subhepatic, intrahepatic, and suprahepatic.

can ensure that any small remaining fragments of thrombus are flushed free from the vena cava. When the tumor thrombectomy is completed, the cavotomy incision is repaired with a continuous 5-0 vascular suture (Fig. 13–14G).

In occasional cases, there is direct caval invasion of the tumor at the level of the entrance of the renal vein and for varying distances. This requires resection of a portion of the vena caval wall. Narrowing of the caval lumen by up to 50% will not adversely affect maintenance of caval patency. If further narrowing appears likely, caval reconstruction can be performed with a free graft of pericardium.

In some patients, more extensive direct growth of tumor into the wall of the vena cava is found at surgery. The prognosis for these patients is generally poor, particularly when hepatic venous tributaries are also involved, and the decision to proceed with radical surgical excision must be carefully considered. Several important principles must be kept in mind when undertaking en bloc vena caval resection. Resection of the infrarenal portion of the vena cava usually can be done safely, because an extensive collateral venous supply will have developed in most cases. With right-sided kidney tumors, resection of the suprarenal vena cava is also possible provided the left renal vein is ligated distal to the gonadal and adrenal tributaries, which then provide collateral venous drainage from the left kidney with left-sided kidney tumors. The suprarenal vena cava cannot be resected safely owing to the paucity of collateral venous drainage from the right kidney. In such cases, right renal venous drainage can be maintained by preserving a tumor-free strip of vena cava augmented, if necessary, with a pericardial patch; alternatively, the right kidney can be autotransplanted to the pelvis or an interposition graft of saphenous vein may be placed from the right renal vein to the splenic, inferior mesenteric, or portal vein.

Radical Nephrectomy with Intrahepatic or Suprahepatic Vena Caval Involvement

In patients with renal cell carcinoma and an intrahepatic or suprahepatic IVC thrombus, the difficulty of surgical excision is significantly increased. In such cases, the operative technique must be modified because it is not possible to obtain subdiaphragmatic control of the vena cava above the tumor thrombus. Several different surgical maneuvers have been used to provide adequate exposure, prevent severe bleeding, and achieve complete tumor removal in this setting.[5,7,19–21]

One described technique for obtaining vascular control involves temporary occlusion of the suprahepatic and intrapericardial portion of the IVC. To reduce hepatic venous congestion and troublesome backbleeding, the porta hepatis and superior mesenteric artery are also temporarily occluded.[7] A disadvantage of this approach is that occlusion of the latter vessels can be safely tolerated for only 20 minutes. This approach is also not applicable in cases of tumor extension into the right atrium. At the Cleveland Clinic, we have preferred to employ cardiopulmonary bypass with deep hypothermic circulatory arrest for most patients with supradiaphragmatic tumor thrombi and for all patients with right atrial tumor thrombi. We initially reported a favorable experience with this approach in 43 patients,[5] and a subsequent study has shown excellent long-term cancer-free survival following its use in patients with right atrial thrombi.[9] The relevant technical aspects are subsequently described.

A bilateral subcostal incision is used for the ab-

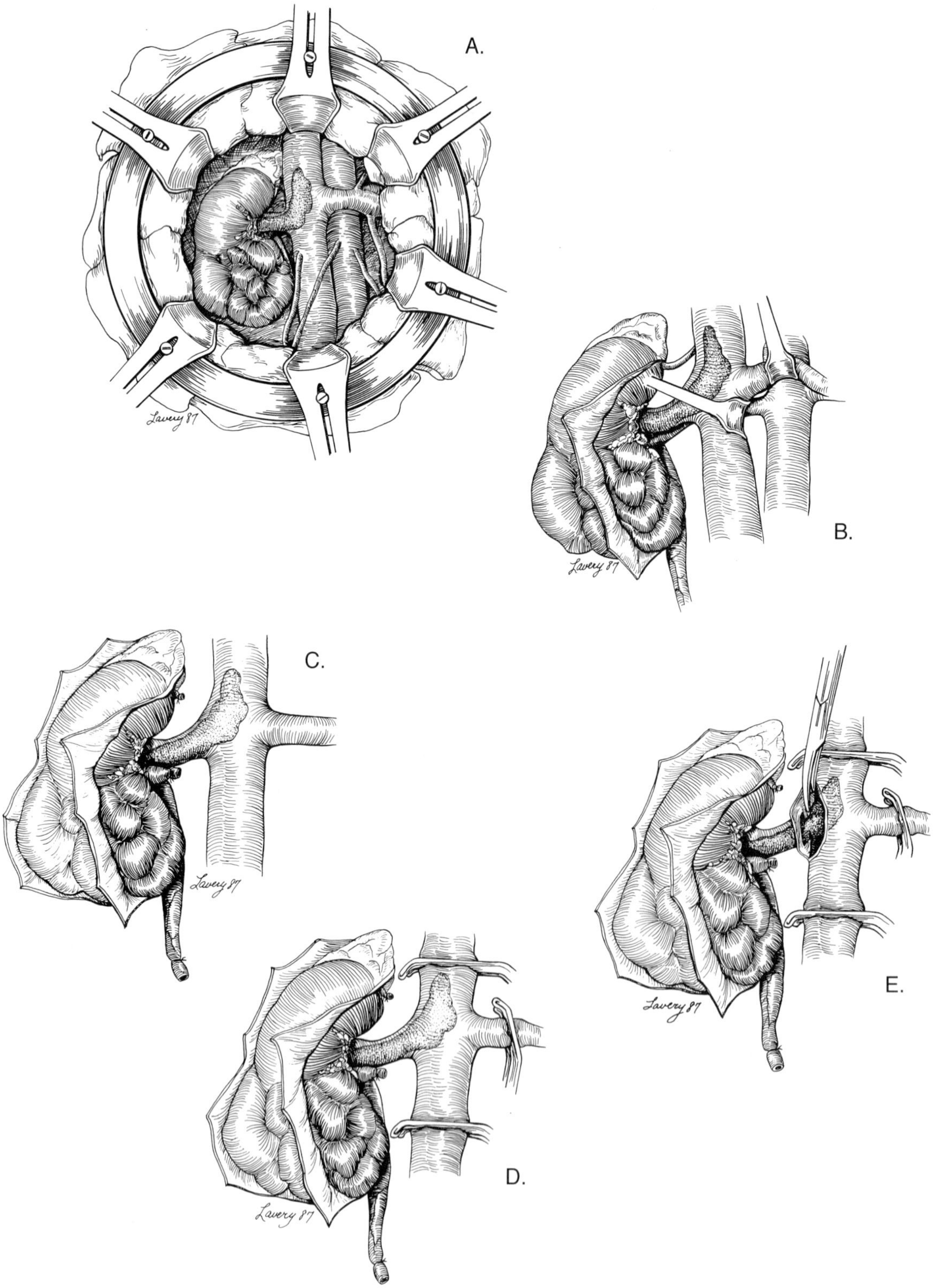
A.
B.
C.
D.
E.

FIGURE 13–14. Technique of radical nephrectomy and vena cava thrombectomy with infrahepatic tumor thrombus. (From Novick AC: Stewart AC [ed]: Stewart's Operative Urology. Baltimore, Williams & Wilkins, 1989, with permission.) *Illustration continued on opposite page*

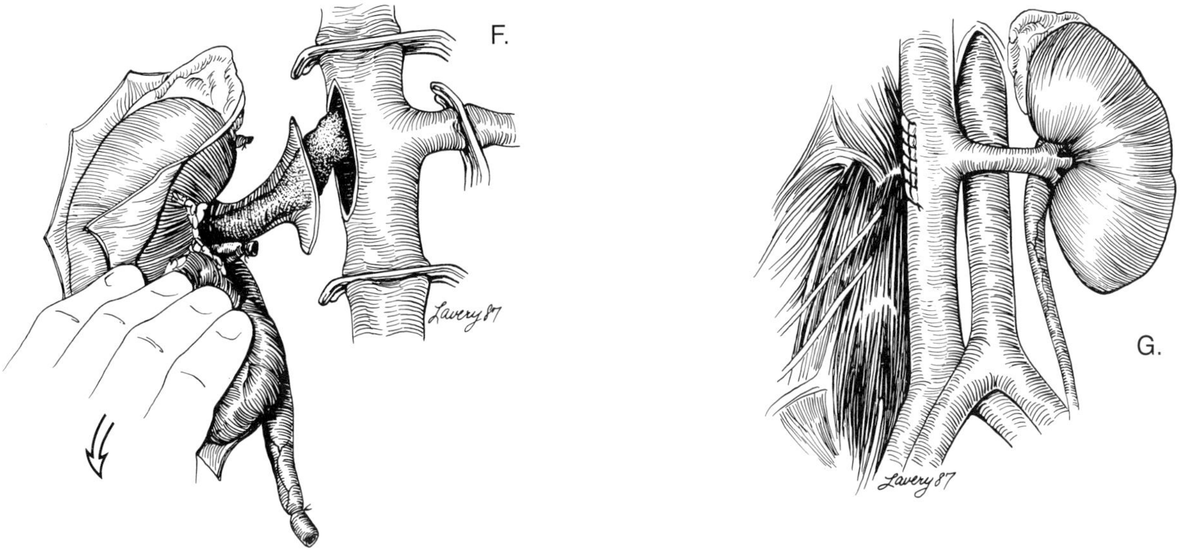
F.
G.

FIGURE 13–14. *Continued*

dominal portion of the operation. After confirming resectability, a median sternotomy is made (Fig. 13–15). Intraoperative monitoring is accomplished with an arterial line, a multiple-lumen central venous pressure catheter, and a pulmonary artery catheter. Nasopharyngeal and bladder temperatures are monitored. Anesthesia is induced with either fentanyl, sufentanil, or thiopental and maintained with a narcotic inhalation agent.[22]

The kidney is completely mobilized outside Gerota's fascia with division of the renal artery and ureter, such that the kidney is left attached only by the renal vein. The infrarenal vena cava and contralateral renal vein are also exposed. Extensive dissection and mobilization of the suprarenal vena cava are not necessary with this approach. Adequate exposure is somewhat more difficult to achieve for a left renal tumor. Simultaneous exposure of the vena cava on the right and the tumor on the left is not readily accomplished simply by reflecting the left colon medially. We have dealt with this by transposing the mobilized left kidney anteriorly through a window in the mesentery of the left colon while leaving the renal vein attached. This maneuver yields excellent exposure of the abdominal vena cava with the attached left renal vein and kidney. Precise retroperitoneal hemostasis is essential before proceeding with cardiopulmonary bypass due to the risk of bleeding associated with systemic heparinization.

The heart and great vessels are now exposed through the median sternotomy. The patient is heparinized, ascending aortic and right atrial venous cannulae are placed, and cardiopulmonary bypass is initiated (Fig. 13–16). When the heart fibrillates, the aorta is clamped and crystalloid cardioplegic solution is infused. Under circulatory arrest, deep hypothermia is initiated by reducing arterial inflow blood temperature as low as 10°C. The head and abdomen are packed in ice during the cooling process. After approximately 15 to 30 minutes, a core temperature of 18° to 20°C is achieved. At this point, flow through the perfusion machine is stopped and 95% of the blood volume is drained into the pump with no flow to any organ.

The tumor thrombus can now be removed in an essentially bloodless operative field. An incision is made in the inferior vena cava at the entrance of the involved renal vein, and the ostium is circumscribed. When the tumor extends into the right atrium, the atrium is opened at the same time (Fig. 13–17). If possible, the tumor thrombus is removed intact with the kidney. Frequently, this step is not possible because of the friability of the thrombus

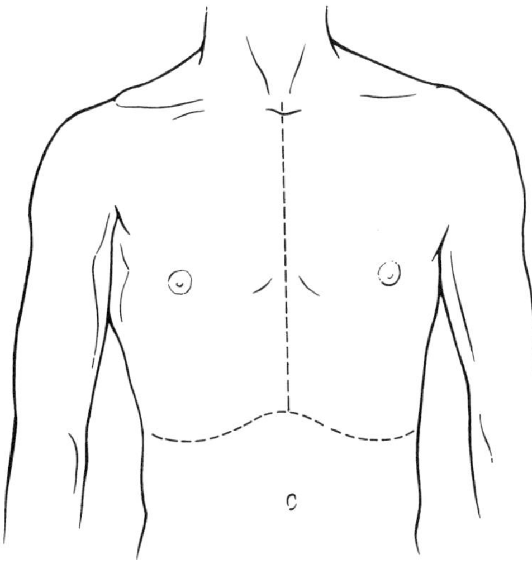

FIGURE 13–15. Surgical incision for performing radical nephrectomy with removal of suprahepatic vena caval tumor thrombus. (From Novick AC: Stewart AC [ed]: Stewart's Operative Urology. Baltimore, Williams & Wilkins, 1989, with permission.)

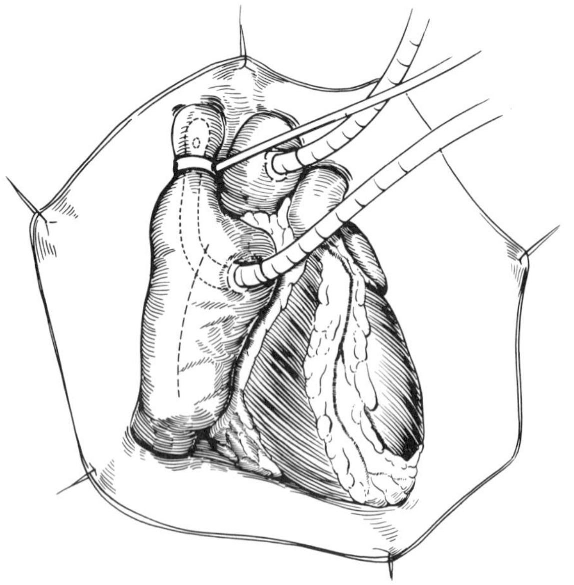

FIGURE 13–16. Cannulae are placed in the ascending aorta and right atrium in preparation for cardiopulmonary bypass. (From Novick AC: Stewart AC [ed]: Stewart's Operative Urology. Baltimore, Williams & Wilkins, 1989, with permission.)

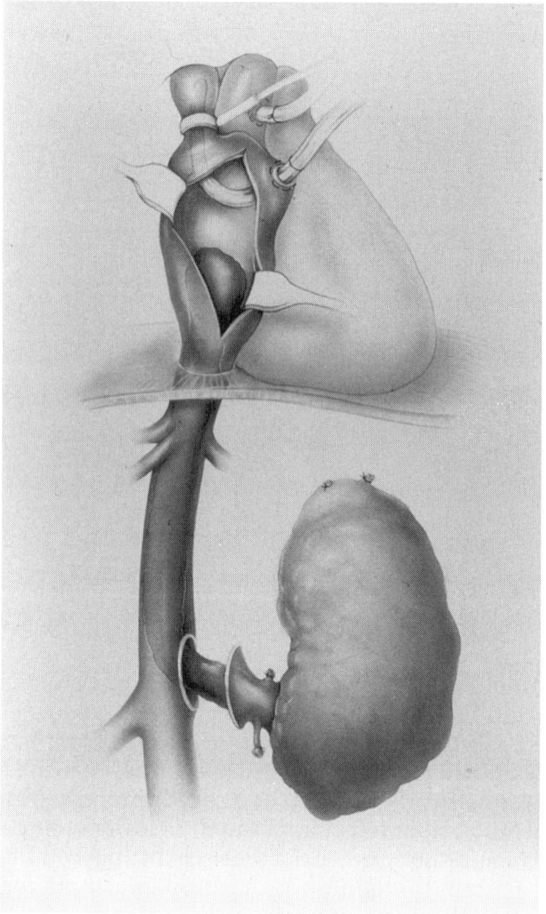

FIGURE 13–17. The ostium of the renal vein is circumferentially incised and the right atrium is opened. Following removal of the tumor thrombus, the atriotomy and vena cavotomy incisions are closed.

and its adherence to the vena caval wall. In such cases, piecemeal removal of the thrombus from above and below is necessary. Occasionally, a venous Fogarty catheter can be inserted into the vena cava to assist in extraction of the thrombus. Under deep hypothermic circulatory arrest, the entire interior lumen of the vena cava can be directly inspected to ensure that all fragments of thrombus are completely removed. Hypothermic circulatory arrest can be safely maintained for at least 40 minutes without incurring a cerebral ischemic event.[23] In difficult cases, this interval can be extended either by maintaining "trickle" blood flow at a rate of 5 to 10 ml/kg/min[24] or by adjunctive retrograde cerebral perfusion.[25]

Following complete removal of all tumor thrombus, the vena cava is closed with a continuous 5-0 vascular suture and the right atrium is closed. As soon as the vena cava and right atrium have been repaired, rewarming of the patient is initiated. If coronary artery bypass grafting is necessary, this procedure is done during the rewarming period. Rewarming takes 20 to 45 minutes and is continued until a core temperature of approximately 37°C is obtained. Cardiopulmonary bypass is then terminated. Decannulation takes place, and protamine sulfate is administered to reverse the effects of the heparin. Platelets, fresh-frozen plasma, desmopressin acetate, or their combination may be provided when coagulopathy is suspected.[26] Aprotinin has also proven effective in reversing the coagulopathy associated with cardiopulmonary bypass[27] but may induce thrombotic complications. Mediastinal chest tubes are placed but the abdomen is not routinely drained.

In patients with supradiaphragmatic vena caval tumor thrombi that do not extend into the right atrium, venovenous bypass in the form of a caval-atrial shunt may be employed.[21,22] In this approach, the intrapericardiac vena cava, infrarenal vena cava, and opposite renal vein are temporarily occluded. Cannulas are then inserted into the right atrium and infrarenal vena cava. These cannulas are connected to a primed pump to maintain adequate flow from the vena cava to the right heart (Fig. 13–18). This avoids the obligatory hypotension associated with temporary occlusion alone of the intrapericardiac and infrarenal vena cava. Following the initiation of venovenous bypass, the abdominal vena cava is opened and the thrombus is removed. If bleeding from the hepatic veins is troublesome during extraction of the thrombus, the porta hepatis may also be occluded (Pringle maneuver). After removal of the thrombus, repair of the vena cava is performed as previously described. This technique is simpler than cardiopulmonary bypass with hypothermic circulatory arrest but may entail more operative bleeding.

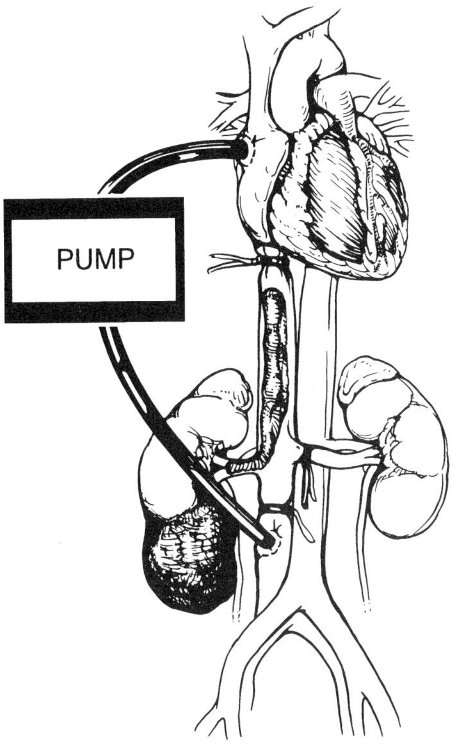
PUMP

FIGURE 13–18. Technique of venovenous bypass for removal of supradiaphragmatic vena caval tumor thrombus.

PARTIAL NEPHRECTOMY

Recent interest in partial nephrectomy or nephron-sparing surgery for renal cell carcinoma has been stimulated by advances in renal imaging, improved surgical techniques, the increasing number of incidentally discovered low-stage renal cell carcinomas and good long-term survival in patients undergoing this form of treatment. Partial nephrectomy entails complete local resection of a renal tumor while leaving the largest possible amount of normal functioning parenchyma in the involved kidney.

Accepted indications for partial nephrectomy include situations in which radical nephrectomy would render the patient anephric with subsequent immediate need for dialysis. This encompasses patients with bilateral renal cell carcinoma or renal cell carcinoma involving a solitary functioning kidney. The latter circumstance may be present due to unilateral renal agenesis, prior removal of the contralateral kidney, or irreversible impairment of contralateral renal function represented by patients with unilateral renal cell carcinoma and a functioning opposite kidney, when the opposite kidney is affected by a condition that might threaten its future function, such as calculus disease, chronic pyelonephritis, renal artery stenosis, ureteral reflux, or systemic diseases such as diabetes and nephrosclerosis.[28]

Recent studies have clarified the role of partial nephrectomy in patients with localized unilateral renal cell carcinoma and a normal contralateral kidney. The data indicate that radical nephrectomy and partial nephrectomy provide equally effective curative treatment for such patients who present with a single, small (<4 cm), and clearly localized renal cell carcinoma.[29] The results of partial nephrectomy are less satisfactory in patients with larger (>4 cm) or multiple localized renal cell carcinomas, and radical nephrectomy remains the treatment of choice in such cases when the opposite kidney is normal. The long-term renal functional advantage of partial nephrectomy with a normal opposite kidney requires further study.

The technical success rate with partial nephrectomy for renal cell carcinoma is excellent, and several large studies have reported 5-year cancer-specific survival rates of 87 to 90% in such patients.[30–32] These survival rates are comparable to those obtained after radical nephrectomy, particularly for low-stage renal cell carcinoma. The major disadvantage of partial nephrectomy for renal cell carcinoma is the risk of postoperative local tumor recurrence in the operated kidney which has been observed in 4 to 6% of patients.[30–32] These local recurrences are most likely a manifestation of undetected microscopic multifocal renal cell carcinoma in the renal remnant. The risk of local tumor recurrence after radical nephrectomy has not been studied, but it is presumably very low.

Evaluation of patients with renal cell carcinoma for partial nephrectomy should include preoperative testing to rule out locally extensive or metastatic disease. For most patients, preoperative renal arteriography to delineate the intrarenal vasculature aids in excising the tumor with minimal blood loss and damage to adjacent normal parenchyma. This test can be deferred in patients with small peripheral tumors. Selective renal venography is performed in patients with large or centrally located tumors to evaluate for intrarenal venous thrombosis secondary to malignancy.[33] The latter, if present, implies a more advanced local tumor stage and also increases the technical complexity of tumor excision. Preoperative hydration and mannitol administration are important adjuncts to ensure optimal renal perfusion at operation.

In patients with bilateral synchronous renal cell carcinoma, the kidney most amenable to a partial nephrectomy is usually approached first by the author. Then, approximately 1 month after a technically successful result has been documented, radical nephrectomy or a second partial nephrectomy is performed on the opposite kidney. Staging surgery in this fashion obviates the need for temporary dialysis if ischemic renal failure occurs following nephron-sparing excision of renal cell carcinoma.

It is usually possible to perform partial nephrectomy for malignancy in situ by using an operative approach that optimizes exposure of the kidney and by combining meticulous surgical technique with an understanding of the renal vascular anatomy in relation to the tumor. We employ an extraperitoneal flank incision through the bed of the eleventh or twelfth rib for almost all of these operations; we occasionally use a thoracoabdominal incision for very large tumors involving the upper portion of the kidney. These incisions allow the surgeon to operate on the mobilized kidney almost at skin level and provide excellent exposure of the peripheral renal vessels. With an anterior subcostal transperitoneal incision, the kidney is invariably located in the depth of the wound, and the surgical exposure is simply not as good.

When performing in situ partial nephrectomy for malignancy, the kidney is mobilized within Gerota's fascia while leaving intact the perirenal fat around the tumor. For small peripheral renal tumors, it may not be necessary to control the renal artery. In most cases, however, partial nephrectomy is most effectively performed after temporary renal arterial occlusion. This measure not only limits intraoperative bleeding but, by reducing renal tissue turgor, also improves access to intrarenal structures. In most cases, we believe that it is important to leave the renal vein patent throughout the operation. This measure decreases intraoperative renal ischemia and, by allowing venous backbleeding, facilitates hemostasis by enabling identification of small transected renal veins. In patients with centrally located tumors, it is helpful to occlude the renal vein temporarily to minimize intraoperative bleeding from transected major venous branches.

When the renal circulation is temporarily interrupted, in situ renal hypothermia is used to protect against postischemic renal injury. Surface cooling of the kidney with ice slush allows up to 3 hours of safe ischemia without permanent renal injury. An important caveat with this method is to keep the entire kidney covered with ice slush for 10 to 15 minutes immediately after occluding the renal artery and before commencing the partial nephrectomy. This amount of time is needed to obtain core renal cooling to a temperature (~20°C) that optimizes in situ renal preservation. During excision of the tumor, invariably large portions of the kidney are no longer covered with ice slush and, in the absence of adequate prior renal cooling, rapid rewarming and ischemic renal injury can occur. Cooling by perfusion of the kidney with a cold solution instilled via the renal artery is not recommended due to the theoretical risk of tumor dissemination. Mannitol is given intravenously 5 to 10 minutes before temporary renal arterial occlusion. Systemic or regional anticoagulation to prevent intrarenal vascular thrombosis is not necessary.

A variety of surgical techniques are available for performing partial nephrectomy in patients with malignancy.[34] These include simple enucleation, polar segmental nephrectomy, wedge resection, transverse resection, and extracorporeal partial nephrectomy with renal autotransplantation. All of these techniques require adherence to basic principles of early vascular control: avoidance of ischemic renal damage; complete tumor excision with free margins; precise closure of the collecting system; careful hemostasis; and closure or coverage of the renal defect with adjacent fat, fascia, peritoneum, or Oxycel. Whichever technique is employed, the tumor is removed with at least 1-cm surrounding margin of grossly normal renal parenchyma. Intraoperative ultrasound is very helpful in achieving accurate tumor localization, particularly for intrarenal lesions that are not visible or palpable from the external surface of the kidney.[35,36] The argon beam coagulator is a useful adjunct for achieving hemostasis on the transected renal surface.[37] If possible, the renal defect created by the excision is closed as an additional hemostatic measure. A retroperitoneal drain is always used as an additional hemostatic measure. A retroperitoneal drain is always left in place for at least 7 days. An intraoperative ureteral stent is placed only when major reconstruction of the intrarenal collecting system has been performed.

In patients with renal cell carcinoma, partial nephrectomy is contraindicated in the presence of lymph node metastasis, because the prognosis for these patients is poor. Enlarged or suspicious-looking lymph nodes should be biopsied before initiating the renal resection. When partial nephrectomy is performed, after excision of all gross tumor, absence of malignancy in the remaining portion of the kidney should be verified intraoperatively by frozen-section examinations of biopsy specimens obtained at random from the renal margin of excision. It is usual for such biopsies to demonstrate residual tumor but, if so, additional renal tissue must be excised.

Segmental Polar Nephrectomy

In a patient with malignancy confined to the upper or lower pole of the kidney, partial nephrectomy can be performed by isolating and ligating the segmental apical or basilar arterial branch while allowing unimpaired perfusion to the remainder of the kidney from the main renal artery. This procedure is illustrated in Figure 13–19 for a tumor confined to the apical vascular segment. The apical artery is dissected away from the adjacent structures, ligated, and divided. Often, a corresponding venous branch is present, which is similarly ligated and divided. An ischemic line of demarcation will then generally appear on the surface of the kidney and will outline the segment to be excised. If this area is not obvious, a few milliliters of methylene blue can be directly injected distally into the ligated apical artery to better outline the limits of the involved renal segment. An incision is then made in the renal cortex at the line of demarcation, which should be at least 1 cm away from the visible edge of the cancer. The parenchyma is divided by sharp

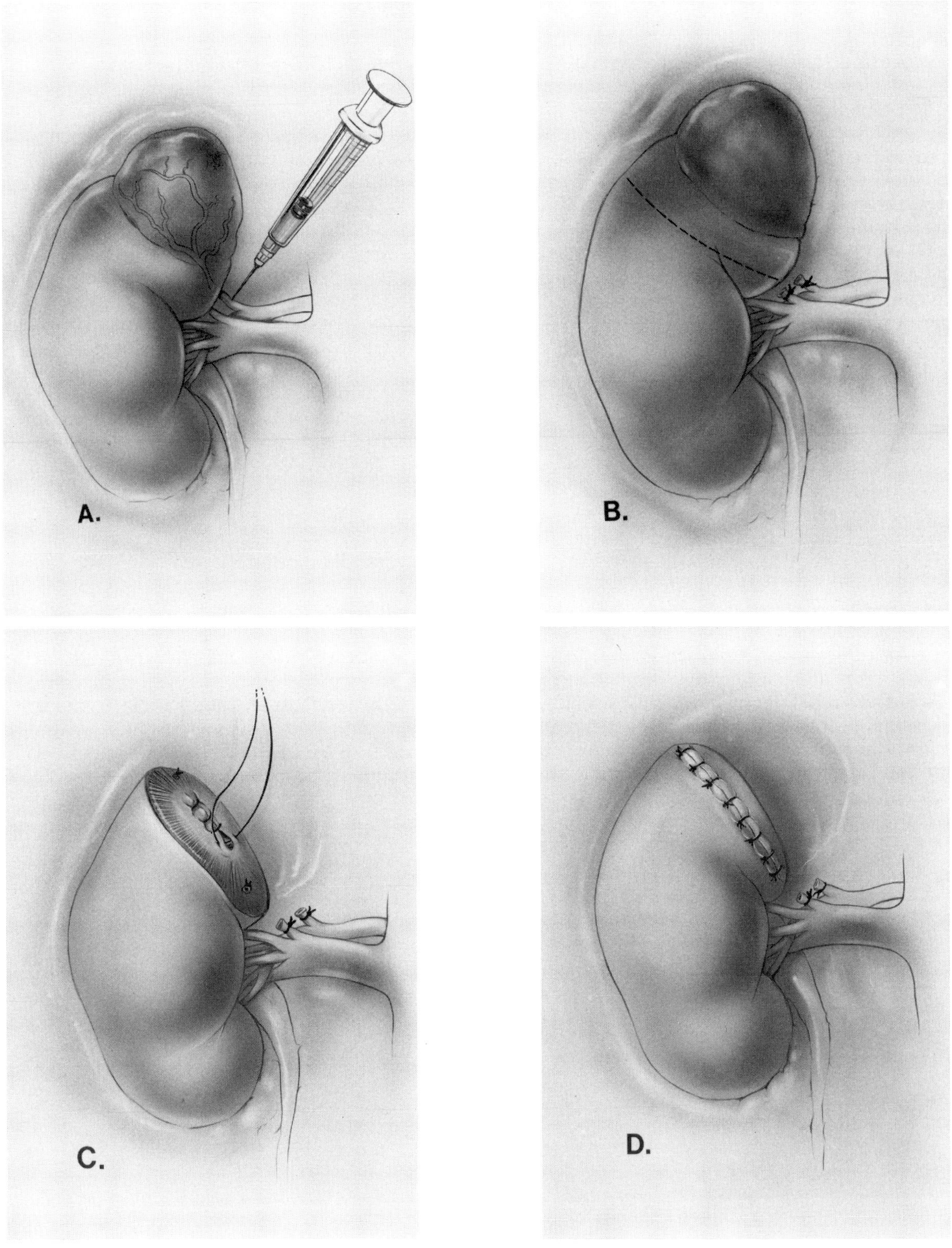
A.
B.
C.
D.

FIGURE 13–19. Technique of segmental (apical) polar nephrectomy with preliminary ligation of apical arterial and venous branches. (From Novick AC: Partial nephrectomy for renal cell carcinoma. Urol Clin North Am 1987; 14:419, with permission.)

and blunt dissection, and the polar segment is removed. In cases of malignancy, it is not possible to preserve a strip of capsule beyond the parenchymal line of resection for use in closing the renal defect.

Often a portion of the collecting system will have been removed with the cancer during a segmental polar nephrectomy. The collecting system is carefully closed with interrupted or continuous 4-0 chromic sutures to ensure a watertight repair. Small transected blood vessels on the renal surface are identified and ligated with shallow figure-of-eight 4-0 chromic sutures. The edges of the kidney are reapproximated as an additional hemostatic measure, using simple interrupted 3-0 chromic sutures inserted through the capsule and a small amount of parenchyma. Before these sutures are tied, perirenal fat or Oxycel can be inserted into the defect for inclusion in the renal closure. If the collecting system has been entered, a Penrose drain is left in the perinephric space.

Wedge Resection

Wedge resection is an appropriate technique for removing peripheral tumors on the surface of the kidney, particularly ones that are larger or not confined to either renal pole. Because these lesions often encompass more than one renal segment, and because this technique is generally associated with heavier bleeding, it is best to perform wedge resection with temporary renal arterial occlusion and surface hypothermia.

In performing a wedge resection, the tumor is removed with a 1-cm surrounding margin of grossly normal renal parenchyma (Fig. 13–20). The parenchyma is divided by a combination of sharp and blunt dissection. Invariably, the tumor extends deeply into the kidney, and the collecting system is entered. Often, prominent intrarenal vessels are identified as the parenchyma is being incised. These may be directly suture-ligated at that time, while they are most visible. After excision of the tumor, the collecting system is closed with interrupted or continuous 4-0 chromic sutures. Remaining transected blood vessels on the renal surface are secured with figure-of-eight 4-0 chromic sutures. Bleeding at this point is usually minimal, and the operative field can be kept satisfactorily clear by gentle suction during placement of hemostatic sutures.

The renal defect can be closed in one of two ways. The kidney may be closed upon itself by approximating the transected cortical margins with simple interrupted 3-0 chromic sutures, after placing a small piece of Oxycel at the base of the defect. If this is done, there must be no tension on the suture line and no significant angulation or kinking of blood vessels supplying the kidney. Alternatively, a portion of perirenal fat may simply be inserted into the base of the renal defect as a hemostatic measure and sutured to the parenchymal margins with interrupted 4-0 chromic. After closure or coverage of the renal defect, the renal artery is unclamped and circulation to the kidney is restored. A Penrose drain is left in the perinephric space.

Transverse Resection

A transverse resection is done to remove large tumors that extensively involve the upper or lower portion of the kidney. This technique is performed using surface hypothermia after temporary occlusion of the renal artery (Fig. 13–21). Major branches of the renal artery and vein supplying the tumor-bearing portion of the kidney are identified in the renal hilus, ligated, and divided. If possible, this should be done before temporarily occluding the

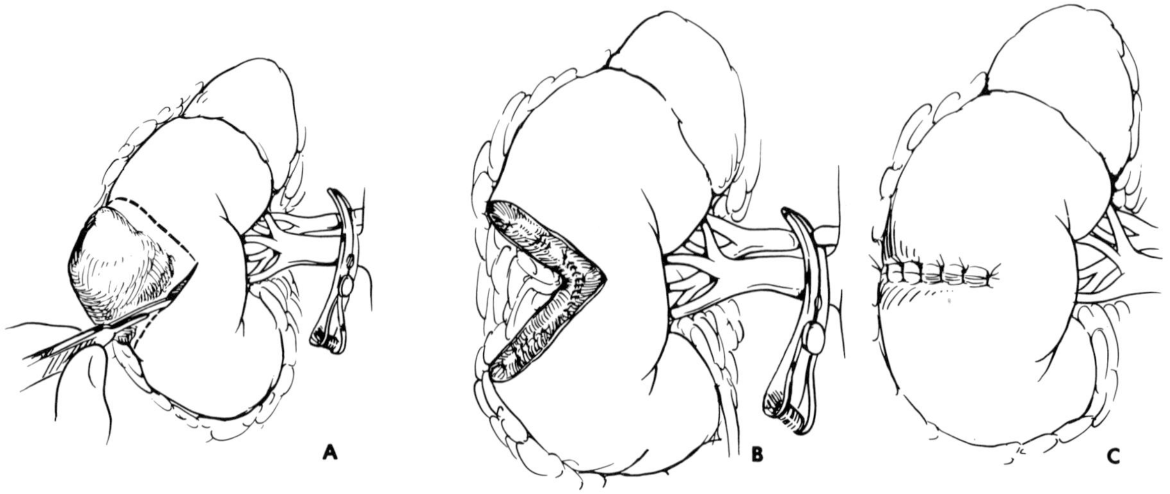
A
B
C

FIGURE 13–20. Technique of wedge resection for a peripheral tumor on the surface of the kidney. The renal defect may be closed upon itself or covered with perirenal fat.

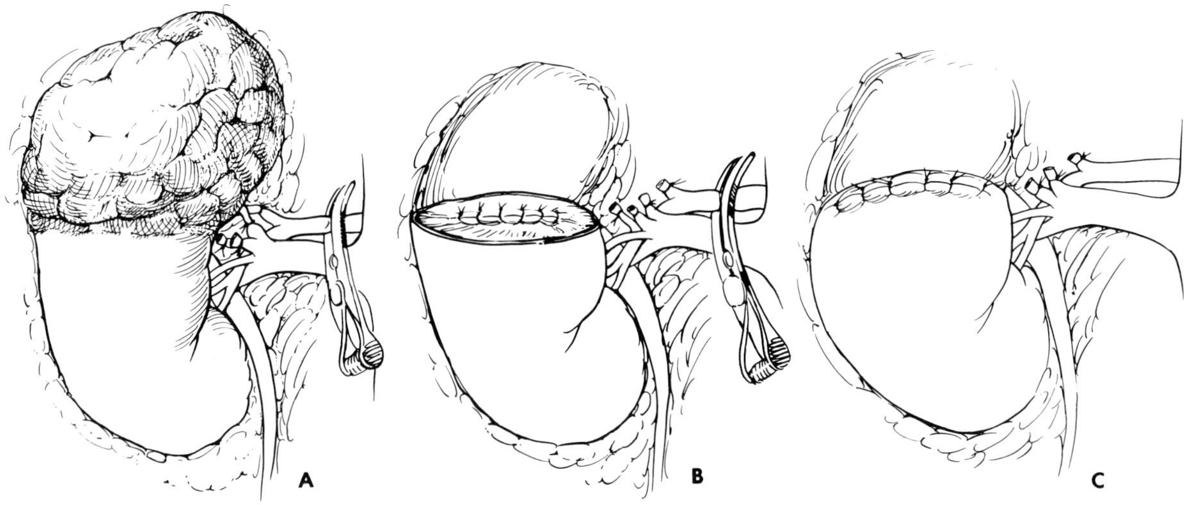
A
B
C

FIGURE 13–21. Technique of transverse resection for a tumor involving the upper half of the kidney.

renal artery to minimize the overall period of renal ischemia.

After occluding the renal artery, the parenchyma is divided with blunt and sharp dissection, leaving a 1-cm margin of grossly normal tissue around the tumor. Transected blood vessels on the renal surface are secured as previously described, and the hilus is inspected carefully for remaining unligated segmental vessels. An internal ureteral stent may be inserted if extensive reconstruction of the collecting system is necessary. If possible, the renal defect is sutured together with one of the techniques previously described. If this suture cannot be placed without tension or without distorting the renal vessels, a piece of peritoneum or perirenal fat is sutured in place to cover the defect. Circulation to the kidney is restored, and a Penrose drain is left in the perirenal space.

Simple Enucleation

Some renal cell carcinomas are surrounded by a distinct pseudocapsule of fibrous tissue.[38] The technique of simple enucleation implies circumferential incision of the renal parenchyma around the tumors simply and rapidly at any location, often with no vascular occlusion and with maximal preservation of normal parenchyma.

Initial reports indicated satisfactory short-term clinical results after enucleation with good patient survival and low rate of local tumor recurrence.[39,40] However, most recent studies have suggested a higher risk of leaving residual malignancy in the kidney when enucleation is performed.[41–43]

These latter reports include several carefully done histopathologic studies that have demonstrated frequent microscopic tumor penetration of the pseudocapsule that surrounds the neoplasm. These data indicate that it is not always possible to be assured of complete tumor encapsulation prior to surgery. Local recurrence of tumor in the treated kidney is a grave complication of partial nephrectomy for renal cell carcinoma, and every attempt should be made to prevent it. Therefore, it is the author's view that a surrounding margin of normal parenchyma should be removed with the tumor whenever possible. This provides an added margin of safety against the development of local tumor recurrence and, in most cases, does not appreciably increase the technical difficulty of the operation. The technique of enucleation is currently employed only in occasional patients with von Hippel-Lindau disease and multiple low-stage encapsulated tumors involving both kidneys.[44]

Extracorporeal Partial Nephrectomy and Autotransplantation

Extracorporeal partial nephrectomy for renal cell carcinoma with autotransplantation of the renal remnant was initially described to facilitate excision of large complex tumors involving the renal hilus. Reconstruction of kidneys with renal cell carcinoma as well as renal artery disease may also be facilitated with this approach.[45] The advantages of an extracorporeal approach include optimum exposure, a bloodless surgical field, the ability to perform a more precise operation with maximum conservation of renal parenchyma, and a greater protection of the kidney from prolonged ischemia. Disadvantages of extracorporeal surgery include longer operative time with the need for vascular and ureteral anastomoses and an increased risk of temporary and permanent renal failure[46]; the latter presumably reflects a more severe intraoperative ischemic insult to the kidney. While some urologic surgeons have found that almost all patients undergoing partial nephrectomy for renal cell carcinoma can be managed satisfactorily in situ,[32] others have continued to recommend an extracorporeal approach for selected patients.[30]

Extracorporeal partial nephrectomy and renal autotransplantation are generally performed through a single midline incision. The kidney is mobilized and removed outside Gerota's fascia with ligation and division of the renal artery and vein as the last steps in the operation (Fig. 13–22*A*). Immediately after dividing the renal vessels, the removed kidney is flushed with 500 ml of a chilled intracellular electrolyte solution and is submerged in a basin of ice slush saline solution to maintain hypothermia. Under these conditions, if warm renal ischemia has been minimal, the kidney can safely be preserved outside the body for as much time as is needed to perform extracorporeal partial nephrectomy.

If possible, it is best to leave the ureter attached in such cases to preserve its distal collateral vascular supply, particularly with large hilar or lower renal tumors in which complex excision may unavoidably compromise the blood supply to the pelvis, ureter, or both. When this procedure is done, the extracorporeal operation is performed on the abdominal wall. If the ureter is left attached, it must be occluded temporarily to prevent retrograde blood flow to the kidney when it is outside the body. Often, unless the patient is thin, working on the abdominal wall with the ureter attached is cumbersome because of the tethering and restricted movement of the kidney. If these are observed, the ureter should be divided and the kidney placed on a separate workbench. This practice will provide better exposure for the extracorporeal operation and, as this is being done, a second surgical team can be simultaneously preparing the iliac fossa for autotransplantation. If concern exists about the adequacy of ureteral blood supply, the risk of postoperative urinary extravasation can be diminished by restoring urinary continuity through direct anastomosis of the renal pelvis to the retained distal ureter.

Extracorporeal partial nephrectomy is done with the flushed kidney preserved under surface hypothermia. The kidney is first divested of all perinephric fat to appreciate the full extent of the neoplasm. Because such tumors are usually centrally located, dissection is generally begun in the renal hilus with identification of major segmental arterial and venous branches. Vessels clearly directed to-

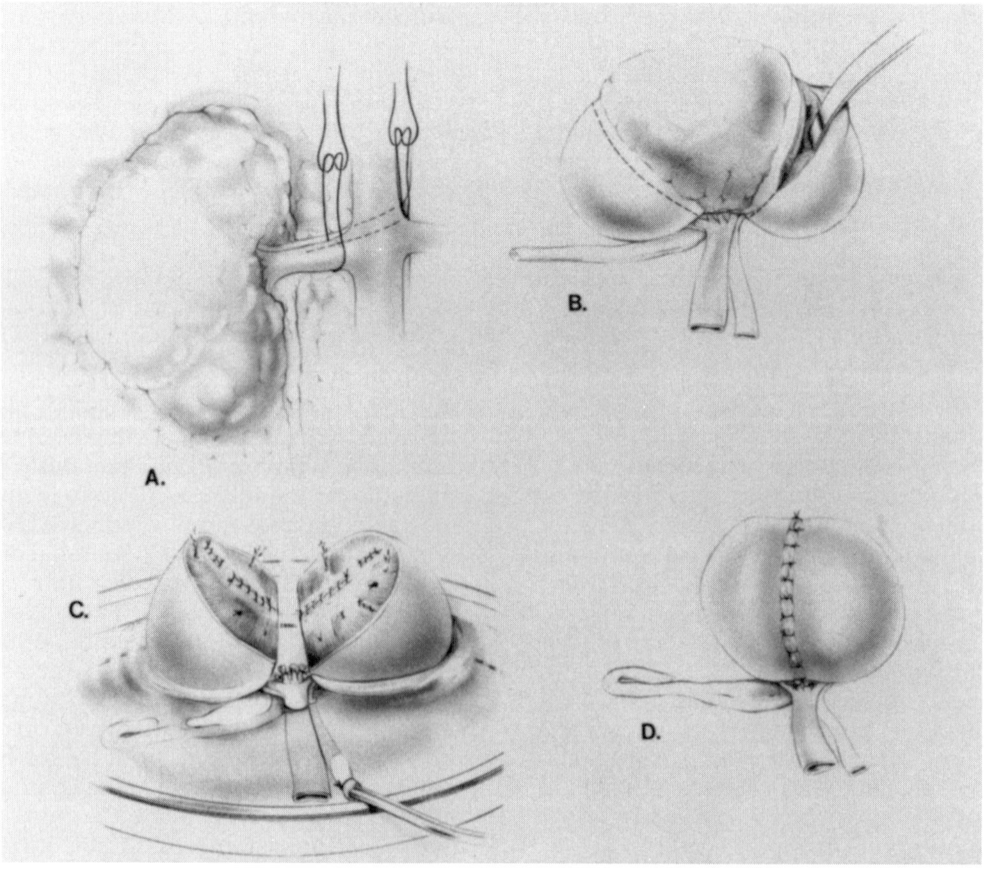
A.
B.
C.
D.

FIGURE 13–22. Technique of extracorporeal partial nephrectomy for a large central tumor. *A,* The kidney is removed outside Gerota's fascia. *B,* The tumor is excised extracorporeally while preserving the vascular branches to involved parenchyma. *C,* Pulsatile perfusion or reflushing are used to identify transected blood vessels. *D,* The kidney is closed upon itself. (From Novick AC: Partial nephrectomy for renal cell carcinoma. Urol Clin North Am 1987; 14:419, with permission.)

ward the neoplasm are secured and divided, and those supplying uninvolved renal parenchyma are preserved. The tumor is then removed by incising the capsule and parenchyma to preserve a 1-cm surrounding margin of normal renal tissue (Fig. 13–22*B*). Transected blood vessels visible on the renal surface are secured, and the collecting system is closed as described for in situ partial nephrectomy.

At this point, the renal remnant may be reflushed or placed on the pulsatile perfusion unit to facilitate identification and suture ligation of remaining potential bleeding points (Fig. 13–22*C*). The kidney can be alternatively perfused through the renal artery and vein to ensure both arterial and venous hemostasis. Because the flushing solution and perfusate lack clotting ability, there may continue to be some parenchymal oozing, which can safely be ignored. If possible, the defect created by the partial nephrectomy is closed by suturing the kidney upon itself to further ensure a watertight repair (Fig. 13–22*D*).

Autotransplantation into the iliac fossa is done, employing the same vascular technique as that in renal allotransplantation. Urinary continuity may be restored with ureteroneocystostomy or pyeloureterostomy, leaving an internal ureteral stent in place. When removal of the neoplasm has necessitated extensive hilar dissection of vessels supplying the renal pelvic, an indwelling nephrostomy tube is also left for postoperative drainage. After autotransplantation, a Penrose drain is positioned extraperitoneally in the iliac fossa away from the vascular anastomotic sites.

REFERENCES

1. Robson CJ, Churchill BM, Anderson W: The results of radical nephrectomy for renal cell carcinoma. J Urol 1969; 101: 297.
2. Skinner DG, Colvin RB, Vermillion CD, et al: Diagnosis and management of renal cell carcinoma: a clinical and pathological study of 309 cases. Cancer 1971; 28:1165.
3. Schefft P, Novick AC, Straffon RA, Stewart BH: Surgery for renal cell carcinoma extending into the vena cava. J Urol 1978; 120:28.
4. Libertino JA, Zinman L, Watkins E: Long-term results of resection of renal cell cancer with extension into inferior vena cava. J Urol 1987; 137:21.
5. Novick AC, Kaye M, Cosgrove D, et al: Experience with cardiopulmonary bypass and deep hypothermic circulatory arrest in the management of retroperitoneal tumors with large vena caval thrombi. Ann Surg 1990; 212:472.
6. Neves RJ, Zincke H: Surgical treatment of renal cancer with vena cava extension. Br J Urol 1987; 59:390.
7. Skinner DG, Pritchett TR, Lieskovsky G, et al: Vena caval involvement by renal cell carcinoma: surgical resection provides meaningful long-term survival. Ann Surg 1989; 210:387.
8. Cherrie RJ, Goldman DG, Linder A, deKernion JG: Prognostic implications of vena caval extension of renal cell carcinoma. J Urol 1982; 128:910.
9. Glazer AA, Novick AC: Long-term follow-up after surgical treatment for renal cell carcinoma extending into the right atrium. J Urol 1996; 155:448.
10. Pritchett TR, Raval JK, Benson RC, et al: Preoperative magnetic resonance imaging of vena caval tumor thrombi: experience with 5 cases. J Urol 1987; 138:1220.
11. Goldfarb DA, Novick AC, Lorgi R, et al: Magnetic resonance imaging for assessment of vena caval tumor thrombi: a comparative study with vena cavography and CT scanning. J Urol 1990; 144:1110.
12. Treiger BFG, Humphrey LS, Peterson CV, et al: Transesophageal echocardiography in renal cell carcinoma: an accurate diagnostic technique for intracaval neoplastic extension. J Urol 1991; 145:1138.
13. McGahan JP, Blake LC, DeVere White R, et al: Color flow sonographic mapping of intravascular extension of malignant renal tumors. J Ultrasound Med 1993; 12:403.
14. Belis JA, Pae WE, Rohner TJ, et al: Cardiovascular evaluation before circulatory arrest for removal of vena cava extension of renal carcinoma. J Urol 1989; 141:1302.
15. Sagalowaky AI, Kadesky KT, Ewalt DM, Kennedy TJ: Factors influencing adrenal metastasis in renal cell carcinoma. J Urol 1994; 151:1181.
16. Marshall FF, Powell KC: Lymphadenectomy for renal cell carcinoma: anatomical and therapeutic considerations. J Urol 1982; 128:677.
17. Giuliani L, Giberti C, Martorama G, Rovida S: Radical extensive surgery for renal cell carcinoma. J Urol 1990; 143: 468.
18. Novick AC, Streem SB: Surgery of the kidney. *In* Walsh PC, Retik AB, Stamey TA, Vaughan ED Jr (eds): Campbell's Urology, 6th edition, pp 2413–2500. Philadelphia, WB Saunders Co, 1992.
19. Cummings KB, Li WI, Ryan JA, et al: Intraoperative management of renal cell carcinoma with supradiaphragmatic caval excision. J Urol 1979; 122:829.
20. Foster RS, Mahomed Y, Bihrle RR, Strup S: Use of caval-atrial shunt for resection of a caval tumor thrombus in renal cell carcinoma. J Urol 1988; 140:1370.
21. Burt M: Inferior vena caval involvement by renal cell carcinoma: use of venovenous bypass as adjunct during resection. Urol Clin North Am 1991; 18:437.
22. Welch M, Bazaral MG, Schmidt R, et al: Anesthetic management for surgical removal of renal cell carcinoma with caval or atrial tumor thrombus using deep hypothermic circulatory arrest. J Cardiothorac Anesth 1989; 3:580.
23. Svenson L, Crawford E, Hess K, et al: Deep hypothermia with circulatory arrest. J Thorac Cardiovasc Surg 1993; 106: 19.
24. Mault J, Ohtake S, Klingensmith M, et al: Cerebral metabolism and circulatory arrest: effects of duration and strategies for protection. Ann Thorac Surg 1993; 55:57.
25. Pagano D, Carey JA, Patel RL, et al: Retrograde cerebral perfusion: clinical experience in emergency and elective aortic operations. Ann Thorac Surg 1995; 59:393.
26. Harker LA: Bleeding after cardiopulmonary bypass. N Engl J Med 1986; 314:1446.
27. Bisstrup BP, Royston D, Sapsford RN, et al: Reduction in blood loss and blood use after cardiopulmonary bypass with high dose aprotinin (Trasylol). J Thorac Cardiovasc Surg 1989; 97:364.
28. Licht MR, Novick AC: Nephron-sparing surgery for renal cell carcinoma. J Urol 1993; 145:1–7.
29. Butler BP, Novick AC, Miller DP, et al: Management of small unilateral renal cell carcinomas: radical versus nephron-sparing surgery. Urology 1995; 45:34.
30. Morgan WR, Zincke H: Progression and survival after renal conserving surgery of renal cell carcinoma: experience in 104 patients and extended follow-up. J Urol 1990; 144: 857–858.
31. Steinbach F, Stockle M, Muller SC, et al: Conservative surgery of renal tumors in 140 patients: 21 years of experience. J Urol 1992; 148:24–30.
32. Licht MR, Novick AC, Goormastic M: Nephron-sparing surgery in incidental versus suspected renal cell carcinoma. J Urol 1994; 152:39–42.

33. Angermeier KW, Novick AC, Streem SB, Montie JE: Nephron-sparing surgery for renal cell carcinoma with venous involvement. J Urol 1990; 144:1352.
34. Novick AC: Partial nephrectomy for renal cell carcinoma. Urol Clin North Am 1987; 14:419.
35. Assimos DG, Boyce WH, Woodruff RD, et al: Intraoperative renal ultrasonography: a useful adjunct to partial nephrectomy. J Urol 1991; 146:1218.
36. Campbell S, Novick AC, Steinbach F, et al: Intraoperative evaluation of renal cell carcinoma: a prospective study of the role of ultrasonography and histopathological frozen sections. J Urol 1996; 155:1191.
37. Hernandez AD, Smith JA Jr, Jeppson KG, Terreros DA: A controlled study of the argon beam coagulator for partial nephrectomy. J Urol 1990; 143:1062.
38. Vermooten V: Indications for conservative surgery in certain renal tumors: a study based on the growth pattern of clear cell carcinoma. J Urol 1950; 64:200.
39. Graham SD Jr, Glenn JF: Enucleation surgery for renal malignancy. J Urol 1979; 122:546.
40. Jaeger N, Weissbach L, Vahelensieck W: Valve of enucleation of tumor in solitary kidneys. Eur Urol 1985; 11:369.
41. Rosenthal CL, Kraft R, Zingg EJ: Organ-preserving surgery in renal cell carcinoma: tumor enucleation versus partial kidney resection. Eur Urol 1984; 10:222.
42. Marshall FF, Taxy JB, Fishman EK, Chang R: The feasibility of surgical enucleation for renal cell carcinoma. J Urol 1986; 135:231.
43. Blackley SK, Ladaga L, Woolfit RA, Schellhammer PF: Ex situ study of the effectiveness of enucleation in patients with renal cell carcinoma. J Urol 1988; 140:6.
44. Spencer WF, Novick A, Montie JE, et al: Surgical treatment of localized renal carcinoma in von Hippel-Lindau disease. J Urol 1988; 139:507.
45. Campbell SC, Novick AC, Streem SB, Klein EA: Management of renal cell carcinoma with coexistent renal artery disease. J Urol 1993; 150:808.
46. Campbell SC, Novick AC, Streem SB, et al: Complications of nephron-sparing surgery for renal tumors. J Urol 1994; 151:1177.

14

TRANSITIONAL CELL CARCINOMA OF THE RENAL PELVIS AND URETER: DIAGNOSIS, STAGING, MANAGEMENT, AND PROGNOSIS

S. MACHELE DONAT, M.D. *and* HARRY W. HERR, M.D.

Transitional cell carcinoma (TCC) of the upper urinary tract was first reported in 1841 by Rayer.[1] It has remained a relatively uncommon tumor and accounts for only 6 to 7% of all primary tumors of the kidney.[2–5] Eighty-two to 90% of upper urinary tract tumors are of epithelial (transitional cell) origin (82 to 90%), followed by squamous cell or epidermoid carcinoma in 10 to 17%, and adenocarcinoma in less than 1%.[2,6,7] It is estimated that the incidence of these tumors is increasing about 3% per year[4]; however, this may be a reflection of improved diagnostic techniques and surveillance methods.

Renal pelvis and ureteral tumors have a two- to threefold preponderance in men as compared to women and are most common in the sixth and seventh decade of life. The mean age of presentation is similar for males and females.[2,8–10] It is extremely rare in children, with only about six cases having been reported in children under 20 years old.[10,11]

Transitional cell carcinoma of the upper tract occurs more commonly in the renal pelvis and calyces (66%) than the ureter (34%), and when the ureter is involved it tends to be the distal one third most frequently.[7,10,12,13] The tumors may be unifocal but are more commonly multifocal (16 to 47%) in nature[8–10,14,15] and in the kidney arise from the membranous pelvis or from the urothelium of the calyces overlying the renal parenchyma.[2] Bilateral involvement is estimated to occur in 2 to 4% of patients, but may be as high as 10% in patients in high-risk groups such as Balkan nephropathy.[2,10,16,17] Although the probability of developing upper tract tumors in patients with bladder cancer is only 2 to 4%,[18–21] the risk of developing bladder cancer subsequent to an upper tract tumor is 15 to 50%.[2,5,16,22–25] Following radical cystectomy for bladder cancer, patients have a 1 to 9% risk of developing an upper tract tumor over the ensuing 10 years.[26,27] The majority arise within the first 3 years, with a reported range of 8 months to 20 years.[17,20,26–29] An increased incidence (14 to 18%) of upper tract transitional cell carcinoma has also been reported in patients with a history of recurrent carcinoma in situ of the bladder[30,31] managed with intravesical bacille Calmette-Guérin (BCG), with distal ureteral or prostatic urethral involvement, or high-grade multifocal carcinoma in situ in the bladder at the time of cystectomy.[18,20,27,32] The incidence of unsuspected carcinoma in situ in the distal ureters at the time of cystectomy ranges from 1% (4 of 425) in Zincke's series[27] to 10% in a series reported by Wallace.[33] Culp[34] also reported a 17% incidence of "epithelial aberrations" in juxtavesical ureters of patients undergoing cystectomy. Neither the duration of bladder involvement nor the number of recurrences appear to have any significant relationship to the incidence of ureteral carcinoma in situ at cystectomy.[32] Approximately 19% of patients will have metastatic disease at their initial presentation.[35]

The standard of treatment for transitional cell carcinoma of the renal pelvis and ureter remains nephroureterectomy with a cuff of bladder; however, improvements in percutaneous and retrograde endourologic techniques and a better understanding of the natural history of the disease have provided avenues for more conservative management in appropriate cases. Most of the data and management decisions of transitional cell carcinoma of the upper tract have been derived from retrospective analysis of patients. This is largely due to the rarity of the condition making prospective data difficult to accumulate in any one institution.

ETIOLOGY

There have been several environmental factors identified that correlate with an increased risk of developing transitional cell carcinoma of the upper tracts. The identification of most of these factors was delayed by the long latency period between the first exposure and the development of the tumor. The first correlation was suggested in 1895 by Rehn when he suspected an association between workmen in factories exposed to aniline dyes.[33] Hueper in 1938 showed there was also a relationship between upper tract tumors and B-naphthylamine, an intermediate compound of dyes. This aroused suspicion that there might be other chemical compounds in industry that exposure to could result in the development of tumors of the urinary tract.

In 1949 the Imperial Chemical company in England felt the relationship was so strong that they voluntarily stopped the production and withdrew all stocks of B-naphthylamine.[36] Virtually 100% of workers exposed to the distillation of the chemical developed tumors, and benzidine exposure increased the risk of tumors to 70 times that of the general population. By 1966 the manufacture of benzidine and A-naphthylamine were also stopped in England, but the United States did not follow suit until several years later.[37] Retrospective reviews of workers and health problems revealed an average delay of 18 years between exposure and the development of a tumor.[38] Since that time correlations between the development of upper tract TCC and cigarette smoking; chemicals in rubber, petroleum, textile, cable, and plastics industries; increased consumption of phenacetin-containing analgesics; a contrast agent, thorium dioxide; and cyclophosphamide therapy have been identified[21,39–43] (Table 14–1).

Industrial agents including benzidine, B-naphthylamine, 4-aminobiphenyl, and 4,4′-diaminobiphenyl have more effect on the lower urinary tract and are believed to exert their effect through the process of malignant transformation. The fact that there is a greater effect on the lower tract is hypothesized to be secondary to the rapid transit time of the agent through the upper tract, relative stasis in the bladder, and that the agents may be converted to a conjugated active form capable of promoting tumor development in the bladder.[39]

TABLE 14–1. ETIOLOGIC FACTORS IN THE DEVELOPMENT OF UPPER TRACT TRANSITIONAL CELL CANCER

Cigarette smoking	
Chemicals in manufacture of:	
Analine Dyes	B-Naphthylamine
Rubber	Benzidine
Petroleum	A-Naphthylamine
Textile	4-Aminobiphenyl
Plastics	4-4′-Diaminobiphenyl
Phenacetin-containing analgesics	
Thorium dioxide (contrast agent Thorotrast)	
Cyclophosphamide therapy	
Balkan nephropathy	
Molecular genetic alterations	
Chromosomes 9, 17, 13, and 3	
p53	
Idiopathic	

On the other hand, analgesic abuse and Balkan nephropathy are conditions associated with the almost exclusive development of upper tract TCC.[39,41]

Hultengen et al.[41] reported the first association with excessive consumption of phenacetin-containing analgesics and the development of renal pelvis TCC in 1965. Only phenacetin-containing analgesics are unequivocally associated with the development of tumors; however, there is a weak association with paracetamol, the chief intermediate metabolite of phenacetin.[8,39–41] The exact mechanism of tumorigenesis is unknown, but it is hypothesized that the main metabolite of phenacetin, "4-acetoaminoprophenol," is similar structurally to known carcinogens and exerts its effect by directly acting as a carcinogen, and indirectly by causing papillary necrosis, "analgesic nephropathy," which acts as a local promoter of urothelial carcinogenesis.[8,16,39–41] It is believed to affect the renal pelvis (82 to 90%) preferentially because of the short half-life of the metabolites; therefore, by the time it reaches the bladder it is in a detoxified form and has little effect.[39,44,45] The risk of developing upper tract TCC in patients with histologic and radiologic evidence of analgesic nephropathy has been reported to be 150 times that of patients without them. The risk of tumor development has a reported mean induction time of 22 years with a range of 20 to 34 years[39,42] and a history of consumption lasting a mean of 17 years. Most of the studies demonstrating the association have been performed retrospectively and have not controlled well for the confounding effect of smoking, but the association was felt to be strong enough that in New South Wales, where renal pelvic TCC is more prevalent than in any other Western society, the sale of nonprescriptive compound analgesic preparations was prohibited by legislation passed in 1979.[42] When the risk of smoking has been controlled for, analgesics still conferred a risk of cancer four to eight times in men and 10 to 13 times in women.[42]

Petkovic reported the association of upper tract TCC in patients with Balkan nephropathy, also known as Danuvian endemic familial nephropathy.[46] The incidence in the inhabitants of the Balkan regions (Yugoslavia, Rumania, Bulgaria, and Greece) is 100 to 200 times that of other populations despite similar incidences of bladder cancer between the regions. In addition, family members who leave the area are unaffected, suggesting an environmental cause and making a hereditary component less likely. The etiology of the nephropathy is unknown but develops slowly over 20 years. The tumors that develop are usually low grade but have a 10% incidence of bilaterality. The patients usually succumb to renal failure secondary to the nephropathy rather than the tumors.

Perhaps the most common cause of upper tract TCC that has been identified is cigarette smoking. In 1991 McLaughlin et al.[4] reported the results of a large case-controlled study involving 502 cases and 496 controls that showed a 2.6- to 6.5-fold increased risk of developing upper tract TCC in men and a 1.6- to 2.4-fold increase in women dependent on their current or previous history of smoking. In general, smoking-related risk appeared to be higher for the development of ureteral tumors. There appeared to be a strong relationship between the amount smoked per day, the number of years smoked, and the pack-year history of use with the development of upper tract tumors. The duration of smoking appeared to be a stronger indicator of risk than the amount smoked, and the risk of tumor development did decrease 60 to 70% relative to the number of years from the cessation of smoking. This has also been found to be true of bladder cancer.[47] Patients that have smoked greater than 25 years have been found to have a relative risk of 4.5 ($p < .0001$) of developing upper tract tumors compared to nonsmokers.[40] Also of note was that cigar and pipe smoking did increase the risk but not significantly. Eight prior case-controlled studies in the United States,[40,48,49] England,[50] Denmark,[51] and Australia[42,52,53] that evaluated smoking and the relative risk of developing TCC of the upper tract confirm a 4- to 11-fold increased risk when compared to nonsmokers.

Cigarette smoke is known to contain a large number of carcinogens, but it is unclear whether these concentrate in the upper tract, if the upper tract urothelium is more susceptible, or if they are degradated or diluted enough in the bladder so that they do not exert as great of an effect there. Others have suggested that although cigarette smoking has not been shown to significantly alter the kinds of mutations sustained in the p53 gene, it may act to increase the extent of DNA damage per mutagenic event.[54]

About six cases of upper tract TCC have been reported in patients following cyclophosphamide therapy, with an average induction time of 5 years.[43] Cyclophosphamide is an alkylating agent widely used in the treatment of carcinomas of B-cell origin such as lymphoma and multiple myeloma. Most urologic oncologists are familiar with the more immediate complications of the therapy including hemorrhagic cystitis and bladder fibrosis.

Another substance that is highly associated with the development of upper tract TCC is a contrast agent called thorium dioxide (Thorotrast), which was used in the 1930s and 1940s for retrograde pyelograms.[39] The latency period to the development of tumors is about 20 years.[55] The agent is no longer used but was hypothesized to produce vascular insufficiency with a subsequent foreign body reaction that predisposed the patient to the development of tumor, most of which occurred in the renal pelvis.

Attempts to locate molecular genetic alterations in transitional cell carcinoma have identified some abnormalities on chromosome 9 and 17 near the p53 locus, on chromosome 13 near the retinoblastoma locus, and on chromosome 3 near the kidney cancer gene locus, although a specific gene associated with transitional cell carcinoma has not been identified.[56–59] Orphali et al.[60] and Frisher et al.[61] reported on nine kindreds exhibiting a familial pattern in the development of transitional cell carcinoma with 22% having upper tract tumors alone, 18% with both upper and lower tract tumors, and 59% with carcinoma of the bladder alone.

PATHOLOGY

As previously discussed, transitional cell carcinoma is the most common tumor of the upper tract. The predominant histologic pattern is a papillary tumor with stratified epithelium and nonkeratinizing epithelium supported on a thin fibrovascular core.[2,10] Tumors may occur singly or more commonly multifocally. Studies of nephroureterectomy specimens have documented the multifocal nature of the urothelial changes.[39,62] McCarron et al.[62] demonstrated a parallel relationship between the grade of the tumor and the degree of epithelial changes in macroscopically normal appearing areas. As previously reported by Heney et al.,[63] McCarron also found that grade 1 tumors tended to have no associated atypia, whereas grade 2 to 3 tumors had significant changes in the surrounding mucosa ranging from atypia to carcinoma in situ. In addition, 62% of high-grade tumors of the renal pelvis also had moderate to severe atypia in the ureter.[62] Figure 14–1 demonstrates the multifocal nature and gross appearance of papillary tumors of the renal pelvis and ureter.[2]

Transformation of the adjacent mucosa may present as a flat or micropapillary carcinoma in situ (Fig. 14–2). In fact, flat carcinoma in situ may be found in 7 to 25% of patients undergoing cystectomy for an invasive carcinoma of the bladder. It is more commonly found in patients with multiple recurrences over time or multifocal disease and may represent an extension of the bladder cancer into the distal ureter.[2,18,32,64] The panurothelial nature of

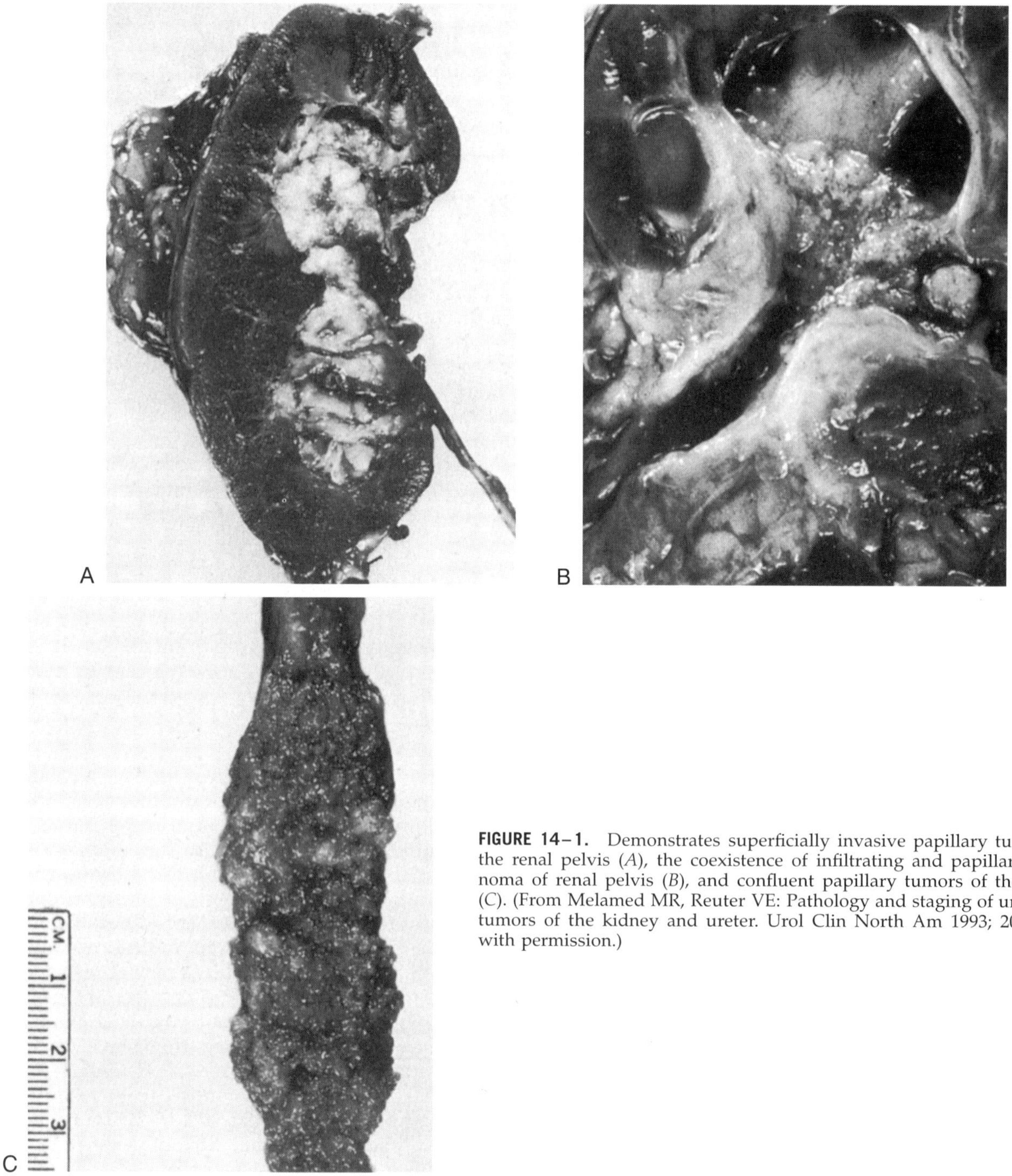
A
B
C.M. 1 2 3
C

FIGURE 14–1. Demonstrates superficially invasive papillary tumors of the renal pelvis (*A*), the coexistence of infiltrating and papillary carcinoma of renal pelvis (*B*), and confluent papillary tumors of the ureter (*C*). (From Melamed MR, Reuter VE: Pathology and staging of urothelial tumors of the kidney and ureter. Urol Clin North Am 1993; 20[2]:333, with permission.)

carcinoma in situ is further emphasized by the finding of increased risk (20%, 26 of 128 patients) of the development of upper tract tumors in patients whose bladders have been preserved by successful intravesical BCG therapy.[30,64] Such tumors have been detected as late as 15 years or more after treatment of the initial bladder tumor, mandating surveillance of the upper tracts probably for the lifetime of the patient.

Flat carcinoma in situ may also develop in the ureter or renal pelvis unrelated to the condition of the bladder and is usually asymptomatic and found incidentally on work-up of a positive urine cytology. It is difficult to define grossly, as the mucosal appearance may vary from being slightly thickened and pale white when epithelial hyperplasia is present, to an erythemic congested appearance when there is an increase in subepithelial vascularity.[2]

Theories on multifocality and recurrent disease have been published as early as 1890 when Housemann first proposed the concept of multicentric origin.[65] Reuter et al. propose that there is a sequence in tumor development progressing from mucosal hyperplasia to, finally, an invasive papillary carci-

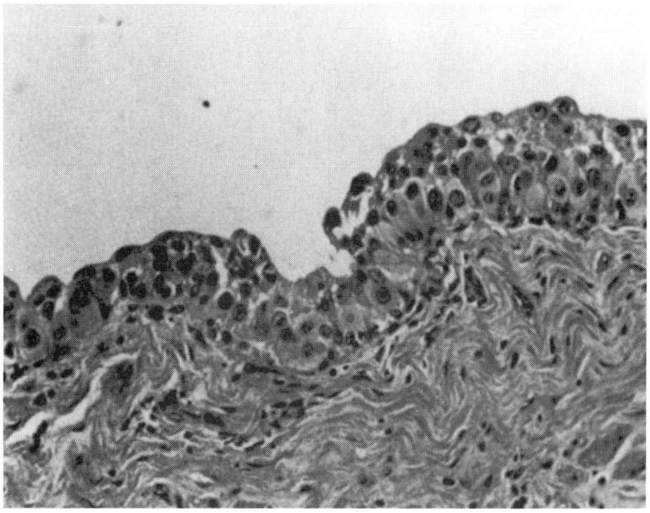

FIGURE 14–2. Flat carcinoma in situ. Malignant enlarged epithelial cells with large nuclei and abundant cytoplasm replacing urothelium (hematoxylin and eosin). (From Melamed MR, Reuter VE: Pathology and staging of urothelial tumors of the kidney and ureter. Urol Clin North Am 1993; 20:[2]: 333, with permission.)

noma as seen in Figure 14–3.[2] This progression is suggested by the not uncommon finding of areas of carcinoma in an otherwise benign appearing papilloma and is described as papilloma with carcinoma in situ. This suggests that the pathogenesis of papillary carcinoma is through the transformation of a pre-existing papilloma, although it is also possible for some patients to develop an invasive carcinoma from the accompanying flat carcinoma in situ and not from the papillary tumor.[66] It is still unclear whether the development of new tumors represents the multifocality in a carcinoma-prone urothelium or if it represents the dissemination of cells from the initial tumor.[2,10,21,67,68] Arguments favoring the multifocal origin of tumors are the occurrence of bilateral upper tract tumors, and the common finding of separate areas of carcinoma and carcinoma in situ in cystectomy series. Arguments supporting the theory of dissemination are the high incidence of the development of bladder cancer subsequent to the appearance of upper tract tumors as opposed to the very low incidence of the reverse occurring, the decreasing likelihood of developing subsequent tumor in the bladder over time after a nephroureterectomy, the reported cases of percutaneous tract and retroperitoneal seeding after pyelotomies for renal pelvis tumors,[69,70] the recent demonstration of common genetic markers in what appear to be separate urinary tract tumors,[67,71] the increased risk (15 to 20 times) of bladder cancer patients with vesicoureteral reflux developing upper tract tumors,[72,73] and the experimental animal evidence that tumor has the potential to spread by dissemination.[74]

DIAGNOSIS

Presenting Symptoms

Upper tract tumors are often discovered incidentally on surveillance testing for lower tract tumors and are asymptomatic in up to 29% of patients.[39,68] Patients who are symptomatic frequently present with gross hematuria or symptoms of obstruction, hydronephrosis, or pyelonephritis.[2,39,68] Only 10% of patients present with the classic triad of flank pain, abdominal mass, and gross hematuria, but when present this usually indicates advanced disease.[75]

Mucosal Hyperplasia

⇓

Papilloma

⇓

Atypical Papilloma

⇓

Papilloma with Focal CIS

⇓

Non-invasive Papillary Carcinoma

⇓

Papillary Carcinoma with Invasion

FIGURE 14–3. Proposed transformation of urothelium from hyperplasia to invasive papillary carcinoma. (From Melamed MR, Reuter VE: Pathology and staging of urothelial tumors of the kidney and ureter. Urol Clin North Am 1993; 20:[2]:333, with permission.)

Hematuria is by far the most common initial symptom, with a reported occurrence of 56 to 98%.[10,39,68,75] Flank pain occurs in 10 to 40% of patients and usually is an indication of more advanced disease. It is usually dull in nature and secondary to obstruction or invasion into adjacent organs, but can be similar to acute renal colic in patients with significant upper tract bleeding.[10,39,68,75] About 10 to 15% of patients will present with associated weight loss, anorexia, and lethargy, which are ominous indicators of metastatic disease.[39,68,75]

Radiographic Appearance and Evaluation

Radiographic errors in diagnosis of upper tract transitional cell carcinoma have been reported in up to 15% of cases, with the most frequent error being mistaken adenocarcinoma of the kidney in 24%, followed by lithiasis in 16%, hydronephrosis in 13%, pyonephrosis in 10%, urinary tuberculosis in 9%, extrinsic compression in 5%, and other miscellaneous causes in 13%.[6]

Classic urographic findings for upper tract transitional cell carcinoma include the "goblet or Bergmann" sign, which is a meniscus-shaped ureteral filling defect, and the "stipple sign" produced by contrast trapping in the fronds of a papillary tumor. Filling defects may be the result of the parietal implantation of tumor, the uneven jagged contours of papillary fronds, or obstruction of a ureter with proximal dilation.[10] Figures 14–4 through 14–6 demonstrate the radiographic evaluation of a patient with gross hematuria during an episode of severe acute pyelonephritis requiring a 2-week hospitalization and intravenous antibiotics to resolve. He subsequently was found to have an invasive TCC of the renal pelvis.

An *intravenous pyelogram* (IVP) is abnormal in 47 to 98% of patients with upper tract tumors and is the initial radiographic study of choice.[5,10,13,68,75,76] About 50% of patients will have a filling defect either in the renal pelvis or ureter and may have an associated hydronephrosis, hydroureter, or nonvisualization of the kidney secondary to obstruction.[10,39] Nonvisualization is usually seen in more advanced disease and is frequently associated with invasion of tumor into the renal parenchyma indicating a poorer prognosis.[5,25,39] Stenosis is a specific sign of infiltrating disease and is more commonly seen in the renal pelvis than ureter.[10] If no abnormalities are found on intravenous pyelogram and a tumor is present on other studies, it will be low grade in 85% of cases.[39]

Retrograde pyelogram (RPG) can be used to further delineate anatomically the exact nature and extent of the problem seen on intravenous pyelogram.[39,76] This is well demonstrated in Figures 14–4 and 14–5, where the IVP has subtle findings of an incomplete upper pole calyx, but on the retrograde pyelogram there is clear evidence of an infiltrative process in the upper pole consistent with tumor. It allows for complete visualization of the upper tracts, which may not have been adequate by IVP, or in patients with renal insufficiency or allergic reactions to contrast agents prohibiting the use of IVP.

A *loopogram* is a type of retrograde study used in patients following radical cystectomy to visualize the upper tracts and to evaluate the normally refluxing ureteroileal anastomosis for stenosis. It is performed by placing a Foley catheter into the ileal conduit stoma and inflating the balloon just enough to obstruct the stoma prior to instillation of contrast under fluoroscopy. If visualization is adequate this study may negate the need for an intravenous contrast and may also be used in patients with renal failure or contrast allergies.

Ultrasound and *computed tomography (CT) scan* can be helpful in distinguishing nonopaque calculi from soft tissue filling defects. In this instance a noncontrast study is needed to detect the high-attenuation coefficients of calculi and the CT is more sensitive in distinguishing the sometimes slight increase in radiodensity than any other study.[76,77] Transitional cell carcinomas may calcify; however, these are usually in a stippled or curvilinear pattern and usually associated with masses. In this case, a 3- to 5-mm thin-cut CT (helical or standard) through the suspicious area with and without contrast may be helpful in making the diagnosis.[78]

When CT demonstrates direct tumor extension through the renal pelvis or ureteral wall it is a sensitive indicator of high-stage disease; however, in the absence of these findings it is of limited value in staging tumors. Without definite evidence of direct extension, CT only has a 43% specificity, 75% sensitivity, and 77% accuracy in detecting parenchymal invasion, and only 44% specificity, 67% sensitivity, and 72% accuracy in detecting periureteral or perirenal fat invasion.[76,77]

Angiography has not been found to be useful in differentiating ureteral lesions due to the fact that most transitional cell carcinomas do not show abnormal vascular patterns.[10,79]

Urine Cytology and DNA Ploidy Analysis

Urine cytology is frequently used to follow patients with transitional cell carcinoma of both the lower and upper tracts. Positive cytologies in patients with no evidence of disease in the bladder often lead to discovery of upper tract disease in an otherwise asymptomatic patient on further evaluation. Its greatest value is in the diagnosis of carcinoma in situ, where it has a sensitivity of about 90%. Unfortunately, urine cytologies have an overall false-negative rate of 65% in diagnosing upper tract TCC,[10,80–83] and as high as 96% in low-grade upper tract tumors and therefore are of limited

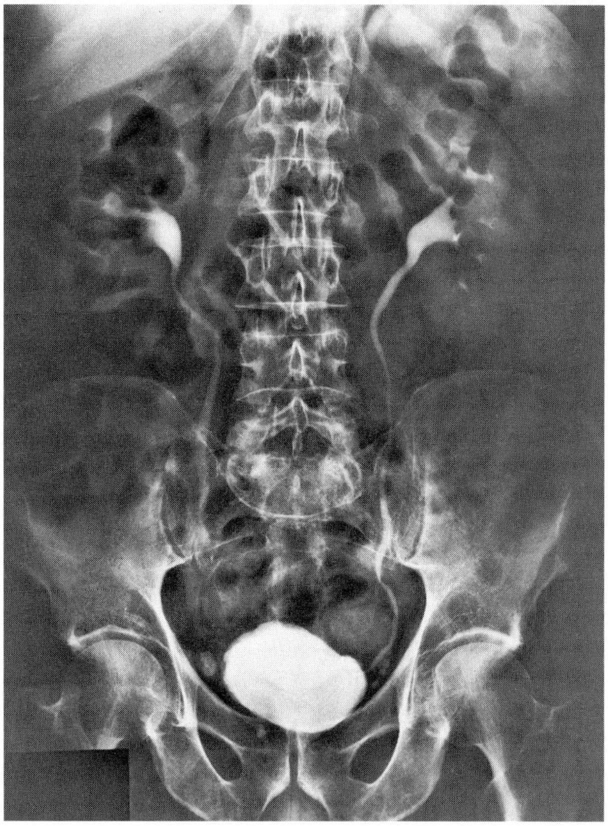

A

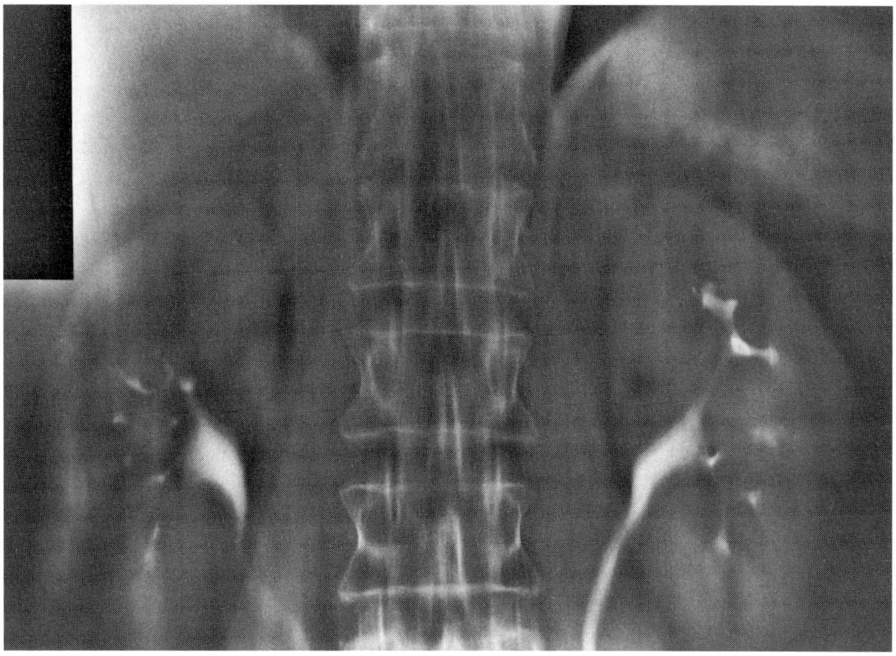

B

FIGURE 14–4. Intravenous pyelogram with tomogram in patient with invasive TCC of right upper pole presenting with gross hematuria and pyelonephritis.

value for the diagnosis of these tumors.[7,24,80] In fact, urine cytologies are negative in up to 80% of patients with low-grade tumors.[7] This is thought to be because lower grade tumors have fewer morphologic alterations leading to loss of intercellular attachments and adhesiveness to make them identifiable on cytologic analysis. When they are exfoliated, low-grade tumors are usually shed in

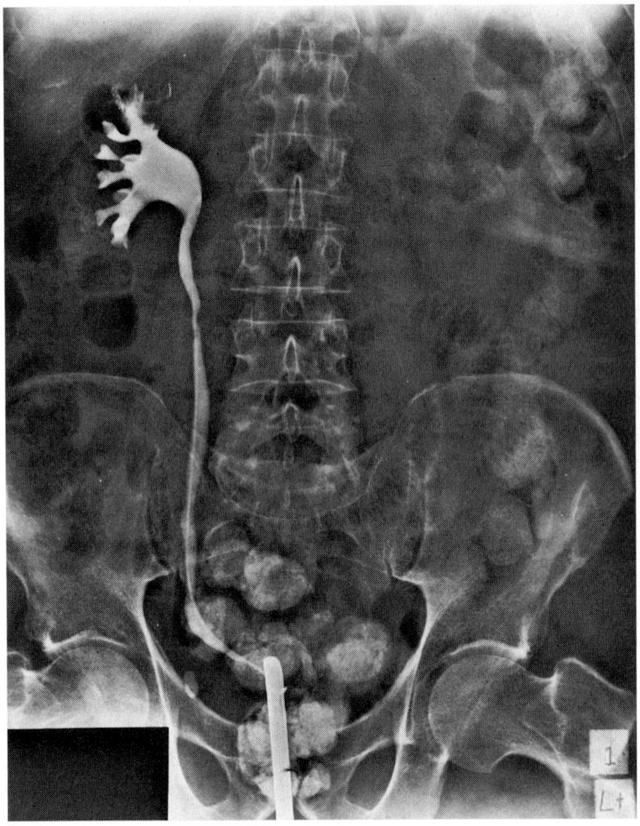
1
Lt

FIGURE 14–5. Retrograde pyelogram (in same patient as seen in Fig. 14–4) demonstrating clearly an infiltrative TCC of the upper pole.

large papillary fragments (Fig. 14–7). Cells tend to be uniform in size with minimal changes in nuclear/cytoplasmic ratio and have small or absent nucleoli. High-grade tumors, on the other hand, tend to have greater morphologic changes leading to exfoliation and discovery on cytologic examination. High-grade tumor cells tend to be more isolated in loose clusters and elongated with marked pleomorphism and increased nuclear/cytoplasmic ratios (Fig. 14–8). Nucleoli are variable in size.

If the cytology is positive and there is no discernible upper tract lesion, selective ureteral and renal pelvis washings (the diagnostic accuracy of which is still debated because of possible contamination from the bladder) may be performed. Some investigators, however, report an accuracy rate of up to 80% in detecting carcinoma in situ of the upper tract with appropriate barbotage methods.[39]

Some of the diagnostic inaccuracy of urine cytologies is caused by poor specimen collection technique and handling. Catheterized specimens can denude normal surface epithelial cells, which can coalesce in papillary groups and be misinterpreted as low-grade TCC. Voided specimens with prolonged exposure to concentrated urine or specimens from female patients contaminated with vaginal, cervical, endometrial, or epithelial cells can also be misinterpreted.[39] Chronic urinary tract infections, inflammatory conditions, and stone disease can result in degenerative changes and atypia in cells. And finally, the ability of the cytopathologist to interpret the specimen plays some role.

DNA ploidy analysis has been used to evaluate the DNA content of transitional cell tumors. DNA content of tumors may currently be measured by flow cytometry or quantitative fluorescence image analysis. Flow cytometry allows the analysis of up to 1000 cells/sec, but it is impossible to assign DNA content to the morphology of a specific cell. Image analysis, on the other hand, is a slower method, but it permits the DNA measurement of cells already diagnosed visually as tumor cells.[15] Both are being studied not just for the identification of abnormal DNA content but what this may mean prognostically to the individual patient in terms of survival and progression of disease. Tumor heterogeneity, individual cell cycle phases of tumors, morphology, and DNA content may all be determined by these methods.

Biochemical and Immunologic Evaluation

Several biochemical and immunologic markers have been studied but none have demonstrated reliable diagnostic results to date.[80] Urinary enzymes for *lactate dehydrogenase* and *alkaline phosphatase* do not appear to be specific or reliably increased in patients with transitional cell carcinoma.[84] *Carcinoembryonic antigen* (CEA) levels are detectable in urine and serum and can be elevated at levels proportional to the mass and surface area of the tumor; however, they may also simply reflect tissue breakdown secondary to infection or other tissue-destructive lesions and therefore are also nonspecific and unreliable.[85] *Tumor-specific* or *-associated antigens* in the serum or urine of patients with TCC have also not been found to be specifically or reliably increased.[84]

Endoscopic Evaluation

Radiographic and cytologic evaluations of renal pelvic and ureteral tumors can often be indeterminate in differentiating between benign and malignant etiologies of upper tract abnormalities (Table 14–2). In addition, patients may present with positive urine cytologies but no discernable radiographic etiology. *Cystoscopic examination* should be a routine part of the work-up of patients with suspected upper tract TCC.

Limitations in cytologic evaluations led to the development of brush biopsies in the evaluation of upper tract TCC.[86,87] Gill et al.[80] described the technique of *brush biopsy* in the upper tracts through open-ended catheters using fluoroscopy and contrast to localize the tumor. They reported the correct diagnosis of upper tract TCC, renal cell carcinoma,

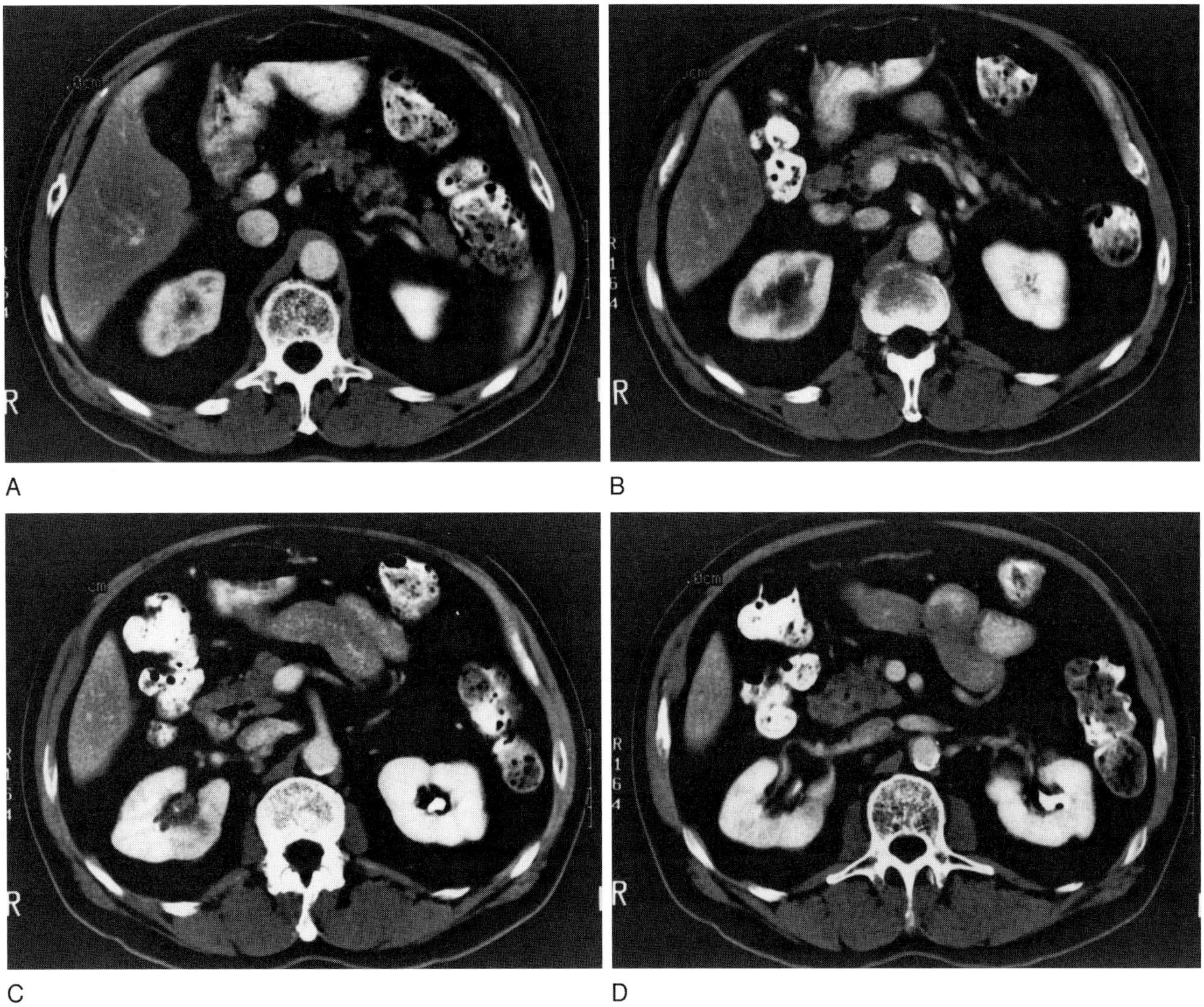
A
B
C
D

FIGURE 14–6. Computed tomography scan demonstrating nonspecific process in right upper pole of the kidney (same patient as in Figs. 14–4 and 14–5).

and multiple myeloma as well as benign conditions including stones, polyps, sloughed papillae, and ureteritis cystica using this technique. Cells and tissue fragments are entrapped in the bristles of the brush, which are then touch prepped onto glass slides for analysis. The diagnostic accuracy of brush biopsies is reported at 80 to 89% with a sensitivity of 90% and a specificity of 88%.[7,70,88] The morbidity of the technique appears to be minimal[80] but may include bacteremia, perforation of renal pelvis or ureter, renal colic from transient ureteral edema, mucosal flap injury, and bleeding. This technique may also be performed under direct vision using flexible or rigid ureteroscopy as well. In 1964, Marshall pioneered the technique of *ureteroscopy* through a ureterotomy. Lyon et al. then reported on the use of a rigid pediatric cystoscope to evaluate the lower 4 to 6 cm of the ureter in female patients. By 1980, a long rigid ureteroscope came in to use

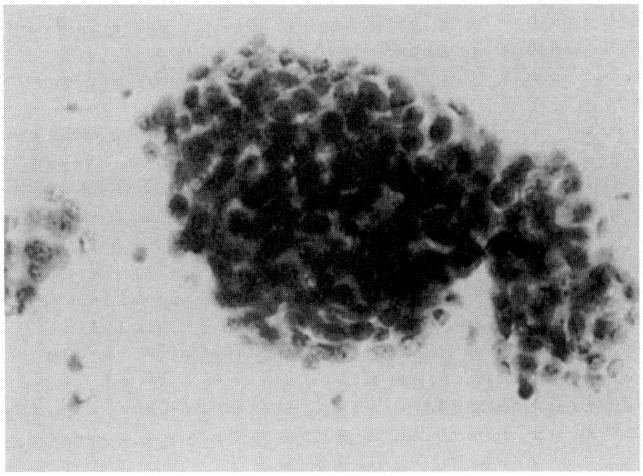

FIGURE 14–7. Urine cytology, low-grade papillary TCC. (Modified from Kleer E, Osterling JE: Transitional cell carcinoma of the upper tracts. Prob Urol 1992; 6[3]:531, with permission.)

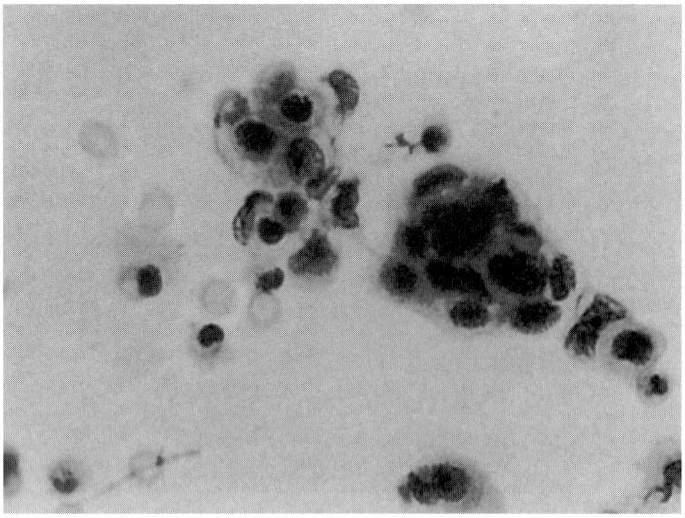

FIGURE 14–8. Urine cytology, high-grade papillary TCC. (Modified from Kleer E, Osterling JE: Transitional cell carcinoma of the upper tracts. Prob Urol 1992; 6[3]:531, with permission.)

for evaluation of the entire upper tract under direct vision.[39,89] The use of ureteroscopy has improved our ability to diagnose upper tract lesions reliably (86% sensitivity in renal pelvis tumors and 90% in ureteral tumors) and should be used in conjunction with radiographic examination when indicated.[70] Both direct vision brush biopsies or cold forceps biopsies may be obtained through the ureteroscope. Since 1980 there have been many refinements made in the instrumentation, making both endoscopic evaluation and treatment of some upper tract tumors possible. However, even with these advancements endoscopic evaluation can be hampered by the inability to pass the scope into the orifice and intramural tunnel despite dilation, the inability to cross over the iliac vessels or ureteropelvic junction, a tortuous ureter, and the inability to maneuver the scope to visualize the lower pole infundibulum. Reported complications of ureteroscopy have included acute pyelonephritis, ureteral stenosis and fibrosis, perforation with extravasation, tumor implantation, perioperative ureteral edema and obstruction, and febrile episodes.[39,89]

TABLE 14–2. ENTITIES TO CONSIDER IN DIFFERENTIAL DIAGNOSIS OF RADIOLUCENT DEFECTS OF THE UPPER TRACTS

Malignant urothelial tumors
- Transitional cell carcinoma
- Renal cell carcinoma
- Squamous cell carcinoma
- Secondary metastasis

Benign polyps
Calculi
- Uric acid or matrix stones

Blood clots
Sloughed papillae
Ureteritis and pyelitis cystica
Extrinsic compression
- Blood vessels
- Tumor in adjacent nodes

Urinary tuberculosis

STAGING, GRADE, AND PROGNOSIS

Staging

Staging systems for renal pelvis and ureteral transitional cell carcinoma have been based on the bladder cancer models because they are both urothelial malignancies. In 1971, Grabstald et al. described a staging system for renal pelvic tumors based on the Jewett-Marshall bladder model. Two different but related staging systems have since emerged and are generally accepted for staging both renal pelvic and ureteral tumors, the tumor-nodal-metastasis (TNM) of the Interrelated Union Against Cancer (UICC), which is most commonly used (Table 14–3), and the American Joint Committee on Cancer (AJCC) staging system (see Fig. 14–9 for a comparison of the staging systems).

TNM is derived from the three components of the staging system. "T" denotes the tumor size and extent, "N" denotes regional lymph node involvement (i.e., renal hilar, abdominal para-aortic, paracaval, iliac nodes), and "M" denotes metastasis to distant sites. Transitional cell carcinoma may spread by direct invasion, vascular or lymphatic invasion, and by mucosal seeding. The most common sites of metastasis in decreasing frequency are lung, bone, and liver.[2] Lymph node involvement at initial clinical staging is about 7%, but the true pathologic incidence is about 18%.[90] Superficial tumors rarely metastasize to nodes; however, T3 and T4 tumors have a 48% and 78% incidence of nodal involvement, respectively, which is consistent with their poorer prognosis.[90]

TABLE 14–3. UICC STAGING SYSTEM FOR TUMORS OF RENAL PELVIS AND URETER

T or pT (primary tumor)	
TX	Primary tumor is occult and cannot be assessed; for example, positive cytology findings in ureteral urine without (or prior to) demonstration of tumor
TO	No evidence of primary tumor
Tis	Carcinoma in situ (flat or nonpapillary carcinoma in situ)
Ta	Noninvasive papillary carcinoma
T1	Carcinoma involves subepithelial connective tissue
T2	Carcinoma invades muscularis
T3	Carcinoma invades beyond muscularis into periureteric or peripelvic fat; carcinomas invading into renal parenchyma are also classified T3 in the UICC system*
T4	Carcinoma invades adjacent organs or extends through kidney into perinephric fat
N or pN (regional lymph nodes)	
NX	Regional lymph nodes cannot be assessed
NO	No regional lymph node metastasis
N1	Metastasis in a single lymph node 2 cm or less in diameter
N2	Metastasis in a single lymph node 2–5 cm in diameter or metastases to multiple lymph nodes, none more than 5 cm in diameter
N3	Metastasis in a lymph node more than 5 cm in diameter
M (distant metastasis)	
MX	Presence of distant metastasis cannot be assessed
MO	No distant metastasis
M1	Distant metastasis

*See Guinan P, Vogelzang NJ, Randazzo R, et al: Renal pelvic transitional cell carcinoma: the role of the kidney in tumor-nodes-metastasis staging. Cancer 1992; 69:1773–1775.

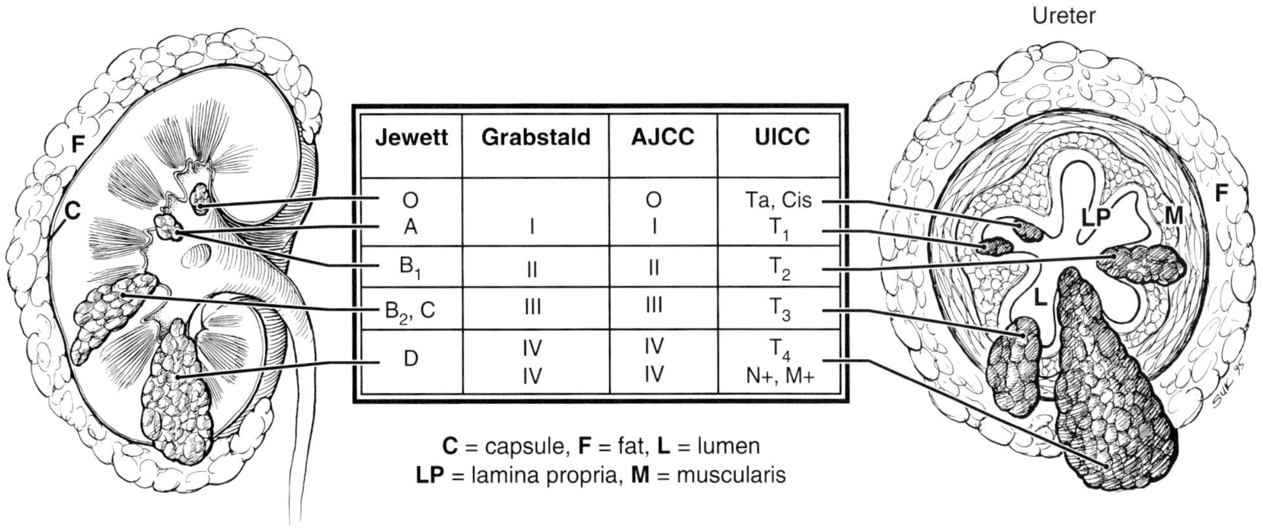
Ureter
F
C
F
LP
M
L
Jewett
Grabstald
AJCC
UICC
O
A
I
O
I
Ta, Cis
T1
B1
II
II
T2
B2, C
III
III
T3
D
IV
IV
IV
IV
T4
N+, M+
C = capsule, F = fat, L = lumen
LP = lamina propria, M = muscularis

FIGURE 14–9. Comparison of staging systems for renal pelvis and ureteral TCC.

Stage O, Ta, Cis	Noninvasive
Stage A, I, T_1	Subepithelial invasion
Stage B_1, II, T_2	Invasion muscularis but not through renal capsule or adventitia of pelvis or ureter.
Stage B_2, C, III, T_3	Invades renal parenchyma, into peripelvic or periureteral fat.
Stage D, IV, T_4, N+, M+	Extends through kidney into perinephric fat, with or without invasion of adjacent organs or lymph nodes.

(Modified from Kleer E, Osterling JE: Transitional cell carcinoma of the upper tracts. Prob Urol 1992; 6[3]:531, with permission.)

Grading

The two most commonly used grading systems were introduced by Ash and Mostofi. In 1940, Ash proposed an adaption of Broders' cytologic grading system for papillary transitional cell carcinoma, dividing tumors into grades 1 through 4 based on the degree of nuclear anaplasia present.[2,39] Grade 1 is equivalent to a papilloma, which is a papillary lesion on a thin fibrovascular core covered by normal appearing mucosa. Grade 2 tumors comprise the majority of tumors and are well differentiated, with a thickened urothelium containing more than seven layers of cells exhibiting only slight pleomorphism or anaplasia. Grade 3 is composed of solid masses of pleomorphic cells on a wider fibrovascular core with hyperchromatic, irregular, disproportionately large nuclei. Grade 4 are highly anaplastic undifferentiated or sarcomatoid appearing cells.[2] Mostofi later modified this system by separating out papillomas, leaving papillary grades 1 through 3 (World Health Organization).

Prognosis

Many investigators feel that although renal pelvis and ureteral cancers are histologically similar, they are anatomically and biologically dissimilar because transmural invasion of the ureteral urothelium is associated with a poorer survival prognosis than the same depth of invasion in the renal pelvis.[5,91,92] The retrospective review by Guinan et al. of renal pelvis and ureteral TCC patients at multiple institutions indicates that the renal parenchyma may serve as an anatomic barrier to the spread of tumor. For example, a T3 tumor (invasion beyond the muscularis into the peripelvic or periureteral fat) of the renal pelvis has a 5-year survival of 54% compared to 24% at the same depth of invasion in the ureter.[10,75,91] Once the tumor invades the perinephric fat, however, survival is virtually equivalent with periureteral fat invasion.[5,9,75,93,94] This correlation with tumor stage and survival was reported as early as 1971 by Whitmore et al.,[95] who showed a progressive decrease in survival of patients with increasing stage (Table 14–4) with the most striking difference again being the involvement of perirenal or periureteral (T3) fat. Although ureteral tumors are often diagnosed earlier (63% versus 45% of renal pelvic tumors) due to associated symptoms when corrected for stage, there is no significant survival difference.[96] Other retrospective reviews have also demonstrated correlations with tumor grade, multifocality of disease, concomitant bladder carcinoma, and ploidy, although tumor stage has the highest correlation.[8–10,16,17,25,39,96–98]

DNA ploidy, although providing no additional prognostic information in high-grade high-stage tumors, may be of benefit in predicting disease-free survival in low-grade low-stage upper tract tumors.[15,99] Al-Abadi and Nagel[15] demonstrated that grade 2 tumors are heterogenous with respect to DNA ploidy even though they have the same histomorphologic degree of differentiation, and therefore can be subclassified as diploid/tetraploid (biologically less aggressive) or aneuploid (biologically aggressive) tumors. Figure 14–10 demonstrates this correlation found between DNA ploidy and histologic staging and grade of renal pelvis and ureteral tumors very well.[15] In addition to this correlation between DNA ploidy and tumor stage and grade, ploidy has also been found to be a significant predictor of survival.[15,39,99] Blute et al. reported 5- and 10-year survivals for diploid tumors to be 79% and 70%, tetraploid tumors 55% and 44%, and aneuploid tumors 25% and 0%, respectively.[100]

Metastatic upper tract transitional cell carcinoma to the soft tissue, lymph nodes, viscera, or bone carries an extremely poor prognosis, with the majority not surviving 3 years, and a 5-year survival of 0% despite adjuvant treatment.[39,96]

MANAGEMENT

The type of surgical management a patient receives can affect the likelihood of recurrences, progression of disease, and survival, so it is important that they receive appropriate management early on. Stage, grade, multifocality, and location of tumor must all be taken into consideration when deciding on treatment options. Overall medical condition, renal function, and whether they have a solitary kidney or not also have an impact on the decision. Figures 14–11 and 14–12 provide a proposed algorithm for the management of renal pelvis and ureteral TCC.

Understaging of ureteral and renal pelvic tumors is estimated to occur 35% of the time primarily because of the fear of perforation in endoscopic biopsies or resection and the inherent inadequacies of radiologic evaluation (CT 43% specificity, 67 to 77% sensitivity).[101,102] Retrospective analysis of conservative surgical approaches led to the current standards in treatment and provided some indication of the natural history of the disease.

Open Radical Versus Conservative Surgery

The first nephroureterectomy was performed in 1895 by Dr. Howard Kelly. At that time it was regarded as a "formidable procedure," and simple nephrectomy remained the standard treatment until 1929. The risk of ipsilateral ureteral recurrences after simple nephrectomy were reported in 30 to 84%,[10,14,103,104] and subsequent bladder tumors were noted to occur most frequently around the ipsilateral ureteral orifice.[105] Nephroureterectomy with a cuff of bladder was again advocated as the treat-

TABLE 14–4. STAGE VERSUS SURVIVAL (MONTHS) FOR RENAL PELVIC TUMORS*

Diagnosis	Stage	No. of Patients	Dead of Tumor	Without Tumor	
				Alive	Dead†
Papilloma	Noninvasive	7‡	—	5 (40–220)	1 (304)
Papillary carcinoma	O (noninvasive) A (superficial invasion)	9‡	—	4 (36–186)	4 (13–104)
Papillary carcinoma	B (deep invasion into but not through kidney or membranous pelvis)	2	—	2 (33–48)	
Papillary carcinoma	C (invasion of perirenal or peripelvic tissue)	15	13 (1–22)	1 (11)	1 (25)

*Adapted from Grabstald H, Whitmore WF Jr, Melamed MR: Renal pelvic tumors. JAMA 1971; 218:845–854. Copyright 1971, American Medical Association, with permission.

†All deaths from causes other than tumor.

‡One tumor was an incidental finding at autopsy.

ment of choice for renal pelvic and ureteral tumors,[5,14,74,102,106] and currently remains the standard of therapy because of the multifocal nature of the disease, the high risk of ipsilateral recurrence when conservative operations are performed, and the low incidence of contralateral involvement.[5,9,10,14,17] It wasn't until 1945 that investigators again began to question the need for radical surgery in all cases, and with recent advances in endoscopic abilities it remains a point of discussion today.[2,102,107] The same argument is used for justification of radical surgery and conservative surgery—that is, the tendency of the tumors to recur.

There have been several studies demonstrating a strong correlation between tumor recurrence and the stage and grade of the original tumor.[10,92,108,109] For low-grade low-stage tumors there are no statistical differences in survival between patients treated with local therapies such as distal or segmental ureterectomy, endoscopic resection, fulguration, or laser. Relapse rates range from 22 to 65% for renal pelvis tumors[10,110] and 8 to 17% for distal

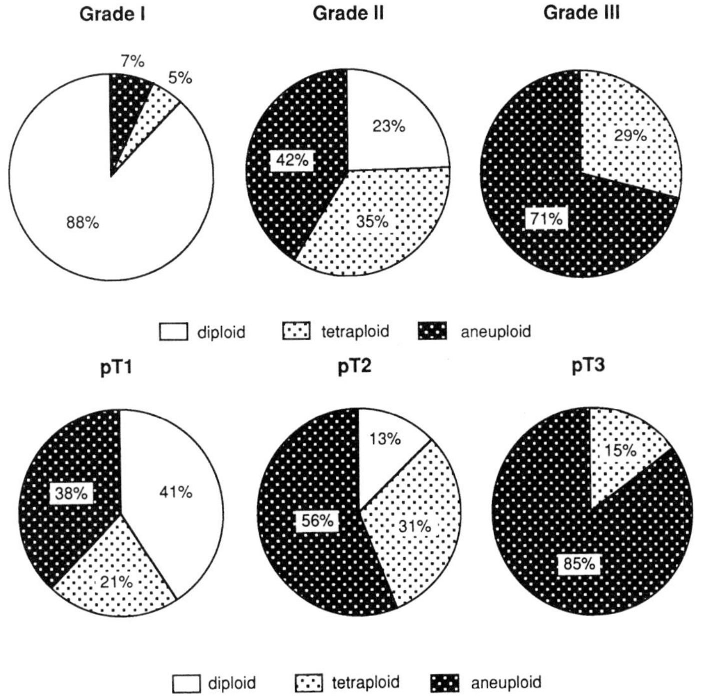

Grade I
Grade II
Grade III
7%
5%
88%
23%
42%
35%
29%
71%
diploid
tetraploid
aneuploid
pT1
pT2
pT3
38%
41%
21%
13%
56%
31%
15%
85%
diploid
tetraploid
aneuploid

FIGURE 14–10. Demonstrates the correlations seen between DNA ploidy and tumor grade and histologic staging in TCC. (From Al-Abadi H, Nagel R: Transitional cell carcinoma of the renal pelvis and ureter: prognostic relevance of nuclear deoxyribonucleic acid ploidy studied by slide cytometry: an 8-year survival time study. J Urol 1992; 148:31, with permission.)

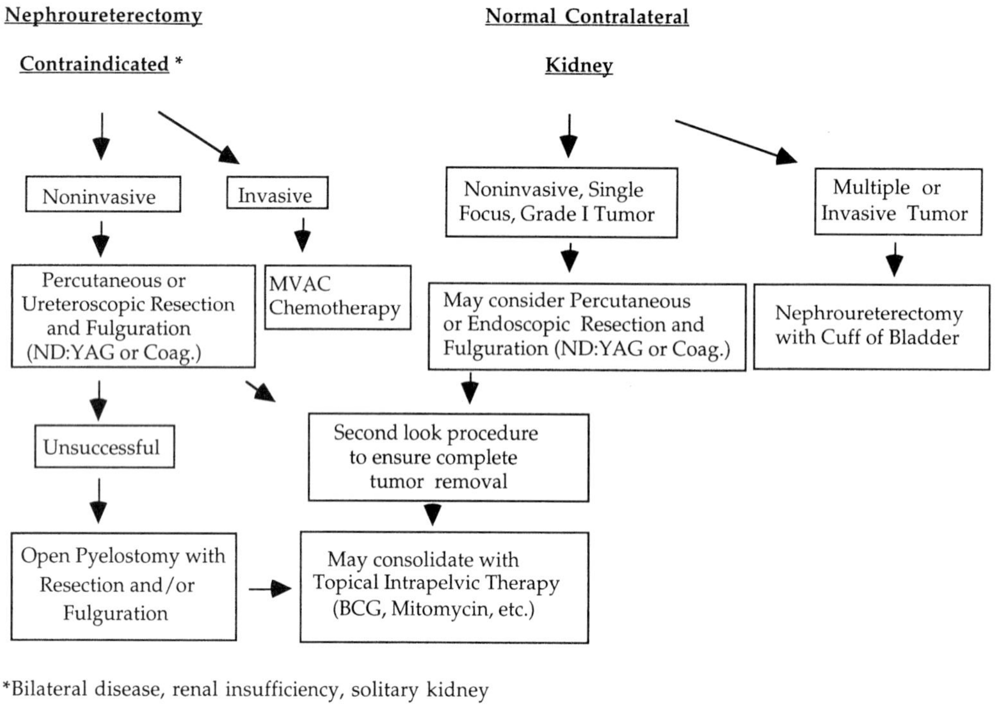
Nephroureterectomy Contraindicated *
Normal Contralateral Kidney
Noninvasive
Invasive
Noninvasive, Single Focus, Grade I Tumor
Multiple or Invasive Tumor
Percutaneous or Ureteroscopic Resection and Fulguration (ND:YAG or Coag.)
MVAC Chemotherapy
May consider Percutaneous or Endoscopic Resection and Fulguration (ND:YAG or Coag.)
Nephroureterectomy with Cuff of Bladder
Unsuccessful
Second look procedure to ensure complete tumor removal
Open Pyelostomy with Resection and/or Fulguration
May consolidate with Topical Intrapelvic Therapy (BCG, Mitomycin, etc.)
*Bilateral disease, renal insufficiency, solitary kidney

FIGURE 14–11. Algorithm for management of renal pelvis TCC.

ureteral tumors.[10,106] The efficacy of segmental or distal ureterectomy for tumors of the lower ureter has been well established[8,10,14,98,102,106]; however, this cannot be translated to the upper ureter or renal pelvis.[9,10,39] The incidence of tumor in the ureteral remnant appears proportional to the length of the remaining stump.[64,111,112] There have been several studies comparing the outcome of patients treated conservatively to those undergoing the standard nephroureterectomy. Zincke et al.[92] proposed that both tumor grade and location (renal pelvis versus ureter) were important variables in determining patient outcome with conservative treatment. In his series, 52% of low-grade renal pelvis tumors recurred versus 100% of high-grade tumors, and ureteral recurrence rates were 15% overall compared to 62% in the renal pelvis. Furthermore, no ureteral cancer treated conservatively had a systemic recurrence, whereas 19% of renal pelvic tumors treated conservatively did. Zincke attributed this difference to the higher incidence of atypical adjacent urothelium and the greater difficulty in excising all the tumor in the renal pelvis. As suspected, radical surgery resulted in higher tumor-

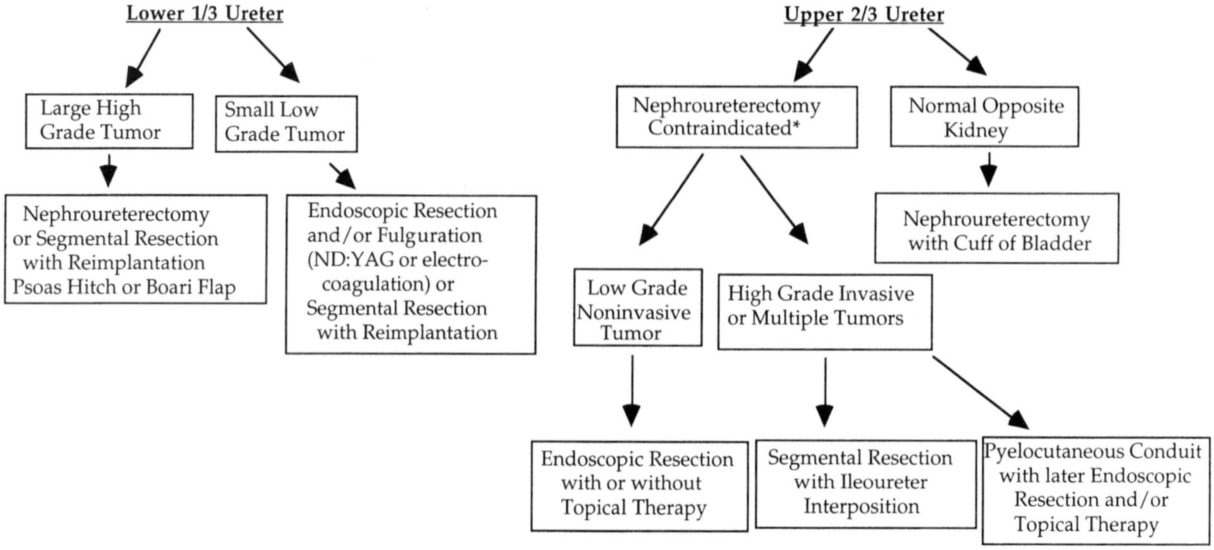
Lower 1/3 Ureter
Upper 2/3 Ureter
Large High Grade Tumor
Small Low Grade Tumor
Nephroureterectomy Contraindicated*
Normal Opposite Kidney
Nephroureterectomy or Segmental Resection with Reimplantation Psoas Hitch or Boari Flap
Endoscopic Resection and/or Fulguration (ND:YAG or electro-coagulation) or Segmental Resection with Reimplantation
Nephroureterectomy with Cuff of Bladder
Low Grade Noninvasive Tumor
High Grade Invasive or Multiple Tumors
Endoscopic Resection with or without Topical Therapy
Segmental Resection with Ileoureter Interposition
Pyelocutaneous Conduit with later Endoscopic Resection and/or Topical Therapy

FIGURE 14–12. Algorithm for management of ureteral pelvis TCC.

specific survival rates in patients with high-stage tumors than conservative treatment did (90% versus 46% 2-year survival in stage 3 and 50% versus 25% in stage 4), supporting the argument that radical surgery is more effective for higher stage, higher grade tumors.[9] Therefore, distal ureterectomy with reimplantation should be considered only in patients with papillary tumors confined to the lower one third of the ureter.[98] Where doubt exists, nephroureterectomy is the preferred approach. The development of subsequent bladder carcinoma has been reported in 30 to 64% of patients following upper tract tumors; therefore, both preoperative and follow-up cystoscopies should be performed on a routine basis.[5,16,92,96,102,111] Recurrences in the upper tract following conservative management have been noted to be of a higher grade and stage than the original tumor in 25 to 66%.[10,14] Charbit et al.'s review of 108 patients with upper tract TCC supported Zincke's findings and in addition demonstrated the multifocal nature of the disease, the inability to define all tumors preoperatively, and the higher ipsilateral recurrence rates in patients with higher grade and stage disease.[14] These findings, in addition to few studies offering 10-year follow-up with conservative treatment of upper tract tumors, make it difficult to extend the current criteria for conservative management.

Conservative Endoscopic Management

Endoscopic conservative management is currently reserved for patients with a solitary kidney, bilateral disease, renal insufficiency, preoperative evidence of a single low-grade tumor, or poor surgical candidates.[16,23,94,109,113] Treatment from the endoscopic approach may consist of resection, diathermy, or laser.[40] Risks of endoscopic procedures in the upper tract include perforation with extravasation into the retroperitoneum, pyelovenous or pyelolymphatic backflow, intrapelvic explosions with diathermy, bleeding requiring transfusion, embolization or nephrectomy, and seeding of percutaneous tract or areas of perforation.[39,94,107,114] When feasible, a transureteral approach is preferred over the percutaneous approach to lessen the chances of tumor seeding, although there have been few documented cases of tract seeding.[39,107] Others contend that tumor seeding may also occur in areas where mucosal injury has been caused by instrumentation and advocate that ureteroscopy not be performed in patients with a recognized bladder tumor.[89] An advantage of the percutaneous approach to renal pelvis tumors is the easy access to calyceal tumors and the ability to use a wide variety of instruments through the large port not available through the ureteroscopic approach.[94,115] Woodhouse et al.[116] have reported local irradiation of the percutaneous tract via iridium-192 (^{192}Ir) wire left in place for a few days postoperatively to avoid the detrimental effects of radiation nephropathy seen with external beam therapy. Other methods advocated to decrease the risk of tract seeding include the use of sterile H_2O as irrigating fluid because of its cytolytic effect, maintaining the intrapelvic pressure between 15 and 40 cm H_2O, and the development of the nephrostomy tract and resection of tumor in one stage.[102,117] Still others would argue that the larger experience with transurethral management of bladder tumors indicates that the risk of local tumor implantation even with wall perforation is of no clinical significance and may be related to grade and stage.[94] As with TCC of the bladder, high-grade upper tract tumors are associated with positive urine cytologies.[16,23] A positive urine cytology in a patient with upper tract disease would therefore be a contraindication to conservative management if the patient was capable of undergoing more radical surgery.

Table 14–5 shows some of the published series of endoscopically managed upper tract tumors and recurrences.[39] Smith et al. recently reported their 9-year follow-up of 34 patients with upper tract TCC managed endoscopically.[107] When tumors were small and easily accessed, a retrograde ureteroscopic approach was utilized; otherwise, a percutaneous approach was used. Second-look procedures were used to ensure complete removal of tumors. Likelihood of recurrences could be predicted in patients with multifocal high-grade or invasive tumors, mucosal abnormalities on random biopsy, positive preoperative cytologies, or history of TCC in other segments of the urothelium. As previously reported, tumor grade was the strongest predictor of tumor recurrence and cancer-related deaths.[39,94] Patients with higher grade tumor suffered more serious bleeding complications related to the need for more aggressive resection. In fact, patients with grade 3 tumors tended to suffer from tumor understaging and higher complication rates, and their procedures tended to be noncurative, with most requiring a nephroureterectomy at some point. This resulted in the conclusion that percutaneous management of upper tract tumors is of no benefit in patients with grade 3 tumors, but may be of benefit in patients with grade 1 disease provided they are willing to comply with rigorous follow-up and in grade 2 patients who are at definite risk from a major open operation or renal failure requiring dialysis. Several investigators have explored the use of topical therapies following percutaneous or ureteroscopic removal of tumors.[107,118–122] Methods of delivery have included percutaneously, through a retrograde external ureteral catheter, and via reflux around a double J stent. Responses have been variable and patient numbers too small to come to any conclusion as to its benefit, but durable responses up to 31 months[122] have been reported with both mitomycin and BCG instillations.

TABLE 14–5. SUMMARY OF SELECTED CASES FOR ENDOUROLOGIC MANAGEMENT OF UPPER URINARY TRACT TCC*

Series	Year	No. of Patients	Tumor Location	Tumor Grade	0% Recurrences†	Dead of Disease	Mean Follow-up (Months)	Nd:YAG Laser	Topical Agent Instilled	Tract Seeding	Complications	Required‡ Nephrectomy
Huffman et al.[58]	1985	8	Ureter	I (7) II (0) III (1)	50	0	21	No	Mitomycin (1)	—	Stricture (1)	0
Smith et al.[29]	1987	9	Renal pelvis	I (3) II (4) III (2)	44	2	9.5	Yes (6)	Mitomycin (1) BCG (5)	0	Bleeding (1) Stricture (1) Fever (1)	2
Schmeller et al.[80]	1989	20	Ureter	I (6) II (10) III (4)	19	0	13.8	Yes (16)	—	—	Stricture (4)	1
Blute et al.[27]	1989	13 8	Ureter Renal pelvis	I (7) II (11) III (3)	15 20	0 0	20.5 24.5	Yes (11) Yes (3)	—	0	Perforation (3) Fever (2)	2
Nurse[28]	1989	13	Renal pelvis	I (9) II (4) III (0)	38	2	23.5	—	Mitomycin (2) Thiotepa (1)	0	Bleeding (3) DVT (1) Perforation (4) Urinary fistula (1) Death (1)	1
Tasca et al.[103]	1990	4	Renal pelvis	I (2) II (2) III (0)	0	0	16.5	No	—	—	0	0
Schoenberg et al.[102]	1991	9 1	Renal pelvis Ureter	I (1) II (7) III (1)	56	1§	24	Yes	Mitomycin (2) BCG (9)	—	Bleeding Fever (1)	0
Grossman et al.[26]	1992	7 1	Ureter Renal pelvis	I (4) II (3) III (1)	63	0	12.5	Yes	—	—	—	1
Smith et al.[101]	1995	36	Renal pelvis	I (11) II (12) III (13)	33	6	56.4	Yes	BCG (19)	0	Bleeding 6‖ (18) Renal failure (2) Hemothorax (2) Abscess (1) Stricture (2)	11

*Modified from Kleer E, Oesterling JE: Transitional cell carcinoma of the upper tracts. Prob Urol 1992; 6(3):531–551, with permission.
†Majority of recurrences occurred in patients with high grade (II–III) tumors.
‡Required nephroureterectomy either in perioperative period due to complications or advanced disease (24 hours to 12 months).
§One dead of disease and one alive with metastatic disease.
‖Required transfusion, embolization, or nephrectomy to stop.
TCC, transitional cell carcinoma; Nd:YAG, neodymium:yttrium-aluminum-garnet; BCG, bacille Calmette-Guérin; DUT, deep venous thrombosis.

Adjuvant Therapy

Once the tumor has infiltrated into the renal parenchyma or extrarenal soft tissue, there is a marked deterioration in survival regardless of the procedure performed.[5,8,16,25] This is demonstrated by the high local recurrence rates seen with surgery alone. *Adjuvant radiation therapy* can markedly reduce this risk but does not address distant disease that occurs in at least 50% of patients.[16,92,123] Cozad et al.[123] recommend adjuvant radiation in patients with high-grade or -stage disease, close surgical margins, or microscopic residual disease with fields encompassing the tumor bed and regional nodes with a dose of 45 Gy followed by a boost to the primary site to 50 Gy. This is unchanged from the recommendations of 6000 rads by Batata et al. in 1975. Bergman and Hotchkiss,[124] on the other hand, recommend radiation therapy only for symptomatic metastatic disease.

Cisplatin-based combination chemotherapy has been found to be effective against metastatic transitional cell carcinoma of the urinary tract,[125,126] and its role in the adjuvant or neoadjuvant settings is still being defined. Freiha et al.[90] report a 50% (four of eight patients) durable response of 3 to 6 years using a CMV (cisplatin, methotrexate, vinblastine) regimen in the neoadjuvant setting for advanced or metastatic transitional cell carcinoma of the upper tract. The remaining four patients died of disease, with two progressing on treatment and two recurring at 6 and 8 months. There are currently no large institutional experiences because of the rarity of the condition.

SUMMARY

Transitional cell carcinoma of the renal pelvis and ureter is a relatively rare tumor, accounting for only 7% of all primary tumors of the kidney; therefore, most management decisions have been made on retrospective reviews of patient outcomes. Arguments for conservative management are the same as for radical surgery (i.e., the tendency for tumors to recur). It has been well established that for low-grade low-stage tumors, conservative surgical resection in the distal ureter by segmental or distal ureterectomy with reimplantation or endoscopic resection offers the same survival rates as radical nephroureterectomy. New advances in endoscopic and percutaneous abilities and equipment have expanded the possibilities of conservative treatment to the renal pelvis as well. High-grade high-stage tumors are still best managed by radical nephroureterectomy with a cuff of bladder. Endoscopic or percutaneous management in this group is not recommended and is reserved only for those unable medically to undergo more radical surgery (e.g., in those with renal insufficiency or solitary kidneys). With multiple recurrences and failed conservative therapy and the inherent difficulty in accurate staging of upper tract tumors, some patients should be considered for complete nephroureterectomy (with or without cystectomy) and dialysis. Failure to do so risks metastatic disease and outweighs the risk of death from dialysis. The value of regional lymphadenectomy has not been well established but is useful for staging purposes and determining the need for adjuvant therapies. Radiation therapy appears to provide some improvement in local control in patients but does not alter the risk of distant metastasis. Neoadjuvant or adjuvant cisplatin-based combination chemotherapy has shown some promise in the treatment of advanced and metastatic transitional cell carcinoma of the bladder, but because of the rarity of transitional cell carcinoma of the upper tract its effectiveness in this setting is yet to be defined. Patients at higher risk for the development of upper tract disease include diffuse carcinoma in situ in the bladder or prostatic urethra, and long-term BCG patients. Such patients should have their upper tracts imaged at least annually. All patients with upper tract disease require preoperative cystoscopy (to rule out concomitant bladder cancer) and follow-up cystoscopies to detect subsequent bladder tumors.

REFERENCES

1. Rayer PFO: Traites des maladies du reins, Vol 3, p 699. Paris, JB Baillier, 1841.
2. Melamed MR, Reuter VE: Pathology and staging of urothelial tumors of the kidney and ureter. Urol Clin North Am 1993; 20(2):333.
3. Boring CC, Squire TS, Montgomery S, et al: Cancer statistics, 1994. CA Cancer J Clin 1994; 44:7.
4. McLaughlin JK, Silverman DT, Fraumeni JF, et al: Cigarette smoking and cancers of the renal pelvis and ureter. Cancer Res 1992; 52:254.
5. Rubenstein MA, Walz BJ, Bucy JG: Transitional cell carcinoma of the kidney: 25-year experience. J Urol 1978; 119:594.
6. Bennington JL, Beckwith JB: Tumors of the kidney, renal pelvis, and ureter. *In* Atlas of Tumor Pathology, Second Series, Fasicle 12. Washington, DC, Armed Forces Institute of Pathology, 1975.
7. Vicente J, Pilar L, Sole-Balcells FJ, et al: Transitional cell carcinoma in the upper urinary tract: diagnosis and management. Urol Int 1995; 2(1):7.
8. Mufti GR, Gove JR, Blandy JP, et al: Transitional cell carcinoma of the renal pelvis and ureter. Br J Urol 1989; 63: 135.
9. Booth CM, Cameron KM, Pugh RCB: Urothelial carcinoma of the kidney and ureter. Br J Urol 1980; 52:430.
10. Mazeman E: Tumours of the upper urinary tract calyces, renal pelvis and ureter. Eur Urol 1976; 2:120.
11. Yanase M, Tsukamoto T, Kondo N, et al: Transitional cell carcinoma of the bladder or renal pelvis in children. Eur Urol 1991; 19:312.
12. Petkovic SD: Conservation of the kidney in operations for tumors of the renal pelvis and calyces. Br J Urol 1972; 44:1.
13. Murphy DM, Zinke H, Furlow WL: Management of high grade transitional cell cancer of the upper tract. J Urol 1980; 125:25.
14. Charbit L, Gendreau MC, Cukier J, et al: Tumors of the

upper urinary tract: 10 years of experience. J Urol 1991; 146:1243.
15. Al-Abadi H, Nagel R: Transitional cell carcinoma of the renal pelvis and ureter: prognostic relevance of nuclear deoxyribonucleic acid ploidy studied by slide cytometry: an 8-year survival time study. J Urol 1992; 148:31.
16. Huben RP, Mounzer AM, Murphy GP: Tumor grade and prognostic variables in upper tract urothelial tumors. Cancer 1988; 62:2016.
17. Krogh J, Kvist E, Rye B: Transitional cell carcinoma of the upper urinary tract: prognostic variables and post-operative recurrences. Br J Urol 1991; 67:32.
18. Zincke H, Garbeff PJ, Beahrs RJ: Upper urinary tract transitional cell cancer after radical cystectomy for bladder cancer. J Urol 1984; 131:50.
19. Schellhammer PF, Whitmore WF: Transitional cell carcinoma of the urethra in men having cystectomy for bladder cancer. J Urol 1976; 115:56.
20. Schwartz CB, Bekirov H, Melman A: Urothelial tumors of upper tract following treatment of primary bladder transitional cell carcinoma. Urology 1992; 40(6):509.
21. Shinka T, Uekado Y, Ohkawa T, et al: Occurrence of uroepithelial tumors of the upper urinary tract after initial diagnosis of bladder cancer. J Urol 1988; 140:745.
22. Seaman EK, Slawin KM, Benson MC: Treatment options for upper tract transitional cell carcinoma. Urol Clin North Am 1993; 20(2):349.
23. Reitelman C, Sawczuk IS, Benson MC: Prognostic variables in patients with transitional cell carcinoma of the renal pelvis and proximal ureter. J Urol 1987; 138:1144.
24. Holmang S, Hedelin H, Johansson SL, et al: The relationship among multiple recurrences, progression and prognosis of patients with stages ta and t1 transitional cell cancer of the bladder followed for at least 20 years. J Urol 1995; 153:1823.
25. Williams CB, Mitchell JP: Carcinoma of the renal pelvis: a review of 43 cases. Br J Urol 1973; 45:370.
26. Oldbrig J, Glifberg I, Pawel M, et al: Carcinoma of the renal pelvis and ureter following bladder carcinoma: frequency, risk factors and clinicopathological findings. J Urol 1989; 141:1311.
27. Malkowicz SB, Skinner DG: Development of upper tract carcinoma after cystectomy for bladder cancer. Urology 1990; 36:20.
28. Hastie KJ, Hamdy FC, Collins MC, et al: Upper tract tumors following cystectomy for bladder cancer: is routine intravenous urography worthwhile? Br J Urol 1991; 67:29.
29. Mufti GR, Gove JR, Riddle PR: Nephroureterectomy after radical cystectomy. J Urol 1988; 139:588.
30. Hudson M, Herr HW: Carcinoma in situ of the bladder (review article). J Urol 1995; 153:564.
31. Herr HW, Wartinger DD, Oettgen HF: Bacillus Calmette-Guérin therapy for the superficial bladder cancer: a 10 year followup. J Urol 1992; 147:1020.
32. Sharma TC, Melamed MR, Whitmore WF: Carcinoma in-situ of the ureter in patients with bladder carcinoma treated by cystectomy. Cancer 1970; 26(3):583.
33. Wallace D: Cancer of the bladder. AJR 1968; 102(3):581.
34. Culp OS, Utz DC, Harrison EG: Experience with ureteral carcinoma in-situ detected during operations for vesical problems. J Urol 1967; 97:679.
35. Akaza H, Koiso K, Niijima T: Clinical evaluation of urothelial tumors of the renal pelvis and ureter based on a new classification system. Cancer 1987; 59:1369.
36. Case RAM: Tumors of urinary tract as an occupational disease in several industries. Ann R Coll Surg 1966; 39: 213.
37. Lieben J: An epidemiological study of occupational bladder cancer. Acta Unio Int Contracancrum 1963; 19:749.
38. Davies JM: Bladder tumours in electric-cable industry. Lancet 1965; 2:143.
39. Kleer E, Oesterling JE: Transitional cell carcinoma of the upper tracts. Prob Urol 1992; 6(3):531.
40. Ross RK, Paganini-Hil A, Henderson BE: Analgesics, cigarette smoking, and other risk factors for cancer of the renal pelvis and ureter. Cancer Res 1989; 49:1045.
41. McCredie M, Stewart JH, Day NE: Different roles for phenacetin and paracetamol in cancer of the kidney and renal pelvis. Int J Cancer 1993; 53:245.
42. McCredie M, Ford JM, Stewart JH, et al: Analgesics and cancer of the renal pelvis in New South Wales. Cancer 1982; 49:2617.
43. Levine E: Transitional cell carcinoma of the renal pelvis associated with cyclophosphamide therapy. AJR 1992; 159:1027.
44. Bengtsson U, Johansson S, Angervall L: Malignancies of the urinary tract and their relation to analgesic abuse. Kidney Int 1978; 13:107.
45. Mahony JF, Storey BG, Stewart JH, et al: Analgesic abuse, renal parenchymal disease and carcinoma of the kidney or ureter. Aust N Z J Med 1977; 7:463.
46. Petkovic SD: Epidemiology and treatment of renal pelvic and ureteral tumor. J Urol 1975; 114:858.
47. Hartge P, Silverman D, West D, et al: Changing cigarette habits and bladder cancer risk; a case-control study. J Natl Cancer Inst 1987; 78:1119.
48. McLaughlin JK, Blot WJ, Fraumeni JF: Etiology of cancer of the renal pelvis. J Natl Cancer Inst 1983; 71:287.
49. Schmauz R, Cole P: Epidemiology of cancer of the renal pelvis and ureter. J Natl Cancer Inst 1974; 52:1431.
50. Armstrong B, Garrod A, Doll R: A retrospective study of renal cancer with special reference to coffee and animal protein consumption. Br J Cancer 1976; 33:127.
51. Jensen OM, Knudsen JB, Sorensen BL, et al: The Copenhagen case-control study of renal pelvis and ureter cancer: role of smoking and occupational exposures. Int J Cancer 1988; 41:557.
52. McCredie M, Stewart JH, Ford JM: Analgesics and tobacco as risk factors for cancer of the ureter and renal pelvis. J Urol 1983; 130:28.
53. McCredie M, Stewart JH, MacLennan RA: Phenacetin-containing analgesics and cancers of the bladder and renal pelvis in women. Br J Urol 1983; 55:220.
54. Spruck CH, Rideout WM, Jones PA, et al: Distinct pattern of p53 mutations in bladder cancer: relationship to tobacco. Cancer Res 1993; 53:1162.
55. Verhaak RLOM, Harmsen AE, Van Urink AJM: On the frequency of tumor induction in a thorotrast kidney. Cancer 1974; 34:2061.
56. Tsai YC, Nichols PW, Skinner DG, et al: Allelic losses of chromosomes 9, 11, and 17 in human bladder cancer. Cancer Res 1990; 50:44.
57. Presti JC, Reuter VE, Cordon-Cardo C, et al: Molecular genetic alterations in superficial and locally advanced human bladder cancer. Cancer Res 1991; 51:5405.
58. Ishikawa J, Xu H, Hu S, et al: Inactivation of the retinoblastoma gene in human bladder and renal cell carcinomas. Cancer Res 1991; 51:5736.
59. Oka K, Ishikawa J, Saya H, et al: Detection of loss of heterozygosity in the p53 gene in renal cell carcinoma and bladder cancer using the polymerase chain reaction. Mol Carcinogen 1991; 4:10.
60. Orphali SLJ, Shols GW, Palmer JM: Familial transitional cell carcinoma of renal pelvis and upper ureter. Urology 1986; 27:394.
61. Frischer Z, Waltzer WC, Gonder MJ: Bilateral transitional cell carcinoma of the renal pelvis in the cancer family syndrome. J Urol 1985; 134:1197.
62. McCarron JP, Chasko SB, Gray GF: Systemic mapping of nephroureterectomy specimens removed for urothelial cancer: pathological findings and clinical correlations. J Urol 1982; 128:243.
63. Heney NM, Nocks BN, Parkhurst EC, et al: Prognostic factors in carcinoma of the ureter. J Urol 1981; 125:632.
64. Herr HW, Whitmore WF: Ureteral carcinoma in situ after successful intravesical therapy for superficial bladder tumors: incidence, pathogenesis and management. J Urol 1987; 138:292.

65. Housemann D: Veber asymetrische zelltheilung in epithel krebsan und deren biologische bedeutung. Virchows Arch Pathol Anat 1890; 119:299.
66. Holtz F: Papillomas and primary carcinoma of the ureter: report of 20 cases. J Urol 1962; 88:380.
67. Lunec J, Challen C, Neal DE, et al: c-erbB-2 amplification and identical p53 mutations in concomitant transitional carcinomas of the renal pelvis and urinary bladder. Lancet 1992; 339:439.
68. Raabe NK, Fossa SD, Bjerkehagen B: Carcinoma of the renal pelvis. Scand J Urol Nephrol 1992; 26:357.
69. Studer UE, Casanova G, Zingg EJ, et al: Percutaneous bacillus Calmette-Guérin perfusion of the upper urinary tract for carcinoma in-situ. J Urol 1989; 142:975.
70. Blute ML, Segura JW, Zincke H, et al: Impact of endourology on diagnosis and management of upper urinary tract urothelial cancer. J Urol 1989; 141:1298.
71. Sidransky D, Frost P, von Eschenbach A, et al: Clonal origin of bladder cancer. N Engl J Med 1992; 326:737.
72. Amar AD, Das S: Upper urinary tract transitional cell carcinoma in patients with bladder carcinoma and associated vesicoureteral reflux. J Urol 1985; 133:468.
73. DeTorres-Mateos JA, Banus Gassol JM, Morote Robles J, et al: Vesicorenal reflux and upper urinary tract transitional cell carcinoma after transurethral resection of recurrent superficial bladder carcinoma. J Urol 1987; 138:49.
74. Soloway MS, Masters BS: Urothelial susceptibility to tumor cell implantation. Cancer 1980; 46:1158.
75. Guinan P, Vogelzang NJ, Sylvester J, et al: Renal pelvic cancer: a review of 611 patients treated in Illinois 1975–1985. Urology 1992; 40(5):393.
76. McCoy JG, Honda H, Williams RD, et al: Computerized tomography for detection and staging of localized and pathologically defined upper tract urothelial tumors. J Urol 1991; 146:1500.
77. Badalament RA, Bennett WF, Perez J, et al: Computed tomography of primary transitional cell carcinoma of upper urinary tracts. Urology 1992; 40(1):71.
78. Dinsmore BJ, Pollach HM, Banner MP: Calcified transitional cell carcinoma of the renal pelvis. Radiology 1988; 167:401.
79. Kincaid OW, Davis GD: Renal angiography. *In* Renal Cell Carcinoma, pp 203–205. Chicago, Year Book Medical Publishers, Inc, 1966.
80. Gill WB, Lu C, Bibbo M: Retrograde brush biopsy of the ureter and renal pelvis. Urol Clin North Am 1979; 6(3): 573.
81. Grace DA, Taylor WN, Taylor JN: Carcinoma of the renal pelvis: a 15 year review. J Urol 1967; 98:566.
82. Hawtrey CE: Fifty-two cases of primary ureteral carcinoma: a clinical-pathologic study. J Urol 1971; 105:188.
83. Sarnacki CT, McCormack LJ, Kiser WS, et al: Urinary cytology and the clinical diagnosis of urinary tract malignancy: a clinicopathologic study of 1400 patients. J Urol 1971; 106:761.
84. Wacker WEC: Lactic dehydrogenase and alkaline phosphatase activities in the diagnosis of renal cell cancer. *In* King JS (ed): Renal Neoplasia, p 87. Boston, Little, Brown & Co, 1967.
85. Guinan P, John T, Sandoughi N: Urinary carcinoembryonic-like antigen levels in patients with bladder carcinoma. J Urol 1974; 111:350.
86. Bibbo M, Gill WB, Harris MJ: Retrograde brushing as a diagnostic procedure of ureteral, renal pelvic, and renal calyceal lesions. Acta Cytol 1974; 18:137.
87. Gill WB, Bibbo M, Thomsen S, et al: Evaluation of renal masses: including retrograde renal brushing. Surg Clin North Am 1976; 56:149.
88. Sheline M, Amendola MA, Pollack HM, et al: Fluoroscopically guided retrograde brush biopsy in the diagnosis of transitional cell carcinoma of the upper urinary tract: results in 45 patients. AJR 1989; 153:313.
89. Huffman JL, Bagley DH, Whitmore WF: Endoscopic diagnosis and treatment of upper-tract urothelial tumors. Cancer 1985; 55:1422.
90. Freiha FS: Renal, renal pelvis and ureteral tumors: should retroperitoneal nodes be treated? *In* Meyer JL (ed): The Lymphatic System and Cancer, Vol 28, p 155. Basel, Karger, 1994.
91. Guinan P, Volgelzang NJ, Sener S, et al: Renal pelvic transitional cell carcinoma: the role of the kidney in tumor-node-metastasis staging. Cancer 1992; 69(7):1773.
92. Zincke H, Neves RJ: Feasibility of conservative surgery for transitional cell carcinoma of the upper tract. Urol Clin North Am 1984; 11:717.
93. Huffman JL: Ureteroscopic management of transitional cell carcinoma of the upper urinary tract. Urol Clin North Am 1988; 15:419.
94. Smith AD, Orihuela E, Crowley AB: Percutaneous management of renal pelvic tumors: a treatment option in selected cases. J Urol 1987; 137:852.
95. Grabstald J, Whitmore WF, Melamed MR: Renal pelvic tumors. JAMA 1971; 218:845.
96. Das AK, Culley CC, Paulson DF, et al: Primary carcinoma of the upper urinary tract: effect of primary and secondary therapy on survival. Cancer 1990; 66:1919.
97. Davis BW, Hough AJ, Gardner WA: Renal pelvic carcinoma: morphological correlates of metastatic behaviour. J Urol 1987; 137:857.
98. Johnson DE, Babaian RJ: Conservative surgical management for noninvasive distal ureteral carcinoma. Urology 1979; 13(4):365.
99. Badalament RA, O'Toole RV, Drago JR, et al: Prognostic factors in patients with primary transitional cell carcinoma of the upper urinary tract. J Urol 1990; 144:859.
100. Blute ML, Tsushima K, Lieber MM, et al: Transitional cell carcinoma of the renal pelvis: nuclear deoxyribonucleic acid ploidy studied by flow cytometry. J Urol 1988; 140: 944.
101. Braslis KG, Soloway MS: Management of ureteral and renal pelvic recurrence after cystectomy. Urol Clin North Am 1994; 21(4):653.
102. Gerber GS, Lyon ES: Endourological management of upper tract urothelial tumors. J Urol 1993; 150:2.
103. Colston JAC: Complete nephroureterectomy. J Urol 1935; 33:110.
104. Kimball FN, Ferris HW: Papillomatous tumor of the renal pelvis associated with similar tumors of the ureter and bladder. J Urol 1934; 31:257.
105. Droller MJ: Transitional cell cancer: upper tracts and the bladder. *In* Walsh PC, Gittes RF, Perlmutter AD, et al (eds): Campbell's Urology, 5th edition, p 1343. Philadelphia, WB Saunders Co, 1986.
106. Mazeman E, Biserte J: Renal-sparing treatment of upper-tract urothelial tumors. Curr Opin Urol 1994; 4:168.
107. Jarrett TW, Sweetser PM, Smith AD, et al: Percutaneous management of transitional cell carcinoma of the renal collecting system: 9-year experience. J Urol 1995; 154: 1629.
108. McCarron JP, Mills C, Vaughn ED Jr: Tumors of the renal pelvis and ureter: current concepts and management. Semin Urol 1983; 1:75.
109. Wallace DMA, Wallace DM, Wickham JEA, et al: The late results of conservative surgery for upper tract urothelial carcinomas. Br J Urol 1981; 53:537.
110. Catalona WJ: Urothelial tumors of the urinary tract. *In* Walsh PC, Retik AB, Stamey TA, Vaughan ED Jr (eds): Campbell's Urology, 6th edition, p 1094. Philadelphia, WB Saunders Co, 1992.
111. Kakizoe T, Fujita J, Kishi K, et al: Transitional cell carcinoma of the bladder in patients with renal pelvic and ureteral cancer. J Urol 1980; 124:17.
112. Strong DW, Pearse HD, Hodges CV, et al: The ureteral stump after nephroureterectomy. J Urol 1976; 115:654.
113. Nurse DE, Woodhouse CRJ, Dearnley DP, et al: Percutaneous removal of upper tract tumors. World J Urol 1989; 7:131.
114. Andrews PE, Segura JW: Renal pelvic explosion during conservative management of upper tract urothelial cancer. J Urol 1991; 146:407.

115. Grossman HB, Schwartz SL, Konnak JW: Ureteroscopic treatment of urothelial carcinoma of the ureter and renal pelvis. J Urol 1992; 148:275.
116. Woodhouse CRJ, Kellett MJ, Bloom HJG: Percutaneous renal surgery and local radiotherapy in the management of renal pelvic transitional cell carcinoma. Br J Urol 1986; 58:245.
117. Streem SB, Pontes EJ: Percutaneous management of upper tract transitional cell carcinoma. J Urol 1986; 135:773.
118. Herr HW: Durable response of a carcinoma in situ of the renal pelvis to topical bacillus Calmette-Guérin. J Urol 1985; 134:531.
119. Ramsey JC, Soloway MS: Instillation of bacillus Calmette-Guérin into the renal pelvis of a solitary kidney for the treatment of transitional cell carcinoma. J Urol 1990; 143: 1220.
120. Eastham JA, Huffman JL: Technique of mitomycin C instillation in the treatment of upper tract urothelial tumors. J Urol 1993; 150:324.
121. Huffman JL, Morse MJ, Whitmore WF, et al: Consideration for treatment of upper urinary tract tumors with topical therapy. Urology 1985; 26(4)(Suppl):47.
122. Schoenberg MP, Van Arsdalen KN, Wein AJ: The management of transitional cell carcinoma in solitary renal units. J Urol 1992; 146:700.
123. Cozad SC, Smalley SR, Reymond R, et al: Adjuvant radiotherapy in high stage transitional cell carcinoma of the renal pelvis and ureter. Int J Radiat Oncol Biol Phys 1992; 24:743.
124. Bergman H, Hotchkiss R: Ureteral tumors. *In* Bergman (ed): The Ureter, 2nd edition, p 271. New York, Springer, 1981.
125. Harker W, Meyers F, Torti F, et al: Cisplatin, methotrexate and vinblastine (cmv): an effective chemotherapy regimen for metastatic transitional cell carcinoma of the urinary tract. J Clin Oncol 1985; 3:1463.
126. Sternberg C, Yagoda A, Whitmore WF, et al: Preliminary results of M-VAC (methotrexate, vinblastine, doxorubicin, and cisplatin) for transitional cell carcinoma of the urothelium. J Urol 1985; 133:403.

15

SURGERY FOR UPPER TRACT TRANSITIONAL CELL CARCINOMA

JENNY J. FRANKE, M.D. *and* JOSEPH A. SMITH, JR., M.D.

The primary goal of surgical treatment of transitional cell carcinoma of the upper urinary tract is straightforward: excision of all tumor-bearing tissue with an adequate surgical margin. Additionally, though, the surgical strategy frequently involves removal of urothelium in the ipsilateral kidney and ureter, which is at risk for the development of new tumors because of field change or, perhaps, tumor cell implantation. In some situations, though, especially in the face of a compromised or absent contralateral kidney, preservation of some degree of renal function or ureteral integrity is required. Thus, partial excision of the kidney or ureter may be appropriate. Finally, minimally invasive surgical approaches are being applied increasingly for upper tract transitional cell carcinoma.

This chapter reviews various methods for surgical management of transitional cell carcinoma of the ureter and kidney. Technical aspects of the surgical procedures are discussed. In addition, emphasis is placed upon appropriate patient selection for the various surgical techniques.

TUMOR BIOLOGY AND NATURAL HISTORY INFLUENCING SELECTION OF SURGICAL APPROACH

Transitional cell cancers may arise in the upper urinary tract anywhere from the ureterovesical junction to the renal calyces. As with transitional cell carcinoma of the bladder, prognosis is directly related to grade and stage at the time of diagnosis.[1] High-grade and invasive tumors are associated with a poor prognosis, as the thin wall of the ureter and renal pelvis can lead directly to lymphatic or hematogenous dissemination. Thus, adequate excision of the primary tumor is the most important objective in the surgical treatment of upper tract transitional cell cancer.[2]

The multifocal nature of transitional cell cancer is also a major determinant of the selection of surgical therapy.[3] The "field change" frequently observed with transitional cell cancer implies a risk for new tumor occurrence (Fig. 15–1). Urothelial dysplasia or carcinoma in situ may be observed within the ipsilateral upper collecting system at sites remote from the primary tumor. Moreover, new tumors may be observed in the bladder. In most situations, the risk of upper tract tumor in the contralateral kidney or ureter is only a few per cent, but some patients have a panurothelial tumor diathesis associated with multiple tumors throughout the urinary tract.[4,5]

A phenomenon of tumor cell implantation also seems to be operative to some degree. Downstream recurrence distal to an upper ureteral or renal pelvic tumor is observed more frequently than proximal recurrence. However, especially in the presence of high-grade lesions, proximal recurrence may be observed even if a tumor in the distal ureter is adequately excised.

As with transitional cell cancer of the bladder, recurrent tumors usually have histology similar to previously treated ones (i.e., recurrences tend to be low-grade and low-stage in patients with a prior history of similar tumors). This observation can influence the selection of surgical treatment. A more conservative approach may be selected for low-grade tumors. Also, low-stage, papillary tumors are better suited for endoscopic destruction.

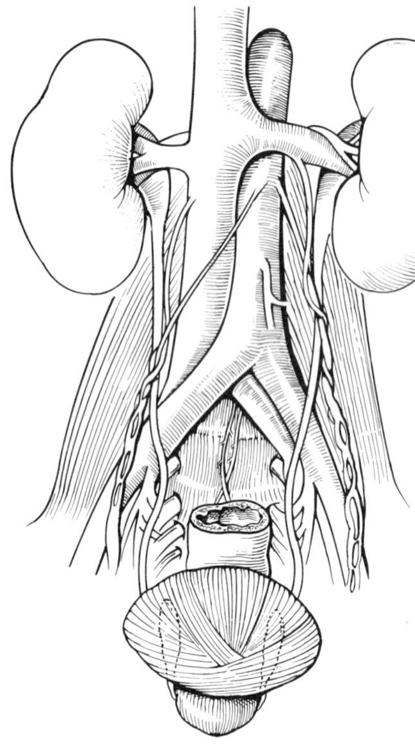

FIGURE 15–1. Anatomy of ureters and kidneys in relation to other retroperitoneal structures. Transitional cell carcinoma may arise at any point within the upper urinary collecting system.

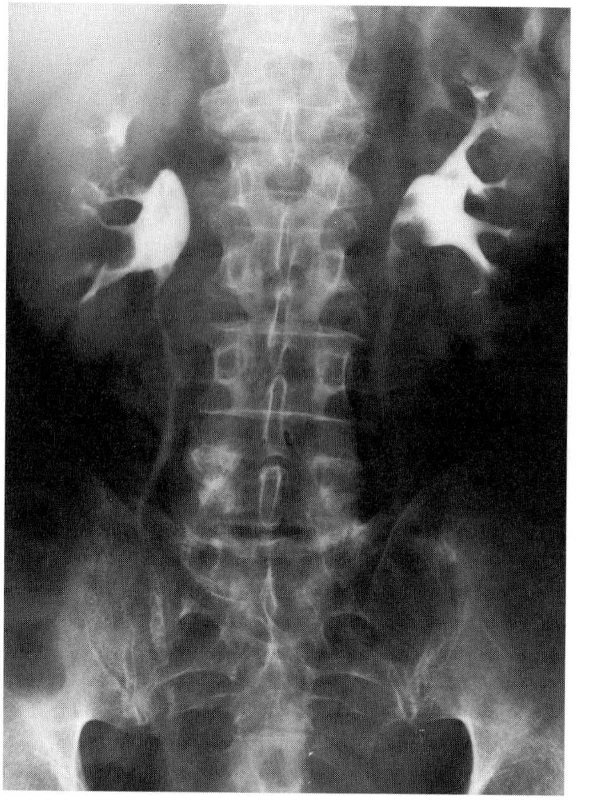

FIGURE 15–2. Multiple filling defects in the ureter and renal pelvis of a patient with multifocal transitional cell carcinoma.

NEPHROURETERECTOMY

Removal of the kidney, the entire ipsilateral ureter, and a cuff of bladder surrounding the ureteral orifice is used commonly for the surgical treatment of transitional cell carcinoma of the upper urinary tract. Nephroureterectomy provides the widest margin of excision of surrounding tissue and removes all ipsilateral urothelium. Nephroureterectomy is the preferred approach for high-grade tumors of any portion of the ureter or intrarenal collecting system in the presence of a normal contralateral kidney. Nephroureterectomy is also appropriate for low-grade tumors in the proximal portions of the ureter or in the intrarenal collecting system when adequate access for endoscopic destruction cannot be obtained (Fig. 15–2).

Hilar lymph nodes may be removed along with the kidney specimen. A separate lymph node dissection usually is not performed. Enlarged or indurated lymph nodes should, however, be sampled for prognostic purposes and to help identify patients who may benefit from adjuvant therapy.

Surgical Technique

Nephroureterectomy may be performed either through a single incision or through two separate ones. The decision is based upon the preference and experience of the surgeon as well as the body habitus of the patient. In either event, en bloc removal of the surgical specimen is usually performed.[6]

Adequate exposure for removal of the kidney and ureter with a single incision can be obtained through a midline abdominal approach or a flank incision with paramedian or midline abdominal extension. When a midline incision is used, the patient is placed in a supine position. The incision generally extends from the pubis to the xyphoid in order to obtain adequate exposure for dissection of the upper pole of the kidney as well as the distal ureter and bladder. Reflection of the peritoneum medially can be accomplished, but the procedure often involves intraperitoneal exposure when performed through a midline approach. The right or left colon is reflected medially. Gerota's fascia is incised and the kidney is sharply dissected from the surrounding perinephric fat. The renal artery is secured first followed by the renal vein. The adrenal gland is left in situ. Dissection around the renal pelvis should encompass as much surrounding fat tissue as possible. The ureter is dissected to the level of the ureterovesical junction. The amount of soft tissue surrounding the ureter that is removed should be as generous as possible. Extra caution is necessary at the point where the ureter crosses the iliac vessels, especially if tumor or inflammation from obstruction has caused the ureter to be adherent to the surrounding tissues.

Classically, the bladder is opened in the midline

in order to perform complete excision of the distal ureter along with a cuff of surrounding bladder mucosa. The extravesical mobilization of the ureter should be as complete as possible in order to facilitate the intravesical dissection. A stent or feeding tube is passed into the ureter and sutured to the bladder mucosa. The contralateral bladder trigone should be visualized in order to avoid compromise of the ureteral orifice during either the dissection or bladder closure. A cuff of bladder mucosa for 1 to 2 cm surrounding the ureteral orifice is circumscribed and removed along with the intramural ureter. An alternative approach for removal of the distal ureter is to perform the entire dissection from an extravesical approach. If this method is used, however, care should be taken to avoid leaving the intramural ureter in situ. In addition, caution is required to avoid entrapping the contralateral ureteral orifice in bladder-closing sutures.

After the surgical specimen has been removed, the defect in the trigone is closed with absorbable suture and the midline cystotomy incision is also closed. Usually, Foley catheter drainage of the bladder postoperatively is sufficient, but a suprapubic catheter may be left indwelling. A closed suction drain is left indwelling in the pelvis for several days.

A complete extraperitoneal approach is used more often when a single incision is performed with paramedian or midline extension of a flank incision. The patient is not placed in a full decubitus position but, usually, at a 45-degree angle in order to obtain adequate access to the abdomen. The incision is made below the twelfth rib and the peritoneum retracted medially. In obese patients, surgical exposure can be somewhat compromised by this approach. Additionally, postoperative laxity of the abdominal muscles is observed frequently.

Nephroureterectomy often is performed through two separate surgical incisions. Usually, a flank incision is accompanied by either a lower abdominal midline or Pfannenstiel incision. Most often, removal of the kidney is performed first. Sometimes, though, the preoperative diagnosis of a transitional cell cancer may not be secure. For example, in the face of distal ureteral obstruction in which the etiology is uncertain despite preoperative diagnostic measures, exploration of the distal ureter is performed first. Palpation of an intrinsic soft tissue mass within the ureter may be considered sufficient for diagnostic purposes depending upon the circumstances. Ureterotomy should be avoided in patients with transitional cell cancers but occasionally is necessary in order to establish the diagnosis.

When the nephrectomy is performed first, the patient is placed in a lateral decubitus position. An incision below the twelfth rib usually provides sufficient access, but rib resection or extension into the intercostal space may be performed for better superior exposure. The kidney is removed as described above and the ureter is dissected as far distally as possible. Usually, the dissection extends to the level of the iliac vessels. Ideally, the surgical specimen is removed en bloc. After the flank incision has been closed, the patient is placed supine and a midline abdominal or Pfannenstiel incision performed. The previously mobilized kidney and upper ureter are brought through the incision and the remaining portion of the distal ureter dissected. Excision of the intramural ureter is performed through either an open cystotomy or an extravesical dissection as described above. En bloc removal of the surgical specimen is performed to avoid spillage of tumor cells through the open urinary tract. If the known primary tumor is located at a site remote from the midportion of the ureter, ligation and division of the ureter is permissible prior to closure of the flank incision, although en bloc removal is preferable.

PARTIAL NEPHRECTOMY

Partial nephrectomy is rarely indicated in the management of transitional cell carcinoma. There is a high risk of tumor recurrence within the remaining ipsilateral intrarenal collecting system. Even in the face of a compromised or absent contralateral kidney, alternative methods of management such as ureteroscopic, percutaneous, or open endoscopic tumor destruction generally are preferable to partial nephrectomy. Occasionally, though, upper or lower pole nephrectomy is used when alternative methods of management fail or are not feasible.[7,8]

Partial nephrectomy may play a role in a patient with a single functioning kidney and a tumor in the upper or lower pole which is too large for endoscopic management. In a relatively young patient, nephrectomy with dialysis and, subsequently, transplantation may be preferred. Despite a high risk for recurrence in the remaining portion of the kidney, though, some patients have prolonged disease-free survival after partial nephrectomy for transitional cell cancer.

Before considering partial nephrectomy, the kidneys should be carefully inspected radiographically and, if possible, endoscopically to make certain that there is no gross tumor in the remaining portion of the kidney. Intraoperative tumor spillage is a concern. Before opening the collecting system, the adjacent retroperitoneal structures should be packed with sponges and a plastic or rubber dam placed around the kidney. This not only shields adjacent tissues from tumor spillage but also facilitates cooling of the kidney with an ice slush.

After renal exposure is obtained through a flank incision, the renal artery and vein are identified and dissected free. The dam is placed around the kidney and the entire kidney cooled with the ice slush. The renal artery and vein are controlled with Rumel or vascular clamps. Depending upon the location of the tumor, an incision is made in the renal capsule. Blunt separation of the renal parenchyma is performed to the level of the collecting system, which is entered sharply. Direct inspection is performed to make certain that adequate incision of the tumor is accomplished. A double-J stent is placed and a nephrostomy tube may be used. The collecting system is closed with a running absorbable suture and large blood vessels are transfixed with interrupted absorbable sutures. The vascular clamps are released and further hemostasis secured. Horizontal mattress sutures placed through the opposing margins of the renal capsule can help provide hemostasis through tamponade. Adjacent perirenal fat may be used to cover the defect in the kidney. A closed suction drain should be placed.

URETEROURETEROSTOMY

Segmental excision of the ureter with a direct ureteroureterostomy is occasionally indicated in the management of transitional cell carcinoma. There is a significant risk of recurrence in the ureter distal to the site of excision. If segmental ureterectomy is to be used, direct anastomosis to the bladder is preferable. Nonetheless, when preservation of the ipsilateral renal unit is mandatory, segmental excision of a portion of the mid or upper ureter with ureteroureterostomy may occasionally be necessary.

The optimal operative approach depends on the level of the ureteral pathology. A flank approach accesses the upper ureter and a Gibson incision is suitable for the mid ureter. The lower ureter can be approached through a lower midline incision or a Pfannenstiel approach. Proximal ureteral dissection may be difficult through a Pfannenstiel incision, however, necessitating cephalad extension of the lateral portion of the incision. Extraperitoneal dissection generally is used.

After an appropriate incision has been made, the retroperitoneal space is developed and the peritoneum mobilized and retracted medially. The ureter is adherent to the posterior peritoneum and is most easily identified as it crosses the iliac vessel. A Penrose drain, vessel loop, or Babcock clamp placed around the ureter can help provide surgical traction. Care must be taken to preserve the adventitia that loosely attaches the blood supply to the ureter.

Ureteral mobilization must be sufficient to allow a tension-free anastomosis, but excessive mobilization should be avoided. The area of tumor involvement usually is palpable. As much margin of ureter around the tumor as is possible should be excised while leaving sufficient length for a tension-free anastomosis. Care should be taken to minimize tumor spillage in the retroperitoneum.

Both ureteral segments are correctly oriented and spatulated for 5 to 6 mm at points 180 degrees apart (Fig. 15–3). A grossly dilated ureter may be transected obliquely and not spatulated in order to match the circumference of the nondilated segment. A fine, absorbable suture is placed in the corner of

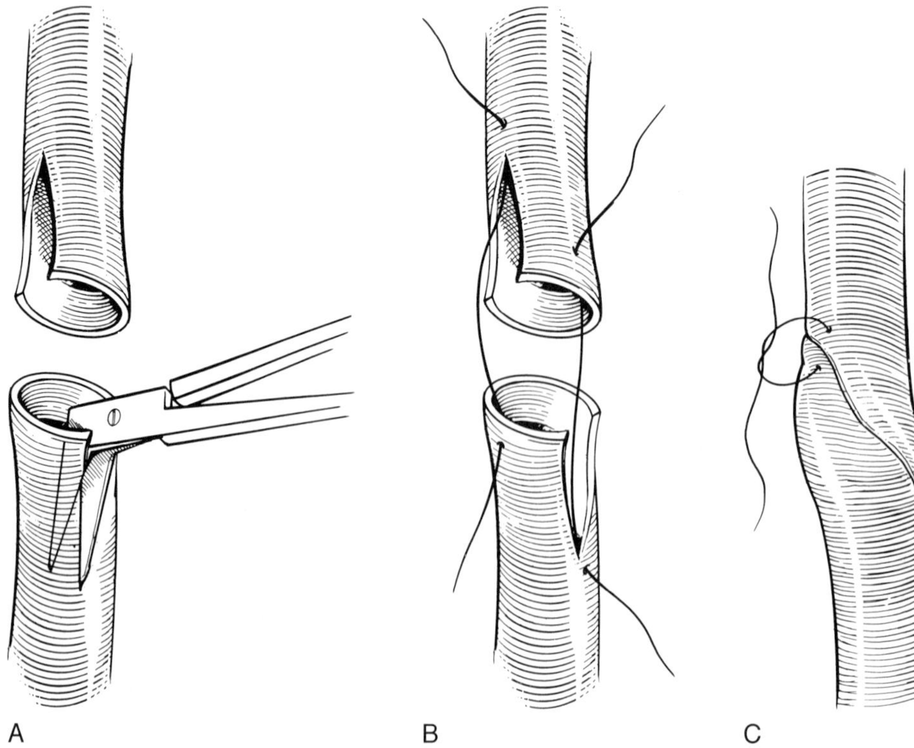
A
B
C

FIGURE 15–3. Technique for ureteroureterostomy. *A*, Ureteral ends are spatulated 180 degrees apart from one another. *B*, Fine, absorbable suture is placed through both ureters. *C*, Ureteral edges are approximated with a running suture.

one ureteral segment and the apex of the other and tied outside the lumen. The opposing corner and apex are similarly approximated. The anastomosis may then proceed by running these two sutures in 2-mm bites and tying them to each other or by placing interrupted sutures. A double-J stent should be placed prior to completion of the closure.[9] Ureteral stents are available in diameters of 4.0 to 8.0 French and lengths of 8 to 30 cm. Stents so large as to fit snugly in the ureter and cause ureteral blanching can significantly compromise ureteral blood supply and lead to stricture formation. Smaller stents with vertical grooves have been suggested to aid in the passage of ureteral stones. Generally, in open ureteral surgery, the largest diameter stent that fits comfortably within the ureter will provide the largest scaffold for healing and adequate diversion without producing ischemia. When using indwelling stents, the length should be tailored to the patient. Ureteral length can be estimated on a plain radiograph or by observing the patient's height and body habitus. A 26- or 28-cm stent is adequate in most adults. Additional length within the bladder may exacerbate irritative voiding symptoms; therefore, precise estimation is preferable.

Retroperitoneal fat or omentum may be mobilized to surround the anastomosis. The retroperitoneum should be drained and a Foley catheter is generally left indwelling postoperatively for 1 or 2 days. The double-J stent is usually removed endoscopically 4 to 6 weeks postoperatively.

DISTAL URETERECTOMY WITH URETERONEOCYSTOSTOMY

Tumors occurring in the distal portion of the ureter may be treated by distal ureterectomy with reimplantation of the ureter into the bladder. This preserves ipsilateral renal function, although there is some risk for tumor recurrence in more proximal segments of the collecting system. The risk for recurrence within the ipsilateral collecting system is greater in the presence of high-grade or invasive tumors.

Exposure to the lower ureter usually is acquired through a lower midline or Pfannenstiel incision. The distal ureter should be excised along with the entire intramural ureter. There should be a generous margin of around 2 cm of normal ureter at the proximal end. The ureter is then mobilized proximally with care taken to preserve the ureteral adventitia and blood supply. Direct ureteroneocystotomy is performed if a tension-free anastomosis is possible. Otherwise, a psoas hitch or Boari flap is used. A direct, nontunnelled anastomosis may be performed without a submucosal tunnel. There is no good evidence that a nonrefluxing anastomosis decreases the risk of pyelonephritis in an adult.

Psoas hitch, when required, is an effective means to decrease tension on the anastomosis after excision of the distal ureter[10,11] (Fig. 15–4). The space of Retzius is developed and the bladder mobilized by freeing its peritoneal attachments. With traction on

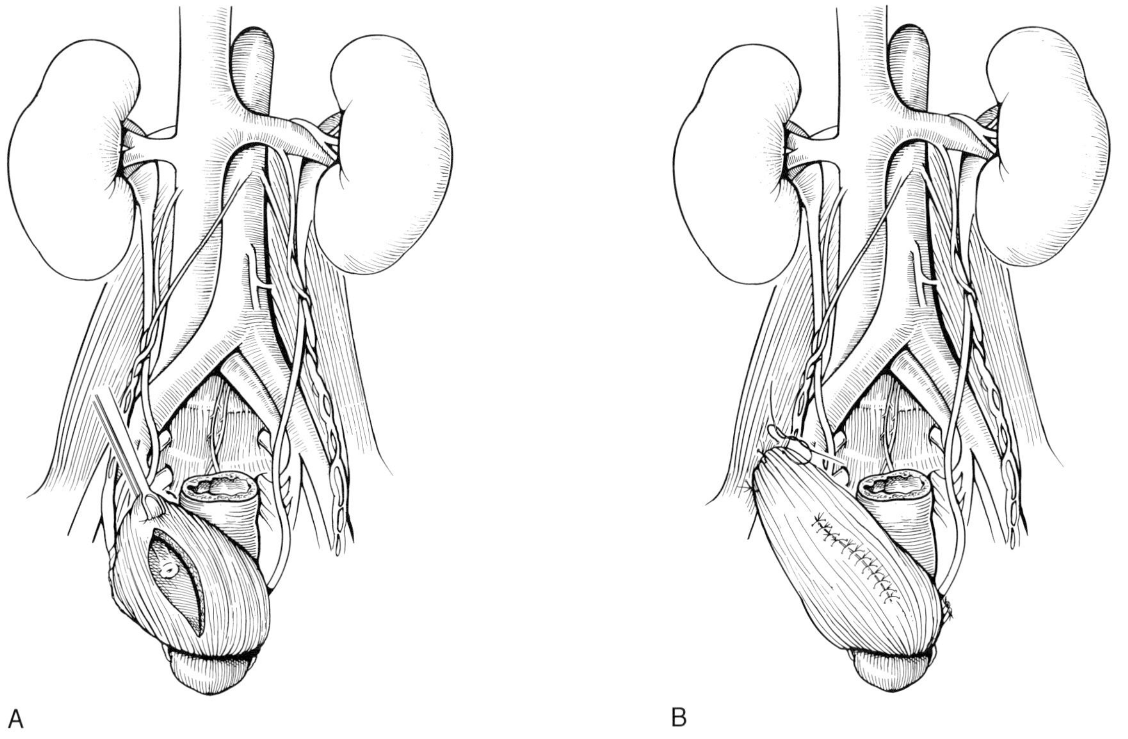

FIGURE 15–4. Psoas hitch ureteral implant. *A*, The open bladder is displaced cephalad to allow ureteroneocystotomy. *B*, Fixation sutures are placed between the bladder and psoas tendon.

the ipsilateral dome, the bladder should be able to reach superior to the iliac vessels. Additional mobility may be gained by dividing the contralateral superior vesical artery. Generally, a vertical or oblique cystotomy incision is used.

The ureter is delivered into the bladder at the superolateral aspect of the dome and the anastomosis performed. The ipsilateral bladder dome is sutured to the psoas minor tendon, if present, or the psoas major muscle using several absorbable sutures.[12] Care should be taken to avoid injury to the genitofemoral nerve when placing the sutures. Alternatively, psoas fixation may be performed prior to ureteral reimplantation.

If there is insufficient ureteral length or bladder mobility to allow a psoas hitch and reimplantation, a Boari flap may be required. Boari flaps can be constructed to bridge 10- to 15-cm defects, while spiraled bladder flaps can reach to the renal pelvis in some circumstances. Bladder capacity should be evaluated preoperatively. The ipsilateral superior vesical artery or one of its branches is identified and a posterolateral bladder flap outlined. The base of the flap should be at least 4 cm in width, depending upon the size of the flap needed. The flap is brought obliquely across the anterior bladder wall with the tip being at least 3 cm in width.

The distal end of the flap is secured to the psoas minor tendon or psoas major muscle with several absorbable sutures. The ureter is delivered to the posterior flap and a standard mucosa-to-mucosa anastomosis carried out after spatulation. The tube is rolled anteriorly and closed using absorbable suture.

A problem with distal ureterectomy and reimplantation is the difficulty that may be encountered in obtaining surveillance of the upper urinary tract postoperatively. Ureteroscopy or even retrograde pyelography may be difficult after any method of ureteral reimplantation, especially when accompanied by a psoas hitch or Boari flap. Intravenous pyelography and urine cytology may be the only available methods for postoperative surveillance for tumor recurrence.

URETEROSCOPIC TREATMENT

Most transitional cell carcinomas of the upper urinary tract are low grade and low stage, making them at least potentially amenable to endoscopic therapy. Certainly, transurethral resection is the preferred surgical therapy for low-grade, low-stage transitional cell tumors of the bladder. Tumors of the upper urinary tract present several problems, however, for endoscopic management.

First of all, there is the issue of diagnosis.[13] While endoscopic treatment for low-grade, low-stage tumors may be indicated in some patients, it rarely is appropriate in those with higher grade or stage lesions. Obtaining adequate tissue for histology and staging of ureteral tumors managed endoscopically is problematic.[14] Undertreatment of a high-grade tumor is a concern.

Undoubtedly, tumors of the ureter and intrarenal collecting system are less accessible than those within the bladder. Flexible ureteroscopes can provide good visualization of most tumors but only instruments of very small caliber can be inserted through ureteroscopes.[15,16] Any bleeding that occurs during the course of treatment can quickly obscure vision.

Another problem is the difficulty in monitoring the upper urinary tract for recurrence after treatment. Radiographic methods are insensitive and multiple repeat ureteroscopic examinations invasive. Long-term monitoring is required, as patients are at risk not only for incomplete destruction of known, existing tumors but also for new tumor occurrence.

A final yet important consideration is that delivery of topical immunotherapy or chemotherapy to the upper urinary tract is difficult and associated with potential hazard.[17] Within the bladder, adjuvant treatment with topical therapy can have a favorable influence on the risk of tumor recurrence. This same advantage is not easily obtained in the ureter or upper collecting system.

Technique

Rigid ureteroscopes provide the best instrument control and afford some expansion of the ureter immediately distal to the tumor that helps in visualization and energy application. However, rigid instruments may be difficult to pass into segments of the ureter proximal to the iliac vessels, so a flexible device may be preferable for tumors in this location. Dilation of the intramural ureter is usually not necessary but may be useful when larger caliber rigid instruments are used.

The visual appearance of the tumor is important. Low-grade, low-stage tumors have a characteristic papillary appearance and often can be seen arising from a small base or stalk. Histologic confirmation of the diagnosis is preferable, depending upon the circumstances, and can be obtained with a cold-cup biopsy forceps. However, it is difficult to obtain adequate tissue from the tumor base for optimal staging.

Small tumors (<1 cm in size) may be treated primarily (Fig. 15–5). Larger lesions generally require some sort of debulking. This may be performed with a cold-cup biopsy forceps to expose the base of the tumor. However, bleeding that occurs as a consequence of cold-cup removal can cause difficulty with visualization as well as with subsequent application of the laser energy.

Most experience with laser destruction has been with an end-fire neodymium:yttrium-aluminum-garnet (Nd:YAG) laser fiber with a small angle of

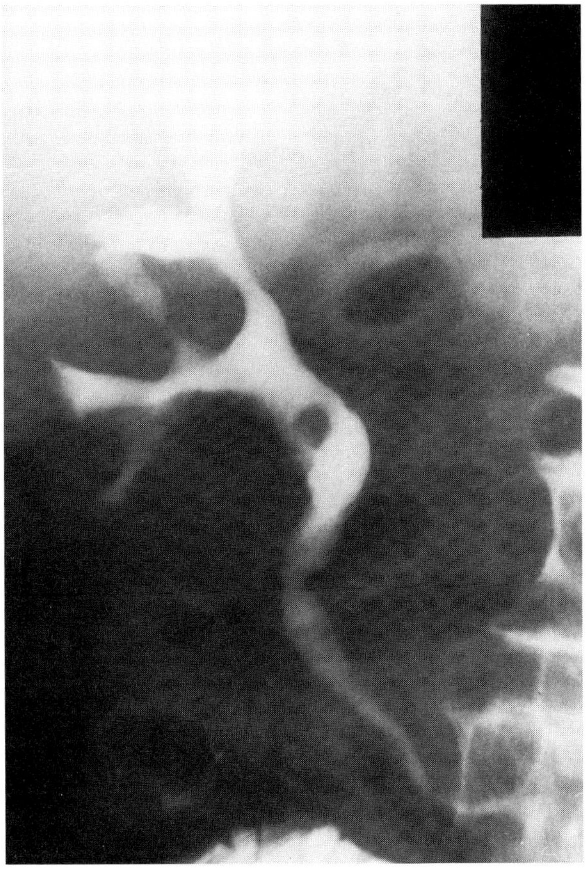

FIGURE 15–5. Small filling defect of the renal pelvis caused by a low-grade, low-stage transitional cell tumor. Endoscopic treatment is feasible for lesions of this size and location.

divergence.[18] The widely divergent fibers as are used with treatment of the prostate provide less specifically directed coagulation. The fibers themselves are of sufficiently small caliber that they can be passed through the working channel of either flexible or rigid ureteroscopes. The tip of the fiber is visualized and positioned several millimeters from the surface of the tumor. Usually, a power output of 25 to 30 watts is used with a continuous pulse duration. The tumor undergoes a characteristic white discoloration that is indicative of adequate thermal necrosis. Coagulated portions of the tumor can be dislodged with the tip of the fiber or ureteroscope to expose deeper areas. Tissue necrosis and coagulation extend beyond the visible changes, so care should be taken to avoid excessive energy application in any given area.

Ideally, a double-J stent should be left indwelling after laser treatment of the ureter. Edema at the site of treatment may otherwise lead to obstruction or perforation of the ureter and result in urinary extravasation. Complete healing and reepithelialization may take several months. Depending upon the circumstances, follow-up ureteroscopic examination of the ureter may be indicated in order to ensure complete eradication of the tumor.

Schmeller and Hofstetter reported on the use of a Nd:YAG laser to treat ureteral tumors.[19] Caution was expressed against the use of a laser for treatment of invasive cancers. Postoperative strictures were felt to be related to the ureteroscopy itself rather than the laser treatment.[20]

Gaboardi and associates treated 18 patients with ureteroscopic Nd:YAG laser irradiation.[21] Eight patients developed recurrence with a mean 15 months of follow-up. Kaufman and Carson reported laser treatment of nine highly selected patients with low-grade papillary transitional cell carcinoma of the ureter and had no recurrences observed during the reported period of follow-up.

PERCUTANEOUS RENAL SURGERY

A percutaneous approach to the kidney can permit endoscopic destruction of some transitional cell tumors of the upper collecting system.[22,23] Nephroscopes are of larger caliber than ureteroscopes and this facilitates access, visualization, and energy delivery.[24] A concern, though, is the potential for implantation of tumor cells along the nephrostomy tract or in the perinephric space.

Renal endoscopy through an open pyelotomy incision is associated with a relatively high rate of tumor cell implantation. In addition, implantation of tumor cells along nephrostomy tracts has been observed. However, controlled nephrostomy tube insertion and percutaneous kidney surgery are associated with less extravasation of the irrigant into the perinephric space. Nonetheless, because of the risk of implantation, percutaneous surgical treatment of transitional cell cancer of the kidney generally is reserved for situations in which there is compromised or absent contralateral renal function and ureteroscopic treatment is not feasible.

Percutaneous access is obtained in the usual fashion as performed for nephrolithotomy. In order to prevent excessive extravasation of urine or irrigating fluid, the nephrostomy tube may be left in site for several days before the surgical treatment in order to allow the tract around the tube to mature and seal somewhat from the surrounding tissues. Dilation of the tract is performed and a nephroscope inserted. The location of the tumor is noted and, if indicated, biopsies obtained for histologic confirmation.

The method of energy chosen for tumor destruction depends upon tumor size, location, and the potential for harmful extension of the energy to adjacent structures. Tumors chosen for percutaneous management often have considerable bulk, and resection of the exophytic portion of the tumor using an electrical loop may help expose the tumor base. Electrical fulguration with a loop or roller electrode may be performed. Caution is particularly necessary in the renal pelvis, as the renal vessels are immediately adjacent.

Laser energy may also be used for tumor destruction.[25] Most often, a Nd:YAG laser is chosen but other wavelengths may provide comparable results. In general, coagulation rather than vaporization seems advisable, since this provides the best hemostasis.

When an end-fire Nd:YAG laser probe with a small angle of divergence is used, 20 to 25 watts of energy usually provides good tissue coagulation. Excellent hemostasis occurs during the treatment, but any ongoing bleeding before the laser application interferes with delivery of the laser energy to the tumor surface. Smith has reported 25 patients with transitional cell cancers of the kidney treated percutaneously.[26] Twelve patients underwent combined electrocautery resection and laser therapy and 13 had resection alone. Recurrences within the collecting system were observed in ten patients but there were no reported incidences of tumor cell implantation along the nephrostomy tract.

Vasavada and associates performed percutaneous resection of transitional cell carcinoma in six patients with anatomically solitary kidneys with a prior history of transitional cell carcinoma elsewhere in the urinary tract.[27] A 6-week course of topical bacille Calmette-Guérin (BCG) was administered postoperatively. Only one patient had evidence of tumor recurrence with a mean 22 months of follow-up. The authors concluded that this approach is useful in a high-risk patient group.

SUMMARY

Surgical therapy remains the primary method of treatment for transitional cell carcinoma of the ureter and upper collecting system. Often, this involves open surgical excision but, increasingly, less invasive treatment methods are being explored.[28] Sometimes, the situation mandates approaches that may provide less optimal treatment results but are required in order to preserve renal function.[29] As with any surgical procedure, appropriate patient selection is a key factor contributing to the outcome of therapy.

REFERENCES

1. Huben RP, Mounzer AM, Murphy GP: Tumor grade and stage as prognostic variables in upper tract urothelial tumors. Cancer 1988; 62:2016.
2. McCarron JP, Mills C, Vaughan ED Jr: Tumors of the renal pelvis and ureter: current concepts and management. Semin Urol 1983; 1:75.
3. Heney NM, Nocks BN, Daly JJ, et al: Prognostic factors in carcinoma of the ureter. J Urol 1981; 125:632.
4. Murphy DM, Zincke H, Furlow WL: Management of high grade transitional cell cancer of the upper urinary tract. J Urol 1981; 125:25.
5. Reitelman C, Sawczuk IS, Olsson CA, et al: Prognostic variables in patients with transitional cell carcinoma of the renal pelvis and proximal ureter. J Urol 1987; 138:1144.
6. Babaian RJ, Johnson DE: Primary carcinoma of the ureter. J Urol 1980; 123:357.
7. Zincke H, Neves R: Feasibility of conservative surgery for transitional cell cancer of the upper urinary tract. Urol Clin North Am 1984; 11:717.
8. Gittes RF: Management of transitional cell carcinoma of the upper tract: case for conservative local excision. Urol Clin North Am 1980; 7:559.
9. Lee CK, Smith AD: Role of stents in open ureteral surgery. J Endourol 1993; 7(2):141–144.
10. Turner-Warwick RT, Worth PHL: The psoas bladder-hitch procedure for the replacement of the lower third of the ureter. Br J Urol 1969; 41:701.
11. Ehrlich RM, Melman A, Skinner DG: The use of vesico-psoas hitch in urologic surgery. J Urol 1978; 119:322.
12. Middleton RG: Routine use of the psoas hitch in ureteral reimplantation. J Urol 1980; 123:352.
13. Blute ML, Segura JW, Patterson DE, et al: Impact of endourology on diagnosis and management of upper urinary tract urothelial cancer. J Urol 1989; 141:1298.
14. Ohigashi T, Baba S, Tachibana M, Hata M: Endourologic management of filling defect in renal pelvis: limited value of cold cup biopsy. Urology 1990; 35:51.
15. Huffman JL: Ureteroscopic management of transitional cell carcinoma of the upper urinary tract. Urol Clin North Am 1988; 15:419.
16. Huffman JL, Bagley DH, Lyon ES, et al: Endoscopic diagnosis and treatment of upper-tract urothelial tumors. Cancer 1985; 55:1422.
17. Ramsey JC, Soloway MS: Instillation of bacillus Calmette-Guérin into the renal pelvis of a solitary kidney for the treatment of transitional cell carcinoma. J Urol 1990; 143: 1220.
18. Kaufman RP Jr, Carson CC III: Ureteroscopic management of transitional cell carcinoma of the uterer using the neodymium:YAG laser. Lasers Surg Med 1993; 13:625–628.
19. Schmeller NT, Hofstetter AG: Laser treatment of ureteral tumors. J Urol 1989; 141:840.
20. Schmeller N, Pensel J: Laser treatment of the ureter. *In* Smith JA Jr (ed): Lasers in Urologic Surgery, 2nd edition, pp 81–91. Chicago, Mosby Yearbook Medical Publishers, 1988.
21. Gaboardi F, Bozzola A, Dotti E, Galli L: Conservative treatment of upper urinary tract tumors with Nd:YAG laser. J Endourol 1994; 8:37.
22. Tasca A, Zattoni F: The case for a percutaneous approach to transitional cell carcinoma of the renal pelvis. J Urol 1990; 143:902.
23. Streem SB: Percutaneous management of upper-tract transitional cell carcinoma. Urol Clin North Am 1995; 22: 221–229.
24. Orihuela E, Smith AD: Percutaneous treatment of transitional cell carcinoma of the upper urinary tract. Urol Clin North Am 1988; 15:425.
25. Sweetser P, Weiss GH, Smith AD: Percutaneous laser treatment of the kidney and ureter. *In* Smith JA Jr (ed): Lasers in Urologic Surgery, 3rd edition, pp 157–170. Chicago, Mosby Yearbook Medical Publishers, 1994.
26. Smith AD, Orihuela E, Crowley AR: Percutaneous management of renal pelvic tumors: a treatment option in selected cases. J Urol 1987; 137:852.
27. Vasavada SP, Streem SB, Novick AC: Definitive tumor resection and percutaneous bacillus Calmette-Guérin for management of renal pelvic transitional cell carcinoma in solitary kidneys. Urology 1995; 45:381–386.
28. Huffman JL: Ureteroscopic management of transitional cell carcinoma of the urinary tract. Urol Clin North Am 1988; 15:419.
29. Schoenberg MP, Van Arsdalen KN, Wein AJ: The management of transitional cell carcinoma in solitary renal units. J Urol 1991; 146:700.

V

BLADDER

16

DIAGNOSIS AND STAGING OF BLADDER CANCER

MICHAEL J. DROLLER, M.D.

Numerous advances have been made in our understanding of the natural history and developmental course of bladder cancer. Correspondingly, methods to diagnose, stage, and characterize particular forms of bladder cancer have advanced from standard histologic evaluation of surgical specimens to application of molecular and genetic methods by which the potential intrinsic biology of a particular form of cancer may be characterized.

This chapter will discuss methods currently used to diagnose and stage bladder cancer. It will also review those features that can be used to assess the intrinsic biologic potential of various forms of bladder cancer and how these may be used in the selection of treatment.

INITIAL DIAGNOSIS OF BLADDER CANCER

Bladder cancer is the fourth most prevalent noncutaneous malignancy in the United States.[1] Recent surveillance information indicates that over 50,000 new cases are diagnosed annually and nearly 10,000 deaths occur.[1]

The diagnosis of bladder cancer is usually occasioned by the appearance of blood in the urine either grossly or microscopically.[2] Although initial and terminal hematuria, as opposed to total hematuria, are usually of prostatic origin, any of these patterns may reflect the presence of a bladder cancer. The degree of hematuria bears no relation either to the size of the tumor or to its grade or stage.

Although generally not causing a change in voiding pattern, the presence of bladder cancer may occasionally be accompanied by irritative symptoms manifested by a sense of increased urgency or frequency. This seems to occur most often in the presence of diffuse flat carcinoma in situ (see below) or when the transitional cell cancer involves the bladder trigone or prostatic urethra.

Since hematuria is not exclusively of bladder origin, evaluation of its cause requires imaging of the entire urinary tract. This generally involves sonography or intravenous pyelography of the kidneys and bladder, with observations reflecting on the ureters and prostate as well. The efficacy of ultrasound in detecting upper tract lesions depends upon both the extent of a specific abnormality and the experience and thoroughness of the radiologist performing the procedure. Sonography is most effective in identifying renal masses and distinguishing between those that are solid and those that are cystic.[3] It may also be useful in detecting upper tract dilatation, which may be indicative of obstruction either from a ureteral lesion or an invasive bladder cancer at the ureteral orifice. Intravenous pyelography (IVP) will generally provide better definition than sonography of abnormalities through the entire collecting system from the outermost calyx and infundibulum through profile of the ureter and bladder.[3] However, it will not permit identification of small lesions of the renal parenchyma or of the renal pelvis. Retrograde pyelography can further define the anatomy of the upper tract and characterize further any areas of the upper tract that may be abnormal or that may have been visualized inadequately on IVP.

Both ultrasound and intravenous pyelography may also be used to image the bladder, albeit with somewhat limited efficacy.[3] Detection of bladder cancer by transabdominal ultrasound depends upon the size of the lesion and the degree to which the bladder is distended to permit assessment of the regularity of the bladder wall during the examination.[4] Sonography may be additionally useful in identifying upper tract dilation due to an invasive bladder tumor located at the ureteral orifice.

Intravenous pyelography is subject to some of the same limitations that affect the efficacy of transabdominal ultrasound in imaging bladder tumors.

The size of the lesion may limit its visualization as the bladder fills with contrast.[5] Limitations on the distensibility of the bladder wall may reflect conditions other than tumor. On the other hand, imaging of the bladder in various positions as it fills with contrast may allow visualization of one or multiple bladder tumors, which may be seen as radiolucent filling defects. In addition, the presence of ureteral obstruction with upper tract dilatation may be associated with muscle-invasive tumors located at or near the ureteral orifice.

Although they may identify upper tract lesions, ureteral dilatation, and masses in the bladder, computed tomography (CT) and magnetic resonance imaging (MRI) are not generally used as initial means of evaluating the cause of hematuria or as first-line methods in diagnosing bladder cancer.

In further assessment of the cause of hematuria, voided urines and/or barbitaged irrigation specimens should also be obtained to determine if abnormal cells are present. The presence of cancer cells in such specimens can be interpreted to represent the shedding of cells from the tumor, from visibly abnormal areas of the bladder mucosa, or from endoscopically normal areas that may also be involved in the cancer diathesis.[6] A positive urine cytology usually suggests the presence of high-grade disease, since individual cells in this setting have an easily recognizable abnormal appearance.[7] However, a normal urinary cytology does not exclude the possible presence of a tumor. Low-grade tumors may produce a negative reading in a voided urinary cytology in as many as 25 to 70% of cases.[8] In these instances, clusters of cells may suggest the presence of a low-grade malignancy, since it is unusual to see such clusters in the absence of cancer or instrumentation. Correspondingly, although a barbitaged specimen may demonstrate a positive reading when a voided specimen has been read as negative, it may also introduce an instrumentation artifact resulting in the dislodgment of clusters of cells that leads to a false-positive reading. Barbitage has generally been used to provide sufficient numbers of cells for flow cytometric analysis, which may detect abnormalities when a urine cytology is interpreted as negative.[9] Under these circumstances, however, low-grade disease may still be interpreted as negative, depending upon the standards that are used to calibrate gated levels of sensitivity and specificity.

A great deal of interest has recently been generated by reports of the ability to diagnose the presence of bladder cancer by detection of certain substances in the urine. These have included bladder tumor antigen (BTA),[10] nuclear matrix protein (NMP-22),[11] DNA fragments (microsatellites),[12] and telomerase activity,[13] each representing the presence of urothelial cancer cells. The value of these tests may ultimately reside in their ability to screen for the presence of bladder cancer in populations that may be at particular risk or in those who have had bladder cancer and are being monitored for recurrence.

After preliminary imaging of the upper tract and bladder and an analysis of urinary cytology has been done, cystoscopic examination is necessary to visualize the urothelium of the urethra and the bladder to determine if a malignancy is present. Characterization of the architecture of the tumor and the multiplicity of tumors or the diffuseness of mucosal involvement will help to assess the nature of the cancer diathesis.

The sine qua non for diagnosis of bladder cancer is transurethral resection of the tumor and pathologic evaluation of the surgical specimen. Selected biopsies, using a cold-cup biopsy forceps, of areas adjacent to the presenting lesion, of areas of mucosal irregularity and erythema, and of areas at the bladder neck and within the prostatic urethra prior to transurethral resection of the tumor may provide information on the extent of the cancer diathesis and the need for adjunctive intravesical treatment. Random biopsies of endoscopically normal areas of the urothelium are no longer advocated as part of the standard diagnostic approach in the initial evaluation of a bladder cancer diathesis.[14] However, these may be useful in those instances when there is no endoscopically visible lesion, upper tracts and urethra are negative for cancer, and urinary cytology is persistently positive. The diagnostic yield from such random biopsies, however, is likely to be low because of the limited sampling that is provided.

The endoscopic configuration of the tumor may suggest whether it is superficial or invasive, and whether the bladder wall is correspondingly likely to be thicker than normal because of the presence of the cancer. A papillary lesion is more likely to be "superficial"; a nodular or solid lesion is more likely to be invasive.[15,16] Papillary tumors should initially be resected flush with the bladder mucosa. Somewhat deeper resection should then be done to permit evaluation of the lamina propria and the superficial level of the muscularis propria. Care should be taken, however, not to resect too deeply to avoid perforation of the bladder wall, which may be quite thin in these cases. In contrast, if the tumor appears to be solid or nodular, it is more likely that the bladder wall is thicker. In these instances, resection of the superficial (or intraluminal) portion of the solid tumor should be recovered separately for pathologic evaluation. Deeper resection should then be done to include the muscularis propria layer to determine the depth of infiltration. Resection to the level of the perivesical fat can be performed if the intent is to incorporate extensiveness of the transurethral resection as a treatment modality (see below).

Bimanual examination of the bladder under anesthesia before and after transurethral resection of the cancer may provide additional information of a tumor's extent.[17] Failure to palpate a tumor mass prior to resection may suggest that the tumor is superficial or less extensive if invasive. Palpation of a mass that is mobile suggests the presence of a nodular, infiltrative cancer that does not involve adjacent structures. Palpation of a mass that is fixed suggests that the cancer may have involved adjacent structures or the pelvic sidewalls. In attempting to assess the extent of invasive disease, bimanual palpation is highly subjective. Its greatest value may be in cases of large tumors that are extensively infiltrative, since these are more likely to be palpable and generally indicate an adverse prognosis, especially if they are palpable after resection.

Transurethral ultrasound, CT, and MRI imaging can also be used to assess tumor extent prior to transurethral resection. Transurethral ultrasound examination has been reported to have a sensitivity of 90% and a specificity of 76% in determining whether a tumor is muscle-invasive.[18] See and Fuller observed that 24% of tumors staged as T1 by transurethral ultrasound had been overstaged and that 10% of tumors staged as T2 by this modality had been understaged.[19] In evaluating corresponding figures for stages T3b–T4 tumors, it appeared that 29% of stage T3b were understaged and that 5% of stage T3a tumors were overstaged by transurethral ultrasound.[19]

The sensitivity of CT scanning in detecting extravesical extension of a bladder cancer has ranged between 60 and 96%, and its specificity has ranged between 66 and 93%.[20] Its cumulative sensitivity and specificity have been calculated at 83% and 82%, respectively, implying that extravesical extension remains undetected in 17% of instances and is overdiagnosed in 18% of patients. CT scanning has had limited success in distinguishing between superficial and muscle-invasive disease. Overstaging has occurred in two thirds of patients with superficial disease, while understaging has been found in 30% of patients with muscle-invasive tumors.[19]

Although MRI has several features that would theoretically make it more accurate than CT scanning in the staging of bladder cancer, MRI provides the ability to obtain images in multiple planes and to demonstrate perivesical fat planes and boundaries of the prostate and seminal vesicles. T1-weighted images of the primary tumor can be contrasted with low-signal-intensity images of urine and high-signal-intensity images of perivesical fat, while T2-weighted images can be used to assess disruption of the muscle wall and invasion of other organs.[21] The sensitivity for MRI in identifying extravesical tumor extension has been found to range between 60 and 100%, with a cumulative average of 73%.[19,22] Specificity has also ranged between 60 and 100%, with a cumulative average of 84%. Recent reports have described improved sensitivity and specificity in detecting muscle invasion (96.2% and 83.3%, respectively) with the use of gadolinium-DTPA–enhanced MRI for tumor staging.[23]

Notwithstanding the advantages provided by these imaging modalities, the staging of bladder cancer by transurethral ultrasound, CT scanning, and MRI is limited by the inability of each modality to discern microscopic extension of disease and the relative dependence of each on disruption of normal "radiographic" tissue planes to identify cancer extension. The former may lead to understaging of disease, since extension of the cancer, even if only microscopic, may be associated with a greater likelihood of metastasis. Correspondingly, the latter can lead to overstaging, since images suggestive of disruption of the muscularis can be created by prior resection, inflammatory processes, or other therapeutic interventions.

Ultimately, the critical element in the characterization of a bladder cancer is its pathologic appearance. The extent to which the cancer has been found on microscopic examination to penetrate the bladder wall,[24] the histologic appearance of the tumor cells,[25] the architectural configuration of the cells (papillary versus nodular),[26] whether or not bladder wall lymphatics or vasculature are involved by the cancer,[27] and the nature of the urothelium adjacent to and at sites distant from the presenting lesion(s)[28] are each important in this regard.

Current convention bases the staging of disease on the depth to which a cancer has penetrated the bladder wall. As such, transurethral resection may not be adequate in providing specimens that permit accurate characterization of the extent of involvement by the cancer of the different layers of the bladder wall.[29] More definitive assessment may be possible by analyzing partial cystectomy or total cystectomy specimens, since these provide a full thickness of the bladder wall for pathologic examination.[30] Recent reports have described the use of transabdominal ultrasound-guided needle biopsies to provide full-thickness bladder wall specimens to evaluate the depth of cancer infiltration with greater accuracy.[31] This technique is still in a developmental stage.

Early attempts to characterize the prognosis of various forms of bladder cancer were based on an analysis of their histologic appearance. Broders described different grades of disease and associated those that were poorly differentiated with a more ominous prognosis[32] than those that were well differentiated. Subsequently, Aschner correlated the increasing depth to which a tumor had penetrated into the bladder wall with a progressively worse prognosis.[33]

In the mid-1940s, Jewett proposed a classification of bladder cancer based upon the degree of involvement of the bladder wall and the "curability" of the tumor by cystectomy.[34,35] His initial observations were based upon an autopsy series in which those tumors that had penetrated deeply into the bladder wall were considered "incurable."[34] In a subsequent study of cystectomy specimens, Jewett proposed that tumors that had invaded only superficially were curable by cystectomy, whereas those that invaded the bladder wall more deeply were not.[35]

Subsequent refinements in staging were based upon more precise correlations between the depth of invasion of a tumor and its prognosis, although the original classifications by Jewett continued to provide the basis of stages that were defined. Currently, the TNM classification as endorsed by the International Union Against Cancer (UICC) has been adopted as the standard staging system for bladder cancer.[36] The objectives of this system are to suggest prognosis, to form a basis for selecting treatment, to provide a standard for evaluating treatment results, and to facilitate the exchange of information on treatment results through standardization of the classification of the disease being treated.

The TNM system currently consists of a pretreatment *clinical* classification and a postsurgical *histopathologic* classification.[36] The pretreatment clinical staging classification is based upon imaging studies and impressions obtained by endoscopic visualization and bimanual examination. The postsurgical histopathologic staging classification is based upon specimens obtained by transurethral resection. Differences between these two classifications within individual categories have been substantial.[37] Moreover, the latter has also been subject to substantial error when compared to assessments of the extent of a tumor in full-thickness bladder wall specimens.[38]

The 1992 TNM classification for bladder tumors was reviewed in the Fourth International Consensus Meeting on Bladder Cancer held in Antwerp, Belgium, in 1993 (Table 16–1). For superficial tumors, specific classifications for carcinoma in situ (Tis), mucosally confined cancers (stage Ta), and cancers that had infiltrated the lamina propria (stage T1) were felt to satisfy staging objectives as described above and were therefore maintained without a change[39] (Fig. 16–1).

Mucosally confined tumors (stage Ta) have repeatedly been found to have the best prognosis of any other form of bladder cancer. Only 2 to 4% of stage Ta tumors progress.[40] Those that do are largely high grade, and high-grade tumors comprise only 1 to 2% of all stage Ta cancers.[41,42] These tumors comprise true papillary tumors and do not include so-called papillomas, which are extensions of urothelium with normal cellularity into the lumen of the bladder, have essentially no malignant activity or apparent malignant potential, and presumably represent a proliferation of cells in response to an inflammatory or irritative stimulus.[43]

In contrast, cancers that have invaded the lamina propria (stage T1) have been found to have a 20 to 30% possibility of progression.[40] High-grade tumors in this category appear most likely to be associated with potential progression.[41] Some have also suggested that those tumors in this category associated with a more diffuse cancer diathesis (carcinoma in situ) are those most likely to progress.[44]

TABLE 16–1. THE TNM CLASSIFICATION OF BLADDER TUMORS*

Primary tumor (T)

The suffix (m) should be added to the appropriate T category to indicate multiple tumors. The suffix (is) may be added to any T to indicate the presence of associated carcinoma in situ.

TX	Primary tumor cannot be assessed
T0	No evidence of primary tumor
Ta	Noninvasive papillary carcinoma
Tis	Carcinoma in situ: "flat tumor"
T1	Tumor invades subepithelial connective tissue
T2	Tumor invades superficial muscle (inner half)
T3	Tumor invades deep muscle or perivesical fat
T3a	Tumor invades deep muscle (outer half)
T3b	Tumor invades perivesical fat
i	microscopically
ii	macroscopically (extravesical mass)
T4	Tumor invades any of the following: prostate, uterus, vagina, pelvic wall, or abdominal wall
T4a	Tumor invades the prostate, uterus, vagina
T4b	Tumor invades the pelvic wall or abdominal wall or both

Regional lymph nodes (N)

Regional lymph nodes are those within the true pelvis: all others are distant nodes

NX	Regional lymph nodes cannot be assessed
N0	No regional lymph node metastasis
N1	Metastasis in a single lymph node, 2 cm or less in greatest dimension
N2	Metastasis in a single lymph node, more than 2 cm but not more than 5 cm in greatest dimension, or multiple lymph nodes, none more than 5 cm in greatest dimension
N3	Metastasis in a lymph node more than 5 cm in greatest dimension

Distant metastasis (M)

MX	Presence of distant metastasis cannot be assessed
M0	No distant metastasis
M1	Distant metastasis

Stage grouping

Stage			
0_a	Ta	N0	M0
0_{is}	Tis	N0	M0
I	T1	N0	M0
II	T2	N0	M0
	T3a	N0	M0
III	T3b	N0	M0
	T4a	N0	M0
IV	T4b	N0	M0
	Any T	N1–3	M0
	Any T	Any N	M1

*Adapted from American Joint Committee on Cancer: Manual for Staging Cancer, 4th edition. Philadelphia, JB Lippincott Co, 1992; and the International Union Against Cancer: *In* Hermanek P, Sobin LH (eds): TNM Classification of Malignant Tumours, 2nd revision, 4th edition. Berlin, Springer-Verlag, 1992, with permission.

In some instances the submucosal connective tissue (lamina propria) contains a prominent "muscularis mucosae."[45] This muscle layer is sometimes confused with the detrusor muscularis (muscularis propria). As a result, penetration of the muscularis mucosae layer by stage T1 tumors has occasionally been interpreted as indicating the presence of true muscle invasion. Some have suggested subdividing stage T1 tumors depending upon whether they have invaded to or through the muscularis mucosae (stage T1a and stage T1b, respectively).[46] This has been based on the possibility that penetration

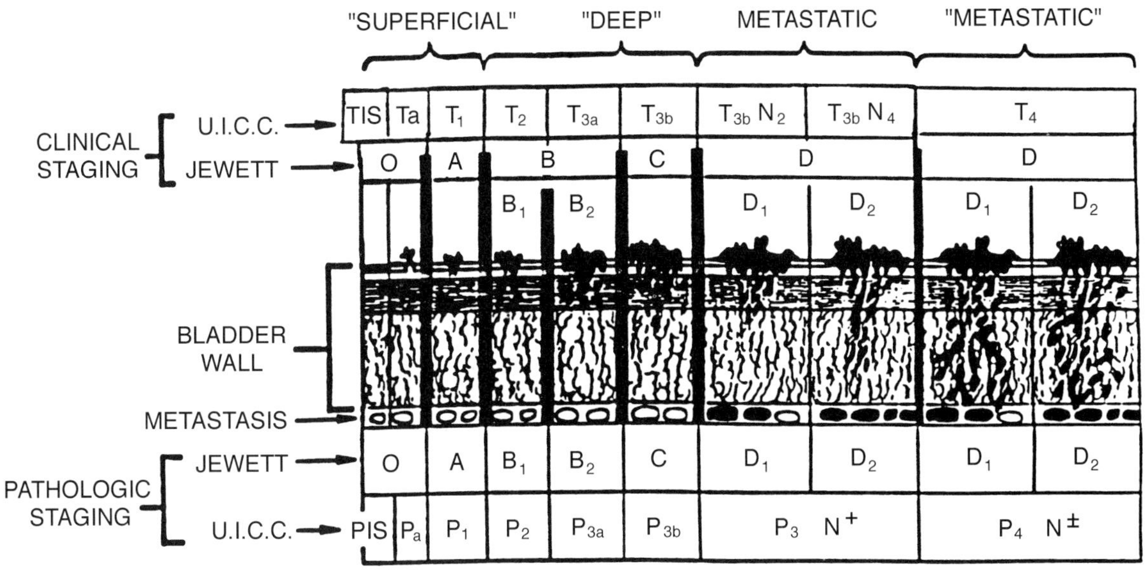
"SUPERFICIAL"
"DEEP"
METASTATIC
"METASTATIC"
CLINICAL STAGING
U.I.C.C.
JEWETT
TIS Ta T1 T2 T3a T3b T3b N2 T3b N4 T4
O A B C D D
B1 B2 D1 D2 D1 D2
BLADDER WALL
METASTASIS
PATHOLOGIC STAGING
JEWETT
U.I.C.C.
O A B1 B2 C D1 D2 D1 D2
PIS Pa P1 P2 P3a P3b P3 N+ P4 N±

FIGURE 16–1. Staging schema for bladder cancer. This schema for staging systems of bladder cancer is a composite of the clinical and pathologic classification of bladder cancer as initially developed by Jewett with subsequent modifications by the American Joint Committee on Cancer and the International Union Against Cancer (see Table 16–1). The schema presents a sequence of stages leading from carcinoma in situ to mucosally confined papillary cancer and progressive invasion through the various layers of the bladder wall. An increasing likelihood of regional and distant metastatic disease is depicted with advancing stage. (From Koss LG: Tumors of the urinary bladder. *In* Atlas of Tumor Pathology, series 2, fasicle 11. Washington, DC, AFIP, 1975. Courtesy of Willet Whitmore, M.D.)

of the muscularis mucosa may represent a more aggressive cancer. Whether this distinction is valid on the basis of the relationship of these tumors to the muscularis mucosae, however, has not been resolved. First, this muscle layer is not always readily defined. Second, many of those tumors that invade more deeply are more extensive and of a more nodular configuration, while those that are more superficial are less extensive and of a more papillary configuration, which in itself may be more indicative of behavioral potential than their relation to the mucosae muscle fibers.[40]

In considering distinctions in the biologic potential of these forms of superficial bladder cancer, the natural history of carcinoma in situ and its influence in the staging of bladder cancer may be of substantial importance. This may be due in part to the variability in the manner in which carcinoma in situ presents, conflicting opinions as to its prognosis, and the heterogeneity of its response to different types of treatment. The most common form is characterized by highly abnormal cells that involve the bladder mucosa diffusely. Other forms may be unifocal and more well differentiated, and may represent a less malignant diathesis.

The ominous prognosis originally ascribed to carcinoma in situ may have been based on its association with concomitant muscle-invasive transitional cell cancer.[47] Thus, the muscle-invasive cancer rather than the carcinoma in situ was suggested to lead to progression and death in the majority of these cases. Subsequent observations of an apparently prolonged and often nonprogressive course of carcinoma in situ when muscle-invasive cancer was not present suggested that this form of cancer by itself might pose little threat.[48] Recent observations have supported the ultimately ominous potential of carcinoma in situ regardless of whether other types of tumor are present.[49] However, this may pertain to diffuse carcinoma in situ; in contrast, a small asymptomatic focus of "carcinoma in situ" that remains unifocal, is asymptomatic, and is not accompanied by other forms of bladder cancer may represent a tumor diathesis that is more benign and does not lead to the development of invasive disease. In one series the incidence of progressive disease in long-term follow-up of carcinoma in situ ranged from 8% when only a small focus of carcinoma in situ was present to 78% in patients who had diffuse disease.[50]

Several additional observations are relevant in this regard. First, carcinoma in situ has been found to have microscopic penetration into the lamina propria in 20 to 30% of cases.[51] Second, high-grade carcinoma in situ appears to be more commonly associated with papillary and papillonodular tumors that are invasive of the lamina propria than with those that are mucosally confined.[52] Since the former have been found to be more likely to become progressive, this form of carcinoma in situ may reflect a more aggressive diathesis. Third, several reports have suggested the development of solid or nodular tumors from foci of carcinoma in situ.[53] If carcinoma in situ is the direct antecedent of nodular tumors, which are more deeply invasive when they become clinically apparent than are papillary tumors, the diagnosis of this type of carcinoma in situ may be interpreted as signifying a particularly ominous neoplastic diathesis.[54]

In view of these considerations, the placement of carcinoma in situ within the generally accepted staging system remains unclear. Clearly, all forms of bladder cancer have their origin in a form of intraepithelial neoplastic transformation that by definition would constitute "carcinoma in situ." However, the schematic sequence of development of various superficial tumors from carcinoma in situ may not accurately reflect the intrinsic biologic potential of the different types of superficial tumor diatheses that occur. As such, carcinoma in situ may have to be factored into the subclassification of other stages of disease in view of how it represents the intrinsic biologic potential of a particular tumor diathesis and how it may consequently affect the prognosis of that tumor diathesis and its response to particular treatments.

Cancers that have traditionally been described as "invasive" have generally comprised those that have penetrated the bladder wall muscle ("muscularis propria"). Progressive depth of penetration has been correlated with an increased likelihood of metastasis.[55] However, the directness of this association is not always maintained. For example, tumors that have penetrated only the superficial muscle (stage T2) and have maintained a papillary configuration have occasionally been found to have a better prognosis than those that have penetrated only the lamina propria (stage T1) but that have manifested a tentacular form of infiltration.[56] Several considerations, however, could affect the validity of these exceptions. Occasionally, cancers staged as T2 have actually been found to be infiltrative of only the muscularis mucosae and not of the muscularis propria. Moreover, such tumors have occasionally been observed only to abut the detrusor muscle and not to be truly infiltrative of that layer. Correspondingly, cancers staged as T1 might occasionally be understaged, such that repeat resection would find residual cancer that was actually more deeply invasive.[57]

At the 1993 Bladder Cancer Consensus Conference in Antwerp, it was proposed that stage T3a tumors (deep muscle invasion) and stage T2 tumors (superficial muscle invasion) be combined in a single stage (stage T2).[58] Stage T2a would then comprise tumors that invaded only the superficial muscle (less than one half of the depth of the muscle layer), and stage T2b would comprise tumors that invaded the deep muscle (greater than one half of the depth of the muscle layer). Stage T3 would then be used to designate tumor involvement of the perivesical tissues.[58] Stage T3a would comprise those tumors that demonstrated only microscopic invasion and stage T3b would comprise those tumors that had more extensive invasion of extravesical tissues.

The rationale for including all muscle-invasive cancers in one category reflected the problem of accurately determining the depth of muscle invasion by transurethral resection, the impression that all cancers invading the muscle wall behaved in a similar aggressive fashion regardless of whether they invaded superficially (less than halfway through the depth of the muscle wall) or deeply, and the suggestion that muscle-invasive tumors did not exhibit the same potential biologic behavior as did tumors that had extended through the full thickness of the bladder wall into the perivesical fat.[58]

However, this proposal failed to take into account several clinical observations. First, those tumors that had penetrated only the superficial muscle appeared less likely to be associated with metastases and were also more likely to be cured by a variety of surgical approaches.[59] Many of these, for example, showed no cancer remaining in the cystectomy specimen after preliminary extensive transurethral resection or radiation therapy, and treatment outcomes were at least twice as successful in terms of time to disease recurrence or survival as they were for more deeply invasive disease. Second, those tumors that had invaded the muscle layer more deeply appeared to have an ominous prognosis similar to that of tumors that had involved the perivesical soft tissues microscopically. Taken together, the stages for muscle-invasive disease as set forth in the TNM system of the UICC (Fig. 16–1; Table 16–1) are currently those that are most commonly used.

Other features that distinguish superficial from deep muscle invasion have included the architecture of the infiltrating cancer, the associated degree of vascular or lymphatic involvement in the bladder wall, and the pattern of invasion. Superficial muscle invasion has been associated with a papillary configuration and a pattern of infiltration described as "broad front," in which tumor cells penetrate the bladder wall muscle in large clusters with a broad infiltrative margin.[60] Such tumors have appeared to involve the bladder wall vasculature and lymphatics in only one third of cases.[61] In contrast, deeply invasive tumors have been associated with a more nodular type of configuration and a pattern of infiltration described as tentacular, in which tumor cells have appeared to percolate through the bladder wall in small clusters or as fingerlike projections. These tumors have been found to involve the bladder wall lymphatics and vasculature in two thirds of instances.[61]

The stage of disease denoted as T4 has been used to indicate invasion of other pelvic organs by the cancer. Stage T4a represents tumor invasion of the prostate, uterus, or vagina; stage T4b represents tumor invasion of the pelvic or abdominal wall. Conflicting observations have made definitive staging in these categories somewhat unclear. For example, as many as 40% of cystectomy specimens have been found on thorough pathologic examination to have tumor involvement of the prostate.[62] Although traditionally thought to indicate an ominous prognosis, prostatic involvement may actually represent a variable outcome. If the cancer involving the prostate has remained mucosally confined (even if it has extended into the prostatic ducts) its effect will be less ominous than if the cancer has infiltrated the prostatic stroma.[63] The situation in women may be similar. If there has been direct penetration only of the anterior vaginal wall, prognosis may be less ominous than if there has been more extensive involvement of the vagina or penetration of the uterus.

Involvement of regional lymph nodes has generally been interpreted to indicate an ominous prognosis. However, several reports have suggested that prognosis may not be as grave when only microscopic metastases (<2 mm) are found to have involved only one or two nodes.[64] Under these circumstances, aggressive surgery has been reported to produce 10 to 15% 5-year survivals, and some have suggested that an extensive and meticulous lymphadenectomy may be curative in as many as 35% of these patients.[65] In contrast, gross involvement of lymph nodes or involvement of more than two lymph nodes has been associated with a poor prognosis.[64,66] Although some have suggested staging subdivisions according to the degree of lymph node involvement, such distinctions based upon either the number of lymph nodes involved or whether involvement is macroscopic or microscopic have not yet been found to be predictably reliable.

Standard schematic depictions of bladder cancer in association with the likelihood of progression have created the impression that the various diatheses represent a sequence of stages in cancer development (Fig. 16–1).[67] This has implied progression from the most superficial histologic appearance to the most extensive invasion with a corresponding increase in the probability for the development of metastatic disease.

A schema that implies a sequence of stages may not be entirely correct. The natural history of various forms of bladder cancer may instead reflect a number of developmental pathways that, although interrelated, may be distinct from one another.[68] A

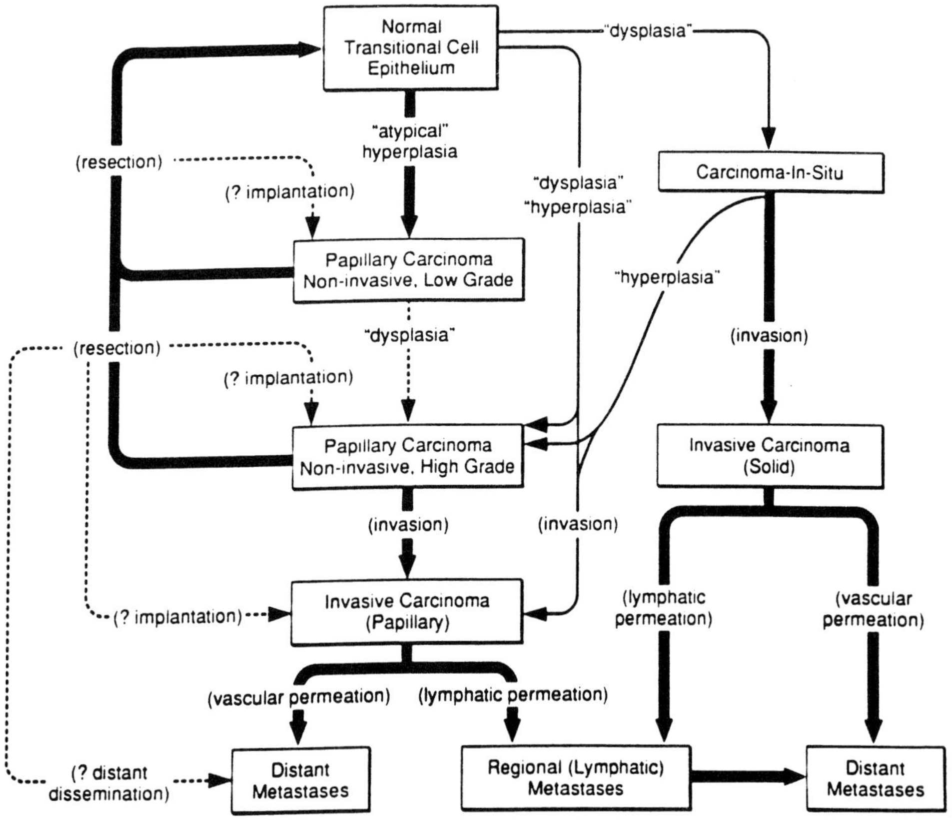
Normal Transitional Cell Epithelium
"dysplasia"
"atypical" hyperplasia
(resection)
(? implantation)
"dysplasia" "hyperplasia"
Carcinoma-In-Situ
Papillary Carcinoma Non-invasive, Low Grade
"hyperplasia"
"dysplasia"
(resection)
(? implantation)
(invasion)
Papillary Carcinoma Non-invasive, High Grade
Invasive Carcinoma (Solid)
(invasion)
(invasion)
(? implantation)
Invasive Carcinoma (Papillary)
(lymphatic permeation)
(vascular permeation)
(vascular permeation)
(lymphatic permeation)
(? distant dissemination)
Distant Metastases
Regional (Lymphatic) Metastases
Distant Metastases

FIGURE 16–2. Pathways of development of bladder cancer. This schema depicts the variety of pathways that may account for the different types of bladder cancer that are seen. The term "atypical hyperplasia" refers to a proliferative process without implying the possibility for motility or invasiveness. The term "dysplasia" implies that enzymatic capacity for cancer cells of more undifferentiated appearance to penetrate the connective tissue stroma. The different phenotypic forms of bladder cancer occupy different steps in these interrelated pathways and suggest that the development of bladder cancer may not necessarily reflect a sequence of stages but may be the manifestation of different chromosomal changes that lead to the development of cancer cells with different biologic capabilities. The size of the arrows represents the likelihood of the development of a particular form of bladder cancer and its progression. (Courtesy of Michael J. Droller, M.D.)

schema that incorporates the concept of a variety of different developmental pathways may complement the standard concept of a sequence of stages (Fig. 16–2). Distinctions in the potential biologic behavior of a cancer at a specific point in time (either at initial diagnosis or at the time of recurrence) may be of use in determining whether aggressive treatment is indicated (even if a tumor appears to be at an "early" stage) or whether conservative treatment may be appropriate (even if a tumor appears to be more advanced).

In considering a schema in which different pathways portray the biology of various types of bladder cancer, a number of developmental terms may be applied to describe the different processes that give rise to various forms of tumor diathesis (Fig. 16–2). For example, papillary tumors may arise through a process described as predominantly "proliferative."[68] Accordingly, transformed epithelial cells proliferate, induce angiogenesis, and produce tumors with a multilayered epithelium in papillary configuration surrounding a central fibrovascular core. The process of proliferation by itself may produce tumors that contain cells with a histologically normal appearance ("low-grade"). Tumors that are comprised of histologically abnormal ("high-grade") cells may occur as the result of a process termed "dysplasia" that is superimposed upon the proliferative process.[68] However, it is unusual to see papillary tumors that are high-grade and truly mucosally confined. In fact, this has been reported to occur in only 1 to 2% of all mucosally confined tumors.[42]

A high-grade histologic appearance in papillary tumors is more commonly seen when penetration of the basement membrane and invasion of the lamina propria has also occurred.[69] This difference in appearance may suggest that the developmental process termed "dysplasia" may have conferred a different biologic capability on these tumors such that they not only proliferate but can also infiltrate other tissues. Although low-grade, mucosally confined tumors could conceivably change during the course of their proliferation to become high-grade tumors that have also acquired the biochemical machinery to penetrate into the subepithelial stroma, it can also be hypothesized that "dysplasia" may have been the primary result of neoplastic transformation in these cases, and may then have led to the development of a papillary high-grade transitional cell cancer that could penetrate the lamina propria.

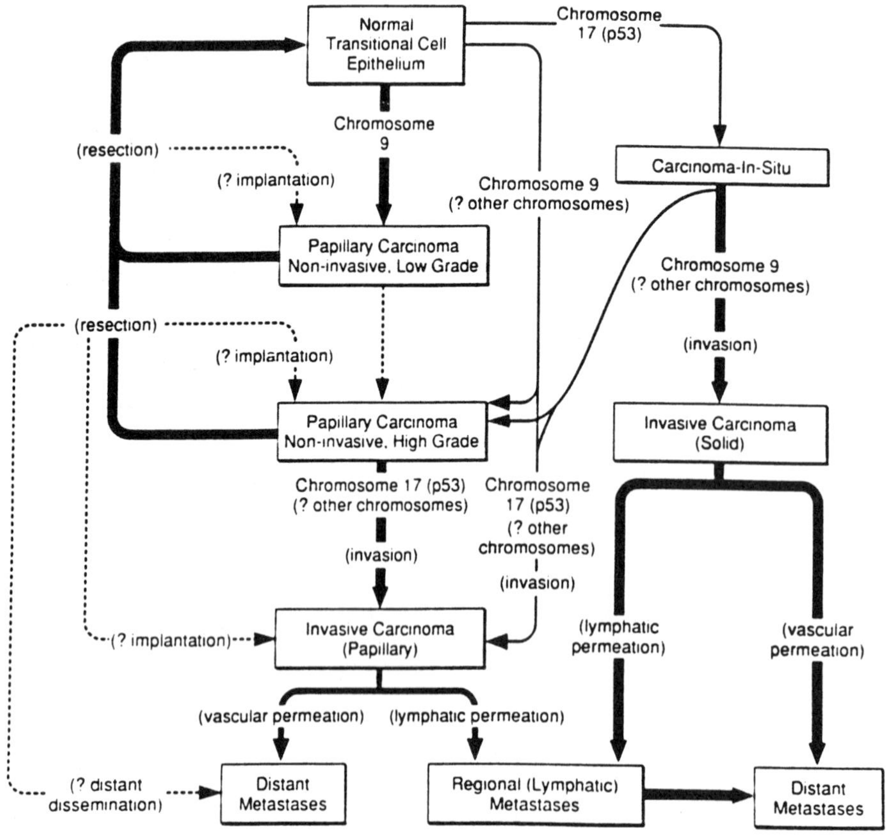
Normal Transitional Cell Epithelium
Chromosome 17 (p53)
Chromosome 9
(resection)
(? implantation)
Chromosome 9 (? other chromosomes)
Carcinoma-In-Situ
Papillary Carcinoma Non-invasive, Low Grade
Chromosome 9 (? other chromosomes)
(resection)
(? implantation)
(invasion)
Papillary Carcinoma Non-invasive, High Grade
Invasive Carcinoma (Solid)
Chromosome 17 (p53) (? other chromosomes)
Chromosome 17 (p53) (? other chromosomes)
(invasion)
(invasion)
(? implantation)
Invasive Carcinoma (Papillary)
(lymphatic permeation)
(vascular permeation)
(vascular permeation)
(lymphatic permeation)
(? distant dissemination)
Distant Metastases
Regional (Lymphatic) Metastases
Distant Metastases

FIGURE 16–3. Chromosomal changes and pathways of bladder cancer development. A number of chromosomal changes have been discovered in various forms of bladder cancer. These can be superimposed upon the schematic clinical pathways for the development of different bladder cancer phenotypes depicted in Figure 16–2. Such findings support the suggestion that different pathways of tumor development and progression may characterize the biology of bladder cancer. (Courtesy of Michael J. Droller, M.D.)

A neoplastic pathway primarily characterized by dysplasia could also lead to the development of flat carcinoma in situ, which could then produce, through proliferation, a high-grade papillary tumor.[68] However, it may be more likely that nodular or solid rather than papillary tumors arise from foci of flat carcinoma in situ and that these penetrate directly into the lamina propria and into the muscularis before they are diagnosed.[70] Microinvasion has been observed in 20 to 30% of cases of flat carcinoma in situ.[51] Moreover, as the cancer cells proliferate they could theoretically form nodules that extend into the bladder wall and infiltrate more deeply before they protrude into the bladder lumen and create symptoms that could lead to their diagnosis.

Recent observations of genetic defects in different types of bladder cancer support the concept that different pathways may account for the development of various forms of bladder cancer[71] (Fig. 16–3). For example, aberrations of chromosome 9 have been seen in both low-grade, low-stage bladder tumors and higher grade, invasive tumors.[72] This has suggested that loss of heterozygosity of chromosome 9 may occur early in the genesis of a variety of bladder cancers. It has also been shown that chromosome 9 was lost in each of several multifocal tumors within an individual patient, supporting the concept of a field change in the genesis of bladder cancer.

Loss of heterozygosity of chromosomes other than chromosome 9 has been observed in high-grade, high-stage tumors.[73] For example, mutations in chromosome 17 with expression of p53 have been identified in approximately half of all high-grade, high-stage bladder cancers.[74] In fact, a specific type of mutation has been seen in bladder cancer in which a genetic change may occur at codon 280 of chromosome 17 with the occurrence of a high proportion of G–C transversions. These specific changes are relatively rare in the p53 gene in other kinds of human cancers.[74] This suggests that the initial change of chromosome 9 may be followed by multiple sequential changes of other genes, which may then lead to an invasive and potentially metastatic phenotype.

Several studies have also shown that carcinoma in situ does not contain a high frequency of loss of heterozygosity of chromosome 9 but does express p53 mutations.[71] Moreover, recent studies have demonstrated that only those lamina propria invasive tumors that express p53 have been found to progress to muscle invasion.[75] Other studies have shown that p53-positive tumors are more likely to be associated with incurability.[76,77]

Ultimately, a molecular profile for a particular cancer may be superimposed upon the stage of a tumor as determined by pathologic analysis of a surgical specimen to determine not only the type of therapy that may be effective in a particular cancer diathesis, but also to predict the outcome of particular treatment regimens in the context of the natural history of that diathesis.[78]

REFERENCES

1. Parker SL, Tong T, Bolden S, Wingo PA: Cancer statistics, 1996. CA Cancer J Clin 1996; 46:5.
2. Messing EM, Young TB, Hunt VB, et al: Urinary tract cancers found by home screening with hematuria dipstick in healthy men over 50 years of age. Cancer 1989; 64:2361.
3. Resnick MI: Overview: imaging of the genitourinary tract. *In* Droller MJ (ed): Surgical Management of Urologic Disease, An Anatomic Approach, p 69. St Louis, Mosby-Yearbook, 1992.
4. Denkhaus H, Crone-Munzebrock W, Huland H: Non-invasive ultrasound in detecting and staging bladder carcinoma. Urol Radiol 1985; 7:121.
5. Hatch TR, Barry JM: The value of excretory urography in staging bladder cancer. J Urol 1986; 135:49.
6. Badalament RA, Fair WR, Whitmore WF Jr, et al: The relative value of cytometry and cytology in the management of bladder cancer. Semin Urol 1988; 6:22.
7. Billerey C, Lamy B, Bettard H, et al: Flow cytometry versus urinary cytology in the diagnosis and follow-up of bladder tumors: critical review of a 5-year experience. World J Urol 1993; 11:156.
8. Kannan V, Bose S: Low grade transitional cell carcinoma and instrument artifact. A challenge I urine cytology. Acta Cytol 1993; 37:899.
9. Murphy WM: DNA flow cytometry in diagnostic pathology of the urinary tract. Hum Pathol 1987; 18:317.
10. Sarosdy MF, deVere White R, White MS, et al: Results of a multi-center trial using the BTA test to monitor for and diagnose recurrent bladder cancer. J Urol 1995; 154:379.
11. Soloway MS, Briggman JV, Carpinito GA, et al: Use of a new tumor marker, urinary NMP22, in the detection of occult or rapidly transitional cell carcinoma of the urinary tract folowing surgical treatment. J Urol 1996; 156:363.
12. Mao L, Schoenberg MP, Scicchitano M, et al: Molecular detection of primary bladder cancer by microsatellite analyses. Science 1996; 271:659.
13. Kim NW, Piatyszek MA, Prowse KA, et al: Specific association of human telomerase activity with immortal cells and cancer. Science 1994; 266:2011.
14. Heney NM, Daly J, Prout JR Jr: Biopsy of apparently normal epithelium in patients with bladder carcinoma. J Urol 1978; 120:57.
15. Kakizoe T, Tobisu K, Takai K, et al: Relationship between papillary and nodular transitional cell carcinoma in the human urinary bladder. Cancer Res 1988; 48:2299.
16. Friedell GN, Parija GC, Nagy K, et al: The pathology of human bladder cancer. Cancer 1980; 45:1823.
17. Herr HW: A proposed simplified staging system of invasive bladder tumors. Urol Int 1993; 50:17.
18. Holm HH, Juul N, Torp-Pedersen S, et al: Bladder tumor staging by transurethral ultrasonic scanning. Eur Urol 1988; 15:31.
19. See WA, Fuller JR: Staging of advanced bladder cancer: current concepts and pitfalls. Urol Clin North Am 1992; 19:663.
20. Bryan PJ, Butler HE, Lipuma JP, et al: CT and MR imaging in staging bladder neoplasms. J Comput Tomogr 1987; 11: 96.
21. Husband JE, Olliff JFC, Williams MP, et al: Bladder cancer staging with CT and MR imaging. Radiology 1989; 173: 435.
22. Nishimura K, Hido S, Nishio Y, et al: The validity of MRI in the staging of bladder cancer: comparison with CT and transurethral US. Am J Clin Oncol 1988; 18:217.
23. Tanimoto A, Yuasa Y, Imai Y, et al: Bladder tumor staging: comparison of conventional and gadolinium-enhanced dynamic MR imaging and CT. Radiology 1992; 185:741.

24. Husband JE: Staging bladder cancer (Review). Clin Radiol 1992; 46:153.
25. Jordan AM, Weingarten J, Murphy WM: Transitional cell neoplasms of the urinary bladder. Can biological potential be predicted from histologic grading? Cancer 1987; 60: 2761.
26. Slack NH, Prout GR Jr: Heterogeneity of invasive bladder carcinoma and different responses to treatment. J Urol 1980; 123:644.
27. Frazier HA, Robertson JE, Dodge RK, et al: The value of pathologic factors in predicting cancer specific survival among patients treated with radical cystectomy for transitional cell cancer of the bladder and prostate. Cancer 1993; 71:3993.
28. Aprikan AG, Sarkis AS, Reuter V, et al: Biological markers of prognosis in transitional cell carcinoma of the bladder: current concepts. Semin Urol 1993; 11:137.
29. Klan R, Loy V, Huland H: Residual tumor discovered in routine second transurethral resection in patients with stage T1 transitional cell carcinoma of the bladder. J Urol 1991; 146:316.
30. Cummings KB: Clinical versus pathologic staging and classification of bladder cancer. Urology 1984; 23(Suppl 4): 55.
31. Malmstrom PU, Lonnemark M, Busch C, Magnusson A: Staging of bladder carcinoma by computer tomography-guided transmural core biopsy. Scand J Urol Nephrol 1993; 27:193.
32. Broders AC: Epithelioma of the genitourinary organs. Ann Surg 1922; 75:574.
33. Aschner PW: The pathology of vesical neoplasms. Its evaluation in diagnosis prognosis. JAMA 1928; 91:1697.
34. Jewett HJ, Strong GH: Infiltrating carcinoma of the bladder: relation of depth of penetration of the bladder wall to incidence of local extension and metastases. J Urol 1946; 55:366.
35. Jewett HJ, Lewis E: Infiltrating carcinoma of bladder: curability by total cystectomy. J Urol 1948; 60:107.
36. Hermanek P, Sobin LH: International Union Against Cancer: TNM Classification of Malignant Tumours, 2nd revision, 4th edition. Berlin, Springer-Verlag, 1992.
37. Fuller WA Jr: Staging of advanced bladder cancer. Current concepts and pitfalls (Review). Urol Clin North Am 1992; 19:663.
38. Herr HW: Staging invasive bladder tumors (Review). J Surg Oncol 1992; 51:217.
39. Kotake T, Flanigan RC, Kirkels W, et al: The current TNM-classification of bladder carcinoma: is it as good as we need it to be. Int J Urol 1995; 2:36.
40. Heney NM, Nocks BN, Daly JJ, et al: Ta and T1 bladder cancer; location, recurrence, and progression. Br J Urol 1982; 54:152.
41. Heney NM, Ahmed S, Flanagan MJ, et al: Superficial bladder cancer: progression and recurrence. J Urol 1983; 130: 1083.
42. Jakse G, Loidle W, Seeber G: Stage T1, grade 3 transitional cell carcinoma of the bladder: an unfavourable tumor? J Urol 1987; 137:39.
43. Green LF, Hanash KA, Farrow GN: Benign papilloma or papillary carcinoma of the bladder. J Urol 1973; 110:205.
44. Vicente J, Laguna MP, Duarte D, et al: Carcinoma in situ as a prognostic factor for G3pT1 bladder tumors. Br J Urol 1991; 68:380.
45. Engel P, Anagnostaki L, Braendstrup O: The muscularis mucosae of the human urinary bladder. Implications for tumor staging on biopsies. Scand J Urol Nephrol 1992; 26(Suppl):249.
46. Pagano F, Garbeglio A, Milani C, et al: Prognosis of bladder cancer. I. Risk factors in superficial transitional cell carcinoma. Eur Urol 1987; 13:145.
47. Melicow M: Histological study of vesical epithelium intervening between gross neoplasms in total cystectomy. J Urol 1952; 68:261.
48. Weinstein R, Miller AW III, Pauli BV: Carcinoma in situ: comments on the pathology of a paradox. Urol Clin North Am 1980; 18:523.
49. Herr HW: When is a cystectomy necessary in carcinoma in situ? *In* Murphy GP, Khoury S (eds): Therapeutic Progress in Urologic Cancers, p 511. New York, Alan R Liss, 1989.
50. Lamm DL: Carcinoma in situ. Urol Clin North Am 1992; 19:499.
51. Farrow GM, Utz DC: Observations on microinvasive transitional cell carcinoma of the urinary bladder. Clin Oncol 1982; 1:609.
52. Rubben H, Lutzeyer W, Fischer N, et al: Natural history and treatment of low and high risk superficial bladder tumors. J Urol 1988; 139:283.
53. Kakizoe T, Matumoto K, Nishio Y, et al: Significance of carcinoma in situ in association with bladder cancer. J Urol 1985; 133:395.
54. Kakizoe T, Tobisu K, Takai K, et al: Relationship between papillary and nodular transitional cell carcinoma in the human urinary bladder. Cancer Res 1988; 48:2299.
55. Schroder FH, Cooper EH, Debruyne FMJ, et al: TNM classification of genitourinary tumors 1987-position of the EORTC Genitourinary Group. Br J Urol 1988; 62:502.
56. Abel PD, Hall RR, Williams G: Should P_1 transitional cell carcinoma of the bladder still be classified as superficial? Br J Urol 1988; 62:235.
57. Koloszy Z: Histopathological "self-control" in transurethral resection of bladder tumours. Br J Urol 1991; 67:162.
58. Herr HW: A proposed simplified staging system of invasive bladder tumors. Urol Int 1993; 50:17.
59. Jewett HJ: Comments on the staging of invasive bladder cancer: two B's or not two B's: that is the question (apologies to Shakespeare, Hamlet, act 2, sc I, lines 1056) (Editorial). J Urol 1978; 119:39.
60. Friedell GN, Parija GC, Nagy K, et al: The pathology of human bladder cancer. Cancer 1980; 45:1823.
61. Soto EA, Friedell GH, Tiltman AJ: Bladder cancer as seen in giant histologic sections. Cancer 1977; 39:447.
62. Schellhammer PF, Bean MA, Whitmore WF: Prostatic involvement by transitional cell carcinoma: pathogenesis, patterns and prognosis. J Urol 1977; 118:399.
63. Wood DP, Montie JE, Pontes JE, et al: Transitional cell carcinoma of the prostate in cysto-prostatectomy specimens removed for bladder cancer. J Urol 1989; 141:346.
64. Smith JA Jr, Whitmore WF Jr: Regional lymph node metastases from bladder cancer. J Urol 1981; 126:591.
65. Skinner DG: Management of invasive bladder cancer: a meticulous pelvic lymph node dissection can make a difference. J Urol 1982; 128:34.
66. Roehborn CG, Sagalowsky AI, Peters PC: Long-term patient survival after cystectomy for regional metastatic transitional cell carcinoma of the bladder. J Urol 1991; 146:36.
67. Hendry WF, Rawson NSB, Turney L, et al: Computerization of urothelial carcinoma records: 16 years' experience with the TNM system. Br J Urol 1990; 65:583.
68. Droller MJ: Bladder cancer. Curr Probl Surg 1981; 18:205.
69. Kaubisch S, Lum BL, Reese J, et al: Stage T1 bladder cancer: grade is the primary determinant for risk of muscle invasion. J Urol 1991; 146:28.
70. Jones PA, Droller MJ: Pathways of development and progression in bladder cancer: new correlations between clinical observations and molecular mechanisms. Semin Urol 1993; 11:177.
71. Spruck CH, Ohneseit PF, Gonzalez-Zulueta M, et al: Two molecular pathways to transitional carcinoma of the bladder. Cancer Res 1994; 54:784.
72. Miyao N, Tsai YC, Lerner SP, et al: The role of chromosome 9 in human bladder cancer. Cancer Res 1993; 53:4066.
73. Tsai YC, Nichols PW, Hiti AL, et al: Allelic losses of chromosome 9, 11 and 17, in human bladder cancer. Cancer Res 1990; 50:44.
74. Fujimoto K, Yamada Y, Okajima E, et al: Frequent association of p53 gene mutations in invasive bladder cancer. Cancer Res 1992; 52:1393.
75. Sarkis AS, Dalbagni G, Cordon-Cardo C, et al: Nuclear

overexpression of p53 protein in transitional cell bladder carcinoma: a marker for disease progression. J Natl Cancer Inst 1993; 85:53.
76. Sidransky D, Messing E: Molecular genetics and biochemical mechanisms in bladder cancer: oncogenes, tumor suppressor genes and growth factors. Urol Clin North Am 1992; 19:629.
77. Olumi AF, Tsai YC, Nicholes PW, et al: Allelic loss of chromosome 17p distinguishes high grade from low grade transitional cell carcinomas of the bladder. Cancer Res 1990; 50:7081.
78. Theodorescu D: Commentary on genetic prognostic markers for transitional carcinoma of the bladder: from microscopes to molecules. J Urol 1996; 155:2.

17

SUPERFICIAL TRANSITIONAL CELL CARCINOMA OF THE BLADDER: MANAGEMENT AND PROGNOSIS

HOWARD J. KORMAN, M.D., ROGER B. WATSON, M.D.,
and MARK S. SOLOWAY, M.D.

Superficial transitional cell carcinoma (TCC) of the urinary bladder—that is, tumor confined to the mucosa (Ta, Tis) or submucosa (T1)—is a heterogeneous disease with a variable natural history. At one end of the spectrum, low-grade Ta tumors require initial endoscopic treatment and surveillance, but rarely represent a threat to the patient. At the other extreme, high-grade T1 tumors have a high malignant potential with significant progression and cancer death rates.

Many characteristics of TCC have been studied in an attempt to predict this variable tumor behavior. These include pathologic features, cytologic analysis, and biologic and molecular markers. Although thorough endoscopic tumor resection remains the principal treatment, intravesical agents have become important in the subgroup of tumors that are at risk of progression. In order to tailor treatment appropriately, the urologist should review the various prognostic factors and define the behavior of the tumors as precisely as possible.

INITIAL EVALUATION

Patient evaluation begins with a thorough history (including exposure to known carcinogens), physical examination, and urine analysis. Endoscopic assessment of the entire urethra and urinary bladder remains the most important diagnostic procedure. Modern flexible endoscopes with high-quality optics allow this to be performed safely, with minimal patient discomfort, as an office examination.[1] The anterior bladder wall and bladder neck regions are well visualized with flexible cystoscopy. Cold-cup biopsy is possible, although sufficient tissue to determine depth of invasion is difficult to obtain with small forceps. Thus we reserve biopsy for endoscopy under anesthesia.

Upper tract radiologic visualization should be performed in all cases. Intravenous urography is sensitive in detecting papillary tumors, as well as in providing functional and anatomic information. Ultrasound has also been used for upper tract assessment, with the advantages of avoiding contrast reactions, radiation, and intestinal preparation. However, ultrasound is less sensitive in detecting small tumors. Retrograde ureteropyelography, with cytologic washings at the time of tumor resection, is useful to further assess suspicious or poorly imaged areas.

If there is suspicion of a high-grade tumor, cytologic assessment is important. Bladder washings have a better yield than voided urine cytologies.[2] Gentle barbotage using 50 ml of sterile saline with prompt cytology evaluation is suggested.

ENDOSCOPIC MANAGEMENT

Well-performed transurethral resection (TUR) remains the most important method of managing primary and recurrent bladder tumors, despite the evolving role of intravesical therapy. Technological improvements have dramatically improved this procedure.[3]

Videoendoscopy has been a major advance in all areas of endourology, but particularly for bladder tumor resection. In addition to minimizing the surgeon's exposure to body fluids, it allows all areas of the bladder, including the dome and anterior wall, to be resected with greater ease and improved magnification. It also provides documentation and improved teaching opportunities. Continuous-flow resection allows the urologist to control the degree of bladder filling, thus reducing the risk of perforation and obturator nerve excitation.

Adequate anesthesia is important for safe, controlled resection and patient comfort. We believe that this is best achieved with regional anesthesia, allowing pelvic floor, abdominal wall, and bladder relaxation. In males, we prefer beginning the procedure with an optical dilator that provides calibration and dilation of the urethra with visual assessment prior to placement of the resectoscope.[4] Saline barbotage for cytologic analysis should be performed first if high-grade tumor is suspected. The entire bladder should be examined using the 70-degree lens. The number, location, and size of any papillary lesions or suspicious areas should be noted.

Papillary tumors should be systematically resected with a right-angle or bladder wall loop, as appropriate. The bladder wall or angled loop is designed for resecting tumors located on the high lateral or posterior walls. The aim is to achieve complete resection of all tumor. This includes sampling the tumor base, which may involve resection into muscle. Specimens should be retrieved for histopathology. Suspicious mucosal areas should be biopsied with a cold-cup forceps to minimize cautery artifact. The roller ball electrode is used to fulgurate all suspicious areas and to achieve hemostasis.

A history or the presence of a high-grade tumor necessitates transurethral biopsy of the prostatic urethra. This is best performed with the resectoscope, as opposed to cold-cup forceps. One should sample the mucosa and underlying stroma from the bladder neck to the verumontanum. A bimanual examination should be performed. Catheter drainage is necessary if there is bleeding requiring irrigation, or if a deep resection has been performed. The majority of procedures can be performed on an outpatient or overnight basis.

PATHOLOGIC PROGNOSTIC FACTORS

After complete endoscopic resection, approximately 30 to 80% of patients will develop additional tumors, usually of similar grade and stage. The majority of these lesions are new occurrences, as opposed to true recurrences, reflecting a generalized instability of the urothelium. Although close follow-up with endoscopic management of recurrences is appropriate for most cases, the adjuvant use of intravesical chemotherapeutic and immunotherapeutic agents is sometimes appropriate. In order to identify patients at higher risk of progression and recurrence, who may benefit from such therapy, numerous prognostic factors have been proposed (Table 17–1). These include well-established pathologic features such as grade and stage, endoscopic features, cytologic characteristics, tumor cell products, and molecular genetic markers such as p53. Although some of these prognostic factors have an established clinical role, some of the newer markers remain investigational.

TABLE 17–1. PROGNOSTIC FACTORS FOR SUPERFICIAL BLADDER CANCER

Number of tumors
Tumor size
Tumor grade
Tumor T stage
Lymphatic invasion
Carcinoma in situ
Urine cytology
DNA ploidy
Blood group antigens
Tumor cell products—EGFR, AMFR, PCNA
Molecular genetic markers—p53; c-*erb* B-2; c-*myc*

Histologic Grade

Tumor grade is well established as an important prognostic factor for both new tumor occurrence and progression to invasion.[5,6] Mostofi et al.[7] introduced a World Health Organization (WHO) classification system for grading TCC as grades 1, 2, and 3, based on the degree of cellular differentiation. In an attempt to simplify tumor grading, Murphy et al.[8] proposed two categories based upon cytologic features. Low-grade carcinoma, corresponding to WHO grade 1, describes a well-differentiated tumor. These are predominately papillary in architecture and confined to the mucosa. Only 6% have lamina propria invasion.[5] High-grade carcinoma describes moderate to poorly differentiated neoplasms corresponding to WHO grades 2 and 3. This simplified system has been proposed to reduce interobserver error. Not infrequently there are areas of variable grade within one tumor, and the pathologist reports the highest.

A solitary papillary tumor with a fibrovascular core and no more than either seven or eight normal appearing cell layers is regarded by some as a papilloma.[9] Others include these with grade 1 papillary carcinomas.

The WHO grading system takes into account the degree of anaplasia as determined by increased cellularity, nuclear crowding, disturbance of cellular polarity, the absence of differentiation from base to surface, pleomorphism, variations in nuclear shape and chromatin pattern, mitotic counts, and the presence of giant cells.[7] This pattern is reproducible at the extremes (grades 1 and 3), but leaves grade 2 as a heterogeneous intermediate group.[10,11]

There is a strong correlation between higher grade and invasion, disease progression, metastases, and survival.[5,6] Mortality from progression of grade 1 tumors is low (0 and 4% at 10 years).[6,12] Another 3% recur as grade 3 tumors.[6] Grade 3 tumors frequently progress to muscle invasion, however. This has been documented in 50% and 62% of cases,[6,12] with a 35% 10-year actuarial survival rate.[6]

Predicting the behavior of grade 2 tumors is less well defined. For all grade 2 tumors, between 18 and 33% are reported to progress, with a 10-year actuarial survival of 87%.[5,6] In an attempt to clarify the behavior of these heterogeneous tumors, Carbin et al.[11] subclassified them into 2a and 2b based on nuclear pleomorphism and the number of mitoses. When progression was assessed, grade 2a tumors faired much better, with a 92% 5-year survival compared with 43% for grade 2b. This prognostic discrimination has been demonstrated elsewhere.[13] Nuclear size (area) has also been used to stratify intermediate-grade tumors.[14]

The major criticism of multiple subclassifications for clinical application has been subjectivity. The subclassification of Carbin et al.[10] was demonstrated to be highly reproducible, with an interobserver agreement of 90%. However, inter- and intraobserver errors ranging from 50 to 87% have been reported for grade using reference pathologists in controlled trials.[15]

The categorization of grade becomes increasingly important for T1 tumors. This group has a much higher risk of progression to muscle invasion than Ta tumors. In a series of T1 tumors, 50% of grade 3 and 22% of grade 2 tumors progressed.[12]

Histologic Stage

Depth of tumor invasion was first included as a marker of outcome by Jewett and Strong.[16] It is now commonly used as a prognostic indicator and incorporated into staging systems including the current American Joint Committee on Cancer (AJCC) system.[17]

There is a significant difference in prognosis between Ta tumors, which are confined to the mucosa (not penetrating the basement membrane), and T1 tumors, which infiltrate the lamina propria. This difference has been documented for both tumor recurrence and progression. The difference in recurrence risk between the two stages is minimal. Grade, multiplicity, and size are more important in determining the recurrence rate.[18] However, the risk of stage progression is clearly higher for T1 tumors. Between 0 and 4% of Ta tumors and 27 to 46% of T1 tumors will progress to muscle invasion at 3 years.[12,19–22]

Long-term survival for Ta tumors is excellent. Ten-year survival rates are 95% for grade 1, 89% for grade 2, and 84% for grade 3 tumors.[23] Twenty-year cancer-specific survival for Ta tumors is 89%, compared with 30% for T1 tumors.[24]

Clearly, careful evaluation for lamina propria invasion is important. Muscularis mucosa is identifiable as a landmark in 70 to 80% of TUR specimens.[25] When absent, the larger arteries of the deep lamina propria are a useful landmark. The surgeon should attempt to minimize cautery artifact by using cold-cup biopsies or reducing the coagulation current. With papillary disease, the tumor base should be sampled carefully, submitting the underlying tissue as a separate specimen if necessary.

The significance of the depth of lamina propria invasion has varied mainly due to difficulties in identifying the muscularis mucosae. In a series with three review pathologists, the concurrence rate for depth of invasion was only 50%.[26] Despite this interobserver error, two series have used T1 subclassification and found it useful for prognostic discrimination. Younes and associates[27] used the presence of invasion to, and beyond, the muscularis mucosae to subclassify T1 tumors. Superficial invasion, termed T1a, had a 75% 5-year survival compared with 14% for deep invasion (T1b). Using the same classification system, Hassui and colleagues[25] reported a 7% progression rate for T1a, and 53% for T1b, independent of tumor grade, number, and size. The deep lamina propria is rich in lymphatics, and this may explain why it is an important factor in progression to deep muscle invasion. The practical role of T1 subclassification needs further study to clarify its clinical application.

Vascular and lymphatic invasion in general confer a poorer prognosis. In a study including Ta and T1 tumors, 7% had documented vascular or lymphatic invasion, with a 30% 6-year survival. These results were independent of grade.[23] Clearly, it is important to exclude muscularis propria invasion. If there is any doubt the urologist should re-resect the tumor site to be certain of the stage. In a series of 46 patients who had a second TUR within 2 weeks of their first resection, 43% demonstrated residual tumor in the deep resection.[28] Given the implication of muscle invasion, adequate tissue sampling to include muscle is essential.

Reproducibility of Grade and Stage

As indicated, there are limitations with the current staging and grading system for superficial tumors. This has implications for tailoring treatment for an individual patient, and for the analysis of prognostic factors in clinical trials.

Oomes et al.,[15] with seven review pathologists, reported a high inter- and intraobserver error of grade. A similar discrepancy in stage, with an intraobserver error of 50% has also been demonstrated.[18,29–31]

In reviewing a series of multicenter trials by the Dutch Uro-Oncology Group, which utilized review pathology, the error of grading was 30%, with a tendency for local pathologists to undergrade.[32] The error in T stage was 20%, with a tendency for local pathologists to overstage.

The same problem has been reported in interpreting biopsies of normal-appearing urothelium in patients with superficial tumors. In one study, biopsies reported as "dysplasia" were reproduced only 60% of the time.[33]

In randomized trials, such distortion of pathologic results is balanced in both treatment and control arms and hence does not have a major impact on the outcome of a study.[32] This variation becomes more significant, however, when comparing results between studies of "similar" pathologic stage. It also has an important implication in the management of an individual patient, particularly when identifying muscle-invasive disease. These limitations in staging and grading must be recognized. The important lesson is for the clinician to review the slides with the pathologist prior to any major treatment decision.

Status of Bladder Mucosa Distant from the Tumor

Any abnormality of the mucosa distant from the primary tumor provides prognostic information on recurrence rates. Recently, there has been increasing support for tumor cell implantation as one explanation for high recurrence rates.[34,35] In general, any abnormal appearing mucosa should be biopsied. A cold-cup technique is preferable, as it allows adequate tissue sampling without diathermy artifact. More controversial is the role of biopsy of normal-appearing mucosa. The incidence of associated changes in normal-appearing mucosa is between 10 and 50%.[5,36,37] Dysplasia is reported in approximately 15%,[38] with carcinoma in situ more variable (10 to 50%).[37] In general, CIS is more common with grade 3 tumors.[37] The incidence of concurrent CIS in the prostatic urethra is reported to be between 16 and 30%.[39,40] We believe that the magnification associated with videoendoscopy lessens the likelihood of CIS being found in "normal"-appearing bladder mucosa.

Less well defined is the accuracy and reproducibility of dysplasia reported in a biopsy, and the true risk of progression for dysplasia.[41–44] Progression for Ta and T1 tumors has been shown to increase from 8% to 30% when moderate or severe mucosal dysplasia was also present on biopsy.[5] Others have suggested that moderate dysplasia like mild dysplasia is not a risk factor.[41]

More widespread use of cytology and improved endoscopic optics, particularly video magnification, have reduced the role of mucosal biopsies. In an attempt to define the role of random biopsies in predicting recurrence and progression, Kiemeney et al.[38] demonstrated that random biopsies did not significantly influence patient outcome. Biopsies gave no additional information to predict tumor behavior beyond stage, grade, tumor size, and number.

Most patients with high-grade tumor will receive adjuvant treatment, regardless of the information from mucosal biopsies. Therefore, we infrequently perform mucosal bladder biopsies outside of clinical trials.

ENDOSCOPIC FEATURES

The number of primary tumors is a strong predictor of recurrence. The presence of two or more tumors increases the recurrence rate approximately twofold, and decreases the time to first recurrence.[5,45–48] Heney et al.[5] showed that the recurrence rate for multiple tumors increased from 18% to 43% for Ta disease and from 33% to 46% for T1 disease. Multiple primary tumors are also associated with a tendency for increasing grade with recurrence.[48] There is an approximately 1.5-times increased risk of progression for multiple tumors.[12,45] Tumor size is also a predictor of recurrence and progression.[48,49] The risk of stage progression increases from 9% to 35% for tumors greater than 5 cm.[5]

The time to first recurrence is also prognostic. A recurrence or new occurrence at 3 months has been shown to increase the risk of subsequent recurrence from 20% to between 70% and 85%.[47,48] This emphasizes the importance of the disease status at the first follow-up cystoscopy.[18]

CYTOLOGIC PROGNOSTIC FACTORS

Urine Cytology

Urinary cytology performed on exfoliated urothelial cells in urine or bladder washings can be used to detect TCC. Care must be taken with specimen collection and handling to preserve exfoliated cells and avoid bacterial contamination.

The yield for diagnosis of low-grade tumors is low, generally less than 30%.[50] Recognition of subtle malignant features requires a skilled cytopathologist. However, cytology is highly sensitive for high-grade disease for both CIS and papillary tumors. Greater than 60% of papillary tumors and 90% of cases of CIS have positive cytology. The reduced cellular adherence of high-grade tumors results in a higher proportion of cells shed into the urine and thus detectable with cytology. This complements cytoscopy in the detection of high-grade TCC. Bladder wash cytology may provide more information on the presence or absence of CIS than random biopsies.

It is important to provide relevant clinical history for accurate interpretation by the cytopathologist.

In addition to identifying the method of specimen collection, it is important to note any history of previous treatment (radiation, chemotherapy, or immunotherapy), urinary infection, stones, recent surgery, or catheterization. All of these conditions may produce cells with nuclear features that may be confused with malignancy.[51]

The interpretation of a positive urine cytology requires knowledge of tumor status of the bladder. The absence of cancer in the bladder requires exclusion of CIS or high-grade disease in the upper tracts or prostatic urethra. Cytology also has a valuable role in follow-up of high-grade superficial tumors.

DNA Ploidy

DNA ploidy as assessed by flow cytometry has been used to assess transitional cell carcinoma. In general, all grade 1 and most grade 2 tumors are diploid. Some grade 2 tumors are tetraploid, while others, and most grade 3 tumors, are nontetraploid aneuploid.[52] Variation in DNA content within a tumor is a significant limitation in the application of ploidy studies.

There is a correlation between ploidy and tumor behavior. Of 229 grade 1 and 2 superficial tumors, Gustafson et al.[53] showed that none of the diploid tumors progressed, while 35% of the aneuploid tumors progressed with a 21% death rate. Aneuploid tumors have also been shown to recur more frequently.[54]

There is conflicting evidence as to the ability of ploidy to independently predict progression over grade alone.[55,56] Ploidy remains expensive, and has yet to establish a clinical role. We do not use this in decision-making.

BIOLOGIC PROGNOSTIC MARKERS

Blood Group Antigens

There has been long-standing recognition of the prognostic importance of the loss or absence of blood group antigens from the tumor cell surface.[57,58] This can be assessed by immunohistochemistry or red-cell adherence tests. However, the results are usually qualitative and the methodology subjective. The result is also dependent on the patient's blood group, with group O being prone to false-negative results.

An increased risk for progression has been documented with loss of antigen expression.[58] This information appears to be independent of grade and stage.[59] There is also an association with tumor recurrence rate[60] and response to bacille Calmette-Guérin (BCG) treatment.[61]

Other cell surface antigens have also been correlated with prognosis. These include the Lewis surface antigens and the Thompson-Friedenreich antigen.[62,63] Advances in immunostaining with monoclonal antibodies have allowed assessment of these antigens in urine, with improved sensitivity and specificity.[64] They have not as yet found a role in clinical practice.

Tumor Cell Products

There have been numerous cell proteins that appear to correlate with tumor behavior. They perform various functions, but often act as cell receptors. These include desmosomal glycoprotein[65]; transferrin receptor[66]; and human milk fat globulin.[67] Epidermal growth factor (EGF) receptor and basement membrane tissues have been more extensively studied.

EGF receptor is reported to be an independent predictor for stage progression in Ta and T1 tumors.[68] In addition, an increased recurrence rate from 7% to 17% has been noted for receptor-positive patients.[69] This marker would appear to have potential clinical application on the basis of results to date.

Various connective tissue components of the basement membrane have been studied as potential markers. The loss of laminin and type IV collagen in the basement membrane underlying noninvasive tumors correlates with increasing tumor progression.[70]

Cytogenic and Molecular Genetic Markers

Although the majority of invasive bladder tumors commonly contain nondiploid and morphologically abnormal DNA, most superficial tumors are near diploid. Sandberg[71] first identified abnormal DNA in Ta and T1 tumors, and demonstrated a relationship with risk of recurrence and progression. Chromosomal analysis for solid tumors has been simplified with the development of specific probes such as fluorescent in situ hybridization (FISH) for DNA sequence analysis. RNA amino acid sequencing with polymerase chain reaction (PCR) has also contributed to the understanding of TCC. Both FISH and PCR can be performed on paraffin sections.

Specific chromosomal abnormalities for bladder cancer have been identified on chromosomes 1, 5, 7, 9, 11, and 17.[72–75] Abnormalities of chromosome 7 include alteration to the c-*erb* B oncogene, which codes for the EGF receptor.

Loss of heterozygosity at chromosomes 9q, 11p, and 17p correlates with known tumor suppressor genes, namely the Wilms' tumor gene (WTG) and p53.[73,76,77] Studies on the role of oncogenes and carcinogenesis have traditionally used rodent tumors, particularly the *ras* family.[78–80] Unfortunately, it has not proven useful in the study of human TCC.

Promising results have been demonstrated

through molecular genetic work with oncogenes. The p53 oncogene (17p13-1 locus) codes for a nuclear phosphoprotein whose major role appears to be in transcriptional regulation. p53 is involved in DNA repair or induction of apoptosis for irreversibly damaged DNA. Hence, it is thought to function as a tumor suppressor gene.[81] There are two forms of this gene product—the wild, or unaltered type, and the mutant form.[82] Mutation of wild type results in the accumulation of mutant p53 protein within the tumor cell nucleus, due to a prolonged half-life. This leads to alterations in modulating activity.[83] Mutant p53 can be easily detected immunohistochemically using monoclonal antibodies on fresh or fixed tumor specimens.[84] Immunohistochemical changes have been shown to correspond to abnormalities with DNA sequence analysis.[85–88] It must be recognized that the limitation of monoclonal immunohistochemistry is false-negative results,[89] although this is reduced with the monoclonal antibody Pab-1801.[89]

Changes in p53 are the most commonly recognized genetic alterations in human malignancy, and correlate with tumor behavior.[90] Mutations have been observed in 50% of high-stage bladder tumors.[85–87,91]

However, p53 changes and their relationship to tumor behavior in superficial tumors are less clear. Studies have utilized both immunohistochemistry and nucleic acid sequence analysis for assessment of Tis, Ta, and T1 tumors. Mutations have been observed in up to 65% of biopsies of primary Tis (pTis).[92] Positivity for p53 has been demonstrated as an independent predictor of progression in a series of 33 pTis patients followed for 124 months.[89]

The results for Ta and T1 disease are more variable. Positive mutant p53 staining has ranged between 8 and 95%,[85,93–97] with a strong correlation between positivity and tumor grade.[94,95,98] Several recent institutional reviews of Ta and T1 tumors utilizing multivariate analysis have demonstrated p53 status as a statistically significant prognostic factor for progression-free and overall survival.[99,100] The disparity between numerous investigators is difficult to explain. Technical factors may play a role. In summary, the oncogene p53 is an encouraging prognostic marker for bladder cancer. Its clinical role in superficial disease will remain unclear until further large series with multivariate analyses are performed.

The overexpression of other oncogenes, c-*erb* B-2 and c-*myc*, has also been observed and is more frequently in high-grade, high-stage TCC.[101–103] Their role in superficial TCC has not been defined.

INTRAVESICAL THERAPY

Rationale

The high incidence of subsequent tumors after initial TUR, whether true recurrences or new occurrences, has led to the use of intravesical instillation of antineoplastic agents. This form of treatment can be used either therapeutically, to eradicate residual tumor after an incomplete TUR, or prophylactically, after all visible tumor has been resected and urinary cytology, if performed, is negative. Intravesical therapy can be subdivided into chemotherapy and immunotherapy. The decision to use intravesical treatment is dependent on numerous factors including tumor stage, grade, size and multiplicity; the presence of CIS or positive urinary cytology; the side-effect profile of each agent; and other patient-specific factors (Table 17–2). Economic factors may also play a part in the decision process.

The ideal intravesical agent would have an antitumor effect against TCC, show no phase specificity in the cell cycle, and have limited systemic and local toxicity on an acute and chronic basis. Much of the systemic toxicity associated with intravesical therapy is due to drug absorption. Factors associated with increased absorption include low molecular weight of the instilled drug, temporal relationship to the TUR, and extent of resection. Local toxicity with intravesical therapy is frequent and usually consists of irritative voiding symptoms or hematuria.[104] Delaying the initiation of intravesical therapy for 10 or more days after resection will allow healing of the resected urothelium and may lessen the local side effects.

Increasing exposure of the urothelium to the intravesical agent would seem to be important. This can be done by increasing the concentration and contact time of the drug. Some advocate asking the patient to lie in the prone position for part of the treatment.[105] Others suggest that sterile water, instead of saline, as the diluent decreases the osmolality of the solution, thereby increasing the intracellular concentration of the drug.[106]

Recommended dosages, administration schedule, and duration of intravesical therapy have varied and are largely based on empiric data. Patients who receive intravesical therapy should be monitored for response. This includes endoscopy and bladder wash cytology. Appropriate end-points include recurrence, time to recurrence, progression in grade or stage, and time to progression. Patients are monitored for response 3 months after initiation of treatment. A complete response to treatment is defined as no tumor on endoscopy, negative cytology, and negative bladder biopsies. Anything less than a

TABLE 17–2. INDICATIONS FOR INTRAVESICAL THERAPY

Cumulative tumor size >5 cm
Multiple tumors
Multiple recurrences
Stage T1 or high-grade TCC
CIS or positive cytology
Incomplete tumor resection

complete response is considered a treatment failure, as partial responders have the same incidence of progression as nonresponders.[107]

If any question exists as to the persistence of tumor, resection or biopsy is performed. In the face of a positive biopsy or cytology after intravesical treatment, it is less likely that another course with the same agent will be effective, and an alternative treatment should be used. BCG may be an exception, as a second 6-week course is beneficial in some instances.[108,109] The stage and grade of the tumor recurrence will ultimately be the determinant of future treatment (e.g., cystectomy, TUR alone).[110]

Intravesical Chemotherapy

Thiotepa

Thiotepa is an antineoplastic alkylating agent related to nitrogen mustard that has been shown to eradicate existing tumors and delay the development of new tumors.[111] The usual dosage is 30 to 60 mg in 30 to 60 ml of distilled water. The National Bladder Cancer Study Group found that the complete response rate for 30 mg was equal to that for 60 mg. Hence the lower dose is recommended.[112] Duration of treatment is usually weekly for 6 to 8 weeks when given therapeutically and weekly for 4 to 6 weeks when given prophylactically. If maintenance is given, a monthly schedule is usually selected. A randomized cooperative study by the Medical Research Council found no statistically significant difference in tumor recurrence rates in patients receiving (1) no intravesical therapy, (2) a single instillation of thiotepa at the time of resection, or (3) a single thiotepa instillation at the initial resection and 3-month intervals for a total of five treatments in a year. Median follow-up was almost 9 years.[113] Thus, it appears that it is necessary to give more than five treatments of thiotepa in a year to make a significant difference in tumor recurrence.

When used as a therapeutic agent, complete response rates of 35 to 45% have been reported.[114,115] Long-term use of thiotepa prophylaxis was evaluated by the National Bladder Cancer Collaborative Group.[112] They reported that 53% of patients were tumor free at 2 years compared to only 27% of untreated patients. The benefits were only noted in patients with grade 1 lesions (51% treated with thiotepa were tumor free at 2 years versus 14% of the control group). Recurrence rates of grade 2 and 3 tumors were not significantly different than controls, suggesting that thiotepa is most effective in treating patients with low-grade tumors.

Due to thiotepa's low molecular weight (189 Da), it is absorbed more than any other intravesical agent. Myelosuppression occurs in up to 9% of patients, usually in the form of leukopenia or thrombocytopenia. Thus, white blood cell and platelet counts must be monitored during the course of therapy. In a study of 670 patients, Soloway and Ford found that only 4% of patients suffered this side effect and none of the consequences were severe.[116] Cystitis is relatively rare, but as with other intravesical agents, can be severe. Overall, thiotepa is relatively safe and inexpensive, and is most effective for low-grade tumors. We believe it is a reasonable choice for prophylaxis in patients with multiple, recurrent grade 1, Ta bladder tumors.

Mitomycin C

Mitomycin C (MMC) is a 329-kDa antitumor antibiotic. There has never been a thorough dose-response study with MMC. Most studies have used from 20 to 40 mg in 20 to 40 ml of water, weekly, for 8 weeks. Many studies have used MMC for residual TCC after incomplete resection (i.e., treatment rather than prophylaxis). Most patients in these studies were at high risk for recurrence, having a history of prior TCC. A study by the National Bladder Cancer Group involved treatment with 40 mg of MMC for 8 consecutive weeks.[117] The study included 117 patients with CIS or grade I to III Ta or T1 disease. Each patient had failed a course of intravesical thiotepa. At 3 months, 27% of patients had a complete response as defined by negative endoscopy, biopsy, and cytology. Another 9% had negative endoscopy and cytology but were not rebiopsied. Despite a negative endoscopy, an additional 12% were not considered complete responders, since their cytology was positive. Overall, 18% of patients with T1 disease, 29% with Ta disease, and 35% with CIS were rendered tumor free.

The National Bladder Cancer Collaborative Group also compared MMC and thiotepa for treatment of TCC.[118] Study participants received either 40 mg of MMC in 40 ml or 30 mg of thiotepa in 30 ml of sterile water weekly for 8 weeks. MMC patients had a statistically significant higher complete response rate (39% versus 27% with thiotepa, $p = .02$). Ta grade 1 tumors responded best as in previously reported thiotepa studies.

Soloway[119] reported a series of 80 patients who received 8 weekly 40-mg instillations of MMC for treatment with evaluation for response at 12 weeks. All complete and some partial responders received monthly MMC for 1 year. Average follow-up was 40 months. Complete responses were noted in 37% (15 of 41) of Ta patients, 33% (7 of 21) of CIS patients, and 44% (8 of 18) of T1 patients. Twenty-six per cent of patients eventually had a cystectomy and 15% developed muscle invasion. Nine per cent (7 of 80) of the patients eventually died of bladder cancer.

The initial response to MMC was predictive of the patient's eventual outcome. Of those who had persistent TCC at 3 months, 34% later required cystectomy compared to only 13% of initial complete responders. Death from carcinoma of the bladder occurred in 12% of early treatment failures compared to only 3% of initial complete responders. It thus may be prudent to consider cystectomy for patients with high-grade TCC who do not have a complete response with intravesical treatment.

Huland et al.[120] reported a randomized prospective study of MMC used for prophylaxis. Patients received either 20 mg of MMC in 20 ml every other week for up to 18 months or had a TUR alone. Only 10% of MMC-treated patients recurred compared to 51% of controls.

Maier et al.[121] reported a study of 63 patients who received MMC prophylaxis over a 2-year period. The mean follow-up was 50 months. Fifty-two per cent developed a recurrence. One third (21 of 63) failed while receiving MMC. Of the remaining 42 patients, 26% recurred at an average of 14 months after MMC was discontinued. The remaining 31 patients (48% of the original 63) remained tumor free at a mean 26 months after MMC was completed.

The Medical Research Council has recently reported the 7-year follow-up of a 502-patient randomized multicenter trial involving the use of early instillation of MMC. After complete resection of Ta and T1 tumors, patients were randomized to receive either no further treatment until the next endoscopy, a single instillation of 40 mg MMC within 24 hours of resection, or an instillation within 24 hours of resection and at 3-month intervals for 1 year (five total doses). They found that the overall recurrence rates were lower and the interval to recurrence prolonged in patients receiving one or five instillations of MMC compared to controls. The estimated 5-year reduction in recurrence risk was 15% and 23% for the one- and five-dose regimens, respectively.[122]

Due to MMC's molecular weight, systemic toxicity is rare. Local symptoms, primarily chemical cystitis, are relatively common (10 to 17%).[117,120,123] A desquamating rash of the palms and genitalia is unique to MMC. It occurs in approximately 5% of patients and is thought to be a form of contact dermatitis.[104,119] Occasionally, the rash is diffuse. Severe bladder contracture requiring cystectomy (4%) has also been reported.[120] Myelosuppression is rare.[104,119,124]

In summation, MMC appears to be more effective than thiotepa. The toxicity of MMC is acceptable. The widespread use of MMC as a first-line therapy, however, is limited in the United States by its cost.

Doxorubicin

Best known as a systemic chemotherapeutic drug, this antitumor antibiotic has been shown to be an active intravesical agent. Doxorubicin is a 580-kDa intercalating agent. The vast majority of the literature comes from Japan, where doxorubicin is the most frequently used intravesical agent. The doses varied widely from 10 to 100 mg at various intervals. Therefore, there is no standard dose.

There have been a number of randomized studies using doxorubicin for prophylaxis. Niijima et al. reported findings from a randomized study of doxorubicin (30 mg in 30 ml twice weekly for 4 weeks) plus TUR versus TUR alone.[125] At a minimum 12 months' follow-up, 70% (104 of 149) of patients receiving doxorubicin were recurrence free compared to 55% (77 of 139) who had a TUR alone. Kurth et al.[126] found that 64% (58 of 86) of patients randomized to receive doxorubicin (50 mg in 30 ml weekly for 1 month then monthly for 1 year) in addition to TUR were recurrence free versus 52% (39 of 69) in the control group. Doxorubicin was not shown to be superior to thiotepa for prevention of superficial tumor recurrence in other controlled double-blind studies.[127,128]

In a randomized trial comparing the efficacy of doxorubicin and BCG for CIS, Lamm et al. reported a 34% complete response (CR) rate for doxorubicin. Median length of time to failure was 5 months. BCG was superior for treatment of CIS.[129] Others have demonstrated up to a 70% CR rate with doxorubicin, but follow-up was short.[130]

Due to doxorubicin's high molecular weight, absorption is low and myelosuppression rare. Cystitis is the primary toxicity, occurring in 25% of patients.[104,124,131] Diminished bladder capacity occurs in up to 9% of patients and anaphylactic reactions have been seen.[104,130] Overall, doxorubicin has been shown to be an effective agent for treatment and prophylaxis of TCC.

AD-32

AD-32 (*N*-trifluoroacetyladriamycin-14-valerate), an anthracycline derivative, is a semisynthetic analogue of doxorubicin. AD-32 (MW 723) differs from doxorubicin (Adriamycin) in that it lacks cardiotoxicity, is associated with less local toxicity, and it is lipophilic. AD-32 does not bind DNA but is an active inhibitor of DNA and RNA synthesis.[132] Preliminary studies have focused on treating patients with CIS or superficial disease who failed BCG. Phase 1 trials of patients treated with AD-32 have been completed. Of the 35 courses given, 69% had some local toxicity, 31% grade 2 or 3. Irritative voiding symptoms accounted for all but three adverse events. Reducing the alcohol content in the diluent decreased these symptoms. Three patients had hematuria, one severe. There was negligible systemic absorption.[133]

The first treatment group consisted of 32 patients, 7 with CIS, 25 with papillary TCC. At a mean follow-up of 24 months (range 12 to 27), 2 of 7 (29%) patients with CIS and 7 of 24 (29%) patients with TCC had a complete response. One patient was lost to follow-up.[133] Further trials for patients with BCG-refractory CIS are in progress.

Immunotherapy

Bacille Calmette-Guérin

Since BCG was initially identified as an effective intravesical agent for superficial bladder cancer, much has been learned about its actions. Still more remains to be elucidated.[134] BCG is a live attenuated tuberculosis organism first developed from cultures at the Pasteur Institute of Lille.[135] Its mechanism of action remains ill defined, but at least part of its effectiveness is due to an immunologic host response. T-cell–deprived animals do not respond to BCG. Furthermore, BCG must bind to urothelial cells to be active and binds by attaching to fibronectin.[136] An immunologic cascade of events occurs causing a strong inflammatory response. The inflammatory response itself may have a deleterious effect on tumor cells. In addition, various cytokines are released including interleukins, which have known antineoplastic activity.[134,136]

The urologic literature is replete with reports on the efficacy of BCG. There is marked variability. This variability may be due to differences in the completeness of resection, tumor stage and grade, prior history of TCC, prior intravesical therapy, associated CIS, the number of instillations, the BCG substrain used, host immunologic factors, and length of follow-up.

The optimal schedule for BCG administration has yet to be established. The number of milligrams per colony count differs among the numerous BCG substrains. The concept of six weekly instillations is arbitrary. An induction phase is necessary for the development of the immunologic response in the bladder. While most patients develop an inflammatory response with six instillations, some will require fewer and some may require more.[137] Studies have shown that 19 to 26% of patients treated who do not respond to an initial 6-week course of BCG will respond to six additional weekly doses.[108,109] Maintenance therapy is also controversial. Early studies showed no clear benefit to maintenance BCG to justify the increased risk of side effects.[137] However, Lamm et al. recently reported results of a randomized, prospective Southwest Oncology Group (SWOG) trial of maintenance BCG for CIS, Ta, and T1 disease. After a 6-week induction course, patients received BCG in three weekly doses at 3 months, 6 months, and every 6 months for 3 years. In this study, maintenance therapy further reduced the tumor recurrence rate.[138] However, the optimal timing of these maintenance doses whether monthly, 3-monthly, or even yearly has not been established.

BCG for CIS

The literature strongly supports the use of BCG for treatment of CIS. Complete response rates of 70% have been reported.[139–142] Dejager et al. reported on 123 patients from six phase II studies. Patients received at least six weekly instillations of Tice BCG and 12 monthly maintenance doses. A 76% complete remission rate was reported, including a 71% (45 of 63) CR rate for patients who failed intravesical chemotherapy. A durable CR was seen in 50% of responders at a mean follow-up of 48 months. Only 11% of responders subsequently required cystectomy, versus 55% of nonresponders. However, no survival difference was noted between responders and nonresponders.[141] Lamm et al., in the aforementioned randomized study of BCG versus doxorubicin for CIS, reported a 70% CR rate for BCG versus 34% for doxorubucin. The mean interval to treatment failure was 39 months for BCG compared to 5 months for doxorubicin.[129]

BCG for Prophylaxis

Several randomized studies have compared the efficacy of TUR alone versus TUR plus BCG. Herr recently summarized the results of five such studies encompassing 437 patients. Overall, 70% of patients who received BCG prophylaxis were tumor free compared to 31% of patients who had TUR alone. Follow-up ranged from 12 to 60 months.[142]

To address the impact of BCG on disease progression, Herr et al. reviewed the 10-year follow-up of 86 patients with recurrent Ta, T1, and Tis disease, who were randomized to either TUR plus 6 weeks of Armand-Frappier BCG or TUR alone. Crossover was available for patients in the TUR group who recurred. The 10-year progression-free and overall survival were 62% and 75%, respectively, for patients who received BCG and 37% and 55% for patients who had a TUR alone. The median progression-free survival was not reached for the BCG group and was 46 months for the "control" group. Fifteen of 18 patients who crossed over and received BCG did not have tumor progression. The authors concluded that BCG delayed both tumor progression and death in patients with superficial bladder cancer.[143]

BCG has also been compared to the most commonly used intravesical chemotherapeutic agents. Brosman and Martinez-Pineiro, in separate studies, found BCG to be superior to thiotepa in reducing tumor recurrence.[109,144,145] Lamm et al. reported the results of a Southwest Oncology Group comparison of BCG and doxorubicin in patients with rapidly recurring superficial TCC. The mean interval to recurrence in the patients with papillary tumors receiving BCG was 22 months versus 10 months in patients receiving doxorubicin.[146]

Vegt et al.[147] recently reported the results of a randomized prospective study of 435 patients with pTa or pT1 disease comparing the efficacy of Tice BCG, RIVM-BCG, and mitomycin C. Mean follow-up was 36 months. Patients underwent TUR followed by either 6 weeks of Tice or RIVM-BCG or 4 weeks of MMC followed by monthly doses for 6 months. Results are shown in Table 17–3. They concluded that MMC was equivalent to BCG in efficacy. Drug-induced cystitis, the most common local toxicity, and systemic side effects were significantly less in the MMC group.

In regard to T1 disease, Eure et al.[109] reported a series of 30 patients with high-grade T1 disease treated with a 6-week course of Armand-Frappier

TABLE 17–3. RANDOMIZED TRIAL OF TICE AND RIVM BCG AND MMC*

	Tice BCG	RIVM-BCG	MMC
Recurrence Ta/T1	75 of 117 (64%)	62 of 134 (46%)	58 of 136 (43%)
Recurrence CIS	17 of 23 (74%)	9 of 15 (60%)	8 of 12 (67%)
Progression at recurrence	7 (5%)	8 (6%)	8 (6%)

*From Vegt PDJ, Witjes JA, Witjes WPJ, et al: A randomized study of intravesical mitomycin C, bacillus Calmette-Guérin Tice and bacillus Calmette-Guérin RIVM treatment in pTa-pT1 papillary carcinoma and carcinoma in situ of the bladder. J Urol 1995; 153:929, with permission.

BCG. After one course, 47% (14 of 30) had a negative cytology and biopsy at 6 months. Another six patients responded to a second 6-week course, for an overall CR rate of 66%. Four patients required a cystectomy for progression or recurrent T1 tumor, and one patient had metastasis. All had failed a first course of BCG. Thus, the overall progression rate was 17%.

Cookson and Sarosdy studied BCG for T1 disease in 86 patients. Patients underwent TUR prior to receiving a 6-week course of Pasteur BCG. Some patients received booster doses at 3, 6, and 12 months. Patients with recurrence had a repeat TUR followed by additional BCG either weekly or monthly. At a median follow-up of 59 months (range 9 to 149), 91% were disease free. Of the 91%, 69% responded to the initial induction course and 22% were recurrence free after re-resection and additional BCG. Progression to T2 disease occurred in only 7% of patients. They concluded that BCG was effective in the treatment of T1 tumors.[148] Some patients in their study, however, were listed as having grade 1, T1 tumors. Grade 1, T1 disease rarely, if ever, exists. This underscores the importance of pathology review.

Nadler et al.[149] reported that 23 of 66 (35%) patients who were disease free 2 years after treatment with BCG had tumor recurrence after 2 to 11 years of follow-up. Thus, lifelong monitoring after BCG is essential even with an excellent initial response to treatment.

Cystitis is the most common side effect of BCG, occurring in up to 90% of patients. Hematuria occurs in up to one third of patients and can be problematic. Major adverse reactions include fever over 103°F (3%), granulomatous prostatitis (0.9%), and pneumonitis or hepatitis (0.7%). BCG sepsis, the most serious complication, occurs in 0.4% of patients. Thus far, ten deaths from BCG sepsis have been reported. Caution should be used in administering BCG to patients who are immunocompromised or have liver disease. Treatment depends on the clinical situation but includes isoniazid 300 mg and rifampin 600 mg daily. In advanced cases, ethambutol 1200 mg daily is useful. Cycloserine 250 to 500 mg twice daily in combination with isoniazid and rifampin should be used if the patient is septic. In addition, the coadministration of antituberculin agents with BCG to lessen side effects of treatment has been proposed.[150]

Interferon

Interferons (IFN) are biologic response modifiers that are integrally associated with the immunologic cascade. IFN has antiproliferative and antiviral properties. It stimulates macrophage function, enhances natural killer (NK) cell cytolytic activity, and activates B and T lymphocytes.[151]

The success of IFN alfa-2b has been limited in several previously reported series of superficial TCC.[152] The Northern California Oncology Group reported that 4 of 16 patients (25%) with superficial TCC had a CR with intravesical recombinant IFN alfa-2b. In the same study, 6 of 19 patients with CIS had a CR. Of the ten CRs in the study, five were durable at 18 to 37 months.[153]

Glashan reported on a series of 87 patients with CIS. Patients received either high-dose (100 million units) or low-dose (10 million units) IFN alfa-2b, weekly for 12 weeks, then monthly up to a year. In the high-dose group, 20 of 47 (43%) had a CR compared to only 2 of 38 (5%) in the low-dose group. Interestingly, six of nine patients who failed a course of BCG had a CR with IFN alfa-2b. Seven patients in each group eventually required a cystectomy, 13 for disease progression. The median interval to cystectomy was 32 weeks for the high-dose group and 18 weeks for the low-dose group. The primary toxicity was a flulike syndrome occurring in 17% of high-dose and 8% of low-dose patients. Local symptoms did not occur and no patient discontinued therapy due to side effects.[154] The expense of high-dose intravesical interferon, however, has limited its use.

Keyhole-Limpet Hemocyanin

Keyhole-limpet hemocyanin (KLH) is a high-molecular-weight immunogenic protein collected from the hemolymph of the mollusk *Megathura crenulata*. In humans, KLH induces both cell-mediated and humoral responses. KLH was initially used as a skin test to evaluate delayed-type hypersensitivity responses in humans.[152]

Olsson first reported the use of KLH immunotherapy for superficial TCC of the bladder. Patients immunized with KLH were noted to have fewer tumor recurrences.[155] In a prospective trial of 19 patients with a history of superficial TCC, prophylactic KLH injections were given after TUR. Of the nine immunized patients, only one had a recurrence over 204 patient-months. In the nonimmunized group, seven of ten had a recurrence over 228 patient-months.

In a randomized controlled study, Jurinic et al. found that KLH was more effective than MMC in prophylaxis against recurrent TCC. KLH (10 mg) was given intravesically following a 1-mg intracutaneous dose. Twenty-three patients received 20 mg of intravesical MMC. Fourteen per cent of KLH patients recurred compared to 39% in the MMC group.[156] In a subsequent nonrandomized single-arm study, Jurinic reported that 17 of 81 patients (21%) had recurrence of TCC after the same KLH regimen. No adverse effects were reported.[152,156]

Bropirimine

Bropirimine is a pyrimidinone that induces interferon, presumably leading to antineoplastic and immunomodulatory activity.[157] Bropirimine is a unique agent for urothelial neoplasms, since it can be given orally. In a phase I trial for treatment of CIS and papillary TCC, Sarosdy et al. reported that 6 of 26 evaluable patients had a CR at 3 months. Five of 11 patients with CIS had a CR. The drug was most effective when given at high doses, 3 g/day for 3 consecutive days, weekly for 12 weeks. Only one of ten papillary tumors regressed completely.[158]

In a subsequent phase II trial using high-dose bropirimine, 20 of 39 patients (51%) with CIS had a CR. This included 6 of 13 patients (46%) who were BCG failures. CRs lasted as long as 17 months. Flulike symptoms were the most common adverse effect, occurring in 62% of patients.[159] Further phase II trials of bropirimine alone and in combination with BCG are in progress.

Recommendations

From the above data it is clear that BCG plus TUR is more beneficial than TUR alone for patients with high-grade TCC and T1 disease. Furthermore, BCG has been shown to prolong the interval to progression, while intravesical chemotherapy has not. BCG or MMC appears to be the agent of choice for CIS.

For recurrent, low-grade Ta tumors, the optimal treatment is less clear. The likelihood of progression to muscle-invasive disease is very low (<5%). We recommend either no adjuvant therapy or intravesical chemotherapy. In this situation, the role of intravesical chemotherapy would be to prolong the tumor-free interval and decrease the cost and morbidity of frequent surgical procedures. Some studies show no significant difference between BCG and chemotherapy for low-grade, low-stage disease,[139] and as described above, the side-effect profile of BCG is not insignificant. Thus we do not suggest BCG for grade 1 TCC.

For grade 2 or 3 Ta tumors treatment should be individualized based on recurrence patterns. Either BCG or intravesical therapy may be appropriate in these situations. If intravesical chemotherapy fails, BCG would be a reasonable next step. If a patient were to fail a course of BCG, a second 6-week course could be considered. This may help avoid the morbidity of cystectomy in a subgroup of patients. Yet, this delay may allow disease progression and loss of curability with radical treatment. Herr et al. reported a series of 61 patients with high-grade superficial bladder cancer who were initially treated with BCG. At a follow-up ranging from 10 to 13 years, 12 patients (20%) died of metastatic urothelial cancer.[160] Thus in many cases, despite diligent follow-up, patients progress and die of bladder cancer.

Biologic immune response modifiers other than BCG have been used to treat TCC. These cytokines can be administered orally or intravesically. Their mechanisms of action are not clearly defined. A host response appears to be central to their efficacy. Further elucidation of the mechanism of action of these agents, as well as controlled studies of various drug combinations at various doses, will better define their role in the treatment of Ta and T1 TCC and CIS.

TRANSITIONAL CELL CARCINOMA OF THE PROSTATIC URETHRA

TCC of the prostatic urethra is usually found concomitant with or subsequent to TCC of the bladder. It is rarely primary.[161] Analysis of cystoprostatectomy specimens has identified TCC of the prostate in 10 to 50% of cases.[162,163] Involvement is more common with high-grade bladder tumors, occurring in 70% of men with primary CIS of the bladder.[164] Since the presence of TCC of the prostate may alter the treatment strategy, a TUR biopsy of the floor of the prostatic urethra should be performed in all men with high-grade TCC of the bladder.[162]

The management and prognosis of TCC of the prostatic urethra depend on stage and grade. Although the UICC staging system indicates that all TCC of the prostate is stage T4, it seems prudent to substratify patients based upon involvement of the prostatic urethra, ducts, or stroma.[165] The prognosis for prostatic mucosal CIS and ductal involvement differs from that of stromal invasion.

Treatment of TCC of the prostatic urethra must take into consideration the status of the bladder (i.e., current TCC or prior history of TCC and treatment). Therapeutic options include intravesical chemotherapy, immunotherapy, or cystoprostatectomy (Fig. 17–1). BCG has been the most widely

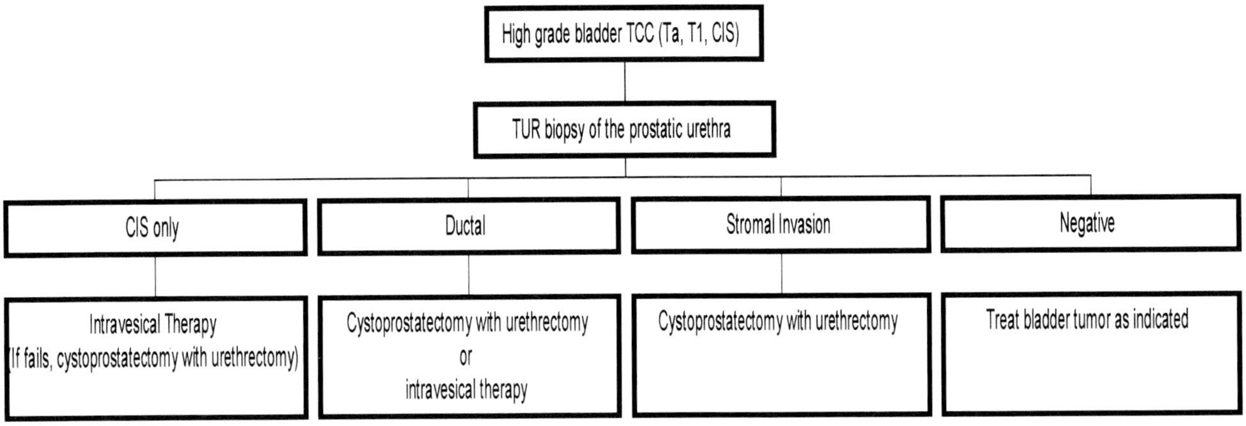
High grade bladder TCC (Ta, T1, CIS)
TUR biopsy of the prostatic urethra
CIS only
Ductal
Stromal Invasion
Negative
Intravesical Therapy
(If fails, cystoprostatectomy with urethrectomy)
Cystoprostatectomy with urethrectomy
or
intravesical therapy
Cystoprostatectomy with urethrectomy
Treat bladder tumor as indicated

FIGURE 17–1. Algorithm for evaluation and treatment of prostatic urethral TCC. (From Matzkin H, Soloway MS, Hardeman S: Transitional cell carcinoma of the prostate. J Urol 1991; 146:1210, with permission.)

studied agent for topical therapy. Initial concerns about obtaining effective contact with the prostatic urethra arose from observations of recurrence in the prostatic urethra after BCG therapy for TCC of the bladder.[166,167] However, bladder neck incompetence following TUR would seem to allow adequate tissue contact for treatment. For disease confined to the prostatic urethra, several series have documented CRs using BCG.[168,169]

Cystoprostatectomy is recommended for most cases of TCC involving the prostatic ducts or stroma.[162] Concurrent urethrectomy is recommended because there is a 30 to 50% risk of urethral recurrence.[170] The prognosis for urethral involvement relates to disease stage,[171] with high-T-stage lesions associated with a grim outcome.

PARTIAL AND RADICAL CYSTECTOMY

With the current efficacy of quality endoscopic instruments and multiple intravesical agents, the majority of patients with superficial bladder cancer will not require radical surgery. The indications for cystectomy include failed intravesical therapy for high-grade disease (papillary or CIS), persisting or recurrent high-grade tumor, or progression to bladder muscle or prostatic stromal invasion (Table 17–4). Persistently positive urine cytology after intravesical treatment requires a thorough re-evaluation of the bladder, in addition to reassessment of the upper tracts and the prostatic urethra in men. Localization and accurate restaging is necessary before considering cystectomy.

TABLE 17–4. INDICATIONS FOR CYSTECTOMY FOR SUPERFICIAL BLADDER CANCER

Persistent or recurrent high-grade papillary tumor
Persistent or recurrent CIS
Progression to muscularis propria or prostatic stromal invasion
TCC involving prostatic ducts

Cystectomy should also be strongly considered when pathologic understaging is suspected. Hydronephrosis associated with a bladder tumor usually indicates muscle invasion. Staging error rates as high as 55% have been reported for T2 tumors.[172,173] This reinforces the importance of careful pathologic review of all biopsy material.

Consideration should be given to concurrent urethrectomy with cystectomy if there is widespread multifocal CIS, involvement of the prostatic urethra in men, or bladder neck and trigone in women. This probably precludes orthotopic urinary reconstruction to the urethra for these individuals, although some suggest that this is not an absolute contraindication with limited prostatic urethral involvement.

Partial cystectomy has a limited role. There is a subgroup of superficial tumors in which this may be considered, such as tumors within bladder diverticulae. Diverticulectomy should be performed with care to obtain adequate surgical margins and avoid tumor cell spillage.

Surgery alone achieves a high cure rate for superficial TCC. Amling et al.[174] reported cancer-specific 5-year survival rates of 88% for Ta, 76% for T1, and 100% for CIS. Pelvic lymph node metastases were present in 5.9%. Similar survival figures have been reported in other large series.[175–177]

FOLLOW-UP

Since 30 to 80% of tumors will recur, close follow-up is important to diagnose and treat recurrence early. Flexible endoscopy and urinary cytology (for high-grade disease) are essential for follow-up. Historically this has been performed at 3-month intervals, then tailored according to patterns of recurrence. The disease status at the initial 3-month cystoscopy is important in predicting future tumor behavior, and has become the basis of follow-up protocols.[18,48]

TABLE 17–5. FOLLOW-UP FOR SUPERFICIAL BLADDER CANCER*

Risk Category	Recommended Follow-up
1. Single tumor with no recurrence at 3 months	Annual cystoscopy
2. Single tumor with recurrence at 3 months, or multiple tumors with no recurrence	3-monthly cystoscopy
3. Multiple tumors with recurrence at 3 months	Adjuvant treatment

*From Parmer MKB, Freedman CS, Hargreave TB, et al: Prognostic factors for recurrence and followup policies in the treatment of superficial bladder cancer: report from the BMRC subgroup on superficial bladder cancer (Urological Cancer Working Party). J Urol 1989; 142:284–288, with permission.

Treatment of papillary recurrence, or suspicious areas, is ideally performed under anesthesia, with rigid instrumentation, allowing adequate biopsies and thorough visual assessment. The mucosa distant from the tumor and the prostatic urethra in males should be sampled as previously outlined for high-grade primary tumors.

Laser ablation via flexible endoscopy under topical anesthesia has been used to manage recurrences in selected cases.[178,179] Laser is well tolerated, although there is a recognized risk of bowel injury.[178] Diathermy has also been used[180]; 4-French electrodes are available to treat small lesions. Care must be taken to pass the electrode at least 1 cm beyond the tip of the endoscope to avoid thermal damage to the fiberoptic system. Both techniques require a cooperative patient. There is considerable cost benefit for this strategy in appropriate individuals. It must be emphasized that representative histopathology is necessary to avoid undertreatment of innocent-appearing high-grade lesions.[181]

Protocols for cystoscopic follow-up have been proposed based upon known prognostic factors such as tumor size, number, histologic grade and stage, urine cytology, and DNA ploidy. Parmar et al.[18] concluded that the likelihood of recurrence, and hence the need for follow-up cystoscopy, could be predicted simply and accurately by the number of tumors at initial presentation and the presence of recurrent tumor at the first 3-month cystoscopy. Risk categories and appropriate follow-up are summarized in Table 17–5. The power of this classification lies in the objectivity and reliability of these two prognostic factors. The safety and efficacy of this protocol have been demonstrated in a retrospective review of 232 patients.[182]

The duration of endoscopic follow-up for patients free of recurrence for many years has been debated. Morris et al.,[183] in a longitudinal follow-up study of 179 patients with Ta and T1 TCC, documented recurrence risk over time. They reported that after a tumor-free interval of 2, 5, and 10 years, the risk of recurrence is 43, 22, and 2%, respectively. No patient had a recurrence after remaining tumor free for 12 years. No patient free of recurrence for 2 years progressed to muscle invasion or metastases. Holmang et al.[24] reported that only 1 of 59 patients tumor free for 5 years progressed. They also observed that patients who had recurrences on ten or more cystoscopic studies, or multiple recurrences over more than 4 years, continued to have recurrences until death or cystectomy.

Urinary markers and cytology may have a role in long-term follow-up. Table 17–6 lists sensitivities and specificities for potentially useful urinary markers. The ideal noninvasive bladder tumor

TABLE 17–6. URINARY MARKERS FOR FOLLOW-UP OF SUPERFICIAL BLADDER CANCER

Marker	Technique	No. of Patients	Sensitivity (%)	Specificity (%)
Lewis X antigen[64]	Immunocytology	101	81	86
Lewis X antigen[184]	Immunocytology (Bladder wash)	89	85	85
Basement membrane complex (Bard BTA)[185]	Latex agglutination	499	40	82
Autocrine motility factor (AMF) receptor[186]	Qualitative immunoassay	70	80	75
Nuclear matrix protein (NMP-22)*	Quantitative immunoassay	69	74	78
Hyaluronidase†	Quantitative ELISA assay	104	63 (High grade—99)	94

*Data derived from Soloway MS, Briggman J, Carpinito G, et al: Use of a new tumor marker, urinary NMP22, in the detection of occult or rapidly recurring transitional cell carcinoma of the urinary tract following surgical treatment. Personal communication, 1995.

†Data derived from Lokeshwar BI: Personal communication, November, 1995.

ELISA, enzyme-linked immunosorbent assay.

marker would need to be nearly 100% sensitive before replacing follow-up cystoscopy. Further prospective multicenter assessment for all these markers is necessary.

The frequency of radiologic follow-up depends on the individual's risk of developing upper urinary tract tumors. This risk varies from 0.5% with low-grade bladder tumors[24,187] to 15% with CIS.[188] Intravenous pyelography should be performed every 2 to 5 years, accordingly.

CASE HISTORIES

Case 1

A 74-year-old female presented with a 4-cm papillary bladder tumor. TUR confirmed a grade 3 T1 tumor with invasion to the level of the muscularis mucosae but not involving deep muscle (stage T1a).

CASE 1 DISCUSSION. Accurate staging is important when evidence of lamina propria invasion is present on initial biopsy. Confirmed lamina propria invasion and high grade puts this patient at high risk for both recurrence and progression. Intravesical BCG was administered weekly for 6 weeks, without evidence of recurrence.

Case 2

A 48-year-old woman presented with a 2-cm papillary tumor on the bladder trigone, near the ureteric orifice, with negative mucosal biopsies. Pathology confirmed a grade 3 Ta lesion that was strongly positive for p53 on immunohistochemical staining. Small papillary recurrences were resected at 13 and 21 months, all of which remained grade 3 Ta and p53-positive. Intravesical mitomycin (20 mg weekly for 5 weeks) was administered. The patient remains tumor free at 10 months following the last TUR.

CASE 2 DISCUSSION. Recent data suggest p53-positive papillary tumors may be at increased risk for progression. These tumors initially recurred as high-grade noninvasive lesions, although they appear to have responded to a prophylactic course of mitomycin. BCG would have been an equally reasonable alternative and will be used with recurrence. Intravesical therapy could have been used at the time of diagnosis given the high tumor grade.

Case 3

A 66-year-old male underwent a TUR of the prostate for symptoms associated with benign prostatic hyperplasia. Surprisingly, the pathology noted grade 3 TCC involving the prostatic ducts. No bladder disease was detected on biopsy at a subsequent cystoscopy. The patient declined further treatment. A TUR biopsy at 24 months again demonstrated CIS involving prostatic ducts with no stromal invasion and no TCC of the bladder.

CASE 3 DISCUSSION. The management options for prostatic ductal involvement include intravesical BCG or cystoprostatectomy. A cystoprostatectomy with urethrectomy was performed confirming prostatic ductal CIS with extensive CIS of the bladder and one focus of lamina propria invasion. This demonstrates the problems of disease understaging, which is the major concern with intravesical treatment for both bladder and prostatic urethral TCC.

Case 4

A 65-year-old male presented with a 1-cm grade 3 Ta tumor involving the left wall of the bladder, which was completely resected. A large, wide-mouthed bladder diverticulum located on the right wall of the bladder was filled with a second grade 3 papillary tumor. Random bladder and prostatic urethral biopsies were negative. A TUR biopsy at 8 weeks revealed no evidence of tumor in the left wall. A partial cystectomy removing the bladder diverticulum was performed, confirming a grade 3 Ta tumor with associated CIS but negative surgical margins.

CASE 4 DISCUSSION. Residual or high-grade noninvasive tumor involving a bladder diverticulum could be managed with diverticulectomy or cystoprostatectomy. Care must be taken to exclude and treat other foci of tumor, if bladder preservation is chosen.

Case 5

A 74-year-old female presented with a history of CIS and T1 grade 3 TCC of the bladder. After resection she was treated with 6 weeks of BCG.

CASE 5 DISCUSSION. This case prompts consideration as to whether to give maintenance BCG. Early randomized studies showed no clear-cut advantage to giving maintenance BCG over a standard 6-week inductive course. Lamm et al. recently reported that not only can maintenance therapy reduce tumor recurrence but may also increase survival.[138] The optimal timing of maintenance doses has not been clearly established. Given the patient's age and risk of side effects, no maintenance therapy was given in this case.

Case 6

A 77-year-old woman was diagnosed with multifocal CIS in 1990. She was treated with 6 weekly doses of intravesical MMC. At that time she had frequency and urgency as well as perineal discomfort. In 1993, she had a right distal ureter stricture treated with distal ureterectomy and reimplantation. In follow-up she had a positive cytology but no evidence of tumor on bladder biopsy. She received 6 weeks of BCG. Her irritative symptoms worsened. She later had dysplasia in the bladder documented by biopsy and received another 6-week course of MMC. She remained tumor free but presented with incapacitating irritative voiding symptoms and incontinence and a severely contracted bladder. She underwent a cystectomy and ileal conduit for severe bladder contracture. There was no cancer in the specimen.

Case 6 Discussion. This is a classic case of overtreatment with intravesical therapy and incapacitating iatrogenic morbidity. While intravesical agents may prolong recurrence-free survival, the side effects of treatment should not be underestimated.

Case 7

A 75-year-old woman presented with a history of superficial, low-grade TCC in 1983. She had been treated previously for interstitial cystitis. In 1988, she underwent a left nephroureterectomy for T1, grade 2 TCC of the ureter. In 1991 she was found to have CIS in the bladder and superficial tumor in the right distal ureter. A stent was placed and she received intravesical MMC. Four months later she had a resection of a T1, grade 3 bladder tumor. She was given a second 6-week course of BCG. Nine months later she had a TURBT, with pathology revealing a high-grade, muscle-invasive tumor with involvement of the right ureteral orifice and invasion of the bladder neck and urethra. Cystectomy with urinary diversion was performed. Pathology revealed a grade 3 T3 TCC. No adjuvant chemotherapy was given.

Case 7 Discussion. This case illustrates the progression of a superficial lesion to a high-grade invasive tumor despite intravesical MMC, BCG, and close surveillance.

REFERENCES

1. Soloway MS: Flexible cystourethroscopy: alternative to rigid instruments for evaluation of the lower urinary tract. Urology 1985; 25:472.
2. Matzkin H, Moinuddin S, Soloway MS: Value of urine cytology versus bladder washing in bladder cancer. Urology 1992; 39(3):201.
3. Soloway MS, Patel J: Surgical techniques for endoscopic resection of bladder cancer. Urol Clin North Am 1992; 19(3):467.
4. Soloway MS: An optical dilator to obviate blind urethral dilation prior to endoscopic resections. Urol 1988; 31:427.
5. Heney NM, Ahmed S, Flanagan MJ, et al: Superficial bladder cancer: progression and recurrence. J Urol 1983; 130:1083.
6. Jordan AM, Weingarten J, Murphy WM: Transitional cell neoplasms of the urinary bladder: can biological potential be predicted from histological grading? Cancer 1987; 60: 2766.
7. Mostofi FK, Sobin LH, Torlini H: Histological typing of urinary bladder tumors. International Histological Classification of Tumors No. 10. Geneva, World Health Organisation, 1973.
8. Murphy WM, Beckwith JB, Farrow G: Tumors of the Kidney, Bladder and Related Urinary Structures, pp 198–224. Washington, DC, Armed Forces Institute of Pathology, 1994.
9. Ayala AG, Ro JY: Premalignant lesions of the urothelium and transitional cell tumors. *In* Young RH (ed): Pathology of the Urinary Bladder, pp 65–101. New York, Churchill Livingstone, 1989.
10. Carbin BE, Elkman P, Gustafson H, et al: Grading of human urothelial neoplasms based on nuclear atypia and mitotic frequency I: histological description. J Urol 1991; 145:968.
11. Carbin BE, Elkman P, Gustafson H, et al: Grading of human urothelial neoplasms based on nuclear atypia and mitotic frequency II: prognostic importance. J Urol 1991; 145:972.
12. Kaubisch S, Lum BL, Reese J, et al: Stage T1 bladder cancer: grade is the primary determinant for risk of muscle invasion. J Urol 1991; 146:28.
13. Pauwels RP, Schapers RFM, Smeets AWGB, et al: Grading in superficial bladder cancer I: morphological criteria. Br J Urol 1988; 61:129.
14. Blomjous CEM, Vos W, Schipper NW: The prognostic significance of selective nuclear morphometry in urinary bladder carcinoma. Hum Pathol 1990; 21:409.
15. Ooms ECM, Anderson WAD, Alons CL, et al: Analysis of the performance of pathologists in the grading of bladder tumors. Hum Pathol 1983; 14:140.
16. Jewett HJ, Strong GH: Infiltrating carcinoma of the bladder: relation of depth of penetration of bladder wall to incidence of local extension and metastases. J Urol 1946; 55:366.
17. Beahrs OH, Henson DE: The Manual for Staging of Cancer. AJCC. Philadelphia, Lippincott-Raven, 1993.
18. Parmar MKB, Friedman LS, Hargreave TB, et al: Prognostic factors for recurrence follow-up policies in the treatment of superficial bladder cancer: report from the British Medical Research Council Subgroup on superficial bladder cancer. J Urol 1989; 142:284.
19. Abel PD, Hall RR, Williams G: Should pT1 transitional cell carcinoma of the bladder still be classified as superficial? Br J Urol 1988; 62:235.
20. Heney NM, Nocks BN, Daley JJ, et al: Ta and T1 bladder cancer: location, recurrence, and progression. Br J Urol 1982; 54:152.
21. Williams JL, Hammonds JC, Saunders N: T1 bladder tumors. Br J Urol 1977; 49:663.
22. Birch BRP, Harland SJ: The pT1 G3 bladder tumor. Br J Urol 1989; 64:109.
23. Anderström C, Johansson S, Nilsson S: The significance of lamina propria invasion on the prognosis of patients with bladder tumors. J Urol 1980; 124:23.
24. Holmäng S, Hedelin H, Anderström C, et al: The relationship among multiple recurrences, progression, and prognosis of patients with stages Ta and T1 transitional cell carcinoma of the bladder followed for at least 20 years. J Urol 1995; 153:18.
25. Hassui Y, Osada Y, Kitada S, et al: Significance of invasion to the muscularis mucosa on the progression of superficial bladder cancer. Urology 1994; 43:782.
26. Dixon JS, Gosling JA: Histology and fine structure of the muscularis mucosa of the human urinary bladder. J Anat 1983; 136:265.
27. Younes M, Sussman J, True LD: The usefulness of the level of muscularis mucosa in the staging of invasive transitional cell carcinoma of the urinary bladder. Cancer 1990; 66:543.
28. Klän R, Loy V, Huland H: Residual tumor discovered in routine second TUR in patients with T1 transitional cell carcinoma of the bladder. J Urol 1991; 146:316.
29. Lynch CF, Platz CE, Jones MP, et al: Cancer registry problems in classifying invasive bladder cancer. J Natl Cancer Inst 1991; 83:429.
30. Abel PB, Henderson D, Bennett MK, et al: Differing interpretations by pathologists of the pT category and grade of transitional cell carcinoma of the bladder. Br J Urol 1988; 62:339.
31. Olsen LH, Overgaard S, Frederiksen P, et al: The reliability of staging and grading of bladder tumors: impact of misinformation of the pathologists' diagnosis. Scand J Urol Nephrol 1993; 27:349.
32. Witjes JA, Kiemeney LALM, Schaafsma HE, et al: The influence of review pathology on study outcome of a randomised multicenter superficial bladder cancer trial. Br J Urol 1994; 73:172.
33. Richards B, Parmar MKB, Anderson CK, et al: Interpre-

tation of biopsies of "normal" urothelium in patients with superficial bladder cancer. Br J Urol 1991; 67:369.
34. Sidransky D, Frost P, Von Eschenbach A, et al: Clonal origin of bladder cancer. N Engl J Med 1992; 326:737.
35. Harris AL, Neal D: Bladder cancer—field versus clonal origin. N Engl J Med 1992; 326:759.
36. Soloway MS, Murphy W, Rao MK, et al: Serial multiple site biopsies in patients with bladder cancer. J Urol 1978; 120:57.
37. Kakizoe T, Matumoto K, Nishio Y, et al: Significance of carcinoma in-situ and dysplasia in association with bladder cancer. J Urol 1985; 133:395.
38. Kiemeney LALM, Witjes JA, Heijbroek RP, et al: Should random urothelial biopsies be taken from patients with primary superficial bladder cancer? A decision analysis. Br J Urol 1994; 73:164.
39. Hardeman SW, Perry A, Soloway MS: Transitional cell carcinoma of the prostate following intravesical therapy for transitional cell carcinoma of the bladder. J Urol 1988; 140:289.
40. Montie JE, Mersky H, Levin HS: Transitional cell carcinoma of the prostate in a series of cystectomies: incidence and staging problems. J Urol 1986; 135:243A.
41. Wolf H, Hojgaard K: Urothelial dysplasia concomitant with bladder tumors as a determining factor for future new occurrences. Lancet 1983; 2(8342):134.
42. Althausen AF, Prout GR, Daly JJ: Non-invasive papillary carcinoma of the bladder associated with carcinoma-in-situ. J Urol 1976; 116:575.
43. Smith G, Elton RA, Beynon LL, et al: Prognostic significance of biopsy results of normal looking mucosa in cases of superficial bladder cancer. Br J Urol 1983; 55:665.
44. Olsen PR, Wolf H, Schoeder T, et al: Urothelial atypia and survival rate of 500 unselected patients with primary transitional cell carcinoma of the urinary bladder. Scand J Urol Nephrol 1988; 22:257.
45. Lerman RI, Hulter RVP, Whitmore WF: Papilloma of the urinary bladder. Cancer 1970; 25:333.
46. Cutler SJ, Heney NM, Friedell GH: Longitudinal study of patients with bladder cancer: factors associated with disease recurrence and progression. *In* Bonney WW, Prout JR (eds), Bladder Cancer, p 35. Baltimore, Williams & Wilkins, 1982.
47. Lutzeyer W, Rubben H, Damm H: Prognostic parameters in superficial bladder cancer: an analysis of 315 cases. J Urol 1982; 127:250.
48. Fitzpatrick JM, West AB, Butler MR, et al: Superficial bladder tumors (stage pTa grades 1&2): the importance of recurrence pattern following initial resection. J Urol 1986; 135:920.
49. Pagano F, Garbeglio A, Milani C, et al: Prognosis of bladder cancer I: risk factors in superficial transitional cell carcinoma. Eur Urol 1987; 13: 145.
50. Murphy WM, Soloway MS, Jukkola AF, et al: Urine cytology and bladder cancer. Cancer 1984; 53:1555.
51. Murphy WM: Current status of urine cytology in the evaluation of bladder neoplasms. Hum Pathol 1990; 21: 886.
52. De Vita R, Forte D, Maggi F, et al: Cellular DNA content and proliferative activity evaluated by flow cytometry versus histopathological staging classifications in human bladder tumors. Eur Urol 1991; 19:65.
53. Gustafson H, Tribukait B, Esposti PL: DNA pattern, histological grade, and multiplicity related to recurrence rate in superficial bladder tumors. Scand J Urol Nephrol 1982; 16:135.
54. Gustafson H, Tribukait B, Esposti PL: DNA profile in tumor progression in patients with superficial bladder tumors. Urol Res 1982; 10:13.
55. Masters JRW, Camplejohn RS, Parkinson MC, et al: DNA ploidy and the prognosis of stage pT1 bladder cancer. Br J Urol 1989; 64:403.
56. Murphy WM, Chandler RW, Trafford RM: Flow cytometry of deparaffinised nuclei compared to histological grading for the pathological evaluation of transitional cell carcinoma. J Urol 1986; 135:694.
57. Newman AJ, Carlton C, Johnson S: Cell surface A,B, O blood group antigen as an indicator of malignant potential in stage A bladder carcinoma. J Urol 1980; 124:27.
58. Richie JP, Blute RD, Waisman J: Immunological indicators of prognosis in bladder cancer: the importance of cell surface antigens. J Urol 1980; 123:22.
59. Blasco E, Tarrado J, Belloso L, et al: T antigen: a prognostic indicator of high recurrence index in transitional cell carcinoma of the bladder. Cancer 1988; 61:1091.
60. Bergman S, Javadpour N: The cell surface antigen as an indicator of malignant potential in stage A bladder cancer. J Urol 1978; 119:49.
61. Sanders H, McCue P, Graham SD: ABO (H) antigens and beta-2 microglobulin in transitional cell carcinoma: predictors of response to intravesical BCG. Cancer 1991; 67: 3024.
62. Juhl BR, Hartzen SH, Hainau B: Lewis A antigen in transitional cell tumors of the urinary bladder. Cancer 1986; 58:222.
63. Langkilde NC, Wolf H, Milgard P, et al: Frequency and mechanism of Lewis antigen expression in human urinary bladder and colon carcinoma patients. Br J Cancer 1991; 63:583.
64. Golijanin D, Scherman Y, Shapiro A: Detection of bladder tumors by immunostaining of Lewis X antigen in cells from voided urine. Urology 1995; 46:173.
65. Conn IG, Vilela MJ, Garrod DR, et al: Immunohistochemical staining with monoclonal antibody 32-2B to desmosomal glycoprotein I: its role in the histological assessment of urothelial carcinomas. Br J Urol 1990; 65:176.
66. Smith NW, Stutton GM, Walsh MD, et al: Transferrin receptor expression in primary superficial bladder tumors identifies patients who develop recurrences. Br J Urol 1990; 65:339.
67. Conn IG, Crocker J, Emtage LA, et al: Human milk fat globulin-2 as a prognostic indicator in superficial bladder cancer. J Clin Pathol 1988; 41:1191.
68. Neal DE, Scharples L, Smith K, et al: The epidermal growth factor receptor and the prognosis of bladder cancer. Cancer 1990; 65:1619.
69. Mellow K, Wright C, Kelly P, et al: Long term outcome related to epidermal growth factor receptor status in bladder cancer. J Urol 1995; 153:919.
70. Schapers RFM, Pauwels RPE, Havenith MG, et al: Prognostic significance of type IV collagen and laminin immunoreactivity in urothelial carcinomas of the bladder. Cancer 1990; 66:2583.
71. Sandberg AA: Chromosome markers and progression in bladder cancer. Cancer Res 1977; 37:2950.
72. Waldman FM, Carroll PR, Kerschmann R, et al: Centromeric copy number of chromosome 7 is strongly correlated with tumor grade and labelling index in human bladder cancer. Cancer Res 1981; 51:3807.
73. Fearon ER, Feinberg AP, Hamilton SH, et al: Loss of genes on the short arm of chromosome 11 in bladder cancer. Nature 1985; 318:377.
74. Hopman A, Moesker O, Smeets A, et al: Numerical chromosome 1, 7, 9, 11 aberrations in bladder cancer detected by in-situ hybridisation. Cancer Res 1991; 51:644.
75. Summers JL, Falor W, Ward R: A 10 year analysis of chromosomes in non-invasive papillary carcinoma of the bladder. J Urol 1981; 125:177.
76. Tsai YC, Nichols PW, Hiti AL, et al: Allelic losses of chromosomes 9, 11, and 17 in human bladder cancer. Cancer Res 1990; 50:44.
77. Olumi AF, Tsai YC, Nichols PW, et al: Allelic loss of chromosome 17p distinguishes high grade from low grade transitional cell carcinoma of the bladder. Cancer Res 1990; 50:7081.
78. Agnantis NJ, Constantinidou A, Poulios C, et al: Immunohistochemical study of the *ras* oncogene expression in human bladder endoscopy specimens. Eur J Surg Oncol 1990; 16:153.

79. Viola MV, Fromowitz F, Oravez S, et al: *Ras* oncogene p21 expression is increased in premalignant lesions and high grade bladder cancer. J Exp Med 1985; 161:1213.
80. Feinberg AP, Vogelstein B, Droller MJ, et al: Mutation affecting the 12th amino acid of the c-Ha-*ras* oncogene product occurs infrequently in human cancer. Science 1983; 220:1175.
81. Lane DP: p53 guardian of the genome. Nature 1991; 358: 15.
82. Kasten MB, Onyekwere O, Sidransky D, et al: Participation of p53 protein in the cellular response to DNA damage. Cancer Res 1991; 51:6304.
83. Reich NC, Oren M, Levine AJ: Two distinct mechanisms regulate the levels of cellular tumor antigen p53. Mol Cell Biol 1993; 3:2143.
84. Harris AL: Telling change of base. Nature 1990; 350:377.
85. Fujimoto K, Yamada Y, Okajima E, et al: Frequent association of p53 gene mutation in invasive bladder cancer. Cancer Res 1992; 52:1393.
86. Sidransky D, von Eschenbach A, Tsai YC: Identification of p53 gene mutations in bladder cancers and urine samples. Science 1991; 252:706.
87. Lunec J, Challen C, Wright C, et al: c-erb B-2 amplification and identical p53 mutations in concomitant transitional carcinoma of the renal pelvis and urinary bladder. Lancet 1992; 339:439.
88. Iggo R, Gatter K, Bartek J, et al: Increased expression of mutant forms of p53 oncogene in primary lung cancer. Lancet 1990; 335:675.
89. Sarkis A, Dalbagni G, Cordon-Cardo C, et al: Association of p53 nuclear overexpression and tumor progression in carcinoma-in-situ of the bladder. J Urol 1994; 152:388.
90. Sidransky D, Mikkelsen T, Schwechheimer K, et al: Clonal expansion of p53 mutant cells is associated with brain tumor progression. Nature 1992; 355:846.
91. Oka K, Ishikana J, Bruner JM, et al: Detection of loss of heterozygosity in p53 gene in renal cell carcinoma and bladder carcinoma using the polymerase chain reaction. Mol Carcinog 1991; 4:10.
92. Spruck CH, Ohneseit PF, Gonzales-Sulueta M, et al: Two molecular pathways to transitional cell carcinoma of the bladder. Cancer Res 1994; 54:784.
93. Yoskimura I, Kudoh J, Saito S: p53 gene mutation in recurrent superficial bladder cancer. J Urol 1995; 153:1711.
94. Uchida T, Wada C, Ishida H, et al: p53 mutations and prognosis in bladder tumors. J Urol 1995; 153:1097.
95. Lipponen PK: Overexpression of p53 nuclear oncoprotein in transitional cell bladder cancer and its prognostic value. Int J Cancer 1993; 53:365.
96. Gardiner RA, Walsh MD, Allen S, et al: Immunohistological expression of p53 in primary pT1 transitional cell bladder cancer in relation to tumor progression. Br J Urol 1994; 73:526.
97. Sarkis A, Dalbagni G, Cordon-Cardo C, et al: Nuclear overexpression of p53 protein in transitional cell bladder carcinoma: a marker of disease progression. J Natl Cancer Inst 1993; 85:53.
98. Esrig D, Spruck C, Nichols P, et al: p53 nuclear protein accumulation correlates with mutations in the p53 gene, tumor grade, and stage, in bladder cancer. Am J Pathol 1993; 143:1389.
99. Dalbagni G, Cordon-Cardo C, Reuter V, et al: Tumor suppressor gene alterations in bladder carcinoma translational correlates to clinical practise. Surg Oncol Clin North Am 1995; 4:231.
100. Esrig D, Elmajian D, Groshen S, et al: Accumulation of nuclear p53 and tumor progression in bladder cancer. N Engl J Med 1994; 331:1259.
101. Sato K, Moriyama M, Mori S, et al: An immunohistological evaluation of c-*erb* B-2 gene product in patients with urinary bladder carcinoma. Cancer 1983; 70:2493.
102. Moriyama M, Akiyama T, Yamamoto T, et al: Expression of c-*erb* B-2 gene product in urinary bladder cancer. J Urol 1991; 145:423.
103. Masters JR, Vessey SG, Minn CF: C-*myc* oncoprotein levels in bladder cancer. Urol Res 1988; 16:341.
104. Lamm DL, Lamm LM: Benefits of intravesical chemotherapy for superficial disease. Contemp Urol 1989; June/July:3.
105. Walker MC, Masters JR, Parris CN, et al: Intravesical chemotherapy: in vitro studies on the relationship between dose and cytotoxicity. Urol Res 1986; 14:137.
106. Goos E, Masters JR: Intravesical chemotherapy: studies on the relationship between osmolality and cytotoxicity. J Urol 1986; 136:399.
107. Cant JD, Murphy WM, Soloway MS: Prognostic significance of urine cytology on initial follow up after intravesical mitomycin C for superficial bladder cancer. Cancer 1986; 57:2119.
108. Haaf EO, Dresner SM, Ratliff TL, et al: Two courses of intravesical bacillus Calmette-Guérin for transitional cell carcinoma of the bladder. J Urol 1986; 136:820.
109. Eure GR, Cundiff MR, Shellhammer PF: Bacillus Calmette-Guérin therapy for high risk stage T1 superficial bladder cancer. J Urol 1992, 152:376.
110. Soloway MS, Perito PE: Superficial bladder cancer: diagnosis, surveillance and treatment. J Cell Biochem 1992; 161(Suppl):120.
111. Soloway MS: Surgery and intravesical chemotherapy in the management of superficial bladder cancer. Semin Urol 1983; 11:23.
112. Prout GR Jr, Koontz WW Jr, Coombs LJ, et al: Long-term fate of 90 patients with superficial bladder cancer randomly assigned to receive or not to receive thiotepa. J Urol 1983; 130:677.
113. MRC Working Party on Urological Cancer, Subgroup on Superficial Bladder Cancer: The effect of intravesical thiotepa on tumour recurrence after endoscopic treatment of newly diagnosed superficial bladder cancer. A further report with long-term follow-up of a Medical Research Council randomized trial. Br J Urol 1994; 73:632.
114. Soloway MS: Rationale for intensive intravesical chemotherapy for superficial bladder cancer. J Urol 1980; 123: 461.
115. Soloway MS, Jordan AM, Murphy WM: Rationale for intravesical chemotherapy in the treatment and prophylaxis of superficial transitional cell carcinoma. Prog Clin Biol Res 1989; 310:215.
116. Soloway MS, Ford KS: Thiotepa-induced myelosuppression: review of 670 bladder instillations. J Urol 1983; 130: 889.
117. Koontz WW Jr, Heney NM, Barton B, et al: Intravesical effects of mitomycin C in patients with superficial bladder carcinoma who have previously failed therapy with thiotepa. Urology 1985; 26:30.
118. Heney NM: First-line chemotherapy of superficial bladder cancer: mitomycin C versus thiotepa. Urology 1985; 26:27.
119. Soloway MS: Diagnosis and management of superficial bladder cancer. Semin Surg Oncol 1989; 5:247.
120. Huland H, Otto J, Droese M, et al: Long-term mitomycin C instillation after transurethral resection of superficial bladder carcinoma: influence on recurrence, progression, and survival. J Urol 1984; 132:27.
121. Maier U, Hobarth K: Long-term observation after intravesical metaphylaxis with mitomycin C in patients with superficial bladder tumours. Urology 1991; 37(5):481.
122. Tolley DA, Parmar MKB, Grigor KM, et al: The effect of intravesical mitomycin C on recurrence of newly diagnosed superficial bladder cancer: a further report with 7 years' follow-up. J Urol 1995 (in press).
123. Nissenkorn I, Herrod H, Soloway MS: Side effects associated with intravesical mitomycin. J Urol 1981; 126:596.
124. Batts CN: Adjuvant intravesical therapy for superficial bladder cancer. Ann Pharmacother 1992; 26:1270.
125. Niijima T, Koiso K, Adaza H: Randomized clinical trial for chemoprophylaxis of recurrence in superficial bladder cancer. *In* Spitzy KH, Karrer K (eds): Proceedings of the

13th International Congress of Chemotherapy, pp 240–246, Vienna, 1983.

126. Kurth KH, Debruyne FJM, Senge T, et al: Adjuvant chemotherapy of superficial transitional cell carcinoma: an E.O.R.T.C. randomized trial comparing doxorubicin hydrochloride, ethoglucid and TUR-alone. Prog Clin Biol Res 1985; 162A:135.
127. Zincke H, Utz DC, Taylor WF, et al: Influence of thiotepa and doxorubicin instillation at time of transurethral surgical treatment of bladder cancer on tumor recurrence: a prospective, randomized, double-blind, controlled trial. J Urol 1983; 129:505.
128. Llopis B, Gallego J, Mompo JA, et al: Thiotepa versus Adriamycin versus cis-platinum in the intravesical prophylaxis of superficial bladder tumors. Eur Urol 1985; 11: 73.
129. Lamm DL, Blumenstein BA, Crawford ED, et al: A randomized trial of intravesical doxorubicin and immunotherapy with bacille Calmette-Guérin for transitional cell carcinoma of the bladder. N Engl J Med 1991; 325:1205.
130. Jackse G, Hofstadter F, Marsberger H: Topical doxorubicin hydrochloride therapy for carcinoma in situ of the bladder: a follow-up. J Urol 1984; 131:41.
131. Ausfield A, Beer M, Muhlethale J, et al: Adjuvant intravesical chemotherapy of superficial bladder cancer with monthly doxorubicin of intensive mitomycin: a comparison of two consecutive series. Eur Urol 1987; 13:10.
132. Sweatman TW, Parker RF, Israel M: Pharmacologic rationale for (AD-32): a preclinical study. Cancer Chemother Pharmacol 1991; 28:1.
133. Greenberg R, O'Dwyer P, Patterson L, et al: Intravesical AD-32 (N-trifluoroacetyladriamycin-14-valerate) in the treatment of patients with refractory bladder carcinoma—clinical efficacy, pharmacology, and safety. J Urol 1995; 153:233A.
134. Morales AM, Eidinger D, Bruce AW: Intracavitary bacillus Calmette-Guérin in the treatment of superficial bladder tumors. J Urol 1976; 116:180.
135. Guerin C: The history of BCG. *In* Rosenthal SR (ed): BCG Vaccination Against Tuberculosis, p 35. Boston, Little, Brown & Co, 1957.
136. Ratliff TL, Haaff EO, and Catalona WJ: Interleukin 2 production during intravesical bacillus Calmette-Guérin therapy for bladder cancer. Clin Immunol Immunopathol 1986; 40:375.
137. Brosman S: Bacillus Calmette-Guérin immunotherapy: techniques and results. Urol Clin North Am 1992; 19(3): 557.
138. Lamm DL, Crawford ED, Blumenstein B, et al: Maintenance BCG immunotherapy of superficial bladder cancer: a randomized prospective Southwest Oncology Group Study (Abstract 242). J Urol 1992; 147(part 2):274A.
139. Lamm DL: BCG in carcinoma-in-situ and superficial bladder tumors. EORTC Genitourinary Group. Monogr 1988; 5:497.
140. Herr HW, Laudone VP, Whitmore WF: An overview of intravesical therapy for superficial bladder tumors. J Urol 1987; 138:1363.
141. DeJager R, Guinan P, Lamm D, et al: Long-term complete remission in bladder carcinoma in situ with intravesical Tice bacillus Calmette-Guérin: overview analysis of six phase II clinical trials. Urology 1991; 38:507
142. Herr HW: Intravesical BCG: current results, natural history and implications for urothelial cancer prevention. J Cell Biochem 1992; 161(Suppl):112.
143. Herr HW, Schwalb DM, Zhang ZF, et al: Intravesical bacillus Calmette-Guérin therapy prevents tumor progression and death from superficial bladder cancer: ten-year follow-up of a prospective randomized trial. J Clin Oncol 1995; 13:1404.
144. Brosman SA: Experience with bacillus Calmette-Guérin in patients with superficial bladder carcinoma. J Urol 1982; 128:27.
145. Martinez-Pineiro JA: BCG vaccine in superficial bladder tumors: eight years later. Eur Urol 1989; 142:719.
146. Lamm DL, Crissinan J, Blumenstein BA, et al: Adriamycin versus BCG in superficial bladder cancer: a Southwest Oncology Group study. *In* Debruyne FMJ, van der Meijden APM (eds): BCG in Superficial Bladder Cancer, p 123. New York, Alan R Liss, 1989.
147. Vegt PDJ, Witjes JA, Witjes WPJ, et al: A randomized study of intravesical mitomycin C, bacillus Calmette-Guérin Tice and bacillus Calmette-Guérin RIVM treatment in pTa-pT1 papillary carcinoma and carcinoma in situ of the bladder. J Urol 1995; 153:929.
148. Cookson MS, Sarosdy MF: Management of stage T1 superficial bladder cancer with intravesical bacillus Calmette-Guérin therapy. J Urol 1992; 148:797.
149. Nadler RB, Catalona WJ, Hudson MA, et al: Durability of the tumor-free response for intravesical bacillus Calmette-Guérin therapy. J Urol 1994; 152:367.
150. Lamm DL: Complications of bacillus Calmette-Guérin immunotherapy. Urol Clin North Am 1992; 19:565.
151. Nelson B, Borden E: Interferons: biological and clinical effects. Semin Surg Oncol 1989; 5:391.
152. Sargent ER, Williams RD: Immunotherapeutic alternatives in superficial bladder cancer: interferon, interleukin 2 and keyhole limpet hemocyanin. Urol Clin North Am 1992; 19(3):581.
153. Torti F, Shortliffe L, Williams R, et al: Alpha-interferon in superficial bladder cancer: a Northern California Oncology Group study. J Clin Oncol 1988; 6:476.
154. Glashan RW: A randomized controlled study of intravesical α-2b-interferon in carcinoma in situ of the bladder. J Urol 1990; 144:658.
155. Olsson D, Rao C, Menzoian J, et al: Immunologic unreactivity in bladder cancer patients. J Urol 1972; 107:607.
156. Jurinic C, Engelmann U, Gasch J: Immunotherapy in bladder cancer with keyhole-limpet hemocyanin: a randomized study. J Urol 1988; 139:723.
157. Wierenga W: Antiviral and other bioactivities of pyrimidinones. Pharmacol Ther 1985; 30:67.
158. Sarosdy MF, Lamm DL, Williams RD, et al: Phase 1 trial of oral bropirimine in superficial bladder cancer. J Urol 1992; 147:31.
159. Sarosdy MF, Lowe BA, Schellhammer PF, et al: Bropirimine immunotherapy of bladder CIS: positive phase II results of an oral interferon inducer. J Urol 1994; 13:304A.
160. Herr HW, Wartinger DD, Fair WR, et al: Bacillus Calmette-Guérin therapy for superficial bladder cancer: a ten year follow-up. J Urol 1992; 147:1020.
161. Zinke H, Utz DC, Farrow GM: Review of Mayo Clinic experience with carcinoma-in-situ. Urology (Suppl) 1985; 26:39.
162. Matzkin H, Soloway MS, Hardeman S: Transitional cell carcinoma of the prostate. J Urol 1991; 146:1207.
163. Wood D, Montie J, Pontes J, et al: Transitional cell carcinoma of the prostate in cystoprostatectomy specimens removed for bladder cancer. J Urol 1989; 141:346.
164. Seemayer TA, Knaack J, Thelmo W, et al: Further observations on carcinoma-in-situ of the urinary bladder: silent but extensive intraprostatic involvement. Cancer 1975; 36: 514.
165. Hardeman S, Soloway M: Transitional cell carcinoma of the prostate: diagnosis, staging and management. World J Urol 1988; 6:170.
166. Hardeman S, Perry A, Soloway MS: Transitional cell carcinoma of the prostate following intravesical therapy for transitional cell carcinoma of the bladder. J Urol 1988; 140: 289.
167. Herr H, Pinsky C, Whitmore W, et al: Long term effect of intravesical bacillus Calmette-Guérin on flat carcinoma-in-situ of the bladder. J Urol 1986; 135:265.
168. Bretton P, Herr H, Whitmore W, et al: Intravesical bacillus Calmette-Guérin therapy for in-situ transitional cell carcinoma of the prostatic urethra. J Urol 1989; 141:853.
169. Hillyard R, Ladaga L, Schellhammer P: Superficial transitional cell carcinoma of the bladder associated with mucosal involvement of the prostatic urethra: results of treat-

ment with intravesical bacillus Calmette-Guérin. J Urol 1988; 139:290.
170. Hardeman S, Soloway MS: Urethral recurrence following radical cystectomy. J Urol 1990; 144:666.
171. Schellhammer P, Bean M, Whitmore W: Prostatic involvement by transitional cell carcinoma: pathogenesis, patterns, and prognosis. J Urol 1977; 118:399.
172. Hudson M: When intravesical measures fail: indications for cystectomy in superficial disease. Urol Clin North Am 1992; 19:601.
173. Soloway MS, Lopez A, Patel J, et al: Results of radical cystectomy for transitional cell carcinoma of the bladder and the effect of chemotherapy. Cancer 1994; 73:1926.
174. Amling C, Thraser J, Frazier H, et al: Radical cystectomy for stages Ta, Tis, & T1 transitional cell carcinoma of the bladder. J Urol 1994; 151:31.
175. Bracken RB, McDonald WW, Johnson DE: Cystectomy for superficial bladder cancer. Urology 1981; 18:459.
176. Malkowicz SB, Nicols P, Lieskovsky G, et al: The role of radical cystectomy in the management of high grade superficial bladder cancer (pA, p1, pis, & p2). J Urol 1990; 144:641.
177. Pagano F, Bassi P, Galetti TP, et al: Results of contemporary radical cystectomy for invasive bladder cancer: a clinicopathological study with an emphasis on the inadequacy of tumor, nodes and metastases classification. J Urol 1991; 145:45.
178. Smith JA: Laser surgery for transitional cell carcinoma. Technique, advantages and limitations. Urol Clin North Am 1992; 19(3):473.
179. Tarantino A, Aretz T, Libertino J, et al: Is the neodymium YAG laser effective therapy for invasive bladder cancer? Urology 1991; 38:514.
180. Herr H: Outpatient flexible cystoscopy and fulguration of recurrent superficial bladder tumors. J Urol 1990; 144: 1365.
181. Bianchi G, Nevelli P, Beltrami P, et al: Small urothelial carcinoma: diagnosis and treatment by cold cup forcep biopsy. J Urol 1990; 144:872.
182. Reading J, Hall RR, Parmar MKB: The application of prognostic factor analysis for Ta/T1 bladder cancer in routine urological practise. Br J Urol 1995; 75:604.
183. Morris SB, Gordon EM, Shearer RJ, et al: Superficial bladder cancer: how long should a tumor-free patient have check cystoscopies? Br J Urol 1995; 75:193.
184. Sheinfeld J, Reuter VE, Melamed MR, et al: Enhanced bladder cancer detection with the Lewis X antigen as a marker of neoplastic transformation. J Urol 1990; 143:285.
185. Sarosdy MF, De Vere White RW, Soloway MS, et al: Results of a multicenter trial using the BTA test to monitor for and diagnose recurrent bladder cancer. J Urol 1995; 154:379.
186. Korman HJ, Peabody JO, Cerny JC, et al: Autocrine motility factor receptor as a possible urine marker for transitional cell carcinoma of the bladder. J Urol 1996 (in press).
187. Booth CM, Kellett MJ: Intravenous urography and the follow-up of carcinoma of the bladder. Br J Urol 1981; 53: 246.
188. Miller EB, Eure GR, Schellhammer PF, et al: Upper tract transitional cell carcinoma following treatment of superficial bladder cancer with BCG. Urology 1993; 42(1):26.

18

INVASIVE TRANSITIONAL CELL CARCINOMA OF THE BLADDER: PROGNOSIS AND MANAGEMENT

LEE B. PRESSLER, M.D., DANIEL P. PETRYLAK, M.D., *and* CARL A. OLSSON, M.D.

In memory of Alan Yagoda, M.D.

Transitional cell carcinoma (TCC) of the bladder is the second most common genitourinary malignancy. In 1996, it is estimated that 50,500 patients will be diagnosed with bladder cancer and 11,200 will die from the disease, making it the fifth most common cause of cancer deaths in patients over 75 years old. Men have a higher incidence of the disease by a ratio of almost 3:1. Improvements in the diagnosis, staging, and treatment of bladder cancer have resulted in an increase in the 5-year survival from 53% to 81% among whites and from 24% to 60% among blacks over the past 40 years.[1]

Fortunately, 75% of patients present with superficial disease limited to the mucosa. Of these 75% will recur, however, only 10 to 15% will advance to muscle invasion.[2,3] A review of cystectomy specimens by Soto and associates revealed that papillary tumors invade along a broad front and tend to remain superficial, while solid carcinomas invade with long tentacles and are more deeply invasive.[4] Treatment of superficial disease usually consists of local transurethral resection or fulguration with the addition of intravesical chemotherapy and immunotherapy in selected cases. The management of superficial TCC has already been discussed.

Invasive bladder cancer includes tumors with invasion of the detrusor muscle (T2) and extends to invasion of the perivesical fat (T3) or adjacent organs (T4), with and without local and distant metastases. In the past, T1 lesions have been treated as superficial disease with radical cystectomy reserved for muscle-invasive cancer (T2 or greater). However, in some patients with high-grade T1 lesions, the tumors behave more like invasive cancer. In fact, as many as 50% of T1 grade 3 lesions will progress to muscle-invasive disease.[2,5] Therefore, clinicians should attempt to identify which T1 lesions will progress in order to treat these patients more aggressively with the hopes of cure.

The treatment of invasive bladder cancer should be focused upon control of local disease versus metastatic disease. Of those cancers that are muscle invasive on initial evaluation, 50% are associated with distant micrometastases at the time of presentation. In addition, while urologists have improved upon the local control of invasive bladder cancer, 50% of invasive bladder cancer patients eventually die of metastatic disease.[3,6] Therefore, localized therapy alone (radical cystectomy) may not be curative and combination chemotherapy may be required in an effort to control metastases. Great advances have been made in the treatment of distant disease with the advent of platinum-based combination chemotherapy such as M-VAC (methotrexate, vinblastine, Adriamycin, and cis-platinum) in the neoadjuvant and adjuvant setting.

Presently, patients with muscle-invasive disease (T2 or greater) are treated with radical cystectomy. Radical cystectomy should be considered the "gold standard" against which all other therapies are compared. With improvements in preoperative and postoperative care and the development of continent urinary diversion, the morbidity and social stigmata associated with radical cystectomy have greatly improved.

Over the years a variety of "radical" therapies other than cystectomy have been attempted for treating invasive bladder cancer, including aggressive transurethral resection, definitive radiotherapy, definitive chemotherapy, or combinations of the three.

A comparison of the multitude of clinical trials attempting different treatment strategies performed over the past 50 years is difficult because of differences in patient selection, preoperative staging (before and after the computed tomography [CT] scan era), operative techniques, preoperative and postoperative care, and patient follow-up. Stage migration has probably occurred in contemporary studies versus those prior to the advent of CT scan and magnetic resonance imaging (MRI). Our ability to detect enlarged lymph nodes and diffuse metastatic disease presently allows some patients to migrate toward a higher pretreatment stage. Thus, survival is improved in the lower stage patient because he/she is less likely to have metastatic disease. Furthermore, the survival of the higher stage patient is also improved because he/she is more likely to have subclinical metastases only.[2]

In this chapter we will review the current issues surrounding the treatment of invasive transitional cell carcinoma and we will try to identify prognostic factors that will help urologists optimize treatment of their patients.

DIAGNOSIS AND PREOPERATIVE STAGING

The initial evaluation of patients with suspected bladder cancer includes routine urinalysis, urine culture, urine cytology, and intravenous urography (IVU) to rule out upper tract pathology. IVU should be performed prior to cystoscopy so that a retrograde pyelogram can be performed simultaneously if the upper tracts were not adequately visualized on the IVU. Once the diagnosis of bladder cancer has been made either by cytology or by visualization of a tumor on cystoscopy, the depth of invasion and the presence of metastasis must be evaluated by both transurethral resection (TUR) and CT scan or MRI. If an invasive lesion is suspected it is beneficial to perform imaging prior to transurethral resection to avoid artifact from the resection on the imaging study. Routine preoperative tests should include complete blood count, electrolytes, liver function tests, coagulation profile, urinalysis and culture, and chest x-ray. In addition to TUR of the obvious lesion, multiple biopsies of the rest of the bladder and the prostatic urethra (in men) must be performed to rule out occult carcinoma in situ or neoplastic change in other areas of the urothelium. In pursuing a positive urine cytology where cystoscopy and biopsies are totally negative, selective cytology of each kidney and ureter must be obtained to localize the lesion.

TABLE 18–1. 5-YEAR SURVIVAL RATES FOR INVASIVE BLADDER CANCER TREATED WITH TURBT

Author(s)	No. of Patients	T2	T3a	T2 + T3a
Flocks[8]	142	56	43	47
Milner[9]	88	57	23	53
Barnes et al.[10]	114			40
O'Flynn et al.[13]	123	59	20	52
Barnes et al.[10]	75			31
Herr[15]	45	70	57	68
Henry et al.[14]	43	63	38	52

MANAGEMENT OF INVASIVE TCC

Transurethral Resection of Bladder Tumor

Traditionally, transurethral resection of bladder tumors (TURBT) has been used for diagnosis and local staging of bladder cancer. While radical cystectomy is the standard treatment modality for invasive bladder cancer, many clinicians have tried to identify patients who can be managed with transurethral resection alone, thereby sparing them bladder loss and urinary diversion.[7] These studies were originally prompted by the high morbidity and mortality associated with radical cystectomy in the early part of this century and later by the occasional finding of no residual tumor (pT0) in radical cystectomy specimens following TURBT.

In 1951, Flocks[8] reviewed his experience with TURBT as the primary therapy for 167 stage A (Jewett) and 126 stage B tumors (Table 18–1). Seventy-seven per cent of the stage A tumors were controlled compared to 54% of the stage B tumors. Poor prognosticators in his report included the presence of multiple tumors, tumor at the dome, anterior bladder neck (due to incomplete resection), and prostatic urethra.[8] Flocks, however, did not differentiate between stage B1 and B2 lesions, nor did he report overall survival data. Milner[9] reported a 36% 5-year survival of 190 patients with "infiltrative" TCC managed with TURBT alone. However, more than half the patients had only stage A or B1 (Marshall) lesions. Of patients treated conservatively by TURBT or TURBT plus radon seed implants, only 57% of B1 lesions and 23% of B2 lesions were totally eradicated.[9]

In 1967, Barnes et al.[10] compared the results with transurethral resection of 410 bladder tumors to the results of radical cystectomy series previously reported by Whitmore (1962)[11] and Jewett (1964).[12] For stage B cancer, Barnes achieved a 41% 5-year survival compared to 17% (B2) and 28% in the Whitmore and Jewett series, respectively. He concluded that TURBT was the treatment of choice for invasive bladder cancers.[10] Examination of his data demonstrates that 95 patients with more extensive disease were not deemed candidates for TURBT, resulting in a significant selection bias, compared to the Whitmore and Jewett series, where all patients underwent radical surgery.[10] O'Flynn et al.[13] reported 5-year survival rates of 54% for stage B1 and 20% for stage B2 tumors in 800 patients treated by TURBT.[13]

More recently, Henry and associates[14] retrospectively evaluated 114 patients with stage B1 and B2 TCC. Patients were separated into four groups according to treatment modality: group 1, TURBT alone (*n* = 43); group 2, 6500 to 7000 rads, (*n* = 16); group 3, radical cystectomy alone (*n* = 15); and group 4, 4000 to 6000 rads followed by radical cystectomy (*n* = 40). Patients with B1 tumors treated by TURBT alone had improved 5-year survival when compared to the three other "radical" therapies. The 5-year cancer-specific survival rates for B1 and B2 tumors, respectively, were 63 and 38% in group 1, 53 and 11% in group 2, 25 and 33% in group 3, and 48 and 54% in group 4. Patients with B2 tumors were best treated by preoperative external radiation therapy (XRT) and radical cystectomy. However, it should be emphasized that the selection of treatment was not randomized. As a consequence, group 1 patients had a greater proportion of B1 lesions than the other three groups and the tumors tended to be smaller in size.[14]

Restaging with TURBT of the tumor bed may identify patients who will benefit from aggressive TURBT alone. Herr was able to identify 20 of 217 patients (9%) who had complete response (pT0) after TURBT alone as shown by the lack of tumor on repeat resection. Two-hundred seventeen patients were evaluated for conservative surgical therapy by examination under anesthesia and repeat TUR of the bladder including the scar from the original resection. Forty-five patients were considered candidates for conservative management, being either pT0 (20), Pcis (17), P1 (4), or P2 (4). Of the 45, 30 remained disease free with their bladders intact.[15]

Can one predict a good outcome in a TURBT sampling resulting in pT0 status? Thrasher et al., in a retrospective analysis of 433 patients undergoing cystectomy with stage pT0 on final pathology, determined that stage pT0 does not confer a survival advantage. They compared the survival of 66 patients with pathologic stage pT0 to the survival of patients with the same pathologic stage as clinical stage. Of the 54 cTis/Ta patients, the 11 pT0 and the 24 pTis/Ta patients had an identical 5-year survival of 78%. Of the 166 cT1 patients, 32 pT0 and 78 pT1 had the same 73% 5-year survival and of the 213 cT2 patients the 23 pT0 and the 71 pT2 patients had a 5-year survival of 63%. They concluded that pT0 does not translate to increased survival.[16]

While TURBT alone may be curative for a highly select group of patients, it may result in withholding definitive therapy in the majority of patients. In a retrospective review of 240 patients, Pollack et al.[17] found that the actuarial 5-year freedom from metastases rate for those with local control was 77% compared to 29% for those with local failure. Distant metastases occurred in 56% of patients with local failure.[17] Therefore, patients may have one best first chance to control local disease that may be denied them with conservative management. Certainly, in elderly patients with significant comorbidity TURBT is a reasonable palliative measure to control local disease. However, in otherwise healthy individuals the results of TURBT alone are inferior to radical cystectomy.

Hall and associates[18] studied the role of aggressive TURBT and adjuvant chemotherapy in the management of invasive bladder. They reviewed their experience with 63 patients who underwent complete TURBT followed by four cycles of high-dose methotrexate. At 6 months 59% were tumor free and 12% had only superficial recurrence. A total of 43 patients (68%) were without evidence of invasive tumor. Fifteen patients (24%) still had invasive tumor present and three progressed to stage T4. Two patients developed metastases and three died as a result of treatment. At 3-year follow-up, 31 (57%) of the 54 evaluable patients were alive and disease free, 15 (28%) had invasive bladder cancer, 4 were tumor free after receiving radiotherapy, and 4 underwent salvage cystectomy.[18]

In another review of 36 patients with stage T3 bladder cancer treated with TURBT followed by two cycles of methtrexate and cis-platinum, Hall demonstrated a 56% 36-month disease-free survival. Twenty-two per cent of the patients had invasive cancer and 22% had metastases.[19]

Partial Cystectomy

Partial or segmental cystectomy is a surgical option in about 2 to 10% of patients with newly diagnosed invasive TCC.[3,20,21] At the Cleveland Clinic, only 50 of 2000 (2.5%) patients seen over a 10-year period were deemed candidates for segmental resection.[21] Similarly, at the Mayo Clinic only 6% of 3454 patients evaluated over 20 years met the criteria for partial cystectomy.[20] Criteria for partial cystectomy include the presence of a solitary lesion in an area amenable to partial resection such as within a diverticulum or at the dome or side wall of the bladder where a 2-cm margin around the lesion may be obtained. There must be no other lesions or carcinoma in situ as demonstrated by random mucosal biopsies. In men, the prostatic urethra must also be free of disease. Optimally, a 2-cm margin should be obtained and margins free of cancer should be confirmed at the time of surgery. Finally, there must be enough bladder remaining after resection to be functionally useful.[2,20-22]

Unfortunately, there have been no published series of prospective randomized trials to evaluate the efficacy of partial cystectomy for the treatment of invasive bladder cancer. Rather, the series published to date result from the random experience of mostly large tertiary care centers. Table 18–2 summarizes these series. Novick and Stewart, in a review of 50 patients who had partial cystectomy at

TABLE 18–2. 5-YEAR SURVIVAL AFTER PARTIAL CYSTECTOMY*

Arthur	Stage 0–A (%)	Stage B (%)	Stage C (%)	Stage D (%)	Overall (%)
Riches	58	36	0	0	59.5
Magri	80	38	26	0	42
Jewett	58	30	16	0	
Masina	82	50	38	0	
Cox	61	27	17	0	42
Long	73	33	9	0	38
Utz	68	44	29	0	43
Evans	69	31	0	0	60
Novick	67	53	17	25	50
Kaneti	68	40	33	0	50
Resnick	71	77	12.5	20	35

*Modified from Novick AC, Stewart BH: Partial cystectomy in the treatment of primary and secondary carcinoma of the bladder. J Urol 1976; 116:570, with permission.

TABLE 18–3. RATE OF TUMOR RECURRENCE AFTER PARTIAL CYSTECTOMY*

Source	Percent Recurrence
Resnick and O'Conor	76
Evans and Texter	40
Novick and Stewart	50
Cummings et al.	49
Schoberg et al.	70
Faysal and Frieha	78
Jardin and Vallencien	78
Lindahl et al.	58
Kaneti	38

*From Sweeney P, Kursh ED, Resnick MI: Partial cystectomy. Urol Clin North Am 1992; 19:701, with permission.

the Cleveland Clinic between 1960 and 1972, further defined the criteria listed above.[21] The 5-year survival rates for patients with stage B and stage C lesions treated with partial cystectomy were 53 and 17%, respectively. They correlated survival with tumor size, location, the presence of multifocality, and negative surgical margins. Clearly, patients with unifocal disease and negative margins had improved 5-year survival of 59 and 57%, respectively, compared to patients with multifocal tumors and positive margins whose 5-year survivals were 31 and 0%, respectively. Smaller tumors (<2 cm) had improved 10-year survival. For unclear reasons, tumors located on the posterior bladder wall fared better while patients with dome lesions fared worse.[21]

Schoberg et al.[23] reported a 5-year survival rate of only 40% for stage B tumors and 12% for stage C tumors. The fact that patients with stage B2 tumors lived longer than patients with stage B1 tumors is curious.[23] Kaneti reported 5-year survival rates of 40 and 33% for stage B and stage C tumors, respectively.[24]

Obviously, after partial cystectomy, local recurrence or new tumors can develop. The recurrence rates in numerous series have been reviewed by Sweeney and can be seen in Table 18–3.[22] Most of the recurrences appear to occur within the first 2 years after surgery.[22,25,26] Since the recurrence rate is higher in patients with a prior history of bladder tumors, partial cystectomy should be reserved for patients presenting with their initial tumor.

A worrisome complication of partial cystectomy is the implantation of tumor cells within the pelvis and/or wound at the time of surgery. Implantation of spilled tumor cells has been reported to occur in as high as 20% of patients.[27] Novick and Utz achieved a 0 and 1.5% implantation rate, respectively, by packing off the bladder and irrigating the field with distilled water prior to closure.[20,21] Van Derwerf Messing observed a 0% recurrence rate in patients receiving preoperative radiation prior to suprapubic insertion of radium seed implants compared to 14% in those who did not, suggesting that preoperative radiation in doses of 1000 to 1200 cGy the week prior to surgery decreases the chance of implantation.[28] At our institution Adriamycin is instilled into the bladder prior to surgery. The Adriamycin remains in the bladder for 1 hour, after which the bladder is emptied and serial irrigations are used to remove the drug from the bladder before formal cystotomy. When using suprapubic tubes, persistent drainage from the suprapubic tube tract has been reported in up to 14% of patients.[29,30] These patients appear to be at increased risk for tumor seeding of the tract.[22,29] Sweeney and associates advocate the use of Foley catheter drainage only postoperatively to avoid this complication.[22]

The effect of partial cystectomy on functional bladder capacity is controversial. Baker and associates[31] found that bladders subjected to subtotal cystectomy eventually regained functional bladder capacity, while Merrel et al. suggest that no more than 50% of the bladder be removed.[32] Cummings and associates[33] found an association between both preoperative radiotherapy (XRT) and multiple prior TURBT with voiding dysfunction after partial cystectomy.[33]

Survival rates for partial cystectomy are comparable to radical cystectomy in properly selected patients. Predictors of failure include multifocality, recurrence in new locations within the bladder, and positive surgical margins. Therefore, it is essential to rule out occult TCC and to achieve negative surgical margins in patients undergoing partial cystectomy for invasive bladder cancer. Most importantly, because of the multifocal nature of transitional cell carcinoma, patients having partial cystectomy must be followed aggressively with interval cystoscopy and cytology to rule out tumor recurrence.

Radical Cystectomy

Clinical Prognostic Factors

Numerous studies over the past 40 years have clearly demonstrated that tumor stage and grade are the primary clinical predictors of outcome in patients with bladder cancer.[34–38] Narayana et al. reported that clinical tumor stage, grade, and size were the most important clinical prognosticators in 468 patients with bladder cancer.[34] In an effort to identify additional indicators of prognosis, Thrasher and associates recently reviewed their experience in 531 patients who underwent radical cystectomy as the primary form of treatment for bladder cancer at Duke University. Patient age, sex, clinical stage, presenting signs and symptoms, past medical history, and admission labs were all evaluated. Clinical stage greater than T2, age greater than 65 years, irritative voiding symptoms, high-grade tumor, anemia (Hb < 12 g/dl), history of nephroureterectomy, creatinine greater than 1.5 mg/dl, and history of definitive XRT were all indicators of poor prognosis on univariate and multivariate analysis in decreasing order. Patients who had failed definitive XRT had a median survival of 2.7 years; this compared to those who underwent cystectomy with or without prior XRT who had an 8.7-year median survival. The 156 patients who had preoperative XRT showed no improved survival. Obstructive hydronephrosis was a significantly poor prognosticator on univariate but not multivariate analysis.[38]

Pathologic Prognostic Factors

The use of radical cystectomy for the treatment of invasive bladder cancer prior to 1950 originated from the observations of Jewett and Strong that correlated the depth of penetration into the bladder wall with local extension, lymph node metastases, and potential curability. They determined that lesions confined to the mucosa (stage A), with infiltration into the muscle (stage B) and into the perivesical fat (stage C), were associated with pelvic lymph node metastases in 0, 13, and 74%, respectively.[39] Jewett later reported the 5-year survival of superficial muscle invasion to be 76% compared to 3% for deep muscle and perivesical invasion and postulated that increased lymph node involvement was the reason for the poor survival associated with deep muscle invasion.[40] More recent studies have found lymph node metastases in 20 to 30% of organ-confined tumors (P2 and P3a) and in 30 to 66% of tumors extending into the perivesical fat and beyond (P3b or greater).[41–49,71]

Numerous studies have found that overall disease-free survival correlated best with pathologic stage rather than clinical stage.[49] In patients with organ-confined invasive cancer (P2 and P3a), pelvic lymph node involvement is the most important prognosticator.[46,47,50–52] In fact, in the absence of lymph node metastases the survival rates for stage P2 and P3a bladder cancer are comparable. In a series of 141 patients (Figs. 18–1 through 18–3), Pagano et al. demonstrated 70% 5-year survival rates for stage T1, T2, and T3a lesions without nodal disease compared to a less than 30% survival in patients with positive lymph nodes.[50] In a follow-up

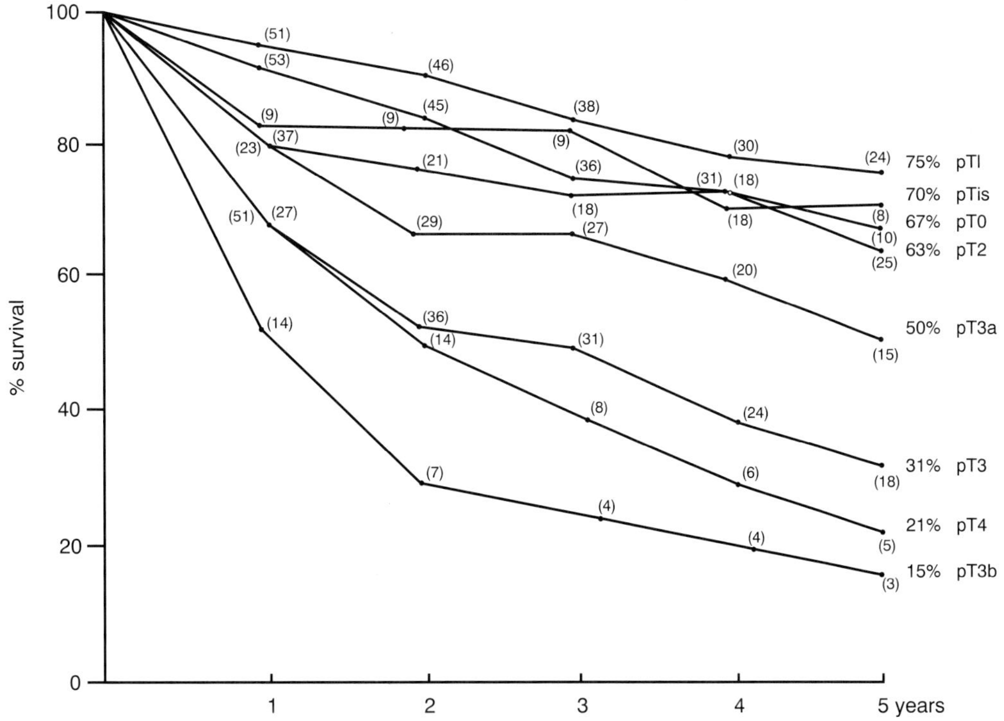
100
80
60
40
20
0
% survival
1
2
3
4
5 years
75% pTI
70% pTis
67% pTO
63% pT2
50% pT3a
31% pT3
21% pT4
15% pT3b
(51)
(53)
(46)
(45)
(38)
(9)
(9)
(9)
(37)
(23)
(30)
(24)
(21)
(36)
(31)
(18)
(51)
(27)
(29)
(18)
(27)
(18)
(8)
(10)
(25)
(20)
(14)
(36)
(14)
(31)
(15)
(8)
(24)
(7)
(6)
(18)
(4)
(4)
(5)
(3)

FIGURE 18–1. Overall 5-year survival according to pathologic stage. (From Pagano F, Pierfrancesco B, Galetti TP, et al: Results of contemporary radical cystectomy for invasive bladder cancer: a clinicopathologic study with emphasis on the inadequacy of the tumor, nodes and metastases classification. J Urol 1991; 145:45, with permission.)

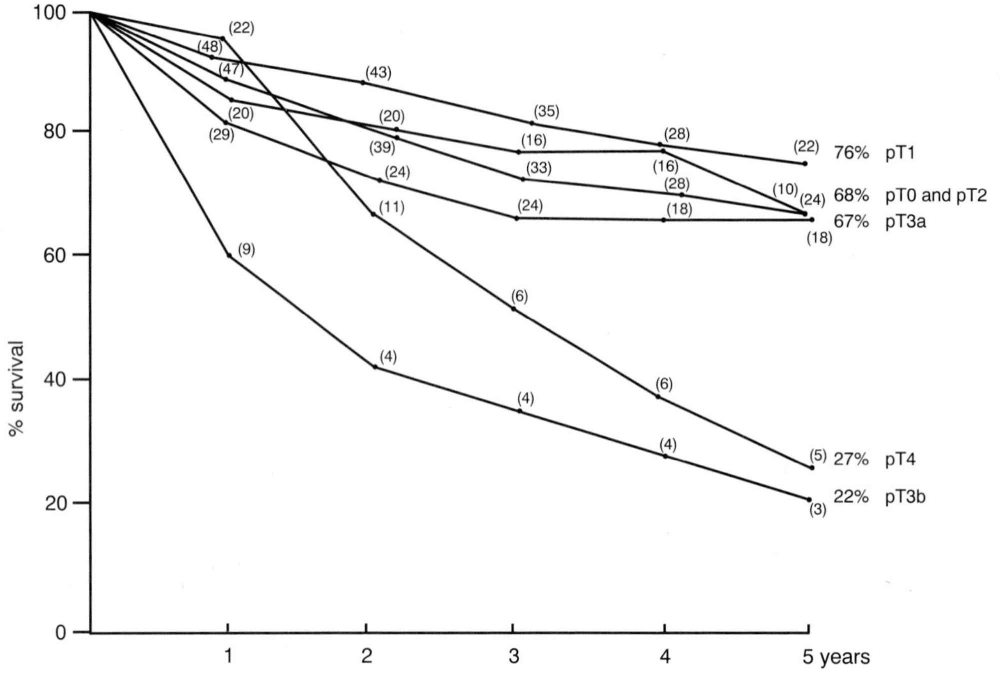
100
80
60
40
20
0
% survival
1
2
3
4
5 years
(22) 76% pT1
(24) 68% pT0 and pT2
67% pT3a
(18)
(5) 27% pT4
(3) 22% pT3b

FIGURE 18–2. Overall 5-year survival according to pathologic stage in N– patients. Patients with stage P2 and P3a tumors have comparable survivals. (From Pagano F, Pierfrancesco B, Galetti TP, et al: Results of contemporary radical cystectomy for invasive bladder cancer: a clinicopathologic study with emphasis on the inadequacy of the tumor, nodes and metastases classification. J Urol 1991; 145:45, with permission.)

study of 261 patients, they later reported 5-year survival rates of 60 and 4% for node-negative versus node-positive disease, respectively.[51] In Skinner and Lieskovsky's experience, patients whose primary tumor was confined to the bladder had a 5-year survival of at least 69% compared to all patients with node-positive, disease who had a 5-year survival of only 33%.[46]

The decreased 5-year survival associated with extravesical extension of the tumor is only partially

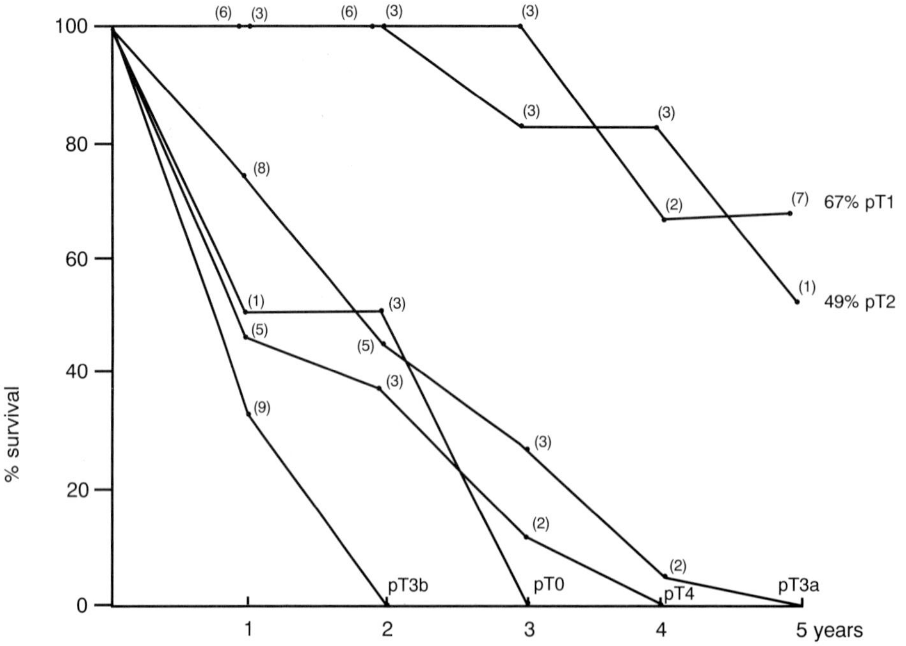
100
80
60
40
20
0
% survival
1
2
3
4
5 years
(7) 67% pT1
(1) 49% pT2
pT3b
pT0
pT4
pT3a

FIGURE 18–3. Overall 5-year survival according to pathologic stage in N+ patients. (From Pagano F, Pierfrancesco B, Galetti TP, et al: Results of contemporary radical cystectomy for invasive bladder cancer: a clinicopathologic study with emphasis on the inadequacy of the tumor, nodes and metastases classification. J Urol 1991; 145:45, with permission.)

due to increased incidence of lymph node metastases. Lerner et al. found that 5-year survival was significantly better in patients with organ-confined cancer with positive lymph nodes (50%) compared to those with extravesical extension and positive lymph nodes (18%).[41,42] These results have recently been confirmed by Vieweg and associates' review of the experience at Memorial Sloan-Kettering Cancer Center (MSKCC). They found that patients with stage P3a N+ or less had a 52.6% 5-year survival compared to 23.4% for those with extravesical extension (P3b, N+ or greater) (Fig. 18–4).[52] These results may reflect a higher incidence of distant metastases via hematogenous routes in patients with cancer beyond the confines of the bladder.

In a review of 188 patients with muscle-invasive bladder cancer treated by radical cystectomy with and without adjuvant chemotherapy at M.D. Anderson Cancer Center, the disease-free survivals for stage D visceral and stage D nodal patients were almost identical, implying that distant micrometastasis was the important prognostic factor in these patients. Furthermore, patients with stage D nodal disease without vascular invasion fared much better than those with, with disease-free survivals of 100 and 40%, respectively.[53] While the results were statistically significant, the number of patients was quite small. Clearly, the poorer prognosis associated with deeper invasion into the bladder muscle and perivesical structures is the result of many factors including the likelihood of lymphatic as well as hematogenous metastases. Once the cancer has extended beyond the bladder (P3b and P4), the presence of positive lymph nodes is of little consequence, with all patients having a dismal prognosis.

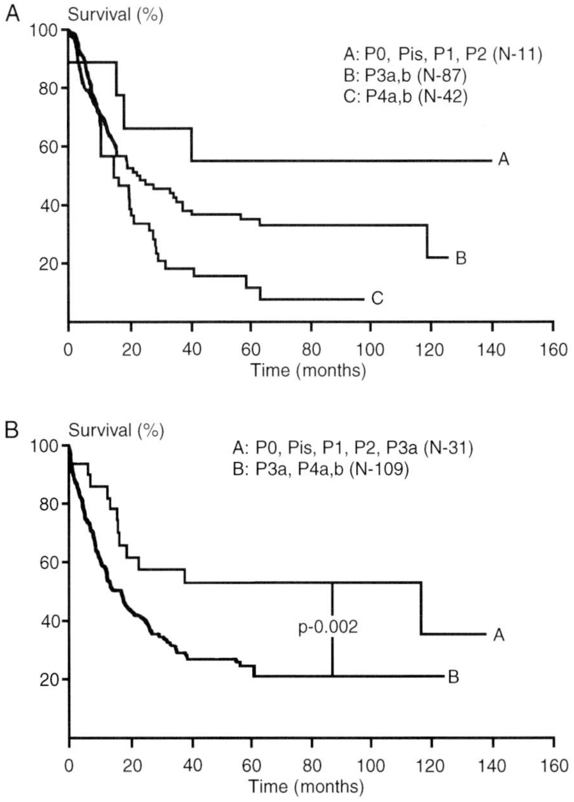
A
Survival (%)
100
80
60
40
20
A: P0, Pis, P1, P2 (N-11)
B: P3a,b (N-87)
C: P4a,b (N-42)
A
B
C
0
20
40
60
80
100
120
140
160
Time (months)
B
Survival (%)
100
80
60
40
20
A: P0, Pis, P1, P2, P3a (N-31)
B: P3a, P4a,b (N-109)
p-0.002
A
B
0
20
40
60
80
100
120
140
160
Time (months)

FIGURE 18–4. *A*, Long-term survival of 140 patients with N+ bladder cancer according to pathologic stage. *B*, Differences between tumors confined to the bladder P3a and tumors extending beyond the confines of the bladder P3b were statistically significant (p = .02). (From Vieweg J, Whitmore WF, Herr HW, et al: The role of pelvic lymphadenectomy and radical cystectomy for lymph node positive bladder cancer. Cancer 1994; 73:3020. Copyright American Cancer Society, 1994, with permission.)

In their review of 531 patients, Frazier and associates also correlated survival with tumor grade, involvement of the ureter, and prostatic urethra. As would be expected, patients with high-grade lesions (grades 3 and 4) fared worse than those with low-grade lesions; however, carcinoma in situ (CIS) was not an adverse prognostic indicator. Ureteral involvement conferred a 40% 5-year survival compared to those without, who had a 60% 5-year survival. Finally, 33 patients with involvement of the prostatic stroma had a markedly decreased 5-year survival (20%).[48]

Involvement of the prostate is a particularly ominous prognostic factor. Invasion of the prostate from a bladder neoplasm occurs in 10 to 51% of cases, of which 23 to 46% will invade the prostate stroma.[54] These patients generally die from distant metastatic disease, with 5-year survival rates less than 20%.[41] Patients with CIS of the prostatic urothelium without stromal invasion have survival rates dependent upon the stage of the primary bladder tumor.[41,49]

Radical Cystectomy for NO Disease

The results of early radical cystectomy series were extremely poor because of operative mortality rates as high as 15 to 40% and 5-year survival rates as low as 11%.[40,55–61] However, more contemporary series of patients treated with radical cystectomy and pelvic lymph node dissection (PLND) without XRT yield 5-year survival rates as high as 88, 69, and 40% for stages P2, P3A, and P3b, respectively.[2,3,46,53,62–66] In fact, the operative mortality rate for radical cystectomy is now less than 2%.[41]

Over the past 20 years, radical cystectomy has become the standard therapy for invasive bladder cancer. While long-term survival is related to the presence or absence of lymph node or distant metastases, wide excision of the tumor by radical cystectomy and pelvic lymphadenectomy provides the patient with the best chances for local control and, it is hoped, cure. Table 18–4 summarizes the results of series of radical cystectomy and pelvic lymphadenectomy as the primary treatment of invasive bladder cancer over the past 20 years. Montie and associates in 1984 reported on 157 patients treated at the Cleveland Clinic between 1960 and 1979, of whom 99 underwent radical cystectomy without

TABLE 18–4. SURVIVAL RATES FOR RADICAL CYSTECTOMY*

Author(s)	Year	Percent Survival				
		P2	P2/P3a	P3a	P3a/P3b	P3b
Brice et al.[55]	1956				9	
Jewett[40]	1964	50		16		12
Poole-Wilson and Bernard[56]	1971		25			12
Long et al.[57]	1972		36			24
Bredael et al.[64]	1980	52		36		11
Mathur et al.[63]	1981	88		57		40
Montie et al.[62]	1982	50		63		29
Skinner and Lieskovsky[46]	1988	83		69		29
Freiha[65]	1990		83			47
Pagano et al.[51]	1991	63		50		15
Frazier et al.[48]	1993	64			39	

*Series prior to 1980 (*top*) had poorer survival rates compared to contemporary series (*bottom*).

preoperative XRT. Patients treated with radical cystectomy with and without XRT faired much better than those treated with XRT alone, with 10-year survival rates of 50 and 10% respectively.[62] In the 99 patients treated with radical cystectomy and PLND alone, there was a 9% pelvic recurrence rate and 5-year survival rates for stages P2, P3a, and P3b of 62, 74, and 57%, respectively. In addition, patients operated on after 1976 did much better than those treated prior to 1976, probably due to increased experience in performing the operation as well as caring for patients postoperatively.[62] Mathur and associates reported the 5-year survival of 58 patients treated with radical cystectomy alone between 1967 and 1974 to be 88, 57, and 40% for stage P2, P3a, and P3b, respectively.[63] Pagano et al.[51] and Freiha[65] have published similar results.

Skinner and associates reported the 5-year survival rates on 189 patients treated with radical cystectomy and PLND with stages P2 and P3a to be 83 and 69%, respectively. Patients with significant extravesical disease experienced a much shorter 5-year survival. Patients with stage P3b and P4 tumors had 5-year survivals of only 29 and 22%, respectively. As mentioned above, high-stage lesions with positive lymph nodes did not alter survival, with all patients doing uniformly poorly (33% 5-year survival).[46,66] Radical cystectomy should be performed on all patients with cancer clinically localized to the pelvis. Pelvic lymph node dissection will accurately stage these patients, possibly cure some with minimal nodal disease, and identify candidates for adjuvant chemotherapy.

Nerve-sparing radical cystoprostatectomy does not appear to affect either local pelvic recurrence or 5-year survival. In a review of 76 patients, Brendler and Walsh reported an actuarial 5-year pelvic recurrence rate of only 7.5% (3.9% at 38 months) and a 5-year survival of 78%. Sixty-four per cent of the 42 men who did not have urethrectomy were potent compared to 17% of those with urethrectomy.[68] Certainly, in potent men not requiring urethrectomy a nerve-sparing approach is appropriate as long as it does not compromise excision of the entire lesion.[66,67]

Radical Cystectomy for N+ Disease

Cancer involving the pelvic lymph nodes occurs in as many as 20 to 35% of patients with invasive bladder cancer and may be as high as 66% in patients with stage P3b or greater disease. This has led many urologists to advocate either nihilism or an extensive PLND in association with radical cystectomy for the treatment of invasive bladder cancer.[46,69–71] The primary lymphatic drainage of the bladder is the obturator and external iliac lymph nodes. In a review of 134 patients with positive lymph node metastases, obturator (74%) and external iliac (65%) were most often involved.[72] While many groups have demonstrated little or no added morbidity to the operation with the addition of PLND, the dismal prognosis of patients with N+ bladder cancer has led many urologists to question the role of "curative" radical cystectomy and PLND in these patients.[46,69–71]

Table 18–5 summarizes the incidence and sur-

TABLE 18–5. 5-YEAR SURVIVAL RATE FOLLOWING RADICAL CYSTECTOMY AND PLND IN PATIENTS WITH NODAL INVOLVEMENT

Author	Date	N+	Percent	Percent 5-Year Survival
Whitmore and Marshall[58]	1962	46	20	4
Dretler et al.[73]	1973	54	13	17
Bredael et al.[64]	1980	26	15	4
Smith and Whitmore[72]	1977	134	20	7
Skinner et al.[70]	1982	36	24	36
Wishnow and Tenney[53]*	1985	32	15	52
Roehrborn et al.[74]	1991	42	15	19
Lerner et al.[41]	1992	132	22	29
Vieweg et al.[52]	1993	140	26	29

*28 of 32 patients received adjuvant chemotherapy.

vival of patients with nodal disease treated by radical cystetectomy over the past 50 years. In 1973, Dretler and associates found that 33% of patients with only one or two involved lymph nodes survived 5 years, suggesting that PLND may cure a subset of patients with minimal nodal disease.[73] Smith and Whitmore performed a retrospective analysis of 134 N+ patients who underwent radical cystectomy and PLND between 1966 and 1977. All patients had preoperative XRT and 89% of the lesions were stage P3 or greater. Of the nine patients who survived 5 years, five had minimal nodal involvement (17% 5-year survival). There was a statistically significant trend towards increased time to recurrence and survival in patients with less extensive nodal disease. Patients with minimal nodal disease (N1) had a median survival of 22 months compared to 7 months for patients with more extensive nodal disease. Patients with minimal to moderate nodal disease (N1 and N2) tended to recur at distant sites rather than locally. They suggested that extensive PLND may help with local cancer control which, when coupled with systemic chemotherapy to control distant metastases, may provide patients with enhanced survival.[72]

In a more contemporary review of 36 patients with nodal involvement, Skinner found the rate of lymph node metastases in patients with P1, P2–P3a, and P3b–P4 to be 10, 35, and 66%, respectively. The 5-year survival rate for the entire group was 36% and only two patients recurred in the pelvis.[71] Roehrborn and associates found similar results in 42 patients operated on between 1971 and 1987. Patients with pN1 and pN2 (TNM) stage disease experienced 30 and 18% 3-year survivals, respectively. Patients with stage pT3b, N0 disease in the same series had a 36% 3-year survival. The authors concluded that because pT3b, N0 versus N1 patients had similar 3-year survival rates, some patients with minimal nodal disease may actually be cured of their local disease by extensive PLND.[74]

The largest series to date has been reported from MSKCC. In a retrospective review, the results of 140 N+ patients treated by radical cystectomy and PLND were analyzed. Fifty-three per cent of the patients received adjuvant or neoadjuvant chemotherapy and 74% had prior XRT. In these patients, P stage was the most significant prognostic factor. Neither XRT nor chemotherapy seemed to confer a survival advantage. Seventy-nine per cent of the N+ patients had extravesical extension of the cancer and experienced an average survival of 15.7 (±2.6) months compared to patients with organ-confined disease (21%), who demonstrated a survival of 119 (±69) months. The extent of nodal disease did not impact on long-term survival but was significant for predicting local recurrence and disease-free survival. Median time to recurrence was 2.5 months for stage N3, and 8.6 and 7.9 months for N1 and N2, respectively. The studies cited above imply that radical cystectomy and PLND for organ-confined bladder cancer with minimal nodal disease does have therapeutic value.[52]

While PLND appears to be of therapeutic benefit in patients with organ-confined tumors, the high incidence of distant microscopic metastatic disease associated with stage P3b or greater cancer and in patients with gross lymphadenopathy on staging CT scan or MRI may make the addition of PLND to standard cystectomy unnecessary except for staging purposes.

Urethrectomy

Urethral CIS on autopsy specimens has been detected in as high as 31% of patients who die of bladder cancer.[41,75,76] Furthermore, the risk of urethral recurrence is approximately 17% at 10 years and may be as high as 40% for patients with CIS.[77] Hardeman and Soloway determined the risk for anterior urethral recurrence was 37% for tumor involving the prostate stroma or ducts and only 4% for tumors not involving the prostate.[78]

Patients with urethral recurrence usually present with bloody urethral discharge, urethral pain, and/or mass and inguinal adenopathy.[41] The indication for urethrectomy at the time of the initial surgery is involvement of the prostatic urethra or stroma by either direct tumor extension or with CIS. Delayed urethrectomy should be performed when the final pathology demonstrates tumor in the prostatic urethra. In patients where the urethra is left behind (and not in continuity with the urinary tract), saline barbotage cytology is indicated at interval. In patients with an orthotopic neobladder, the urethra may be monitored closely with urethroscopy and urethral cytologic washings every 3 months. At the first sign of recurrence, a urethrectomy should be performed and the continence mechanism converted to a catheterizable stoma.[41]

Definitive Radiation Therapy

Because of the high morbidity and mortality associated with radical cystectomy, definitive radiation therapy (DXRT) followed by salvage cystectomy in nonresponders played an important role in the treatment of bladder cancer prior to the 1960s. However, better patient selection, staging, and operative and anesthetic techniques have decreased the morbidity and operative mortality of radical cystectomy to less than 2% in most series. When compared to contemporary surgical series, radiation therapy is clearly inferior to radical cystectomy in the treatment of patients with invasive bladder cancer.

The urologist should be aware of conditions in which radiation therapy is contraindicated. Patients with inflammatory bowel disease, prior pelvic irradiation, extensive pelvic surgery, chronic pelvic infections, and irritable voiding symptoms are not candidates for XRT.[79] In addition, patients with large atonic bladders and with diverticula do poorly because of irregular dosing and often will have a deterioration of bladder function after treatment.[79]

PREOPERATIVE RADIATION THERAPY

The generally poor local control and survival of patients treated by both radical cystectomy alone and DXRT in the 1940s and 1950s led to a combined approach of preoperative XRT (PO-XRT) followed by radical cystectomy. The rationale for PO-XRT was threefold: (1) prevention of intraoperative seeding of cancer cells, (2) local treatment of microscopic extravesical disease, and (3) tumor downstaging. PO-XRT has been given in doses ranging from 2000 cGy over 1 week followed by immediate cystectomy and PLND to 5000 cGy over 5 weeks with cystectomy 4 weeks later.[80] While higher doses appear to have improved local control, they are associated with increased toxicity.

Whitmore and associates at MSKCC treated all patients with stage T3 TCC with 4500 cGy preoperative XRT followed by radical cystectomy 4 weeks later. They observed a 12% local recurrence rate and a 37% 5-year survival rate compared to a 40% local recurrence rate and 17% 5-year survival rate found in historical controls.[81] In a later review they found a 42 versus 33% 5-year survival and a 20 versus 37% pelvic recurrence rate for patients treated by XRT followed by cystectomy compared to historical controls treated by cystectomy alone.[82] A meta-analysis of numerous nonrandomized studies with 1185 patients found that preoperative XRT in patients with T3 tumors results in a 15 to 20% survival advantage over cystectomy alone.[83] While these early studies suggested local control and survival advantages with preoperative XRT, the studies were nonrandomized and used historical surgical controls, which are inferior to contemporary surgical series.[2]

In the 1970s, two prospective trials conducted to determine the efficacy of PO-XRT were unable to show any benefit to PO-XRT. The Veterans Administration Cooperative Urological Research Group randomized 72 patients with stage T2, N0 and T3, N0 to one of three groups: (1) DXRT, (2) PO-XRT plus surgery, and (3) surgery alone. The 3-year survival for all three groups was 40%, with no difference between the groups. Of note, 25% of the patients entered into the study did not finish.[84] Slack and Prout reporting for the National Surgical Adjuvant Bladder Project Group also reported no differences between treatment groups and also suffered from an exceedingly high dropout rate (50%).[85,86] In a 5-year follow-up Slack and associates reported that patients who had a complete response to PO-XRT had a 55% 5-year survival compared to 32% for those who did not.[86] The authors use this result as an argument for the benefits of PO-XRT. However, we suggest that their results were due to the fact that those patients who responded to XRT had inherently less aggressive tumors and therefore had a prolonged survival. A prospective randomized trial from the Southwest Oncology Group (SWOG) also demonstrated no survival advantage associated with PO-XRT.

Contemporary series of PO-XRT combined with radical cystectomy have reported similar recurrence and survival rates compared to cystectomy alone. Fossa and associates reported no difference in survival of 122 patients treated either by high-dose PO-XRT or low-dose PO-XRT followed by radical cystectomy or by radical cystectomy alone.[88] In a series of 197 patients, Skinner and Lieskovsky also found similar outcomes between patients receiving PO-XRT versus cystectomy alone. One hundred patients were treated with 1600 cGy over 4 days followed by immediate cystectomy and 97 were treated with cystectomy and PLND alone. The 5-year survivals for P2–P3a, P3a–P3b, and P4, N+ were 75, 43, and 35%, respectively, for both groups. In addition, no differences were observed in local pelvic failure (9% in PO-XRT group and 7% in the radical cystectomy group). The use of adjuvant chemotherapy also showed no benefit after 18 months. The surgery-only group was later expanded to 197 patients. When compared to the 100 patients who received PO-XRT, no survival benefit was observed (Table 18–6). While this was not a prospectively randomized study, both groups of patients were treated by the same urologists over the same period of time.[46,66]

TABLE 18–6. ACTUARIAL 5-YEAR SURVIVAL FOR PATIENTS WITH INVASIVE BLADDER CANCER TREATED BY CYSTECTOMY AND PLND ALONE VERSUS PREOPERATIVE XRT FOLLOWED BY CYSTECTOMY AND PLND*†

	Stage P2	Stage P3a	Stage P3b	Stage P4	Stage N(+)
Cystectomy	83%	69%	29%	22%	32%
Preoperative XRT	53%	48%	39%	25%	36%

*Data from Skinner DG, Lieskovsky G: Management of invasive and high grade bladder cancer. *In* Skinner DG, Lieskovsky G (eds): Diagnostic and Management of Genitourinary Cancer, pp 295–312. Philadelphia, WB Saunders Co, 1988, with permission.

†Differences were not statistically significant.

Most recently, Cole and associates reviewed the experience at M.D. Anderson Cancer Center with 338 patients treated with PO-XRT (4900 cGy) and cystectomy between 1960 and 1983 and 232 patients treated with cystectomy alone between 1985 and 1990. For patients with T3b lesions, the actuarial 5-year local control for the PO-XRT group was 91% compared to 72% for the cystectomy-alone group. The PO-XRT group also showed slightly better freedom from distant metastases, disease freedom, and overall survival, but the results were not statistically significant. Furthermore, the relationship was not significant for other clinical stages. They conclude that PO-XRT should be considered for patients with clinical stage T3a bladder cancer.[89] One problem with this study was the use of clinical rather than pathologic staging; the understaging rate for bladder cancer approaches 50%. Another problem, of course, is that the study was not randomized and covered different time frames when patterns of institutional referral may have differed.

Bloom and associates carried out a British Institute of Urology study reporting a significant benefit from PO-XRT compared to DXRT in men under age 60 years. The 5-year survival rates were 45 and 29% for the PO-XRT versus DXRT groups, respectively.[90] The Danish Vesical Group found a statistically insignificant survival advantage in 183 patients randomized to PO-XRT and cystectomy compared to DXRT and salvage cystectomy in those with incomplete response or tumor recurrence.[91]

While preoperative radiation therapy may slightly improve local control of invasive bladder cancer, it does not appear to confer an increase in survival. This makes biologic sense, since most patients die from distant metastases rather than local recurrence. However, recently Pollack reviewed 240 patients treated with radical cystectomy and PLND with and without chemotherapy and concluded that local failure correlated with distant failure. His conclusions may be flawed because 49% of the patients (61% T2–T3a and 81% T3b–T4) received combination chemotherapy.[17] The patients who received adjuvant chemotherapy were those with a poor surgical outcome (margin-positive or node-positive). Therefore, these patients most likely had microscopic distant metastases at the time of diagnosis, and the relationship between local and distant failure was not causal.

CURRENT CHEMOTHERAPY

As mentioned previously, despite effective local therapy, half of all patients with muscle-invasive TCC of the bladder die not from local failure but rather from distant metastases. Consequently, improvement in survival can best be obtained from directing therapy toward micrometastases. A goal then is the integration of systemic chemotherapy with cystectomy or radiation. Effective single and combination chemotherapeutic agents have been evaluated as neoadjuvant or adjuvant therapy. Cytotoxic therapy has also been administered sequentially or concurrently with radiation. Controversy reigns as to the exact role of chemotherapy in the treatment of locally advanced bladder cancer. Despite a 30% local complete response rate observed in some neoadjuvant trials and a suggestion of improved disease-free survival in adjuvant trials, clear proof of benefit is yet to be conclusively demonstrated.

The most clinically active and extensively studied agents against transitional cell carcinoma include platinum-based compounds and antifols. Cisplatin at a dose of 70 mg/m^2 every 3 to 4 weeks demonstrated a response rate (complete [CR] and partial [PR]) of 30% in 320 previously untreated patients (95% confidence intervals [CI] 25 to 35%).[92] Active analogues of cisplatin include carboplatin (CR and PR, 13%) and iproplatin (CR and PR, 18%). Although it would appear that these analogues have less activity than cisplatin, cooperative group studies have demonstrated statistically similar response rates.[93] Methotrexate in doses of 30 to 40 mg/m^2 results in a reported response rate of 29% (95% CI, 23 to 35%). The antifolates trimetrexate (CR and PR, 17%; 95% CI, 7 to 30%) and piretrexam (CR and PR, 30%) have also shown significant activity.[93]

Recent studies of Taxol administered at a dose of 250 mg/m^2 with granulocyte colony-stimulating factor (G-CSF) support demonstrated a 42% response rate in 26 nonpretreated patients.[94] Taxotere, a water-soluble analogue of Taxol, was found to induce responses in 20% (95% CI, 6 to 44%) of platinum-resistant patients.[95] Gemcitibine, a cytodine analogue, has also demonstrated considerable activity in seven of nine unpretreated cases. Of note, complete responses are rare with single-agent therapy and the median duration of response is usually only 3 to 5 months.[96]

Phase II studies of combinations of agents have generally demonstrated higher response rates (CR and PR, 41 to 69%) than achievable with single drugs.[92] These regimens include CA (cisplatin, + Adriamycin), CISCA or CAP (cisplatin, Adriamycin, cyclophospamide), CMV (cisplatin, methotrexate, vinblastine), and M-VAC (methotrexate, vinblastine, Adriamycin, cisplatin). Of these multidrug regimens, however, only the M-VAC regimen has proven to be superior to single-agent therapy.[97]

Two prospective randomized phase III studies in over 350 cases documented superiority of M-VAC in response and in survival ($p < .0001$) when compared to either cisplatin alone or to the CISCA regimen. Median survival for patients treated with M-VAC was 54 and 82 weeks versus 36 weeks for cisplatin and 40 weeks for CISCA.[98] While the response rate in the cisplatin randomized trial was lower than that reported in both the original M-VAC and the CISCA randomized studies, most patients were unable to receive the standard M-VAC dosage schedule, and dosages were either eliminated or modified. In contrast, about 80% of the cases in the randomized study against CISCA did receive the complete cycles, which may explain the better survival statistics. Such data support the contention that a combination chemotherapy regimen is statistically superior to a single agent.[98,99]

ADJUVANT CHEMOTHERAPY

Delivery of effective cytotoxic agents administered after definitive local therapy has an advantage over neoadjuvant therapy; pathologic staging helps select only those patients at high risk for relapse (T3b, T4 or N+ disease), enabling those at lower risk to avoid unnecessary treatment with resultant side effects. On the other hand, removal of the primary tumor prior to treatment does limit the measure of outcome to progression-free and overall survival and abrogates ability to assess in vivo chemosensitivity. Furthermore, administration of therapy may be limited by the patient's physical condition after surgery or radiation therapy; some refuse treatment, and others may receive inadequate doses.

Nonrandomized phase II trials have suggested a survival benefit for those patients receiving adjuvant therapy after definitive local treament. In a study of 339 patients undergoing radical cystectomy at M.D. Anderson Cancer Center from 1981 to 1986, Logothetis et al.[100] identified patients at high risk for relapse as those with extravesicular involvement (T3b or T4), nodal metastases, or lymphatic or vascular invasion. Of the 133 high-risk patients, 72 received CISCA treatment within 6 weeks of cystectomy, whereas 62 either refused or were deemed unsuitable for treatment. Seventy-one low-risk patients were treated, while 206 were observed. Of patients treated, 67% received the full intended five courses. No difference in survival was noted between treated and untreated low-risk patients, whereas the treated high-risk patients had a significantly higher ($p = .0012$) 2-year disease-free survival (70%) when compared to observed high-risk patients (37%). Subset analysis of high-risk patients treated demonstrated benefit in those having extravesical or nodal disease, while those patients who had lymphatic or vascular invasion alone showed no benefit from adjuvant treatment.[100] In another phase II study, Wei et al. treated 56 pT2–pT4 N+/− patients with adjuvant CMV: 1- and 3-year survival rates of 66 and 28%, respectively, were observed.[101]

To date, only two randomized phase III trials have employed proven active combinations in the adjuvant setting; these studies have been criticized because of incomplete patient compliance and methodology. Two earlier trials using adjuvant doxyrubicin and 5-fluorouracil after RT or cisplatin singly after cystectomy resulted in no survival benefit, probably due to the marginal activity of these regimens.[102,103]

The first reported randomized study to evaluate a proven active multidrug regimen was performed at the University of Southern California (USC). Over an 8-year period, 498 patients had an attempted radical cystectomy, 91 (18%) of whom were eligible for randomization to either observation or combination therapy. Of the 44 patients randomized to receive chemotherapy, only 33 (75%) were treated, 32 of whom received cisplatin. Several treatment regimens and doses were employed; the majority of patients received CAP. Despite a change in treatment regimens, as well as an inability to administer full doses in some patients randomized to treatment, a significant delay in time to progression was demonstrated in patients receiving therapy, with 70 versus 46% of untreated patients remaining disease free at 3 years ($p = .001$). Median survival in patients receiving chemotherapy was 4.3 years, compared to 2.4 years in patients observed. Multivariate analysis revealed the effect of chemotherapy was abrogated in patients having two or more lymph nodes positive for transitional cell carcinoma; however, this analysis was hampered by the small numbers in each subgroup.[104] Stockel et al. randomized 49 patients who had extravesicular transitional cell carcinoma of the bladder (pT3b, T4a, pN1, pN2) at cystectomy to observation versus three cycles of M-VAC or M-VEC (E = epirubicin). A significant increase in relapse-free survival was detected in patients randomized to the chemotherapy group compared to those who were observed ($p < .0015$). Overall, the relapse rate for patients randomized to treatment versus observation was 26.9 versus 81%, respectively, at a median of 19.7 and 11.6 months, respectively.[105] Of note, reanalysis of this study to account for the eight patients who refused chemotherapy or were inadequately treated improved the relapse rate of the treatment group to 17%, with a median follow-up of 13.6 months. Unfortunately, the initial highly significant difference in relapse-free survival necessitated the early termination of this trial, thus limiting the number of cases entered and followed-up. Still, when the treated and untreated patients were followed to a median of 54 and 57 months, respectively, only 42% of patients treated relapsed compared to 87% of the untreated patients.[106]

NEOADJUVANT CHEMOTHERAPY

Neoadjuvant therapy refers to the administration of chemotherapy prior to definitive local treatment. Several advantages are imparted by this approach. Patients with unresectable bladder lesions who respond to treatment may become candidates for cystectomy. Complete responders may have their bladders preserved. Preoperative therapy also provides an in vivo test of chemosensitivity, potentially guiding future treatment. This is based on the assumption that primary tumors and micrometastases have similar drug-resistance profiles. Moreover, a higher dose intensity may be delivered to the tumor, as the overall tumor burden of these patients is lower.

Some patients will not clinically benefit from neoadjuvant therapy. Not all patients harbor micrometastases; thus, they are exposed to unnecessary treatment. Patients with tumors that are intrinsically resistant to treatment, or acquire resistance during chemotherapy, may evidence tumor growth such that they become inoperable. Although P-glycoprotein, a membrane protein responsible for multidrug resistance, has been identified in 13% of untreated bladder cancer specimens, its value as a marker of drug-resistant bladder tumors has yet to be demonstrated.[107]

Neoadjuvant Therapy Impact on Survival

Despite many phase II trials that have demonstrated complete pathologic responses, a paucity of randomized data exists to study whether neoadjuvant therapy prolongs survival.[108,109] Completion of randomized neoadjuvant trials has been difficult, in part due to the physician's reluctance to enter patients, resulting from a desire that a patient receive the best therapy. Additionally, completion of early single-agent trials has also been hampered by the concomitant evolution of more effective chemotherapeutic regimens. Six randomized trials have thus far been published; only one employed a combination (cisplatin plus doxorubicin) prior to local therapy, while four administered single-agent cisplatin and one administered single-agent methotrexate. Definitive local treatment included cystectomy alone in one trial, radiotherapy alone in two, radiotherapy followed by cystectomy in one, and radiotherapy with salvage cystectomy in one. Only one trial, which administered cisplatin plus doxorubicin prior to radiation therapy, demonstrated a minimal survival benefit for those receiving chemotherapy prior to cystectomy.[110–114] A meta-analysis of four trials demonstrated a minimal reduction (9%) in the rate of death in those patients receiving chemotherapy, with the greatest benefit being conferred on those patients who were younger than 60 years of age.[115] Currently, SWOG is near completion of a randomized trial of three cycles of neoadjuvant M-VAC versus cystectomy alone.

Effect of Response on Survival

Schutz and colleagues perfomed a 5-year analysis of 111 patients with transitional cell carcinoma of the bladder treated with neoadjuvant M-VAC, 81 of whom were pathologically staged. After undergoing a diagnostic TURBT, patients received a median of four cycles of M-VAC. The overall median survival of this group was 59.9 months, with a 5-year survival of 48%, similar to that which one would observe in patients treated with surgery alone. Of the pretherapy variables examined, only the initial T stage, presence of ureteral obstruction, and presence of a palpable mass were significant to survival; the mulivariate analysis demonstrated the two most important variables to be the initial T and P stage. In correlating response with survival, an association was observed in only those patients with initial extravesical disease who were downstaged to pT2 or less. An association between survival and downstaging was not detected in those patients whose disease was initially confined to the bladder.[116] These results contrast with the findings of a meta-analysis performed by Splinter et al., who analyzed the patterns of response and survival of 147 patients treated with neoadjuvant therapy at eight centers. Ninety per cent of patients received either cisplatin plus methotrexate or M-VAC. A survival advantage was demonstrated in all patients who were downstaged regardless of their initial clinical stage; patients whose cystectomy specimens were staged pT2 or less had a 5-year survival of 75%.[109] In both these studies, although it would appear that the response to neoadjuvant therapy allows the clinician to stratify patients into prognostic groups based on response to chemotherapy, it cannot be determined whether this effect is due to a biased selection of patients with less aggressive tumors, rather than destruction of micrometastases.

Bladder Preservation Protocols

Chemotherapy can not only treat distant metastases but, when administered with external beam radiation, can also increase the rate of local tumor control. This effect can be additive or synergistic and may be sequence dependent. The optimal agents and sequence of administration are subjects of active investigation. Increases in the therapeutic index of radiation by chemotherapy result from destruction of radiation-resistant cells as well as inhibition of repair of radiation-induced DNA damage.

Phase II trials have demonstrated high CR rates (61 to 71%) from the combined administration of single agents such as cisplatin or 5-fluorouracil with 4000 to 6500 cGy of radiation therapy.[114,117] Although these local response rates appear to be superior to radiation therapy alone, randomized trials have not demonstrated a significant difference in survival.[118] The failure of this approach seems to relate to the use of inadequate chemotherapy, as the pattern of relapse is distant rather than local. Multidrug regimens, when administered with radiation, may not have a higher rate of complete response, but may also serve to more effectively treat distant metastases. Kaufman et al. used the three-drug regiment MCV (methotrexate, 30 mg/m^2; vinblastine, 3 mg/m^2; cisplatin, 70 mg/m^2) to treat 53 patients with muscle-invasive transitional cell carcinoma of the bladder.[119] All patients first underwent a complete TURBT, followed by two cycles of MCV therapy. Of the 53 patients entered, 49 went on to have consolidation therapy with cisplatin and 4000 cGy of radiation therapy. Patients were then reevaluated by cystoscopy; those who continued to respond were consolidated with further radiation therapy and cisplatin. Ten patients who did not respond underwent cystectomy. At a median follow-up of 48 months, 45% of patients were alive without evidence of disease. Twenty-eight patients had a complete response in the bladder after treatment; 89% had functioning tumor-free bladders. Long-term follow-up is necessary to determine whether this approach is comparable to cystectomy or neoadjuvant chemotherapy and cystectomy. These results are being actively studied in a national trial by the Radiation Therapy Oncology Group (RTOG).

Alternating radiation and chemotherapy has also been attempted.[120] The rationale for this approach was derived from preclinical data that suggest prior exposure to chemotherapy may inactivate cellular mechanisms responsible for radiation resistance. Twenty-one patients were treated with a modified M-VAC regimen, with the Adriamycin dose reduced to 25 mg/m^2 to minimize hematologic toxicity. M-VAC was administered every 4 weeks, with radiation (ten fractions of 180 to 200 cGy) delivered on weeks 2, 5, and 8 of treatment. Of 18 evaluable patients, all retained their bladders, with 83.5% retaining normal function. One toxic death occurred. The observed 3-year survival rate of 60% appears to be compatible with some cystectomy series.[121]

SUMMARY

As mentioned previously in this chapter, the gold standard for management of invasive bladder cancer in the United States is radical cystoprostatectomy in the male or radical cystectomy in the female. Inclusion of the anterior urethra in the male or the entire urethrectomy in the female is appropriate in selected circumstances; alternatively, bladder replacement procedures can be carried out, decreasing the psychosocial burden once attributed to radical cystectomy.

Unfortunately, not all patients are salvageable by this treatment. Although local recurrence rates have dropped remarkably with increased understanding of appropriate surgical technique, the frequent incidence of subclinical micrometastases requires that systemic treatment in addition to surgery will be necessary for optimum patient survival. It is the authors' prejudice that neoadjuvant or adjuvant mutidrug treatments, along with surgery, will provide the greatest patient survival.

For those patients (and surgeons) interested in bladder salvage, it is clear that a small number of patients are candidates for partial cystectomy. When partial cystectomy is not applicable, there are complicated and as yet unproven treatment options available. Provided hydronephrosis is not present, protocols combining radiation therapy with systemic chemotherapy may be attempted. The authors' prejudice, however, is that similar survivability might be achieved with repetitive TURBT along with chemotherapy in these instances.

REFERENCES

1. Wingo PA, Tong T, Bolden S: Cancer statistics, 1995. CA Cancer J Clin 1995; 45:8.
2. Thrasher JB, Crawford ED: Current management of invasive and metastatic transitional cell carcinoma of the bladder. J Urol 1993; 149:957.
3. Catalona WJ: Urothelial tumors of the urinary tract. *In* Walsh PC, Retik AB, Stamey TA, Vaughan ED Jr (eds): Campbell's Urology, 6th edition, p 1094. Philadelphia, WB Saunders Co, 1992.
4. Soto EA, Friedell GH, Tiltman AJ: Bladder cancer as seen in giant histologic sections. Cancer 1977; 39:447.
5. Heney NM, Ahmed S, Flanagan MJ, et al: Superficial bladder cancer: progression and recurrence. J Urol 1983; 130:1083.
6. Whitmore WF: Management of invasive bladder neoplasms. Semin Urol 1983; 1:4.
7. Herr HW: Transurethral resection in regionally advanced bladder cancer. Urol Clin North Am 1992; 19:695.
8. Flocks RH: Treatment of patients with carcinoma of the bladder. JAMA 1951; 145:295.
9. Milner WA: The role of conservative surgery in the treatment of bladder tumors. Br J Urol 1954; 26:375.
10. Barnes RW, Bergman RT, Hadley HL: Control of bladder tumors by endoscopic surgery. J Urol 1967; 97:864.
11. Whitmore WF, Marshal VF: Radical total cystectomy for cancer of the bladder: 230 cases five years later. J Urol 1962; 87:853.
12. Jewet HJ: Prognosis of bladder tumors based on anatomical and pathologic study. *In* Fergusson FD (ed): XIII Congres de la Societe Internationale d'Urologie, Vol 1, p 138. London, E and S Livingstone Ltd, 1964.
13. O'Flynn JD, Smith JD, Hanson JS: Transurethral resection for the assessment and treatment of vesical neoplasms. A review of 800 consecutive cases. Int J Radiat Oncol Biol Phys 1975; 1:38.
14. Henry K, Miller J, Mori M: Comparison of transurethral resection to radical therapies for stage B bladder tumors. J Urol 1988; 140:964.
15. Herr HW: Conservative management of muscle infiltrating bladder cancer: prospective experience. J Urol 1987; 138:1162.
16. Thrasher JB, Frazier HA, Robertson JE: Does a stage pT0 confer a survival advantage in patients with minimally invasive bladder cancer? J Urol 1994; 152:393.
17. Pollack A, Zagars GK, Cole CJ, et al: Relationship of local control to distant metastases in muscle invasive bladder cancer. J Urol 1995; 154:2059.
18. Hall RR, Newling PW, Ramsden PD, et al: Treatment of invasive bladder cancer by local resection and high dose methotrexate. Br J Urol 1984; 56:668.
19. Hall RR, Robert TJ, Marsh MM: Radical TUR and chemotherapy aiming at bladder preservation. Prog Clin Biol Res 1990; 553:163.
20. Utz DC, Schmitz SE, Fulgeso PD: A clinicopathologic

evaluation of partial cystecomy for carcinoma of the urinary bladder. Cancer 1973; 32:1075.
21. Novick AC, Stewart BH: Partial cystectomy in the treatment of primary and secondary carcinoma of the bladder. J Urol 1976; 116:570.
22. Sweeney P, Kursh ED, Resnick MI: Partial cystectomy. Urol Clin North Am 1992; 19:701.
23. Schoborg TW, Sapolsky JL, Lewis CW Jr: Carcinoma of the bladder treated by segmental resection. J Urol 1979; 122:473.
24. Kaneti J: Partial cystectomy in the management of bladder carcinoma. Eur Urol 1986; 12:249.
25. Resnick MI, O'Conor VJ: Segmental resection for carcinoma of the bladder: review of 102 patients. J Urol 1973; 109:1007.
26. Faysal MH, Frieha FS: Evaluation of partial cystectomy for bladder cancer. Urology 1979; 14:352.
27. Magri J: Partial cystectomy: a review of 104 cases. Br J Urol 1962; 34:74.
28. van der Werf-Messing: Cancer of the urinary bladder treated by interstitial radium implant. Int J Radiat Oncol Biol Phys 1978; 4:373.
29. Peress JA, Waterhouse K, Cole AT: Complications of partial cystectomy in patients with high grade bladder carcinoma. J Urol 1977; 118:761.
30. Brannan W, Ochsner MG, Feuslier HA, et al: Partial cystectomy in the treatment of transitional cell carcinoma of the bladder. J Urol 1978; 119:213.
31. Baker R, Kelly T, Tehan T, et al: Subtotal cystectomy and total bladder regeneration in the treatment of bladder cancer. JAMA 1958; 168:1178.
32. Merrell RW, Brown HE, Rose JF: Bladder carcinoma treated by partial cystectomy: a review of 54 cases. J Urol 1979; 122:471.
33. Cummings KB, Mason JT, Correa RJ, et al: Segmental resection in the management of bladder carcinoma. J Urol 1978; 119:56.
34. Narayana AS, Loening SA, Slymen DJ, et al: Bladder cancer: factors affecting survival. J Urol 1983; 130:56.
35. Lipponen PK, Eskenlien MJ, Kiviranta J, et al: Prognosis of transitional cell cancer of the bladder: a multivariate prognostic score for improved prediction. J Urol 1991; 146:1535–1540.
36. Nilsson B, Wahren B, Espositi PL, et al: Prediction of survival and recurrence in bladder carcinoma. Urol Res 1982; 10:109–113.
37. Pryor JP: Factors influencing the survival of patients with transitional cell tumors of the urinary bladder. Br J Urol 1973; 45:586–592.
38. Thrasher JB, Frazier HA, Robertson JE, et al: Clinical variables which serve as predictors of cancer specific survival among patients treated with radical cystectomy for transitional cell carcinoma of the bladder and prostate. Cancer 1993; 73:1708–1715.
39. Jewett HJ, Strong GH: Infiltrating carcinoma of the bladder: relation of depth of penetration of the bladder wall to incidence of local extension and metastases. J Urol 1946; 55:366–372.
40. Jewett HJ: Carcinoma of the bladder: influence of depth of invasion on the 5 year results following complete extirpation of the primary growth. J Urol 1952; 67:672.
41. Lerner SP, Skinner E, Skinner DG: Radical cystectomy in regionally advanced bladder cancer. Urol Clin North Am 1992; 19:713–723.
42. Lerner SP, Skinner DG, Lieskovsky G, et al: The rationale for en bloc lymph node dissection for bladder cancer patients with nodal metastases: long term results. J Urol 1992; 147:402A.
43. Skinner DG: Management of invasive bladder cancer: a meticulous lymph node dissection can make a difference. J Urol 1982; 128:34.
44. Giulani L, Giberti C, Martorana G, et al: Results of radical cystectomy for primary bladder cancer: retrospective study of more than 200 cases. Urology 1985; 26:243.
45. Prout GR Jr, Griffin PP, Shipley WU: Bladder carcinoma as a systemic disease. Cancer 1979; 45:2532.
46. Skinner DG, Lieskovsky G: Management of invasive and high grade bladder cancer. In Skinner DG, Lieskovsky G (eds): Diagnosis and Management of Genitourinary Cancer, pp 295–312. Philadelphia, WB Saunders Co, 1988.
47. Wishnow KI, Johnson DE, Ro JY, et al: Incidence, extent and location of unsuspected pelvic lymph node metastases in patients undergoing radical cystectomy for bladder cancer. Cancer 1987; 137:408.
48. Frazier HA, Robertson JE, Dodge MS, et al: The value of pathologic factors in predicting cancer specific survival among patients treated with radical cystectomy for transitional cell carcinoma of the bladder and prostate. Cancer 1993; 71:3993.
49. Paulson DF: Critical review of radical cystectomy and indicators of prognosis. Semin Urol 1993; 11:205.
50. Pagano F, Guazzieri S, Artibani W, et al: Prognosis of bladder cancer: the value of radical cystectomy in the management of invasive bladder cancer. Eur Urol 1988; 15:166–170.
51. Pagano F, Pierfrancesco B, Galetti TP, et al: Results of contemporary radical cystectomy for invasive bladder cancer: a clinicopathologic study with emphasis on the inadequacy of the tumor, nodes and metastases classification. J Urol 1991; 145:45.
52. Vieweg J, Whitmore WF, Herr HW, et al: The role of pelvic lymphadenectomy and radical cystectomy for lymph node positive bladder cancer. Cancer 1994; 73:3020.
53. Wishnow KI, Tenney DM: Will Rogers and the results of radical cystectomy for invasive bladder cancer. Urol Clin North Am 1991; 18:529–537.
54. Matzkin H, Soloway MS, Hardeman S: Transitional cell carcinoma of the prostate. J Urol 1991; 146:1207.
55. Brice M II, Marshall VF, Green JL, et al: Simple total cystectomy for carcinoma of the urinary bladder. Cancer 1956; 9:572.
56. Poole-Wilson DS, Barnard RJ: Total cystectomy for bladder tumors. Br J Urol 1971; 43:16.
57. Long RTL, Grummon RA, Spratt JS Jr, et al: Carcinoma of the urinary bladder: comparison with radical, simple and partial cystectomy and intravesical formalin. Cancer 1972; 29:98.
58. Whitmore WF, Marshall VF: Radical surgery for carcinoma of the urinary bladder. One hundred consecutive cases 4 years later. Cancer 1956; 9:596.
59. Leadbetter WF, Cooper JF: Regional gland dissection for carcinoma of the bladder: technique for one stage cystectomy, gland dissection and bilateral uretero-enterostomy. J Urol 1950; 63:242.
60. Whitmore WF Jr, Grabstald H, MacKensie AR, et al: Preoperative irradiation with cystectomy in the management of bladder cancer. AJR 1968; 102:570.
61. Morabito RA, Kandzari SJ, Milam DF: Invasive bladder carcinoma treated by radical cystectomy. Urology 1979; 14:478.
62. Montie JB, Straffon RA, Stewart BH: Radical cystectomy without radiation therapy for carcinoma of the bladder. J Urol 1984; 131:477.
63. Mathur VK, Krahn HP, Ramsey EW: Total cystectomy for bladder cancer. J Urol 1981; 125:784.
64. Bredael JJ, Croker BP, Glenn JF: The curability of invasive bladder cancer treated by radical cystectomy. Eur Urol 1980; 6:206.
65. Freiha FS: Open bladder surgery. *In* Walsh PC, Retik AB, Stamey TA, Vaughan ED Jr (eds): Campbell's Urology, 6th edition, p 2750. Philadelphia, WB Saunders Co, 1992.
66. Skinner DG, Lieskovsky G: Contemporary cystectomy with pelvic lymph node dissection compared to preoperative radiation therapy plus cysectomy in the management of invasive bladder cancer. J Urol 1984; 131:1069.
67. Walsh PC, Mostwin JL: Radical prostatectomy and cystoprostatectomy with preservation of potency. Results using new nerve sparing technique. Br J Urol 1984; 56: 694.

68. Brendler CB, Steinberg GD, Marshall FF, et al: Local recurrence and survival following nerve sparing radical cystoprostatectomy. J Urol 1990; 144:1137.
69. Skinner DG: Current perspectives in the management of high grade invasive bladder cancer. Cancer 1980; 45:1866.
70. Skinner DG, Tift JP, Kaufman JJ: High dose, short course preoperative radiation therapy and immediate single stage radical cystectomy with pelvic lymph node dissection in the management of bladder cancer. J Urol 1982; 127:671.
71. Skinner DG: Management of bladder cancer: a meticulous pelvic lymph node dissection can make a difference. J Urol 1982; 128:34.
72. Smith JA Jr, Whitmore WF Jr: Regional lymph node metastases from bladder cancer. J Urol 1981; 126:591.
73. Dretler SP, Ragsdale BD, Leadbetter WF: The value of pelvic lymphadenectomy in the surgical treatment of bladder cancer. J Urol 1973; 109:414.
74. Roehrborn CG, Sagalowsky AI, Peters PC: Long term patients survival after cystectomy for regional metastatic transitional cell carcinoma of the bladder. J Urol 1991; 146: 36.
75. Gowing NFC: Urethral carcinoma associated with cancer of the bladder. Br J Urol 1960; 32:428.
76. Hendry WF, Gowing NFC, Wallace DM: Surgical treatment of urethral tumors associated with bladder cancer. Proc R Soc Med 1974; 67:304.
77. Beahers JR, Fleming TR, Zincke H: Risk of local recurrence after cystectomy for bladder cancer. J Urol 1984; 131:264.
78. Hardeman SW, Soloway MS: Urethral recurrence following radical cystectomy. J Urol 1990; 144:666.
79. Gospodarowicz MK, Warde P: The role of radiation therapy in the management of transitional cell carcinoma of the bladder. Hematol Oncol Clin North Am 1992; 6:147.
80. Wesson MF: Radiation therapy in regionally advanced bladder cancer. Urol Clin North Am 1992; 19:725.
81. Whitmore WF, Grabstald HA, MacKenzie AR, et al: Preoperative irradiation and cystectomy in the management of bladder cancer. AJR 1968; 102:570.
82. Whitmore WF, Batata M: Status of integrated irradiation and cystectomy for bladder cancer. Urol Clin North Am 1984; 11:681.
83. Parsons JT, Millon RR: Planned preoperative irradiation in the management of clinical stage B2-c (T3) bladder carcinoma. Int J Radiat Oncol Biol Phys 1988; 14:797.
84. Blackbard CE, Byar DP: Veterans Administration Cooperative Urologic Research Group: Results of a clinical trial of surgery and radiation in stages II and III carcinoma of the bladder. J Urol 1972; 108:875.
85. Prout GR, Slack NH, Bross IDJ: Preoperative irradiation as an adjuvant in the surgical management of invasive bladder carcinoma. J Urol 1971; 105:223.
86. Slack NH, Bross IDJ, Prour GR: Five year follow-up results of a collaborative study of therapies for carcinoma of the bladder. J Surg Oncol 1977; 9:393.
87. Crawford ED, Das S, Smith JA Jr: Preoperative radiation therapy in the treatment of bladder cancer. Urol Clin North Am 1987; 14:781.
88. Fossa SD, Ous S, Tveter K, et al: Treatment of T2/T3 bladder carcinoma: total cystectomy with and without preoperative irradiation. Eur Urol 1986; 12:158.
89. Cole CJ, Pollack A, Zagars GK, et al: Local control of muscle invasive bladder cancer: preoperative radiotherapy and cystectomy versus cystectomy alone. Int Radiat Oncol Biol Phys 1995; 32:331.
90. Bloom HJG, Hendry WF, Wallace DM: Treatment of T3 bladder cancer: controlled trial of pre-operative radiotherapy and radical cystectomy versus radical radiotherapy. Second report and review (for the clinical trials group, Institute of Urology). Br J Urol 1982; 54:136.
91. Sell A, Jakobsen A, Nerstrom B, et al: Treatment of advanced bladder cancer category T2 T3 and T4. Scand J Urol Nephrol Suppl 1991; 138:193.
92. Yagoda A: The role of cisplatin-based chemotherapy in advanced urothelial tract cancer. Semin Oncol 1989; 16(Suppl 6):98–104.
93. Trump DL, Elson R, Madajewicz S, et al: Randomized phase II comparison of carboplatin and CHIP in advanced transitional cell carcinoma of the urothelium: the Eastern Cooperative Oncology Group. J Urol 1990; 144: 1119–1122.
94. Roth BJ, Dreicer R, Einhorn LH, et al: Paclitaxel in previously treated, advanced transitional cell carcinoma of the urothelium: a phase II trial of the Eastern Cooperative Oncology Group (ECOG). Proc ASCO 1994; 13:320.
95. Sadan S, Bajorin D, Amersterdam A, et al: Docetaxel in patients with advanced transitional cell cancer (TCC) who failed cisplatin-based chemotherapy: a phase II trial (Abstract 761). Proc ASCO 1994; 13:244.
96. Stadler W, Kuzel T, Raghavan D, et al: A phase II study of gemcitabine in the treatment of patients with advanced transitional cell carcinoma. Proc ASCO 1995; 14:241.
97. Sternberg CN, Yagoda A, Scher HI, et al: M-VAC for advanced transitional cell carcinoma of the urothelium: efficacy and patterns of response and relapse. Cancer 1989; 64:2448–2458.
98. Logothetis CJ, Dexeus FH, Finn L, et al: A prospective randomized trial comparing MVAC and CISCA chemotherapy for patients with metastatic urothelial tumors. J Clin Oncol 1990; 8:1050–1055.
99. Loehrer PJ, Einhorn LH, Elson PJ, et al: A randomized comparison of cisplatin alone or in combination with methotrexate, vinblastine, and doxorubicin in patients with metastatic urothelial carcinoma: a cooperative group trial. J Clin Oncol 1992; 10:1066–1073.
100. Logothetis CJ, Johnson DE, Dexeus FH, et al: Adjuvant cyclophosphamide, doxorubicin and cisplatin chemotherapy for bladder cancer: an update. J Clin Oncol 1988; 6: 1590–1596.
101. Wei CH, Hsich RK, Chiou JJ, et al: Adjuvant methotrexate, vinblastine and cisplatin chemotherapy for invasive transitional cell carcinoma. Taiwan experience. J Urol 1996; 155:118.
102. Richards B, Bastable JR, Freedman L, et al: Adjuvant chemotherapy with doxorubicin (Adriamycin) and 5-fluorouracil in T3, NX, M0 bladder cancer treated with radiotherapy. Br J Urol 1983; 55:386.
103. Studer UE, Bacchi M, Biedermann C, et al: Adjuvant cisplatin chemotherapy for bladder cancer: results of a prospective randomized trial. J Urol 1994; 152:81.
104. Skinner DG, Daniels JR, Russell CA, et al: The role of adjuvant chemotherapy following cystectomy for invasive bladder cancer: a prospective comparative trial. J Urol 1991; 145:459.
105. Stockle M, Meyenburg W, Wellek S, et al: Advanced bladder cancer (stages pT3b, PT4a, pN1, and pN2): improved survival after radical cystectomy and 3 adjuvant cycles of chemotherapy. Results of a controlled prospective study. J Urol 1992; 148:302–307.
106. Stockle M, Meyenburg W, Wellek S, et al: Adjuvant polychemotherapy of nonorgan confined bladder cancer after radical cystectomy revisited: long term results of a controlled prospective study and further clinical experience. J Urol 1995; 153:47.
107. Petrylak DP, Scher HI, Reuter V, et al: P-glycoprotein expression in primary and metastatic transitional cell carcinoma of the bladder. Ann Oncol 1994; 5:835.
108. Scher H, Yagoda A, Herr H, et al: Neoadjuvant M-VAC (methotrexate, vinblastine, doxorubicin, and cisplatin) effect on the primary bladder lesion. J Urol 1988; 139:470–474.
109. Splinter TAW, Scher HI, Denis L, et al: The prognostic value of the pathological response to combination chemotherapy before cystectomy in patients with invasive bladder cancer. J Urol 1992; 147:606–608.
110. Rintala E, Hannisdahl E, Fossa SD, et al: Neoadjuvant chemotherapy in bladder cancer: a randomized study. Nordic cystectomy trial 1. Scand J Urol Nephrol 1993; 27: 355.

111. Martinez-Piniero JA, Gonzalez Martin M, Arocena F, et al: Neoadjuvant cisplatin chemotherapy before radical cystectomy in invasive transitional cell carcinoma of the bladder: a prospective randomized phase III study. J Urol 1995; 153:964–973.
112. Wallace DM, Raghavan D, Kelly KA, et al: Neoadjuvant cisplatin therapy in invasive transitional cell carcinoma of the bladder. Br J Urol 1991; 67:608.
113. Shearer RJ, Chilvers CF, Bloom HJ, et al: Adjuvant chemotherapy in T3 carcinoma of the bladder. A prospective trial: preliminary report. Br J Urol 1988; 62:558.
114. Copin C, Gospodarowicz M, Dixon P, et al: Improved local control of invasive bladder cancer by concurrent cisplatin and preoperative or radical radiation. Proc ASCO 1992; 11:198.
115. Anonymous: Does neoadjuvant cisplatin based chemotherapy improve the survival of patients with locally advanced bladder cancer: a meta-analysis of individual patient data from randomized clinical trials. Advanced bladder cancer overview collaboration. Br J Urol 1995; 75:206.
116. Schultz PK, Herr HW, Zhang ZF, et al: Neoadjuvant chemotherapy for invasive bladder cancer: prognostic factors for survival of patients treated with M-VAC with 5 year follow-up. J Clin Oncol 1994; 13:300.
117. Chauvet B, Brewer Y, Felix-Faure C, et al: Combined radiation therapy and cisplatin for locally advanced carcinoma of the urinary bladder. Cancer 1990; 72:2213.
118. Rotman M, Macchia R, Silverstein R, et al: Treatment of advanced bladder cancer with irradiation and concomitant 5-fluorouracil infusion. Cancer 1987; 59:710.
119. Kaufman DS, Shipley WU, Griffin PP, et al: Selective bladder preservation by combination treatment of invasive bladder cancer. N Engl J Med 1993; 329:1377.
120. Vikram B, Malamud, Silverman P, et al: A pilot study of chemotherapy alternating with twice a day accelerated radiation as an alternative to cystectomy in muscle infiltrating (stage T2 and T3) cancer of the bladder: preliminary results. J Urol 1994; 151:602.
121. Housset M, Maulard C, Chretien Y, et al: Combined radiation and chemotherapy for invasive transitional cell carcinoma of the bladder: a prospective study. J Clin Oncol 1993; 11:2150.

19

TRANSURETHRAL SURGERY OF BLADDER TUMORS

YVES FRADET, M.D., F.R.C.S.(C.) *and*
MIREILLE GRÉGOIRE, M.D., F.R.C.S.(C.)

Cancers originating from the urothelium are responsible for 8% of all diagnosed tumors in men and 4% in women. In the United States alone, this corresponds to more than 50,000 new cases yearly,[1] transitional cell carcinoma (TCC) accounting for approximately 90% of all cases.[2] At the time of diagnosis, about 80% of bladder tumors are superficial and limited to the mucosa or submucosa (Ta, T1), while 20% invade the muscular layer of the bladder wall. In recent cohort studies of patients newly diagnosed with Ta, T1 tumors, a 55% recurrence rate was observed within 3 years,[3,4] but previous studies had reported up to 70% recurrence within 5 years of the initial diagnosis.[5] The majority of these recurrent tumors will remain superficial, and progression to muscle-invasive or metastatic cancer will occur in less than 10% of recurrent cases. These statistics underscore the overall importance of transurethral surgery as the primary and often only treatment modality for bladder cancer. Obviously, intravesical immunotherapy and chemotherapy have become important therapeutic modalities to prevent recurrence and progression of superficial bladder tumors. Nevertheless, the quality of the transurethral surgery has an important influence on the risk of tumor recurrence, since up to 41% of recurrent tumors were reported to occur at the site of the original resection in the National Bladder Cancer Collaborative Group study.[6]

Endoscopic resection or fulguration of bladder tumor is usually effective, has low morbidity, and is associated with a rapid postoperative recovery. Transurethral resection (TUR) is the standard method for the initial diagnosis and staging of bladder cancer as well as for the eradication of low-stage bladder tumor. Some infiltrating bladder cancers can also be treated primarily by TUR, with or without adjuvant radiotherapy or systemic chemotherapy. Laser therapy, either as thermocoagulation of bladder tumors or photodynamic therapy, is an alternative that has become part of the treatment armamentarium. This chapter will review the indications, techniques, and outcomes of transurethral resection, laser thermocoagulation, and photodynamic therapy in the management of bladder cancer.

TRANSURETHRAL RESECTION

Preparation

The diagnosis of bladder cancer is usually made by flexible or rigid cystoscopy. Before TUR of the first tumor, it is advisable to evaluate the upper urinary tract by excretory urography to rule out an associated transitional cell carcinoma of the renal pelvis or ureter, or more commonly, hydroureteronephrosis created by the bladder tumor. The presence of ureteral obstruction is usually indicative of invasive bladder carcinoma and is associated with increased risk of lymph node metastasis and poorer clinical outcome. On the other hand, the knowledge of absence of secondary hydronephrosis is useful in the resection of bladder tumors masking the ureteral orifice. If the bladder tumor appears sessile rather than papillary at diagnostic cystoscopy, it is important to obtain a computed tomography (CT) scan evaluation of the abdomen and pelvis before TUR to help better determine the extent of bladder wall invasion, since this information may alter the anticipated transurethral resection of the tumor. A urine culture must be obtained and appropriate antimicrobial therapy initiated before surgery if urine is infected.

In order to proceed to surgical resection of bladder tumors, optimal analgesia and lower abdomi-

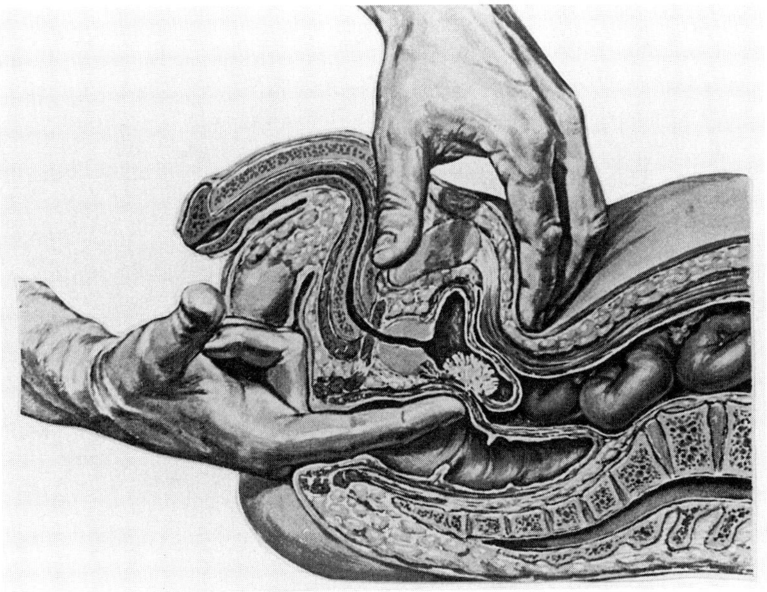

FIGURE 19–1. Bimanual examination.

nal muscle relaxation is usually obtained by either spinal or general anesthesia. However, Engbert et al. reported resecting superficial bladder tumors under topical urethral anesthesia and infiltration of the tumor base with local anesthetic.[7] Intravesical anesthesia using an electromotive drug administration (EMDA) system, which facilitates bladder wall penetration of lidocaine, may prove to be an important tool in association with less painful microwave energy for cost-effective TUR of bladder tumors on an outpatient basis.[8]

Before introducing the instruments into the urethra, a bimanual examination of the pelvis should be performed (Fig. 19–1).[9] This allows determination of whether a mass is palpable and whether it is fixed or not to the adjacent organs or the pelvis walls. In the case of a palpable mass before TUR, a repeat examination after surgery will help to determine the completeness of resection in cases where it was attempted.

TUR is best achieved using a large-bore resectoscope, size 24 French or larger. The different types of resectoscopes available are basically variations of the Stern-McCarthey type (operated with two hands) or based on Iglesias, Nesbit, or Baumrucker (operated with one hand). Either a continuous- or noncontinuous-flow resectoscope may be used. The continuous-flow system offers the advantage of maintaining a relatively constant volume of bladder distention to facilitate resection of tumors occurring in a nonfixed portion of the bladder. The resectoscope should be examined before surgery to prevent loss of time and complications because of malfunctioning instrument. In particular, it is wise to ensure that the electrical wire loop is firmly attached to the resectoscope. A blended current is not recommended for bladder tumor resection. The irrigation fluid should be nonelectrolytic. Sterile water may be used but only for the resection of very small tumors. Most commonly, 1.5% glycine or sorbitol isotonic solutions are used for the resection of larger bladder tumors.

Surgical Technique

The resectoscope is inserted gently through the urethra in order not to induce bleeding, which will diminish visibility and ease of surgery. A careful cystoscopic examination of all surfaces of the bladder as well as the prostatic urethra is of the utmost importance before beginning tumor resection. This examination should determine the gross appearance and the number, size, and position of tumors in reference to bladder neck and ureteral orifices. The bladder mucosa away from the tumor should be carefully examined to detect velvety erythematous area or punctuated whitish lesions that may be suggestive of carcinoma in situ (CIS). This evaluation allows the planning of surgery. In cases of multiple tumors, it is usually safer to resect the smaller tumors first, since it is easier to ensure a proper hemostasis to maintain clear visibility all along the procedure. The resection usually starts from the posterior portion of the tumors located on the lateral walls, anteriorly or on the trigone, and on top of the tumors located on the posterior wall (Fig. 19–2).[9] The resecting loop should be passed beyond the tumor and then pulled back toward the viewing eye while applying the electrocautery. At some point, however, it is necessary to maintain the resectoscope loop in an extended fixed position and to move the resectoscope downward with a rocking motion parallel to the base of the tumor, similar to scraping a wall. Constant orientation is necessary during these maneuvers. With papillary tumors,

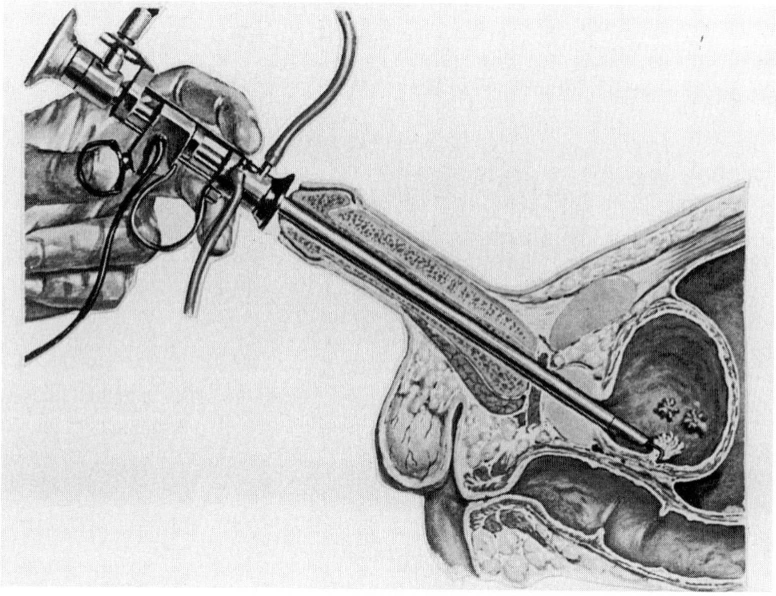

FIGURE 19–2. Transurethral resection of a bladder tumor.

the resecting loop is often used to elevate the tumor off the bladder wall before application of the electric current. The base of bladder tumors with small pedicle can often be resected at once. In larger tumors, however, early attempt at transecting its base will result in a nonfixed tumor that may be difficult to resect. Resection of tumors should ideally be performed in two steps: resection of the tumor and resection of the tumor base, which must include bladder wall muscle. Care should be taken to limit coagulation of the specimen to allow better preservation for histologic interpretation. Loops using microwave energy instead of electricity may improve the quality of the surgical specimen in the future.

Muscle fibers should be visible once a tumor is fully resected. It is advisable to avoid overdistention of the bladder during this phase of the resection to reduce chances of bladder perforation, particularly in women that usually have a thinner bladder wall. However, it is occasionally necessary to purposely resect down to the perivesical fat for tumors considered to be deeply invasive when healthy-appearing muscle fibers are not visible during resection of the tumor base. Because of the importance of TUR on tumor control, the resection should be completed by including a 0.5-cm rim of normal surrounding mucosa. Moreover, after coagulating the bleeding vessels, the resection site should be fulgurated extensively. If multiple small tumors form a colony in one area, these should be resected in continuity in order to reduce the chance of recurrence in that area.

In patients with possible invasive cancer or a suspicion of carcinoma in situ, a TUR of the prostatic urethra should be performed to rule out CIS or intraductal neoplasia in the prostate. Such information is of paramount importance in planning intravesical therapy or orthotopic neobladder after cystectomy for invasive cancer. Sampling of the prostatic urethra is best accomplished by superficial resection immediately proximal to the verumontanum on both sides. TUR of the bladder neck may be necessary in cases with prostatic CIS to allow appropriate contact with prostatic mucosa of intravesically administered bacille Calmette-Guérin (BCG) therapy.

After completion of the endoscopic surgery, hemostasis must be meticulous and the bladder cavity carefully emptied of resected tissue. Unless the resection is very limited, an indwelling 22-French Foley catheter is left in place and connected to gravity drainage or to intermittent bladder irrigation. The catheter is left in for a day or two, until the urine is visibly clear. Occasionally, in patients with deep resection, the catheter may be left in for 3 to 5 days. Oral antibiotics may be advisable when catheters are left in place for more than 1 day. A close follow-up is necessary after TUR of bladder tumors. The most standard schedule for check cystoscopies is every 3 months for the first 2 years, every 6 months for up to 5 years, and yearly thereafter if no recurrence is observed. The identification of risk factors for tumor recurrence may allow better adaptation of follow-up schedules for individual patients.

Management of Intraoperative Problems

Tumors on the anterior wall of the bladder, particularly when they are near the bladder neck, may be difficult to resect. These tumors can usually be brought into better visibility by pushing down the lower abdomen with the opposite hand. This manipulation can be carried out by an assistant if the resectionist prefers the two-handed instrument

(Stern-McCarthy). However, even with use of a long resectoscope, such tumors may remain inaccessible in a morbidly obese patient. In this uncommon setting, the resectoscope can be introduced by a perineal urethrostomy performed in the bulbar urethra over a metal sound to circumvent the suspensory ligament of the penis. After TUR, a Foley catheter can be inserted into the penile urethra or through the perineal urethrostomy, which will usually heal within 24 hours of removal of the catheter.

Deep resection in the bladder neck area must be done carefully to avoid complications. In females, resection in such an area can create a vesicovaginal fistula. In men, it may result in trigonal undermining hampering further resection and even bladder catheterization. If an undermined trigone is apparent at the end of surgery, the catheter should be inserted with the help of a catheter guide. If the insertion of a urethral catheter is unsuccessful, a suprapubic cystostomy drainage should be performed.

Tumors involving the ureteral orifice occur in approximately 10 to 15% of cases. Noninvasive tumors should be resected aggressively and resection may be pursued to remove the entire intramural ureter if a papillary tumor is found to extend in this area. Complete resection of a noninvasive papillary tumor will usually leave a bulging ureteral mucosa. In order to prevent stenosis of the orifice, fulguration should be avoided in this area or along the presumed intramural ureter. If extensive fulguration is required or if the ureteral mucosa does not appear to protrude satisfactorily, a ureteral catheter should be placed for a few days to allow initial healing and obviate acute symptoms related to transient obstruction. Resection of a ureteral orifice and the intramural portion of a ureter will usually result in vesicoureteral reflux postoperatively. While reflux may perhaps increase the risk of developing upper tract transitional cell carcinoma,[10] it may also permit passage, and ensuing preventive effect of intravesical immunotherapy or chemotherapy up the ureter.

Transurethral surgery of tumors arising in an acquired bladder diverticulum is limited, since the absence of an underlying muscular component will result in a perforation. Only small, superficial tumors should be resected or fulgurated in a diverticulum with a wide mouth. Otherwise, one may rely on laser therapy or intravesical immunotherapy, and, in case of doubt or persistent tumors, a diverticulectomy by an extravesical approach should be performed after proper control of the other tumors in the bladder has been obtained. The goal of TUR treatment for superficial bladder tumors should be the complete eradication of the tumors. If tumors are too numerous, or if visibility is progressively hampered by uncontrolled bleeding, surgery may be stopped and resumed after 1 or 2 weeks of healing. If the remaining tumors are small, one may rely on laser therapy or intravesical immunotherapy as primary treatment for residual papillary superficial bladder tumors.

Occasionally, concurrent benign prostatic adenoma may be large enough or protruding into the bladder in such a way to impede transurethral resection of vesical neoplasms. Ideally, the bladder tumor should be resected first and allowed to heal before a TUR of the prostate is contemplated to prevent tumor implantation in the prostatic fossa. TUR of the prostate may also be useful to ensure easier follow-up cystoscopies, although the availability of flexible cystoscopes may circumvent this problem. In rare instances, however, it may be necessary to first resect a prostatic lobe before being able to resect the bladder tumor. While no increase in transitional cell tumors of the prostatic urethra has been observed in previous reports of concomitant transurethral resection of vesical neoplasm and prostatic hyperplasia,[11] it may be well advised to use a single instillation of Adriamycin or mitomycin C immediately postoperatively to decrease the risk of viable tumor cell implantation. Indeed, recent reports have shown a reduced bladder tumor recurrence rate when TUR was followed immediately with the instillation of mitomycin C or doxorubicin.[12] In a randomized study of 431 patients with superficial tumors, the 2-year recurrence rate after a single epirubicin instillation given at the time of TUR was significantly less than that noted in patients given placebo.[13] Thiotepa did not induce such a response in patients treated similarly.[14] Immediate postoperative single instillation of chemotherapeutic agents may become a standard adjuvant to TUR of bladder tumors.

Complications

Potential short-term complications of endoscopic resection of bladder tumors include hemorrhage and septicemia. Careful coagulation after TUR will decrease postoperative bleeding. Nevertheless, it is not uncommon to have important postoperative bleeding in patients with crystal-clear irrigation fluid at the end of surgery. Hyponatremia and hypervolemia are extremely rare even after TUR of large bladder tumors.

Obturator nerve reflex may be evoked while resecting lesions on the lateral bladder wall, particularly in thin patients. This reflex will result in adductor spasms of the leg as well as inward movement of the bladder wall during resection, which may result in its perforation and, in extremely rare cases, even in trauma to major pelvic vessels. The obturator reflex may be prevented by lowering the cutting current and avoiding distention of the bladder during resection of this area. If these maneuvers are unsuccessful, it may be necessary to give the patient a general anesthetic and a neuromuscular blocking agent, or to block the nerve with a local anesthetic as described by Augspurger et al.[15]

Extraperitoneal bladder perforation in the perivesical fat can usually be treated conservatively by Foley catheter drainage for 4 to 6 days and use of antibiotics. Intraperitoneal perforations occur in the posterior wall or in the dome of the bladder. In patients under regional anesthesia, this will be accompanied by sudden and severe abdominal pain. At the time of perforation the greater omentum or the small bowel may protrude into the bladder. In smaller defects, one may only notice failure of the irrigation fluid to return completely. Important intraperitoneal perforation must be treated by emergency laparotomy, bladder closure, and drainage. Smaller defects may be treated conservatively.

Hydronephrosis resulting from the stricture of a ureteral orifice or the distal ureter may go clinically unrecognized until severe dilatation and loss of renal parenchyma. Excretory urography should be performed within a few weeks after a TUR that has involved the periureteral area to detect hydronephrosis due to ureteral injury. Prolonged and multiple resections may result in fibrosis and stricture of the urethra, most commonly at the meatus, fossa navicularis, and at the junction of the pendular and bulbar urethra. Most of these strictures are usually easily managed by dilatation. Multiple or very extensive resection of the bladder wall may result in a contracted bladder with small capacity. This may also cause vesicoureteral reflux, which may promote the appearance of upper tract tumors in patients with continued bladder tumor recurrences. In patients with important symptoms due to a severely contracted bladder, a cystoplasty should be considered only if the bladder is free of tumor recurrence. Otherwise, cystectomy and urinary diversion are indicated.

TUR as Primary Treatment of Invasive Cancer

Although the treatment of bladder cancer by TUR has been used mainly for the management of superficial stage Ta and T1 bladder tumors, TUR also has a role as primary curative treatment of selected patients with muscle-invasive bladder cancer. That TUR may effectively cure some patients with invasive bladder cancer is supported by reported 5-year survival rates of approximately 60% after TUR alone in several series of selected patients with muscle-infiltrating cancer.[16,17] Moreover, in most series, up to 10% of patients undergoing radical cystectomy for stage T2 or T3 bladder cancer after TUR will have no tumor (stage P0) found within the surgical specimen. Herr recently reported that 118 (25%) of 466 patients referred to him with a diagnosis of muscle-infiltrating bladder cancer were not treated by radical cystectomy because a second staging TUR failed to document residual muscle invasion.[18] Of these 118 patients, 77 (65%) remained free of invasive disease beyond 5 years with the bladder intact, while the others were treated by radical cystectomy upon failure, resulting in an overall survival of 83%.

Based on this experience, it is possible to identify some criteria for the selection of patients with T2 or T3 cancers more suitable for this conservative approach. Consideration for TUR alone for invasive bladder cancer should be given to patients with good bladder function and in the presence of no more than two tumors not exceeding 2 cm at the base. Tumors should be papillary, well circumscribed, and located at the base or on the lateral walls of the bladder. Tumors at the bladder neck or at the dome of the bladder or high on the posterior wall, where the peritoneum covers the outer surface of the bladder, should be avoided. No mass should be palpated on bimanual examination. A wide and deep TUR down to the perivesical fat should be performed. In cases treated conservatively, a second mandatory TUR of the resected area should be performed within 2 months of the initial resection. In cases selected for conservative follow-up, it may be advisable to perform a laparoscopic or minilaparotomy pelvic lymphadenectomy, since 20 to 30% of patients may have lymph node metastasis and thus may benefit from adjuvant systemic polychemotherapy. In the absence of positive node and with complete TUR, the need for adjuvant radiation therapy or systemic therapy may be more debatable.[19] TUR alone is also a viable and reasonable approach in any patient with an invasive bladder cancer who is otherwise medically unfit or refuses a more aggressive surgery such as radical cystectomy.

LASER THERAPY OF BLADDER CANCER

Technical Considerations

Surgical lasers have several properties of interest for the endoscopic treatment of bladder tumors. Many sources of laser energy are available. However neodymium:yttrium-aluminum-garnet (Nd:YAG) is the most widely used in urologic practice, mainly because of its effectiveness through the water medium required for endoscopic treatment. The wavelength emitted by the Nd:YAG laser (1060 nm) is fully absorbed by body pigments but not by water. The light energy emitted by the laser is transformed into thermal energy leading to coagulation necrosis of tissues. This thermal necrosis is usually only 2 to 3 mm in depth but can attain 7 mm. The probe used for coagulation is flexible and can be introduced through a flexible or rigid cystoscope sheet. When using a rigid cystoscope, a specially designed albarran adaptor must be used. Energy emission is usually controlled with a foot pedal; 35 to 40 watts of power is ample for thermal necrosis.

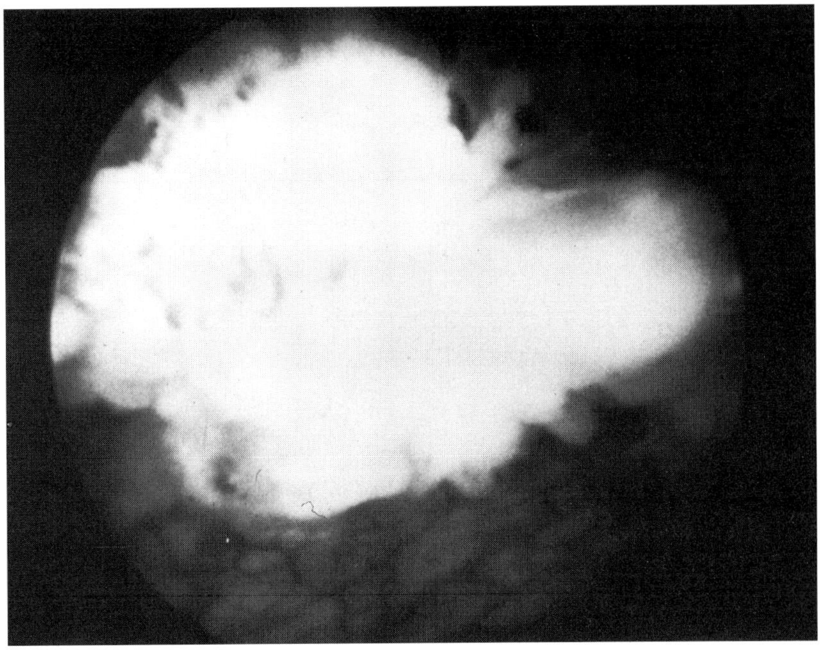

FIGURE 19–3. Nd:YAG laser-induced coagulation necrosis of a bladder tumor. (Courtesy of Dr. Guy Drouin.)

The flexible fiber, through which a visible light beam is carried, is positioned 2 to 3 mm away from the tumor to be treated. However, there is a 5- to 8-degree angle of diversion between the visible spotlight and the actual laser energy emission. This explains why thermal necrosis does not occur quite where the light beam would indicate. Therefore, the flexible fiber rod must be positioned very close to the tumor without touching it, as this would lead to obstruction of the laser energy and overheating and damage of the laser fiber. Bladder tumor necrosis is obtained by painting the tumor with the laser beam until there is a complete tissue necrosis, which is characterized by a white discoloration (Fig. 19–3).

Laser therapy is well suited for superficial papillary recurrent bladder tumors less than 2.5 cm and offers several advantages. This procedure can be done in an outpatient setting, since there is no bleeding and no catheter drainage is necessary. Moreover, unlike electrocautery there is no obturator nerve stimulation and therefore a lessened risk of bladder perforation. Since the laser fiber probe is somewhat flexible, the instrument can be used with a flexible cystoscope. This can be particularly advantageous for areas that are normally difficult to reach with the rigid resectoscope, such as the bladder neck. Moreover, this treatment can be applied to tumors arising in a ureteral orifice without causing sclerosis of the orifice and potential secondary hydronephrosis. When treating an orificial tumor, a metallic guidewire must be introduced in the ureter for ease of anatomic orientation (polymer ureteral catheters will melt during treatment and should not be used). A ureteral catheter should be inserted in the ureter after laser coagulation to prevent significant edema and renal colic. Laser fulguration requires no anesthesia, as the water medium used for bladder distention and visibility cools off the heat that can be felt by the patient. Tumors arising in bladder diverticula can be treated in this fashion without perforating the bladder or damaging the iliac blood vessels if the diverticula are laterally located. Laser thermal coagulation does not alter the overall histologic architecture of the bladder wall, unlike electrocautery.

Disadvantages of laser fulguration are few and include the lack of histopathologic specimens for diagnosis. It is advisable to perform a TUR at first diagnosis to obtain proper grading and staging of the tumor. Another disadvantage of laser is that it is an expensive tool. Moreover, eye protection must be worn to avoid retinal damage by the laser beam. Although rare, perforation of the bladder can occur as well as bowel perforation even in the absence of bladder perforation.[20] Bleeding tumors are not amenable to laser fulguration, as blood absorbs the laser energy.

Results of Treatment

Few studies have compared electrosurgical endoscopic resection and laser thermal coagulation for the treatment of superficial bladder tumors. Several studies have reported a low incidence of tumor recurrence after laser treatment of superficial tumors. However, a randomized, prospective study found no difference in overall recurrence rate between laser-treated patients and those undergoing electrocautery resection. On the other hand, local recurrence at the primary tumor site was found in 19 of 44 patients undergoing TUR alone compared with only 3 of 44 treated with Nd:YAG laser, suggesting that the latter modality may be more effective in eradicating tumors, while obviously not affecting the urothelial instability leading to tumor recurrence in other sites.[21]

Laser photocoagulation has also been used in muscle-invasive bladder tumors in conjunction with TUR in order to extend tumor control 5 to 7 mm deeper. For this procedure, however, some form of anesthesia is required. Results of combined treatment by TUR and laser fulguration were reported by several groups. Smith et al. reported on 34 patients with biopsy-proven infiltrating bladder cancer. In clinical stage T2 and T3a patients, 84 and 54%, respectively, had no recurrence at 6 months, but 68% of stage T3b patients showed persistent tumors.[22] McPhee et al. found no recurrence of the initial tumor in 12 patients treated for T2 cancer and followed for 6 to 78 months, although four patients had a T1 recurrence elsewhere in the bladder. Eight of 14 T3a patients demonstrated tumor persistence.[23] Beisland et al. treated 15 patients with clinical stage T2 bladder cancer, and with a follow-up from 56 to 78 months, 10 patients remained free of recurrence. Thus, although laser fulguration combined with TUR may be effective in selected cases, its clinical application remains limited.

Photodynamic Therapy of Bladder Cancer

Technical Considerations

Photodynamic therapy (PDT) is an original form of laser treatment consisting of an intravenous injection of porphyrin derivatives, which are light sensitive, followed by bladder endoscopic illumination at 630 nm. The most widely used photosensitizing agent is porfimer sodium (Photofrin, QLT Photo Therapeutics, Inc.). When administered intravenously (2 mg/kg) it concentrates in tissues rich in reticuloendothelial cells, such as the liver and kidneys, where it is metabolized. It also accumulates in the skin, probably because of the presence of a significant number of macrophages, mast cells, and Langerhans cells.[24] This agent is mainly carried by serum lipoproteins and has a serum half-life of 22 hours. The product is preferentially taken up by tumor cells, as opposed to adjacent normal bladder cells. Endocytosis and low-density lipoprotein (LDL) receptors have been implicated in the mechanisms of tumoral intracytoplasmic porfimer concentration.[25] Leakage from tumor neovasculature as well as the absence of lymphatic vessels within tumors may also contribute to the selective uptake of porfimer by cancer cells.[26] Tissue peak levels of porfimer are attained within 5 to 10 hours. To allow for maximal clearance of porfimer from normal tissues and therefore for an optimal differential between normal and malignant tissue, it is recommended that 48 to 72 hours elapse between

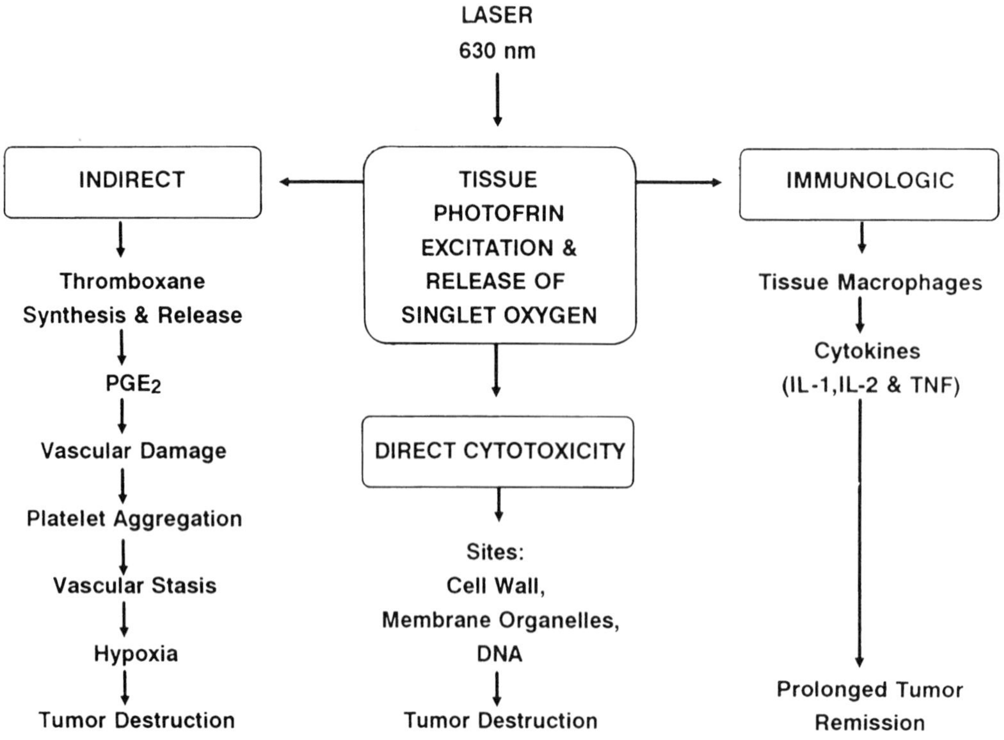
LASER
630 nm
INDIRECT
TISSUE PHOTOFRIN EXCITATION & RELEASE OF SINGLET OXYGEN
IMMUNOLOGIC
Thromboxane Synthesis & Release
PGE2
Vascular Damage
Platelet Aggregation
Vascular Stasis
Hypoxia
Tumor Destruction
DIRECT CYTOTOXICITY
Sites:
Cell Wall,
Membrane Organelles,
DNA
Tumor Destruction
Tissue Macrophages
Cytokines
(IL-1,IL-2 & TNF)
Prolonged Tumor Remission

FIGURE 19–4. Possible mechanisms of tumor destruction by Nd:YAG treatment.

intravenous injection of porfimer and illumination of the bladder.

When a porfimer molecule is excited, optimally with light at 630 nm, it induces a series of chemical reactions, such as the formation of singlet molecular oxygen from O_2. This is probably the most significant phenomenon through which PDT is effective[24,27] (Fig. 19–4). In vitro studies have shown that oxygen-repleted cells treated with PDT show signs of damage, whereas oxygen-deficient cells do not respond to PDT. Moreover, cytokine production and the formation of free radicals, which are toxic to the cell metabolism, may contribute to the therapeutic effect.[28,29] Damage to vascular endothelium has also been suggested as another mechanism.[30]

The 630-nm wavelength light energy is obtained by an argon laser coupled with a dual laser (Kiton Red/rhodamine B). A flexible laser fiber that is attached to the laser apparatus is then introduced through a No. 23 cystoscope. Although a microlens can be introduced for treatment of a specific bladder tumor, the majority of patients undergoing PDT need whole-bladder illumination, which requires a bulb tip fiber. Placement of the optical fiber in the center of the distended bladder is most important for optimal treatment, as the energy administered by the laser fiber decreases according to the square of the distance between bulb tip and the bladder wall. Visual placement has been shown to be inaccurate and abdominal ultrasound should be used to optimize placement of the light source. Adequate distention of the bladder is essential in order to avoid areas unexposed to light, a phenomenon called shadowing[26] (Fig. 19–5). It is also very important to avoid bleeding, as hemoglobin absorbs

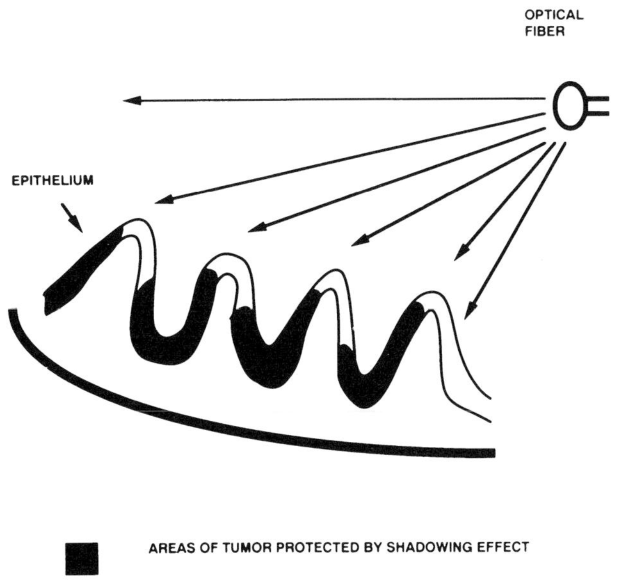
OPTICAL FIBER
EPITHELIUM
AREAS OF TUMOR PROTECTED BY SHADOWING EFFECT

FIGURE 19–5. Schematic representation of uneven surface found in a hollow viscus such as the bladder. Areas of tumor may be protected by shadows. (From Manyak MJ: Photodynamic therapy for urologic malignancy. AUA Update Series 1995; 14:12, with permission.)

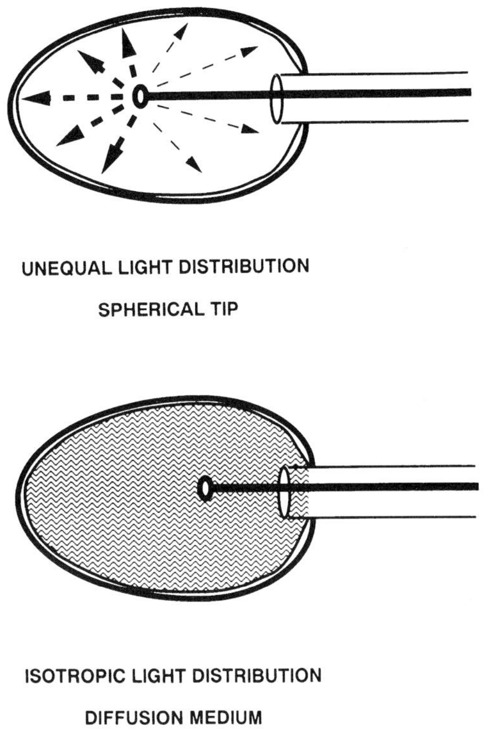
UNEQUAL LIGHT DISTRIBUTION
SPHERICAL TIP
ISOTROPIC LIGHT DISTRIBUTION
DIFFUSION MEDIUM

FIGURE 19–6. Light distribution within the bladder with intravesical instillation of a saline (*above*) and diffusion media (*below*). Diffusion medium compensates for both the unequal light distribution from the bulb tip fiber and shadows cast by irregularities of the epithelial surface. (From Manyak MJ: Photodynamic therapy for urologic malignancy. AUA Update Series 1995; 14:12, with permission.)

light. In order to improve light diffusion, special media such as 0.02% soybean emulsion have been used with success[26] (Fig. 19–6). Total light dose varies according to the type of cancer to be treated and the bladder surface area. Papillary tumors usually require 50 to 300 joules/cm^2, whereas CIS requires between 10 and 50 joules/cm^2. Bladder surface is calculated from bladder volume as measured by abdominal ultrasound.

Results of PDT

Results of PDT studies have shown that it is most effective for CIS and less so for papillary tumors. Poor response of papillary tumors, especially those larger than 2 cm, is probably due to the shallow tissue penetration (3 mm) of the 630-nm light.[31] However, tumors less than 1 cm can respond well to this treatment. One study even reports a cure rate of 83% at 3 months in 23 patients with superficial bladder tumors (Ta, T1).[32] In one recent study, treatment with HPD of 14 patients with diffuse superficial bladder tumors and 5 patients with CIS resulted in complete response at 3 months of 12 of the 19 patients.

As CIS is a noninvasive but highly aggressive form of bladder carcinoma, it has received most of the attention with regards to PDT. A first study reported 11 complete responses and 3 partial responses in 16 patients treated for CIS.[33] Long-term results in patients treated for CIS resistant to intravesical therapy appear particularly promising, as 9 of 15 patients followed for 24 to 54 months after PDT had a sustained complete response.[34] Another study reported 22 complete responses and 11 partial responses in 37 similar patients, although many patients did have bladder tumor recurrences at an average time of 15 months. A more recent report on 34 patients with refractory CIS treated with PDT showed a 73.5% complete response at 3 months. Although 78% of the responders had a recurrence within 2 years, the majority were low-grade papillary tumors successfully treated by TUR. Ten of the 34 patients are alive with intact bladder 64 months after PDT.[35] Similar results were also reported on 15 patients by another group who used in situ dosimetry to measure scatter and nonscatter light energy.[36]

PDT Side Effects

Dermal photosensitivity consisting of first- and second-degree sunburns, when the skin is exposed to sunlight, is the most common side effect of PDT. This phenomenon is variable from patient to patient and is unrelated to dosage.[26] Irritative bladder symptoms are also frequent. Other infrequent side effects include nausea and vomiting, eye photosensitivity, liver toxicity, and a metallic taste after injection.[37] A serious side effect encountered with PDT has been a reduction in bladder capacity secondary to fibrosis. This can occur if a large number of inflammatory cells are present in the bladder wall, therefore increasing the amount of photosensitizing agent retained. For this reason, it is usually recommended that 4 to 6 weeks must elapse between PDT and intravesical chemotherapy, immunotherapy, or endosurgical resection. Contributing factors may include use of intravesical Adriamycin, which has photosensitizing properties,[32] and excessive light administration. The use of 75 joules/cm^2 leads to a 9% rate of bladder fibrosis compared to less than 1% observed with BCG intravesical therapy.[36] Research is currently in progress to identify photosensitizers that may be more selective and that could be administered intravesically rather than systemically. Photodynamic therapy thus remains a second-line treatment that could be used advantageously in patients with resistant CIS to avoid cystectomy in a group of patients.

REFERENCES

1. Wingo PA, Tong T, Bolden S: Cancer statistics, 1995. CA Cancer J Clin 1995; 45:8.
2. Weiss MA, Mills SE: Atlas of Genitourinary Tract Disorders, pp 12.5–12.0. Singapore, Gower Medical Publishing, 1989.
3. Allard P, Fradet Y, Têtu B, et al: Tumor-associated antigens as prognostic factors for recurrence in 382 patients with primary transitional cell carcinoma of the bladder. Clin Cancer Res 1995; 1:1195.
4. Kiemeney LALM, Witjes JA, Heijbroek RP, et al: Predictability of recurrent and progressive disease in individual patients with primary superficial bladder cancer. J Urol 1993; 150:60.
5. Malmstrom PU, Busch C, Norlen BJ: Recurrence, progression and survival in bladder cancer: a retrospective analysis of 232 patients with greater than or equal to 5-year follow-up. Scand J Urol Nephrol 1987; 21:185.
6. National Bladder Cancer Collaborative Group: Surveillance, initial assessment, and subsequent progress of patients with superficial and subsequent bladder cancer in a prospective longitudinal study. Cancer Res 1977; 37:2907.
7. Engberg A, Spanberg A, Urnes T: Transurethral resection of bladder tumors under local anesthesia. Urology 1983; 22:385.
8. Stephen R, Miotti D, Bettaglio R, et al: Electromotive administration of a new morphine formulation: morphine citrate. Artif Organs 1994; 18:461.
9. Netter FH: The CIBA collection of medical illustration; kidneys, ureters, and urinary bladder, pp 210–211. Indianpolis, CIBA, 1973.
10. DeTorres-Mateos JA, Banus Gassol JM, Palou Redorta J, et al: Vesicoureteral reflux and upper urinary tract transitional cell carcinoma after transurethral resection of recurrent superficial bladder carcinoma. J Urol 1987; 138:49.
11. Laor E, Grabstald H, Whitmore WF: The influence of simultaneous resection of bladder tumors and prostate on the occurrence of prostatic urethral tumors. J Urol 1981; 126:171.
12. Bouffioux C, Kurth KH, Bono A, et al: Intravesical adjuvant chemotherapy for superficial transitional cell bladder carcinoma: results of 2 European Organization for Research and Treatment of Cancer randomized trials with mitomycin C and doxorubicin comparing early versus delayed instillations and short-term versus long-term treatment. European Organization for Research and Treatment of Cancer Genitourinary Group. J Urol 1995; 153:934.
13. Oosterlinck W, Kurth KH, Schroder F, et al: A prospective European Organization for Research and Treatment of Cancer Genitourinary Group randomized trial comparing transurethral resection followed by a single intravesical instillation of epirubicin or water in single stage Ta, T1 papillary carcinoma of the bladder. J Urol 1993; 149:749.
14. Medical Research Council Working Party on Urological Cancer, Subgroup on Superficial Bladder Cancer: The effect of intravesical thiotepa on tumour recurrence after endoscopic treatment of newly diagnosed superficial bladder cancer. A further report with long-term follow-up of a Medical Research Council randomized trial. Br J Urol 1994; 73:632.
15. Augspurger R, Donohue RE: Prevention of obturator nerve stimulation during transurethral surgery. J Urol 1980; 123: 170.
16. Herr HW: Transurethral resection in regionally advanced bladder cancer. Urol Clin North Am 1992; 19:695.
17. Hall RR, Newsling PWW, Ramsden PD, et al: Treatment of invasive bladder cancer by local resection and high dose methotrexate. Br J Urol 1984; 56:668.
18. Herr HW, Kata EJ: The role of transurethral resection for muscle invasive bladder carcinoma. J Urol 1993; 149:316A.
19. Hall RR: The role of transurethral surgery alone and with combined modality therapy. *In* Vogelzang NJ, Scardino PT, Shipley WU, Coffey DS (eds): Comprehensive Textbook of Genitourinary Oncology, pp 509–533. Baltimore, Williams & Wilkins, 1996.
20. Greskovich FJ, von Eschenbach AC: Bladder perforation resulting from the use of the neodymium: YAG laser. Lasers Surg Med 1991; 11:5.
21. Beisland HO, Seland P: A prospective randomized study

of Nd:YAG laser irradiation vs TUR in the treatment of urinary bladder cancer. Scand J Urol Nephrol 1986; 20:209.
22. Smith JA: Laser treatment of invasive bladder cancer. J Urol 1986; 135:55.
23. McPhee MC, Arnfield MR, Tulip J, et al: Neodymium: YAG laser therapy for infiltrating bladder cancer. J Urol 1988; 140:44.
24. Nseyo UO: Photodynamic therapy. Urol Clin North Am 1992; 19:591.
25. Dougherty TJ: Photodynamic therapy (PDT) of malignant tumors. Crit Rev Oncol Hematol 1984; 2:83.
26. Manyak MJ: Photodynamic therapy for urologic malignancy. AUA Update Series 1995; 14:12.
27. Weiskaupt KR, Gomer CJ, Dougherty TJ: Identification of singlet oxygen as the cytotoxic agent in photoactivation of a murine tumor. Cancer Res 1976; 6:2326.
28. Nseyo UO, Whalen RK, Duncan MR, et al: Urinary cytokines following photodynamic therapy for bladder cancer. A preliminary report. Urology 1990; 36:167.
29. Foote CS: Definition of type I and type II photosensitized oxidation (Editorial). Photochem Photobiol 1991; 54:659.
30. Selman S, Kerck R, Kreimer-Birnbaum M, et al: Acute blood flow changes in transplantable FANFT-induced urothelial tumors treated with hematoporphyrin derivatives and light. Surg Forum 1983; 34:676.
31. Hisazumi H, Misaki T, Miyoshi N: Photoradiation therapy of bladder tumors. J Urol 1983; 130:685.
32. Nseyo UO, Dougherty TJ, Sullivan L, et al: Photodynamic therapy in the management of lower urinary tract cancer. Cancer 1987; 60:3113.
33. Shumaker BP, Hetzel FW: Clinical laser photodynamic therapy in the treatment of bladder carcinoma. Photochem Photobiol 1987; 46:899.
34. Jocham D, Beer M, Baumgartner R, et al: Long-term experience with integral photodynamic therapy of Tis bladder carcinoma. Ciba Found Symp 1989; 146:198.
35. Uchibayashi T, Koshida K, Kunimi K, et al: Whole bladder wall photodynamic therapy for refractory carcinoma in situ of the bladder. Br J Cancer 1995; 71:625.
36. D'Hallewin MA, Baert L: Long-term results of whole bladder wall photodynamic therapy for carcinoma in situ of the bladder. Urology 1995; 45:763.
37. Manyak MJ, Russo A, Smith PD: Photodynamic therapy. J Clin Oncol 1988; 6:380.

20

PARTIAL CYSTECTOMY AND RADICAL CYSTECTOMY

JOHN A. FREEMAN, M.D. *and* DONALD G. SKINNER, M.D.

Bladder tumors that invade beyond the lamina propria into the muscular wall of the bladder are, with few exceptions, best treated by radical cystectomy. Radical cystectomy, or anterior exenteration, implies the removal of the pelvic organs anterior to the rectum: the prostate, seminal vesicles, and bladder with peritoneal reflection and urachus in males, and the cervix, uterus, ovaries, fallopian tubes, and bladder with peritoneal reflection and urachus in females. The perivesical fat and pelvic lymph nodes are removed en bloc with the specimen. Preservation of a functional urethra is safe and technically possible in the majority of both male[1] and female[2–4] patients, allowing the patient the option of orthotopic neobladder reconstruction.[5,6] Currently, radical cystectomy provides the best results in terms of staging, prevention of local recurrence, and survival for patients with muscle-invasive bladder tumors.

Five fundamental observations support the view that radical cystectomy is optimal therapy for muscle-invasive bladder cancer. First, the morbidity and mortality associated with the procedure have declined in the past three decades due to medical, surgical, and anesthetic advances. Second, the best long-term survival to date is achieved following surgical resection of invasive tumors. Bladder cancer tends to spread progressively from its origin in the mucosa to the lamina propria and then sequentially to the muscularis, perivesical fat, and adjacent pelvic viscera with increasing incidence of lymph node metastases at each site. Wide, en bloc resection of the anterior pelvic viscera, perivesical fat, and pelvic lymph nodes provides negative surgical margins and low local recurrence rates. Third, transitional cell carcinoma is resistant to even high doses of radiation therapy. Fourth, chemotherapy alone or in combination with bladder-sparing surgery has not yielded equivalent long-term survival comparable to radical cystectomy. Finally, surgical reconstruction of the genitourinary tract can return the patient to a satisfactory and functional lifestyle following radical cystectomy. The majority of patients are able to micturate via the urethra, preserve renal function, and resume functional sexual activity.

PARTIAL CYSTECTOMY

In spite of the success of reconstructive surgery, preservation of the native bladder with maintenance of normal sexual function is preferable if it can be achieved with equivalent disease control. An option to radical cystectomy is local resection of the tumor, leaving a functional detrusor in place. Transurethral approaches to muscle-invasive tumors are addressed in Chapters 18 and 19. Open surgical excision of a segment of bladder (partial cystectomy) for the control of muscle-invasive bladder cancer is only rarely appropriate. Unfortunately, this operation continues to be overutilized in an attempt at bladder preservation.

Partial cystectomy should be considered only if an individual patient fulfills strict selection criteria: a unifocal tumor with no evidence of atypia or associated carcinoma in situ (CIS) in the bladder, the ability to obtain a circumferential 2-cm margin, and no prior history of bladder cancer. Relative contraindications include high-grade tumors, since recurrence rates as high as 70% are seen following partial cystectomy in this setting, and patients with tumors of the trigone or bladder neck.[7] If ureteral reimplantation is required, consideration should be given to radical cystectomy instead. In the Mayo Clinic 20-year experience, only 199 of 3454 patients (6%) were considered candidates[8]; similarly, only 50 of 2000 new patients (2.5%) in a 10-year period at the Cleveland Clinic underwent partial cystectomy for invasive bladder cancer.[9] In properly selected patients, however, results are equivalent to more aggressive therapy (e.g., radical cystectomy). The role of pelvic lymphadenectomy is controversial. Because of the availability of effective adjuvant chemotherapy for patients with lymph node metastases at high risk for distant failure, however, it is recommended as a staging procedure.

An additional consideration in patients with bladder tumors undergoing open operation where tumor cells could potentially spill into the wound and implant is high-dose, short-course preoperative radiation. Wound implantation occurs in 10 to 20% of bladder cancer patients undergoing cystotomy without radiation,[10] and this can be prevented by the addition of preoperative radiation.[11] This currently appears to be the only role for radiation in the management of surgically resectable bladder cancer.

RADICAL CYSTECTOMY

Preoperative Preparation

Patients are admitted the morning before surgery for bowel preparation, intravenous hydration, and to be evaluated and instructed by the enterostomal therapist. A clear liquid diet is consumed until midnight, when the patients are made NPO. A standardized modified Nichols bowel prep is utilized that is well tolerated, cleanses and decompresses the small and large bowel, avoids dehydration, obviates the need for enemas, and maintains nutritional support (Table 20–1).[12] Intravenous crystalloid fluid hydration is begun on the evening of admission and maintained overnight to ensure that the patient enters the operating room well hydrated. Patients over the age of 50 years are routinely loaded with digoxin prophylactically on the day of admission unless there is a specific contraindication (0.5 mg orally [PO] at 1200, 0.25 mg PO at 1800, and 0.125 mg PO at 2400; no digoxin is given the morning of surgery) to decrease the risk of perioperative dysrhythmias and congestive heart failure.[13] Broad-spectrum antibiotic coverage is administered intravenously (IV) when the patient is called to the operating room, so the antibiotics will be in the circulation at the time of incision.

TABLE 20–1. MODIFIED NICHOLS BOWEL PREPARATION*

1. Clear liquid diet beginning the morning of the preoperative day (day of admission)
2. 120 ml of Neoloid (caster oil emulsion) PO immediately upon arrival
3. 1 g neomycin PO at 1000, 1100, 1200, 1300, 1600, 2000, and 2400 hours
4. 1 g erythromycin base PO at 1200, 1600, 2000, and 2400 hours

*From Steiner DG, Lieskovsky G: Technique of radical cystectomy. *In* Skinner DG, Lieskovsky G (eds): Diagnosis and Management of Genitourinary Cancer. Philadelphia, WB Saunders Co, 1988, with permission.

An important aspect of the preoperative evaluation is performed by the enterostomal therapist. An appropriate abdominal location is selected for a stoma. Patients who elect to have an orthotopic form of urinary diversion are marked and receive all of the instruction for cutaneous forms of diversion in case intraoperative findings necessitate a cutaneous form of reconstruction. Medical or technical factors may preclude neobladder reconstruction to the urethra, so an abdominal stoma site should always be marked. The stoma site is selected after examining the patient in the supine, sitting, and standing positions. The location of scars, bony prominences, natural belt line, and the tendency of the pannus to shift with position changes is noted when making site selection. Proper stoma site selection is crucial to patient acceptance and technical success of the procedure, should cutaneous diversion be necessary. In general, incontinent stoma sites are located higher on the abdominal wall. Stoma sites for continent stomas, since they are not dependent on an external appliance, can be hidden lower on the abdomen and often below the belt line. If a cutaneous diversion is anticipated, the patient is educated about the use of appliances or catheterization of a cutaneous stoma. If an orthotopic diversion is planned, the patient is also instructed in intermittent catheterization of the urethra.

Operative Technique

Anesthetic Considerations. Typically, a central venous catheter is placed to administer fluid and monitor central venous pressure intraoperatively. This allows assessment of intravascular volume status during the time when the ureters are clipped and urine output is not evaluable. An arterial line allows for minute-to-minute monitoring of blood pressure, critical to the safe performance of controlled hypotensive anesthesia. Preoperative placement of an epidural catheter allows for intraoperative use of lidocaine, reducing the need for depolarizing muscle relaxants, and allowing for controlled hypotensive anesthesia techniques to be used. The proper use of controlled hypotensive anesthesia during the performance of the exenterative portion of the operation diminishes blood loss and transfusion requirements. However, during the reconstructive portion of the procedure (when the urinary diversion is fashioned from bowel) the epidural should not be activated, since it can result in bowel spasm, making manipulation of the intestines more difficult. Postoperatively, the epidural catheter can be used for analgesia, prior to the patient being converted to a patient-controlled analgesia regimen.

Patient Positioning. The patient is placed on the operating table with the iliac crests just below the level of the fulcrum point of the table. The legs

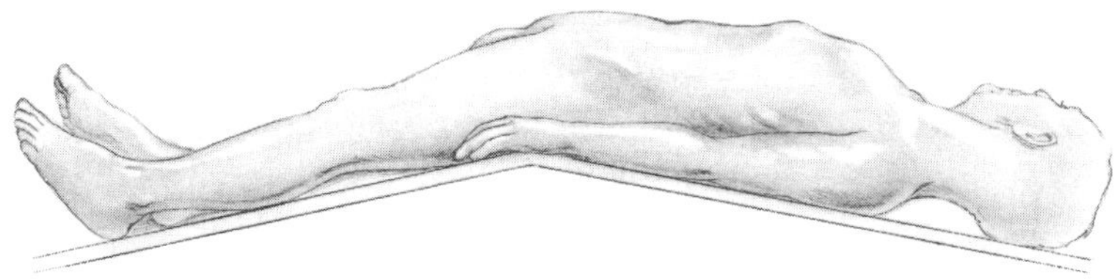

FIGURE 20–1. Position of the patient for radical cystectomy. The legs are abducted, the table is hyperextended, and reverse Trendelenberg position is utilized to bring the abdominal wall parallel with the floor. (From Skinner DG, Lieskovsky G: Technique of radical cystectomy. *In* Skinner DG, Lieskovsky G [eds]: Diagnosis and Management of Genitourinary Cancer. Philadelphia, WB Saunders Co, 1988, with permission.)

are abducted so that the heels are at the corners of the foot of the table, and the table is hyperextended. Reverse Trendelenberg position is used to bring the abdomen parallel to the floor (Fig. 20–1). A nasogastric tube is placed, and the patient is prepped from the nipples to the mid thighs. In female patients the vagina is fully prepped. Once prepared and draped, a 20-French Foley catheter is placed in the bladder and left to gravity drainage. A right-handed surgeon stands on the patient's left hand side of the operating table.

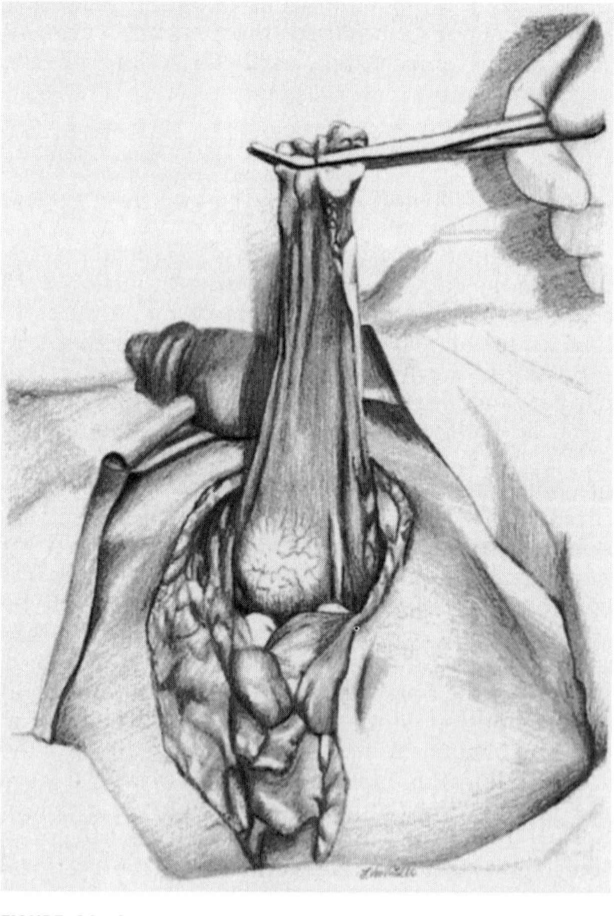

FIGURE 20–2. The urachal remnant is widely excised below the umbilicus and removed en bloc with the bladder specimen. (From Freiha FS: Open bladder surgery. *In* Walsh PC, Retik AB, Stamey TA, Vaughan ED Jr [eds]: Campbell's Urology, 6th edition, vol III. Philadelphia, WB Saunders Co, 1992, with permission.)

INCISION. A vertical midline incision is made from the epigastrium to the symphysis pubis and is carried lateral to the umbilicus on the side opposite of the cutaneous stoma mark. The linea alba is incised and the peritoneal cavity entered in the epigastrium. As the peritoneum is incised inferiorly to the level of the umbilicus, the urachal remnant is identified and circumscribed widely to be removed en bloc with the bladder specimen (Fig. 20–2). This prevents early entry into a high-riding bladder and guarantees complete removal of all bladder remnant tissue. If the patient has had a previous cystotomy or partial cystectomy, the cystotomy tract and cutaneous incision are completely excised en bloc with the bladder.

ABDOMINAL EXPLORATION. The abdominal contents are explored to determine if hepatic metastases, carcinomatosis, gross retroperitoneal adenopathy, or unresectable tumor is present. The abdominal viscera are palpated to rule out unsuspected coexisting abnormalities. If there are no contraindications to proceeding with the procedure, all adhesions are taken down.

BOWEL MOBILIZATION. The bowel is mobilized, beginning with the right colon. A right-angle Richardson retractor elevates the right abdominal wall and the ascending colon is mobilized along the peritoneal reflection (white line of Toldt). The small bowel mesentery is mobilized off of the retroperitoneum toward the ligament of Treitz until the duodenum is exposed. Conceptually, the mobilized mesentery forms an inverted right triangle: the base is formed by the third portion of the duodenum, the right edge represented by the white line of Toldt, the left edge by the medial aspect of the sigmoid and descending colon mesentery, and the apex represented by the ileocecal region (Fig. 20–3, *inset*). This mobilization is an important part of setting up the operative field to perform a cystectomy, and facilitates packing the intestines out of the operative field during the exenterative portion of the operation. The right ureter is exposed, as are the bifurcations of the aorta and inferior vena cava, important landmarks in the operation (Fig. 20–3).

The left colon and sigmoid mesentery are then mobilized by dividing the white line of Toldt lateral to the colon. The sigmoid mesentery is elevated off of the sacrum and iliac vessels up to the level of

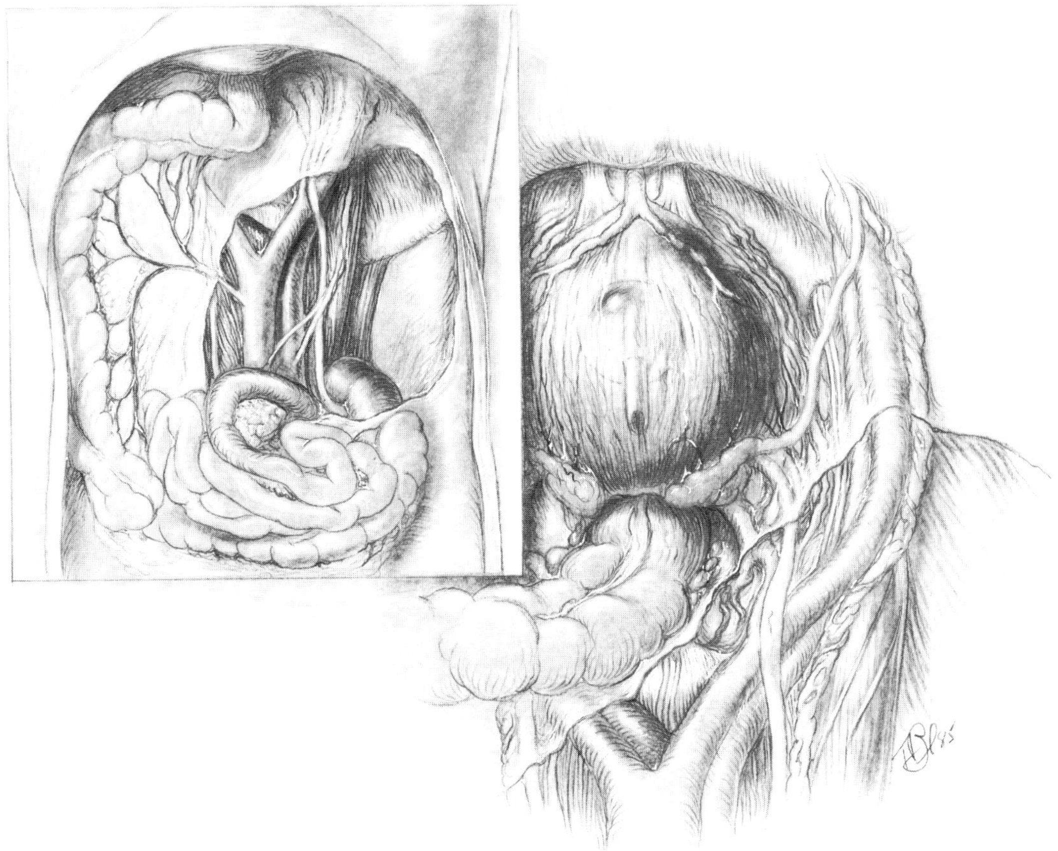

FIGURE 20–3. View of the pelvis following mobilization of the bowel. The ascending colon and small bowel have been mobilized up to the level of the third portion of the duodenum (*inset*). This mobility allows the intestines to be packed in the epigastrium and facilitates exposure of the aortic bifurcation where the lymph node dissection will begin. (From Skinner DG, Lieskovsky G: Technique of radical cystectomy. *In* Skinner DG, Lieskovsky G [eds]: Diagnosis and Management of Genitourinary Cancer. Philadelphia, WB Saunders Co, 1988, with permission.)

the origin of the inferior mesenteric artery on the aorta. This provides a mesenteric window to pass the left ureter through without angulation or tension at the time of ureterointestinal anastomosis for urinary diversion, allows identification of the left ureter, and facilitates the left pelvic lymph node dissection (Fig. 20–4).

With the bowel completely mobilized, a self-retaining retractor is placed; the authors prefer a Finochietto retractor. The right colon and small bowel are then carefully packed in the epigastrium under three open moistened lap pads and a rolled towel. The descending colon is not packed and is left as free as possible, since elevation of the sigmoid is necessary during the ureteral mobilization and left pelvic lymph node dissection. Careful packing of the intestinal contents protects them and prevents their spillage into the operative field during the cystectomy. Packing begins by sweeping the right colon and attached small bowel under one's left hand, along the right sidewall. A moist open lap pad is then swept along the palm of the left hand, under the viscera along the retroperitoneum and right sidewall, and is draped over the top of the bowel, trapping it. Next, the left gutter is packed in a similar fashion, taking care not to pack the left colon. Finally, the central small bowel is packed, and a moist towel rolled to the width of the abdomen is placed horizontally caudal to the lap pads, above the level of the aortic bifurcation. Gentle traction on the rolled towel with a Deaver retractor can facilitate exposure if necessary.

Ureteral Dissection. The ureters are identified in the retroperitoneum and are dissected deep into the pelvis, several centimeters distal to where they cross the iliac vessels. Two hemoclips are placed on each ureter, and the ureter is divided immediately proximal to the distal clip. The ureteral segment distal to the proximal clip (~1 cm in length) is sent for frozen section. The ureter is mobilized proximally and packed beneath the rolled towel to protect it. Typically, an arterial tributary from the common iliac artery or aorta needs to be divided in order to mobilize the ureter adequately. Rich collateral vessels emanate from the male spermatic vessels and the female infundibulopelvic ligament. Ureteral attachments to these vessels are protected to improve vascularity at the subsequent

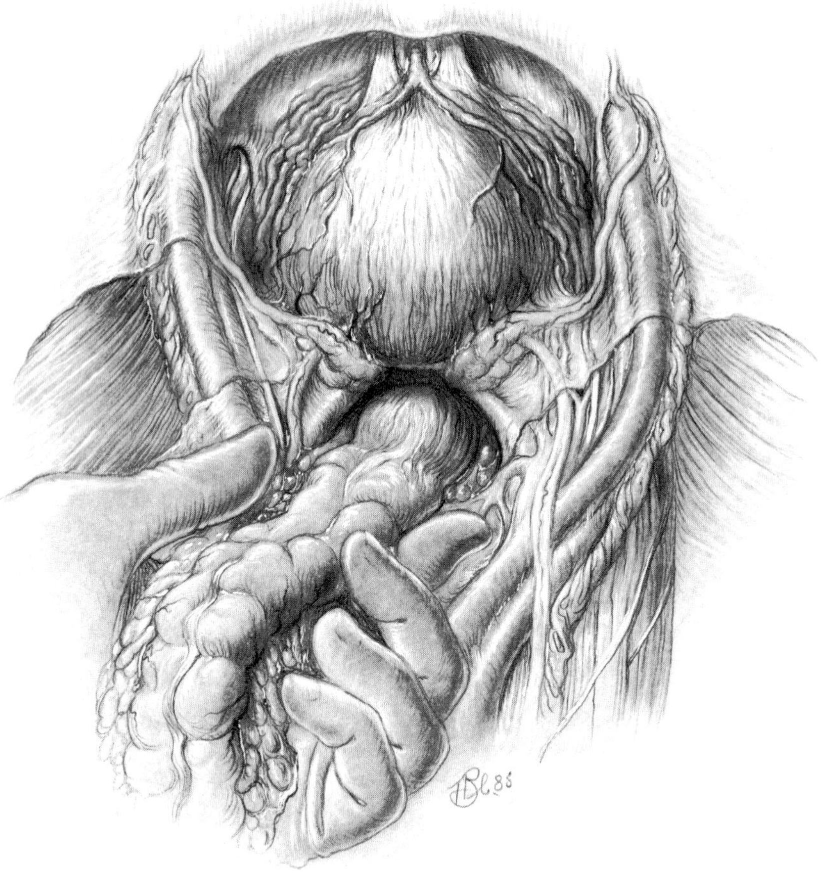

FIGURE 20–4. The sigmoid mesentery has been mobilized from its peritoneal reflection and off of the sacrum up to the origin of the inferior mesenteric artery. The left ureter is identified posterior to the sigmoid and will reach the urinary diversion by passing posterior to the sigmoid in the mesenteric window. (From Skinner DG, Lieskovsky G: Technique of radical cystectomy. *In* Skinner DG, Lieskovsky G [eds]: Diagnosis and Management of Genitourinary Cancer. Philadelphia, WB Saunders Co, 1988, with permission.)

ureteroileal anastomosis. This is particularly important in irradiated patients or those with undilated ureters. Leaving the proximal clip on the divided ureter during the performance of the cystectomy will result in hydrostatic ureteral dilation, facilitating later ureterointestinal anastomosis.

Pelvic Lymph Node Dissection. Overall, some 20 to 35% of patients undergoing cystectomy will be found to have pelvic lymph node metastases. In addition to staging, a therapeutic benefit may be conferred by pelvic lymphadenectomy. Of patients with small-volume nodal metastases, up to one third will be cured by surgery alone.[14,15] Additionally, local pelvic tumor recurrences may be decreased by a carefully performed lymph node dissection.[16] For these reasons we feel that a bilateral pelvic lymph node dissection should be an integral part of the cystectomy in all patients, unless a salvage procedure is being performed for failed radiation treatment in excess of 5000 cGy. In the latter case, pelvic lymphadenectomy is difficult, when possible, and increases the risk of injury to the iliac vessels and obturator nerve.

Pelvic lymphadenectomy is performed en bloc with radical cystectomy. The dissection begins 2 cm above the aortic bifurcation and extends laterally to the genitofemoral nerve, which represents the lateral limit of dissection. Care must be taken not to avulse a consistent anterior tributary to the vena cava just above the bifurcation when initiating the lymphadenectomy. The cephalad side of the lymphatics is ligated with hemoclips, whereas the caudal (specimen) side is ligated only if a significant vessel is identified. In the male, the spermatic vessels are retracted laterally and spared; in the female, the infundibulopelvic ligament with the ovarian vessels is ligated and divided at the pelvic brim, since the ovaries will be removed.

All of the fibroareolar and lymphatic tissue is swept off the aorta, vena cava, and common iliac vessels distally over the sacral promontory. The initial dissection along the common iliac vessels is begun over the arteries, skeletonizing them. As the common iliac veins are dissected medially, care must be taken to control small arterial and venous branches along the anterior surface of the sacrum. Electrocautery is very helpful in this location, since hemoclips tend to become dislodged from the surface of the sacral promontory. Significant bleeding from these presacral vessels can occur if they are not controlled prospectively.

With the proximal iliac vessel dissection complete, a finger is passed between the pelvic peritoneum and the external iliac artery and vein down toward the femoral canal. This blunt dissection joins with the incised transversalis fascia from the inferior aspect of the midline incision. The peritoneum is incised, defining the lateral extent of peritoneum to be removed with the specimen. In male patients the incision lies medial to the spermatic vessels, whereas in female patients it lies lateral to the ovarian vein. The exposed vas deferens or round ligament is divided between hemoclips.

Distal exposure in the area of the femoral canal is facilitated using a large rake (Israel) retractor to elevate the lower abdominal wall and spermatic cord or round ligament remnant. Care should be taken to protect the inferior epigastric vessels in this location. Traction is directed toward the ceiling, not the foot or side of the table, maximally exposing the distal external iliac vessels. The distal limits of dissection are identified: Cooper's ligament medially, the circumflex iliac vein crossing the external iliac artery distally, and the genitofemoral nerve laterally. The lymphatics draining from the thigh, particularly medial to the external iliac vein, are meticulously clipped and divided. The lymph node of Cloquet, or Rosenmüller, represents the distal limit of lymphatic dissection in this location. The distal external iliac artery and vein are circumferentially mobilized, taking care to ligate an accessory obturator vein on the medial inferior aspect of the external iliac vein present in 40% of patients.

Next, the proximal and distal dissections are joined. The proximal external iliac artery and vein are skeletonized circumferentially (Fig. 20–5). The only vessel of consequence in this dissection is a fairly consistent branch to the psoas muscle on the lateral surface of the proximal external iliac vessels. The vessels are retracted medially, and the fascia overlying the psoas is incised medial to the genitofemoral nerve. On the left side, branches of the genitofemoral nerve often pursue a more medial course and may be intimately related to the vessels, in which case they are excised.

At this point the lymphatics surrounding the iliac vessels have been split into compartments medial and lateral to the vessels. The compartments remain attached at their base within the obturator fossa. The lateral compartment, freed medially from the vessels and laterally from the psoas, is swept into the obturator fossa by retracting the iliac vessels medially and passing a small sponge lateral to the vessels along the psoas (Fig. 20–6). The sponge is passed along the course of, and distal to, the internal iliac vein, protecting it; the external iliac vessels are elevated and the sponge withdrawn from the obturator fossa with traction using the left hand (Fig. 20–7). This maneuver facilitates identification of the obturator nerve (Fig. 20–8), which is dissected free from the surrounding lymphatics. The obturator nerve is retracted laterally. The obturator artery and vein are entrapped between the index and middle fingers of the left hand against the pelvic floor at the endopelvic fascia, ligated, and divided. The obturator node packet can then be swept medially, ligating small tributary vessels from the pelvic sidewall musculature, along the lateral bladder wall to be removed en bloc with the cystectomy specimen.

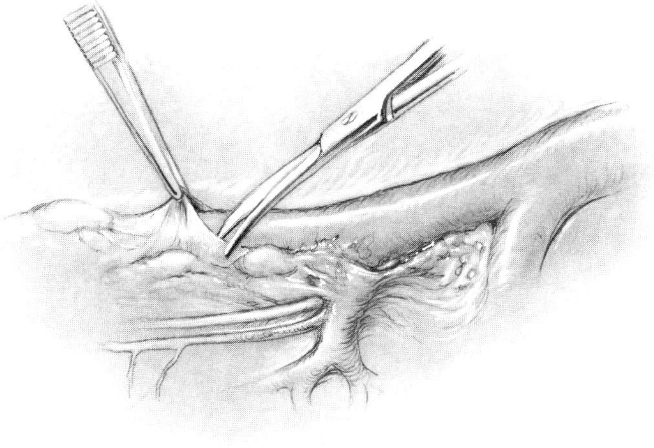

FIGURE 20–5. The external iliac artery and vein are circumferentially skeletonized. Incising over the vessels allows half of the lymphatic material to pass laterally into the obturator fossa, and the other half falls medially toward the bladder. The packets remain attached at the base within the obturator fossa. (From Skinner DG, Lieskovsky G: Technique of radical cystectomy. *In* Skinner DG, Lieskovsky G [eds]: Diagnosis and Management of Genitourinary Cancer. Philadelphia, WB Saunders CO, 1988, with permission.)

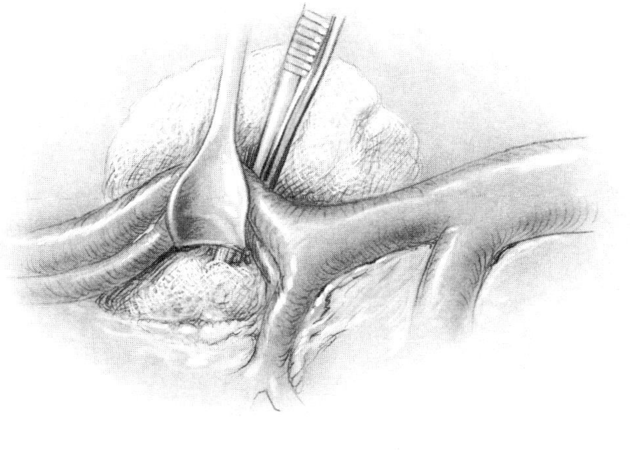

FIGURE 20–6. The lateral external iliac packet is passed into the obturator fossa with a sponge after freeing it medially from the vessels and laterally from the psoas. (From Skinner DG, Lieskovsky G: Technique of radical cystectomy. *In* Skinner DG, Lieskovsky G [eds]: Diagnosis and Management of Genitourinary Cancer. Philadelphia, WB Saunders Co, 1988, with permission.)

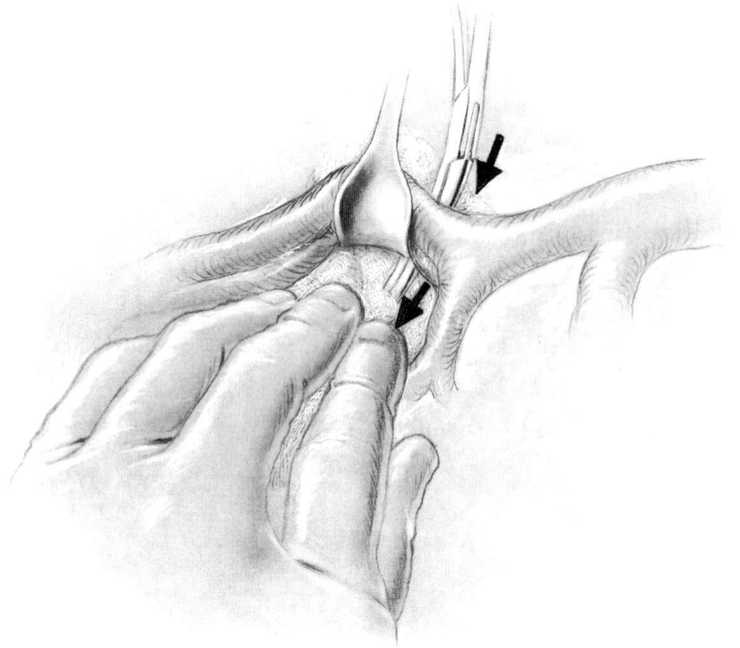

FIGURE 20–7. The sponge is withdrawn from the obturator fossa. Traction with the left hand allows fibroareolar attachments to the underside of the external iliac vessels to be sharply transected. (From Skinner DG, Lieskovsky G: Technique of radical cystectomy. *In* Skinner DG, Lieskovsky G [eds]: Diagnosis and Management of Genitourinary Cancer. Philadelphia, WB Saunders Co, 1988, with permission.)

Ligation of Lateral Bladder Vascular Pedicle. Safe performance of radical cystectomy depends in large part on controlling pelvic hemorrhage. Following dissection of the obturator fossa and ligation of the obturator vessels, the lateral vascular pedicle to the bladder is isolated and divided. Correctly developing the plane that defines this pedicle is perhaps the single most important aspect of the safe performance of a radical cystectomy. When done properly, hemostasis is secured and visualization within the pelvis remains excellent. Identification and isolation of the vascular pedicle is achieved using the left (nondominant) hand. The bladder is retracted toward the left pelvis, placing the branches of the internal iliac (hypogastric) artery on stretch. The left index finger is passed medial to the hypogastric artery, posterior to the pelvic visceral branches. It is directed into the deep pelvis, parallel to the sweep of the sacrum down to the level of the endopelvic fascia (Fig. 20–9). This maneuver defines two major bladder vascular pedicles: the lateral pedicle is anterior to the index finger, composed of branches to the bladder and prostate from the hypogastric artery. The posterior pedicle lies posterior to the index finger, made up of visceral branches between the bladder and rectum.

With the left index finger positioned along the sweep of the sacrum, the lateral pedicle rests between the left index and middle fingers. As traction is applied with the left hand, the pedicle is placed on gentle stretch. The hypogastric artery is skeletonized. The posterior division of the hypogastric artery, composed of the iliolumbar, lateral sacral, and superior gluteal arteries, is spared to prevent gluteal claudication. Distal to this level, the hypogastric artery may be ligated for vascular control but should not be divided, since the pedicle is easier to define if it is left in continuity and on traction. The lateral pedicle is divided between large hemoclips all the way to the endopelvic fascia, or as far as is technically feasible (Fig. 20–9). Right-angle

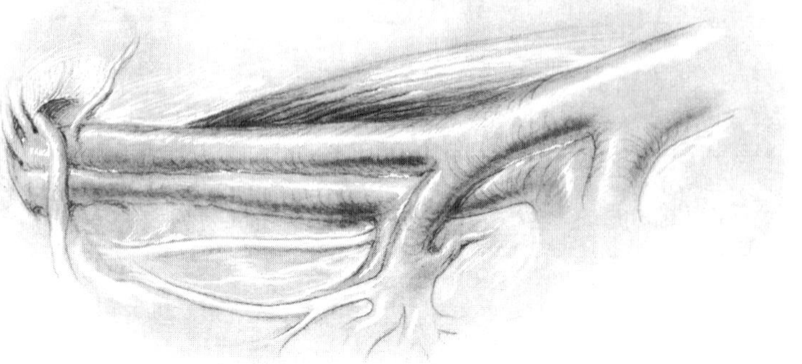

FIGURE 20–8. As the sponge is withdrawn from the obturator fossa the obturator nerve is exposed. The nerve is dissected free from the lymphatic tissue and protected with a vein retractor as all of the lymphatics are removed from the obturator fossa. (From Skinner DG, Lieskovsky G: Technique of radical cystectomy. *In* Skinner DG, Lieskovsky G [eds]: Diagnosis and Management of Genitourinary Cancer. Philadelphia, WB Saunders Co, 1988, with permission.)

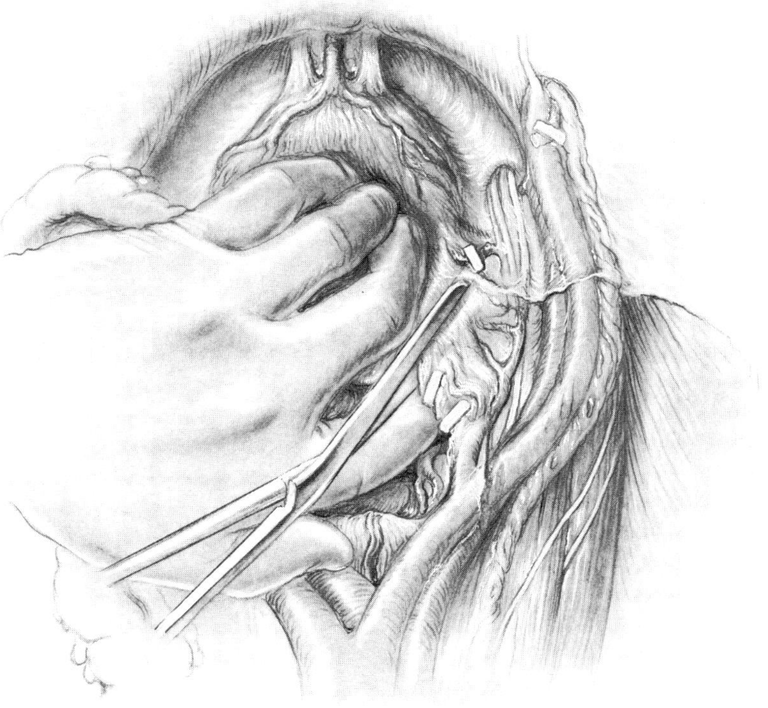

FIGURE 20–9. The lateral pedicle of the bladder extends from the hypogastric artery to the bladder. Here, the right lateral pedicle of the bladder is divided down to the endopelvic fascia deep in the pelvis (see text for description). (From Skinner DG, Lieskovsky G: Technique of radical cystectomy. *In* Skinner DG, Lieskovsky, G [eds]: Diagnosis and Management of Genitourinary Cancer. Philadelphia, WB Saunders Co, 1988, with permission.)

hemoclip appliers are ideally suited for proper placement of hemoclips, and it is important to position the paired set of clips as far apart as possible so that at least 0.5 to 1 cm of tissue projects beyond each clip as the pedicle is divided. This prevents the clips from being dislodged and allowing subsequent bleeding. In obese individuals, the abundant pelvic fat may necessitate dividing the lateral pedicle into two manageable parallel pedicles as dissection proceeds toward the pelvic floor. Incising the endopelvic fascia lateral to the prostate, as is done in radical prostatectomy, helps define the distal limit of the lateral pedicle.

Ligation of Posterior Bladder Vascular Pedicle. After the lateral pedicles have been divided bilaterally, the bladder specimen is retracted anterior and caudal, exposing the rectovesicle space or pouch of Douglas. As the surgeon elevates the bladder with a small sponge under the left hand, the assistant retracts cephalad on the peritoneum overlying the rectosigmoid. This traction and countertraction exposes the recess of the rectovesicle space and places the peritoneal reflection on stretch, facilitating its sharp division. The peritoneum lateral to the rectum is incised first, and then extended into the cul-de-sac to join the contralateral incision (Fig. 20–10). It is important to remember that the anterior and posterior peritoneal reflections meet in the cul-de-sac to form Denonvilliers' fascia, which extends caudally to the urogenital diaphragm (Fig. 20–11, *large arrow*). This is an extremely important anatomic boundary in the male, separating the prostate and seminal vesicles in front from the rectum behind. The plane between the prostate and seminal vesicles and the anterior sheath of Denonvilliers' fascia will not develop easily; in contrast, the plane between the rectum and the posterior sheath of Denonvilliers' fascia (Denonvilliers' space) will develop bluntly. Therefore, the peritoneal incision in the cul-de-sac should be made immediately on the rectal side rather than on the bladder side (Fig. 20–11, *inset, small arrow*). In this way, the plane between the posterior sheath of Denonvilliers' fascia and the anterior rectal wall can be safely developed (Fig. 20–12). A posterior motion with the hand should be used to free the rectum from Denonvilliers' fascia and develop the posterior pedicles down to the prostatic apex where the urethral catheter is palpable.

Several situations make development of the proper plane difficult. Perhaps most common is the erroneous entry into the cul-de-sac too far anteriorly to gain access to Denonvilliers' space. This reiterates the need for incision on the rectal side of the reflection. Other causes include local tumor infiltration or prior high-dose pelvic irradiation. In cases where high-dose irradiation has preceded surgery, consideration should be given to the initial development of this plane from a perineal approach, as in perineal prostatectomy, to avoid rec-

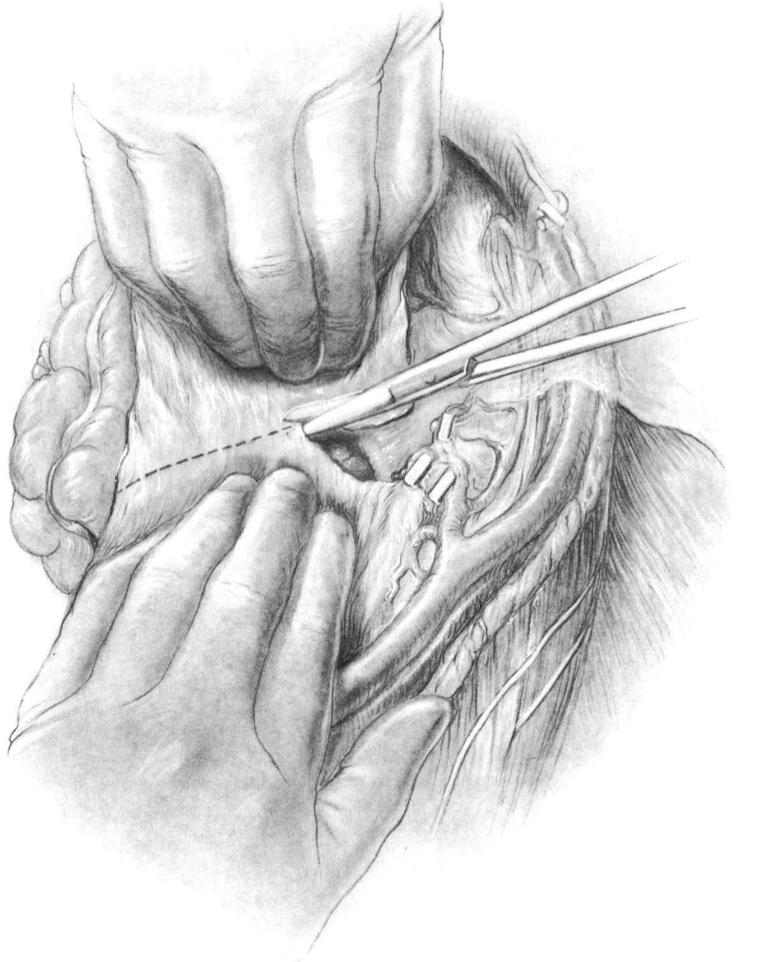

FIGURE 20–10. The peritoneal reflection is divided lateral to the rectum and carried posteriorly into the area of the cul-de-sac where it joins the dissection from the opposite side. This must be performed at the junction with the anterior rectal wall in the midline to facilitate entry into Denonvilliers' space. (From Skinner DG, Lieskovsky G: Technique of radical cystectomy. *In* Skinner DG, Lieskovsky G [eds]: Diagnosis and Management of Genitourinary Cancer. Philadelphia, WB Saunders Co, 1988, with permission.)

totomy.[17] If rectotomy does occur, a two- to three-layer primary closure is recommended. Proximal colostomy is not routinely needed unless the patient has previously received high-dose pelvic irradiation. If vaginal reconstruction or orthotopic urinary diversion is planned, an omental interposition between suture lines is recommended to prevent fistulization.

Once the posterior pedicles have been defined, they are clipped and divided to the endopelvic fascia in the male. If the endopelvic fascia was not previously incised it is done now to facilitate dissection to the prostatic apex. In the female the posterior pedicles including the cardinal ligaments are divided for approximately 4 to 5 cm beyond the cervix. The vaginal apex is identified by cephalad pressure on a sponge stick placed in the vagina, and the posterior vagina is opened. Details of a nerve-sparing approach to the posterior pedicles in the female, preserving a functional urethral sphincter mechanism and allowing neobladder diversion, are outlined below. If the tumor is invading the posterior wall, trigone, or bladder neck, the anterior vaginal wall may be excised with the specimen. If it is desirable to preserve the anterior vaginal wall, the anterior vagina is incised and dissected off of the posterior bladder wall down to the region of the urethra. In this way the posterior pedicle is defined between the bladder and the anterolateral vaginal wall. The pedicles are clipped and divided to the level of the urethra distally. The specimen remains attached only anteriorly at the apex.

Apical Anterior Dissection. The type and extent of anterior dissection varies according to the patient's sex and the type of diversion planned. Since most patients request orthotopic urinary diversion, dissection to facilitate neobladder reconstruction will be described first.

Male Patients. The approach is identical to that for the anterior apical dissection in patients undergoing a retrograde radical prostatectomy.[18] Fibroareolar connections between the anterior bladder wall, prostate, and undersurface of the symphysis pubis are divided. The superficial dorsal vein is identified, ligated, and divided. The prostate is depressed posteriorly, placing the puboprostatic ligaments on stretch. The puboprostatic ligaments are then sharply divided on the undersurface of the pubis, lateral to the dorsal vein complex of the penis (Santorini's plexus). The ligaments need not be clipped prior to division, since no vessels run within them, but care must be taken to avoid the

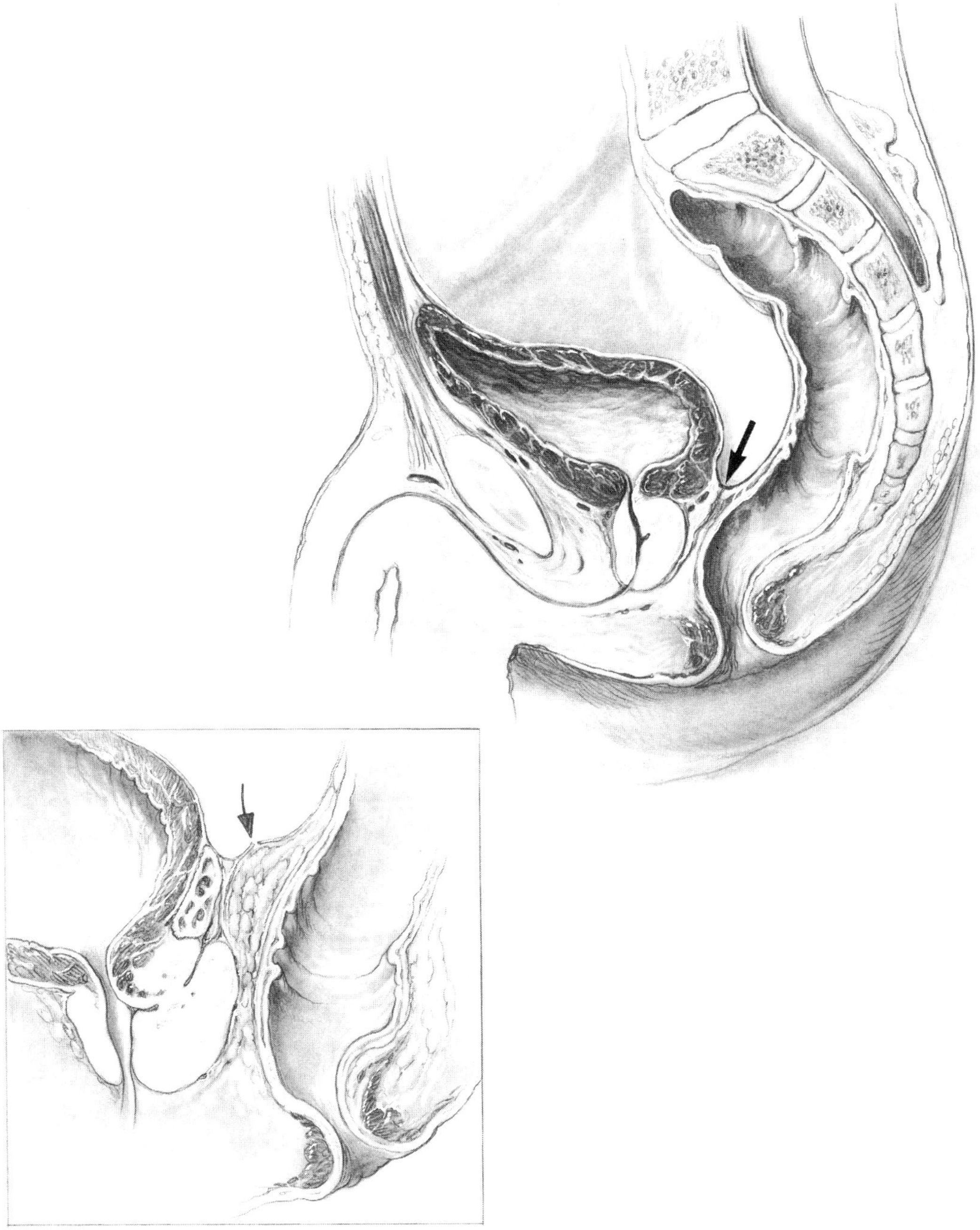

FIGURE 20–11. Diagrammatic representation of the formation of Denonvilliers' fascia. The fascia is formed by a fusion of the anterior and posterior peritoneal reflections behind the bladder, seminal vesicles, and prostate. Denonvilliers' space lies posterior to the fascia, anterior to the rectal serosa (*inset*). Entry into Denonvilliers' space is accomplished by an incision through the posterior peritoneal reflection adjacent to the anterior rectal wall. An incision too close to the bladder will not yield entry into the proper plane and will make this dissection much more difficult. (From Skinner DG, Lieskovsky G: Technique of radical cystectomy. *In* Skinner DG, Lieskovsky G [eds]: Diagnosis and Management of Genitourinary Cancer. Philadelphia, WB Saunders Co, 1988, with permission.)

dorsal vein complex between the paired ligaments (Fig. 20–13). With complete transection of the puboprostatic ligaments and mobilization of the levator fibers from the sides of the prostate, the apex of the prostate and area of the membranous urethra become visible and palpable. Formerly, we passed an angled clamp under direct vision beneath the dorsal vein complex, anterior to the urethra through the region of the urethral striated sphincter and ligated the vein complex with absorbable (0-Vicryl) suture (Fig. 20–14) and subsequently oversewed the area of the dorsal vein and urethral rhabdosphincter with absorbable suture (Fig. 20–15). Recently, we have modified our technique. We cur-

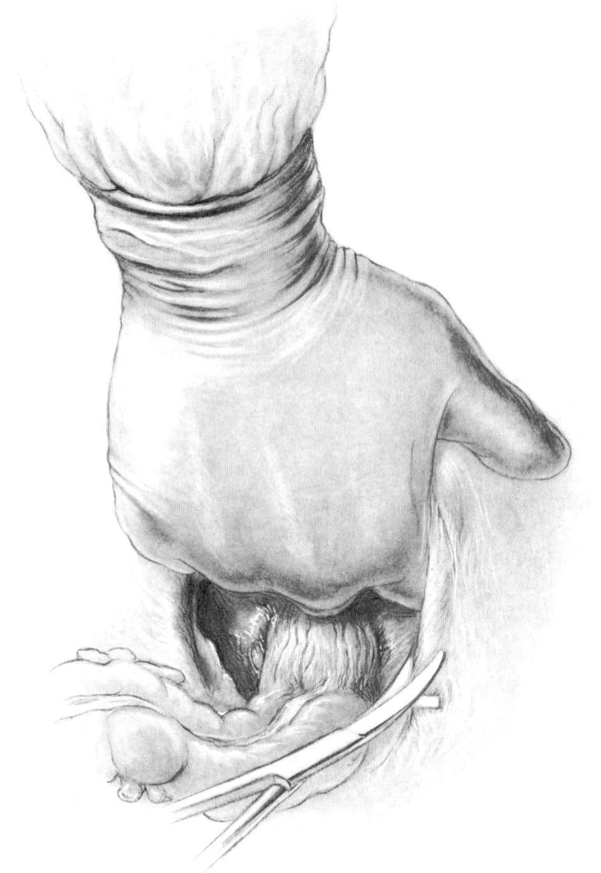

FIGURE 20–12. After entry into Denonvilliers' space is made, the anterior rectal wall is swept off of the posterior leaf of Denonvilliers' fascia using a posteriorly directed sweeping motion. The tissue lateral to the rectum defined by this maneuver constitutes the posterior pedicle of the bladder. (From Skinner DG, Lieskovsky G: Techniques of radical cystectomy. *In* Skinner DG, Lieskovsky G [eds]: Diagnosis and Management of Genitourinary Cancer. Philadelphia, WB Saunders Co, 1988, with permission.)

rently sharply transect the dorsal vein complex without ligation. The anterior surface of the urethra is exposed following division of the dorsal vein complex and the rhabdosphincter is spared the blunt dissection of passing a clamp beneath the dorsal vein complex. This appears to have improved the time to return of continence in patients reconstructed with an orthotopic reservoir.

The prostate is gently retracted cephalad and the anterior two thirds of the urethra is divided, exposing the urethral catheter. This is the optimal time to meticulously place circumferential sutures in the urethra under direct vision for later anastomosis to an orthotopic reservoir. Four 2-0 Vicryl sutures are placed at the 10-, 11-, 1-, and 2-o'clock positions. Placing these sutures at this time allows for direct visualization of the urethral mucosa and lumen, since the attached prostate can be used for gentle cephalad traction on the posterior, undivided urethra. No perineal pressure is required. Placement of these sutures through the rhabdosphincter and dorsal vein complex helps control bleeding as well. The distal (penile) portion of the catheter is then drawn up through the urethrotomy, clamped on the bladder side and divided. Cephalad traction on the bladder side of the divided catheter occludes the bladder neck with the catheter balloon, preventing spill of tumor cells from the bladder lumen. The distal divided end of the catheter is grasped at its tip with a long tonsil clamp; this allows the divided catheter to be telescoped into and out of the distal urethra, exposing the posterior mucosal surface and lumen of the urethra. Four additional 2-0 Vicryl sutures are placed in the posterior surface of the urethra at the 4-, 5-, 7-, and 8-o'clock positions. The posterior urethra and rectourethralis muscle are subsequently divided and the specimen removed. The urethral sutures are tagged to identify their relative location in the urethra and then placed under a protective towel until the selected form of urinary diversion is prepared for urethral anastomosis.

If a cutaneous form of diversion is desired, the levator musculature can be approximated along the pelvic floor with 0-chromic or Vicryl suture to facilitate hemostasis. We generally do not leave a catheter in the urethral remnant to act as a pelvic drain, since this may seed and infect a pelvic hematoma.

Female Patients. In female patients undergoing anterior exenteration, the entire urethra has routinely been removed. Recently, orthotopic urinary reconstruction has been successfully expanded to include female patients.[6,19] Because there are no historical data from which to determine the risk of urethral recurrence in women after cystectomy, extensive research has been done on the location of tumors in patients with recurrent tumors,[2] and on bladder specimens removed from female patients with transitional cell tumors in order to identify risk factors for coexisting bladder neck or urethral tumors.[3,4] Currently, the evidence suggests that there is little risk of leaving tumor or dysplasia in the distal two thirds of the urethra if there is no evidence of carcinoma in the bladder neck or urethra on preoperative evaluation, and the intraoperative frozen section of the urethral margin is free of tumor.

Two separate approaches to urethral preparation are possible when an orthotopic reconstruction is desired in a female patient. Both require developing a surgical plane between the anterior vaginal wall and the bladder. The difference is where that plane is initiated. As described above, the posterior pedicle dissection is begun by incising the posterior vaginal apex distal to the cervix with the assistance of a sponge stick in the vagina. This incision can be carried anteriorly along the lateral and anterior vaginal wall just distal to the cervix, forming a circumferential incision at the vaginal apex. The anterior vagina is then grasped with an Allis or Kelly clamp and depressed posteriorly while the body of the uterus is retracted anteriorly with a double-hooked thyroid tenaculum.

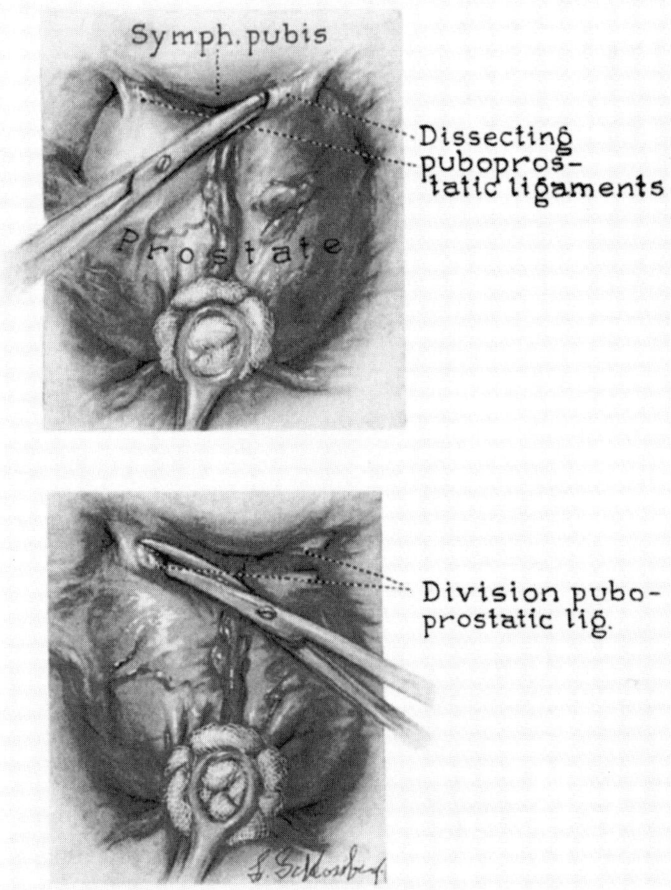
Symph. pubis
Dissecting puboprostatic ligaments
Prostate
Division pubo-prostatic lig.

FIGURE 20–13. The puboprostatic ligaments are divided under direct vision while the prostate is depressed posteriorly. Care must be taken to avoid the dorsal vein of the penis (Santorini's plexus) running between the puboprosatic ligaments. (From Walsh PC: Radical retropubic prostatectomy. *In* Walsh PC, Retik AB, Stamey TA, Vaughan ED Jr [eds]: Campbell's Urology, 6th edition, vol III. Philadelphia, WB Saunders Co, 1992, with permission.)

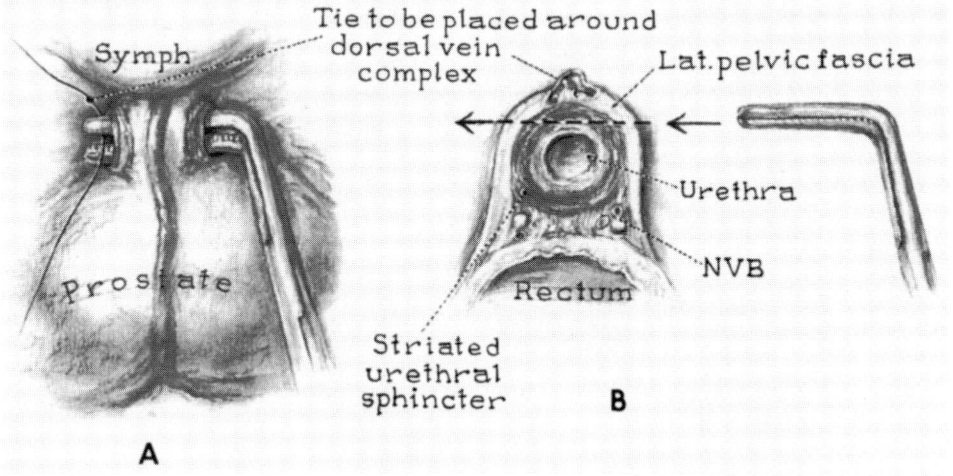
Tie to be placed around dorsal vein complex
Symph
Lat. pelvic fascia
Urethra
NVB
Prostate
Rectum
Striated urethral sphincter
A
B

FIGURE 20–14. We formerly ligated the dorsal vein complex of the penis at the apex of the prostate by bluntly passing a clamp beneath the dorsal vein complex (*A* and *C*). However, the urethral striated sphincter (rhabdosphincter) can be damaged in the blunt passage of the clamp between the dorsal vein complex and the urethra (*B*). We have therefore modified our technique in an attempt to improve the return of continence and currently sharply transect the dorsal vein complex and rhabdosphincter without prior blunt dissection. (From Walsh PC: Radical retropubic prostatectomy. *In* Walsh PC, Retik AB, Stamey TA, Vaughan ED Jr [eds]: Campbell's Urology, 6th edition, vol III. Philadelphia, WB Saunders Co, 1992, with permission.)

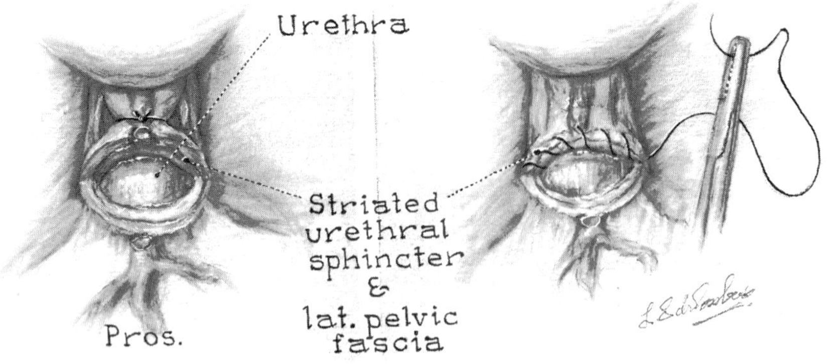
Urethra
Striated urethral sphincter & lat. pelvic fascia
Pros.

FIGURE 20–15. Oversewing the dorsal vein complex after its transection (as depicted here) is usually not necessary. The bleeding is controlled by placing the anterior urethral anastomotic sutures after dividing the anterior urethral wall. (From Walsh PC: Radical retropubic prostatectomy. *In* Walsh PC, Retik AB, Stamey TA, Vaughan ED Jr [eds]: Campbell's Urology, 6th edition, vol III. Philadelphia, WB Saunders Co, 1992, with permission.)

The plane between the anterior vagina and posterior bladder wall is developed. It is often difficult to visualize the anterior vaginal wall site of division until some mobility is gained by sharply dividing the more distal tissue along the lateral vaginal wall toward the endopelvic fascia. A groove can be identified where the posterior bladder wall, anterior vaginal wall, and lateral vaginal wall meet. Ligation and division of the abundant vascular tissue in this groove can greatly facilitate anterior vaginal wall exposure at the apex. In this way the proper retrovesical plane can be developed without inadvertent entry into the posterior bladder wall. With development of the plane between the anterior vagina and the posterior bladder, the posterior pedicles are defined and clipped and divided distally. Traction on the urethral catheter assists in identifying the bladder neck by palpation of the catheter balloon. Dissection continues distally until a 1-cm portion of urethra distal to the bladder neck can be removed. With subsequent closure of the vaginal apex, a functional vagina is preserved. The closed vaginal apex should be suspended to the sacrum or Cooper's ligament to prevent vaginal prolapse or enterocele development postoperatively. The vaginal suture line is distant from the urethroenteric neobladder suture line so an omental interposition is not strictly necessary.

Alternatively, the anterior vaginal wall can be removed en bloc with the bladder specimen. This may be desirable in posteriorly based bladder tumors. After dividing the posterior vaginal apex, the lateral vaginal wall is utilized as the posterior pedicle, leaving the anterior vaginal wall attached to the posterior bladder wall. Again, the catheter balloon facilitates identification of the bladder neck, and a surgical plane between the bladder neck and anterior vaginal wall is developed at this location. A 1-cm length of proximal urethra is mobilized for removal, and the remaining distal urethra is left attached to the anterior vaginal wall. Vaginal closure by clam-shell technique or reconstruction by other means will result in a vaginal suture line in close proximity to the urethroenteric neobladder anastomosis. A vasularized pedicle of omentum is ideal to separate these suture lines to prevent fistulization, and is most often based on the right gastroepiploic artery to avoid filling the left pelvis with both the sigmoid colon and the omental flap.

It is crucial to minimize dissection on the lateral vaginal wall throughout its length, and on the pelvic floor at the distal margin of dissection no matter which approach is utilized in women. Elegant anatomic dissection studies have formed the basis for a nerve-sparing radical cystectomy in the female that allows continent neobladder reconstruction.[20] These studies have revealed that the autonomic nerves that innervate the smooth muscle present throughout the entire length of the urethra course along the lateral vaginal wall until they branch anteriorly at the bladder neck and proximal urethra. In the majority of cases, these autonomic nerves to the smooth muscle component of the urethra can be spared. The entire rhabdosphincter (striated muscle), which is present in the distal half of the urethra, is innervated by the pudendal nerve, which courses beneath the endopelvic fascia. Thus, pelvic floor dissection should be avoided, and the endopelvic fascia should not be disturbed. Damage to these nerves may result in an incompetent distal urethral sphincter mechanism, resulting in incontinence. The rhabdosphincter appears to be the crucial element. Total pelvic exenteration, sacrificing the pelvic autonomic nerves to the smooth muscle of the urethra while sparing the pudendal nerve to the rhabdosphincter, has been successful in the one female patient in whom we have attempted it. We do not routinely attempt to spare the autonomic nerves as they course over the iliac arteries at the time of lymph node dissection.

When this posterior dissection has been completed, attention is directed anteriorly. The fibroareolar tissue between the pubis and the anterior bladder neck region is divided. The pubourethral ligaments are specifically not divided. We avoid the use of electrocautery in the distal dissection, anteriorly and posteriorly, to avoid nerve injury. If a superficial vein complex is identified it is ligated with absorbable suture. A heavy curved pedicle clamp then is placed across the isolated proximal urethral segment, and the urethra is divided 1 cm distal to the bladder neck. One should avoid the urge to make the distal line of transection in the area of the bladder neck or its junction with the proximal one third of the urethra. These structures are denervated in the dissection. Leaving them in place may increase the risk of hypercontinence (urinary retention). The anterior urethra is divided first and the anterior urethral anastomotic sutures placed as described above for male patients. The distal portion of the catheter is drawn into the wound through the urethrotomy, and divided. The pedicle clamp across catheter in the proximal urethra prevents the catheter balloon from deflating and tumor cells from spilling in the pelvis. The distal portion of the catheter is grasped with a long tonsil to facilitate exposure of the lumen and mucosa of the urethra as described above. With the posterior urethra undivided, exposed, and under gentle cephalad traction, the posterior anastomotic sutures are easily and surely placed. The posterior urethra is then transected, completing the anterior exenteration. A frozen section of the urethral margin is obtained to rule out unsuspected tumor.

If a cutaneous diversion is planned, there is no need to protect the autonomic nerves on the lateral surface of the vagina. The posterior pedicles are divided as described above, depending on tumor location and the patient's desire for a functional vagina. The pubourethral ligaments are divided anteriorly and the dorsal vein complex oversewn. If the anterior vaginal wall has been spared, the vagina is opened distally along the urethra to gain access to the catheter. If the anterior vagina has been removed with the bladder specimen, the catheter will be accessible already. The catheter external to the urethral meatus is drawn into the pelvic wound via the vagina, and the anterior and lateral dissection proceeds beyond the meatus. In this way the distal dissection can completely encircle the urethral meatus, ensuring complete removal of the urethra.

Following removal of the specimen, the pelvis is liberally irrigated with warm sterile water. Hemostasis is ensured before the pelvis is packed with a laparotomy pad and attention is directed to formation of the urinary diversion of choice. Hemovac drains are placed at the completion of the operation as necessary. We have found that the routine use of a 20-French Foley catheter as a gastrostomy tube is a simple measure that adequately drains the patient's stomach and is more comfortable than a nasogastric tube while the postoperative ileus resolves.

TABLE 20–2. POSTOPERATIVE CARE PLAN

1. ICU monitoring until stable
2. Maximize patient comfort (epidural catheter or patient-controlled analgesia regimen)
3. Crystalloid/colloid fluid combination on night of surgery
4. Stress ulcer prophylaxis (H_2 blocker)
5. Pulmonary toilet
6. Broad-spectrum antibiotics
7. Anticoagulation (sodium warfarin)
8. Digoxin until discharge
9. Catheter/drain management specific to urinary diversion

POSTOPERATIVE CARE

The goals of postoperative care after cystectomy are to maximize patient comfort and prevent known postoperative complications (Table 20–2). All patients are monitored in a surgical intensive care unit until stable. The extensive pelvic and abdominal dissection is in many ways analogous to an internal thermal injury, in terms of raw surface injury. Third-space fluid losses can be tremendous. We, therefore, administer a combination of crystalloid and colloid fluids on the night of surgery, and convert to crystalloid on the first postoperative day. Prophylaxis against stress ulcers in the form of an H_2 blocker is performed. Pulmonary toilet is encouraged via incentive spirometry, early ambulation, and nursing encouragement toward coughing and deep breathing. Broad-spectrum antibiotics are administered.

Deep venous thrombosis (DVT) prophylaxis is routine. We anticoagulate patients with sodium warfarin to prevent the development of DVT with its attendant risk of pulmonary embolism. An initial dose of 10 mg is given enterally via a nasogastric tube or gastrostomy tube in the recovery room. The daily dose is then adjusted to keep the prothrombin time in the 18- to 22-second range. If the prothrombin time exceeds 24 seconds, 10 mg of vitamin K is administered intramuscularly (IM) as reversal to avoid bleeding complications. An epidural catheter or patient-controlled analgesic regimen is routine. The use of epidural catheters or patient-controlled analgesia regimens allows patient comfort and early ambulation, further decreasing the risk of DVT. If digoxin was administered preoperatively, it is continued until discharge. Wound dressings are removed on the morning of the second postoperative day, and the wound is then left open to the air. The gastrostomy tube is removed at any time after 7 days when the patient tolerates an oral diet. Catheter and drain management is specific to the type of urinary diversion performed.

COMPLICATIONS

Improved medical, anesthetic, and surgical techniques have lessened the morbidity and mortality associated with the performance of radical cystectomy. Still, the operation is an imposing undertaking performed on a population of patients generally older than 50 years at risk for significant coexisting cardiac, pulmonary, and nutritional deficits. A team approach is required for optimal results. Operative mortality from recent large series is in the range of 1 to 3%.[21,22] Identification of early complications related only to the cystectomy (and unrelated to the type of urinary diversion) is an impossible task. Early complications following cystectomy and urinary diversion occur in up to 30% of patients, but are primarily wound related (infection or dehiscence), pulmonary (atelectasis, pneumonia, or embolism), or cardiac. Ileus requiring prolonged hospitalization occurs rarely. Late complications are usually related to the type of urinary diversion performed. Age alone does not independently increase the risk of operative morbidity or mortality, and should not be used as an exclusion criterion for offering patients definitive therapy of their tumors.[23,24]

COMMENTARY

The recent past has seen nerve-sparing surgery, designed to preserve potency, expanded to the treatment of men with invasive bladder cancer. Early results from a series composed primarily of patients with pathologically superficial tumors (<P2N0) are encouraging for their ability to preserve potency and not compromise local recurrence.[25] One of the advantages of the technique here described, however, is the low pelvic recurrence rate, even in the face of extensive pelvic disease including nodal metastases, at the time of cystectomy. In modern series, the pelvic recurrence rate for patients of all pathologic stages following cystectomy is in the range of 10%.[25] In our experience utilizing this technique, only 11% of 132 patients with extensive primary tumors and pelvic nodal metastases were noted to have pelvic recurrence.[14] It remains to be determined what the rate of pelvic recurrence will be following nerve-sparing surgery in these high-stage patients. Since preoperative staging correlates poorly with the final pathologic extent of disease, we are cautious about the broad application of this technique. At this time, pelvic recurrence leads inexorably to distant metastates and death. We are reluctant to trade the chance for cure for a 50% chance to remain potent, particularly with the established options of vacuum erection devices and improved penile prostheses available for male patients. Clearly, however, nerve-sparing surgery will have a role in male patients with bladder cancer. Lack of reliable patient selection criteria limits its use at this time.

In the last three decades, tremendous progress has been made in decreasing the morbidity and mortality associated with radical cystectomy. Currently, it is possible to perform the operation with acceptable morbidity in patients of all ages. The option of continent orthotopic urinary diversion has increased both patient and physician acceptance of the operation. Modern urologic reconstructive techniques allow for the construction of a urinary reservoir with many of the characteristics of the native detruser: large capacity, low pressure, nonrefluxing, continent, permitting volitional voiding per urethra with no abdominal stoma necessary. Patients are able to return to a near normal lifestyle, including the resumption of sexual activity. Hopefully, these advances will encourage both patients and physicians to seek early, appropriate treatment of invasive bladder cancer.

REFERENCES

1. Freeman JA, Esrig D, Stein P, et al: Management of the patient with bladder cancer. Urethral recurrence. Urol Clin North Am 1994; 1(4):645.
2. Stenzl A, Draxl H, Posch B, et al: The risk of urethral tumors in female bladder cancer: can the urethra be used for orthotopic reconstruction of the lower urinary tract? J Urol 1995; 153(2):950.
3. Coloby PJ, Kakizoe T, Tobisu K-I, et al: Urethral involvement in female bladder cancer patients: mapping of 47 consecutive cysto-urethrectomy specimens. J Urol 1994; 152:1438.
4. Stein JP, Cote RJ, Freeman JA, et al: Indications for lower urinary tract reconstruction in women after cystectomy for bladder cancer: pathological review of female cystectomy specimens. J Urol 1995; 154:1329.
5. Skinner DG, Boyd SD, Lieskovsky G, et al: Lower urinary tract reconstruction following cystectomy: experience and results in 126 patients using the Kock ileal reservoir with bilateral ureteroileal urethrostomy. J Urol 1991; 146:756.
6. Stein JP, Stenzl A, Esrig D, et al: Lower urinary tract reconstruction following cystectomy in women using the Kock ileal reservoir with bilateral ureteroileal urethrostomy: initial clinical experience. J Urol 1994; 152:1404.
7. Faysal MH, Frieha FS: Evaluation of partial cystectomy for carcinoma of the bladder. Urology 1979; 14:352.
8. Novick AC, Stewart BH: Partial cystectomy in the treatment of primary and secondary carcinoma of the bladder. J Urol 1976; 116:570.
9. Utz DC, Schmitz SE, Fugelso PD, et al: A clinicopathologic evaluation of partial cystectomy for carcinoma of the urinary bladder. Cancer 1973; 32:1075.
10. Magri J: Partial cystectomy: review of 104 cases. Br J Urol 1962; 32:74.
11. van der Werf-Messing B: Carcinoma of the bladder treated by suprapubic radium implants: the value of additional external irradiation. Eur J Urol 1969; 5:277.
12. Nichols RL, Broido P, Condon RE, et al: Effect of preoperative neomycin-erythromycin intestinal preparation on the incidence of infectious complications following colon surgery. Ann Surg 1973; 178:453.
13. Pinaud MLJ, Blantoeil YAG, Souron RJ: Preoperative prophylactic digitalization of patients with coronary artery disease—a randomized echocardiographic and hemodynamic study. Anesth Analg 1983; 62:865.
14. Lerner SP, Skinner DG, Lieskovsky G, et al: The rationale for en bloc pelvic lymph node dissection for bladder patients with nodal metastases: long-term results. J Urol 1993; 149:758.
15. Dretler SP, Ragsdale BD, Leadbetter WF: The value of pelvic lymphadenectomy in the surgical treatment of bladder cancer. J Urol 1973; 109:414.

16. Skinner DG: Management of invasive bladder cancer: a meticulous pelvic lymph node dissection can make a difference. J Urol 1982; 128:34.
17. Crawford ED, Skinner DG: Salvage cystectomy after irradiation failure. J Urol 1980; 123:32.
18. Walsh PC: Radical retropubic prostatectomy with reduced morbidity: an anatomic approach. NCI Monogr 1988; 7:133.
19. Colleselli K, Strasser J, Moriggl B, et al: Hemi-Kock to the female urethra: anatomical approach to the continence mechanism of the female urethra. J Urol 1994; 151(2):500A.
20. Stenzl A, Colleselli K, Poisel S, et al: Rationale and technique of nerve sparing radical cystectomy before an orthotopic neobladder procedure in women. J Urol 1995; 154:2044.
21. Skinner DG, Lieskovsky G: Technique of radical cystectomy. *In* Skinner DG, Lieskovsky G (eds): Diagnosis and Management of Genitourinary Cancer, pp 607–621. Philadelphia, WB Saunders Co, 1988.
22. Frazier HA, Robertson JE, Paulson DF: Complications of radical cystectomy and urinary diversion: a retrospective review of 675 cases in two decades. J Urol 1992; 148: 1401.
23. Skinner EC, Lieskovsky G, Skinner DG: Radical cystectomy in the elderly patient. J Urol 1984; 131:1065.
24. Leibovitch I, Avigad I, Benn-Chaim J, et al: It is justified to avoid radical cystoprostatectomy in elderly patients with invasive transitional cell carcinoma of the bladder? Cancer 1993; 71:3098.
25. Brendler DB, Steinberg GD, Marshall FE, et al: Local recurrence and survival following nerve-sparing radical cystoprostatectomy. J Urol 1990; 144:1137.

21

TRANSURETHRAL SURGERY PLUS CHEMO-RADIATION FOR SELECTIVE BLADDER PRESERVATION

ALEX F. ALTHAUSEN, M.D., WILLIAM U. SHIPLEY, M.D., *and* DONALD S. KAUFMAN, M.D.

In the United States, the usual treatment of muscle-invasive transitional cell cancer of the bladder is radical cystectomy with the addition, in selected cases, of radiation and chemotherapy. Unfortunately, the overall cure rate is no greater than 50% due to the systemic nature of the invasive transitional cell cancer.[1] The newer surgical techniques of nerve sparing, to help preserve male potency, and the evolution of multiple continent and orthotopic urinary bladder diversions have made cystectomy less "radical" in terms of quality of life. Even the most enthusiastic proponents of orthotopic bladder construction would agree that the natural bladder is preferable. This has led to attempts to use the combined-modality therapy of transurethral resection and chemo-radiation to eradicate the tumor while preserving a normally functioning bladder.

Invasive bladder cancer is a heterogeneous disease. Not all patients are candidates for bladder sparing. Favorable selection criteria include a bladder tumor that can be totally excised by transurethral resection and/or that a complete response to initial chemo-radiation induction as measured by follow-up cytology and cystoscopic biopsies has been achieved. If residual disease is found, immediate cystectomy is recommended. If there is a complete response with induction therapy, prompt consolidation chemo-radiation therapy is provided. Organ-sparing treatments require the judgment of multiple physicians as well as patient understanding of the risks and benefits involved.

Previous chapters in this section on bladder cancers address the various monotherapies of transurethral resection, partial and total cystectomy, as well as definitive radiation and chemotherapy. We have summarized the success rates, all fairly low, of bladder-sparing monotherapies rendering the patients free from recurrence of the initial or from a subsequent invasive tumor (Table 21–1). Barnes et al.[2] reported a 27% 5-year survival in 85 patients with well and moderately differentiated T2 transitional cell carcinomas treated with transurethral resection alone. Sweeney et al.[3] found that 5.8 to 18.9% of patients with muscle-invasive tumors were selected for treatment by partial cystectomy and had a local recurrence rate of 38 to 78%. External beam radiation therapy alone for patients with clinical stage T2 to T4 tumors has a 35 to 45% 5-year local control rate. The prognostic factors that favor good outcomes with radiation as a monotherapy are T2 and T3a tumors that are less than 5 cm and present with no hydronephrosis,[4] as it is well established that patients with hydronephrosis respond poorly to bladder-sparing techniques.

Hall and Roberts reported a 19% 3-year cure rate with chemotherapy alone in 27 patients with localized disease using cisplatin, methotrexate, and Velban with epirubicin.[29]

The cure rates for the monotherapies briefly discussed here are inadequate (Table 21–1) when compared to radical cystectomy, which has a high local cure rate of 85 to 90%. There have been other reports that a combination of transurethral resection followed by radiation or by multidrug systemic chemotherapy achieved a better clinical complete response rate of the primary tumor (Table 21–2).

The results of combined-modality therapy for muscle-invasive bladder cancer have spurred on

TABLE 21–1. BLADDER SPARING WITH MONOTHERAPY

Treatment	No. of Patients	No Recurrence of an Invasive Tumor
Transurethral resection alone[38–39]	331	20%
Radiation alone[4,23,24,40,41]	949	40%
Chemotherapy alone[16,29]	27	19%

TABLE 21–3. RESULTS WITH BLADDER PRESERVATION COMBINED-MODALITY THERAPY

	No. of Patients	5-Year Overall Survival	5-Year Survival with Bladder Preservation
ROTG, 1993[7]	42	52%	42%
Erlangen, 1994[8]	79	52%	41%
MGH, 1995[15]	106	52%	43%
ROTG, 1996[10]*	91	62%	45%
Total of series	318	52%	43% (5 years)

*4-year data.

the ultimate quest for bladder preservation combining transurethral resection, radiation, and chemotherapy. In the last 3 years there have been four studies that give reasonable alternatives to cystectomy in selected patients. They come from the Massachusetts General Hospital,[6] the Radiation Therapy Oncology Group,[7] the University of Erlangen,[8] and the University of Paris[9] (Table 21–3). The Massachusetts General Hospital reported on 53 patients in 1993 with T2 through T4 muscle-invading bladder cancer in a trial of transurethral surgery, combination chemotherapy, and irradiation (4000 cGy) with concurrent cisplatin administration.[6] Cystoscopic evaluation determined further therapy: radical cystectomy in patients with persistent or recurrent disease or additional chemotherapy and radiotherapy (6480 cGy) in patients who achieved a complete response.[6] Accession into the protocol required an attempt at a visually complete transurethral resection of the bladder tumor. Induction chemotherapy is not as effective if a transurethral resection has not been done (Table 21–2). The clinical stage of the primary tumor was T2 in 15 patients, T3 in 29 patients, and T4 in 9 patients. Pathology confirmed that all tumors invaded the muscularis propria. Induction chemotherapy included two 28-day cycles of methotrexate (30 mg/m^2) on days 1, 15, and 22; cisplatin (70 mg/m^2) on day 2; and vinblastine (3 mg/m^2) on days 2, 15, and 22. This was followed by 4000 cGy to the bladder and pelvic lymph nodes with concurrent cisplatin (70 mg/m^2) given on day 1 and day 21 of irradiation. Fatigue, nehrotoxicity, and hematologic toxicity have been the major systemic problems. Eleven of 53 entered patients (21%) did not complete the protocol. The patients' pelvic tissues tolerated the combination therapy well. No patient who received complete treatment with chemo-radiation had a major complication involving the bladder or the rectum. The Radiation Oncology Group results also show that this chemo-radiation induction program does not cause synergistic toxic effects on the bladder or the bowel.[10] With a median follow-up of 4 years, 3 of 28 patients (11%) with complete responses to full courses of chemo-radiation have had local recurrence of invasive tumor. Nine patients (17%) had recurrence of superficial tumors successfully managed in eight of these patients by transurethral resection and intravesical chemotherapy. No invasive bladder tumor has recurred in 31 of the 53 entered patients (58%). This is better than with transurethral resection alone,[11] radiation therapy alone,[12] or systemic chemotherapy alone.[13]

TABLE 21–2. CLINICAL STAGE T2 TO T4 BLADDER CANCER COMPLETE RESPONSE (REBIOPSY AND NEGATIVE CYTOLOGY)

Treatment	No. of Patients	Complete Response
Chemotherapy alone[18,27–31]	301	27%
Radiation alone[23–26]	721	45%
Transurethral resection plus chemotherapy[32–35]	225	51%
Transurethral resection plus chemo-radiation[8–10,36,37]	218	71%

Multivariate analysis of tumor factors influencing survival after this combined-modality treatment showed only the presence or absence of tumor-related hydronephrosis, and tumor stage independently approached statistical significance (p = .07 and p = .09, respectively). The actuarial overall survival rate was 48% at 5 years, consistent with radical cystectomy.[14] The multivariate analysis also showed that the only independent prognostic factor indicating that the bladder would remain free from invasive tumor was the absence of hydronephrosis at the time of initial diagnosis (p = .01). Patients with hydronephrosis should, therefore, not be treated with bladder sparing because their chance of remaining free of tumor is only one in five. These patients should be considered for prompt radical cystectomy.

We recently updated our experience and now report on 106 patients who were treated with combined-modality therapy and selective bladder preservation for invasive bladder cancer from 1986 through 1993.[15] The median follow-up was 4.4 years. Forty patients are alive and under surveillance for 5 or more years. The overall survival at 5 years is 52%, with 43% of these patients retaining their conserved bladders. For T2 patients, actuarial overall survival was 63%, and for T3 and T4, 45%. The 5-year freedom from distant metastases was 66%. No patient required cystectomy for treatment-related morbidity (Table 21–4).

TABLE 21–4. STAGE T2 TO T4 BLADDER CANCER: MASSACHUSETTS GENERAL HOSPITAL TRIALS WITH COMBINED-MODALITY THERAPY*

	No. of Patients	5-Year Overall Survival	Surviving 5 Years with Bladder	Needing Cystectomy
All entered	106	52%	43%	34%
Women	34	54%	50%	30%
Men	72	50%	40%	36%
Stage T2	42	63%	54%	26%
Stages T3–T4	64	45%	35%	39%

*From Kachnic LA, Kaufman DS, Zeitman AL, et al: Bladder preservation by combined modality therapy for invasive bladder cancer. J Clin Oncol 1996 (in press).

The Radiation Therapy Oncology Group reported in 1993 a phase I/II study on 42 patients testing the tolerance and effectiveness of concurrent cisplatin-radiation therapy in stage T2 to T4 invasive bladder cancer.[7] Patients received 4000 cGy of radiation therapy with conventional fractionation and 100 mg/m^2 of cisplatin on days 1 and 22. An additional boost of 2400 cGy was given to the bladder with a third cycle of cisplatin in complete responders as assessed by cystoscopic biopsies and bladder urine cytology. A complete response rate to induction therapy was found in 67% of the patients (28 of 42). Eleven patients remained in remission. Eight relapsed in the bladder as the only site of failure and five of the eight recurrences were noninvasive transitional cell carcinoma. From 1988 to 1990, the Radiation Therapy Oncology Group entered a total of 91 patients in another combined-modality treatment protocol that included two cycles of neoadjuvant chemotherapy prior to concurrent chemo-radiation. The 4-year overall survival was 62% and the 4-year survival with bladder preservation was 45%. Incomplete responders underwent radical cystectomy as did those who developed recurrent invasive tumor.[10]

The University of Erlangen reported their 10-year experience with combined-modality treatment and bladder sparing in 1994.[8] The patients were treated with initial transurethral surgery then 5000 to 5600 cGy in 28 fractions. Cisplatin-based chemotherapy was also given. Transurethral bladder biopsies were then done to assess response. Seventy-nine patients were given this protocol therapy. The 5-year overall survival was 52% and the survival with bladder preservation was 41%.

In 1993, a prospective study from the University of Paris reported the use of chemo-radiation therapy as neoadjuvant treatment prior to cystectomy.[9] This protocol included cisplatin, 5-fluorouracil, and twice-daily 300 cGy on days 1, 3, 15, and 17 of a 3-week induction. One half of the patients also underwent an initial transurethral resection of the tumor. Seventy per cent of these patients had a clinical complete response to this treatment. The first 18 patients who were the complete responders underwent cystectomy and all 18 were found to have no histologic evidence of malignancy in the surgical specimens. This 100% rate of pathologic complete response was a significant improvement over all prior experiences with neoadjuvant chemotherapy without radiation but with transurethral surgery, in which only one half of those patients who are clinical complete responders are found at cystectomy to be pathologic complete responders.[32] This success suggested a real chance for bladder preservation, and their ensuing work with chemo-radiation for bladder preservation has yielded excellent results. Fifty-two of 54 were able to complete induction therapy. In the University of Paris study, 74% of the patients have had complete responses and only 10% of these have subsequently failed within the preserved bladder.

Table 21–3 shows that the 5-year survival following selective bladder preservation ranges from 45 to 54%. Clinical T2 patients did the best, with 64 to 68% 5-year survival. These recent publications supply new overall survival data as good as any reported cystectomy series in comparable patients. This supports the selective use of transurethral surgery, irradiation, and cisplatin-based chemotherapy for patients with clinical T2 to T3a invasive bladder cancers based on a complete response to induction chemo-radiation. Another important aspect of these bladder-sparing protocols is the need to identify the level of response by cystoscopic evaluation 3 to 6 weeks after induction. This allows for prompt cystectomy if local failure occurs.

Deferring immediate cystectomy once the initial diagnosis of muscle-invasive bladder cancer has been made does not appear to compromise survival[13] nor does the addition of induction chemo-radiation increase the morbidity of cystectomy in the hands of well-trained urologic surgeons.[18] In 1991, the Danish Bladder Cancer Group reported a randomized multicenter study of preoperative radiation therapy and cystectomy versus definitive irradiation and early cystectomy for residual tumor. There was no significant difference in overall survival according to randomization with a median follow-up of 50 months.[19] Twenty-seven of 95 patients randomized to receive definitive irradiation underwent salvage cystectomy for recurrent tumor. The incidence of local and/or regional recurrence alone was 7% in the group randomized to preoperative radiation and cystectomy. This was significantly lower than the 36% of the 85 patients ran-

TABLE 21–5. FUNCTION OF THE CONSERVED BLADDER

	Treatment	Patients with Conserved Bladders	Cystectomy for End-Stage Bladders
Lynch et al.[20]	Radiation	69	0%
Dunst et al.[8]	Chemo-radiation	192	1.6%
Kachnic et al.[15]	Chemo-radiation	76	0%

domized to receive definitive radiation. However, the incidence of metastatic disease was similar in both groups, 34 and 32%, respectively. These findings suggest that the 36% of local tumor persistence in patients not randomized to cystectomy did not contribute to an increased risk of metastases.

The quality of life in patients whose bladders have been preserved utilizing combined-modality therapy has been a concern of medical and radiation oncologists and urologic surgeons. It is obvious that once quantity of life has been addressed, quality comes into the picture. The bladder needs to be a conduit as well as a reservoir. Irradiated bladders in the past were not without their problems of marked urinary frequency, urgency with urge incontinence, and significant hematuria. Recent reports following modern radiation techniques have addressed these potential problems. In the Erlangen experience, only three cystectomies were necessary for end-stage irradiated bladders in their series of 192 patients (1.6%). Lynch et al. analyzed bladder function in 72 patients treated with 6000 cGy in 30 fractions. No difference in bladder and bowel function was found when compared with an age-matched and gender-matched control group.[20] Similarly, the Massachusetts General Hospital reported excellent tolerance in 21 women who were successfully treated for bladder conservation by using transurethral resection and chemo-radiation.[21] With a median follow-up of 56 months all patients were continent without dysuria or significant hematuria. Not one of these patients had compromise in bowel or sexual function. In our recent update, 76 of 106 patents were selected for bladder preservation and none has required a cystectomy for the irradiated end-stage bladder syndrome. However, all patients treated by the organ-sparing multimodality therapies must have regular cystoscopic evaluations. Follow-up will reveal a 20 to 30% recurrence of superficial tumors. These patients were well treated by standard management with transurethral resection and intravesical chemotherapy. Based on our recent update of these 76 patients, in the Massachusetts General Hospital series 21 patients (28%) had developed either Ta tumors or carcinoma in situ from the 76 patients with bladder preservation.[15] Fifteen (20%) have been in sustained remission following conservative therapy with 15 to 49 months of follow-up. Salvage cystectomy should be recommended to the patients as soon as a muscle-invasive relapse occurs.

Bladder preservation with extensive transurethral resection and chemo-radiation offers a chance for the same survival outcome as cystectomy while maintaining a normal functioning bladder. About 30% of these bladders will develop noninvasive tumors that usually respond to standard intravesical chemotherapy. Patients who initially present with tumor-related hydronephrosis are not candidates for organ sparing with the available multimodality therapy. There is now enough data to suggest that in selected patients bladder sparing should be offered as a real alternative to pro forma radical cystectomy.

REFERENCES

1. Raghavan D, Shipley WU, Garnick MB, et al: Biology and management of bladder cancer. N Engl J Med 1990; 322: 1129–1138.
2. Barnes RW, Dick AL, Hadley HL, et al: Survival following transurethral resection of bladder carcinoma. Cancer Res 1977; 37:2895–2898.
3. Sweeney P, Kursh ED, Resnick MI: Partial cystectomy. Urol Clin North Am 1992; 2(Suppl 2):75–87.
4. Mameghan H, Fisher R, Mameghan J, et al: Analysis of failure following definitive radiotherapy for invasive transitional cell carcinoma of the bladder. Int J Radiat Oncol Biol Phys 1995; 31:247–254.
5. Hall RR, Roberts JT, Marsh MM: Radical transurethral surgery in chemotherapy aiming at bladder preservation. *In* Splinter AW, Scher HI (eds): Neoadjuvant Chemotherapy in Invasive Bladder Cancer, pp 169–174. New York, Wiley Liss, 1990.
6. Kaufman DS, Shipley WU, Griffen PP, et al: Selective preservation by combination treatment of invasive bladder cancer. N Engl J Med 1993; 329:1377–1382.
7. Tester W, Porter A, Asbell S, et al: Combined modality program with possible organ preservation for invasive bladder carcinoma: results of ROTG protocol 85-12. Int J Radiat Oncol Biol Phys 1993; 25:783–790.
8. Dunst J, Sauer R, Schrott KM, et al: Organ-sparing treatment of advanced bladder cancer. A 10-year experience. Int J Radiat Oncol Biol Phys 1994; 30:261–266.
9. Housset M, Maulard C, Chretlen YC, et al: Combined radiation and chemotherapy for invasive transitional cell carcinoma of the bladder. A prospective study. J Clin Oncol 1993; 11:2150–2157.
10. Tester W, Porter A, Heaney J, et al: Neoadjuvant combined modality therapy with possible organ preservation for invasive bladder cancer. J Clin Oncol 1996; 14:119–126.
11. Henry K, Miller J, Mori M, et al: Comparison of transurethral resection to radical therapies for stage B bladder tumors. J Urol 1988; 140:964–967.
12. Shipley WU, Rose MA, Perrone TL, et al: Full-dose irradiation for patient with invasive bladder carcinoma: clinical and histological factors prognostic of improved survival. J Urol 1985; 134:689–683.
13. Bloom HJG, Hendry WF, Wallace DM, Skeet RG: Treatment of T3 bladder cancer: controlled trial of preoperative radiotherapy and radical cystectomy versus radical radi-

otherapy; second report and review. Br J Urol 1982; 54: 136–151.
14. Skinner DG, Daniels JR, Russell CA, et al: The role of adjuvant chemotherapy following cystectomy for invasive bladder cancer: a prospective comparative trial. J Urol 1991; 145:459–467.
15. Kachnic LA, Kaufman DS, Zeitman AL, et al: Bladder preservation by combined modality therapy for invasive bladder cancer. J Clin Oncol 1996 (in press).
16. Hall RR: Bladder preserving treatment: the role of transurethral surgery alone and combined modality therapy for muscle-invading bladder cancer. *In* Vogelzang NJ, Scardino PT, Shipley WU, Coffey DS (eds): Comprehensive Textbook of Genitourinary Oncology, pp 509–513. Baltimore, Williams & Wilkins, 1995.
17. Rintala E, Hannisdaht E, Fossa SD, et al: Neoadjuvant chemotherapy in bladder cancer: a randomized study. Scand J Urol Nephrol 1989; 64:250–256.
18. Maffezzini M, Torelli T, Villa E, et al: Systemic preoperative chemotherapy with cisplatin, methotrexate and vinblastine for locally advanced bladder cancer: local tumor response and early follow-up results. J Urol 1991; 145:741–743.
19. Sell A, Jackson A, Nerstrom B, et al: Treatment of advanced bladder cancer category T2, T3 and 4a: a randomized multicenter study of preoperative irradiation and cystectomy versus radical irradiation and early salvage cystectomy for residual tumor: DAVECA protocol 8201: Danish Vesical Cancer Group. Scand J Urol Nephrol Suppl 1991; 138:193–201.
20. Lynch WJ, Jenkins BJ, Fowler CG: The quality of life after radical radiotherapy for bladder cancer. Br J Urol 1992; 70: 519–521.
21. Kachnic LA, Shipley WU, Griffen PP, et al: Combined modality treatment with selective bladder conservation for invasive bladder cancer: long term tolerance in the female patient. Cancer J Sci Am 1996; 2:79–84.
22. Cancer Fact and Figures—1995. American Cancer Society, 1599 Clifton Road, Atlanta, GA 30329.
23. Jenkins BJ, Blandy JP, Caulfield MJ, et al: Reappraisal of the role of radical radiotherapy and salvage cystectomy in the treatment of invasive bladder cancer. Br J Urol 1988; 62:343–346.
24. Gospodarowicz MK, Hawkins MV, Rawling GA, et al: Radical radiotherapy for muscle invasive transitional cell carcinoma of the bladder: failure analysis. J Urol 1989; 142: 148–154.
25. Quilty P, Duncan W: Primary radical radiotherapy for T3 transitional cell cancer of the bladder: an analysis of survival and control. Int J Radiat Oncol Biol Phys 1986; 12: 853–860.
26. Smaaland R, Akslen LA, Tonder B, et al: Radical radiation treatment of invasive and locally advanced bladder carcinoma in elderly patients. Br J Urol 1991; 67:61–69.
27. Keating J, Zincke H, Morgan WR, et al: Extended experience with neoadjuvant M-VAC chemotherapy for invasive transitional cell carcinoma of the urinary bladder. J Urol 1989; 141:244a.
28. Kurth KII, Splinter TA, Jacqmin D, et al: Transitional cell carcinoma of the bladder: a phase II study of chemotherapy in T3-4 N0 M0 of the EORTC GU group. *In* Anderson AR, Oliver RT, Hanham IW, Bloom HJ (eds): Urological Oncology Dilemmas and Developments, pp 115–128. New York, Wiley Liss, 1991.
29. Hall RR, Roberts JT: Neoadjuvant chemotherapy, a method to conserve the bladder? (Abstract 144). ECCO 1991:6.
30. Roberts JT, Fossa SP, Richards SB, et al: Results of Medical Research Council phase II study of low dose cisplatin and methotrexate in the primary treatment of locally advanced (T3 and T4) transitional cell carcinoma of the bladder. Br J Urol 1991; 68:162–168.
31. Farah R, Chodak GW, Vogelzang NI, et al: Curative radiotherapy following chemotherapy for invasive bladder carcinoma (a preliminary report). Int J Radiat Oncol Biol Phys 1991; 20:413–417.
32. Scher HI, Herr HW, Sternberg C, et al: Neoadjuvant chemotherapy for invasive bladder cancer. Experience with the MVAC regimen. Br J Urol 1989; 64:250–256.
33. Hall RR, Newling DWW, Ramsden PD, et al: Treatment of invasive bladder cancer by local resection and high dose methotrexate. Br J Urol 1984; 56:668–672.
34. Prout GR, Shipley WU, Kaufman SD, et al: Preliminary results in invasive bladder cancer with transurethral resection, neoadjuvant chemotherapy and combined pelvic irradiation plus cisplatin chemotherapy. J Urol 1990; 144: 1128–1134.
35. Parsons JT, Million RR: Bladder cancer. *In* Perez CA, Brady IW (eds): Principles and Practice of Radiation Oncology, pp 1036–1058. Philadelphia, JB Lippincott Co, 1991.
36. Fung CY, Shipley WU, Young RH, et al: Prognostic factors in invasive bladder carcinoma in a prospective trial of preoperative adjuvant chemotherapy and radiotherapy. J Clin Oncol 1991; 9:1533–1542.
37. Cervak J, Cufer T, Marolt F, et al: Combined chemotherapy and radiotherapy in muscle-invasive bladder carcinoma (Abstract 561). Complete remission results. ECCO 1991:6.
38. Herr HW: Conservative management of muscle-infiltrating bladder cancer: prospective experience. J Urol 1987; 138:1162–1163.
39. Henry K, Miller J, Mort M, et al: Comparison of transurethral resection to radical therapies for stage B bladder tumors. J Urol 1988; 140:964–967.
40. Shearer RJ, Chilvers CE, Bloom HJG, et al: Adjuvant chemotherapy in T3 carcinoma of the bladder. Br J Urol 1988; 62:588–564.
41. DeNeve W, Lybeert ML, Goor C, et al: Radiotherapy for T2 and T3 carcinoma of the bladder: the influence of overall treatment time. Radiol Oncol 1995; 36:183–188.

22

NONCONTINENT URINARY DIVERSION

REGINA M. HOVEY, M.D. *and* PETER R. CARROLL, M.D.

Urinary diversion may be necessary in patients with bladder cancer who undergo cystectomy as well as in patients with severe functional or anatomic abnormalities of the urinary tract. Urinary diversion may be temporary or permanent. Permanent forms of urinary diversion can be accomplished by establishing direct continuity between the urinary tract and the skin or by interposing a segment of bowel between the two. Almost all segments of bowel have been used for urinary diversion. As indicated by the many types of urinary diversion available, no method is ideal for all patients and clinical settings. The method of urinary diversion selected should be dependent on the indication for urinary diversion, as well as individual patient anatomy, renal function, preference, and overall health.

Types of urinary diversion can be categorized into those that are continent and those that are noncontinent. Continent urinary diversion can be achieved with either a continent abdominal stoma or with an orthotopic bladder substitute anastomosed to the urethra. Noncontinent types of urinary diversion generally act as a conduit through which the urine exits the body, requiring the patient to wear an external appliance to collect the urine. Although continent forms of urinary diversion allow freedom from an external appliance, they are technically more difficult to perform and may be associated with a higher complication rate. Continent diversion can, however, be of psychologic benefit to patients concerned with the impact of an external appliance on their self-image and sexuality. In general, there is a high level of satisfaction with both continent and noncontinent forms of urinary diversion.[1] This chapter will emphasize noncontinent forms of permanent urinary diversion. Temporary forms of urinary diversion, such as percutaneous nephrostomy, will be discussed elsewhere.

PREOPERATIVE PREPARATION

Adequate preoperative counseling is essential. The discussion should include the specific goals and complications of the planned procedure as well as what the patient should expect postoperatively in terms of lifestyle changes. In addition, a thorough history should be taken, including previous surgical procedures, associated medical problems, systemic diseases, intestinal disorders, and previous irradiation. The patient should be questioned specifically regarding a history of regional enteritis, ulcerative colitis, diverticulitis, or other gastrointestinal problems, which would help identify what segment of bowel should be used. Preoperative renal function should be determined. The patient's general state of health and fitness for surgery should be evaluated. The upper urinary tracts should be imaged assessing for stone disease, hydronephrosis, and renal scarring. Preoperative evaluation of the bowel by contrast imaging or colonoscopy should be considered in patients with a history of gastrointestinal diseases or symptoms or signs consistent with such diseases.

As the patient will be required to wear an appliance postoperatively, addressing stoma care preoperatively is essential. Prior to surgery, the ability of the patient to perform adequate stoma care should be assessed. Patients who are physically or mentally challenged may require assistance from a family member or a visiting nurse. In general, the collecting device will need to be changed every 4 to 5 days.

The stoma site should be carefully selected prior to surgery. The patient should be evaluated in both the sitting and standing positions. The stoma should be away from any bony prominences, fat folds, and prior abdominal scars that could make securing the appliance difficult. The usual site for stoma location is along a line from the anterior superior iliac spine and the umbilicus, at the lateral edge of the rectus abdominis muscle. It is important to bring the stoma through the rectus muscle to help prevent the formation of a parastomal hernia. An enterostomal therapist may be valuable in helping to select a proper stoma site.

Adequate preoperative bowel preparation is important in reducing infectious complications. Patients should start a mechanical and oral antibiotic bowel preparation and a clear liquid diet 2 days before surgery. Systemic antibiotics are administered perioperatively.

CUTANEOUS PYELOSTOMY

The indications for cutaneous pyelostomy are limited. It was originally reported by Immergut et al. as a method of diverting urine in children with tortuous, dilated ureters.[2] It can be used as a temporizing procedure in children in the presence of gross infection and urinary obstruction, especially if associated with renal failure. This technique requires the presence of an extrarenal pelvis. The relative lack of subcutaneous fat, underdevelopment of flank musculature, and renal mobility in children facilitate this procedure.[3] Pyelostomy can be used as an alternative to percutaneous nephrostomy in small infants, since placement of a nephrostomy tube may be difficult and tube maintenance may pose a problem for parents.[4]

Technique

The renal pelvis is identified and mobilized through a subcostal incision. There is no need to mobilize the ureter or disrupt its collateral circulation. The kidney is rotated anteriorly. The renal pelvis is incised for approximately 3 cm, well away from the ureteropelvic junction (Fig. 22–1*A*). The renal pelvis is brought out to the skin incision and anastomosed to the skin using interrupted absorbable sutures (Fig. 22–1*B*). The remainder of the incision is closed in the usual fashion.

CUTANEOUS URETEROSTOMY

Cutaneous ureterostomy is a simple method of urinary diversion. The first cutaneous ureterostomy was performed by LeDentu in 1889.[5] End-cutaneous ureterostomy can be used as a means of temporary diversion in infants and as a form of palliative diversion in adults.[6,7] Delayed urinary reconstruction can be successfully performed after cutaneous ureterostomy.[8]

The advantages of cutaneous ureterostomy are

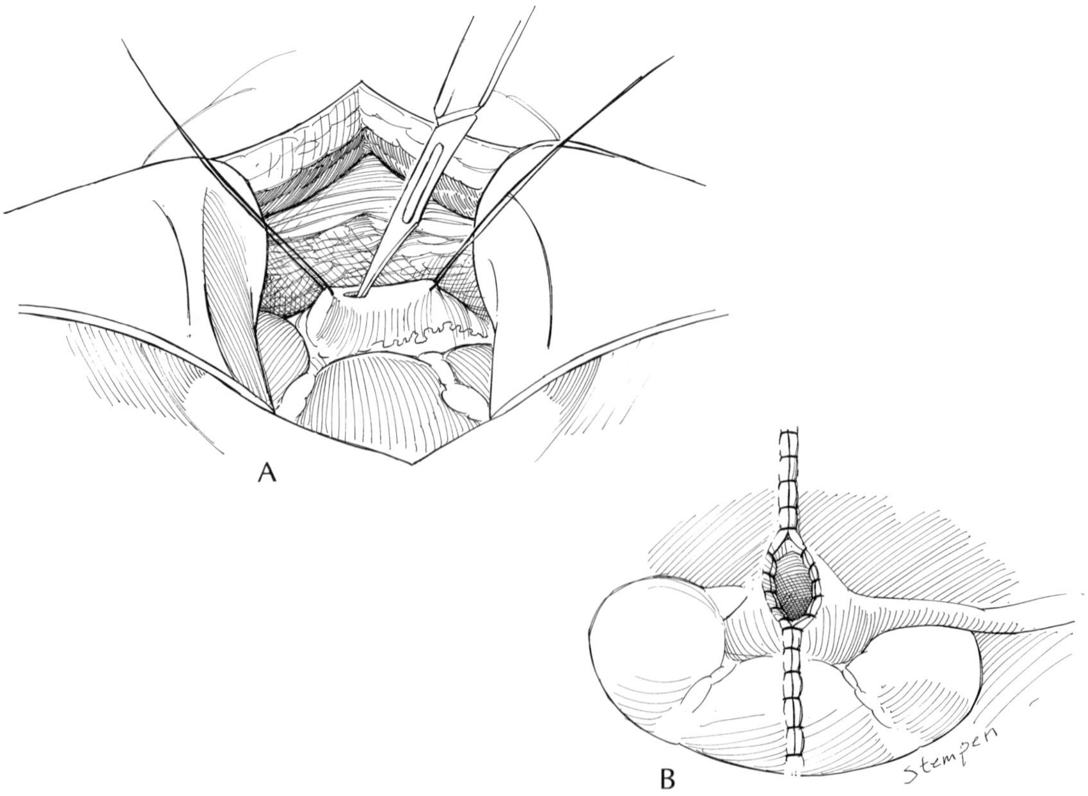
A
B
Stempen

FIGURE 22–1. *A*, The renal pelvis is incised for approximately 3 cm. *B*, The renal pelvis is anastomosed to the skin using interrupted sutures.

decreased operating time, shorter postoperative recovery time, the use of an extraperitoneal approach,[9] as well as the avoidance of bowel surgery. The complications associated with bowel anastomosis and reabsorption of urinary constituents by bowel mucosa can be avoided.[10] Disadvantages of cutaneous ureterostomy are the risk of stomal stenosis, chronic bacteriuria, and stone formation.

A dilated ureter usually is necessary for a successful cutaneous ureterostomy. A thick-walled, well-vascularized ureter facilitates a good outcome.[11] Both ureters can be brought out to the skin if they are both dilated and of adequate length. If only one ureter is dilated, a proximal transureteroureterostomy can be performed, using the dilated ureter as the cutaneous ureterostomy.[8,12]

Technique

If both ureters are dilated, a double stoma cutaneous ureterostomy should be fashioned with the stoma on the side of the shorter ureter. If only one ureter is involved or a transureteroureterostomy is planned, the stoma should be located on the side of the dilated ureter. Whether a single or double stoma is used, only a single stoma site with one appliance is required.

The ureter is mobilized extraperitoneally, carefully preserving its collateral blood supply. The ureter should be freed to the level of the bladder if possible. Prior to transecting the ureter, the ureteral length should be measured to ensure that it is adequate.

If only a single ureter is obstructed, a simple stoma can be created by sewing the end of the ureter flush to the skin at the stoma site. Another option is to perform a V-flap stoma, especially if the diameter of the ureter is marginal (Fig. 22–2). If both ureters are dilated, a simple stoma can be created by suturing the incised ureters together, everting them, and anastomosing the end of the ureters to the skin at the stoma site. Alternatively, a Z-plasty can be performed if the ureters are not adequately dilated[12] (Fig. 22–3).

If a transureteroureterostomy with cutaneous ureterostomy is planned, the smaller ureter should be passed retroperitoneally across to the side of the larger ureter. The ureters should be free of angulation and tension. The larger ureter is incised for 2 cm on its medial aspect. The smaller ureter is trimmed to the appropriate length and spatulated. The ureteral anastomosis is performed using a running absorbable suture. Prior to performing the ureteral anastomosis, ureteral stents may be placed. The stoma is fashioned as previously described for a single ureter.

ILEAL CONDUIT

Seiffert first described ureteroileocutaneous diversion in 1935.[13] However, the procedure was popularized by Bricker in 1950.[14] It remains the most commonly used method of noncontinent urinary diversion in the United States. Important to the success of this procedure are patient selection, stoma location, and careful technique, including the construction of a well-vascularized stoma.

Ileal conduit may be contraindicated in patients with a history of regional enteritis or extensive pelvic irradiation.[15] In this situation a colon conduit may be preferred. The usual stoma location is in the right lower quadrant, meeting the criteria previously outlined. In order to minimize the absorptive surface of the bowel in contact with the urine, as short an ileal segment as appropriate should be utilized. Reabsorption of urinary constituents should not cause a significant problem in those with normal renal function, but may lead to metabolic abnormalities in patients with renal insufficiency.[16]

Technique

The conduit is constructed using a segment of ileum approximately 15 cm proximal to the ileocecal valve. The length of the conduit may vary with patient habitus, but averages 15 cm (Fig. 22–4*A*). As short a segment as possible should be used. Preservation of the vascular supply to the ileal segment is important. Transillumination of the bowel mesentery can help identify the bowel's blood supply. The mesenteric segment supplying blood to the ileal segment should contain at least two major vascular arcades. Once the appropriate segment of ileum is identified and isolated, the mesentery is divided proximally and distally and individual blood vessels are ligated. The bowel is divided either between clamps or using a GIA stapler. The continuity of the bowel is re-established using a stapling device or is sewn by hand. The conduit is placed below the level of the ileoileal reanastomosis. The conduit is positioned caudally, usually in the right lower quadrant of the abdomen in an isoperistaltic direction (Fig. 22–4*B*). The left ureter is brought under the sigmoid mesocolon. The base of the conduit is closed with either a stapling device or with absorbable sutures. The ureters are spatulated and reimplanted into the base of the conduit. The various types of ureteral anastomosis will be discussed later in this chapter. Ureteral stents may be directed into each renal pelvis and brought out through the abdominal stoma to facilitate urinary drainage. The mesentery is closed using nonabsorbable interrupted sutures to prevent internal herniation of bowel.

Next, the stoma is created. A small circle of skin is excised at the preselected stoma site and the underlying fat is removed. The fascia is incised in a cruciate fashion, large enough to accommodate two fingers (Fig. 22–5*A*). The end of the conduit is brought through the rectus abdominis muscle and

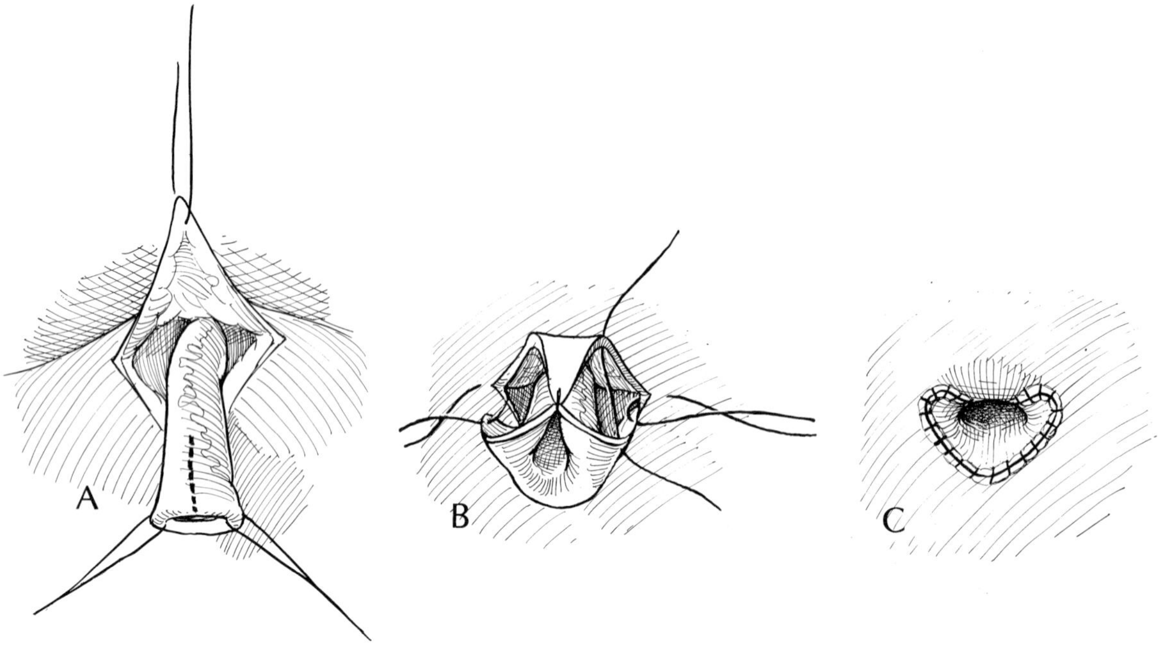
A
B
C

FIGURE 22–2. *A*, The ureter is brought through the skin and spatulated. *B* and *C*, The ureter is everted and the anastomosis is performed using several interrupted absorbable sutures.

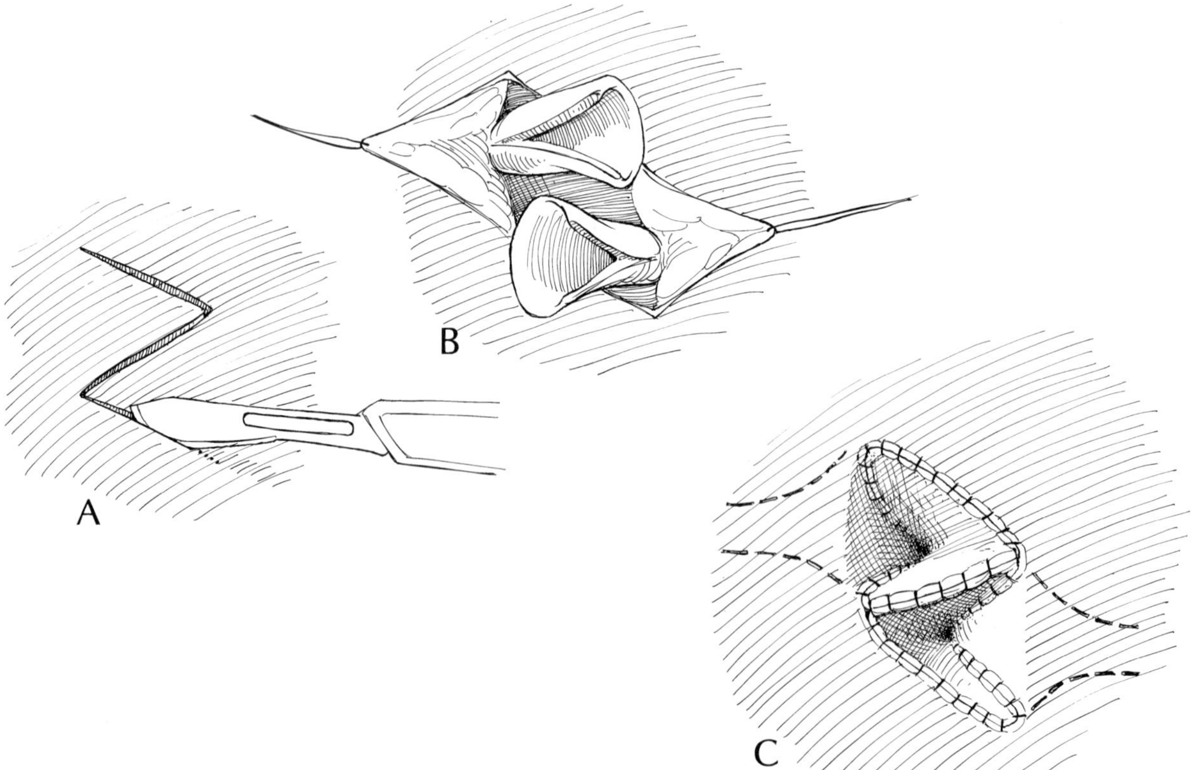
B
A
C

FIGURE 22–3. *A* to *C*, After making a Z-shaped incision, the ureters are spatulated on their lateral aspects and sutured to the skin.

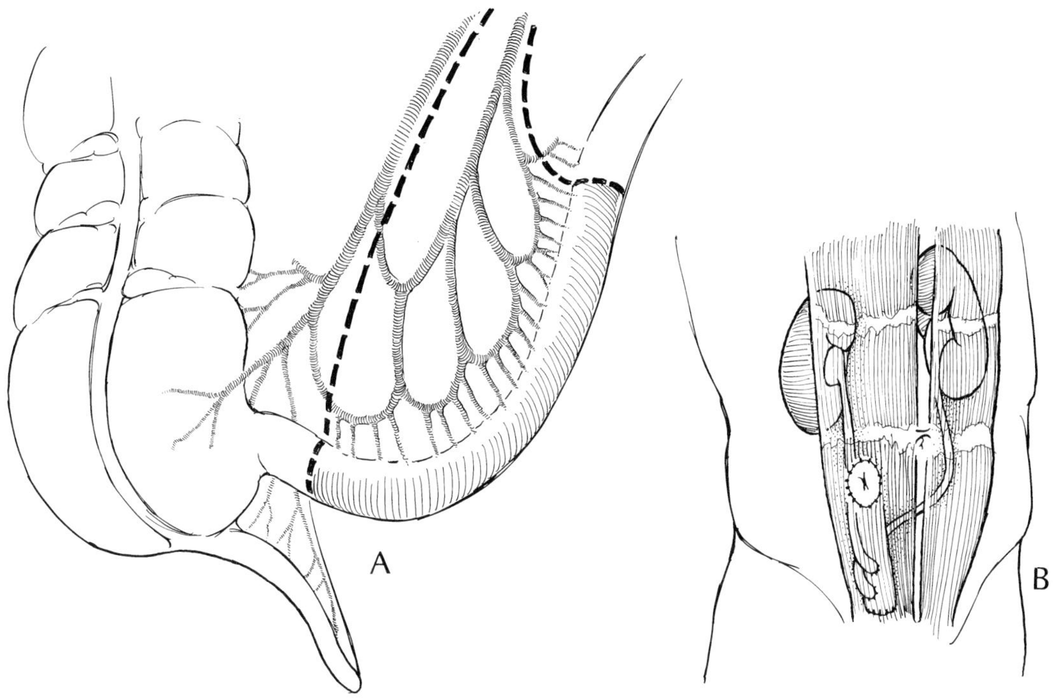
A
B

FIGURE 22–4. *A*, An appropriate segment of ileum is selected, containing two major vascular arcades. *B*, The conduit is positioned in the right lower quadrant and the ureters are reimplanted into the base of the conduit.

anchored to the fascia (Fig. 22–5*B*). The distal staple line, if present, is removed and the stoma is everted using a "rosebudding" technique (Fig. 22–5C). The stoma should protrude, without tension, 2 to 3 cm above the surface of the skin. Alternatively, a Turnbull stoma can be performed in obese patients who have a short mesentery.[17] When properly constructed, both end and loop cutaneous stomas show comparable long-term results in patients with ileal conduits.[18]

JEJUNAL CONDUIT

Jejunal conduit urinary diversion should only be used when other suitable options are not available. Jejunal conduits should be considered in patients who have received previous pelvic irradiation, those with inflammatory bowel disease, or where there has been actual or functional loss of the middle and distal ureters. As will be discussed later, electrolyte disturbances are common when using jejunum as a urinary conduit.[19]

Technique

The length of jejunum used should be as short as possible to reduce metabolic abnormalities. It may be necessary to place the stoma above the umbilicus to help decrease metabolic disturbances. Again, the stoma site should be marked preoperatively after much consideration and should not be situated along the belt line.

Patients who have received significant pelvic irradiation may suffer radiation injury of the distal ureters, requiring transection of the ureters at their point of entry into the true pelvis. The ureters are brought out of the retroperitoneum below the ligament of Treitz.[20] An appropriate segment of jejunum is identified and isolated as previously described for an ileal conduit. Again, the mesentery is divided preserving adequate blood supply to the conduit. The jejunum is divided between clamps or using a GIA stapler, and bowel continuity is restored. The conduit should lie above the restored jejunum. The proximal end of the conduit is directed into the retroperitoneum and the conduit is placed in an isoperistaltic direction. The ureterojejunal anastomoses are performed. Ureteral stents may be useful in decreasing early postoperative electrolyte abnormalities.[15] The mesentery is closed using nonabsorbable sutures. The stoma is created in the same fashion as previously described for an ileal conduit, except that the stoma is usually located in the right upper quadrant.

COLONIC CONDUITS

The colon conduit was popularized by Turner-Warwick in 1960.[21] Urinary conduits constructed of large intestine have several potential advantages

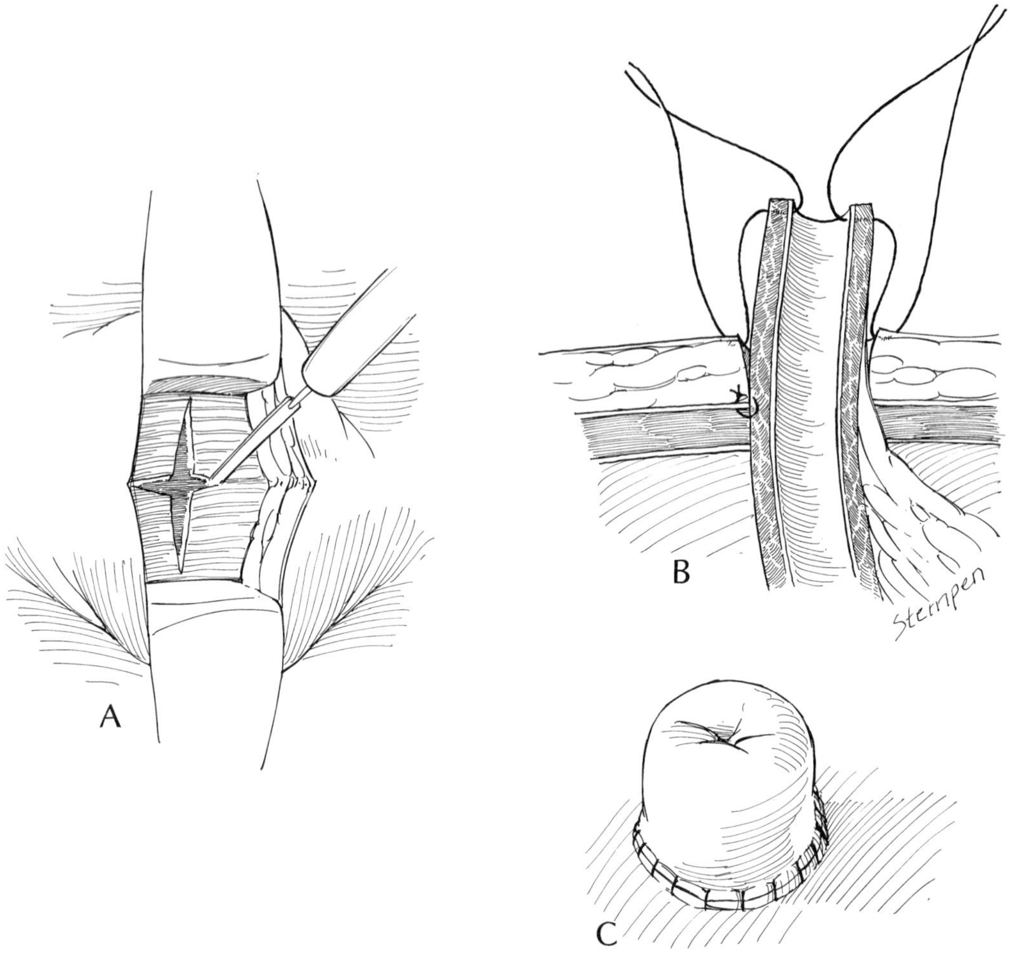
A
B
C
Sternpen

FIGURE 22–5. *A,* The rectus fascia is incised in a cruciate fashion. *B,* The end of the conduit is brought through the rectus muscle and anchored to the fascia. *C,* The stoma is everted and sutured to the skin.

over those constructed of small intestine. A nonrefluxing ureteral anastomosis can be performed by using either a short tunnel through the teniae coli or by using the ileocecal valve. Because of the wide lumen of the colon, stomal stenosis may be less common. A suitable segment of colon can be selected that is outside any field of previous pelvic irradiation. A preoperative contrast study of the large bowel or colonoscopy should be considered when performing a colon conduit.

TRANSVERSE COLON CONDUIT

A transverse colon conduit is well suited for patients who have received extensive pelvic irradiation or where the distal ureters are absent or damaged. The transverse colon segment can be anastomosed directly to the renal pelves in cases where there is inadequate ureteral length.

Technique

A segment of transverse colon approximately 15 cm in length is used for the conduit. The blood supply is based on the middle colic artery (Fig. 22–6*A*). Transillumination of the transverse mesocolon may assist in identifying an appropriate segment. The greater omentum is dissected away from the superior aspect of the transverse colon. The mesentery is incised and individual blood vessels are ligated. The colon is divided both proximally and distally and bowel continuity is restored. The right colon may need to be mobilized to allow for colocolostomy without tension. The proximal end of the colon is closed and fixed posteriorly. After adequate mobilization of the ureters, the ends are spatulated and the ureters are brought through the posterior peritoneum into the abdominal cavity. The ureters are reimplanted into the base of the conduit in either a direct or a nonrefluxing fashion (Fig. 22–6*B*). A

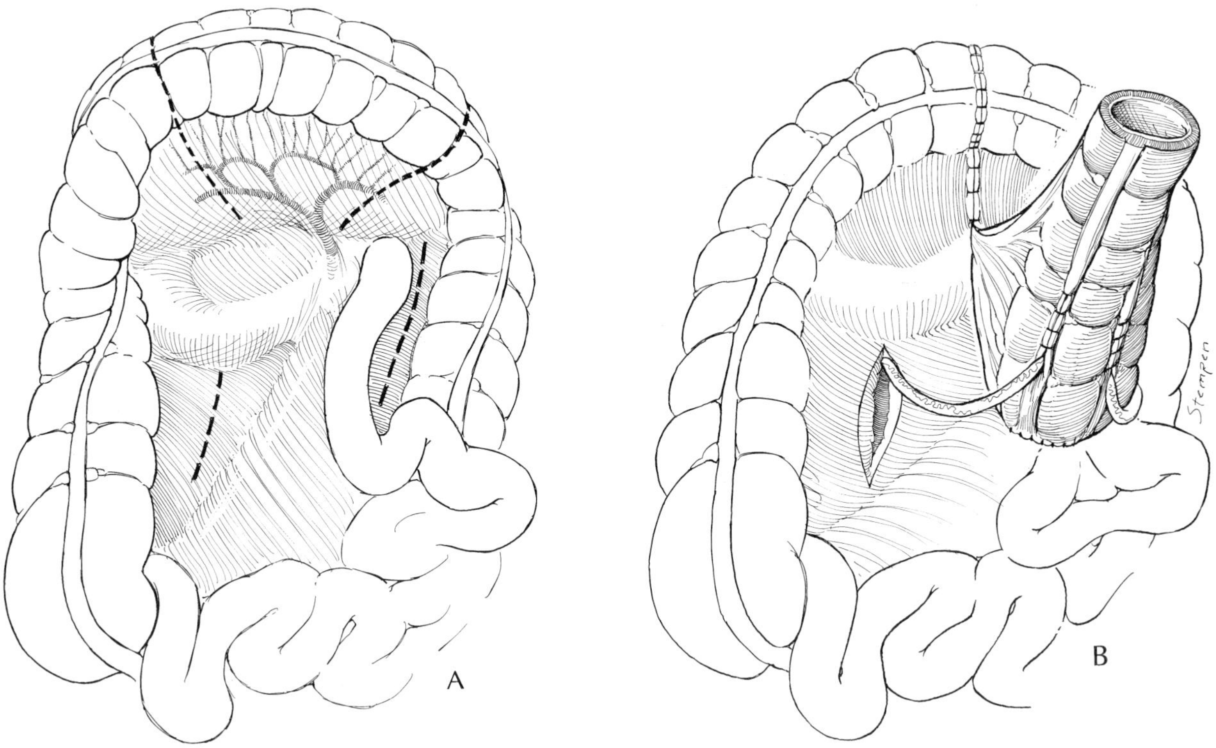
A
B
Stempen

FIGURE 22–6. *A,* An appropriate segment of transverse colon is selected. *B,* After colocolostomy, the ureters are brought into the abdominal cavity and the ureteral anastomoses are performed.

peritoneal flap is fashioned to cover the ureteral anastomoses. Bilateral ureteral stents can be placed. A typical rosebud technique is used to create the stoma. The stoma may be positioned on either the patient's right or left side in the upper or lower quadrants.

SIGMOID COLON CONDUIT

A sigmoid colon conduit should not be used in patients who have had previous pelvic irradiation. The superior hemorrhoidal artery is often injured, leaving inadequate blood supply to the conduit if there has been radiation damage. A sigmoid conduit should also be avoided in patients undergoing cystectomy because the vascular supply to the rectum may be inadequate if the internal pudendal artery is ligated. A sigmoid colon conduit can be used, however, in patients undergoing total pelvic exenteration, alleviating the need for intestinal reanastomosis. A common indication for a sigmoid colon conduit is a patient requiring urinary diversion for management of benign diseases of the lower urinary tract such as a neurogenic bladder.

Technique

The sigmoid colon is mobilized by incising along the white line of Toldt. Adequate mobilization of the colon will allow for easier bowel reanastomosis. An appropriate segment of sigmoid colon, approximately 10 to 12 cm in length, is identified. Care should be taken to preserve adequate blood supply to the conduit. Short mesenteric incisions are made and the colon is divided proximally and distally. The superior hemorrhoidal artery may be divided for increased mobility. Bowel continuity is reestablished and the conduit is placed laterally to the restored bowel. The right ureter is brought under the sigmoid colon. The ureteral anastomosis can be performed using either a direct or a nonrefluxing technique. The preferred stoma site is on the left side of the abdomen. The stoma is created using the previously described rosebud technique.

ILEOCECAL CONDUIT

The ileocecal conduit was first described by Zinman and Libertino in 1975.[22] In this method of urinary diversion the ileocecal valve acts as an antireflux mechanism. Other advantages of this bowel segment are its abundant and constant blood supply and its right lower quadrant location, which facilitates stoma formation.[3] Also, the ileocecal segment is rarely affected by generalized bowel disorders such as diverticulitis, which can affect other colonic segments.

Technique

The blood supply to the ileocecal region is based on the ileocolic artery. The ileocecal segment, including 10 cm of distal ileum, is isolated and divided. An appendectomy is performed. After restoring bowel continuity between the ileum and ascending colon, the ureters are anastomosed in a direct fashion into the ileal segment. The antireflux mechanism depends on the competency of the ileocecal valve. The ileocecal valve can be reinforced by wrapping the redundant cecum around the ileal portion and securing the cecum in place with seromuscular sutures.[22] The proximal portion of the conduit is fixed to the retroperitoneum and the distal cecal portion is brought out to the skin. An everted stoma is created in the standard rosebud fashion.

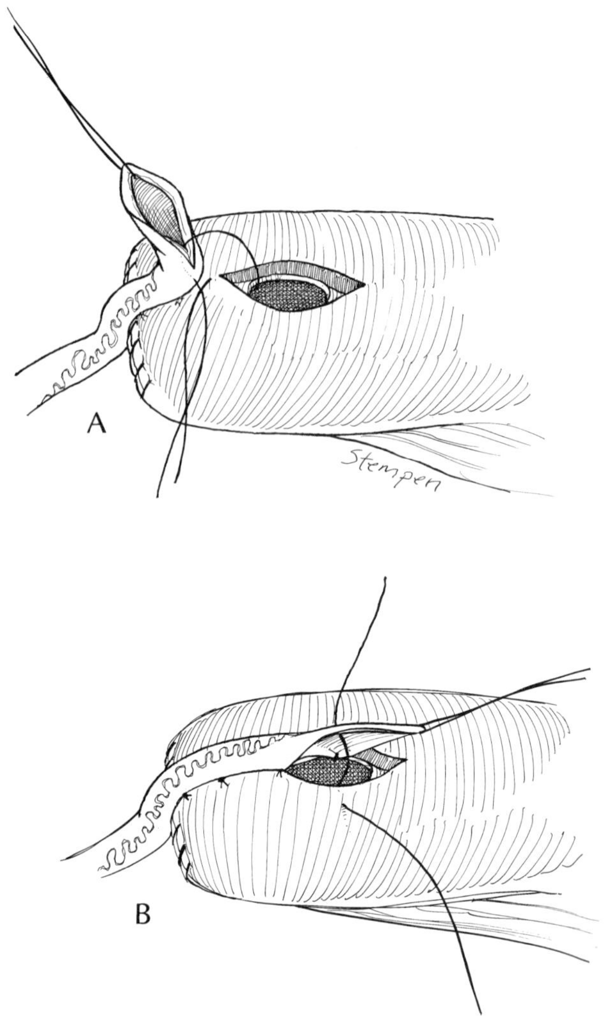
A
B

FIGURE 22–7. *A* and *B*, After removing a small ellipse of bowel, the ureter is spatulated and anastomosed directly to the bowel wall using interrupted absorbable sutures.

URETEROINTESTINAL ANASTOMOSES

The ureterointestinal anastomosis may be performed in either a refluxing or a nonrefluxing fashion. Conceptually, a nonrefluxing anastomosis has the advantage of decreasing upper tract deterioration by preventing intrarenal reflux of infected urine. The subject, however, remains controversial. Nonrefluxing techniques of ureteral anastomosis tend to have a higher stricture rate and renal deterioration occurs not only as a result of reflux but can result from infection, stones, and obstruction as well. Patients with nonrefluxing anastomoses have not been shown to have lower rates of upper tract bacterial colonization.[23] In addition, there is no evidence that patients without reflux have a lower rate of renal deterioration when followed long term.[24]

Both refluxing and nonrefluxing types of anastomoses can be performed on either the large or small bowel. In general, a nonrefluxing anastomosis is easier to perform on the large bowel because of the presence of teniae coli. Numerous techniques for ureterointestinal anastomoses have been described.[25–27] Several common techniques will be discussed.

Ureteral–Small Bowel Anastomoses

Direct Anastomosis

Bricker described his ureteroileocutaneous diversion using a direct end-to-side ureteral anastomosis that is freely refluxing.[14] It is the most simple anastomosis to perform. After spatulating the ureters, a small ellipse of bowel serosa and mucosa are removed from the reimplantation site. The spatulated ureter is anastomosed directly to the bowel (Fig. 22–7). Care should be taken to incorporate both the muscular and mucosal elements of the intestinal wall into the anastomosis. Small segments of the mucosa should be taken to ensure the mucosa will evert and allow a mucosa-to-mucosa anastomosis to be well constructed. The anastomosis can be performed in one or two layers using interrupted absorbable sutures. Prior to completing the anastomosis, the ureters may be stented, especially if the patient is at risk for poor wound healing.

Wallace Technique

When using the Wallace technique, the ureters are joined prior to performing the ureterointestinal anastomosis,[28] potentially decreasing the risk for subsequent ureteral stenosis. Each ureter is spatulated for a length approximately equal to the diameter of the conduit. The ureters are sutured together using a running absorbable suture. The joined ureters are then anastomosed to the open proximal end of the conduit in a refluxing manner (Fig. 22–8). The anastomosis can be performed in one or two layers with absorbable sutures. The ureters may be stented.

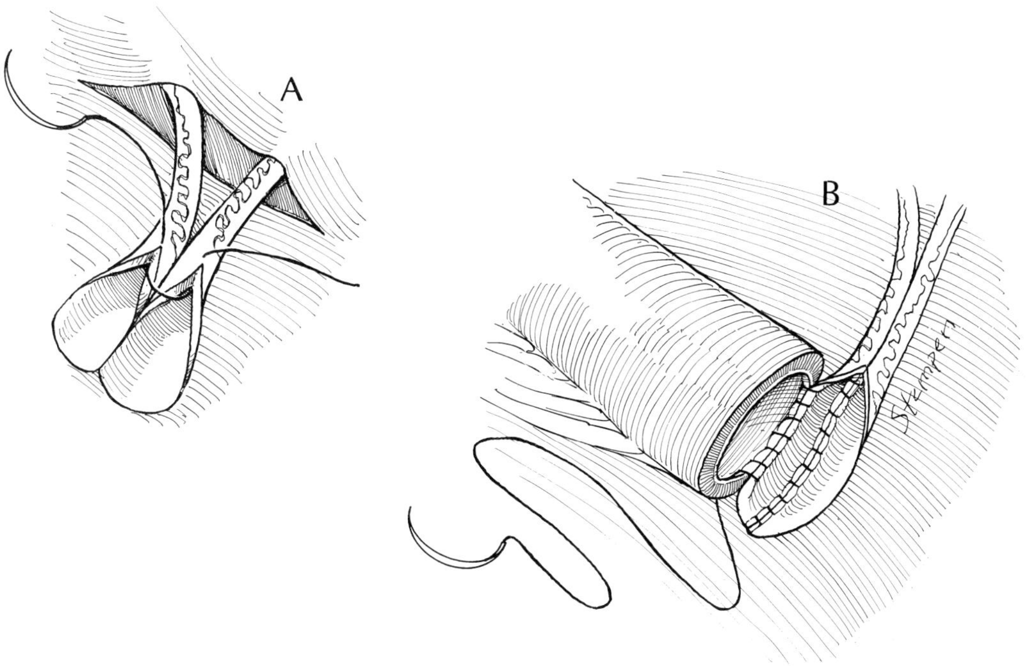
A
B

FIGURE 22–8. *A*, The ureters are spatulated and joined together using a running suture. *B*, The ureters are anastomosed to the open proximal end of the conduit.

Tunneled Ureterointestinal Anastomosis

In this method the ureter is anastomosed to the bowel in a nonrefluxing fashion through a submucosal tunnel.[29] Both ureters are spatulated. A short tunnel is made between the mucosal and seromuscular layers at each anastomotic site. Saline can be injected submucosally into the bowel wall using a small needle to aid with the dissection.[30] A small plug of mucosa is removed from the end of each tunnel, at the site where the ureter will enter the bowel lumen. After advancing each ureter through its tunnel, the ureter is anastomosed to the bowel mucosa.

Ureterocolonic Anastomoses

The ureters can be reimplanted into the large bowel in a direct refluxing fashion as previously described for small bowel or in a nonrefluxing fashion. To perform a nonrefluxing anastomosis, a 3-cm incision is made in a tenia coli (Fig. 22–9*A*). The incision is carried down through the muscular layer, sparing the mucosa. A small ellipse of mucosa is removed at the site where the ureter will enter the bowel lumen. The ureter is anastomosed to the bowel mucosa (Fig. 22–9*B*). The muscular layer of the tenia coli is reapproximated, creating a tunnel through which the ureter travels (Fig. 22–9C).

POSTOPERATIVE CARE

Although the specifics of postoperative care vary with the type of urinary diversion performed, several general principles can be applied. As with most cases of intra-abdominal surgery, paralytic ileus is common after urinary diversion using intestinal segments. A nasogastric tube is routinely placed for gastric decompression and is removed when bowel function returns. Postoperative antibiotics should be continued for only 24 hours in order to decrease the incidence of antibiotic-associated complications. Fluid balance should be monitored and postoperative fluid replacement should be based on maintenance requirements, losses from drains, third-space losses, and systemic conditions leading to hypermetabolism. Serum chemistries should be monitored for electrolyte imbalances. Patients undergoing pelvic surgery are at high risk for venous thromboembolic complications and the risk of thromboembolic event may be reduced with the use of intermittent compression stockings and early postoperative ambulation. The risk of respiratory complications can be reduced by incentive spirometry. If ureteral stents are used they are generally removed after postoperative day 5. Prior to stent removal, a contrast study can be performed to rule out extravasation.

COMPLICATIONS

Numerous complications may occur in all types of urinary diversion. Problems can result from surgical technique, the introduction of intestine into the urinary system, and the patient's underlying disease processes and may appear early or be delayed in onset. Early postoperative complications such as hemorrhage, wound infection, wound de-

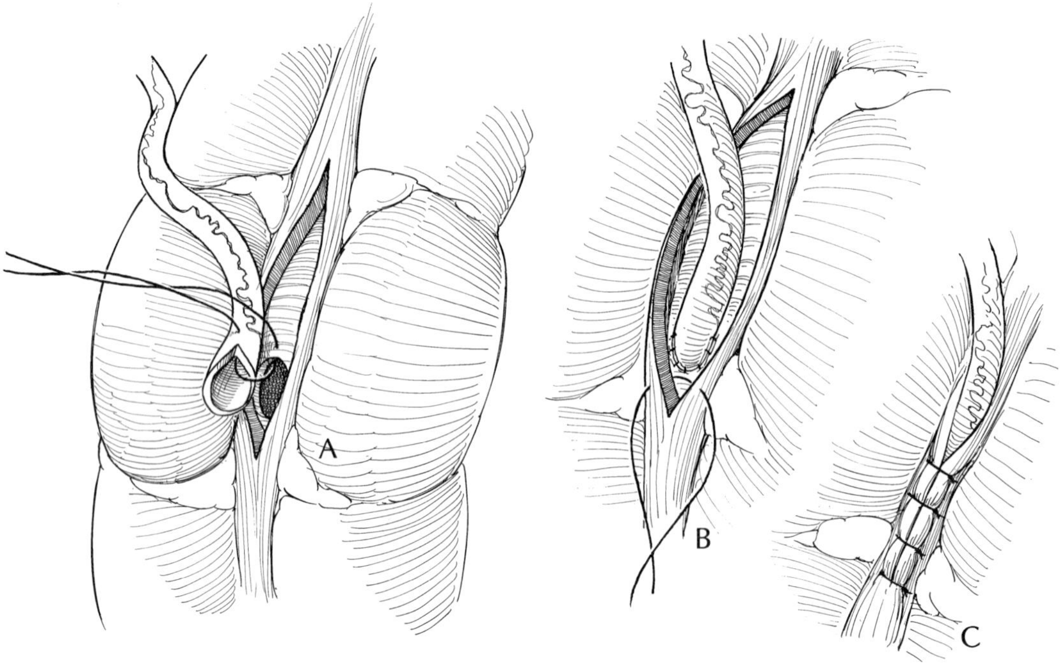
A
B
C

FIGURE 22–9. *A,* A 3-cm incision is made in a tenia coli and a small ellipse of bowel mucosa is removed. *B* and *C,* The ureter is anastomosed to the mucosa and the muscular layer of the tenia is reapproximated.

hiscence, urinary leakage, and bowel obstruction are uncommon. Delayed complications including metabolic abnormalities, stoma problems, renal deterioration, infection, and calculi are more common.

Stoma Complications

Stoma complications are common if patients are followed long enough and can lead to a great deal of patient dissatisfaction. Proper stoma care is important in reducing stoma complications, and training in stomal care should be performed by an enterostomal therapist if possible. Stoma location is important in reducing postoperative problems. Guidelines for selecting a proper stoma site have been previously outlined.

A common late complication of cutaneous ureterostomy is stomal stenosis,[31] occurring in up to 50% of patients. The incidence of stomal stenosis will be lower if only dilated, well-vascularized, thick-walled ureters are used. If the ureter is only marginally dilated, a V-flap technique may be helpful. The treatment of stomal stenosis in cutaneous ureterostomy is surgical, generally requiring urinary intestinal diversion.

Stomal stenosis is seen in all types of intestinal urinary conduits. The risk for developing stomal stenosis increases over time and can be reduced with proper stoma care. In ureteroileal urinary diversion, the incidence of stomal stenosis is as high as 42% in children[32] and 6.7% in adults.[33] Similar rates are present in jejunal conduits.[20] Because colon has a larger lumen, the risk for stomal stenosis should be less. Long-term studies, however, still show a significant incidence of stomal stenosis in patients with colon conduits with rates as high as 61% in children[34,35] (Table 22–1). Stomal stenosis can lead to upper tract obstruction and conduit elongation. The diagnosis can be made by passing a catheter through the stoma and measuring the amount of residual urine present. The treatment of stomal stenosis consists of surgical revision of the stoma.

Parastomal hernia is another delayed complication of intestinal urinary conduit. It is more common in colon conduits (10 to 15%) than in conduits using small bowel. The risk for parastomal hernia is decreased by bringing the bowel through the rectus muscle and removing the excess fat from the mesentery of the distal conduit near the stoma. Significant parastomal hernias should be repaired surgically.

Parastomal skin problems are a common postoperative complication. Parastomal skin problems can be categorized as infectious (fungal), irritative, erosive from mechanical trauma, or pseudoverrucous.[36] The treatment depends on the type of lesion present. In general, parastomal skin problems can be greatly reduced with meticulous and gentle stoma care, the use of nonirritative adhesives, and a properly fitting appliance. The opening in the appliance should be just slightly larger than the stoma to prevent stoma erosion and prolonged contact of the skin with urine.

TABLE 22–1. COMPLICATIONS OF INTESTINAL URINARY CONDUITS

Reference	No. of Patients	Population	% Pyelonephritis	% Ureteral Obstruction	% Stones	% Stomal Stenosis
		Ileal Conduit				
Butcher et al.[33]	307	Adults	13.8	2.3	3.3	6.7
Johnson et al.[47]	181	Adults	5.5	15.5	3.3	3.9
Johnson and Lamy[48]	214	Adults	15.2	18.4	2.5	5.1
Sullivan et al.[37]	336	Adults	19.2	14.7	4.0	5.1
Middleton and Hendren[32]	90	Children	20	10	9	42
Shapiro et al.[40]	90	Children	16.7	22.3	8.9	38
Pitts and Muecke[38]	242	Both	10.7	4.1	5.8	14
		Jejunal Conduit				
Golimbu and Morales[20]	30	Both	—	3.3	—	6.6
		Colon Conduit				
Schmidt et al.[49]	22	Adults	—	4.5	—	0
Morales and Golimbu[34]	46	Both	17	13	4.3	13
Althausen et al.[41]	70	Both	7.1	8.6	4.3	2.8
Elder et al.[35]	41	Children	—	22	16	61.5
		Ileocecal Conduit				
Matsuura et al.[50]	147	Both	13.6	9.5	5.4	2

Renal Complications

Pyelonephritis occurs as both an early and delayed complication in all types of urinary diversion. Pyelonephritis has been reported in 3% of patients with cutaneous ureterostomy.[8] The incidence of pyelonephritis is similar in patients who have ileal conduits and colon conduits (Table 22–1) and has been reported to be as high as 20% in some series.[37] Although many ureterocolonic anastomoses are performed using nonrefluxing techniques, many patients without reflux have upper tract bacterial colonization.[23] Pyelonephritis should be treated with antibiotic therapy directed specifically at the infecting organism(s). A urine sample should be obtained by passing a catheter into the stoma, rather than from the collection device.

Renal deterioration has been associated with all forms of intestinal urinary diversion. Upper tract deterioration can result from pyelonephritis, reflux, or obstruction from either stones or a ureteral stricture. The risk of renal deterioration increases with time and obstruction appears to be the major cause.[38] The reported incidence of renal deterioration is variable but ranges from 18 to 56% in ileal conduits[32,39,40] and 8 to 48% in colon conduits.[34,35,41]

Urinary Calculi

All patients with intestinal urinary diversion are at risk for stone formation. Approximately 5 to 10% of patients with urinary diversion will form stones (Table 22–1). The cause of increased risk for stone formation is multifactorial.[42] Staples used in conduit construction can act as a nidus for stone formation. Bacteriuria exists in most patients with a urinary conduit and colonization with urease-producing bacteria may lead to struvite stones. Metabolic acidosis, commonly found in urinary conduit patients, can promote hypocitraturia and hypercalciuria,[43] increasing the risk for stone formation. Since the terminal ileum plays an important role in bile salt and fat metabolism, patients may suffer from problems with fat malabsorption if this segment is used for urinary diversion as with an ileocecal conduit. Faulty bile salt and fat metabolism may lead to saponification of bile salts with both calcium and magnesium within the gut lumen, resulting in an increase in free gut oxalate and increased oxalate absorption. This may result in hyperoxaluria and calcium oxalate stones.

The management of urinary calculi in patients with urinary diversion may be difficult. Upper tract stones can be successfully treated using a combination of percutaneous and endoscopic retrograde techniques in conjunction with extracorporeal shock wave lithotripsy.[44] Extracorporeal shock wave lithotripsy should be avoided if there is a ureteral stricture distal to the stone.[44] Because the cause is often multifactorial, stone recurrence rate is high. Close follow-up is necessary. Patients with struvite stones may benefit from chronic suppressive antibiotics and treatment with a urease inhibitor.

Metabolic Complications

Metabolic abnormalities are common when bowel is introduced into the urinary tract. The severity of the metabolic disturbance is influenced by the length and segment of bowel used, urinary stasis, renal function, and the concentration of urinary solutes.[16] The metabolic problems associated with urinary solute reabsorption by bowel mucosa are avoided when using cutaneous ureterostomy and pyelostomy. Metabolic abnormalities associated with intestinal urinary diversion include electrolyte problems, altered drug metabolism, osteomalacia, and nutritional disturbances.

Electrolyte Disturbances

The use of jejunum as a urinary conduit may result in hypochloremic, hyponatremic, hyperkalemic metabolic acidosis, which occurs in up to 40% of patients with jejunal conduits.[19] The clinical symptoms of this syndrome are nausea, vomiting, anorexia, weakness, and lethargy. These electrolyte disturbances are a result of normal intestinal physiology. The jejunum is unable to maintain a large solute gradient and there is movement of electrolytes between the extracellular fluid and the conduit lumen. The magnitude and direction of electrolyte absorption and excretion are related to the differential concentration of the electrolytes. Sodium and chloride are excreted into the urine and potassium and urea are reabsorbed. The loss of sodium leads to a decrease in extracellular fluid volume and a reduction in renal blood flow. The reduction in renal blood flow causes activation of the renin-angiotensin system and subsequent stimulation of aldosterone production by angiotensin II. Aldosterone increases reabsorption of hydrogen and excretion of potassium into the distal renal tubule with acidosis and release of intracellular potassium. Reabsorption of urea and dehydration lead to azotemia. Treatment of the jejunal conduit syndrome is with oral sodium chloride replacement.

With the use of ileum or colon as a conduit, metabolic acidosis can occur. Both sodium and chloride are absorbed across the bowel surface, with chloride absorption in excess of sodium. This results in a net loss of bicarbonate into the urine. Renal insufficiency may contribute to the severity of the acidosis. Excess potassium is excreted in the urine as a result of chronic acidosis. Since the ileum is more capable of absorbing urinary potassium than the colon, patients with ileal conduits tend to have normal total body potassium levels and patients with colon conduits tend to be total body potassium depleted. The treatment of choice for electrolyte abnormalities associated with ileal and colon conduits is alkalinization with oral bicarbonate or citrate.

Altered Drug Metabolism

Phenytoin toxicity has been reported in patients with intestinal urinary conduits.[45] Any drug that is excreted unchanged by the kidneys and can be reabsorbed by the intestine has a potential for toxicity in patients with intestinal urinary diversions. Patients with continent urinary diversion who are receiving methotrexate chemotherapy are at risk for toxicity and a catheter should be placed into the reservoir when methotrexate is administered.

Nutritional Disturbances

Use of the distal ileum for urinary diversion can lead to vitamin B_{12} deficiency, resulting in megaloblastic anemia and peripheral neuropathy. Loss of the distal ileum may also impair bile salt absorption leading to fat malabsorption and decreased uptake of fat-soluble vitamins. Fat malabsorption, excess bile salts, and loss of the ileocecal valve can lead to chronic diarrhea. Persistent diarrhea may be treated with cholestyramine and agents that decrease bowel motility. Chronic acidosis can lead to osteomalacia in adults and rickets in children.[46] Bone remineralization can be accomplished with oral alkalinization therapy and supplementation with calcium and vitamin D if necessary.

Surgical Complications

Surgical complications of noncontinent urinary diversion include stomal stenosis, parastomal hernia, urinary extravasation, ureteroanastomotic stricture, bowel obstruction, and wound infection or dehiscence. Stomal complications have been previously discussed. The use of soft Silastic stents may reduce urinary extravasation, which can lead to periureteral scarring and subsequent ureterointestinal anastomotic stricture. In general, ureteral stents should be placed in patients who are at risk for poor wound healing. Nonrefluxing anastomotic techniques tend to have a higher stricture rate. Strictures can occur both at or away from the ureterointestinal anastomosis. Many ureteral strictures can be successfully dilated endoscopically, but some will require open repair. Bowel obstruction after urinary diversion is uncommon and rarely requires exploration.[37] Similar surgical complication rates are seen between ileal and colon conduits in adults.[37] The incidence of ureteral obstruction and stomal stenosis in several different series is summarized in Table 22–1.

REFERENCES

1. Boyd SD, Feinberg SM, Skinner DG, et al: Quality of life survey of urinary diversion patients: comparison of ileal conduits versus continent Kock ileal reservoirs. J Urol 1987; 138:1386–1389.
2. Immergut MA, Jacobson JJ, Culp DA, et al: Cutaneous pyelostomy. J Urol 1969; 101:276–279.
3. Gleeson MJ, Griffith DP: Urinary diversion. Br J Urol 1990; 66:113–122.
4. Rosen MA, Roth DR, Gonzales ET Jr: Current indications for cutaneous ureterostomy. Urology 1994; 43:92–96.
5. Whitmore WF Jr: Ureteral diversion. *In* Bergman HP (ed): The Ureter, p 603. New York, Harper & Row, 1967.
6. Sarduy GS, Crooks KK, Smith JP, et al: Results in children managed by cutaneous ureterostomy. Urology 1982; 19: 486–488.

7. Young JD Jr, Ajedia FT: Further observations on flank ureterostomy and cutaneous transureteroureterostomy. J Urol 1966; 95:327–333.
8. Rainwater LM, Leary FJ, Rife CC: Transureteroureterostomy with cutaneous ureterostomy: a 25-year experience. J Urol 1991; 146:13–15.
9. Persky L, McDougal WS, Kedia KR: Transureteroureterostomy: an adjunct to cystectomy. Urology 1980; 16:20.
10. Chute R, Sallade RL: Bilateral side-to-side cutaneous ureterostomy in the midline for urinary diversion. J Urol 1961; 85:280–283.
11. Rinker JR, Blanchard TW: Improvement of the circulation of the ureter prior to cutaneous ureterostomy: a clinical study. J Urol 1966; 96:44.
12. Straffon RA, Kyle K, Corvalan J: Techniques of cutaneous ureterostomy and results in 51 patients. J Urol 1970; 143: 138–146.
13. Seiffert L: Die "Darm-siphonblase." Arch Klin Chir 1935; 183:569–574.
14. Bricker EM: Bladder substitution after pelvic evisceration. Surg Clin North Am 1950; 30:1511–1521.
15. Benson MC, Olsson CA: Urinary diversion. *In* Walsh PC, Retik AB, Stamey TA, Vaughan ED Jr (eds): Campbell's Urology, 6th edition, p 2654. Philadelphia, WB Saunders Co, 1992.
16. McDougal WS: Metabolic complications of urinary intestinal diversion. J Urol 1992; 147:1199–1208.
17. Turnbull RB Jr, Hewitt CR: Loop-end myotomy ileostomy in the obese patient. Urol Clin North Am 1978; 5:423.
18. Chechile G, Klein EA, Bauer L, et al: Functional equivalence of end and loop ileal conduit stomas. J Urol 1992; 147:582–586.
19. Klein EA, Montie JE, Montague DK, et al: Jejunal conduit urinary diversion. J Urol 1986; 135:244.
20. Golimbu M, Morales P: Jejunal conduits: technique and complications. J Urol 1975; 113:787–795.
21. Turner-Warwick RT: Colonic urinary conduits. Proc R Soc Med 1960; 53:1032–1034.
22. Zinman L, Libertino JA: Ileocecal conduit for temporary and permanent urinary diversion. J Urol 1975; 113:317–323.
23. Gonzalez R, Reinberg Y: Localization of bacteriuria in patients with enterocystoplasty and nonrefluxing conduits. J Urol 1987; 138:1104–1105.
24. Mansson W, Colleen S, Forsberg L, et al: Renal function after urinary diversion. A study of continent caecal reservoir, ileal conduit, and colonic conduit. Scand J Urol Nephrol 1984; 18:307–315.
25. LeDuc A, Camey M, Teillac P: An original antireflux ureteroileal implantation technique: long-term followup. J Urol 1987; 137:1156–1158.
26. Yang W: Yang needle tunneling technique in creating antireflux and continent mechanisms. J Urol 1993; 150:830–834.
27. Hirdes WH, Hoekstra I, Vliestra HP: Hammock anastomoses; a nonrefluxing ureteroileal anastomosis. J Urol 1988; 139:517–518.
28. Wallace DM: Ureteric diversion using a conduit: a simplified technique. Br J Urol 1966; 38:522.
29. Starr A, Rose DH, Cooper JF: Antireflux ureteroileal anastomosis in humans. J Urol 1975; 113:170–174.
30. Menon M, Yu GW, Jeffs RD: Technique for antirefluxing ureterocolonic anastomosis. J Urol 1982; 127:236–237.
31. Feminella JG, Lattimer JK: A retrospective analysis of 70 cases of cutaneous ureterostomy. J Urol 1971; 106:538.
32. Middleton AN Jr, Hendren WH: Ileal conduit in children at the Massachusetts General Hospital from 1955 to 1970. J Urol 1976; 115:591.
33. Butcher HR Jr, Sugg WL, McAfee CA, Bricker EM: Ileal conduit method of ureteral urinary diversion. Ann Surg 1962; 156:682.
34. Morales P, Golimbu M: Colonic urinary diversion: 10 years of experience. J Urol 1975; 113:302.
35. Elder DD, Moisey CU, Rees RWM: A long-term follow-up of the colonic conduit operation in children. Br J Urol 1979; 51:462.
36. Borglund E, Nordstrom G, Nyman CR: Classification of peristomal skin changes in patients with urostomy. J Am Acad Dermatol 1988; 19:623.
37. Sullivan JW, Grabstald H, Whitmore WF: Complications of ureteroileal conduit with radical cystectomy: review of 336 cases. J Urol 1980; 124:797–801.
38. Pitts WR Jr, Muecke EC: A 20-year experience with ileal conduits: the fate of the kidneys. J Urol 1979; 122:154–157.
39. Schwarz GR, Jeffs RD: Ileal conduit urinary diversion in children: computer analysis of follow-up from 2 to 26 years. J Urol 1975; 114:285.
40. Shapiro SR, Lebowitz R, Colodny AH: Fate of 90 children with ileal conduit urinary diversion a decade later: analysis of complications, pyelography, renal function and bacteriology. J Urol 1975; 114:289.
41. Althausen AF, Hagen-Cook K, Hendren WH III: Nonrefluxing colon conduit: experience with 70 cases. J Urol 1978; 120:35.
42. Dretler SP: The pathogenesis of urinary tract calculi occurring after ileal conduit diversion: I. clinical study. II. conduit study. III. prevention. J Urol 1973; 109:204–209.
43. Terai A, Arai Y, Kawakita M, et al: Effect of urinary intestinal diversion on urinary risk factors for urolithiasis. J Urol 1995; 153:37–41.
44. Wolf JS Jr, Stoller ML: Management of upper tract calculi in patients with tubularized urinary diversions. J Urol 1991; 145:266–269.
45. Savarirayan F, Dixey GM: Syncope following ureterosigmoidostomy. J Urol 1969; 101:844.
46. McDougal WS, Koch MO, Shands C III, et al: Bony demineralization following urinary intestinal diversion. J Urol 1988; 140:853–855.
47. Johnson DE, Jackson L, Guinn GA: Ileal conduit diversion for carcinoma of the bladder. South Med J 1970; 63:1115.
48. Johnson DE, Lamy SM: Complications of a single stage radical cystectomy and ileal conduit diversion: review of 214 cases. J Urol 1977; 117:171.
49. Schmidt JD, Buchsbaum HJ, Jacobo EC: Transverse colon conduit for supravesical urinary tract diversion. Urology 1976; 8:542.
50. Matsuura T, Tsujihashi H, Park Y, et al: Assessment of the long-term results of ileocecal conduit urinary diversion. Urol Int 1991; 46:154–158.

23

CONTINENT URINARY DIVERSION

W. SCOTT MCDOUGAL, M.D.

Continent urinary diversion may be conveniently classified according to the location of the urinary outflow (Table 23–1). The three categories of continent diversion include (1) those to the abdominal wall, (2) those anastomosed to the urethra (orthotopic bladder), and (3) those that utilize the rectal sphincter (rectal diversion). There are some attributes common to all and some that are unique to the type of diversion. Both general and specific aspects of the diversion may be subclassified as metabolic, neuromechanical, or surgical. These attributes are used for selecting the most appropriate type of diversion for each individual patient. Thus, for some patients one type of diversion might be appropriate, whereas for another individual that type might be ill-advised.

In the following paragraphs, attributes specific to each type of continent diversion are discussed as well as contraindications to their use. Finally, complications both general and specific categorized as to metabolic, neuromechanical, and surgical are discussed.

ABDOMINAL WALL DIVERSIONS

Continent diversions to the abdominal wall require a valve, constructed of bowel or a foreign body (artificial sphincter). The Koch pouch requires the use of 70 to 80 cm of ileum and employs an intussuscepted portion of ileum as the continence mechanism. This mechanism also is used to prevent reflux into the upper tracts. When right colon is employed the ileal cecal valve is utilized and may either be plicated or intussuscepted to achieve continence. In this type of diversion the right colon to the level of the hepatic flexure and 10 to 15 cm of distal ileum are utilized. The right colon may also be used exclusively employing the appendix submucosally implanted as described by Mitrofanoff as the continence valve. Another methodology utilized employs a hydraulic valve as described by Benchekroun that is fashioned from ileum and made to be patched either to ileum and/or colon. Finally, an artificial sphincter may be employed to achieve continence. (Usually an artificial sphincter is utilized when the enteric segment is anastomosed to the urethra. It has been used most extensively in females and is placed about a segment of right colon.)

ORTHOTOPIC DIVERSION

Orthotopic continent diversions involve an anastomosis to the urethra and utilize the indigenous sphincter as the continence mechanism. Either colon or ileum may be used. When small bowel is the segment employed, 50 to 70 cm of ileum is detubularized and anastomosed directly to the urethra. The antireflux mechanism utilized for ureteral implantation is a submucosal, paramucosal (LeDuc), or paraserosal type of antireflux valve. These segments have been fashioned into a U, N, or W shape to increase capacity. Studer described the use of a long segment of ileum with no specific valve implantation to prevent reflux. Finally, Camey described a nondetubularized ileal segment that may be anastomosed directly to the urethra. Ileal colonic, right colon, and sigmoid segments have also been utilized for urethral enteric reconstruction. These are usually detubularized to increase capacity.

RECTAL DIVERSION

The use of the rectum for the continence valve was perhaps one of the earliest successful forms of continent urinary diversion. The classic example is

TABLE 23–1. TYPES OF CONTINENT DIVERSION

Abdominal
Ileum: Koch
Right colon: Indiana, Mitrofanoff, Benchekroun
Orthotopic:
Ileum: Hemi Koch, Camey, Hautmann, Studer
Ileocolon: Mainz, LeBag
Right colon
Sigmoid
Gastric
Rectum
Ureterosigmoidostomy
Rectal pull-through
Ileal and colonic add-ons
Mainz II

a ureterosigmoidostomy, but because of the significant metabolic and upper tract infectious complications, other modifications of this technique have been utilized. The Mainz II pouch is an attempt to enlarge the rectal reservoir and prevent reflux to the upper tracts. Perhaps the most complete method of excluding the fecal stream from the urinary tract is to perform an end colostomy and anastomose the ureters to the rectal segment, thus creating a rectal bladder. A modification of this technique is to use a portion of rectosigmoid and pull it through the rectal sphincter, thus giving two outlets on the perineum, both of which traverse through the rectal sphincter, one of which excretes feces and the other urine. These types of rectal urinary diversions have not gained great popularity in this country owing to the fact that there is a significant incidence of fecal/urinary incontinence and upper tract infectious complications resulting in upper tract deterioration.

INDICATIONS

Patients who require urinary diversion generally require it because their bladders have been removed for cancer; there is significant vesical dysfunction in which the bladder no longer serves as a storage vessel; there is progressive upper tract deterioration due to an inadequate bladder; the patient has severe vesical pain; or there has been extensive trauma either in the form of blunt, penetrating, or x-ray therapy to the bladder, rendering it dysfunctional. Whether a continent diversion or a conduit is utilized is dependent in large part upon (1) renal function, (2) life expectancy, (3) ability to self-catheterize, (4) risk of urethral recurrence, (5) risk of pelvic recurrence, (6) amount of functional bowel in the enteric tract, (7) body image, and (8) patient willingness to assume some additional operative risk. The simplest type of urinary diversion and that associated with the least immediate postoperative complications is an ileal conduit. However, there are many disadvantages to this type of urinary diversion over the long term with respect to social acceptance and body image. Whether or not continent urinary diversions are any worse or better in preserving renal function is unknown at this time. It is likely, however, that metabolic complications of continent diversion will exceed those of a simple conduit.

In order to utilize large segments of bowel in the urinary tract, a minimal amount of renal function is necessary. In general, patients who have a creatinine level below 2 mg/dl will tolerate continent diversions quite well. However, occasionally it is desirable to perform a continent urinary diversion in patients whose creatinine exceeds 2 mg/dl. Under these circumstances a more extensive evaluation of renal function is mandatory. If complications are to be minimized, such patients must at a minimum meet the following criteria. They must be able to acidify their urine to a pH below 5.5 and increase the urinary osmolality with water deprivation to above 600 mOsm/kg. They must not have excessive proteinuria (exceeding 1 g/day) and have an inulin clearance that exceeds 35 ml/min in the adult. If these criteria are met, patients with significantly diminished renal function will tolerate a continent diversion quite well. The use of stomach in such patients does not obviate the need for the above renal function.

Another factor that should be taken into account when one considers continent diversion is life expectancy. Someone with a markedly limited life expectancy is generally better served by having a urinary diversion that has the least complications and requires the least retraining. This generally means an ileal conduit.

The patient must have the ability to self-catheterize, as virtually everyone with a continent urinary diversion except for a rectal diversion will need to utilize this methodology at some point in the postoperative period, many of whom will be required to perform this throughout their remaining years.

Those individuals who have had cancer must be at low risk for both urethral and pelvic recurrence. In general, the pelvic recurrence rate is 5 to 10% in patients who, at the time of urinary diversion, do not have any evidence of gross disease in the pelvis. Similarly, the incidence of urethral recurrence is about 5 to 10% when all comers are taken into account. These recurrences can be minimized if in the former the pelvic nodes are negative at the time of cystectomy, and in the latter if the prostatic urethra is not involved with carcinoma in situ or invasive transitional cell carcinoma and the bladder neck is not involved with invasive cancer in the female.

A small group of patients with decreased absorptive capacity of the intestine, be it large or small bowel who have had significant gut removed previously, should not in general be candidates for continent urinary diversions, as the harvesting of large portions of additional bowel would cause significant nutritional problems.

Those individuals whose body image is so important to them that an external collecting device is abhorrent should be considered candidates. They must be made aware, however, that there is an increased risk of reoperation when continent diversions are constructed and they must be willing to assume the risk. Most patients, particularly those in whom an orthotopic bladder is being considered, are quite willing to assume the additional risk.

SURGICAL COMPLICATIONS

Complications of urinary intestinal diversions may be divided into three areas: surgical, metabolic, and neuromechanical. Surgical complications include those in the immediate postoperative period as well as those over the long term and may be general, which are associated with all types of urinary diversions, and those more specific to each individual type. Surgical complications of a general nature that include all types of urinary diversion include bowel obstruction, renal failure, upper gastrointestinal bleed, wound infection, thrombophlebitis, myocardial infarction, pneumonia, sepsis, ureteral obstruction, failure of the valve mechanism of the reimplanted ureter, acute pyelonephritis, urine leak, bowel leak, renal calculi, and pouch calculi (Table 23–2). Diarrhea is a general complication and usually occurs in patients who have had significant portions of their enteric tract removed, particularly when the ileal cecal valve has been removed and a major portion of right colon and ileum have been excluded from the fecal stream.

Those complications that are specific to the type of urinary diversion are as follows: individuals with a Koch pouch urinary diversion have a 15% early complication rate and a 13% late complication rate. Valve failure resulting in incontinence occurs in about 7%. Urine leak, stones, and ureteral ileal stenosis comprise the majority of the remaining complications occurring in this group. Individuals in whom the right colon is utilized have an early reoperation rate of about 4% and a late reoperation rate of about 14%. Incontinence occurs in 4%. Difficulty catheterizing the stoma, and stones account for the remaining complications. Use of the Mittrofanoff mechanism has a 4 to 14% incontinence rate with a significant number of patients developing stomal stenosis. The hydraulic valve of Benchekroun carries with it a 24% complication rate. Septic shock and fistula, both urinary and fecal, account for a significant portion of the complications. Approximately 23% of patients require reoperation due to either valve necrosis or failure of the valve. About 7% are incontinent.

METABOLIC COMPLICATIONS

Those complications that are of a metabolic nature include electrolyte abnormalities, altered sensorium, abnormal drug metabolism, osteomalacia, growth retardation, persistent and recurrent infection, formation of renal and reservoir calculi, problems ensuing from removal of portions of the gut from the intestinal tract to include B_{12} malabsorption, diarrhea and nutritional deficiency, and the development of urethral and/or intestinal cancer (Table 23–3). The factors that influence the occurrence of these complications and determine the amount of solute and the type of absorption are the segment of bowel utilized, the surface area of the bowel, the amount of time the urine is exposed to the bowel, the concentration of solutes in the urine, renal function, and the pH of the fluid.

Electrolyte abnormalities are dependent upon both the amount of intestine used and the portion of intestine used. If stomach is employed, a hypochloremic metabolic alkalosis may occur. If jejunum is the segment used, hyponatremia, hyperkalemia, and metabolic acidosis will occur, whereas with ileum and colon a hyperchloremic metabolic acidosis occurs. Virtually all individuals with significant segments of intestine in the urinary tract experience these complications; however, they may

TABLE 23–2. SURGICAL COMPLICATIONS OF A GENERAL NATURE OF CONTINENT URINARY DIVERSION

	Early	Late
Urine leak	10%	
Wound dehiscence	5%	
Acute pyelonephritis		10%
Electrolyte abnormalities		15–50%
Bowel obstruction		5–10%
Fecal leak	2%	
Ureteral stricture		10–15%
Reflux		15–20%
Loss of continence mechanism		15–20%
Prolonged ileus	6%	
Wound infection	5%	
Stones, upper tract		5%
Pouch calculi		5–15%

TABLE 23–3. METABOLIC COMPLICATIONS OF CONTINENT DIVERSION

- Electrolyte abnormalities
  - Acidosis
  - Hypokalemia
  - Hypocalcemia
  - Hyperammonemia
- Osteomalacia
- Growth retardation
- Cancer
- Short Gut
  - B_{12} malabsorption
  - Diarrhea
- Altered sensorium
- Drug intoxication
- Infection
- Stones

be exceedingly subtle and in many they are not clinically relevant. Perhaps the most common segments utilized are the ileum and colon, and it is in these segments where hyperchloremic metabolic acidosis occurs. The mechanism of this acidosis is the substitution of ammonium for sodium in the sodium hydrogen exchanger, with the concomitant absorption of chloride and excretion of bicarbonate by the chloride bicarbonate exchanger. This in essence results in the absorption of ammonium chloride and the secretion into the lumen of CO_2 and water. Those patients with continent urinary diversions utilizing ileum have a 10 to 15% incidence of electrolyte problems, whereas when colon or ileum and colon are used, approximately 65% of patients develop a clinically apparent acidosis. Untreated, patients may develop symptoms of easy fatigability, anorexia, weight loss, polydypsia, and lethargy. The treatment of this disorder involves the administration of alkalinizing agents and/or blockers of chloride transport. Perhaps the most efficacious method is to provide the patient with bicarbonate; however, bicarbonate tablets may cause considerable intestinal gas. Potassium citrate solutions may be used in those who have difficulty taking bicarbonate. The use of chlorpromazine or nicotinic acid to help ameliorate the acidosis by blocking the chloride absorption may be helpful. Hypokalemia, with total-body depletion of potassium, may also be a problem. This is more common when colon is utilized rather than small bowel. Finally, large losses of water may result in dehydration at the most or merely frequent voiding at the very least. This occurs because the bowel is not tight to water movement and therefore it re-equilibrates according to its osmotic gradient. Attempts to water-deprive such patients are inappropriate. It should be avoided and patients should be instructed to keep their fluid intake up, particularly in the summer months of the year.

Altered sensorium may occur as a consequence of either magnesium deficiency, drug intoxication, or abnormalities in ammonia metabolism. As noted above ammonia is reabsorbed, and if the liver is able to detoxify the ammonia, then hyperammonemia does not occur. On the other hand, infections that produce an excessive amount of ammonia in the urinary tract and/or liver dysfunction may result in hyperammonigenic coma. This complication is particularly worrisome in those patients with cirrhosis in whom large portions of bowel have been utilized for urinary diversion. The treatment of this disorder involves ridding the patient of their infection and decreasing the urea-splitting bacteria in the urinary diversion.

Certain drugs are reabsorbed by the bowel and excreted intact in the urinary stream and when reabsorbed by the interposed intestine may lead to drug intoxication. Finally, magnesium deficiency, because of nutritional deprivation and/or lack of significant absorptive bowel, may occur.

Osteomalacia may in fact be a problem, particularly in patients who have had urinary intestinal diversion for long periods of time. Problems of growth and development and bone healing have also been reported in individuals with long-standing urinary intestinal diversion. However, many patients with urinary diversions and in particular male patients who are in the fifth and sixth decades of life suffer no clinically untoward consequences of their urinary diversion with respect to bone mineralization. The individuals most prone to this complication are postmenopausal women and children who have had their urinary diversion for a number of years. Patients who develop osteomalacia generally complain of lethargy, joint pain (especially in the weight-bearing joints), and proximal myopathy. The disorder is generally due to chronic acidosis; however, abnormalities of vitamin D metabolism have also been described.

There is an increased incidence of bacteriuria and bacteremia. Moreover, there is an increased incidence of septic episodes in patients who have urinary intestinal diversions. The reason that septic episodes occur is unclear. However, the intestinal mucosa through the secretion of certain immunoglobulins serves as a protective barrier under normal circumstances. When intestine is interposed in the urinary tract, some of these defense mechanisms may be abrogated, allowing for translocation of bacteria across the bowel wall.

There is an increased incidence of stones, both in the upper tracts (3 to 4%) and in the pouch. Pouch calculi may occur in as many as 15 to 20% of patients depending on what is used to construct the pouch and its type. The use of staples in pouch reconstruction leads to a higher incidence of stones. Marlex erosion into the pouch also leads to a higher incidence of calculi.

Complications of short bowel are of two types: diarrhea and nutritional problems. An example of a nutritional problem is B_{12} absorption abnormalities. This has been documented in a number of patients and results in megaloblastic anemia. Long-track neurologic signs may become evident. When these occur, correction of the B_{12} abnormalities does not correct the neurologic deficit. Thus, those with long-term urinary diversions need to have careful attention paid to B_{12}. When the ileal cecal valve or large segments of ileum are removed, lack of reabsorption of bile acids and salts may occur. This may result in an irritative diarrhea with subsequent nutritional abnormalities.

Although the incidence of cancer development in segments utilized for urinary diversion is exceedingly low, when it does occur it usually occurs in those cases in which the urine, urothelium, and intestinal mucosa are not separated from the fecal stream. Thus, in urinary diversions in which the fecal stream is excluded there is an exceedingly low incidence of intestinal malignancy. On the other hand, individuals who have urothelial mucosa, urine, intestinal mucosa, and feces juxtaposed (classically ureterosigmoidostomies) have a higher incidence of malignancy. The type of malignancy that develops is either an adenocarcinoma or transitional cell carcinoma. These tumors are often exceedingly malignant and generally metastatic by the time they are discovered. It is therefore important that these patients have scheduled periodic examinations of the anastomotic site for the early detection of the development of cancer.

NEUROMECHANICAL COMPLICATIONS

Small bowel and large bowel have been utilized extensively in continent urinary reconstructions. Of some controversy has been whether or not such intestinal segments require detubularization. In the early development of continent diversions, both ileum and right colon were utilized in nondetubularized form. In reviewing the arguments for and against detubularization, the one thing with which all agree is that by reconfiguring the bowel the volume initially achieved is increased. Others suggest that continence is improved. In general, the pressure waves are 10 to 20 cm higher when a tubular structure is maintained as opposed to a detubularized structure. However, it should be pointed out that over a period of time coordinated intestinal contractions do occur even though the segment has been detubularized. The trade-off is a higher incidence of retention in the detubularized segment as opposed to the tubularized segment. In one study the incidence of flaccidity following reconstruction occurred in no patients in whom a tubular segment was utilized and occurred in one quarter of patients in whom the segment was detubularized.

REFERENCES

1. McDougal WS: Metabolic complications of urinary intestinal diversion. J Urol 1992; 147:1199–1208.
2. McDougal WS, Stampfer DS, Kirley S, et al: Intestinal ammonium transport by the sodium hydrogen exchanger. J Am Coll Surg 1995; 181:241–248.
3. Webster GD, Goldwasser B (eds): Urinary Diversion. Oxford, Isis Medical Media, 1995.

24

ORTHOTOPIC BLADDER SUBSTITUTION IN THE MALE AND FEMALE

RICHARD E. HAUTMANN, M.D.

The evolution of urinary diversion has been remarkable, especially during the last decade. At the 4th International Consensus Conference on Bladder Cancer, the consensus was that in the properly selected male bladder cancer patient orthotopic bladder reconstruction to the urethra is the procedure of choice.[1] This recommendation has meanwhile been extended to female patients.[2,3]

Bladder replacement by a variety of small and large bowel segments has become the standard method of re-establishing voiding per urethram. Currently, we are witnessing a change from the use of ileal conduit as well as stomal continent urinary diversions to the increasing frequent use of replacement cystoplasties.

The primary goal of bladder replacement procedures is not to improve survival, impact on cancer prognosis, or decrease renal and metabolic complications but rather an attempt to improve the quality of life. The ultimate degree of success is translated mostly into continence status. Normal micturition and reliable continence are, indeed, the ideals shared by patients and reconstructive urologic surgeons. During the last 10 years, we have witnessed a remarkable resurgence of enthusiasm in orthotopic urinary reconstruction in patients undergoing radical cystectomy for bladder cancer. As a result, the ileum conduit will be reserved for poor-risk candidates or those who are not motivated for continent diversion.

INDICATIONS AND CONTRAINDICATIONS FOR BLADDER SUBSTITUTION IN THE ERA OF ORTHOTOPIC BLADDER REPLACEMENT

In general, anyone who is a surgical candidate for cystectomy is a potential candidate for orthotopic bladder substitution. Currently, at selected urologic centers up to 90% of male patients requiring cystectomy and up to 75% of women undergoing cystectomy for transitional cell carcinoma of the bladder may be appropriate candidates for orthotopic lower urinary tract reconstruction.

Absolute Contraindications

Compromised renal function due to long-standing obstruction or chronic renal failure with serum creatinine greater than or equal to 1.5 to 2.0 mg% are usually considered contraindications to bladder substitution. However, some patients with significant creatinine elevations due to primary bladder cancer can recover sufficient function to allow bladder replacement once the obstruction is relieved. A percutaneous nephrostomy placed before surgery may give a better indication of the true renal function.

Patients with compromised intestinal function, particularly inflammatory bowel disease, may be better helped by a conduit. Prior radiation therapy or chronologic age should not be considered a contraindication to orthotopic reconstruction. Elderly patients without good home help or support are probably better off managing an external appliance. Thick or fat abdominal walls also have difficulty in maintaining an external appliance. These patients may be best managed by lower urinary tract reconstruction in males and females.

Contraindications to this procedure exist in all patients who are candidates for simultaneous urethrectomy based on their primary tumor. The true risk of urethral recurrence in these patients has recently been defined by Stein et al.[4] in the female.

The Risk of Urethral Tumors in Female Bladder Cancer

Incidence, clinical significance, and risk factors for urethral recurrences in men with transitional cell carcinoma of the bladder are well understood. Little is known about urethral recurrences in women with bladder cancer. Reasons include: (1) women have a lower incidence of transitional cell carcinoma of the bladder; (2) routine urethrectomy is performed in women undergoing cystectomy; and (3) before the advent of bladder replacement study of the urethra may not have added any significant information, since it was entirely removed. However, with increasing interest in orthotopic reconstruction in women following cystectomy for carcinoma of the bladder, detailed knowledge of the retained urethra becomes significant in terms of cancer and reconstructive surgery. In a retrospective study with a pathologic review of female cystectomy specimens, Stein et al. showed that all patients with carcinoma involving the urethra had concomitant evidence of carcinoma involving the bladder neck.[4] Those with an uninvolved bladder neck also had an uninvolved urethra. The association between the presence of tumor in the bladder neck and the urethra was highly significant. Tumor involving the bladder neck and urethra tended to be more commonly associated with high-grade and high-stage tumors, and node-positive disease. Consequently, the detection of tumor in the bladder neck is a sensitive and specific measure of urethral involvement, and could have significant impact on the decision to perform orthotopic reconstruction in women after cystectomy. In addition to bladder neck involvement, Stein et al. found that anterior vaginal wall involvement by tumor is another major risk factor for urethral involvement. Patients with tumor extending into the anterior vaginal wall also had bladder neck involvement and 50% of these specimens had urethral involvement as well.[4]

Urethral Recurrence in Male Patients with Ileal Neobladders

Increasing interest in ileal neobladders and in preserving sexual potency after radical cystectomy for transitional cell carcinoma of the bladder has emphasized the need to identify accurately those men who are at high risk for urethral recurrences. In a large study, Freeman et al.[5] compared urethral recurrence between patients who underwent cutaneous urinary diversion and patients who underwent Kock ureteroileal urethrectomy. Kaplan-Meier estimates of time to recurrence were plotted, and the log rank test for censored data was used to test for statistical significance. The probability of urethral recurrence at 5 years is 12% in the cutaneous diversion group and 5% in the Kock urethrostomy group. The 5-year probability of urethral recurrence with carcinoma in situ is 12.7% in the cutaneous diversion group and 4% in the Kock urethrostomy group. Of the patients with prostatic invasion, 25% in the cutaneous diversion group recurred, whereas none in the Kock urethrostomy group has recurred. These results indicate that reconstruction to the urethra following cystectomy for transitional cell cancer is associated with a lower risk of urethral recurrence and that patients with a high risk (Tis and pT4a) may safely be followed with physical examination, urethral cytology, and, if indicated, urethroscopy. Patients with cutaneous diversion and high-risk pathology should undergo prophylactic urethrectomy.

Our indication for orthotopic bladder replacement in Ulm is relatively generous: only when the frozen section of the distal urethral margin is not clear do we refrain from orthotopic bladder replacement in both sexes.

Relative Contraindications

Controversy exists in patients with multifocal, high-grade transitional cell carcinoma and those with multifocal carcinoma in situ.

The presence of positive lymph nodes causes a dilemma. Some investigators feel these patients should not undergo lower urinary tract reconstruction of any type because of short survival and a high incidence of pelvic recurrence. However, recent comprehensive studies of node-positive patients reveal a 30% 5-year survival in several studies.[1] In addition, there is a psychologically damaging stigma to the patient who enters surgery expecting lower urinary tract reconstruction but awakens with a stoma. Unless the tumor directly involves the urogenital diaphragma or the distal urethral margin is positive, lower urinary tract reconstruction can be performed with anticipated good results under palliative intention. However, the patients should be informed that diversion to the skin by an ileal conduit may be necessary due to unexpected tumor extent and there should be an appropriate stoma site marked on the abdominal wall before entering surgery. Age per se should not be an important criterion against lower urinary tract reconstruction. Elderly patients, as part of their informed consent, need to be aware that they may have a greater chance of enuresis or nocturnal incontinence than younger men, but age by itself should not be a contraindication.

Prior radiation therapy does not appear to be a contraindication if the external sphincter mechanism remains intact. In our patients, the postoperative course including hospital stay, perioperative complications, and early functional results did not differ from the nonirradiated patients. There was no perioperative mortality. For patients who underwent combined external and afterloading radiotherapy the indication for orthotopic bladder replacement should be considered critically.

External sphincter dysfunction is a relative contraindication unless simultaneous placement of an artificial sphincter is considered. Patients with significant benign urethral disease, such as recurrent urethral strictures, are probably better managed by diversions to the skin.

TECHNICAL CONSIDERATIONS

Basic Principles, Physics, Mathematics, and Hydraulics

Before a discussion of the functioning of neobladders as high-compliance, low-pressure, continent, nonrefluxing reservoirs allowing for an adequate capacity and preservation of the upper urinary tract, a certain number of basic principles related to physics, mathematics, and hydraulics of various shapes of closed structures should be reviewed. The ideal principles of a neobladder, including configuration, accommodation, viscoelasticity, and contractility have been comprehensively reviewed by Hinman in 1988.[6]

The interested reader is referred to the excellent review article by Martins et al.[7] Configuration determines geometric capacity:

$$\text{Volume} = \text{height} \times \text{radius}^2 \times \pi$$

Accommodation relates pressure and volume to mural tension (law of Laplace); viscoelasticity (compliance) depends on the physical characteristics of the wall and contractility depends on the motor functions of the bowel. The concepts of geometric capacity of a reservoir, and detubularization and rearrangement of a bowel segment leading to volume duplication and consequently greater capacity, have markedly added to our understanding and improvement of the mechanical properties and functional behavior of neobladders.

The law of Laplace states that:

$$T = P \times r$$

where T = wall tension, P = pressure, and r = radius. Knowing that as reservoir capacity and radius increase, wall tension increases in proportion. However, reservoir pressure remains constant until the elastic limits of the wall are reached. ($P = h/r^2$, where h = height). An enlarged reservoir will accommodate larger volumes at pressures identical to those in smaller reservoirs but with generation of a higher wall tension. Another important physical concept is the interrelationship among resistance, pressure, and flow as stated in the equation:

$$R = P/F$$

For the neobladder outlet, flow across the continence zone is intended to be zero. Unlike theoretical models, the pressure generated by biologic models is opposed by only finite resistance. Thus continence cannot be an absolute achievement. How do these principles fit in the behavior of biologic models?

The crucial improvement accomplished by a folded, detubularized spherical shaped reservoir lies in the larger diameter, greater capacity with significantly lower internal pressure and the absence of coordinated contraction of its wall, generated early during bladder filling. Lower pressure within the reservoir allows for the achievement of a better degree of resistance across the continence zone, resulting in improved dryness.

Based on a theoretical in-depth analysis of mathematical models, Colding-Jörgensen et al.[8] concluded that spherical reservoirs will produce half of the pressure produced by a cylindric reservoir for the same wall tension allowing for generation of higher expansile forces with a lesser degree of elastic recoil or coordinated contractions by the wall.[8]

The clinical and urodynamic success of any orthotopic bladder replacement is associated with reservoir geometry. The bowel segments are opened along the antimesenteric border and remodeled into various shapes, such as U, S, or W. These different reservoir shapes produce different relationships among length of bowel, radius, and volume. Furthermore, it becomes apparent that the relationship between volume and length is curved for the spherical but linear for the nonspherical reservoirs (Fig. 24–1). Undoubtedly, the more spherical (detubularized) and composite the reservoir, the better its accommodating capacity in response to

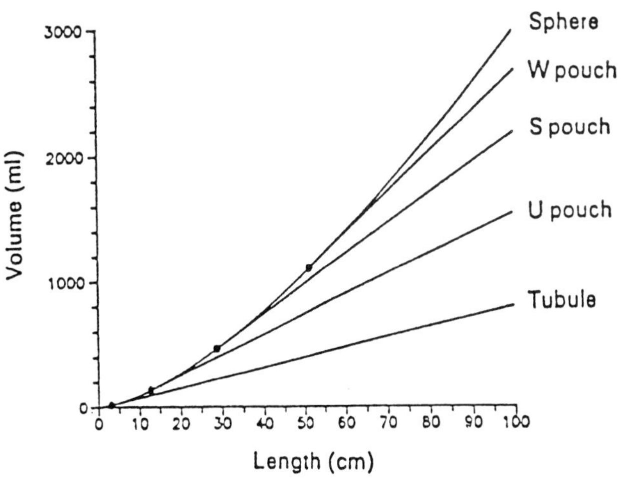
Sphere
W pouch
S pouch
U pouch
Tubule
Volume (ml)
3000
2000
1000
0
0
10
20
30
40
50
60
70
80
90
100
Length (cm)

FIGURE 24–1. Volumes of different types of ileal reservoirs each calculated as a function of length of bowel used for construction. (From Colding-Jörgensen M, Poulsen AL, Steven K: Mechanical characteristics of tubular and detubularized bowel for bladder substitution: theory, urodynamics and clinical results. Br J Urol 1993; 72:586 and Blackwell Science Ltd, with permission.)

increasing volumes, which will be reflected by the resultant pressure increase. Advantages of detubularization consist of a delay in the onset and a decrease of the magnitude of the pressure increase caused by segmental reservoir contractions, higher volumes at lower pressures, and improved nocturnal continence. A relative drawback is the need for a pressure to aid neobladder emptying, which may predispose both to residual urine, thus the need for intermittent catheterization. Overdistention of the neobladder should be avoided, since it potentially leads to urinary retention and ultimately to upper tract dilatation. The knowledge of these concepts and principles has enabled us to understand better the clinical and urodynamic features of neobladders.

Detubularization using the laws of physics is the key to the construction of a quiet, low-pressure reservoir. To date, the ileum has been the most widely utilized segment of bowel for lower urinary tract reconstruction, but acceptable results have been reported using the ileocecal segment, right colon, and sigmoid colon. The ileal neobladder developed by Hautmann and modified by others uses approximately 60 to 65 cm of ileum; the ileal reservoir developed by Kock and modified by Skinner uses approximately 70 to 80 cm of ileum; the Mainz reservoir and other variations use the terminal ileum and various lengths of colon, in some cases up to the middle colic artery.[9–11] Sigmoid reservoirs require approximately 40 to 50 cm of sigmoid with or without ileal patches for detubularization. Gastric pouches do not use small bowel but have generally been used in bladder augmentation only since construction of a reservoir of suitable size totally from stomach is difficult.

It must be pointed out at this point that for all types of reservoirs detubularization remains the key to success. The theoretical results are consistent with clinical observations showing that detubularization increases reservoir capacity substantially, delays the onset, and reduces the amplitude of the pressure rise produced by contractions. These findings account for the markedly improved nocturnal continence rates (see below), the longer voiding intervals, and the predisposition to urinary retention with detubularized bladder substitutes. Altering the shape of a reservoir from spherical to ellipsoid causes only a slight effect on its mechanical characteristics. Consequently, the essence of detubularization is to create a reservoir of high capacity, while shape is of secondary importance. This interrelationship is demonstrated in Figure 24–2, where nocturnal enuresis (one or more voids per night) is plotted versus geometric capacity. Since all types of reservoirs plotted are double-folded, geometric capacity in this case corresponds to the length of the gut segment used for reservoir construction.

The dilemma with the reservoir stems from the fact that all the authors of 45 modifications of reservoirs claim the same success figures as far as continence is concerned. This is absolutely incorrect! Daytime continence is of no concern. Even substitution with closed tubular bowel segments allows normal micturition and reliable daytime continence but results invariably in nighttime incontinence. Some degree of nocturnal leakage is a consistent finding in most reports even despite a technically sound operation. Nevertheless, as outlined in Figure 24–2, nocturnal incontinence varies greatly between the different types of reservoirs and frankly spoken is *the* difference between the available types of reservoirs. Nocturnal incontinence is caused by peristaltic contractions occurring at an early stage during filling. The reduced level of consciousness during sleep makes it impossible to increase the

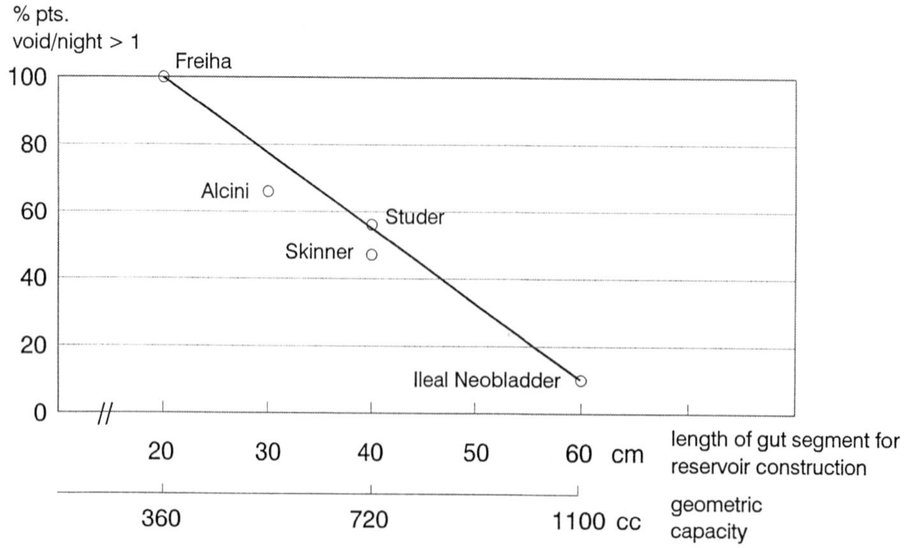
% pts.
void/night > 1
Freiha
Alcini
Studer
Skinner
Ileal Neobladder
100
80
60
40
20
0
20
30
40
50
60 cm
length of gut segment for reservoir construction
360
720
1100 cc
geometric capacity

FIGURE 24–2. Percentage of patients that void once or more per night as an estimate of nocturnal enuresis versus geometric capacity of the reservoir. Continence rate improves linear to the increase in geometric capacity. (Data from Studer et al.,[30] Flohr et al.,[32] Elmajian et al.,[36] Alcini et al.,[37] and Freiha.[38])

urethral closing pressure in response to these contractions. Furthermore, the capacity of tubular bowel substitutes or even detubularized reservoirs constructed from gut segments shorter than 60 cm in length is insufficient to store the overnight urine production, resulting in overflow incontinence, even in the absence of contractions. It is, however, proven (Figs. 24–1 and 24–2) that bladder substitution using perfectly detubularized bowel has an improved nighttime continence.

FUNCTIONAL/URODYNAMIC DATA OF RESERVOIRS CONSTRUCTED FROM DIFFERENT GUT SEGMENTS

Until recently there was no agreement as to which is the ideal form of orthotopic bladder replacement, either in terms of surgical technique or type of bowel segment used. Indeed, the gastrointestinal point of view does not favor a gut segment over the other. However, the urodynamic point of view in terms of bowel compliance favors the small bowel as shown by most urodynamic studies.[12] In a comparative study, Koraitim et al. compared the volume and pressure changes with time in detubularized and nondetubularized neobladders constructed from an intact ileocecal segment, detubularized sigmoid, and detubularized ileum. With time, the capacity of the neobladder increased in all three groups. Concomitantly, while intact ileocecal bladders showed an increase in intrareservoir pressure and persistence of involuntary contractions, detubularized sigmoid and ileal bladders showed a decrease in intrareservoir pressure and involuntary contractions. Detubularized intestinal neobladders not only offer a high-capacity, low-pressure, high-compliance reservoir but these characteristics also are increased with time.[13] An excellent overview on urodynamic characteristics of orthotopic reservoirs has recently been presented by Martins et al.[7]

ORTHOTOPIC ILEAL RESERVOIR CONSTRUCTION (ILEAL NEOBLADDER)

Most pioneering procedures described for bladder replacement incorporate small bowel segments exclusively. We believe that the ileal neobladder almost ideally covers the most salient technical features described above and that advantages and disadvantages of the most commonly used neobladders can be compared with this technique. The ileal neobladder consists of a completely detubularized, low-pressure, high-capacity and highly compliant urinary reservoir made up of reconfigured ileum. An ileal segment 60 to 70 cm long and 15 cm proximal to the ileocecal valve is completely detubularized while preserving the area chosen for the ileourethral anastomosis. The bowel segment is then refashioned in a W or M shape, connecting its

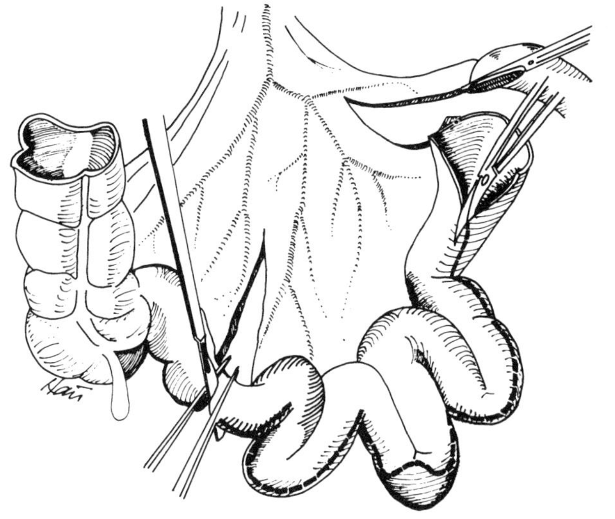

FIGURE 24–3. Operative technique for ileal neobladder. Selection of ileal segment with appropriate vascular supply and antimesenteric splitting of ileum are shown, except for U-shaped flap, when ileourethral anastomosis is planned.

antimesenteric borders with 3-0 polyglycolic acid running sutures. An orifice of approximately the size of a fingertip is then created at the bottom of the U-shaped flap where the ileourethral anastomotic site has been previously selected. A 22-French Foley catheter is placed through it and the ileourethral anastomosis is completed by tying the six sutures placed previously at the urethral remnant, leaving the knots on the inside of the reservoir. The ureters are sutured into the posterior aspect of the reservoir using the nonrefluxing technique of Le Duc. The bowel plate is then closed as a sphere[14–19] (Figs. 24–3 to 24–6).

PRESERVING THE EXTERNAL SPHINCTER MECHANISM IN THE MALE

Continence is determined by sphincteric competence and reservoir behavior. In the male population the absolute precondition for successful orthotopic bladder replacement is experience with radical prostatectomy—in other words, experience with the approach to the membranous urethra, the external sphincter mechanism, and the pelvic floor. This factor depends largely on the urethral preparation, the maintenance of the innervation of the urogenital diaphragm, and the external sphincter mechanism. There is no doubt that the entire prostate should be removed and that the urethra, on the other hand, must be prepared as carefully as in radical prostatectomy. The smooth muscle component receives parasympathetic, cholinergic, and sympathetic noradrenergic nerves with predominance of the latter. The striated muscle component incorporates fast- and slow-twitch fibers, with the latter predominating. The innervation of this muscle component includes the pelvic nerve, pudendal

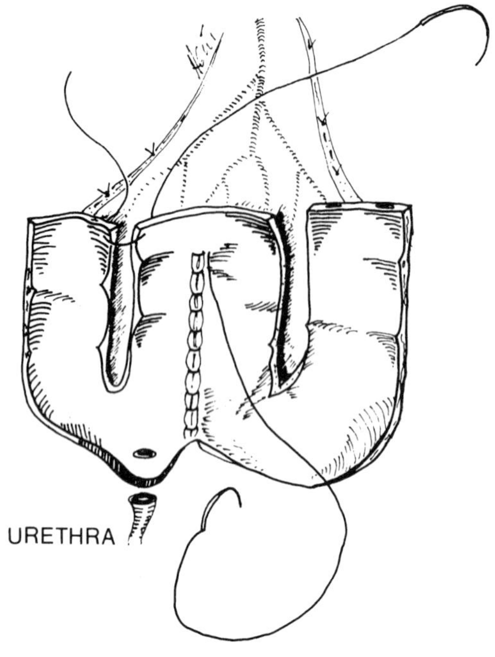
URETHRA

FIGURE 24–4. Creation of ileal sheet by side-to-side anastomosis of in-sized ileum following arrangement in W-shape. Note position of U-shaped flap for ileourethral anastomosis.

nerve, and a combination of autonomic and somatic nerves; that is, a triple innervation. In the male population this important part of the operation consists of the following steps:

1. The superficial dorsal vein is ligated.
2. The puboprostatic ligaments are partly divided to include only the portion that inserts on the prostate—most of the ligament can be left intact.
3. The avascular triangle between membranous urethra, pelvic floor, and venous complex is perforated using a right-angle clamp above the membranous urethra way down to the pelvic floor without jeopardizing the external sphincter mechanism. This step of the operation is critical and must always be done without bleeding (Fig. 24–7).
4. The dorsal vein complex is ligated and transected. This provides ideal exposure of apex and membranous urethra. The anterior half of the urethra is now opened just distal to the apex, the catheter is lifted, grasped with two Kocher clamps, and cut.
5. By gentle traction on the two catheter segments the anastomotic stitches are placed at the 1-, 3-, 9-, and 11-o'clock positions, respectively, including the periurethral tissue.
6. A right-angle clamp is placed under the dorsal urethra including Denonvilliers' fascia. The posterior wall of the urethra is now easily and safely divided close to the prostate.
7. The remainder of the operation is essentially as described by others.

APPROACH TO THE FEMALE URETHRA

When considering female patients for orthotopic lower urinary tract reconstruction three important criteria must be fulfilled:

1. The external sphincter mechanism must remain intact to provide continence and allow for volitional voiding per urethram.
2. Urethral support and pelvic floor undoubtedly play an important role in the urinary continence mechanism and must remain intact.
3. Cancer surgery must not be compromised by orthotopic reconstruction at the ileourethral anastomosis, retained urethra, or at the surgical margins.

If these criteria can be safely guaranteed, the patient may be considered an appropriate candidate for orthotopic lower urinary tract reconstruction.

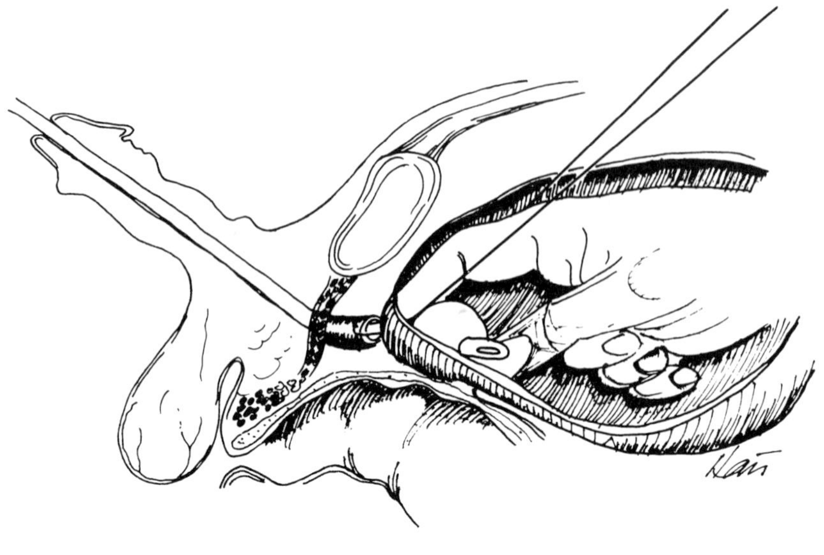

FIGURE 24–5. Anastomosis of ileal sheet to urethral remnant with six mattress sutures tied from inside neobladder (sagittal view of anastomosis).

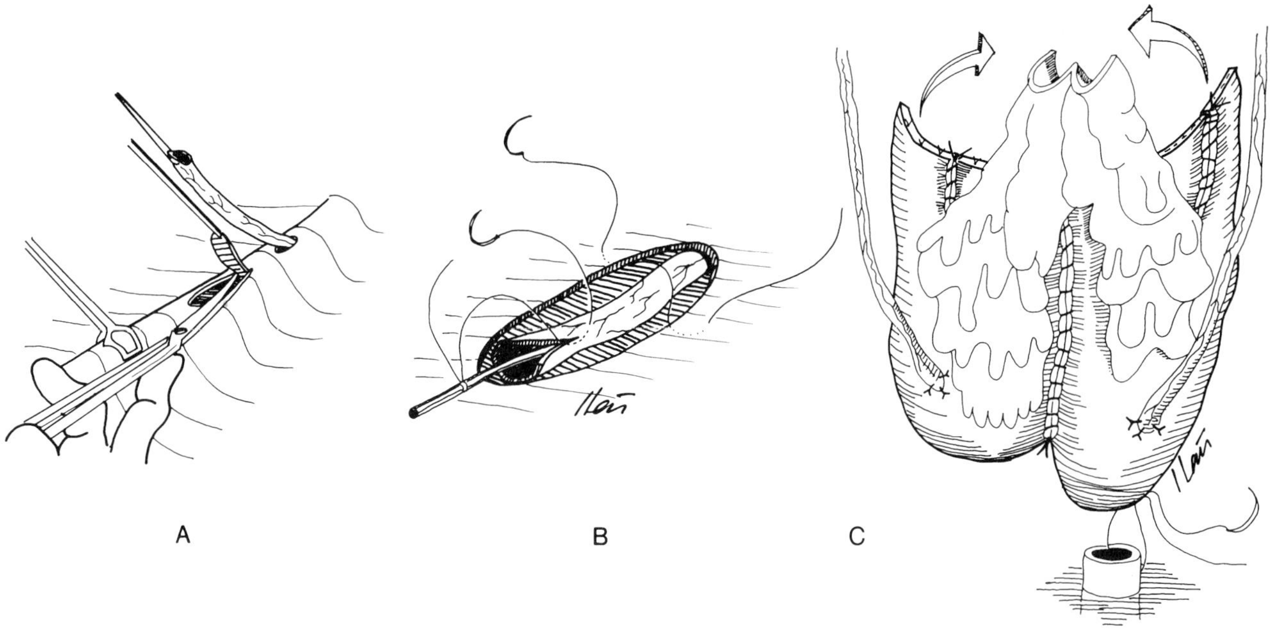
A
B
C

FIGURE 24–6. Ureteroileal anastomosis. *A*, The ureter is pulled through a small incision in the ileal wall at a convenient site. The mucosa is incised to create a sulcus approximately 3 cm long. *B*, The ureter is spatulated and fixed to the ileal wall with two sutures. The ileal mucosa is then closed above the ureter by two or three sutures. A 7-French ureteral catheter is placed and secured by a 4-0 plain catgut suture. *C*, Posterior view of the ureteroileal anastomosis. Note that both the ureters are implanted in the lateral segment of the W.

External Sphincter Mechanism

In the proximal two thirds of the urethra, three layers of smooth muscle can be identified. The innervation of this proximal urethral segment can be traced back to the pelvic plexus running along the lateral aspects of the uterus, vagina, and bladder neck. A gradual transition with intermingling smooth muscle to striated muscle can be identified in the midportion to lower third of the urethra. The striated muscle (rhabdosphincter) has its major portion on the ventral aspect of the urethra in the classic omega shape, with its innervation from the pudendal nerve that runs below the pelvic floor and is not at risk during surgery. Preservation of the musculature at the lower two thirds of the urethra together with a nerve supply potentially are of significance for urinary continence in females.[2]

Urethral Support

The position of the vesical neck is not static but mobile. Its support depends upon connections of the urethrovaginal endopelvic fascia to the medial aspects of the levator ani. In addition, these fasciae are attached to the arcus tendineus fasciae pelvis, which supports the urethra during levator relaxation, and probably during stress. Levator contraction supports the proximal urethra and also pulls the vesical neck anteriorly against a band of endopelvic fascia that is suspended between the arcus tendineus, compressing it closed. Relaxation of the muscles allows the vesical neck to descend and facilitates its opening.[20]

Oncologic Aspects

Although the fate of the retained urethra following cystectomy for bladder cancer in women is un-

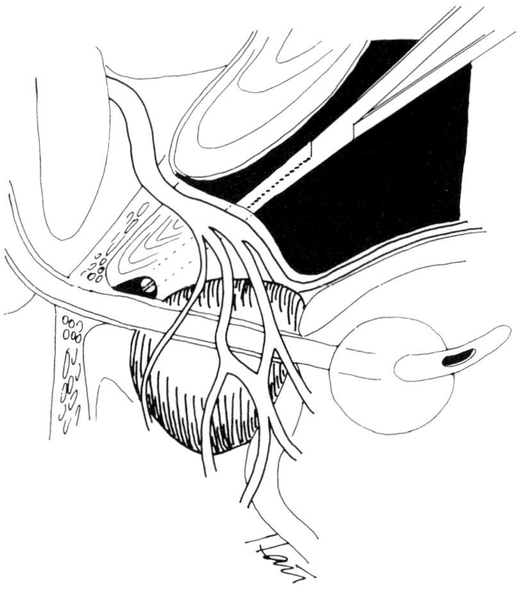

FIGURE 24–7. Avascular triangle between membranous urethra, pelvic floor, and dorsal vein complex is perforated way down to the pelvic floor without jeopardizing the external sphincter mechanism.

known, the results of Stein et al. show that women with transitional cell carcinoma of the bladder without evidence of tumor involving the bladder neck are at low risk for urethral malignancy.[4,21] All patients with carcinoma involving the urethra had concomitant evidence of carcinoma involving the bladder neck. Those with an uninvolved bladder neck also had an uninvolved urethra. The association between the presence of tumor in the bladder neck and urethra was highly significant. Tumors involving the bladder neck and urethra tended to be more commonly associated with high-grade, high-stage tumors and node-positive disease. Patients with a noninvolved urethra may be offered lower urinary tract reconstruction that includes preservation of and diversion through the urethra.

Variations of Surgical Technique for Female Cystectomy[22]

Nerve fibers from the pelvic plexus run along the lateral walls of the vagina to bladder neck and urethra. Standard anterior exenteration and en bloc lymphadenectomy result in transection of most if not all the autonomic nerves to the urethra in women. However, if the entire vagina (or at least the lateral walls of it) remains intact, the majority of plexus fibers to the urethra and the entire urethral support can be preserved. In a modified pelvic lymphadenectomy, dissection of the region of the upper hypogastric nerve where it crosses the common iliac artery must be minimized. Following the mobilization of the ovaries, tubes, and uterus, the ligation and division of the cardinal ligaments is performed. The cervix can be easily palpated so that a circumferential incision can be made into the vagina. To help identify the vagina, it should be packed with sponges. Usually, the cleavage plane between anterior vaginal wall and bladder can be entered easily. Once the posterior dissection is almost completed, the anterior dissection of the bladder neck and the proximal urethra is commenced and is analogous to the dissection in the male. Ligation and division of the dorsal vein complex is done. The endopelvic fascia is incised immediately lateral to the posterior urethra at the urethrovesical junction (Fig. 24–8). As much as possible of the urethropelvic ligament and paraurethral vascular and nerve plexus must be saved. The urethrovesical junction and the proximal urethra are dissected off the anterior vaginal wall and down to the posterior bladder wall until the posterior dissection plane has been reached (Fig. 24–9). The next step of the operation transects the inferior pedicles of the bladder. The nerve fibers leading to the bladder must be transected, but the fibers towards vagina and urethra are left untouched (Figs. 24–10 and 24–11). As the proximal urethra or urethrovesical junction is transected, six interrupted 2-0 polyglycolic acid sutures are placed circumferentially in the urethra.

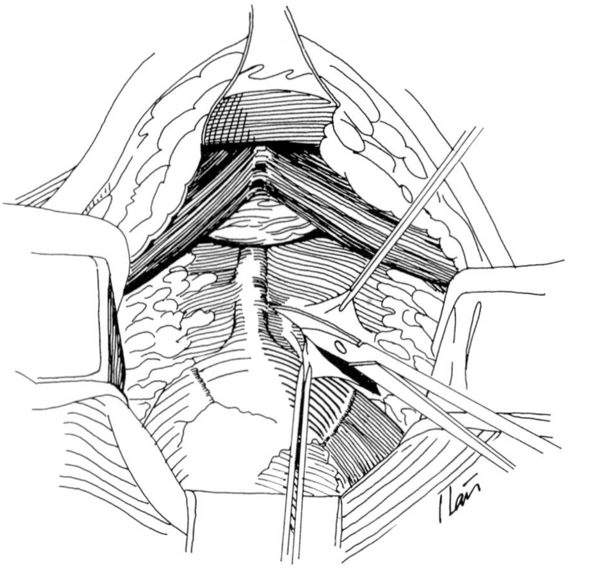

FIGURE 24–8. Nerve-sparing cystectomy in women. Incision of endopelvic fascia is parallel to posterior urethra and urethrovesical junction.

Frozen sections for pathologic examination are taken from the transected end of the urethra/bladder neck to identify overt carcinoma, which would result in subsequent urethrectomy.

ILEOURETERAL MANAGEMENT

Controversy continues as to the optimal ileoureteral management. Is reflux prevention necessary

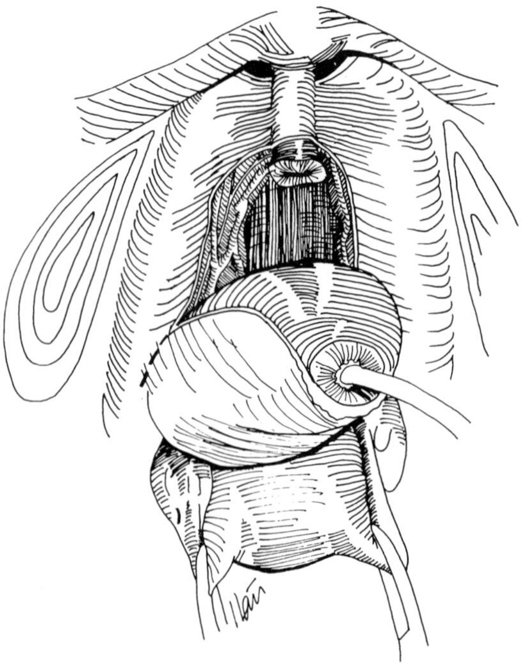

FIGURE 24–9. Transection of posterior urethra. Bladder neck is carefully dissected off anterior vaginal wall. Autonomic fibers are particularly at risk at urethrovesical junction.

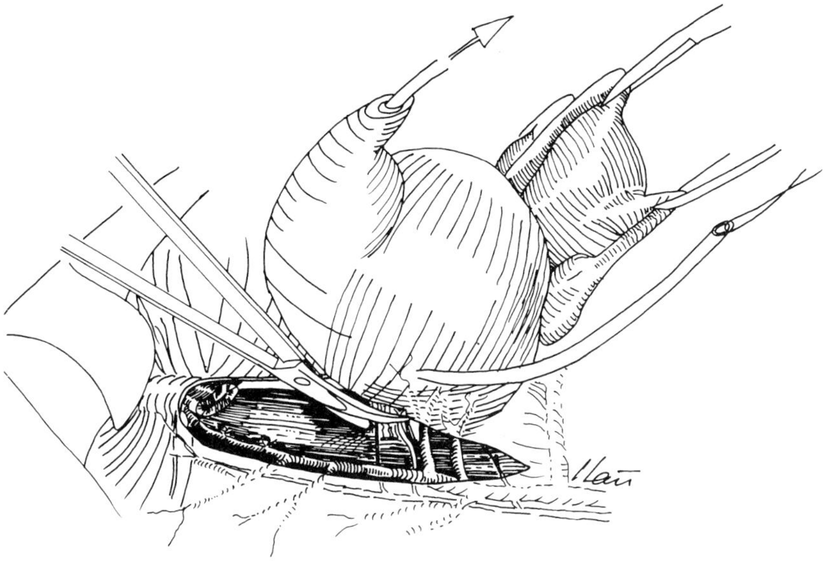

FIGURE 24–10. Upward traction of specimen facilitates dissection between lateral bladder wall and vascular plexus. Autonomic nerve fibers run lateral to vascular plexus. Nerve fibers leading to bladder that run between perivesical plexus must be transected. Fibers traveling parallel to pelvic viscera down towards vagina and urethra are saved.

and/or desirable in the light of low-pressure intestinal reservoirs without major coordinated contractile activity?

In contrast to the danger of renal function deterioration from reflux in patients with an ileal conduit or neuropathic voiding dysfunction associated with intermittent, high-intravesical-pressure peaks, this issue of detubularized low-pressure intestinal neobladders remains an open question to date. It well may be that the late stenosis rate from the various antireflux techniques may outweigh their theoretical advantage. Short-term results appear comparable, but it must be remembered that renal deterioration in patients diverted by an ileal conduit with refluxing ureteroileal anastomoses were seldom seen until patients were followed for at least 5 to 10 years. All the reported antireflux techniques are effective, but the tunnel techniques may have a higher incidence of late stenosis than the direct ureteroileal anastomoses protected by a nipple valve to prevent reflux. Table 24–1 gives an overview of reflux and obstruction rates of ureterointestinal anastomoses in the different types of neobladders.[14] Apparently, surgical experience plays a major role. In all the large series irrespective of the type of ureteroileal anastomosis used the complication rates are surprisingly low, while in smaller series where the learning curve is reflected, complications with the ileoureteral anastomoses tend to be significantly higher. The intussuscepted afferent nipple valve mechanism Skinner is using is a reproducible, highly effective antireflux mechanism preventing pyelonephritis in more than 95% of the patients with only a 3% stenosis rate of the ureteroileal anastomosis.[23] Studer, in his large series, is using a tubularized isoperistaltic afferent ileal loop.[30] With almost 400 cases of ileal neobladder, the Hautmann group is using the original Le Duc technique and reports an obstruction rate of the ureterointestinal anastomoses in the same range.[31] Just recently, Sagalowski reported on the split-cuff-nipple technique of ureteroenteric anastomosis as a versatile addition to the armamentarium for many forms of urinary diversion, including orthotopic bladder replacement.[32] The primary essential feature for any successful method clearly is a low rate of obstruction at the ureteroenteric anastomosis. All of these results are excellent and justify continued application of this technique. Enthusiasm must, however, be tempered by the modest number of cases and duration of follow-up to date. Clearly, long-term follow-up in a larger number of cases is necessary to establish the value of the procedure compared to all the other forms of ureteral implantation in urinary diversion. It will be interesting to see long-term data and the clinical experience of the ileal W-neobladder using the serous-lined extramural ureteroileal implantation technique as described by Abol-Enein and Ghoneim.[33] This serous-lined extramural ureteroileal implantation technique is technically simple, suitable for normal and dilated ureters, saves the use of an extra bowel segment, allows nonobstructed unidirectional urine flow, and the use of staples is not required. Furthermore, all the retrograde endoscopic manipulations including ureteroscopy are feasible.

COMPLICATIONS

An excellent overview of complications of continent cutaneous reservoirs and neobladders using contemporary techniques has been presented by Rowland recently.[34] The data for his comparison have been obtained from the two large series, which are approaching 400 patients from Ulm and Los Angeles.

Experience from the series from Bern and from a combined Lund group (Mansson/Goldwasser) has

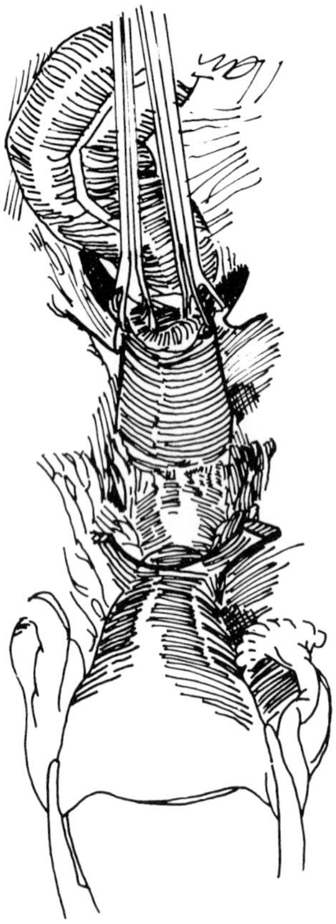

FIGURE 24–11. Uterosacral ligaments on both sides are divided. Edges of transverse incision in posterior fornix of vagina are held under gentle traction with Allis clamps. Posterior bladder wall is dissected off anterior vaginal wall down to bladder neck. Autonomic nerve fibers (inferior hypogastric plexus), which run laterally to vessels, are separated from lateral wall of bladder and vagina.

been added. In each series, patients have been followed for a minimum of 2 years after their procedure. Complications are reported as major early, if they occurred within 30 days of the procedure and either prolonged hospitalization or necessitated an interventional procedure. These were subdivided into those related to formation of the reservoir or neobladder and those that were not related to the formation of the reservoir or neobladder. Major "late" complications were reported in the same manner for all complications related to reservoir or neobladder formation and those not related to reservoir or neobladder formation.

During the first postoperative month, 2.6% of the patients experienced neobladder leaks but only 0.4% required surgical treatment. Another 2.6% had ureteral obstruction; 0.2% required open surgery, while 2.0% were treated endoscopically; 0.4% developed neobladder urethral strictures, which were treated endoscopically; and a total of 6.4% had an episode of pyelonephritis.

Major early complications not related to the neobladder included 3.0% with wound infections; 1.1% required surgical drainage; and 0.2% had percutaneous drainage of an abscess. Prolonged reduction of the gastrointestinal function of 7 days or more occurred in 12.7% of the patients; 2.0% required surgical treatment for bowel obstruction; and 0.7% had gastrointestinal bleeding. A pulmonary embolism was diagnosed in 1.5% of the patients.

Major late complications related to the reservoir included hypertonic bowel requiring surgical correction in 0.2% of the patients, ureteral obstruction in 12.2% of patients, with 3.1% requiring open surgery and 2.0% requiring endoscopic treatment, and neobladder-urethral strictures in 5.2% with 3.0% requiring surgical or endoscopic intervention. A total of 2.8% of the patients experienced an episode of acute pyelonephritis.

Major late complications not related to neobladder construction included 3.9% of patients with wound hernias, 1.5% of the patients with small bowel obstruction, and 3% of patients with deteriorating renal function; 2.4% of the patients had pulmonary embolism; and 1.1% required surgery for some other reason.

The four series of patients had a reoperation rate of 2.8% for major early complications related to neobladder formation and 4.0% for complications not related to the neobladder. The total early reoperation rate was 6.8%.

TABLE 24–1. REFLUX AND OBSTRUCTION RATES OF URETEROINTESTINAL ANASTOMOSIS IN THE DIFFERENT TYPES OF NEOBLADDERS

Type of Neobladder	Type of Ureterointestinal Anastomosis	Reflux	Obstruction
Ileal reservoirs			
Ileal neobladder[17]	Le Duc (pseudotunnel)	2%	4%
Urethral Kock[23]	Intussuscepted ileal nipple valve	0%	3%
Ileal bladder substitute[24]	Tubularized isoperistaltic, afferent ileal loop	0%	2%
Remodeled ileocolonic reservoirs			
Orthotopic Mainz[25]	Submucosal tunnel	2%	2%
Le Bag pouch[26]	—	—	—
Colonic reservoirs			
Detubularized right colon			
Goldwasser et al.[27]	Submucosal tunnel/Le Duc	0%	2/5%
Mansson and Colleen[28]	Le Duc (pseudotunnel)	0%	2%
Sigmoid neobladder[29]	Submucosal tunnel	4%	4%

The late reoperation rates for complications related to the neobladder and those not related to the neobladder were 9.5 and 3.0%, respectively. The total late reoperation rate was 12.5%. The grand total reoperation rate for the neobladder series was 19.3%.

Of particular interest is the question after the risk of bowel dysfunction with diarrhea after continent urinary diversion. Most studies suggest that the risk of bowel dysfunction with diarrhea following resection of an ileocecal segment is twice as high as after ileal resection alone. However, almost all patients respond well to symptomatic therapy with cholestyramine or loperamide. Therefore, it is our belief that diarrhea is an acceptable risk in patients undergoing orthotopic bladder replacement with ileal or ileocecal segments and should not be an excluding factor in the decision for this type of operation. Nevertheless, patients must be informed that chronic diarrhea may be a sequela of the operation. Ileal segments would appear preferable for orthotopic bladder substitution due to the increased risk of chronic diarrhea following ileocecal resection.

Although the technique for orthotopic bladder replacement is still evolving, these procedures can be performed on properly selected patients with acceptable complication rates. The neobladder reoperation rate of 19.3% compares favorably to the exceedingly high reoperation rate of the continent urinary reservoirs mainly because of the unacceptably high reoperation rate of the intussuscepted nipple valve (efferent valve).

In the Ulm experience, one third of our patients at 10-year follow-up are absolutely trouble-free. One third of our patients undergo minor complications with no need for a prolonged hospital stay or readmission to the hospital during the postoperative follow-up. The type of complications to be included into this group is prolonged reduction of the gastrointestinal function in the immediate postoperative course in up to 20% of the patients and some form of metabolic disease in minor form (see below). One third of our patients during the 10-year follow-up undergo open or endoscopic surgery for some form of complication, mainly of an infectious nature or obstruction in the ileoureteral or ileourethral anastomosis.

Evolution based on clinical experience will probably reduce the complication rates further yet. Certainly, the neobladder reoperation rates have always reached reoperation rates of noncontinent urinary diversion series.

CONTINENCE IN THE MALE

As mentioned above, continence is determined by sphincteric competence and reservoir behavior. Reporting of continence in men and women undergoing lower urinary tract reconstruction remains a considerable problem, since most authors accept significant leakage volumes, find excuses for nocturnal awakenings in different cultures, and individual patient psychological preferences. However, surgeons in general are too frequently ready to accept shortcomings of their procedure, while their victims have significant difficulties in tolerating them. For example, it is self-evident that patients would rather sleep a solid 8 hours instead of going to the bathroom several times during the night or setting an alarm clock. However, sleeping for the rest of one's life in a wet bed or a dampened protecting pad cannot be a desirable goal. There is no standard time from surgery in reporting continence. Hautmann has shown that continence continues to improve as long as 4 years after surgery.[17] Daytime continence, however, does not appear to be an issue and is easy to define. The patient is either dry without protection, wears a pad for occasional stress incontinence, or is wet. Another factor is the method of determining continence—by questionnaire; telephone survey; personal interview by an outside, nonbiased questionnaire; or simply by reviewing what the surgeon reports in his follow-up office notes. It is hoped that the "ICS-standardization of assessment and terminology of functional characteristics of intestinal urinary reservoirs" produced by the International Continence Society Committee on standardization of terminology will continue its work and end up with standardized definitions for the quantification of urine loss, particularly during nighttime. The definitions we are using are simple and straightforward:

I. Daytime continence
   A. Dry without protection
   B. Pads for occasional stress incontinence
   C. Wet

II. Nighttime continence
   A. Dry without protection (no awakenings because of uncontrolled micturition)
   B. Dry with one awakening
   C. Wet, leakage, incontinence during sleep, more than one awakening/night, dampness, need for alarm clock

As shown in Figure 24–2, the absolute reservoir capacity and consequently the length of the gut segment used for reservoir construction have significant impact on the continence result. Each surgeon or each technique can extrapolate from the reservoir capacity and the length of the gut segment being used the respective nocturnal continence data. If the surgeon is unable to accommodate the results on the line shown in Figure 24–2, the surgeon must have difficulties in reporting results. Detubularization and refashioning of bowel segments are compulsory steps in orthotopic bladder replacement and result in abrogation of the directional peristaltic activity of the bowel segment used, leading to a low-pressure, high-compliance, large-capacity reservoir, and improvement of the continence status, in particular nocturnal continence. Nocturnal incontinence following orthotopic bladder replacement is more common and lasts longer than daytime incontinence. It is correct that for the male population this feature is shared by all forms of neobladder. However, it is also correct that depending on the geometric reservoir sizes, dramatic differences in the nocturnal continence rates can be observed. Due to the laws of physics, the reservoir with the largest capacity and the most extensive detubularization which includes all the gut segment used into the reservoir must achieve the best results (Fig. 24–2).

Further factors contributing to continence include the decrease in urethral closing pressure, relaxation of the pelvic floor musculature, loss of the urethral sphincter recruitment reflex in response to contractions in the neobladder during sleep, and the fact that the total 24-hour urinary output in patients with an intestinal neobladder exceeds that of normals.

Acceptable reasons for nocturnal incontinence are previous surgery and radiation-induced injuries to the external sphincter mechanism, and damage to the pelvic nerves associated with bladder removal. The nocturnal fluid shift associated with secretion of a hypertonic acidic urine and the resultant influx of water into the neobladder is a well understood fact and must be considered preoperatively by selecting the proper size of the reservoir.

The percentage of patients requiring intermittent catheterization is low (2%). Currently, this phenomenon is not well understood despite extensive interest and diligent functional and urodynamic examination.

CONTINENCE IN THE FEMALE FOLLOWING ORTHOTOPIC BLADDER REPLACEMENT

Just recently, the enthusiasm for orthotopic urinary diversion in men has been extended to women (Fig. 24–12). The initial experience with two large series[2,3] has shown high patient acceptance and perfect continence rates, and must be rated an overwhelming success. In our series, a total of 13 patients were available for complete follow-up as of March 1995. At 3 months postoperatively, excellent continence was achieved in eight patients, while two had grade I stress incontinence and three were hypercontinent. As of March 1995, only four patients voided to completion, while nine required intermittent catheterization (continuously in five and twice daily for residual urine in four). The development of hypercontinence in 70% of the patients with time demonstrates that our current understanding of the functional and anatomic basics of the voiding process is too limited to allow bladder replacement with a perfect functional result in all female patients. Our long-term experience, which is different from initial reports, justifies creation of an ileal neobladder in select female patients as long as they accept a 70% risk of clean intermittent catheterization in the long term. Overall patient satisfaction, including sexual life, is exceptional. However, disappointment is considerable when the clean intermittent catheterization is required after periods of successful voiding per urethram. Our ongoing experience has, however, shown in ten additional patients, all with an anastomosis of the neobladder to the proximal urethra, that the continence rate continues to be exceedingly high (i.e., 100%) and the hypercontinence rate is decreasing to approximately 30%.

METABOLIC IMPLICATIONS AND ELECTROLYTE DISTURBANCES

Since intestine was not meant to serve as either a conduit or a storage vehicle for urine, the use to which it is put in urology, numerous complications may occur in both the short and long term. Those complications that have been noted in patients with

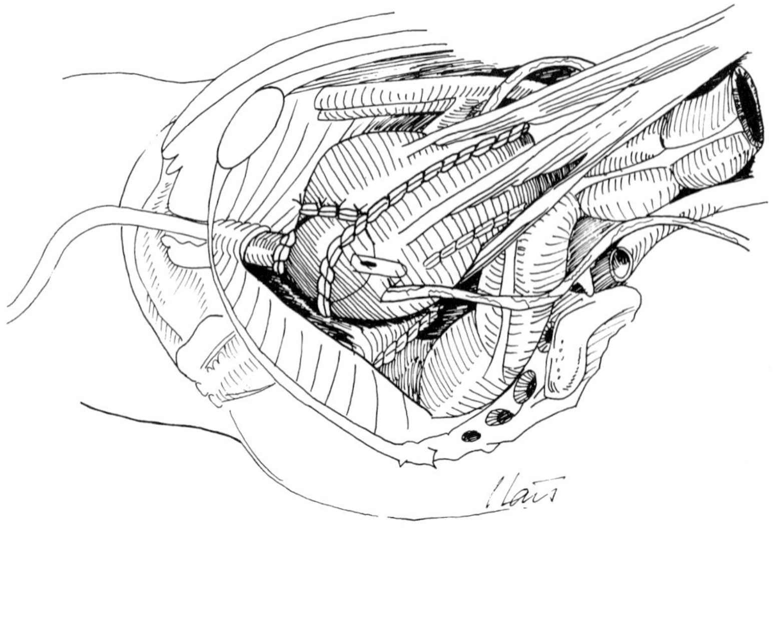

FIGURE 24–12. Ileal neobladder to the female urethra. Situation after completion of the urethroileal anastomosis. Note intact urethrovaginal support.

urinary intestinal diversion occur as a consequence of metabolic abnormalities in disordered electrolyte metabolism, impaired sensorium, altered hepatic metabolism, abnormal drug metabolism, infection, calculus formation, nutritional disturbances, growth retardation, osteomalacia, and cancer.

Many of these metabolic complications are influenced by the degree to which solute absorption occurs across the bowel segment. The factors that influence solute absorption include (1) the segment of bowel employed, (2) the surface area of the bowel utilized, (3) the time of retention of urine, (4) the concentration of solutes in the urine, (5) renal function, and (6) the pH and osmolality of the fluid.

These factors influence the amount of solutes absorbed and, as such, influence the type of metabolic complications and their severity. The length of time the intestinal segment has been in the urinary tract has also been suggested as a determinant of solute absorption. It has been suggested that the activity of transport processes diminishes over time.

Histologic changes occur in the intestinal mucosa when it is placed in contact with urine over extended periods of time. Loss of villous height and areas of atrophy have been reported in portions of ileum exposed to urine. Whether these result in an altered ability of the mucosal cell to transport solute is unclear.

Serum electrolyte complications and their severity are dependent upon the segment of bowel used in the urinary intestinal diversion. If stomach is employed, a hypokalemic, hypochloremic metabolic alkalosis can occur. This is rarely significant in the presence of normal renal function, but in the anephric state or with severely limited renal function a marked hypochloremic metabolic alkalosis can ensue. When jejunum is used, a hyponatremic, hypochloremic, hyperkalemic metabolic acidosis occurs in approximately 25 to 40% of patients. The more proximal the segment, the more likely these electrolyte abnormalities are to occur. If ileum is the segment of choice, a hyperchloremic metabolic acidosis may occur in up to 70% of patients. A significant persistent acidosis that requires therapy occurs in approximately 10% of patients with ileal conduits, and about 20% of patients with ileal conduits who have normal electrolyte values on routine follow-up will have periodic episodes of hyperchloremic metabolic acidosis. When the colon is the segment used as a conduit, about 10 to 15% of patients will exhibit an acidosis. The incidence of these abnormalities is increased in patients who have continent urinary diversions. In those with ureterosigmoidostomies, up to 80% will demonstrate hyperchloremic metabolic acidosis, and in the other types of continent diversions utilizing either ileum, colon, and/or both the incidence is variously reported between 10 and 65%. If careful metabolic studies are performed and arterial blood gases analyzed, the incidence is significantly higher.

Since a comprehensive review of the metabolic complications of urinary intestinal diversion is beyond the scope of this article, the interested reader is referred to the excellent state-of-the-art lecture of McDougal.[35] Since a disordered electrolyte metabolism in some form is the metabolic complication most frequently seen, it will be discussed here:

All patients who have had urinary intestinal diversions have demonstrable decreases in serum bicarbonate when compared to preoperative levels, 20% of patients with normal serum bicarbonate levels have episodes of severe acidosis, and 6 to 33% of diverted patients have severe chronic acidosis. These patients also may have elevated serum solutes such as phosphate and sulfate that result in demineralization of bone and excessive loss of calcium by the kidney. These serum abnormalities, which promote calciuria, decrease the calcium-phosphate product for remineralization, and interfere with vitamin D metabolism, work in concert to cause subtle bone mineral content changes in the majority of patients with urinary intestinal diversion and severe abnormalities of bone mineral content in a few. Since bicarbonate and vitamin C are essential for normal bone growth, and since these two substances in the animal model prevent bone demineralization, it would be prudent to consider administering an alkali and vitamin C to all patients with urinary intestinal diversion who are in the growth phase at a time when new bone is being actively laid down. In patients who present with osteomalacia or rickets, correction of acid base abnormalities with alkali should be the first order of treatment. If rapid remineralization does not occur, consideration should be given to adding calcium supplements and the activated form of vitamin D.

CONCLUSIONS

In 1996, there are few contraindications to orthotopic bladder replacement in the male as well as in the female. All patients considered appropriate surgical candidates for cystectomy should be informed of the option of orthotopic bladder replacement as part of their informed consent. There can be no doubt that for both sexes orthotopic bladder replacement has evolved into the diversion of choice in most centers around the world following cystectomy for patients with primary bladder cancer. Up to 90% of the male cystectomy candidates and up to 75% of the female cystectomy candidates must be considered candidates for orthotopic bladder reconstruction.

REFERENCES

1. Skinner DG, Studer UE, Okada K, et al: Which patients are suitable for continent diversion or bladder substitution following cystectomy or other definitive local treatment? Int J Urol 1995; 2:105.

2. Stein JP, Stenzl A, Esrig D, et al: Lower urinary tract reconstruction following cystectomy in women using the Kock ileal reservoir with bilateral ureteroileal urethrostomy: initial clinical experience. J Urol 1994; 152:1404.
3. Hautmann RE, Paiss T, de Petriconi R: The ileal neobladder in women: 9 years of experience with 18 patients. J Urol 1996; 155:76.
4. Stein JP, Cote RJ, Freeman JA, et al: Indications for lower urinary tract reconstruction in women after cystectomy for bladder cancer: a pathological review of female cystectomy specimens. J Urol 1995; 154:1329.
5. Freeman JA, Esrig D, Tarter TH, et al: Urethral recurrence in patients with ileal neobladders. Abstract Book, Second International Meeting on Continent Urinary Reconstruction, p 59. 1995.
6. Hinman F Jr: Selection of intestinal segments for bladder substitution: physical and physiological characteristics. J Urol 1988; 139:519.
7. Martins FE, Bennett CJ, Skinner DG: Options in replacement cystoplasty following radical cystectomy: high hopes or successful reality. J Urol 1995; 153:1363.
8. Colding-Jörgensen M, Poulsen AL, Steven K: Mechanical characteristics of tubular and detubularized bowel for bladder substitution: theory, urodynamics and clinical results. Br J Urol 1993; 72:586.
9. Hautmann RE, Egghart G, Frohneberg D, et al: The ileal neobladder. J Urol 1988; 139:39.
10. Skinner DG, Boyd SD, Lieskovsky G, et al: Lower urinary tract reconstruction following cystectomy: experience and results in 126 patients using the Kock ileal reservoir with bilateral ureteroileal urethrostomy. J Urol 1991; 146:756.
11. Thüroff J, Alken P, Riedmiller H, et al: 100 cases of Mainz-pouch: continuing experience and evolution. J Urol 1988; 140:283.
12. Lytton B, Green DF: Urodynamic studies in patients undergoing bladder replacement surgery. J Urol 1989; 141: 1394.
13. Koraitim MM, Atta MA, Foda MK: Early and late cystometry of detubularized and nondetubularized intestinal neobladders: new observations and physiological correlates. J Urol 1995; 154:1700.
14. Hautmann RE, Kirkels WJ: Continent urinary diversion: the ileal neobladder. Prob Urol 1992; 6:510.
15. Bachor R, Frohneberg D, Miller K, et al: Continence after total bladder replacement: urodynamic analysis of the ileal neobladder. Br J Urol 1990; 65:462.
16. Bachor R, Hautmann RE: Options in urinary diversions: a review and critical assessment. Semin Urol 1993; 11:235.
17. Hautmann RE, Miller K, Steiner U, et al: The ileal neobladder: 6 years of experience with more than 200 patients. J Urol 1993; 150:40.
18. Miller K, Wenderoth UK, de Petriconi R, et al: The ileal neobladder: operative technique and results. Urol Clin North Am 1991; 18:623.
19. Hautmann RE, Wenderoth UK: Ileal neobladder. Prob Urol 1991; 5:336.
20. DeLancey JOL: Anatomy and physiology of urinary continence. Clin Obstet Gynecol 1990; 33:298.
21. DeLancey JOL: Functional anatomy of the female lower urinary tract and pelvic floor. Neurobiology of Incontinence, p 57. Chichester, Wiley, (Ciba Foundation Symposium 151) 1990.
22. Hautmann RE: The ileal neobladder to the female urethra. Urol Clin North Am 1996 (in press).
23. Skinner DG, Boyd SD, Lieskovsky G, et al: Lower urinary tract reconstruction following cystectomy: experience and results in 126 patients using the Kock ileal reservoir with bilateral ureteroileal urethrectomy. J Urol 1991; 146:756.
24. Studer UE, Ackermann D, Casanova GA, et al: Three-years' experience with an ileal low-pressure bladder substitute. Br J Urol 1989; 63:43.
25. Thüroff JW, Alken P, Riedmiller H, et al: 100 cases of Mainz pouch: continuing experience and evolution. J Urol 1988; 140:283.
26. Marks JL, Anderson DJ, Light JK: Continence following Le Bag. J Urol 1988; 139:335.
27. Goldwasser B, Ramon J: Total bladder replacement using detubularized right colon. *In* Webster G, Kirby R, Kind L, Goldwasser B (eds): Reconstructive Urology, Vol 1, p 477. Boston, Blackwell Scientific Publications, 1993.
28. Mansson W, Colleen S: Experience with a detubularized right colonic segment for bladder replacement. Scand J Urol Nephrol 1990; 24:53.
29. Reddy J, Lange PK, Fraley EE: Total bladder replacement using detubularized sigmoid colon: technique and results. J Urol 1991; 145:51.
30. Studer UE, Danuser H, Merz VW, et al: Experience in 100 patients with an ileal low pressure bladder substitute combined with an afferent tubular isoperistaltic segment. J Urol 1995; 154:49.
31. Sagalowsky AI: Early results with split-cuff nipple ureteral reimplants in urinary diversion. J Urol 1995; 154:2028.
32. Flohr P, Hefty R, Paiss T, et al: The ileal neobladder—updated experience after 306 patients. World J Urol 1996; 14:22.
33. Abol-Enein H, Ghoneim MA: A novel uretero-ileal reimplantation technique: the serous lined extramural tunnel. A preliminary report. J Urol 1994; 151:1193.
34. Rowland RG: Complications of continent cutaneous reservoirs and neobladders—series using contemporary techniques. AUA Update Series, lesson 25, vol XIV, p 202. 1995.
35. McDougal WS: Metabolic complications of urinary intestinal diversion. J Urol 1992; 147:1199.
36. Elmajian DA, Esrig D, Freeman JA, et al: Orthotopic lower urinary tract reconstruction utilizing the Kock ileal reservoir: updated experience in 266 patients. World J Urol 1996; 14:40.
37. Alcini E, D'Addessi A, Racioppi M, et al: Experience of 14 years in bladder replacement using our own three different personal techniques. Abstract Book, Second International Meeting on Continent Urinary Reconstruction, p 79. 1995.
38. Freiha FS: The Stanford pouch: a simple and effective method of bladder substitution. J Urol 1990; 143:397A.

VI

PROSTATE GLAND AND SEMINAL VESICLES

25

CANCER OF THE PROSTATE: DIAGNOSIS AND STAGING

CHERYL T. LEE, M.D. *and* JOSEPH E. OESTERLING, M.D.

EPIDEMIOLOGY

Incidence/Prevalence

In 1996, an estimated 317,100 new cases of prostate cancer will be diagnosed in the United States.[1] This represents 41% of all newly diagnosed cancers in men. An estimated 41,400 patients with prostate cancer will die this year; only lung cancer has a higher mortality (~94,400).[1] The chance of a man developing invasive prostate cancer during his lifetime is 1 in 6 or 15.4%, though it is clear that the risk increases with age, as from birth to age 39 the chances are 1 in 10,000; from 40 to 59, 1 in 103; from 60 to 79, 1 in 8. At the age of 50, a man has a 42% chance of developing prostate cancer, and a 2.9% chance of dying from his disease.[2] Clearly, cancer of the prostate is an important disease process that deserves the attention of clinicians and researchers alike.

Predilection for prostate cancer is still not clearly understood. It affects ethnic groups differently and has international biases. This creates the notion that this disease must, in part, be affected by environmental and/or genetic factors. For example in the United States, African-Americans have a higher presenting stage, tend to have higher grade tumors, and have lower survival rates than their European-American counterparts or their African counterparts. From 1983 to 1990, African-Americans had a 66% 5-year survival rate versus an 81% 5-year survival rate for European-Americans when all stages were examined.[1]

ETIOLOGY/RISK FACTORS

Etiology

Neoplastic growth of human prostate tissue is the result of multifactorial interactions.[3] These factors include genetic influences, endogenous hormonal changes, exposure to environmental substances, and exposure to inflammatory/infectious (possibly sexually transmitted) agents. Genetic factors likely play a role as indicated by the increased incidence of prostate cancer among relations of afflicted individuals, and the recent observation of familial clustering of breast and prostate cancers.[4] In addition, much study has generated from observing important tumor suppressor genes and oncogenes, chromosomes, and other biomodulators in other cancer processes. Speculation continues as to whether in utero influences on the developing prostate predispose to the disease.[5] Unfortunately, our knowledge regarding the specific etiologies of prostate cancer is speculative at best. As in most disease processes, a combination of factors almost certainly leads to carcinogenesis.

Risk Factors

Current risk factors for prostate cancer include age, ethnicity, and family history. Other speculative factors include previous vasectomy or a high-saturated-fat diet.

Age

Age is the most important epidemiologic factor,[6] with estimates of 70% of men over 80 years of age having some histologic evidence of cancer.

Ethnicity

Reports have demonstrated that African-Americans have a higher incidence of prostate cancer, and when diagnosed with prostate cancer present with a higher stage, and overall have a poorer survival compared with European-Americans.[7,8] Pienta et al. examined the impact of age, race, and disease stage on survival in men diagnosed with prostate cancer.[8] This examination was performed utilizing the Surveillance, Epidemiology, and End Results (SEER) program database, which included 12,907 men (9339 European-Americans, 3568 African-Americans) diagnosed from 1973 to 1987. Their results demonstrated that African-American men have a poorer survival than whites for all stages of prostate cancer when the cancer is diagnosed at younger ages. These differences in survival were not demonstrated for men diagnosed with prostate cancer after age 70.

Japanese tend to have a much lower incidence of prostate cancer, whereas members of Scandinavian countries have a higher incidence.[2] From 1988 to 1991, Switzerland, Sweden, and Norway all experienced a prevalence of prostate cancer greater than or equal to 20 per 100,000 men in comparison to the United States with 16.8 per 100,000 men in comparison to Hong Kong with 2.6, Japan 3.8, or Singapore with 4.2 per 100,000.

Family History

Several authors have demonstrated an increased risk with familial aggregation. Aprikian et al.[9] evaluated 2968 men who were referred for prostate cancer detection. Cancer was detected in 133 of 329 (40.4%) patients with a family history and in 769 of 2639 (29.1%) with no family history. The difference was statistically significant ($p < .001$) and resulted in an odds ratio of 1.7. Interestingly, when ethnicity was considered as a second factor, there was no difference between African-Americans, European-Americans, or Asians in the increased risk with family aggregation. Whittemore et al.[10] examined the family history as a risk for prostate cancer in African-American, European-American, and Asian men in the United States and Canada. They found that a positive family history was associated with a statistically significant two- to threefold increase in risk in each of the three ethnic groups. The increased risk was 2.5, which did not vary with the age or ethnicity of the participant. Hayes and colleagues[11] also looked at family history as a risk of prostate cancer in African-Americans and European-Americans. They found a similarly elevated risk for African-Americans and European-Americans with a family history. The overall odds risk in someone with a father or brother with prostate cancer was 2.5 and 5.3, respectively. The similarity of familial risks demonstrated in these studies suggest that ethnic disparity in incidence of prostate cancer is influenced at least in part by environmental factors.

The epidemiology and features of family and hereditary prostate cancer were described by Carter et al.[12] The familial type was characterized by increased risk of prostate cancer, increased number of affected relatives, and earlier age of disease onset. The hereditary type, a subset of the familial group, was characterized by autosomal dominant inheritance from either parent, predisposing men to early development of prostate cancer. They postulated that the hereditary type causes up to 9% of prostate cancer.

Nutrition

When the issue of nutrition is considered with ethnicity, evidence is provided again supporting an environmental factor discrepancy in prostate cancer incidence. Whittemore and colleagues[13] studied international and ethnic differences in prostate cancer incidence in relation to diet, physical activity, and body size in African-Americans, European-Americans, and Asians in the United States and Canada. A total of 1655 African-American, European-American, Chinese-American, and Japanese-American patients diagnosed with prostate cancer from 1987 to 1991 were compared to 1645 control subjects matched to case patients by age, ethnicity, and region of residence. They found a statistically significant association of prostate cancer risk and total fat intake for all ethnic groups. After adjusting for saturated fat, risk was associated only weakly with monounsaturated fat and was unrelated to protein, carbohydrate, polyunsaturated fat, and total food energy. Saturated fat intake was associated with higher risks for Asian-Americans than for African-Americans and European-Americans. Among foreign-born Asian-Americans, risk increased independently with years of residence in North America and with saturated fat intake. Crude estimates suggested that difference in saturated fat intake accounted for 10% of African-American/European-American differences and 15% of European-American/Asian-American differences in incidence. Risk was not consistently associated with body mass, physical activity patterns, or intake of micronutrients. Their results suggested that saturated fats may have a causal role in prostate cancer incidence.

Vasectomy

The increased incidence of prostate cancer in patients who have undergone vasectomy has not been clearly demonstrated, though there have been some reports of this phenomenon, suggesting an increased incidence of 1.56 to 1.66 times.[14–16] Other studies have noted an increased incidence in prostate cancer with a greater than 20-year time span since vasectomy.[15–18] Most recently, John et al.[19] have revisited this issue by analyzing 1642 prostate cancer patients and 1636 control subjects of African-American, European-American, Chinese-American, and Japanese-American descent. They obtained a history including events regarding the vasectomy and age at the time of vasectomy. Their results showed no statistically significant increase in prostate cancer incidence in any of the ethnic groups, although there were trends towards increased incidence up to 1.9 times in the Japanese-Americans.

In accordance with this, a panel convened by the National Institutes of Health reviewed available information regarding causal relationship between vasectomy and prostate cancer. They concluded that data regarding vasectomy and prostate cancer were inconsistent, as were associations between the two.[20] The present authors concur that there is no obvious relationship between vasectomy and prostate cancer, and therefore it should not be considered a risk factor.

CLINICAL PRESENTATION

The presentation of prostate cancer will be varied. As 70% of prostate cancers are in the peripheral zones of the prostate away from the urethra, most men will not have symptoms until the disease progresses. Therefore a lesion within the peripheral zone may produce no symptoms. If this tumor progresses or if a tumor is present in the transition zone (15 to 20% of cancers), symptoms of bladder outlet obstruction may develop. These symptoms may be both obstructive (urinary hesitancy, dribbling, and a decreased force of stream) owing to encroachment of the tumor onto the urethra, or irritative (urinary frequency, urgency, dysuria, nocturia) due to detruser instability and noncompliance from prolonged bladder outlet obstruction. These symptoms are indistinguishable from those of the patient with benign prostatic hypertrophy (BPH). Since BPH and prostate cancer develop in similar patient populations, men presenting with irritative or obstructive voiding symptoms should be evaluated for prostate cancer in addition to BPH.

With further progression of the tumor, local structures (ejaculatory ducts, neurovascular bundles, urethra, bladder, ureters) may be invaded or impinged upon, resulting in hematospermia or decreased ejaculate volume, impotence, hematuria, urinary discharge of necrotic tissue, or ureteral obstruction, respectively. Patients presenting with advanced disease may have bone pain from bony metastases (usually in the axial and appendicular skeleton), lymphadenopathy, or shortness of breath due to lung metastases. A thorough physical examination should be performed particularly evaluating the patient for cervical, supraclavicular, or inguinal adenopathy. Suprapubic fullness may represent bladder outlet obstruction, with a full bladder versus a suprapubic mass present in the patient with locally progressive disease. The digital rectal examination (DRE) is the most important aspect of the exam and should never be deferred. The prostate should be palpated from its apex to the seminal vesicles (cephalad) and laterally onto the pelvic sidewalls. The prostate may be nodular, indurated, asymmetric, firm, or normal appearing. If an abnormality is palpated, its size, shape, and local extension should be noted. One must be cautious of the abnormal exam that is of a benign origin (i.e., prostatitis, prostatic calculi, or prostatic abscess). Urinalysis should be performed to aid in making these distinctions.

DIAGNOSTIC EVALUATION

Tools of Detection

Commonly used tests in the early detection and diagnosis of prostate cancer include DRE, prostate-specific antigen (PSA) measurement, transrectal ultrasonography (TRUS), and transrectal needle biopsy of the prostate (TRNB). For primary care–based case finding and mass screening, TRUS and TRNB would be logistically difficult to include as primary screening tests. Moreover, there is only a marginal value of TRUS above combined DRE and PSA,[21–23] and the risk, discomfort, and cost of TRNB would seem to obviate its use as a primary screening modality.[24] Table 25–1 shows the sensitivity, specificity, and positive predictive value for PSA, DRE, and TRUS. TRUS has been eliminated as a primary screening test because of its lack of sensitivity.

The role of PSA was recently prospectively evaluated as a detector of early prostate cancer.[25] Serum PSA was found to have an overall sensitivity of 46% and specificity of 91%, and to offer an estimated mean lead time for all cancers of 5.5 years. 40% of cancers detected more than 5 years from baseline were nonaggressive.

Many physicians feel that DRE and PSA alone may be adequate to screen patients. Catalona et al.,[26] in a large multicenter clinical trial involving 6630 men, compared DRE and serum PSA in the early detection of prostate cancer. Patients underwent quadrant prostatic biopsies if they had an elevated PSA (> 4 ng/ml) or a suspicious lesion was seen by TRUS. Cancer detection rate was 3.2% for DRE, 4.6% for PSA, and 5.8% for the two combined methods. Positive predictive value was 32% for PSA and 21% for DRE. In those patients who went on to have definitive surgical therapy, PSA had detected 75% of organ-confined disease and DRE detected 56%. The ability of DRE to detect organ-confined disease was increased by 78% when the two methods were used. In addition, had biopsies only been performed on suspicious lesions during TRUS, 39% of carcinomas would have been missed. This is clear evidence for utilizing DRE and PSA together in early detection as well as performing quadrant

TABLE 25–1. REPRESENTATIVE SENSITIVITY, SPECIFICITY, POSITIVE PREDICTIVE VALUE (PPV), AND DETECTION RATES OF DRE, SERUM PSA, AND TRUS*

Method	Sensitivity	Specificity	PPV	Detection Rate
DRE	69–89%	84–98%	26–35%	1.3–1.7%
PSA	57–79%	59–68%	40–49%	2.2–2.6%
TRUS	36–85%	41–79%	27–36%	2.6%

*From Cupp M, Oesterling J: Prostate-specific antigen, digital rectal examination, and transrectal ultrasonography: their roles in diagnosing early prostate cancer. Mayo Clin Proc 1993; 68:297–306, with permission.

or sextant biopsies in patients regardless of actual lesions seen on TRUS.

Smith and Catalona[27] have presented evidence to suggest that PSA-based screening produces a dramatic shift towards earlier stage prostatic cancer in which 96 to 99% of the tumors are clinically localized, 40% are not palpable, and 70% are pathologically organ confined. Also, 97% of these detected cancers have histologic features associated with aggressive cancer, affirming that PSA screening detects clinically important and potentially life-threatening prostate cancer.[27]

Currently, it is unclear whether screening or early detection of prostate cancer will significantly impact patient survival. The prostate, lung, colorectal, and ovarian (PLCO) cancer screening trial of the National Cancer Institute[28] will include 74,000 men and 74,000 women 60 to 74 years of age. This study is designed to determine whether screening for prostate cancer followed by appropriate treatment will save lives. It has a design power of 90% to determine a 20% reduction of prostate cancer mortality with screening efforts. The PLCO protocol has been criticized because the selection of men for 4 years of prostate testing (starting from age 60 to 74) would not catch early cancers at a "young" age, which is where cancers need to be caught to ensure organ confinement and therefore potentially enact a cure. Others have criticized the follow-up period of 4 years as too short.

PSA and Diagnosis

The Glycoprotein

PSA was originally identified in seminal plasma in 1971 by Hara and associates,[29] and was later isolated and purified by Li and Beling.[30] In 1979, Wang and coworkers[31] isolated the same glycoprotein from human prostate tissue and were the first to refer to it as "prostate-specific antigen." In 1980, Papsidero et al.[32] developed a serologic test to measure human serum levels of PSA.

The quantity of PSA in the serum is determined by commercial immunoassays that use monoclonal antibodies (MAbs) to identify epitopes on the PSA molecule. The most frequently used assays in the United States are the Tandem-R PSA and Tandem-E PSA assays (Hybritech, Inc, San Diego, CA) with 16% usage, and the IMx PSA assay (Abbott Laboratories, Abbott Park, IL) with 82% usage. The TOSOH PSA (AIA-PACK) assay (TOSOH Corporation, Tokyo, Japan) recognizes 2% usage. The TOSOH assay is an automated two-site immunoenzymometric assay. The Tandem-R PSA and Tandem-E PSA assays both use two murine monoclonal antibodies directed at separate epitopes on the PSA molecule. The IMx PSA assay is a monoclonal-polyclonal assay. For all assays, the age-specific reference ranges (see Table 25–2) are applicable.[33] Most recently, an enhanced reverse-transcriptase polymerase chain reaction (RTPCR) assay[34] has also been described as a more sensitive and specific means of serum PSA detection. This type of assay may prove to be an effective modality for detecting micrometastases that are not identifiable by standard methods.

TABLE 25–2. AGE-SPECIFIC REFERENCE RANGES FOR SERUM PROSTATE-SPECIFIC ANTIGEN*

Age (years)	Serum PSA† (ng/ml)	PSA Density† (ng/ml/ml)
40–49	0.0–2.5	0.0–0.08
50–59	0.0–3.5	0.0–0.10
60–69	0.0–4.5	0.0–0.11
70–79	0.0–6.5	0.0–0.13

*Modified from Oesterling J, Jacobsen S, Chute C, et al: Serum prostate-specific antigen in a community-based population of healthy men: establishment of age-specific reference ranges. JAMA 1993; 270(7):860–864. Copyright 1993, American Medical Association, with permission.

†Upper limits are defined as the 95th percentile.

The half-life of PSA was determined by Stamey et al.[35] to be 2.2 ± 0.8 days, and later by Oesterling et al.[36] to be 3.2 ± 0.1 days. Because of the long half-life of this glycoprotein, it may take several weeks for serum levels to return to baseline levels after prostatic manipulation or to an undectable value after retropubic radical prostatectomy. Oesterling et al.[37] showed that neither flexible nor rigid cystoscopy significantly changes serum PSA. In the same study, they showed that prostate biopsy causes an immediate median elevation in serum PSA of 7.9 ng/ml and requires a median of 15 days to return to baseline levels. In addition, TURP causes a median elevation in PSA of 5.9 ng/ml and a median of 17 days is required for the PSA value to return to baseline following this procedure. Neal et al.[38] have shown that prostatitis causes elevations in serum PSA, possibly as a result of cell death and inflammatory disruption of epithelial cells and the normal physiologic barriers that routinely keep PSA within the prostatic ductal system.

Effect of DRE on Serum PSA

In a prospective, randomized controlled trial, Chybowski et al.[39] showed that the median serum PSA (Hybritech assay) elevation caused by digital rectal examination (DRE) was 0.4 ng/ml. This represented a statistically but not clinically significant increase in the serum PSA level. The authors concluded that the serum PSA concentration in the immediate post-DRE period is accurate and would not compromise clinical use of the marker. Yuan et al.[40] similarly found that DRE had no significant effect on PSA. Prostatic massage produced serum PSA elevations in 3 of 20 (15%) patients and TRUS produced elevations above pre-TRUS serum PSA in 4 of 36 (11%) patients; the elevations, however, were not statistically significant. The authors concluded that DRE, prostatic massage, and TRUS all have minimal effects on serum PSA levels in most patients.

These studies show that the serum PSA value is accurate and reliable after DRE, TRUS, prostatic massage, or cystoscopic examination. However, PSA is significantly elevated after prostatic needle biopsy, TURP, or episodes of prostatitis. Therefore, clinicians should delay obtaining serum PSA levels for at least 4 to 6 weeks after such procedures/events to avoid spurious results. There appears to be no diurnal variation of PSA or significant PSA changes after ejaculation,[41] although the latter is the subject of ongoing studies by several investigators.

PSA Density

Because PSA is not specific to prostate cancer, there can be considerable overlap in the serum PSA concentrations between patients with early prostate cancer and BPH. The sensitivity of serum PSA ranges from 57 to 79%, and the specificity ranges from 59 to 68%[42]; thus, it can be difficult to distinguish patients with BPH from prostate cancer. Benson and coworkers[43,44] have described the concept of prostate-specific antigen density (PSAD), which represents the serum PSA concentration divided by the volume of the prostate gland as determined by TRUS. They have presented evidence to support a role for PSAD in the differentiation of BPH from prostate cancer.[43] As well, they have shown that PSAD can be used to stratify the risk of cancer in patients with mild elevations of serum PSA (4.1 to 10.0 ng/ml, Hybritech assay).[44]

In another review,[45] 3140 men between the ages of 50 and 89 underwent prostatic evaluation with DRE, TRUS of the prostate, and serum PSA. The authors concluded that PSAD or routine prostatic biopsy is not warranted in patients with a PSA less than 4.0 ng/ml and a normal DRE. As well, if the PSA is greater than 20.0 ng/ml, the patient should undergo prostatic biopsy regardless of the DRE, given a 65% cancer detection rate. (PSAD does not contribute significantly to the detection rate in men with these higher PSA values and is therefore not recommended.) They do advocate the use of PSAD in patients with a PSA value between 4.1 and 20. The prostate volume determination is felt to be important in this group, since there were statistically significant differences noted in PSAD values, but not PSA values, between cancer and BPH groups. Seemingly, the PSAD would allow the clinician to make an informed decision as to whether a biopsy is warranted.

Figure 25–1 is a probability plot that uses PSAD to predict the likelihood of a positive biopsy. The authors recommend clinical observation, DRE, and serial serum PSA for a patient with a PSAD less than or equal to 0.15 and normal DRE. For patients with a normal DRE and a PSA greater than 0.15, the authors advocate proceeding with a prostate biopsy.

In contrast to this report, Brawer and colleagues[46] reviewed 218 men (median age 67 years) undergoing systematic random prostatic needle biopsy. They examined the ability of PSA and PSAD to distinguish benign and malignant disease; in addition, they studied the ability of the two to predict biopsy results. They were unable to show any advantage of PSAD over PSA alone in predicting the presence of prostate cancer. In fact, PSA was superior to PSAD in predicting biopsy results in patients with a normal DRE. Neither test was able to reliably distinguish benign disease from malignant disease in patients with serum PSA values between 4.1 and 10.0 ng/ml.

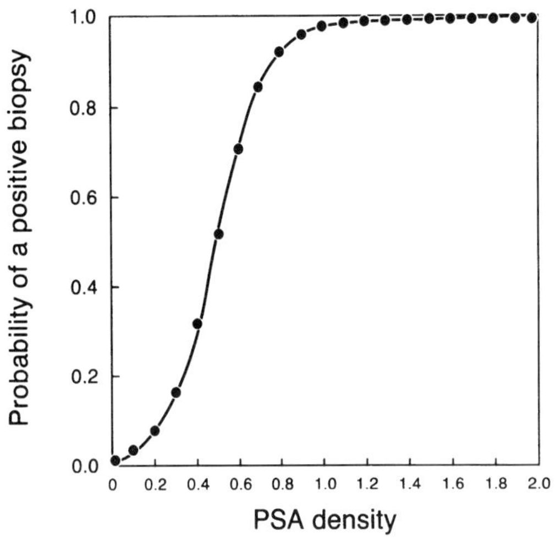
Probability of a positive biopsy
1.0
0.8
0.6
0.4
0.2
0.0
0
0.2
0.4
0.6
0.8
1.0
1.2
1.4
1.6
1.8
2.0
PSA density

FIGURE 25–1. Discriminant analysis of PSAD values for patients whose PSA values are between 4.1 and 10.0 ng/ml. Examines only those patients who underwent prostate biopsy (either abnormal transrectal ultrasound or digital rectal examination). (Adapted from Seaman E, Whang M, Olsson C, et al: PSA density [PSAD]: role in patient evaluation and management. Urol Clin North Am 1993; 20[4]:653–663, with permission.)

Catalona and associates[47] have questioned the suggested PSAD upper limit of normal (0.15). They prospectively studied 4962 men, average age 63 years. Subjects were evaluated by DRE and PSA. If the serum PSA was greater than 4 ng/ml and/or DRE was suspicious, the patient underwent four (quadrant) TRUS-guided prostatic biopsies in addition to biopsies of suspicious areas on DRE and/or TRUS. In evaluating the PSAD for patients with intermediate PSA levels (4.1 to 9.9), a PSAD cutoff of 0.15 had a specificity of 81% and an unacceptably low sensitivity of 52%. The majority (93%) of the tumors missed with this PSAD cutoff were clinically significant. If a PSAD cutoff of 0.15 had been used as an indication for prostatic biopsy, nearly half of the tumors would have been missed. The authors recommended that men in this group should undergo biopsy based upon PSA concentration rather than the PSAD determination.

PSAD appears to have some utility in distinguishing BPH from prostate cancer and in identifying those patients with prostate cancer who have mildly elevated or intermediate PSA levels and normal DRE. However, Oesterling et al.[48] have shown that PSAD does not provide additional clinical information over PSA when age-specific reference ranges are used. Despite the ability of PSAD to identify unapparent but clinically significant cancers in some patients, there still remain concerns regarding reproducibility of density determinations with regard to volume measurements with TRUS, variations in normal prostate sizes, as well as the significant differences in stromal/epithelial ratios between prostates. Currently, we conclude that there is no significant role for PSAD in the early detection of prostate cancer, especially when age-specific reference ranges are used.

PSA Velocity

PSA velocity (PSAV) is defined as the change in serum PSA over time. This concept was developed in an effort to improve the ability of the clinician to distinguish benign prostatic disease from malignant prostatic disease, in addition to improving the identification of men with prostate cancer destined to progress. The rationale for developing such a concept would be to use serial PSA concentrations in a meaningful way to evaluate a patient, thus avoiding the interrelated variables of PSA concentration, BPH volume, cancer volume, and cancer differentiation.[49] As the amount of benign epithelium increases or the cancer volume increases, the PSA concentration increases. However, poorly differentiated cancers produce less PSA than well-differentiated cancers when equal volumes of each are compared.[49] Thus, these variables may make the interpretation of a single PSA somewhat difficult.

In a retrospective study, Carter and associates[50,51] reviewed prostatic evaluation and treatment in 54 men who were part of the Baltimore Longitudinal Study of Aging. A group of 20 men with a histologic diagnosis of BPH and a group of 20 men with a histologic diagnosis of prostate cancer were compared to a control group of 16 men without prostatic disease. When the PSAV was calculated, the investigators found a significant difference in the age-adjusted rate of change in PSA between the groups, with cancer greater than BPH greater than controls ($p < .01$). (Fig. 25–2 shows the exponential changes in the cancer group, and the nonlinear changes in the BPH group. The mean change in PSA for the control group was not significantly different from zero.) A PSAV of ≥0.75 ng/ml/year resulted in correct identification of 72% of the cancer subjects (sensitivity 72%) and correct identification of 92% of the BPH subjects (specificity 90%). The authors concluded that PSAV was a potentially useful tool in distinguishing benign and malignant prostate disease. In addition, PSAV might be helpful in much earlier detection of prostate cancer in men with a normal DRE and a normal PSA.

In a prospective study of 376 cancer-free men, Oesterling and associates[52] examined the rate of change in serum PSA over a period of at least 12 months. They found a tremendous variation in both the serum PSA concentration and PSAV across all

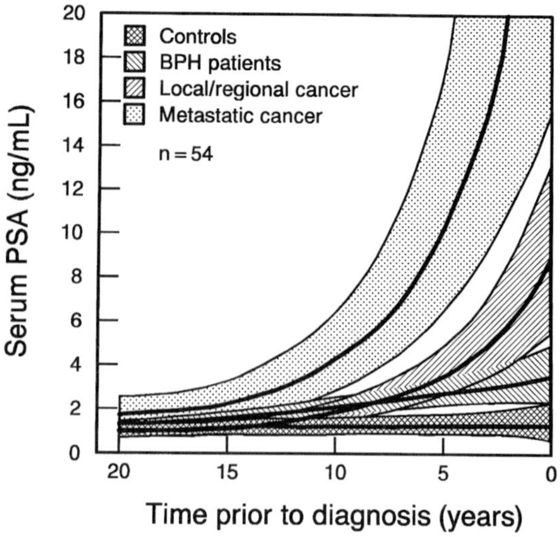
Serum PSA (ng/mL)
20
18
16
14
12
10
8
6
4
2
0
Controls
BPH patients
Local/regional cancer
Metastatic cancer
n = 54
20
15
10
5
0
Time prior to diagnosis (years)

FIGURE 25–2. Average curves (±95% confidence intervals) of PSA levels (ng/ml) as a function of years before diagnosis for three diagnostic groups; based on observed data. (From Carter HB, Pearson J, Metter J, et al: Longitudinal evaluation of prostate specific antigen levels in men with and without prostate disease. JAMA 1992; 267[16]:2215–2220, with permission. Copyright 1992, American Medical Association.)

age ranges; in addition, approximately 25 to 33% of patients without clinical evidence of cancer had more than a 20% increase in the serum PSA concentration during one year. Similarly, Carter and associates[53] suggested that there is great variability in PSA measurements made within a few months apart. Therefore, if PSAV is to have clinical value, we advocate obtaining PSA determinations at least 1 year apart, and using at least three determinations to calculate the velocity value.

Age-Specific Reference Ranges of PSA

Clinicians have used a general PSA reference range of 0.0 to 0.4 ng/ml as a normal result. If an elevated level has returned, further evaluation by TRUS and/or prostate biopsy has been carried out. This may not be the appropriate range for all men, as this single range does not account for age difference or normal variations in prostatic volume.

The normal aging prostate undergoes histologic hyperplastic changes of the epithelial cells. These changes result in increased prostate size and increased levels of PSA production, as 1 g of BPH gives rise to 0.2 ng/ml of PSA in the serum.[35] As well, increased PSA levels in aging prostates may be influenced by prostatic ischemia or infarction, chronic subclinical prostatitis, prostatic intraepithelial neoplasia, and loss of normal physiologic barrier integrity and a leakage of PSA into capillaries and lymphatics.

Oesterling and coworkers[33] critically reviewed this issue in a prospective study of 471 white men aged 40 to 79 years who had no evidence of prostatic cancer by DRE, PSA determination (Tandem-R PSA), or TRUS. These investigators attempted to

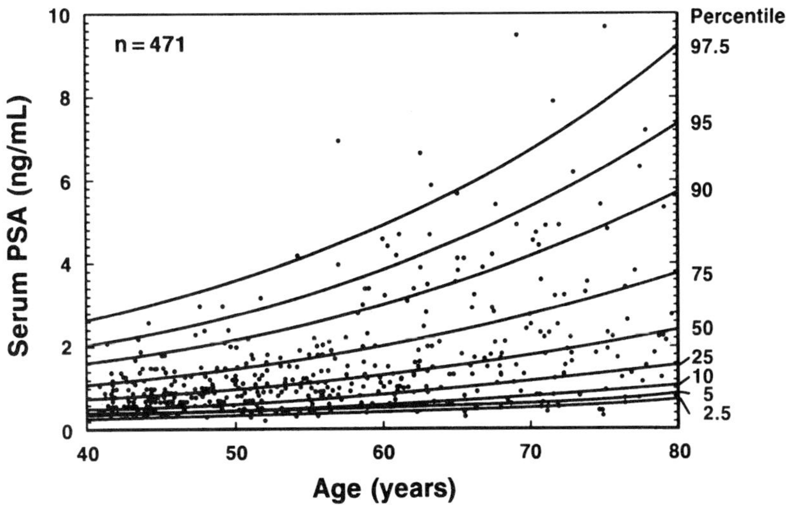
n=471
Serum PSA (ng/mL)
Age (years)
Percentile
97.5
95
90
75
50
25
10
5
2.5
0
2
4
6
8
10
40
50
60
70
80

FIGURE 25–3. Serum PSA concentration as a function of patient age. Scattergram of the individual serum PSA values for all 471 men, with the curves for the 2.5th, 5th, 10th, 25th, 50th, 75th, 90th, 95th, and 97.5th percentiles. (From Oesterling J, Jacobsen S, Chute C, et al: Serum prostate-specific antigen in a community-based population of healthy men: establishment of age-specific reference ranges. JAMA 1993; 270[7]:860–864, with permission. Copyright 1993, American Medical Association.)

define a relationship between serum PSA concentration, prostatic volume (as determined by TRUS), PSAD, and patient age. Pearson product-moment correlation coefficients were used to measure associations between serum concentration PSA and age, prostate volume and age, PSA and prostate volume, and PSAD and age. The Pearson product-moment correlation (r) is a parametric statistical method designed to measure the extent to which pairs of measurements are associated. There were direct correlations between PSA and age (r = .43; p < .0001) (Fig. 25–3); prostatic volume and age (r = .43; p < .0001); PSA and prostatic volume (r = .55; p < .0001), and PSAD and age (r = .25; p = .001). Age ranges were grouped via 10-year intervals from 40 to 79 years of age. The 95th percentile was used as the upper limit of normal for PSA concentration and PSAD, and the 2.5 to 97.5th percentile range was considered normal for prostate volume, within each 10-year range. Table 25–3 reflects the age-specific median values and ranges for serum PSA, prostate volume, and PSAD.

Dalkin and associates[54] have defined upper limits of normal PSA levels after examining 5220 men without evidence of prostate cancer. They determined normal serum PSA levels to be 3.7 ng/ml for men 50 to 54 years, 4.0 ng/ml for 55–59 years, 5.4 ng/ml for 60–64 years, 6.2 ng/ml for 65–69 years, and 6.6 ng/ml for 70–74 years. Feneley and colleagues[55] studied 200 men with symptoms of bladder outlet obstruction using DRE, serum PSA determination, and TRUS. Patients without evidence of prostate cancer demonstrated a statistically significant correlation between prostate volume and age, and PSA and age. These authors favored the use of an age-adjusted PSA reference range applied to the investigation of symptomatic prostatic disease.

TABLE 25–3. MEDIAN VALUES OF SERUM PSA CONCENTRATION, PROSTATE VOLUME, AND PSA DENSITY, BY AGE*

	Age Group			
Parameter	40–49 Years	50–59 Years	60–69 Years	70–79 Years
No of Patients	165	144	94	68
Serum PSA	0.7	1.0	1.4	2.0
(ng/ml)	(0.5, 1.1)†	(0.6, 1.4)	(0.9, 3.0)	(0.9, 3.2)
Prostatic Vol	23.5	30.7	34.6	35.4
(ml)	(20.4, 29.0)	(23.0, 37.1)	(28.0, 43.7)	(29.6, 51.4)
PSA Density	0.03	0.03	0.05	0.05
(ng/ml)	(0.02, 0.04)	(0.02, 0.05)	(0.03, 0.07)	(0.03, 0.08)

*From Oesterling J, Jacobsen S, Chute C, et al: Serum prostate-specific antigen in a community-based population of healthy men: establishment of age-specific reference ranges. JAMA 1993; 270(7):860–864, with permission. Copyright 1993, American Medical Association.

†Numbers in parentheses indicate the 25th and 75th percentiles.

Collins et al.[56] examined the relationship between PSA levels, prostate volume, and age in 472 men (40 to 79 years, mean age 60) who underwent PSA determination, DRE, and TRUS as part of a survey of BPH. None of these subjects had prostate cancer. The authors noted that age and prostate volume influenced PSA levels independently. They concluded that further study was needed to determine the sensitivity and specificity of age-adjusted PSA levels in association with DRE and TRUS in the detection of prostate cancer. Additional evidence in support of age-adjusted reference ranges has been proposed by Crawford and colleagues[57] upon examination of data obtained during Prostate Cancer Awareness Week, 1993. Similarly, Dalkin and associates[58] have also provided additional evidence to support this concept.

Recently, the selection of optimal PSA cutoffs for early detection of prostate cancer was reviewed. Catalona and associates[59] conducted a multicenter prospective clinical trial involving 6630 men 50 years or older. These men underwent serum PSA determination and DRE. Biopsies were performed if the PSA level was greater than 4.0 ng/ml or if DRE was suspicious for cancer. Sensitivity, specificity, and positive and negative predictive values were compared in varying age groups and varying PSA ranges. They did not find a significant difference in total cancers detected and total biopsies avoided. Although there were differences in the number of cancers detected in varying age populations, the authors concluded that there is no need for age-adjusted PSA reference ranges.

The current authors advocate the use of age-specific reference ranges for PSA determinations. Prostate cancer does not have the same clinical significance for men of all ages. In view of this, a constant predictive value for PSA across all ages need not be maintained and should not be an objective. For prostate cancer, the biologic threat to life diminishes with advancing age while its prevalence increases. As a result, the true goal is to increase the sensitivity of PSA in younger men with an extended life expectancy (men who can truly benefit from definitive treatment) and to increase the specificity of PSA in older men with a limited life expectancy (men who are less likely to benefit from aggressive medical intervention). The age-specific reference ranges for serum PSA do exactly this, making PSA a more clinically useful tumor marker for the detection of early prostate cancer.

Molecular Forms of PSA (Free Versus Complexed PSA)

Discrepancies in serum PSA levels between different immunoassays can quickly make the evaluation process quite confusing. Discrepancies may be due to different forms of PSA in circulation or the ability of assays to detect these different forms. Whether an assay utilizes monoclonal or polyclonal antibody conjugates may also impact selection of varying forms.[60] In addition, protein-binding kinetics may favor smaller molecules and, therefore, rapid assay may tend to detect these molecules preferentially.

PSA exists in serum predominantly in a complexed form, bound to either α_1-antichymotrypsin (ACT; MW 58 kDa), or to α_2-macroglobulin (AMG; MW 725 kDa).[61,62] Figure 25–4 shows the free and complexed forms of PSA. ACT and AMG are two major extracellular protease inhibitors, referred to as serpins. Purified PSA is known to form stable complexes with ACT and AMG in vitro.[61] The complexed form of PSA and ACT (PSA-ACT) inactivates the protease effects of PSA. This complex does not prevent immunoassays from detecting PSA, because the ACT molecule does not cover important PSA epitopes. In contrast, when PSA forms a complex with AMG, its epitopes become covered by the enclosing action of the AMG. This enclosure of PSA prevents exposure of its epitopes and therefore inactivates its protease function as well as pre-

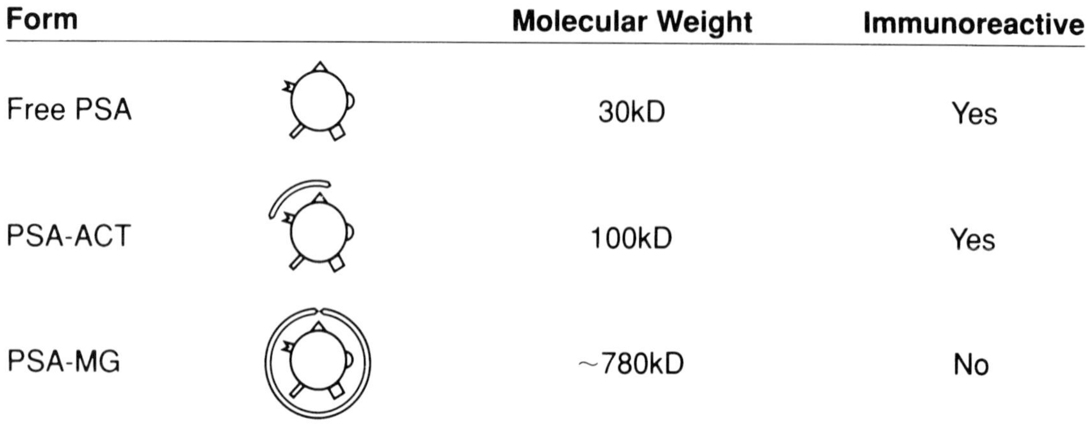
Form
Molecular Weight
Immunoreactive
Free PSA
30kD
Yes
PSA-ACT
100kD
Yes
PSA-MG
~780kD
No

FIGURE 25–4. Forms of PSA in serum. PSA-ACT, PSA complexed to α_1-antichymotrypsin (ACT). PSA-MG, PSA complexed to α_2-macroglobulin (MG). (From Hybritech, Incorporated: Why might different PSA assays yield discrepant results on the same patient? Prostate-Specific Antigen Clinical Brief 1994; 3[1], with permission.)

vents its detection by immunoassays. Thus, free PSA and PSA-ACT are able to be detected by assays.

Antibodies are used in commercial assays to identify epitopes of PSA. Monoclonal antibodies recognize a specific epitope that is present on free and complexed PSA. Polyclonal antibody conjugates, however, may include a subpopulation that binds to the same region of PSA to which ACT binds. Thus, free PSA would only be bound by the subpopulation, as ACT would block the epitope, resulting in preferential binding of free PSA and a skewed response.[63] Differences in kinetics between commercial assays can also lead to discrepancy in detection. Because of its small size, PSA (~30 kDa) may have the potential to react faster than PSA-ACT (~100 kDa). Thus, in rapid nonequilibrium assays, there might be a higher response to free PSA.[63]

Graves[64,65] has described PSA assays that have equimolar response and skewed response. The equimolar assay is dependent on the concentration of PSA present. A skewed-response assay is dependent upon PSA concentration and the ratio of free PSA to PSA-ACT in the sample. Therefore, the skewed response may measure PSA forms disproportionately. The clinical significance of these differences is yet to be determined, but because of assay discrepancies, many currently advocate the standardization of PSA detection.[63]

There has been speculation concerning heterogeneity of PSA among pathologic conditions, which might be manifest as differing patterns of serum binding of PSA forms. Christensson et al.[67] examined serum samples from 265 consecutive patients with prostatic disease; 121 had prostate cancer (mean age 74 years) and 144 had BPH (mean age 72 years). They used three different assays to study free and complexed levels of PSA in the serum of both categories of patients. One assay measured free PSA, a second measured complexed PSA (PSA-ACT), and a third measured total PSA (free plus complexed). They found that complexed PSA was the predominant form in all sera. In addition, the complexed/total ratio was significantly ($p < .0001$) higher in patients with prostate cancer than in patients with BPH. Free PSA constituted a significantly smaller fraction in cancer patients than in patients with BPH ($p < .0001$). They were unable to find a direct correlation between serum PSA and serum α_1-antichymotrypsin.

Similarly, Lilja and coworkers[68] found a median of 18% free PSA in carcinoma and 28% free PSA in BPH. Stenman and coworkers[69] reported 40% free PSA in prostate cancer in comparison to 60% in BPH, as well as a significantly higher proportion of serum PSA complexed to ACT in patients with prostate cancer as opposed to those with BPH. These corroborating observations support the concept that there is a lower free/total (F/T) PSA ratio or a higher complex/total (C/T) PSA ratio in the serum of prostate cancer patients. This concept may create a mechanism to further improve the diagnostic specificity of PSA by examining its various forms.

Using newly developed, monoclonal-monoclonal immunofluorometric assays, Oesterling et al.[70] have established age-specific reference ranges for free, complexed, and total PSA, seen in Table 25–4. Ratios of free/total, complexed/total, and free/complexed (F/C) PSA did not correlate with patient age in their studies. As a result, the appropriate upper limit of normal is constant for men of all ages. The normal range of free/total PSA is greater than 0.15; for complexed/total PSA it is less than 0.70, and for free/complexed PSA it is greater than 0.25. The lack of correlation with age is due to the fact that each molecular form increases 3% per year with advancing age, and the age dependency is lost when the concentration of molecular form is divided by another to generate the ratio. These investigators are prospectively studying a cancer-free cohort of 426 men in order to determine the clinical utility of free and complexed PSA forms in the detection of early prostate cancer.

Currently, the clinical utility remains to be defined, though it appears that the ratio of the molecular forms, F/T, C/T, and F/C, will have clinical importance in view of the above studies. The free PSA/total PSA ratio may particularly increase the ability of PSA to accurately distinguish early prostate cancer from BPH[67]; therefore, improving its

TABLE 25–4. AGE-SPECIFIC REFERENCE RANGES FOR FREE, COMPLEXED, AND TOTAL PSA*

Molecular Form of PSA	Age-Specific Reference Range (ng/ml)			
	40–49 Years	50–59 Years	60–69 Years	70–79 Years
Free (F)	0.5	0.70	1.0	1.2
Complexed (C)	1.0	1.5	2.0	3.0
Total (T)	2.0	3.0	4.0	5.5
PSA ratios				
F/T	>0.15	>0.15	>0.15	>0.15
C/T	<0.7	<0.7	<0.7	<0.7
F/C	>0.25	>0.25	>0.25	>0.25

*From Oesterling J, Jacobsen S, Klee G, et al: Free, complexed, and total serum prostate specific antigen: the establishment of appropriate reference ranges for their concentrations and ratios using newly developed immunofluorometric assays (IFMA). J Urol 1995; 154:1090–1095, with permission.

specificity from 55% to 73% in this study by Christensson et al. When only patients with a serum PSA level between 4.0 and 20.0 ng/ml were considered, the F/T ratio increased the specificity of PSA significantly without a concomitant loss of sensitivity. When a cutoff level of 0.18 for F/T ratio was used in men with a mildly elevated serum PSA level, the specificity increased to 95% with a sensitivity of 71%. Oesterling and colleagues[70] speculate that in view of these results, the complexed forms and ratios of PSA will likely be most valuable in cases where the PSA is between 2.0 and 10.0 ng/ml. This issue will likely be clarified with the use of a recently designed dual-label, monoclonal-monoclonal, immunofluorometric assay for the simultaneous measurement of both free and total PSA serum levels as well as the value of the F/T PSA ratio.[71,72]

Effect of Finasteride on Serum PSA

In the quest to find medical treatment for BPH, finasteride was developed. Finasteride is a synthetic 4-azasteroid compound that competitively inhibits 5α-reductase, an enzyme that converts testosterone to dihydrotestosterone (DHT).[73]

In general, the effect of finasteride is a median decrease of 20% in the size of the prostate gland after 6 months of treatment.[74,75] As well, Gormley and coworkers[76] analyzed the effect of finasteride on BPH and serum PSA level in 895 men from 40 to 83 years of age in a multicenter, double-blinded study. They noted a 50% decrease in PSA levels in patients receiving 5 mg/day by 3 months, and a 48% decrease in those receiving 1 mg/day, also by 3 months. The PSA levels of the placebo group did not change significantly.

Guess and coworkers[77] undertook further review of the North America Phase III multicenter clinical trial of finasteride in the treatment of men with symptomatic BPH. The authors determined that percentage reduction in PSA induced by finasteride did not appear to be influenced by the age of the patient. They reviewed the men found to have prostate cancer while receiving a 5-mg daily dose of finasteride, either during the initial 12 months (n = 1) or during the subsequent 12 months, when all patients were administered 5 mg of finasteride daily (n = 14). The median decrease in PSA concentration (from initiation of therapy to cancer diagnosis) was 36%. Finasteride did not appear to have a greater effect on PSA of malignant origin than PSA of benign origin.

Clinicians should have an increased suspicion for prostate cancer when a patient on finasteride therapy has not had the expected 50% decline from their baseline serum PSA level. There are, however, patients whose PSA levels may not be appropriately decreased secondary to noncompliance. A serum DHT level can provide objective evidence of compliance and should reflect a 60% decrease after 6 months of finasteride therapy.[74] It is important to have a baseline level prior to initiation of finasteride therapy.

Diagnostic Algorithm for the Detection of Prostate Cancer

In view of the recent developments in PSA, regarding its complexed forms and its use as a diagnostic marker, Oesterling and colleagues[48,70] have proposed a diagnostic algorithm to aid clinicians in providing the most thorough yet cost-effective evaluation of the prostate gland. As well, they have proposed an alternative algorithm as assays for F/T PSA ratios become available. They recommend restricting evaluation of the prostate to men 50 years of age or older with a life expectancy of 10 years or more, in view of the slow-growing nature of prostate cancer. That recommendation implies that elderly or debilitated patients with a less than 10-year life expectancy should not be subjected to either a serum PSA determination or a DRE for the purpose of detecting early prostate cancer. In contrast, they advocate aggressive and early evaluation, beginning at age 40, for individuals at high risk for the development of prostate cancer, including African-American men and men with a family history of prostate cancer.

Figure 25–5 demonstrates the current algorithm. If the serum PSA is less than or equal to the age-specific range (see Table 25–2) and the patient has an unremarkable DRE, the patient should be followed with yearly PSA levels and DRE. If the PSA level is greater than the age-specific range, and the DRE is unremarkable, TRUS should be performed along with accompanying biopsy of visible lesions; in addition, a systematic, sextant biopsy of remaining prostatic tissue, taking care to gain tissue from the transition zone, should be performed. If the DRE is remarkable, the patient should undergo TRUS, regardless of the PSA level; at the time of TRUS, a biopsy of the palpable nodules and hypoechoic lesions should be performed; in addition, a systematic, sextant biopsy of the remaining prostate gland should be carried out. Figure 25–6 demonstrates the alternative algorithm when F/T assays become available.

HISTOPATHOLOGY

Local Extension

Prostate cancer may spread via local extension, lymphatic spread, or hematogenous spread. Often, local extension precedes distinct metastatic spread. Local extension tends to be into and through the prostatic capsule, the bladder base, and seminal vesicles, whereas extension into the urethra and rectum is uncommon. Denonvilliers' fascia helps to separate the prostate from the rectum. Cancers involving the apex and base are more likely to have early extracapsular extension due to weakness of the capsule at these sites.[78] Capsular defects occur where adjoining organs meet the prostate, or where neurovascular structures enter or exit the prostate

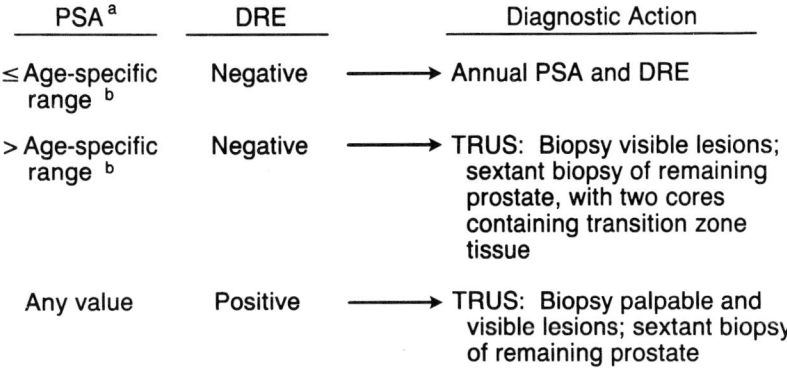

PSA[a]	DRE		Diagnostic Action
≤ Age-specific range[b]	Negative	⟶	Annual PSA and DRE
> Age-specific range[b]	Negative	⟶	TRUS: Biopsy visible lesions; sextant biopsy of remaining prostate, with two cores containing transition zone tissue
Any value	Positive	⟶	TRUS: Biopsy palpable and visible lesions; sextant biopsy of remaining prostate

[a] Tandem-R or IMx PSA assay
[b] 40-49 years: 0-2.5 ng/mL; 50-59 years: 0-3.5 ng/mL
60-69 years: 0-4.5 ng/mL; 70-79 years: 0-6.5 ng/mL

FIGURE 25–5. Algorithm for the use of age-specific PSA reference ranges and digital rectal examination (DRE) to detect clinically significant prostate cancers at an early, curable stage. (Data from Oesterling J, Cooner W, Jacobsen S, et al: Influence of patient age on the serum PSA concentration: an important clinical observation. Urol Clin North Am 1993; 20[4]:671–680.)

including the prostatourethral junction, the bladder neck junction and the entry of the ejaculatory ducts into the prostate.[78] These sites are illustrated in Figure 25–7. Perineural invasion on biopsy samples may correlate with capsular penetration noted after pathologic examination of postprostatectomy samples.[79]

Lymphatic Spread

Metastases occur most often in the obturator lymph nodes followed by the presacral, presciatic, and internal and external iliac nodes.[80] Spread to supradiaphragmatic nodes is uncommon.[81] Figure 25–8 displays lymphatic drainage of the prostate.

Vascular Spread

Generally, metastatic tumors are of the same histology as the primary lesion. Prostatic carcinomas metastasize to bone (most commonly), lung, liver, or brain. Metastases to bone have been observed in up to 80% of patients who die from prostate cancer, as a result of vascular spread and systemic dissemination.[82] Bony metastases are usually osteoblastic as opposed to osteolytic, though both types have been reported.[83] The spine is most frequently involved, followed by the femur, pelvis, rib cage, skull, and humerus. Hematogenous spread is thought to be in part secondary to access through Batson's plexus of presacral veins, which communicate with the preprostatic and periprostatic venous complex.[84,85]

DRE	PSA	Diagnostic Action
Positive	Any value	TRUS-guided biopsy
Negative	≤ 2.0 ng/ml	Annual evaluation
Negative	>10.0 ng/ml	TRUS-guided biopsy
Negative	2.1-10.0 ng/ml	Calculate f-PSA/t-PSA ratio; if ≤ 0.15, TRUS-guided biopsy; if > 0.15, annual evaluation

FIGURE 25–6. Algorithm for the use of F/T PSA, DRE, and TRUS with prostatic biopsy to detect clinically significant prostate cancer.

Anatomy

Figure 25–9 demonstrates the anatomic relationship of the adult prostate within the pelvis. The prostate is composed of tubuloalveolar glands arranged in lobules surrounded by a stroma.[86,87] The gland is rich in nerves, smooth muscle, collagen, and lymphatics. The function of the prostate gland is not clearly understood. Though, it produces 20% of seminal fluid and other substances that may facilitate sperm motility and penetration, they are not essential for fertility. In addition, hormones and enzymes produced by the prostate are not crucial to the maintenance of homeostasis.

This fibromuscular and glandular organ is made up of five regions,[88,89] demonstrated in Figure 25–10. The transition zone surrounds the prostatic urethra and compresses 5% of the glandular tissue. BPH arises here, in addition to 20% of prostate cancers. The central zone surrounds the ejaculatory ducts as they course from the base of the prostate to the verumontanum. It comprises 20 to 25% of the gland and gives rise to 5 to 10% of prostatic cancers. The peripheral zone lies posteriorly and laterally in the prostate, comprises 70 to 75% of the gland, and surrounds the central zone. Seventy per cent of adenocarcinomas arise from this area. The

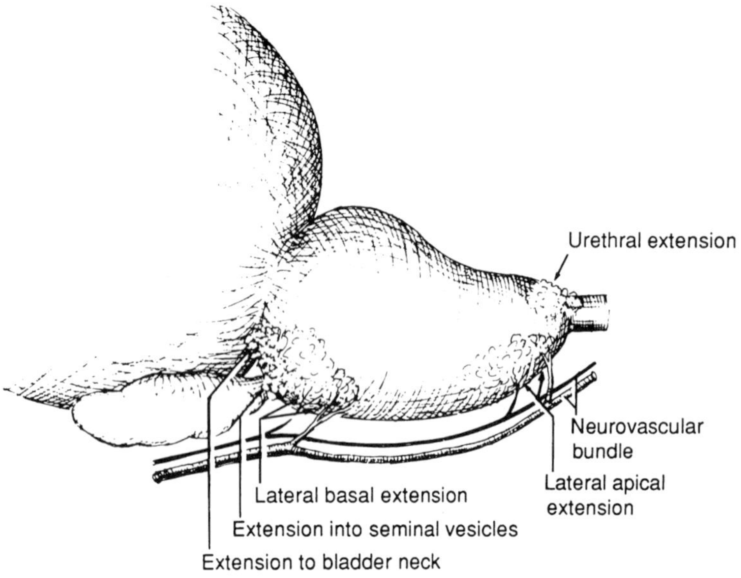
Urethral extension
Neurovascular bundle
Lateral apical extension
Lateral basal extension
Extension into seminal vesicles
Extension to bladder neck

FIGURE 25–7. Areas of capsular weakness of the prostate, depicting sites where extracapsular extension is likely. (From Narayan P: Neoplasms of the prostate gland. *In* Tanagho EA, McAninch JW [eds]: Smith's General Urology, 14th edition, p 392. Norwalk, Appleton & Lange, 1995, with permission.)

peripheral zone is the palpable portion of the prostate on DRE. Periurethral glands lie adjacent to the urethra and are surrounded by the proximal sphincter. Carcinoma does not arise from these glands. The fibromuscular stroma occupies the anterior surface of the prostate and is principally comprised of smooth muscle.

Primary Prostatic Tumors

Prostatic tumors may originate from epithelial cells, germ cells, or mesenchymal cells and comprise a wide variety of pathologic types as seen in Table 25–5. Nonetheless, over 99% of prostate tumors are carcinomas and almost all of these are glandular neoplasms (adenocarcinoma).[90] Non-adenocarcinomatous tumors represent less than 2% of cases. Adenocarcinomas grossly appear pale yellow (see Fig. 25–11) or with gray flecks of tissue coalesced into a firm, poorly defined mass. From a histologic standpoint, these tumors are quite heterogeneous, with nearly all lesions containing at least some areas of acinar/terminal duct differentiation. Intralobular acinar carcinomas are characterized by focal crowding of irregularly shaped glands, associated with budding, cell necrosis, attenuation of cytoplasm with loss of a regular nuclear arrangement, and large nucleoli.[90] Most adenocarcinomas grow in sheets, cords, or isolated compressed glands. Histologic variants of adenocarcinomas include small cell or schirrhous pattern, clear cell variant resembling renal cell carcinoma (RCCa), ductal carcinoma, and mucinous carcinoma. Pure ductal and mucinous variants may represent 0.4 to 1.3% of all adenocarcinomas. Ductal carcinomas may appear in patterns reminiscent of comedocarcinomas of the breast and are likely to be more aggressive, as a poorly differentiated cancer might behave.

Small cell tumors of the prostate are typically large, heterogeneous tumors with dissemination at diagnosis, therefore lending a poor prognosis. These tumor cells are small, round, and generally undifferentiated.[91,92] These tumors may be difficult to differentiate from lymphomas or round cell sarcomas. Transitional cell carcinoma of the prostate gland tends to be confined to periurethral ducts rather than peripheral sites. These tumors often present with obstructive uropathy, and tend to coexist with bladder cancers. They characteristically metastasize early, leaving the patient with a much poorer prognosis than adenocarcinoma.[93] Prostatic intraepithelial neoplasia (PIN) grade III (also known as severe atypical hyperplasia or hyperplasia with anaplasia) is neoplastic by cytologic parameters[94] and is strongly associated with coincidental prostatic carcinomas[95]; however, the true biologic potential is not well known. PIN grades I and II do not express these cytologic features and do not share a strong association with coincidental prostate carcinomas.[94]

Carcinosarcoma is defined as the coexistence of histologically differentiated carcinoma plus malignant mesenchymal elements that have differentiated into recognizable chondrosarcoma, osteosarcoma, myosarcoma, liposarcoma, or angiosarcoma.[90,96] Tumors are often quite firm and large at presentation. Glandular and stromal elements may metastasize[97] and the prognosis is poor, with a mean survival of less than 2 years.

Malignant mesenchymal tumors make up less than 0.3% of prostatic neoplasms. The most recognized histologic patterns are rhabdomyosarcoma and leiomyosarcoma, with rhabdomyosarcoma being seen more commonly in younger and leiomyosarcomas being seen in older patients. Tumors tend to grow locally and are usually at a high stage at diagnosis. As the prognosis depends heavily on stage at presentation, these patients generally have

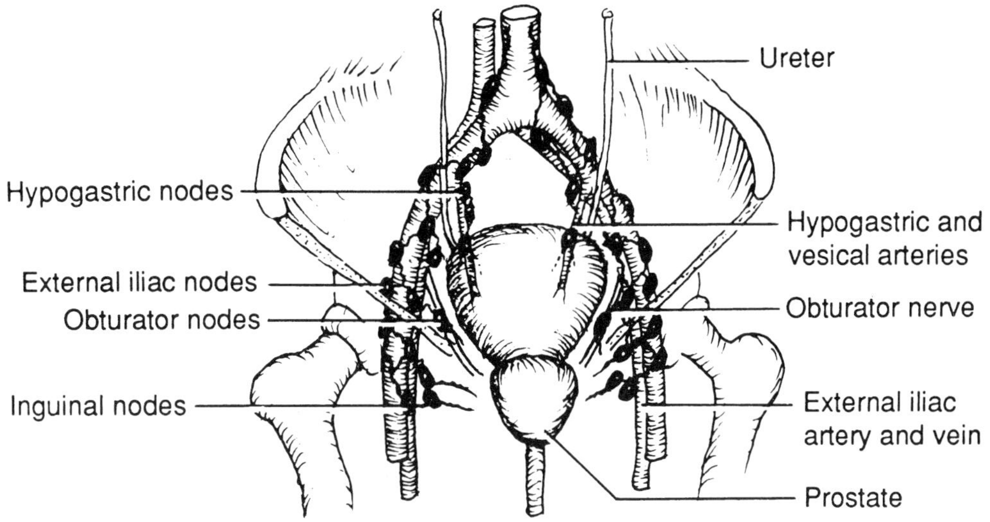
Ureter
Hypogastric nodes
Hypogastric and vesical arteries
External iliac nodes
Obturator nodes
Obturator nerve
Inguinal nodes
External iliac artery and vein
Prostate

FIGURE 25–8. Lymphatic drainage of the prostate. Primary drainage is to obturator and hypogastric nodal areas. Secondary drainage is to external iliac and inguinal nodal areas. (From Narayan P: Neoplasms of the prostate gland. *In* Tanagho EA, McAninch JW [eds]: Smith's General Urology, 14th edition, p 392. Norwalk, Appleton & Lange, 1995, with permission.)

a poor outcome. Rhabdomyosarcomas, in particular, tend to progress rapidly. Leiomyosarcomas grow more slowly, but tend to recur more frequently.

Secondary Prostatic Tumors

Lymphomas rarely represent primary neoplasms of the prostate.[98] They are, however, along with leukemias, the most frequent metastatic tumors to the prostate. Other metastatic neoplasms have included adenocarcinomas of the gastrointestinal tract, lung, melanoma, seminoma, malignant rhabdoid tumor, and granulocytic sarcoma.[90]

GRADING

Epithelial neoplasms are graded by the histologic appearance of the cells. Many grading systems have been proposed, including the Gleason system,[99] the Mostofi system,[100] the Gaeta system,[101] the Bocking system,[102] the Broders system,[103] and the M.D. Anderson Hospital system.[104] Today, the Gleason system is most commonly utilized and is widely accepted. The Gleason system utilizes glandular configuration and the amount of tumor showing specific histologic patterns to develop a scoring system (from 1 to 5) that lends equal weight to the dominant and secondary areas making up the neoplasm. In addition, Gleason has proposed augmenting the scoring with the inclusion of clinical stage,[105] although this component of his system is not widely utilized. Figure 25–12 displays examples of Gleason grades.

STAGING

DRE

Digital rectal examination represents the traditional means of staging prostate cancer patients. In fact, the most commonly used staging systems today (TNM and Whitmore-Jewett systems, see Table 25–6) are based on the palpation of the prostate. There is a subjectivity to this examination, which relies on the experience of the examiner to note the size of the lesion and its extracapsular spread.

Clinical staging by rectal examination provides valuable prognostic information, but this examination regularly underestimates and sometimes overstates the local extension of the tumor, frequently misjudges its location, and correlates poorly with the actual volume of cancer or even the pathologic extent of tumor.[106] Nevertheless, DRE continues to remain an integral part of cancer staging, particularly because it costs little and is easy to perform.

PSA

Kleer and Oesterling[107] have demonstrated a direct relationship between serum PSA and tumor volume. However, overlap in serum PSA levels between stages has resulted in the inability of PSA to reliably predict pathologic stage on an individual basis. The predictive power of PSA, however, can be enhanced with the combination of other factors such as clinical stage (assessed by DRE) and tumor grade (via prostatic biopsy).

Most recently, in a retrospective study of 945 untreated prostate cancer patients with a mean age of 66 years, Kleer and colleagues[108] used multivariate regression analysis to show that local clinical stage and tumor grade significantly enhance the predic-

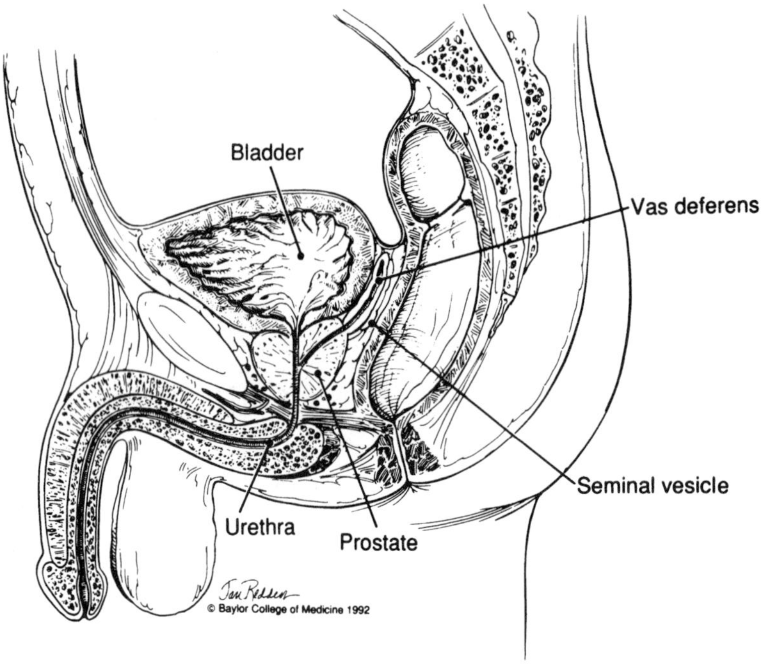
Bladder
Vas deferens
Seminal vesicle
Urethra
Prostate
© Baylor College of Medicine 1992

FIGURE 25–9. Regional anatomy of the pelvis. The prostate is located at the outlet of the urinary bladder and is accessible to palpation through the rectum. (From Hanks GE, Myers CE, Scardino PT: Cancer of the prostate. *In* De Vita VT Jr, Hellman S, Rosenberg SA [eds]: Cancer: Principles and Practice of Oncology, 4th edition, p 1073. Philadelphia, JB Lippincott Co, 1993, with permission.)

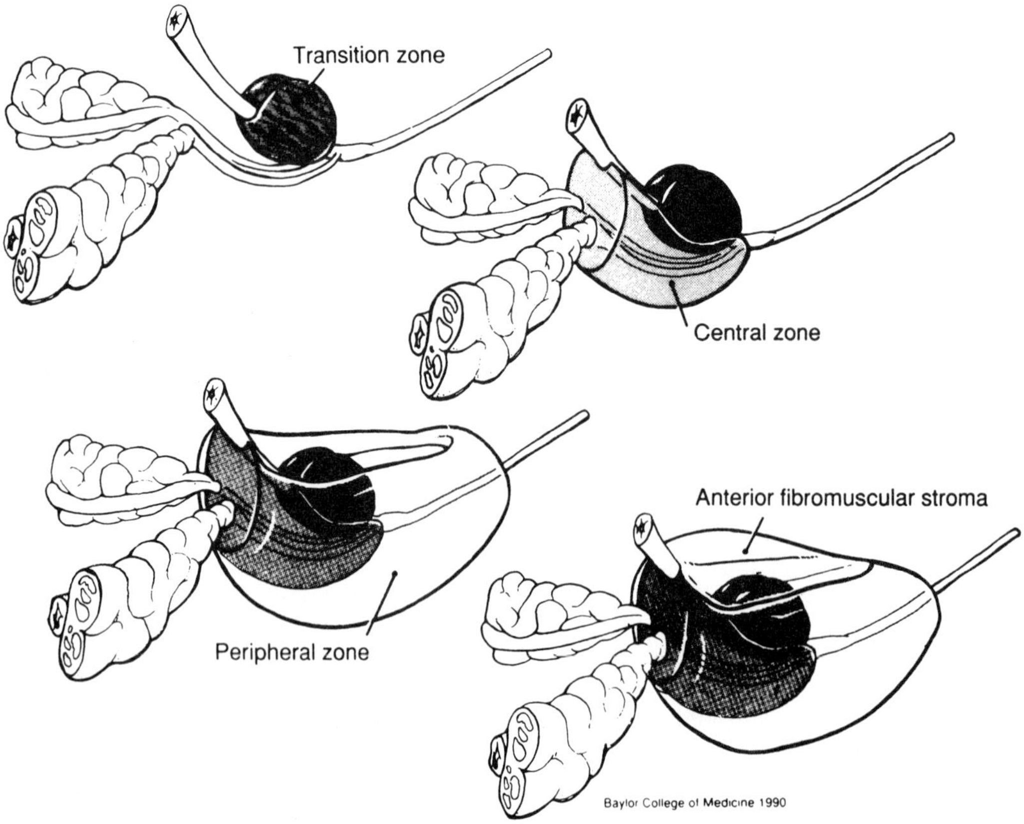
Transition zone
Central zone
Peripheral zone
Anterior fibromuscular stroma
Baylor College of Medicine 1990

FIGURE 25–10. Zonal anatomy of the prostate. There are three glandular zones and the anterior fibromuscular stroma. In the young adult prostate, the transition zone is composed of 10% of the glandular tissue, the central zone 25% and the peripheral zone 65%. (From Hanks GE, Myers CE, Scardino PT: Cancer of the Prostate. *In* De Vita VT Jr, Hellman S, Rosenberg SA [eds]: Cancer: Principles and Practice of Oncology, 4th edition, p 1073. Philadelphia, JB Lippincott Co, 1993, with permission.)

TABLE 25–5. PATHOLOGIC CLASSIFICATION OF PROSTATIC NEOPLASMS*

Epithelial neoplasms
Adenocarcinoma
Pure ductal
Mucinous
Small cell tumors
Transitional cell carcinoma
Carcinoma in situ (intraepithelial neoplasia) and precursors of neoplasia
Rare epithelial neoplasms
Carcinosarcoma
Nonepithelial neoplasms
Mesenchymal—benign and malignant
Lymphoma
Germ cell tumors

*From Murphy WM, Gaeta JF: Diseases of the prostate gland and seminal vesicles. *In* Murphy WM, Bernstein J, McC Chesney T, et al (eds): Urological Pathology, p 147. Philadelphia, WB Saunders Co, 1989, with permission.

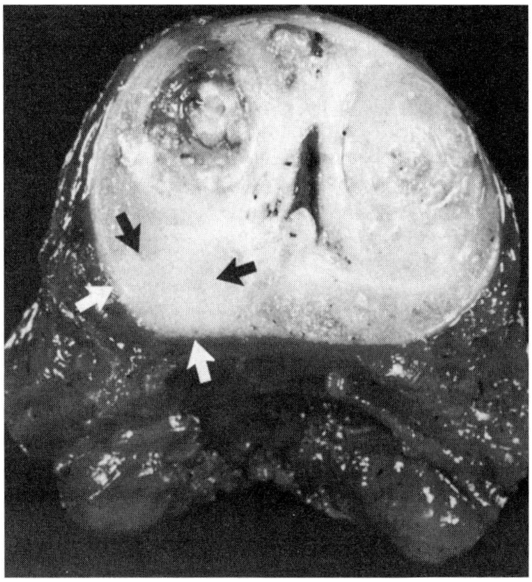

FIGURE 25–11. Adenocarcinoma of the prostate gland appears as a poorly defined, pale gray mass at the periphery of the gland (*arrows*). (From Murphy WM, Gaeta JF: Diseases of the prostate gland and seminal vesicles. *In* Murphy WM, Bernstein J, McC Chesney T, et al [eds]: Urological Pathology, p 147. Philadelphia, WB Saunders Co, 1989, with permission.)

tive power of PSA to determine pathologic stage. They used these preoperative parameters to construct probability plots that would estimate the likelihood of an individual having histologic disease that displayed organ confinement, capsular penetration, seminal vesicle invasion, positive surgical margins, or lymph node involvement. They concluded that these estimations would assist clinicians in recommending the most appropriate therapy and also planning surgical approaches to ensure complete tumor resection with reduced compromise to normal function. Similarly, Partin and coworkers[109] also used logistic regression analysis to show that serum PSA (Hybritech assay), preoperative Gleason score, and clinical stage, in combination, were able to predict final pathologic stage.

Blackwell and colleagues[110] undertook a prospective analysis of 311 previously untreated men with prostate cancer with clinical stages T1cN0 (n = 19), T2aN0 (n = 271), and T3N0 (n = 21). (See Table 25–6 for the TNM classification system for prostate cancer.) They assessed the PSA cancer density (PSACD) (serum PSA times cancer volume divided by prostate volume) and demonstrated a significantly stronger correlation of PSACD with pathologic stage than PSA level alone or PSAD with stage. However, in this study, the cancer and prostatic volumes were obtained from the surgical specimen after radical retropubic prostatectomy, making the results somewhat difficult to apply to preoperative situations. Nevertheless, these data do suggest that preoperative quantification of cancer volume (currently imprecise using standard imaging methods) and prostate volume (likely by TRUS) may provide a promising combination of variables that will be highly predictive of pathologic stage. The authors do suggest the use of endorectal coil magnetic resonance imaging (MRI) as a future means of more precisely assessing prostatic cancer volume.

Overall, staging based on PSA level alone is inexact. However, the combination of tumor grade (by prostatic biopsy), clinical stage (by DRE), and cancer and prostatic volumes, all enhance the power of PSA to predict final pathologic stage. Therefore, all patients undergoing staging evaluation for prostate cancer should have their serum PSA level assessed.

Radionuclide Bone Scan

In the past, standard staging evaluation for the newly diagnosed prostate cancer patient included the radionuclide bone scan. The bone scintigram is a very sensitive method for assessment of the axial skeleton, with superiority over bone radiographs, serum alkaline phosphatase level, and clinical evaluation.[111–113] Unfortunately, the bone scan is so sensitive, it tends to have a high level of false-positives in the patient undergoing staging evaluation,[113] detecting not only metastatic disease but also healing fractures, arthritides, bony infections, and a multitude of other inflammatory bone conditions.[114] False-negative scans occur in less than 1% of all patients.

More recently, the role of the bone scan in staging was evaluated by Levram et al.[115] Eight of 861 patients (0.9%) who underwent bone scan evaluation had a positive result. None of these men had a PSA below 20 ng/ml. In an era of cost consciousness, it seems futile to have every staging evaluation include bone scan examination. The utility of this test will likely be greatest in newly diagnosed prostate cancer patients with symptomatic bone pain, a PSA above 10,[115–118] or evidence of local or distant metastases.

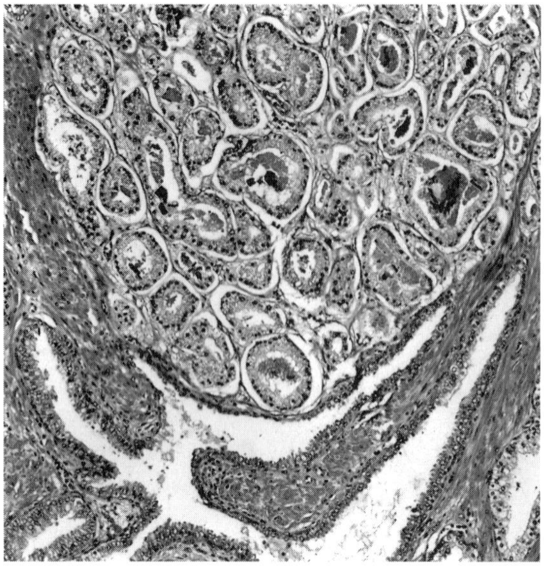

A

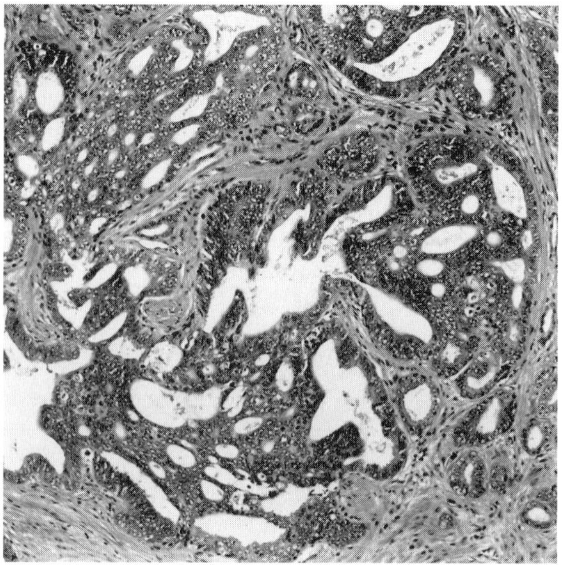

D

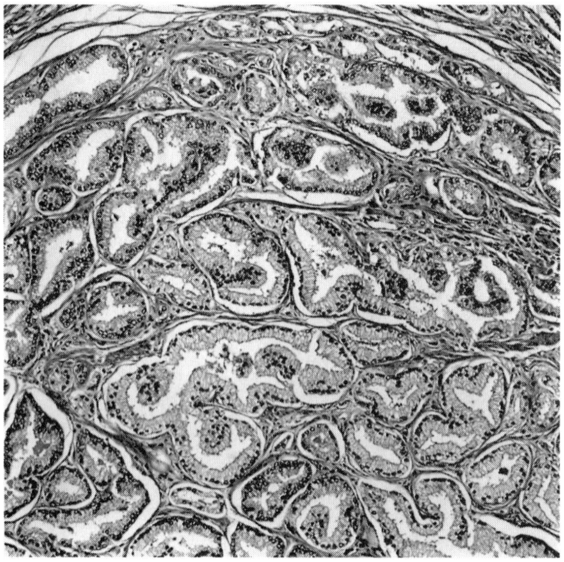

B

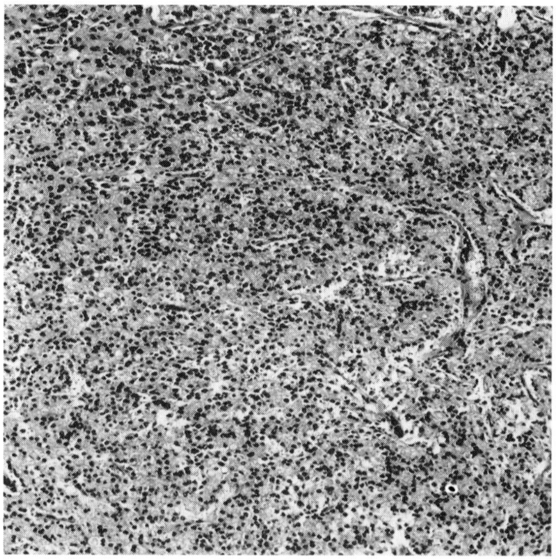

E

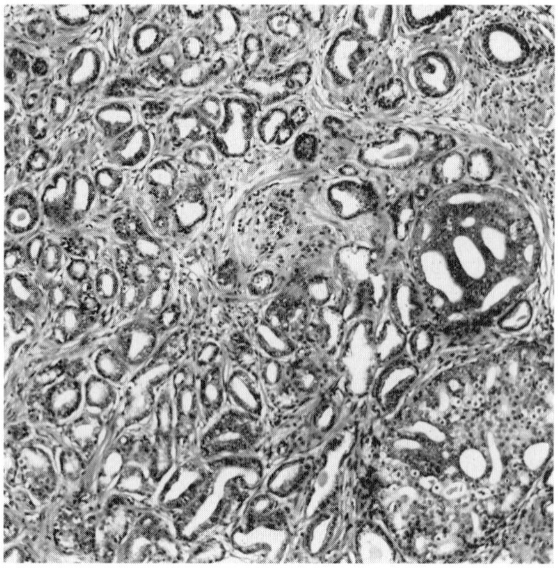

C

FIGURE 25–12. *A*, Gleason 1. Glands are closely packed, single, separate, round, and uniform in appearance. There are well-defined tumor margins. *B*, Gleason 2. Glands are single, separate, and round, but less uniform in appearance. They are separated by stroma, and tumor margins are less well defined. *C*, Gleason 3. Glands are single, separate, and irregular with variable (usually smaller) sizes. Enlarged glandular masses with cribriform patterns are noted, in addition to poorly defined tumor margins. *D*, Gleason 4. Glands are fused in mass with infiltrating cords. Small glands with papillary patterns are seen. *E*, Gleason 5. There are no glands. Solid sheets of tumor cells are seen.

TABLE 25–6. COMPARISON OF TNM AND WHITMORE-JEWETT STAGING SYSTEMS FOR CLINICALLY LOCALIZED PROSTATE CANCER*

Stage		
TNM	Whitmore-Jewett	Description
TX	†	Tumor cannot be assessed
T0	†	No evidence of tumor
T1a	A1	Tumor found incidentally at TURP (<5% of resected tissue)
T1b	A2	Tumor found incidentally at TURP (>5% of resected tissue)
T1c	B0	Nonpalpable tumor identified due to an elevated serum PSA value‡
T2a	B1	Tumor involvement is less than or equal to one half of a lobe
T2b	B1	Tumor involvement is more than one half of a lobe, but not both lobes
T2c	B2	Tumor involves both lobes
T3a	C1	Unilateral extracapsular extension
T3b	C1	Bilateral extracapsular extension
T3c	C2	Tumor invades one or both seminal vesicles
T4a	†	Tumor invades the bladder neck, external sphincter, or rectum
T4b	†	Tumor invades the levator muscles or is fixed to the pelvic sidewall

*From Oesterling J, Suman V, Zincke H, Bostwick D: PSA-detected (clinical stage T1c or B0) prostate cancer: pathologically significant tumors. Urol Clin North Am 1993; 20(4):687–693, with permission.
†No corresponding stage.
‡In the TNM staging system, the tumor should not be visible on transrectal ultrasonography.

Radiography

Plain bone films are quite useful in confirming suspicious lesions on bone scan that might account for metastatic disease. Chest radiography is necessary in initial staging, as 6% of patients will have pulmonary metastases at the time of presentation.[119] The diagnosis of metastatic prostate cancer is often made on the basis of bony abnormalities noted on chest radiograph or lumbar spine series. The diagnosis is based on the finding of diffuse sclerotic lesions.[114]

TRUS

Modern transrectal ultrasound allows for high-resolution images of the prostate, particularly in the peripheral zone. Most neoplasms are hypoechoic, but the degree of hypoechogenicity is variable with the density of cancer cells per unit volume. The variable density and hypoechogenicity are related to the growth and spread of the cancer and not the tumor size.[120] Neoplasms located in the transition zone are difficult to image. In fact, Carter et al.[121] estimate that one half of lesions greater than 1 cm are not visualized by TRUS. TRUS has demonstrated a 66% sensitivity and 46% specificity in its ability to correctly stage advanced and localized disease.[122] Moreover, TRUS identified only 59% of tumors measuring 5 mm or larger on subsequent pathologic analysis.

In view of this and the fact that TRUS cannot visualize pelvic lymph nodes directly, attempts have been made to enhance the staging capabilities of TRUS using prostatic biopsy of the prostate and surrounding tissue including seminal vesicles. One group has noted reasonable efficacy of TRUS-based staging, in combination with Gleason score and PSA.[123] Overall, TRUS is not a useful staging modality at the current time. On the other hand, its ability to direct biopsies in the diagnosis of cancer is extremely useful and important.

Computed Tomography

The sensitivity and accuracy rate of computed tomography (CT) in lymph node staging is conflicting but generally regarded as unacceptably low, with sensitivity ranging from 27 to 75% and specificity from 66 to 100%.[124,125] In addition, CT scan cannot distinguish abnormalities in internal prostatic architecture, although it can detect changes in the size of the gland. Studies have shown poor results in CT assessment of local prostatic cancer progression; therefore, CT is unreliable at distinguishing T2 from T3 disease.[126] It has also been shown to understage[115] and overstage[127] disease. In terms of seminal vesicle size noted on CT, there is a weak correlation between the likelihood of pathologic involvement and seminal vesicle size.[128]

Bearing this in mind, fine-needle aspiration cytology (FNAC) has been studied as an enhancer of CT scan imaging alone. In one study[128] the sensitivity, specificity, and accuracy rates were enhanced from 78, 96.6, and 93.7% to 77.8, 100, and 96.5%, respectively, with FNAC. The enhancement here seems to be little, as the particular sensitivity, specificity, and accuracy were unusually high with CT imaging alone. The current authors do not recommend CT as a routine modality to be used in staging of the newly diagnosed prostate cancer patient with a serum PSA level of 20 or below.

Magnetic Resonance Imaging

Conventional transabdominal MRI has a sensitivity of 77% and a specificity of 57%[122] in its ability to stage advanced and localized disease, respectively. It is able to identify only 60% of all malignant tumors measuring more than 5 mm on pathologic analysis.[122] To improve accuracy, a balloon-mounted endorectal coil was developed to enhance the imaged detail of the prostate and surrounding structures.

A multi-institutional group,[129] looking at 213 patients, assessed the ability of three MRI techniques (imaging with conventional body coil, with fat suppression and a body coil, and with an endorectal coil) to stage prostate cancer. Overall accuracy was 61, 64, and 54%, respectively. They concluded that none of the techniques was highly accurate for staging early prostate cancer. Contrast-enhanced T1-weighted sequences did not improve overall staging accuracy of T2-weighted sequences, which are mandatory for delineation of prostatic carcinoma.[130] At the current time, the cost and inaccuracy of MRI preclude it from having a role in staging prostate cancer; however, with further study, a more sensitive and specific application for this technology may develop.

Pelvic Lymph Node Dissection

Most urologists perform either an open or a laparoscopic pelvic lymphadenectomy for patients with clinically localized prostate cancer to determine the presence or absence of regional nodal metastatic disease before proceeding with definitive therapy. Previously, pelvic lymph nodes were positive in 15% of patients undergoing lymphadenectomy, but today the incidence is reportedly less (0.8% in recent studies).[118,131]

The benefits of laparoscopic pelvic lymphadenectomy for staging purposes involve sparing the patient a large operation which will not be curative in the face of nodal metastases. The patients at risk are those with clinical stage T3 (or C), Gleason sum greater than 6, and PSA greater than 20 ng/ml.[131,132] Laparoscopic pelvic lymphadenectomy offers a reliable, minimally invasive alternative to open node dissection with comparable results.[130]

Molecular Staging

Polymerase chain reaction amplification can detect DNA point mutations or rearrangements, mRNA sequences that are unique to certain cells, or the relative amount of mRNA produced by a cell.[134] This technique allows for the detection of one target cell from a population of 10^6 to 10^7 background cells.[134] Expression of PSA protein by prostate cells makes the PSA mRNA an ideal template for RTPCR, a modification of the PCR technique. RTPCR can therefore detect circulating prostate cancer cells using PSA mRNA. In fact, RTPCR of bone marrow and blood has accurately identified circulating prostate cells in patients with known metastatic disease or lymph node metastases.[135–137] In one study,[135] the presence of circulating cells correlated strongly with the pathologic stage of the patient undergoing a radical retropubic prostatectomy for clinically localized prostate cancer.

The clinical applicability of this test is not yet known. The majority of circulating cancer cells do not have the ability to initiate a metastatic lesion. Therefore, simply identifying circulating cancer cells is not useful. If this technique can predict which patients with circulating cells will experience relapse with recurrent disease, then it will be a beneficial staging tool. A more clinically relevant finding may be a negative RTPCR test, suggesting pathologically organ-confined disease. This may be valuable in encouraging watchful waiting programs for those patients who have a limited life expectancy.[138] At the current time, molecular staging is experimental and is not recommended for routine staging.

SUMMARY

In 1996, prostate cancer continues to be a challenging disease process. There is much controversy surrounding the need for diagnosis, screening or early detection, staging, and treatment of this disorder. Regardless of one's opinions regarding these topics, it is clear that alarming numbers of men are dying from this disease entity each year. This has spurred furious research regarding epidemiology, risk factors, and methods for diagnosis and staging. Within this chapter, the present authors have reviewed pertinent research relevant to these areas, and provided a sensible algorithm for diagnosis (Figs. 25–5 and 25–6), as well as suggestions for cost-efficient staging tools. At this time, there are certain factors that appear to increase the risk of prostate cancer. These factors include age, ethnicity, family aggregation, and nutrition. In the patient with a life expectancy ≥10 years, early detection of prostate cancer is warranted. The diagnosis is best made with a combination of serum PSA determination, DRE, and TRUS-guided sextant biopsies of the prostate. After the diagnosis is made, the patient should undergo appropriate staging studies based on the serum PSA level, clinical stage, and Gleason grade. Many traditional staging studies can be eliminated in the era of serum PSA testing.

REFERENCES

1. Parker SL, Tong T, Bolden S, Wingo PA: Cancer statistics, 1996. CA Cancer J Clin 1996; 46(1):5.
2. Scardino PT, Weaver R, Hudson MA: Early detection of prostate cancer. Hum Pathol 1992; 23:211.
3. Catalona WJ, Scott WW: Carcinoma of the prostate. *In* Walsh PC, Gittes RF, Perlmutter AD, Stamey TA (eds): Campbell's Urology, 5th edition, p. 1463. Philadelphia, WB Saunders Co, 1986.
4. Sellers TA, Potter JD, Rich SS, et al: Familial clustering of breast and prostate cancers and risk of postmenopausal breast cancer. J Natl Cancer Inst 1994; 86(24):1860.
5. Gardner W: Hypothesis: the prenatal origins of prostate cancer. Hum Pathol 1995; 26:1291.
6. Pienta KJ, Esper PS: Risk factors for prostate cancer. Ann Intern Med 1993; 118:793.
7. Natarajan N, Murphy GP, Mettlin C: Prostate cancer in blacks: an update from the American College of Surgeons' patterns of care studies. J Surg Oncol 1989; 40:232.
8. Pienta KJ, Demmers R, Hoff M, et al: Effect of age and race on the survival of men with prostate cancer in the

metropolitan Detroit tricounty area, 1973 to 1987. Urology 1995; 45:93.
9. Aprikian AG, Bazinet M, Plante M, et al: Family history and the risk of prostatic carcinoma in a high risk group of urological patients. J Urol 1995; 154:404.
10. Whittemore AS, Wu AH, Kolonel LN, et al: Family history and prostate cancer risk in black, white, and Asian men in the United States and Canada. Am J Epidemiol 1995; 141:732.
11. Hayes RB, Liff JM, Pottern LM, et al: Prostate cancer risk in U.S. blacks and whites with a family history of cancer. Int J Cancer 1995; 60:361.
12. Carter BS, Bova GS, Beaty TH, et al: Hereditary prostate cancer: epidemiologic and clinical features. J Urol 1993; 150:797.
13. Whittemore AS, Kolonel LN, Wu AH, et al: Prostate cancer in relation to diet, physical activity, and body size in blacks, whites, and Asians in the United States and Canada. J Natl Cancer Inst 1995; 87:652.
14. Honda GD, Bernstein L, Ross RK, et al: Vasectomy, cigarette smoking, and age at first sexual intercourse as risk factors for prostate cancer in middle-aged men. Br J Cancer 1988; 57:326.
15. Giovannucci E, Tosteson TD, Speizer FE, et al: A retrospective cohort study of vasectomy and prostate cancer in US men. JAMA 1993; 269:878.
16. Giovannucci E, Ascherio A, Rimm EB, et al: A prospective cohort study of vasectomy and prostate cancer in U.S. men. JAMA 1993; 269:873.
17. Hayes RB, Pottern LM, Greenberg R, et al: Vasectomy and prostate cancer in U.S. blacks and whites. Am J Epidemiol 1993; 137:263.
18. Rosenberg L, Palmer JR, Zauber AG, et al: The relation of vasectomy to the risk of cancer. Am J Epidemiol 1994; 140:431.
19. John EM, Whittemore AS, Wu AH, et al: Vasectomy and prostate cancer: results from a multiethnic case control study. J Natl Cancer Inst 1995; 87:662.
20. Healy B: From the National Institutes of Health: does vasectomy cause prostate cancer? JAMA 1993; 269(20):2620.
21. Cooner WH, Mosley BR, Rutherford CL, et al: Prostate cancer detection in a clinical urological practice by ultrasonography, digital rectal examination, and prostate specific antigen. J Urol 1990; 143:1146.
22. Littrup PJ, Lee FL, Mettlin C: Prostate cancer screening: current trends and future implications. CA Cancer J Clin 1992; 42:198.
23. Babaian RJ, Dinney CR, Ramirez El, Evans RB: Diagnostic testing for prostate cancer: less is best. Urology 1993; 41: 421.
24. Coley CM, Barry MJ, Fleming C, et al: Should Medicare provide reimbursement for prostate specific antigen testing for early detection of prostate cancer? Part II: Early detection strategies. Urology 1995; 46:125.
25. Gann PH, Hennekens CH, Stampfer MJ: A prospective evaluation of plasma prostate-specific antigen for detection of prostatic cancer. JAMA 1995; 273:289.
26. Catalona WJ, Richie JP, Ahmann FR, et al: Comparison of digital rectal examination and serum prostate specific antigen in the early detection of prostate cancer: results of a multicenter clinical trial of 6,630 men. J Urol 1994; 151: 1283.
27. Smith D, Catalona W: The nature of prostate cancer detected through prostate specific antigen based screening. J Urol 1994; 152(5):1732–1736.
28. Gohagan J, Prork P, Kramer B, Cornett J: Prostate cancer screening in the prostate, lung, colorectal and ovarian cancer screening trial of the National Cancer Institute. J Urol 1994; 152(2):1905–1909.
29. Hara M, Koyanagi Y, Inoue T, Fukuyama T: Some physico-chemical characteristics of gamma-seminoprotein, an antigenic component specific for human seminal plasma. Jpn J Legal Med 1971; 25(4):322–324.
30. Li T, Beling C: Isolation and characterization of two specific antigens of human seminal plasma. Fertil Steril 1973; 24(2):134–144.
31. Wang M, Valenzuela L, Murphy G, et al: Purification of a human prostate specific antigen. Invest Urol 1979; 17(2): 159–163.
32. Papsidero L, Wang M, Valenzuela L, et al: A prostate antigen in sera of prostatic cancer patients. Cancer Res 1980; 40(7):2428–2432.
33. Oesterling J, Jacobsen S, Chute C, et al: Serum prostate-specific antigen in a community-based population of healthy men: establishment of age-specific reference ranges. JAMA 1993; 270(7):860–864.
34. Katz A, Olsson C, Raffo A, et al: Molecular staging of prostate cancer with the use of an enhanced reverse transcriptase-PCR assay. Urology 1994; 43(6):765–775.
35. Stamey T, Yang N, Hay A, et al: Prostate specific antigen as a serum marker for adenocarcinoma of the prostate. N Engl J Med 1987; 317(15):909–916.
36. Oesterling J, Chan D, Epstein J, et al: Prostate specific antigen in the preoperative and postoperative evaluation of localized prostatic cancer treated with radical prostatectomy. J Urol 1988; 139(4):766–772.
37. Oesterling J, Rice D, Glenski W, Bergstralh E: Effect of cystoscopy, prostate biopsy, and transurethral resection of prostate on serum prostate-specific antigen concentration. Urology 1993; 42(3):276–282.
38. Neal D Jr, Clejan S, Sarma D, et al: Prostate specific antigen and prostatitis: effect of prostatitis on serum PSA in the human and nonhuman primate. Prostate 1992; 20: 105–111.
39. Chybowski F, Bergstralh E, Oesterling J: The effect of digital rectal examination on the serum prostate specific antigen concentration: results of a randomized study. J Urol 1992; 148:83–86.
40. Yuan J, Coplen D, Petros J, et al: Effects of rectal examination, prostatic massage, ultrasonography and needle biopsy on serum prostate specific antigen levels. J Urol 1992; 147:810–814.
41. Glenski W, Klee G, Bergstralh E, Oesterling J: Prostate-specific antigen: establishment of the reference range for the clinically normal prostate gland and the effect of digital rectal examination, ejaculation, and time on serum concentrations. Prostate 1992; 21(2):99–110.
42. Cupp M, Oesterling J: Prostate-specific antigen, digital rectal examination, and transrectal ultrasonography: their roles in diagnosing early prostate cancer. Mayo Clin Proc 1993; 68:297–306.
43. Benson M, Whang I, Pantuck A, et al: Prostate specific antigen density: a means of distinguishing benign prostatic hypertrophy and prostate cancer. J Urol 1992; 147: 815–816.
44. Benson M, Whang I, Olsson C, et al: The use of prostate specific antigen density to enhance the predictive value of intermediate levels of serum prostate specific antigen. J Urol 1992; 147:817–821.
45. Seaman E, Whang M, Olsson C, et al: PSA density (PSAD): role in patient evaluation and management. Urol Clin North Am 1993; 20(4):653–663.
46. Brawer M, Aramburu E, Chen G, et al: The inability of prostate specific antigen index to enhance the predictive value of prostate specific antigen in the diagnosis of prostatic carcinoma. J Urol 1993; 150:369–373.
47. Catalona W, Richie J, deKernion, et al: Comparison of prostate specific antigen concentration versus prostate specific antigen density in the early detection of prostate cancer: receiver operating characteristic curves. J Urol 1994; 152:2031–2036.
48. Oesterling J, Cooner W, Jacobsen S, et al: Influence of patient age on the serum PSA concentration: an important clinical observation. Urol Clin North Am 1993; 20(4): 671–680.
49. Partin A, Carter H, Chan D, et al: Prostate specific antigen in the staging of localized prostate cancer: influence of tumor differentiation, tumor volume and benign hyperplasia. J Urol 1990; 143(4):747–752.

50. Carter HB, Pearson J, Metter J, et al: Longitudinal evaluation of prostate specific antigen levels in men with and without prostate disease. JAMA 1992; 267(16):2215–2220.
51. Carter H, Pearson J: PSA velocity for the diagnosis of early prostate cancer: a new concept. Urol Clin North Am 1993; 20(4):665–670.
52. Oesterling J, Chute C, Jacobsen S, et al: Longitudinal changes in serum PSA (PSA velocity) in a community-based cohort of men (Abstract). J Urol 1993; 149:412A.
53. Carter HB, Pearson J, Wacliwew X, et al: PSA variability in men with BPH. J Urol 1994; 151:312A.
54. Dalkin B, Ahmann F, Southwick P, Bottaccini M: Derivation of normal prostate specific antigen (PSA) level by age. J Urol 1993; 149:413A.
55. Feneley M, McLean A, Webb J, Kirby R: Age-corrected prostate-specific antigen in symptomatic benign prostatic hyperplasia. J Urol 1994; 151:312A.
56. Collins G, Lee R, McKelvie G, et al: Relationship between prostate specific antigen, prostate volume and age in the benign prostate. Br J Urol 1993; 71(4):445–450.
57. Crawford E: Report on the 1993 Prostate Cancer Awareness Week. J Urol 1994; 151:71A.
58. Dalkin B, Ahmann F, Kopp J: Prostate specific antigen levels in men older than 50 years without clinical evidence of prostatic carcinoma. J Urol 1993; 150(6):1837–1839.
59. Catalona W, Hudson M, Scardino P, et al: Selection of optimal prostate specific antigen cutoffs for early detection of prostate cancer: receiver operating characteristic curves. J Urol 1994; 152:2037–2042.
60. Vessella R, Lange P: Issues in the assessment of PSA immunoassays. Urol Clin North Am 1993: 20(4):607–619.
61. Christensson A, Laurell CB, Lilja H: Enzymatic activity of prostate-specific antigen and its reactions with extracellular serine proteinase inhibitors. Eur J Biochem 1990; 194:755–763.
62. Lilja H: Significance of different molecular forms of serum PSA: the free, noncomplexed form of PSA versus that complexed to α1-antichymotrypsin. Urol Clin North Am 1993; 20(4):681–686.
63. Hybritech, Incorporated: Why might different PSA assays yield discrepant results on the same patient? Prostate-Specific Antigen Clinical Brief 1994; 3(1).
64. Graves H: Standardization of immunoassays for prostate-specific antigen: a problem of prostate-specific antigen complexation or a problem of assay design? Cancer 1993; 72(11):3141–3144.
65. Graves H: Issues on standardization of immunoassays for prostate-specific antigen: a review. Clin Invest Med 1993; 16(6):416–425.
66. Stamey T: Second conference on international standardization of prostate specific antigen immunoassays: September 1 and 2. Urology 1995; 45:173–184.
67. Christensson A, Bjork T, Nilsson O, et al: Serum prostate specific antigen complexed to α1-antichymotrypsin as an indicator of prostate cancer. J Urol 1993; 150:100–105.
68. Lilja H, Christensson A, Dahlen U, et al: Prostate-specific antigen in serum occurs predominantly in complex with alpha$_1$-antichymotrypsin. Clin Chem 1991; 37(9):1618–1625.
69. Stenman U-H, Leinonen J, Alfthan H, et al: A complex between prostate-specific antigen and alpha-1-antichymotrypsin is the major form of prostate-specific antigen in serum of patients with prostatic cancer: assay of the complex improves clinical sensitivity for cancer. Cancer Res 1991; 51:222–226.
70. Oesterling J, Jacobsen S, Klee G, et al: Free, complexed, and total serum prostate specific antigen: the establishment of appropriate reference ranges for their concentrations and ratios using newly developed immunofluorometric assays (IFMA). J Urol 1995; 154:1090–1095.
71. Lilja H, Bjork T, Abrahamsson P, et al: Improved separation between normals, benign prostatic hyperplasia (BPH) and carcinoma of the prostate (CAP) by measuring free (F), complexed (C) and total concentrations (T) of prostate specific antigen (PSA). J Urol 1994; 151(S):400A.
72. Pettersson K, Mitrunen K, Piironen T, et al: A novel dual-label immunoassay for the simultaneous measurement of the free and total PSA in serum. XIth Congress of the European Association of Urology. July 13–16, 1994.
73. Rasmusson G: Biochemistry and pharmacology of 5α-reductase inhibitors. *In* Furr B, Wakeling A (eds): Pharmacology and Clinical Uses of Inhibitors of Hormone Secretion and Action, pp 308–325. London, Bailliere Tindall, 1987.
74. McConnell J: Current medical therapy for benign prostatic hyperplasia: the scientific basis and clinical efficacy of finasteride and alpha-blockers. *In* Walsh PC, Retik AB, Stamey TA, Vaughn ED Jr (eds): Campbell's Urology, 6th edition, pp 1–12. update no. 3. Philadelphia, WB Saunders Co, 1992.
75. Guess H, Gormeley GJ, Stoner E, Oesterling JE: Effect of finasteride on the serum PSA. J Urol 1996; 155:3.
76. Gormley G, Stoner E, Bruskewitz R, et al: The effect of finasteride in men with benign prostatic hyperplasia. N Engl J Med 1992; 327(17):1185–1191.
77. Guess H, Heyse J, Gormley G, et al: Effect of finasteride on serum PSA concentration in men with benign prostatic hyperplasia: results from the North American phase III clinical trial. Urol Clin North Am 1993; 20(4):627–636.
78. McCormack RT, Rittenhouse HG, Finlay JA, et al: Molecular forms of prostate-specific antigen and the human kallikrein gene family: a new era. Urology 1995; 45:729.
79. Narayan P: Neoplasms of the prostate gland. *In* Tanagho EA, McAninch JW (eds): Smith's General Urology, 14th edition, p 392. Norwalk, Appleton & Lange, 1995.
80. Bastacky SI, Walsh PC, Epstein JI: Relationship between perineural tumor invasion on needle biopsy and radical prostatectomy capsular penetration in clinical stage B adenocarcinoma of the prostate. Am J Surg Pathol 1993; 17: 336.
81. Cho KR, Epstein JI: Metastatic prostate carcinoma to supradiaphragmatic lymph nodes: a clinicopathologic and immunohistochemical study. Am J Surg Pathol 1987; 11: 457.
82. Clinton K: Mortality rates by stage-at-diagnosis. Semin Surg Oncol 1994; 10:7.
83. Jacobs SC: Spread of prostatic cancer to bone. Urology 1983; 21:337.
84. Batson OV: The function of the vertebral veins and their role in the spread of metastases. Ann Surg 1940; 112:138.
85. Dodds PR, Caride VJ, Lytton B: The role of vertebral veins in the dissemination of prostatic carcinoma. J Urol 1981; 126:753.
86. LeDuc IE: The anatomy of the prostate and the pathology of early benign hypertrophy. J Urol 1939; 42:1217.
87. Brandes D, Kirchleim D, Scott W: Ultrastructure of the human prostate. Normal and neoplastic. Lab Invest 1964; 13:1541.
88. NcNeal JE, Redwine EA, Freiha FS, Stamey TA: Zonal distribution of prostatic adenocarcinoma. Am J Surg Pathol 1988; 12:897.
89. Stamey TA, McNeal JE: Adenocarcinoma of the prostate. *In* Walsh PC, Retick AB, Stamey TA, Vaughn ED Jr (eds): Campbell's Urology, 6th edition, p 1159. Philadelphia, WB Saunders Co, 1992.
90. Murphy WM, Gaeta JF: Diseases of the prostate gland and seminal vesicles. *In* Murphy WM, Bernstein J, McC Chesney T, et al (eds): Urological Pathology, p 147. Philadelphia, WB Saunders Co, 1989.
91. Tetu B, Ro JY, Ayala AG, et al: Small cell carcinoma of the prostate. Part I: a clinicopathologic study of 20 cases. Cancer 1987; 59:1803.
92. Ro JY, Tetu B, Ayala AG, Ordonez NG: Small cell carcinoma of the prostate. II. Immunohistochemical and electron microscopic studies of 18 cases. Cancer 1987; 59:977.
93. Bodner DR, Cohen JK, Resnick MI: Primary transitional cell carcinoma of the prostate. J Urol 1986; 92:121.
94. Bostwick DG, Amin MB, Dundore P, et al: Architectural

patterns of high-grade prostatic intraepithelial neoplasia. Hum Pathol 1993; 24:298.
95. Sakr WA, Grignon DJ, Crissman JD, et al: High grade prostatic intraepithelial neoplasia (HGPIN) and prostatic adenocarcinoma between the ages of 20–69; an autopsy study of 249 cases. In Vivo 1994; 8:439.
96. Ginesin Y, Bolkien M, Moskovitz B, et al: Carcinosarcoma of prostate. Eur Urol 1986; 12:441.
97. Haddad JR, Reyes EC: Carcinosarcoma of prostate with metastasis of both elements: case report. J Urol 1970; 103: 80.
98. Bostwick DG, Mann RB: Malignant lymphomas involving the prostate: a study of 13 cases. Cancer 1985; 56:2932.
99. Gleason DF: Classification of prostatic carcinoma. Cancer Chemother Rep 1966; 50:125.
100. Mostofi FK: Grading of prostatic carcinoma. Cancer Chemother Rep 1975; 59:111.
101. Gaeta JF, Asiwartham JE, Miller G, Murphy GP: Histologic grading of primary prostatic cancer. A new approach to an old problem. J Urol 1980; 123:689.
102. Bocking A, Kiehn J, Heinzel-Wach M: Combined histologic grading of prostatic carcinoma. Cancer 1982; 50:288.
103. Broders AC: Epithelium of the genito-urinary organs. Ann Surg 1922; 75:574.
104. Brawn PM, Ayala AG, von Eschenbach AC, et al: Histological grading of prostate adenocarcinoma. The development of a new system and comparison with other methods. Cancer 1982; 49:525.
105. Gleason DF: Histologic grading and clinical staging of prostatic carcinoma. *In* Tannenbaum M (ed): Urologic Pathology: The Prostate, p 171. Philadelphia, Lea & Febiger, 1977.
106. Scardino PT, Shinohara K, Wheeler TM, Carter S: Staging of prostate cancer. Value of ultrasonography. Urol Clin North Am 1989; 16:713.
107. Kleer E, Oesterling J: PSA and staging of localized prostate cancer. Urol Clin North Am 1993; 20(4):695–704.
108. Kleer E, Larson-Keller J, Zincke H, Oesterling J: Ability of preoperative serum prostate-specific antigen value to predict pathologic stage and DNA ploidy: influence of clinical stage and tumor grade. Urology 1993; 41(3):207–216.
109. Partin A, Yoo J, Carter HB, et al: The use of prostate specific antigen, clinical stage and Gleason score to predict pathological stage in men with localized prostate cancer. J Urol 1993; 150:110–114.
110. Blackwell K, Bostwick D, Myers R, et al: Combining prostate specific antigen with cancer and gland volume to predict more reliably pathological stage: the influence of prostate specific antigen cancer density. J Urol 1994; 151: 1565–1570.
111. McGregor B, Tulloch AG, Quinlan MF, Lovegroave F: The role of bone scanning in the assessment of prostatic carcinoma. Br J Urol 1978; 50:178.
112. O'Donoghue EP, Constable AR, Sherwood T, et al: Bone scanning and plasma phosphates in carcinoma of the prostate. Br J Urol 1978; 50:172.
113. Schaffer DL, Pendergrass HP: Comparison of enzyme, clinical radiographic, and radionuclide methods of detecting bone metastases from carcinoma of the prostate. Radiology 1976; 121:431.
114. McCarthy P, Pollack HM: Imaging of patients with stage D prostatic carcinoma. Urol Clin North Am 1991; 18:35.
115. Levran Z, Gonzalez JA, Diokno AC, et al: Are pelvic computed tomography, bone scan and pelvic lymphadenectomy necessary in the staging of prostatic cancer? Br J Urol 1995; 75:778.
116. Chybowski F, Larson-Keller J, Bergstralh E, Oesterling J: Predicting radionuclide bone scan findings in patients with newly diagnosed, untreated prostate cancer: prostate-specific antigen is superior to all other clinical parameters. J Urol 1991; 145:313–318.
117. Oesterling J, Martin S, Bergstralh E, Lowe F: The use of prostate-specific antigen in staging patients with newly diagnosed prostate cancer. JAMA 1993; 269(1):57–60.
118. Oesterling J: Using PSA to eliminate the staging radionuclide bone scan. Significant economic implications. Urol Clin North Am 1993; 20(4):705–711.
119. Lindell MM, Doubleday LC, von Eschenbach AC, et al: Mediastinal metastasis from prostatic carcinoma. J Urol 1982; 128:331.
120. Lee F, Torp-Pedersen S, McLeary: Diagnosis of prostate cancer by transrectal ultrasound. Urol Clin North Am 1989; 16(4):663.
121. Carter HB, Hamper UM, Sheth S, et al: Evaluation of transrectal ultrasound in the early detection of prostate cancer. J Urol 1989; 142:1008.
122. Rifkin MD, Zerhouni EA, Gatsonis CA, et al: Comparison of magnetic resonance imaging and ultrasonography in staging early prostate cancer. Results of a multi-institutional cooperative trial. N Engl J Med 1990; 323:621.
123. Narayan P, Gajendran V, Taylor S, et al: The role of transrectal ultrasound-guided biopsy-based staging, preoperative serum prostate-specific antigen, and biopsy. Gleason score in prediction of final pathologic diagnosis in prostate cancer. Urology 1995; 46:205.
124. Walsh JW, Amendola MA, Konerding KR, et al: Computed tomographic detection of pelvic and inguinal lymph-node metastases from primary and recurrent pelvic malignant disease. Radiology 1980; 137:157.
125. Emory TH, Reinke DB, Hill AL, Lange P: Use of CT to reduce understaging in prostatic cancer: comparison with conventional staging techniques. AJR 1983; 141:351.
126. Hricak H, Theoni RF: Neoplasms of the prostate gland. *In* Pollack HM (ed): Clinical Urography. Philadelphia, WB Saunders Co, 1990.
127. Platt JF, Bree RL, Schwab RE: Accuracy of CT in the staging of carcinoma of the prostate. AJR 1987; 149:315.
128. Larner J, Spencer G, Grizos W, et al: Significance of CT scan detected seminal vesicle enlargement in prostate cancer. A pilot study. Urology 1993; 41:259.
129. Tempany CM, Zhou X, Zerhouni E, et al: Staging of prostate cancer: results of radiology diagnostic oncology group project comparison of three MR imaging techniques. Radiology 1994; 192:47.
130. Huch Boni RA, Boner JA, Lutolf UM, et al: Contrast-enhanced endorectal coil MRI in local staging of prostate carcinoma. J Comput Assist Tomogr 1995; 19:232.
131. Patel M, Katelaris PM: Indications for laparoscopic pelvic lymph node dissection in the staging of prostate cancer. Aust N Z J Surg 1995; 65:233.
132. Maffezzini M, Carmignani G, Perachino M, et al: Benefits and complications of laparoscopic pelvic lymphadenectomy for detection of stage D1 prostate cancer: a multicenter experience. Eur Urol 1995; 27:135.
133. Parra RO, Andrews C, Boullier J: Staging laparoscopic pelvic lymph node dissection: comparison of results with open pelvic lymphadenectomy. J Urol 1992; 147:875.
134. Fey MF, Kulozik AE, Hansen-Hagge TE: The polymerase chain reaction. A new tool for the detection of minimal residual disease in hematological malignancies. Eur J Cancer 1991; 27:89.
135. Wood DP Jr, Banks ER, Humphreys S, et al: Identification of bone marrow micrometastases in patients with prostate cancer. Cancer 1994; 74:2533.
136. Katz A, Olsson C, Raffo A, et al: Molecular staging of prostate cancer with the use of an enhanced reverse transcriptase-PCR assay. Urology 1994; 43:765.
137. Seiden MV, Kantoff PW, Krithivas K, et al: Detection of circulating tumor cells in men with localized prostate cancer. J Clin Oncol 1994; 12:2634.
138. Wood DP Jr: The molecular staging of prostate cancer. Semin Urol 1995; XIII(2):96.
139. Oesterling J, Suman V, Zincke H, Bostwick D: PSA-detected (clinical stage T1c or B_0) prostate cancer: pathologically significant tumors. Urol Clin North Am 1993; 20(4):687–693.
140. Hanks GE, Myers CE, Scardino PT: Cancer of the prostate. *In* De Vita VT Jr, Hellman S, Rosenberg SA (eds): Cancer: Principles and Practice of Oncology, 45th edition, p 1073. Philadelphia, JB Lippincott Co, 1993.

26

CLINICALLY LOCALIZED ADENOCARCINOMA OF THE PROSTATE (STAGE T1a–T2c): MANAGEMENT AND PROGNOSIS

RICHARD G. MIDDLETON, M.D.

Prostate cancer that is clinically localized includes a spectrum of tumors in which there seems to be no extension beyond the capsule of the prostate (Table 26–1). Clinically staging the prostatic tumor relies heavily upon rectal examination to determine whether the process remains within the borders of the prostatic capsule, or breaches that barrier to extend beyond it. Experience and judgment of the examiner play a significant role in clinical staging. Understaging is fairly common; that is, the examiner fails to detect tumor extension beyond the capsule and may not appreciate that induration (representing tumor extension) has reached into the seminal vesicle. Overstaging can occur as well. The examiner notes induration (indicating probable tumor) beyond the prostate capsule; yet a radical prostatectomy specimen ultimately contains only tumor localized within the capsule. Only when a radical prostatectomy is the treatment for localized cancer can one compare the accuracy of clinical staging with definitive pathologic staging, or the histologic assessment of the extent of tumor in the radical prostatectomy specimen. When the prostate-specific antigen (PSA) is over 10 ng/ml (and especially when it exceeds 20 ng/ml), capsular penetration with extracapsular extension is common even if the examiner cannot detect this on digital rectal examination (DRE).[1–3] When the prostatic carcinoma contains high-grade elements (Gleason grade 4 or 5) there is also an increased rate of extraprostatic extension, even if the examiner cannot detect this by DRE.

While PSA level is a rough indicator of whether the tumor is likely confined to the prostate or nonconfined, clinical staging is not significantly improved by imaging studies. Transrectal ultrasound (TRUS), pelvic computed tomography (CT) scanning, and magnetic resonance imaging (MRI) do not reliably identify extraprostatic tumor extension.[4] On occasion, ultrasound-guided biopsies of the seminal vesicles can identify tumor extension to the seminal vesicles, but this is probably best reserved for the patient with an unusually high PSA level or high-grade tumor, or both; that is, when the likelihood of seminal vesicle tumor involvement is high.

Small tumor volume and tumor with low to medium grade (Gleason grade 1 to 3) are factors often associated with a significantly delayed capsular penetration and extracapsular tumor extension. In this situation, the examiner's impression that the tumor is within the capsule by digital rectal examination is likely to be accurate and fairly reliable.

STAGING—TNM SYSTEM (Table 26–1)

T1a and T1b

T1 prostatic cancer is not suspected by rectal examination; there is no nodule or suspicious induration. When the patient undergoes transurethral resection of the prostate (TURP) or simple prostatic enucleation for prostatic obstruction, adenocarcinoma found unexpectedly by the pathologist doing microscopic examination of the removed tissue is termed T1a or T1b cancer. T1a is the designation for histologic tumor that is minimal, occupies less than 5% of the removed tissue, and is also low grade (Gleason 1 and 2). T1b indicates tumor that

TABLE 26–1. LOCALIZED PROSTATE CANCER—TNM STAGING

TNM	Description
Primary Tumor	
T1	Clinically inapparent tumor not palpable or visible by imaging
T1a	Tumor incidental histologic finding in 5% or less of tissue resected
T1b	Tumor incidental histologic finding in more than 5% or tissue resected
T1c	Tumor identified by needle biopsy because of elevated PSA
T2	Palpable tumor confined within prostate
T2a	Tumor involves half of a lobe or less
T2b	Tumor involves more than half of a lobe, but not both sides
T2c	Tumor involves both lobes
T3	Tumor extends through and beyond the prostatic capsule
T3a	Unilateral extracapsular extension
T3b	Bilateral extracapsular extension
T3c	Tumor invades seminal vesicles
T4	Tumor is fixed or invades adjacent structures other than seminal vesicles
Regional Lymph Nodes	
Nx	Regional nodes not assessed
N0	No regional lymph nodes metastasis
N1	Metastasis in a single lymph node, 2 cm or smaller
N2	Metastasis to lymph node 2 to 5 cm in diameter or multiple lymph nodes
N3	Metastasis to lymph nodes more than 5 cm in diameter

involves greater than 5% of the removed tissue and can be any grade. T1b identifies tumors that are more extensive microscopically than T1a lesions.

T1a and T1b tumors are sometimes termed "incidental," "unexpected," or "latent" prostate cancer—actually diagnosed by the surgical pathologist. Tumors of these categories (T1a and T1b) are much less common now than they were a decade or more ago. First, the frequency of TURP has decreased markedly in recent years as alternative treatment measures for benign prostatic hyperplasia (BPH) have been introduced and employed. Second, most men with clinical BPH nowadays have a PSA level determined before treatment is considered. An elevated PSA usually leads to prostatic ultrasound and prostatic biopsies—so the diagnosis is suspected by PSA elevation and confirmed by prostatic biopsy. This leads to far fewer patients who will have tumors termed T1a or T1b.

T1c: Prostate Tumor

T1c is the designation for the tumor that is suspected by PSA elevation and detected by subsequent prostatic biopsies, even though the prostate feels benign by DRE. Specifically, the examiner feels no nodule or suspicious prostatic induration. The incidence of T1c cancers has increased dramatically in the past decade—as the incidence of T1a and T1b tumors has decreased drastically. The wide use of PSA testing in men over the age of 50 is mainly responsible for this change. Also significant is the common use of prostatic ultrasound and the ease of obtaining ultrasound-guided biopsies as an outpatient procedure.

T2 Tumors

T2 cancer is defined as a palpable tumor clinically confined within the prostate. This may be suspicious induration or a definite nodule, and the suspicion of prostate cancer must, of course, be confirmed by prostatic biopsy. Subclassification of T2 cancer varies somewhat in reported series in the urologic literature, but usually it follows this pattern: T2a—palpable tumor involves half of one prostatic lobe or less. T2b—palpable tumor involves more than one half of one lobe but not both lobes. T2c—tumor involves both prostatic lobes.

T3 Tumors

Palpable tumor extension beyond the capsule of the prostate is termed T3 disease, and this stage is often subclassified depending upon whether it passes beyond the capsule on one side (T3a), extends bilaterally beyond the capsule (T3b), or palpably involves one or both seminal vesicles (T3c). Extracapsular tumor is usually detected lateral to the prostate or cephalad into the bladder neck and seminal vesicles. Less common is extracapsular tumor at the apex.

T3 cancer generally is not considered suitable for radical prostatectomy with curative intent because complete extirpation of the cancer is very unlikely. Also, external beam radiation therapy for T3 disease is not very likely to be successful. Therefore, it is important to separate clinical T2 from T3 cancer, and a careful digital rectal examination is a significant factor in this designation.

PROSTATE-SPECIFIC ANTIGEN

PSA determination is a significant item in the evaluation of any man who is suspected to have carcinoma of the prostate. PSA is also commonly obtained as a part of a screening or disease detection process in any man over the age of 50 years. PSA is complementary to DRE. An elevation may often raise the suspicion of prostatic carcinoma in the presence of a benign-feeling prostate—without palpable tumor nodule or even suspicious induration in the prostate. The opposite situation can also occur (i.e., palpable and suspicious induration or nodule in the presence of a normal PSA). Usually, though, palpable tumor will be associated with an elevated PSA level. A high PSA value can also occur in nonmalignant conditions of the prostate. BPH is commonly associated with modest elevation of the PSA (4 to 10 ng/ml), and even higher values occur in prostatitis (especially acute prostatitis), acute urinary retention, and prostatic infarct (virtually impossible to detect clinically). The PSA level is very helpful in prostate cancer detection; it gives one a *rough* idea of tumor volume, stage, and likelihood of extracapsular extension, but one must be aware of the confusion the PSA value may present. Current studies suggest that in the future, ratios of free and protein-bound PSA may help to increase the specificity of PSA in prostate cancer detection and assessment.[5]

PROSTATE CANCER GRADE

Tumor grade indicates the degree of differentiation of tumor cells and also, in the case of prostatic cancer, the relationship of the tumor cells with the adjacent prostatic stroma. Several grading systems have been devised, but most used and generally accepted by pathologists and urologists is the Gleason system of grading. The system is easily understood and highly reproducible from one institution to another. The Gleason grade ranges from 1 to 5, from well-differentiated to highly undifferentiated cancer. The Gleason score takes into account the most common histologic pattern as the first number, followed by a number indicating the grade of the second commonest histologic pattern. The lowest Gleason score possible is 2 (1 + 1), while the highest score possible is 5 + 5 or 10. These are the extremes; the majority of tumors encountered clinically are middle grade (or moderately undifferentiated) tumors. It is helpful to keep in mind that tumors of grade 1, 2, and 3 seem slow to penetrate and extend beyond the prostate capsule. Tumors of grade 4 and 5 are more aggressive generally and are sooner likely to penetrate the capsule and spread beyond the prostate.

TRANSRECTAL ULTRASOUND AND PROSTATIC BIOPSY

Transrectal ultrasonic examination of the prostate has become common and standard among urologists and radiologists in the United States. Previous expectations that prostate tumors and tumorous extension beyond the prostate could be detected by ultrasound imaging alone have been unfulfilled and somewhat disappointing. Some tumors that are hypoechoic can be suspected and detected ultrasonically, but the reliability of imaging alone is unsatisfactory. TRUS has great value for directing biopsies at suspicious areas in the prostate (areas of induration or hypoechoic regions noted ultrasonically) and for obtaining random prostate biopsies. Common practice is the obtaining of sextant biopsies directed by TRUS. Bilateral sextant biopsies include prostate base, midregion, and apex on both sides of the midline. Each biopsy should be submitted individually for histologic examination. The presence of tumor, its grade, and percentage of the biopsy that contains tumor are important items of information.

PELVIC NODAL METASTASIS

In the TNM staging system, N refers to the state of the pelvic lymph nodes—the external iliac and obturator nodes. Tumor that penetrates beyond prostatic capsule and cephalad into the seminal vesicles also can extend to the next level of involvement, pelvic nodes. Nx signifies that the status of the pelvic nodes is unknown. Nx is the rule when patients are treated with radiation or managed by surveillance or treated hormonally. The absence of precise knowledge of pelvic node status in the radiated or surveillance patients makes comparison with radical prostatectomy series difficult.

N0 indicates that pelvic lymph nodes are free of tumor by pelvic lymphadenectomy and histologic examination of the excised nodes. Unfortunately, imaging studies for the detection of tumor-bearing nodes are unreliable. CT scanning, pelvic ultrasound, and pelvic MRI cannot provide reliable data on the status of pelvic nodes. Radical prostatectomy is not a potentially curative effort unless pelvic lymph nodes are free of tumor metastasis. External beam radiation is not particularly effective when there is pelvic lymph nodal extension, and the decision to manage the patient by surveillance only is marred by the unknown state of the pelvic lymph nodes. Staging accuracy historically has been best with radical prostatectomy (compared to external beam radiation and surveillance) because the nodes are removed and examined histologically by frozen section, then later examined by permanent section. The N0 status or absence of node metastasis may be proven by pelvic lymph node dissection with negative histology, or the absence of positive nodes can be presumed or estimated with good accuracy by stage, grade, and PSA level of the patient. The patient with low tumor volume, tumor grade no higher than Gleason grade 3, and PSA under 10 ng/ml has a minimal (<5%) likelihood of pelvic nodal metastasis. With increasing tumor size, the presence of Gleason 4 or 5 tumor, and a PSA above 10 ng/ml, the possibility of positive pelvic nodes increases.

When radical prostatectomy is the proposed therapeutic approach, there are three general clinical situations.

1. T1b, T1c, T2a tumors with no higher than Gleason grade 3 and PSA under 10 ng/ml: Ignoring the pelvic nodes is reasonable, and a radical prostatectomy without pelvic node dissection is appro-

priate. Radical perineal prostatectomy is particularly appealing in the situation because it is quicker to perform, relatively easy for the patient with less blood loss, and allows faster recovery than is the case with a radical retropubic prostatectomy.[6,7] However, the surgeon must be an experienced perineal prostatectomist. Experience with the perineal operation is not so widespread as surgical training and experience with radical retropubic prostatectomy.

2. Stage T2b, T2c tumors, the presence of grade 4 or 5 tumor, and PSA greater than 10 (any one of these factors or any combination): The patient may be "operable" and may be "curable" but the presence of proven negative nodes must be ascertained before embarking upon radical prostatectomy with curative intent. The node dissection can be carried out through lower abdominal incision (as an isolated procedure or in combination with radical retropubic prostatectomy) or it may be accomplished laparoscopically. Also, a preoperative radioisotope bone scan is advisable with high-grade tumor and PSA greater than 10.[8] The presence of bone metastasis virtually ensures the presence of positive pelvic lymph nodes, and clearly radical prostatectomy is unlikely to provide benefit in the patient with distant disease, positive nodes, or bone metastases.

3. Large local tumor, grade 4 to 5 tumor, and a PSA greater than 20: The chances are increasing that nodal metastases have occurred with a large local tumor, high tumor grade, and greater elevation of the PSA. A radioisotope bone scan is mandatory for the staging of this patient. If this is negative, pelvic lymphadenectomy is the next step, and radical prostatectomy should only be considered if the pelvic nodes are free of tumor. Contingency plans must be made for the presence of positive nodes. Since radical prostatectomy is a poor choice here and radiation is of little benefit when pelvic nodes are positive, the only real alternatives are early and late hormonal therapy.

TREATMENT OF LOCALIZED PROSTATE CANCER

Stage 1a and Some Stage 1c Tumors

Stage 1a indicates minimal and low-grade tumor detected by the surgical pathologist in the patient who undergoes TURP or enucleation simple prostatectomy for presumed BPH. To be classified T1a, the tumor is less than 5% of the removed tissue. Five per cent of a large specimen can represent significant tumor volume, but when the tumor amount is truly minimal (just a few local areas) and grade 1 or 2, only tumor surveillance is usually recommended. Surveillance means periodic rectal examination, PSA determination, and future biopsies if any suspicion of tumor recurrence or progression occurs. Most tumors of this category are indolent and have a low likelihood of clinical progression.

The author would include the patient with T1c prostatic carcinoma with minimal focal low-grade tumor in only one biopsy in this general category to be managed by surveillance. However, regular monitoring must be carried out, and future repeat biopsies at periodic intervals are needed. The physician should recognize, and the patient should clearly understand, that prostate tissue sampling is much more extensive by TURP than it is by sextant needle biopsies.

TREATMENT OF ALL OTHER STAGES

The Prostate Cancer Guidelines Committee of the American Urological Association reviewed the medical literature exhaustively on the subject of the outcomes of treatment of localized prostate cancer.[4] The committee noted that there are three definite treatment options for which there is reasonable long-term outcome data. These three are radical prostatectomy, external beam radiation therapy, and surveillance or watchful waiting. While these three are considered therapeutic options, treatment series from the medical literature reveal that reported patients were selected by different and nonstandard methods, staged in different ways with differing follow-up and differing evaluation methods. Reported series of patients who have had radical prostatectomy, radiation, and surveillance are of varying age, have differing patterns of tumor grades, and have not been staged in the same way. On average, patients subjected to radical prostatectomy and reported in the medical literature have been significantly younger than those who have been reported following radiation treatment or surveillance. Reports from surveillance series indicate that patients have been older on average and have lower grade tumors than patients treated by surgery or radiation. Those subjected to radical prostatectomy generally have had staging pelvic lymphadenectomy; those treated with radiation or on surveillance have not had this staging procedure. Thus, treatment outcomes cannot be compared. Furthermore, there are no scientifically randomized studies comparing outcomes from different treatments. The patient with localized carcinoma of the prostate must be informed of these three main treatment methods. There are advantages and disadvantages to each for the patient, and each has its own potential complications. The well-informed patient must be involved in the decision-making process.

There has been much discussion among urologists and much has been written concerning upper age limit for radical prostatectomy for localized prostate cancer. There are those urologic surgeons who emphatically reject radical prostatectomy for the patient of 70 years and beyond. Other urologists extend their upper age limit to 75 years. No data from the prostate cancer literature validate an age limit for radical prostatectomy. More reasonably, the patient considered for radical prostatectomy should have a projected lifespan of 10 years or more and be free of significant life-threatening medical illnesses such as severe coronary artery disease, advanced diabetes mellitus with complications, and severe pulmonary or hepatic disease. Life tables indicate the healthy man of 75 years has an average additional life expectancy of 10 to 12 years; so generally a 75-year age limit makes some sense.

RADICAL PROSTATECTOMY

Radical prostatectomy can be accomplished by the retropubic or perineal route. Retropubic prostatectomy is much more commonly performed, largely because many urologic surgeons are not trained or experienced in the perineal operation. Either operation accomplishes the same goal (i.e., the removal of the total prostate with seminal vesicles, terminal ejaculatory ducts, and a margin of bladder neck). When tumor is localized to the prostate and has not extended beyond the prostatic capsule, radical prostatectomy can be curative. A very appealing aspect is the potential to remove the tumor totally while it is still localized.

Pelvic lymphadenectomy for staging is necessary when the PSA exceeds 10 ng/ml or when there is grade 4 or 5 adenocarcinoma in the biopsy specimens. Pelvic lymphadenectomy is conveniently performed as an early part of the retropubic operation. When the nodes are free of metastasis by frozen section, the surgeon can proceed with radical retropubic prostatectomy with further conviction that the tumor is likely localized or operable—or curable. When lymph nodes are positive (contain metastatic prostatic carcinoma), the tumor has spread beyond its origin, and generally the procedure should be terminated without removal of the prostate. There may be exceptions where radical prostatectomy is performed in the presence of pelvic nodal metastasis, such as a plan to perform radical prostatectomy with combined early hormonal therapy. The benefit of such combined therapy is uncertain, though, and treatment should be discussed thoroughly in advance with the patient.

Pelvic lymphadenectomy can be performed prior to radical perineal prostatectomy by an open operative approach or by laparoscopic node dissection. Commonly, perineal prostatectomy is reserved for the patient with low-grade tumor and a PSA less than 10 ng/ml—in which the incidence of positive nodes is so low that lymphadenectomy can reasonably be eliminated in the treatment plan.

The patient undergoing radical prostatectomy should be in generally good health with a projected life expectancy of 10 years or more. Survival tables tell us that this means the patient should be generally no older than his mid-70s. The mortality rate for radical prostatectomy is under 1%. The major postoperative problems are urinary incontinence and impotence. Incontinence is stress incontinence, common in most men after the catheter is removed (usually 2 to 3 weeks after surgery). Urinary control improves in the early weeks and months following surgery, so that most patients can ultimately eliminate their pads. Long-term and permanent significant incontinence lasting beyond 1 year occurs in 5 to 10% of patients who have undergone radical prostatectomy. In the few who continue with significant incontinence, sphincter exercises, biofeedback methods, and bladder-relaxing medications can be helpful. Ultimately, an artificial urinary sphincter may be the solution for recalcitrant long-term incontinence.

Impotence after radical prostatectomy is to be anticipated if the surgeon removes some of Denonvilliers' fascia and the fat and areolar tissue outside the prostatic capsule. Removal of periprostatic tissue can reduce the incidence of margin-positive disease and is the preferred treatment of cancer (i.e., as wide removal as possible of the organ bearing the tumor).[9] Nerve-sparing or potency-sparing surgery is often a poor choice because the periprostatic tissue is not removed in an attempt to leave intact the nerves controlling penile erection, which course close to the prostatic capsule posteriorly on each side. When tumor is known to be present on both sides of the prostate (on the basis of prostatic sextant biopsies), nerve sparing seems inappropriate. When the tumor clearly lateralizes to one side, unilateral nerve sparing on the contralateral side of the prostate is reasonable. The possibility of postoperative impotence must be discussed with the patient in advance. Often the patient is far less concerned about preserving potency than he is having a wide dissection of the prostate with an improved chance of margin-negative tumor and an increased chance of total eradication of the tumor. Preoperatively, and also after surgery in the event of impotence, the patient should be counseled about intracavernous injection, vacuum devices, and penile prostheses.

Other less common complications from radical prostatectomy are rectal injury, major bleeding, and pulmonary embolus. The patient should be counseled about these complications, and how they can be avoided, and treated if one of these events occurs.

Follow-up after radical prostatectomy emphasizes regular rectal examination (to detect a palpable recurrence anterior to the rectum) and serum PSA determination. Various patterns of follow-up have been advocated. This author favors rectal examination and PSA determination every 3 months for 1 year, every 6 months for the second year, and thereafter yearly and indefinitely.

Total elimination of the tumor is suggested by a persistant PSA of zero. When the PSA rises after surgery, biochemical recurrence is occurring, even though this PSA rise or biochemical recurrence may occur as long as 3 to 4 years before recurrent tumor is detected clinically.

When PSA rises postoperatively, radiation treatment has been advocated, focusing the radiation energy on the bladder neck to urethral anastomotic area, usually the site of recurrence whether this can be proved by anastomotic biopsy or not.[10] External beam radiation in the case of biochemical failure will reduce the PSA in approximately two thirds of patients, but the PSA suppression is temporary, and there is insufficient evidence to know whether postoperative radiation therapy is actually beneficial to patients with a biochemical recurrence.

Another alternative is the introduction of hormonal treatment when the PSA begins to rise. This is effective nearly always in reducing the PSA substantially, but it is not known whether this "early" institution of hormonal therapy is better for the patient than "delayed" hormone therapy.

Randomized therapeutic trials are underway in an attempt to determine whether early postoperative radiation is beneficial in margin-positive disease or in those with seminal vesicle invasion. Also, the use of antiandrogens is being studied in similar types of patients with a high risk of local tumor recurrence.

IRRADIATION THERAPY

External beam radiation treatment for clinically localized prostate cancer can be appealing to some patients with a particular dread of surgery. An operation is avoided, but the treatment schedule can be tedious—usually taking 6 to 7 weeks to deliver the needed radiation energy to the prostate. Improved technology has led to improved targeting of the prostate in recent years, with better sparing of adjacent normal tissues.

The patient treated in this manner should have a relatively long life expectancy. Patients with positive nodes are not likely to benefit from radiation therapy—so a preliminary staging lymphadenectomy is desirable in patients with a PSA above 10 ng/ml and/or grade 4 to 5 tumor. Unfortunately, most patients treated with external beam radiation do not have a preliminary lymph node staging even when they are at high risk of nodal metastasis; thus, results of radiation treatment are difficult to compare with the results of radical prostatectomy, in which pathologic tumor stage, grade, and tumor volume can be determined by the pathologist. When the PSA exceeds 10 to 15 ng/ml and/or there is grade 4 to 5 tumor in the biopsy, patients have not fared well with radiation therapy.[11]

The most common complications of external beam radiation therapy are radiation proctitis and cystitis. Usually these are nuisance symptoms that can be improved with medical treatment and that diminish with time. Impotence also occurs in at least half of the patients treated by external beam radiation.

Follow-up after radiation therapy is similar to that in patients who have had radical prostatectomy. Periodic PSA and rectal examination are the key elements. Interval prostatic biopsy can be useful—especially when the PSA begins to rise. When tumor recurs after radiation treatment, a "salvage" radical prostatectomy is a consideration. Radical prostatectomy performed in an area of radiated tissue can be curative in selected cases, but there is a high risk of anastomotic stricture and urinary incontinence. Hormone treatment initiation is the alternative in this solution.

BRACHYTHERAPY

An alternative method of delivering ionizing radiation to the prostate is the use of brachytherapy, or interstitial radiation. Beads or pellets of isotope material are employed. Early use of radioactive gold (implanted surgically) and iodine-25 (^{125}I) (implanted retropubically) have failed to live up to the expectations of their advocates; neither is in common use today. Other isotopes implanted perineally by ultrasound guidance are currently being employed and evaluated. Early results seem promising, but further time is needed to assess this treatment.

SURVEILLANCE

The bases for surveillance, or the monitoring of a prostate cancer, without aggressive treatment are:

1. Many patients with prostate cancer are elderly and have serious medical problems.
2. Some prostate cancers are slow to progress and may take a number of years to produce significant symptoms to the patient. It is commonly stated that many elderly men die with prostate cancer rather than as a result of prostate cancer.

Surveillance only is reasonable in the elderly man or the patient whose life expectancy seems limited because of serious diabetes, coronary artery disease, pulmonary, renal, liver, or neurologic disease, etc. In these cases progression of the tumor likely can be managed by hormonal measures. When the tumor is low volume and low grade, surveillance is also appropriate. Surveillance is commonly employed in T1a tumor and in T1c cancer with a single low-grade tumor focus.

More controversial would be surveillance in the patient with a T2 tumor of low to medium grade. Age, expected survival, patient's comorbidity, and the patient's informed choice in his treatment are factors to consider. A key factor with surveillance is the need for regular rectal examination and PSA determination. When tumor progression occurs, it is hoped this can be recognized while the tumor is still localized; so reconsideration of other treatment options will be possible.

CRYOTHERAPY

Eradication of localized prostate cancer by freezing, or cryotherapy, is being employed in a number of centers in the United States.[12] Candidates have been those with localized prostate cancer as well as those who have had radiation treatment with local recurrence. Early results look promising, but longer follow-up data will be necessary to truly assess the value of cryotherapy. For now it is considered investigational. There is obvious appeal to the patient because of the brief hospitalization and minimal discomfort he must suffer in the course of cryotherapy.

SUMMARY OF TREATMENT

Radical prostatectomy, radiation therapy, and surveillance are the major management methods for localized prostate cancer. The patient with localized prostate cancer must understand all of these treatments and must have a voice in the ultimate treatment choice. Each method of treatment has its particular complications. Tumor stage, grade, health of the patient, and projected longevity are also factors that enter into the appropriate therapeutic choice.

PROGNOSIS IN THE TREATMENT OF LOCALIZED PROSTATE CANCER

The Prostate Cancer Guidelines Committee of the American Urological Association reviewed extensively outcome experience from the treatment of localized prostate tumors as reported in the medical literature.[4] Roughly two thirds to three fourths of patients treated with radical prostatectomy survived 10 years. Some who died succumbed to causes unrelated to prostatic cancer. Also, some who survived had recurrent tumor at 10 years. Survival rates were highly variable from one reported series to another. Survival was a bit lower after radiation therapy—and a bit lower still in patients on a surveillance protocol.

These survival differences were not statistically significant because of age differences in the patient groups and significant differences in the method of selection of patients for different treatment categories. The committee recognized that 5-year survival data is not of significant value. Ten- to 15-year outcomes are vastly more important, yet most of the reports in the medical literature addressing 10- to 15-year survival actually produce "projected" survivals from Kaplan-Meier curves. Whether the Kaplan-Meier method of projected survival statistics is valid in prostate cancer survival is dubious to this author; yet this has been a standard in the urologic literature for many years.

In the future, PSA follow-up will help to develop answers to the usefulness of our treatment methods. Actual outcomes must be reported and must be important in the assessment of these treatment methods. Radical surgery, radiation, and surveillance can be appropriate, but the value of each approach requires more investigation.

REFERENCES

1. Stamey TA, Kabalin JN, McNeal JE, et al: Prostate specific antigen in the diagnosis and treatment of adenocarcinoma of the prostate. II. Radical prostatectomy treated patients. J Urol 1989; 141:1076.
2. Kleer E, Larson-Keller JJ, Zinke H, Oesterling JE: Ability of preoperative serum prostate-specific antigen value to predict pathologic stage and DNA ploidy. Urology 1993; 41:207.
3. Scaletscky R, Koch MD, Eckstein S, et al: Tumor volume and stage in carcinoma of the prostate detected by elevations in prostate specific antigen. J Urol 1994; 152:129.
4. Middleton RG, Thompson IM, Austenfeld MS, et al: Prostate cancer clinical guidelines panel: report on the management of clinically localized prostate cancer. Baltimore, American Urological Association, Inc, 1995.
5. Oesterling JE, Jacobsen SJ, Klee GG, et al: Free, complexed and total serum prostate specific antigen: the establishment of appropriate reference ranges for their concentrations and ratios. J Urol 1995; 154:1090.
6. Middleton RG: The current role of radical perineal prostatectomy in localized prostate cancer. *In* Middleton RG (ed): Medical and Surgical Management of Prostate Cancer, p 69. New York, Igaku-Shoin, 1996.
7. Parra RO, Isorna S, Perez MG, et al: Radical perineal prostatectomy without pelvic lymphadenectomy: selection criteria and early results. J Urol 1996; 155:612.
8. Oesterling JE, Martin SK, Bergstralh EJ, et al: The use of prostate-specific antigen in staging patients with newly diagnosed prostate cancer. JAMA 1993; 269:57.
9. Stephenson RA, Middleton RG: Radical retropubic prostatectomy using wide excision (non-nerve sparing) or nerve-sparing techniques: improved cancer control vs. potency preservation. *In* Middleton RG (ed): Medical and Surgical Management of Prostate Cancer, p 46. New York, Igaku-Shoin, 1996.
10. Santucci RA, Lange PH: Treatment of the patient with a rising PSA (brachemical failure) following radical prostatectomy. *In* Middleton RG (ed): Medical and Surgical Management of Prostate Cancer, p 54. New York, Igaku-Shoin, 1996.
11. Zietman AL, Shipley WU, Coen JJ: Radical prostatectomy and radical radiation therapy for clinical stages T1 to T2 adenocarcinoma of the prostate: new insights into outcome from repeat biopsy an PSA follow up. J Urol 1994; 152:1806.
12. Connolly JA, Shinohara K, Presti JC Jr, Carroll PR: Role of cryosurgery in the treatment of localized prostate cancer. *In* Middleton RG (ed): Medical and Surgical Management of Prostate Cancer, p 143. New York, Igaku-Shoin, 1996.

27

REGIONALLY ADVANCED ADENOCARCINOMA OF THE PROSTATE (T3a − TNx + M0): MANAGEMENT AND PROGNOSIS

IAN M. THOMPSON, M.D. *and* THOMAS A. ROZANSKI, M.D.

While multiple bodies of data demonstrate excellent outcomes of the management of clinically localized prostate cancer, when there is evidence that the disease is locally advanced, outcomes are substantially less favorable. It is for this reason that the staging and subsequent selection of treatment are paramount in the management of prostate cancer. This chapter will present a comprehensive approach to the staging and treatment of locally advanced prostate cancer.

DEFINITION OF LOCALLY ADVANCED DISEASE

The definition of locally advanced prostate cancer is those stages with which a distinct decrease in cancer control is observed with available treatment. These include clinical T3–T4 (cT3, stage C), nodal-positive (N+) disease, and pathologic T3 disease (pT3) (Table 27–1). Historical data suggest that the incidence of cT3 disease decreased from 17.7% to 12.3% between 1974 and 1983.[1] A recent survey by the American Cancer Society suggested that this rate had increased to 18.5%, but the inclusion of patients with pT3 disease in this category almost certainly confounded this statistic.[2] It is highly probable that the use of prostate-specific antigen (PSA) for screening has led to a significant decrease in the proportion of cases that are locally advanced, and evidence suggests that screening has also reduced the rate of pathologically advanced disease.[3] The utility of the clinical substages of T3 disease has recently been disputed.[4]

Similar to cT3 disease, the rate of positive lymph nodes has also decreased. While previous series found rates of 20 to 40%, more recent series have found rates of 6.7 to 7.7%.[5,6] While not segregated by nodal or T3–T4 status, American Cancer Society data demonstrate that all regionally advanced disease (T3–T4 and nodal-positive disease) has increased only slightly: from 13% in 1980 to 15% in 1995.[7] However, recognizing that the number of cases diagnosed annually has increased from 66,000 in 1980 to 244,000 in 1995, this represents an increase in regionally advanced disease from 8580 cases in 1980 to 36,600 in 1995. A recent study that reanalyzed pelvic lymphadenectomy specimens from 95 patients with pT3N0 using immunocytochemistry for extrinsic epithelial cells found that 16% of patients had unsuspected lymph node metastases.[8] The frequency of the finding of positive pelvic lymph nodes is dependent upon both the clinical stage of the disease as well as tumor grade. In a recent series of 511 patients, nodal disease was found in 8% of patients with B1 nodules compared to 44% of patients with cT3 disease.[9] Similarly, while patients with well-differentiated tumors had a 15% likelihood of positive nodes, those with poorly differentiated tumors had a 62% rate.

Pathologic T3 disease is diagnosed following radical prostatectomy by the demonstration of involvement of the prostatic capsule, evidence of tumor in the surgical margin, or invasion of the seminal vesicles. Involvement of seminal vesicles is uncommon but has been noted in as many as 12% of patients.[10] Conversely, the cumulative rate of extraprostatic disease in all patients undergoing radical prostatectomy is as high as 53%.[11] Several series have demonstrated that there is a stepwise increase in the risk of disease with higher pathologic stage.[12] That

TABLE 27–1. STAGING OF LOCALLY ADVANCED PROSTATE CANCER

AJCC Stage	AUA Stage	Pathologic Stage	Definition
T3a*	C		Unilateral extracapsular extension
T3b*	C		Bilateral extracapsular extension
T3c*	C		Seminal vesicle invasion
T4*	C		
		pT3a† (C1)	Tumor invades or penetrates prostatic capsule
		pT3b† (C2)	Positive margin
		PT3c† (C3)	Invasion of seminal vesicles

*Indicates clinical staging.[85]
†Indicates pathologic staging.
AJCC, American Joint Committee on Cancer; AUA, American Urological Association.

this increasing recognition of pT3 disease is due to an actual increase in risk is doubtful but is more likely due to an increased assiduity in the pathologic examination of radical prostatectomy specimens.

STAGING OF LOCALLY ADVANCED DISEASE

The objective of the accurate staging of prostate cancer is to assist with the determination of optimal treatment. Several clinical, laboratory, and radiographic examinations can be used to assist in the initial evaluation of the patient with newly diagnosed prostate cancer to determine the likelihood that one of the above categories of locally advanced disease is present.

Digital Rectal Examination

A well-performed digital rectal examination (DRE) is essential to local staging. Any evidence of induration beyond the lateral border of the prostate or asymmetry/induration above the prostatic base (in the regions of the seminal vesicles) has a high likelihood of T3 disease. Older studies suggested that as many as 30% of patients with T3 disease actually had pT2 disease, but more recent series suggest that the positive predictive value of a positive DRE is between 91 and 93%.[13–16] These data suggest that if the skillful examiner notes a suggestion of extraprostatic disease on DRE, there is a high likelihood that pathologic examination would confirm this finding.

Prostate-Specific Antigen

PSA is an excellent predictor of all three aspects of staging (cT3, pT3, and nodal-positive disease). While average PSAs for patients with cT1–T2 disease generally range from less than 4 ng/ml to very few patients over 30 ng/ml, series of patients treated for cT3 disease (without evidence of metastatic disease) have ranged from 24 to 204 ng/ml, with most series in the 20- to 30-ng/ml range.[4,15,17–20] Similarly, the initial PSA value relates well to pathologic stage. Partin and associates found that for PSA ranges of less than 4, 4 to 10, 10 to 20, and greater than 20, the risk of pT3 disease was 23, 35, 84, and 87%, respectively.[21] The correlation between PSA and risk of nodal disease is even better documented. Several series have demonstrated that with the combination of PSA, Gleason grade, and clinical stage the risk of lymph node involvement can be determined with considerable precision.[6,22] Figure 27–1 illustrates a nomogram for the risk of positive lymph nodes for patients with cT2a–b disease. Finally, initial PSA value correlates well with outcome of therapy.[23]

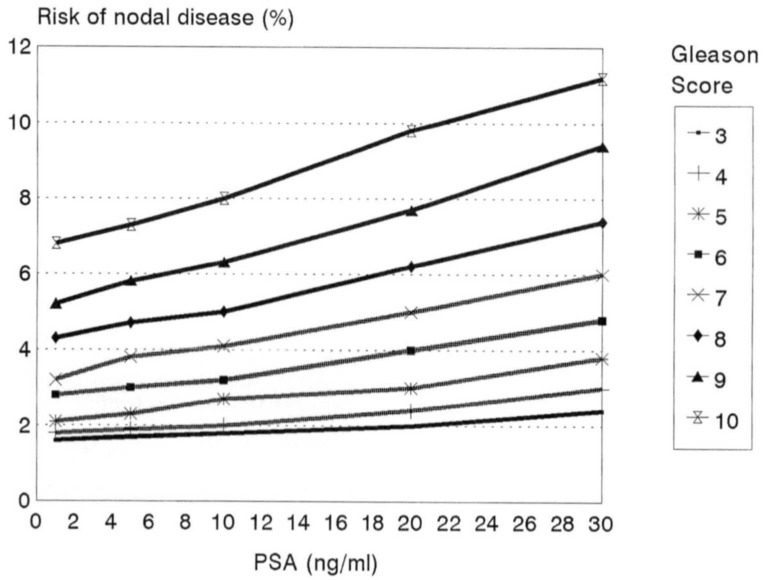

Risk of nodal disease (%)
12
10
8
6
4
2
0
0 2 4 6 8 10 12 14 16 18 20 22 24 26 28 30
PSA (ng/ml)
Gleason Score
3
4
5
6
7
8
9
10

FIGURE 27–1. Risk of positive lymph nodes for patients with T2a–b prostate cancer by Gleason grade and serum prostate-specific antigen.

Transrectal Ultrasonography and Magnetic Resonance Imaging

As the majority of cT3 prostate tumors will be identified by DRE alone, the primary utility of imaging studies for staging would be the assignment of risk of pT3 disease in a patient with a cT2 tumor. Unfortunately, most imaging studies, including transrectal ultrasonography (TRUS) and magnetic resonance imaging (MRI), perform poorly for this purpose. Rifkin et al. found that the sensitivity and specificity of TRUS was 66 and 46%, respectively.[24] By comparison, sensitivity and specificity of MRI was 77 and 57%, respectively. The use of an endorectal coil does not seem to significantly enhance the predictive value of MRI.[25] The reason for this poor performance is undoubtedly the fact that most pT3 disease is truly *microscopic* when examined pathologically—well beyond the resolution of any imaging modality currently available.

Radiographic Imaging of Pelvic Lymph Nodes

Similar to the detection of pT3 disease, imaging of pelvic lymph nodes is hampered by the general stage migration of currently diagnosed disease. As such, most tumors currently diagnosed are of a low volume and, if nodal metastases are present, they are often microscopic deposits in normal-appearing lymph nodes. Data from Bishoff et al. suggest that only a small fraction of currently diagnosed patients are at risk of nodal disease.[6] While some have suggested the utility of preoperative computed tomography (CT) scans to detect the presence of nodal disease, the sensitivity and specificity is quite low and the cost to detect a condition of declining prevalence is substantial.[26] Wolf found the cost of either CT or MRI imaging followed by fine-needle aspiration to be $50,661 per patient who received benefit from this approach.[27] This cost could be reduced by the use of more selective imaging in high-risk patients. Alternatively, laparoscopic pelvic node dissection may afford a higher sensitivity for detection of pelvic nodal metastases yet with even higher costs.[28]

NATURAL HISTORY OF LOCALLY ADVANCED PROSTATE CANCER

Clinical T3NO Disease

As it is a virtual standard of care that androgen deprivation will be provided for all prostate cancer patients if symptomatic disease progression develops, all the studies that provide an insight as to the natural history of the disease reflect the use of hormonal therapy at some point during the patient's course. The Veterans Administration Cooperative Urological Research Group (VACURG) studied the timing of such endocrine therapy and found that while early androgen deprivation delayed the development of metastatic disease, overall survival was not affected.[29] For patients with cT3N0 disease, survival was 50% at 5 years and 20% at 10 years.[30] Subsequent evaluation of VACURG data found that early endocrine therapy enhanced the quality of life when compared with delayed therapy.[31]

Perhaps the largest contemporary series of patients with cT3N0 prostate cancer followed without therapy was that of Adolfsson.[32] With 96% of patients having well-differentiated or moderately differentiated tumors, cancer-specific survival at 5 and 9 years was 88 and 70%, respectively. Crude survival at these two points was 64 and 37%. Two other series have reported similar data on untreated patients but compared to active therapy. Hanno studied a group of cT3N0 patients randomized to receive either external beam radiotherapy or delayed hormone therapy.[30] Comparing these two cohorts of patients, there was no difference in local progression nor in time to first evidence of distant metastasis. The results among patients treated with either early or delayed hormonal therapy in these studies are summarized in Table 27–2. As can be seen, progression rates are substantial and survival rates at 5 and 10 years are between 42 to 64% and 16 to 37%, respectively. Data to estimate the impact of disease progression upon morbidity are lacking. In a series of patients with T2–T4NxM0 disease, 85% required immediate transurethral resection of the prostate (TURP) for obstructive symptoms.[33] With an average follow-up of 4.2 years, 26% had local failure and required either re-TURP (20%), urethrotomy (4%), or nephrostomy (2%), and an additional 46% developed metastatic disease. A recent study of long-term survival in untreated patients with prostate cancer found remarkably pessimistic outcomes. Aus and colleagues studied 158 men with T2b–T3 disease who ultimately died and used the cause of death to determine cause-specific survivals.[34] Contrary to the more optimistic findings of previous authors, 5-, 10-, and 15-year cause-specific survivals were 70, 25, and 12%, respectively.

Pathologic T3 Disease

The natural history of untreated pathologic T3 cancer of the prostate is elusive because of the increased use of adjuvant therapy based upon PSA. Nevertheless, several series attest to the increased risk of disease progression with such locally advanced disease. Paulson and colleagues found that men with specimen-confined (invasion through the prostatic capsule) and margin-positive disease had a 30 and 60% risk, respectively, of treatment failure at 10 years compared to a 12% failure rate for men with organ-confined disease.[35] Several series have reported the natural history of pT3 disease that is

TABLE 27–2. NATURAL HISTORY OF UNTREATED cT3NO PROSTATE CANCER

Reference	Progression-Free Survival		Overall Survival	
	5 Years	10 Years	5 Years	10 Years
Adolfson[32]			64%	37%*
Hanno[30]			50%	20%
Rana et al.[33†]	44%	23%	42%	16%

*9-year follow-up
†Series includes patients with T2–T4 disease.

followed without early adjuvant therapy. These series report 5-, 10-, and 15-year rates of local progression of 11 to 52%, 30 to 70%, and 68%, respectively.[36–40] Survival at these end-points ranged from 68 to 92% at 5 years and 55 to 88% at 10 years of follow-up. The largest series to date was reported from the Mayo Clinic in 1993.[41] In 661 patients who received no adjuvant treatment, progression-free survival at 5, 10, and 15 years was 74, 50, and 42%, respectively, confirming the notion that a significant number of men with pT3 disease will survive for prolonged periods of time disease-free. The importance of the definition of margin positivity compared to a technical violation of the prostate during surgery has been emphasized by Stamey, and recently Ohori has suggested that margin status affected prognosis only in those patients with moderately differentiated tumors.[42,43] The somewhat contrasting findings support the contention that differences in pathologic interpretation may be responsible for many of the variations in outcome.

Nodal-Positive Disease

Only a few series of patients give an insight as to the outcome of untreated nodal-positive prostate cancer. As pelvic lymphadenectomy became commonplace after the advent of hormonal therapy, in all such series, delayed endocrine therapy was used. In three series, encompassing the experience with 71 patients, 5-year survivals of 20 to 29% were noted.[44–46] While some authors have suggested that a lower volume of nodal disease was associated with a longer disease-free survival, an equal number of series have found similar survivals, regardless of the volume or percentage of nodes involved.[9,47]

ACTIVE TREATMENT OF cT3NO PROSTATE CANCER

Radical Prostatectomy

While the general premise that radical prostatectomy affords excellent therapy for the patient with organ-confined disease (cT1–cT2N0M0), it has also been applied with some success for the patient with cT3N0 disease. Early series applying this form of therapy found little difference from the results of observation or hormonal therapy alone.[48] Spaulding and Whitmore, recognizing the poor results with radical prostatectomy alone, applied more exenterative procedures including radical cystectomy.[14] They found that survival at 5 years was 35%. Despite these relatively disappointing results, several recent series have reapplied surgical therapy for such locally advanced disease. It must be emphasized that the improved results may be more related to a stage migration in the definition of disease than an actual improvement in therapy. Van den Ouden studied 100 patients who underwent surgical exploration for cT3 disease with the intent of performance of radical prostatectomy.[16] At the time of surgery, 39 were found to have positive nodes and 2 to have T4 disease and surgery aborted. Of the 59 patients who underwent radical prostatectomy, 9 had positive nodes on final pathology. With a mean follow-up of 43.9 months, 6 patients (10%) died of prostate cancer, 4 died of other causes, and 48 (81%) are alive. A total of 36% of patients have developed clinical progression and 27% have PSA relapse with only 37% of patients remaining free of disease. Thus, of the original group of 100 patients undergoing surgical exploration with intent to perform radical prostatectomy, only 22% are free of disease at 4 years follow-up.

A larger experience was reported from the Mayo Clinic in which 812 patients with cT3 disease underwent radical prostatectomy between 1966 and 1992.[49] Mean follow-up was 4.5 years and adjuvant therapy (radiation, hormonal ablation, or both) was administered in 60% of cases. A total of 74 and 119 patients have developed either local or systemic recurrence, respectively. A combination of both local and systemic recurrence developed in 158 patients. If a PSA above 0.2 ng/ml is added as a criterion for relapse, 296 patients have recurred. Table 27–3 demonstrates both progression and overall survival rates with varying period of follow-up.

Radical Prostatectomy with Hormonal Therapy

The concept that preoperative hormonal therapy may lead to improved cancer control rates is not new; it was first reported in 1944 but popularized in 1969 by Scott and Boyd.[50] Recent reports have suggested that while local tumor response will be noted after neoadjuvant hormonal therapy, long-term response as measured by PSA-negative status is unusual. A multicenter study of 30 patients found that preoperative hormonal therapy led to "downstaging" of T3 disease to clinical T2 disease in 47% of patients but that only 10% of patients ultimately were proven to have pathologic T2 dis-

TABLE 27–3. RESULTS OF RADICAL PROSTATECTOMY FOR cT3NO PROSTATE CANCER

Reference	No. of Patients	Progression-Free Survival			Overall Survival		
		5 Years	10 Years	15 Years	5 Years	10 Years	15 Years
van de Ouden et al.[16]	59	60%					
Lerner et al.[49]*	812		61%	50%	86%	70%	51%

*Adjuvant therapy administered in 491 cases including external beam irradiation in 7%, androgen ablation in 43%, and both in 10%.

ease.[20] Another series of patients so treated found reductions in gland volume of 35% and mean PSA reduction from 29.3 ng/ml to 1.0 ng/ml at the end of 3 months of treatment.[19] Over a mean follow-up of 32.7 months, 72% of patients had disease recurrence. Thus, while neoadjuvant hormonal therapy has been suggested to reduce pathologic T3 disease when given prior to radical prostatectomy for cT2 disease, there is no evidence that this approach for cT3 disease is effective.[18]

External Beam Radiotherapy

A number of series have suggested that external beam radiotherapy may have an impact upon the control of cT3 prostate cancer. Indeed, some of the largest series of patients treated for this disease have received external beam radiotherapy. The experience of Zagars is illustrative.[51] In this series of 602 patients with T3 disease, 5-, 10-, and 15-year rates of local control were 88, 76, and 66%, respectively. Similarly, metastasis-free survivals of 75, 62, and 53% and overall survivals of 77, 49, and 32%, respectively, were achieved. As found in virtually all series, patients with high-grade disease had a dramatically worse prognosis. Despite these seemingly acceptable response rates, when further scrutinized using PSA or posttreatment biopsy as indicators of the durability of the response, the results are considerably worse. Crook and colleagues, in a group of 50 contemporary patients with T3 disease, found only 42% to be without disease at 33 months of follow-up.[52] Of the remainder, 20% had biopsy-proven disease, 4% failed biochemically (PSA), 12% failed locally, 6% had both local and distant failure, and 16% had metastatic disease. Zietman confirmed this observation, finding that at 4 years, radiation yielded *clinical* disease-free survival of 61% compared to only a 15% disease-free survival if PSA failures were considered.[53]

A number of methods have been advocated to enhance radiation therapy as primary treatment for cT3 disease. One approach has been the introduction of three-dimensional conformal radiation therapy (3D-CRT). Using highly sophisticated computerized treatment planning and specialized photon radiotherapy units, a rapid dropoff in the dose delivered to surrounding structures can be achieved.[54] While standard radiotherapy protocols call for tumor doses of 70 to 72 Gy, a number of authors have used conformal radiation to achieve tumor doses as high as 81 Gy. This has been achieved with very low rates of rectal and urinary toxicity.[54] Other authors have conducted studies using fast neutrons in place of standard photon-based radiotherapy. The rationale for this approach lies in the higher amount of energy that can be transferred with neutrons as well as a lesser degree of degradation of effect from tissue hypoxia.[55] In a randomized trial comparing fast neutrons versus standard photon irradiation of 178 patients with either T3–T4 disease or with high-grade T2 disease, the local control rate with neutrons was 89% compared to only 68% with photons.[56] Similarly, PSA failure rates were 17 and 45%, respectively.

Another recent advance in the management of this disease has been the use of neoadjuvant hormonal therapy with radiation therapy. Between 1987 and 1991, the Radiation Therapy Oncology Group conducted a trial comparing radiation therapy alone with radiation therapy and neoadjuvant hormonal therapy.[57] With 456 evaluable patients (219 of which were stage T3–T4) and a median follow-up of 4.5 years, local progression developed in 71% of radiated patients compared to 46% of patients who received both radiation and hormonal therapy. Similarly, the 5-year metastasis-free survival was reduced from 41% to 34% with the addition of hormonal therapy. One further use of neoadjuvant hormonal therapy with radiation is to take advantage of the total size reduction of the prostate (~25 to 30%), thereby reducing the radiation dose received by the bladder and rectum.[58]

Primary Hormonal Therapy

There is no question that immediate hormonal therapy will lead to measurable tumor response in cT3 disease. As demonstrated by neoadjuvant studies, PSA should drop by 95 to 98% and gland volume by 25 to 30%. Indeed, symptom-free survival may be enhanced by early hormonal therapy in locally advanced disease.[59] Review of VACURG studies demonstrated that while overall survival was not affected by early hormonal ablation, a delay in the development of bony metastases and an enhanced quality of life resulted from early hormonal therapy.[29,31] Whether hormonal therapy initiated at the time of diagnosis enhances long-term survival or reduces morbidity is unknown.

Cryotherapy

Cryotherapy for prostate cancer was described as early as 1964.[60] Initially, cryosurgery was performed via a perineal approach in order to monitor the progress of ice ball formation. With the development of transrectal ultrasonography and the recognition that the margin of the ice ball could be monitored ultrasonographically, the renaissance of this technique occurred. For patients with cT3 disease, many investigators have used neoadjuvant hormonal therapy to reduce the prostatic volume and thereby enhance the efficiency of cryotherapy.[61] Initial reports in patients with cT3 disease have suggested that prostate biopsies 3 months following cryotherapy show no detectable cancer in 79% of patients.[62] However, it must be recognized that, unlike radiotherapy, cryotherapy must be held to a higher standard of gland eradication, as it does not have the tumor specificity that radiation is purported to have. With this concept in mind, it is troublesome to recognize that PSA freedom-from-recurrence rates of 91, 80, and 51% are found using PSA cutoffs of less than 4 ng/ml, less than 1 ng/ml, and less than 0.5 ng/ml, respectively.

Also of concern with cryotherapy are the potentially serious complications associated with the potential extension of the ice ball to the rectal wall, the periprostatic region, and the membranous urethra. While Bahn and colleagues reported low complication rates (urethrorectal fistula, 2.4%; incontinence, 2.3%; pelvic pain, 1.5%; stress urinary incontinence, 6.2%; impotence, 41%), Crawford noted a 59% complication rate in 63 patients.[63,64] Complications encountered included urinary retention (29%), urinary incontinence (27%), tissue slough (19%), perineal pain (11%), urethral stricture (3%), and a severe complication rate of 8% (including sepsis, fistula, and ureteral obstruction). At this time, the significant risk of complications with marginal evidence of efficacy mandates that this form of therapy be offered only as a part of an IRB-approved investigative protocol for clinical T3 prostate cancer.

Intermittent Androgen Deprivation

An innovative approach to hormonal management of prostate cancer employs intermittent therapy. Bruchovsky and associates have hypothesized that standard, continuous hormonal therapy eventually leads to a dramatic reduction in the proportion of androgen-dependent stem cells, ultimately resulting in the proliferation of androgen-independent cells.[65] An alternative approach is to initiate hormonal therapy, inducing apoptosis of tumor cells but to terminate the antiandrogen therapy thus allowing hormonally dependent stem cells to proliferate. Thus, when hormonal therapy is reinstituted, it will often be successful.[66] In clinical practice, this can be achieved through the use of a luteinizing hormone releasing hormone (LHRH) agonist (with or without an antiandrogen) for 3 to 8 months until a PSA nadir is reached, followed by cessation of hormonal therapy. Serial PSA examinations are obtained, and when a clinically significant increase is noted, the hormonal therapy is reinstituted. At this time, a prospective trial of intermittent hormonal therapy for metastatic prostate cancer is being conducted by the National Cancer Institute (NCI).

Interstitial Radiation Therapy

Interstitial radiation therapy, popularized in the 1950s and 1960s for clinically localized prostate cancer, has not been used often for clinically advanced disease. The rationale lies in the necessity of providing adequate dosing of radioisotope throughout the prostate. With larger volume tumors and tumors that extend to the bladder base, this becomes technically more difficult and can be associated with a higher rate of local complications.[67] Indeed, Holzman found that 60% of patients suffered one or more adverse events, 69% of which were severe.[68]

One of the methods to determine efficacy of interstitial radiation therapy has traditionally been the determination of durable local control. In the field of external beam radiation, this metric compares well with later end-points as illustrated by Zagars finding that 10-year metastasis-free survival was 64% in patients with local control versus only 41% in patients with local tumor recurrence.[69] In reviewing series with significant duration of follow-up, Thompson found that local control rates with brachytherapy were 15 to 60% lower than seen with external beam irradiation.[48] The use of modern ultrasonographic guidance for implantation, potentially also employing neoadjuvant hormonal therapy, may translate to improvements in outcomes. However, as illustrated by the results of the initial brachytherapy experience, it will require 10 to 20 years to determine the impact of these technological innovations.

TREATMENT OF PATHOLOGIC T3 PROSTATE CANCER

As has been previously discussed, the outcome of patients with capsular invasion, positive margins, or seminal vesicle invasion following radical prostatectomy is distinctly less favorable than patients with organ-confined disease. However, because of the recognition that treatment failure can occur 10 to 15 years following radical prostatectomy, and due to a lack of controlled clinical trials comparing adjuvant therapy with surveillance, it is unknown whether adjuvant therapy will impact upon outcomes of importance to the patient.

Outcomes that have been proposed to evaluate the impact of adjuvant therapy have been (1) local recurrence, (2) PSA recurrence, (3) metastatic disease, (4) disease-free survival, and (5) overall survival. While some authors have used either local recurrence or PSA recurrence as surrogates for later end-points, there is no evidence that improvements in either will translate into a reduced mortality or morbidity from the disease.[70,71] Indeed, adjuvant therapy for breast cancer following breast-conserving surgery, while reducing local recurrences, has not translated into improvements in overall survival.[72–74] Because such clinical trials have not been conducted to ascertain with sufficient power the effect of adjuvant therapy upon pT3 disease, there can only be inferences made on the efficacy and definitive statements must be withheld.

Radiation Therapy

One of the more common adjuvant treatments afforded to men with pT3 disease is external beam radiotherapy. Indeed, no fewer than nine series have reported their results.[41,70,71] The cumulative number of patients in these series, if randomized, would have had sufficient power to detect a significant difference in survival. Unfortunately, because of potential biases in treatment selection, the results must be viewed cautiously. In general, most series have found that adjuvant radiation therapy (ranging from 42 to 72 Gy) to the prostatic bed will reduce the rate of local progression. Nevertheless, as is the case with breast cancer, most series have been unable to detect an improvement in survival. Table 27–4 displays these data.

Of interest regarding adjuvant radiation therapy, in the absence of evidence that an improvement in survival can be demonstrated, is the relative rate of morbidity associated with local recurrence compared to the morbidity associated with radiation. Unfortunately, data are lacking regarding the former. However, it has been the general experience of most urologic surgeons that the fraction of men who are symptomatic from a palpable or ultrasound-detected local recurrence is small. In most such cases, side effects are more common from the treatment of the local recurrence. The only report of a randomized comparison of radiation therapy and observation (INT 0086, a study funded by the National Cancer Institute and about two thirds the way toward reaching the accrual goal of 588 patients) found that in the first 66 patients who received adjuvant radiation, only 3 (5%) had a toxicity greater than grade 2.[75]

This review of adjuvant radiotherapy for pT3 disease suggests the following conclusions: (1) adjuvant radiotherapy will probably reduce local recurrence rates, (2) the rates of morbidity of both local recurrence and radiation therapy are low, and (3) it is unknown if the rates of metastatic disease or survival are affected. Patients with pT3 disease should therefore be provided the above information, offered participation in the NCI INT 0086 study, and if not interested in enrolling, should be encouraged to reach a decision based upon their own priorities regarding treatment efficacies and side effects.

Hormonal Therapy

While a very reasonable option for the management of pT3 prostate cancer, few series have reported on the efficacy of hormonal therapy alone. Cheng and colleagues, among 1035 patients with pT3 disease, employed orchiectomy in 103, radiation in 131, and surveillance in 661.[41] Adjuvant therapy with orchiectomy and radiation was equally effective in increasing the 5-year recurrence-free survival from 84% to greater than 95%, but neither form of adjuvant therapy changed either cause-specific or overall survival. A recent intriguing study randomized patients with elevated PSA following radical prostatectomy (of whom 50% were pT3) to either finasteride 10 mg/day or placebo.[76] Patients who received placebo experienced relentless increases in PSA from a mean of 2.1 to 3.8 ng/ml, while those who received finasteride had a decrease of PSA during the first 6 months followed by a gradual increase back to baseline values during the first year. An interesting observation was that the rate of increase in PSA was slower in patients who received finasteride.

These data suggest that early hormonal therapy

TABLE 27–4. RESULTS OF ADJUVANT RADIOTHERAPY FOR pT3 PROSTATE CANCER*

	Adjuvant Radiation			No Adjuvant Radiation		
	5 Years	10 Years	15 Years	5 Years	10 Years	15 Years
Local progression	0–29%	0–36%	4%	11–52%	30–70%	68%
Survival	76–92%	46–87%		68–92%	55–88%	

*From Thompson IM, Paradelo JC, Crawford ED, et al: An opportunity to determine optimal treatment of pT3 prostate cancer: the window may be closing. Urology 1994; 44:804–811. Copyright Elsevier Science Inc, 1994, with permission.

for pT3 prostate cancer will have an immediate effect upon PSA and may, like radiation therapy, delay local progression. Unfortunately, the impact upon the rate of metastases, the hormonal responsiveness of subsequent metastasis, and survival rate changes are unknown. Recognizing the myriad of side effects of prolonged hormonal therapy (sexual dysfunction, changes in mood and libido, potential for metabolic bone disease) as well as the often low rates of progression for many patients with pT3 disease, it may be a more reasonable option to elect adjuvant radiation therapy for all but those patients who are at the highest risk for early metastatic disease (residual high PSA, high-grade disease, seminal vesicle invasion).

TREATMENT OF NODAL-POSITIVE PROSTATE CANCER

Hormonal Therapy

Hormonal therapy is the cornerstone of the treatment of nodal-positive prostate cancer. The principal question remains the timing of therapy: immediate or delayed. To date, there are no convincing data that one or the other is preferred and all conclusions must be inferred. Kramolowsky reviewed 68 patients with N+ disease who received no therapy for "cure" (e.g., radiation or surgery).[77] Of these, 30 received immediate hormonal therapy. Time to progression was significantly longer in patients who received immediate hormonal therapy (100 versus 43 months). Although an improvement in mean survival was noted (150 versus 90 months), statistical significance was not achieved. It also must be noted that, as this was not a randomized trial, patient selection factors may have caused some of the differences encountered. In general, hormonal therapy is based upon accepted forms of "monotherapy" (orchiectomy or LHRH agonist) or in combination with an antiandrogen. Nevertheless, in a small series of 16 N+ patients, Fleshner and Trachtenberg provided evidence that the combination of finasteride and flutamide will lead to dramatic reductions in PSA in such patients with minimal side effects.[78] It is doubtful, however, that this combination will yield disease-free survival results similar to traditional monotherapy or combined androgen deprivation.

External Beam Radiotherapy

One of the more common treatments of N+ disease is external beam radiotherapy. Data are conflicting as to the efficacy of this form of therapy. Lawton, reviewing 56 patients with N+ disease who received 68 Gy of radiation to the prostate with 50.4 Gy to the pelvis found actuarial 5- and 10-year survivals of 76 and 33%, respectively.[79] Disease-free survivals at 5 and 10 years of follow-up were 61 and 48%, respectively. These results suggest an improvement over delayed hormonal therapy alone compared to the series of Kramer et al., Paulson et al., and Smith et al. but are not substantially different from the untreated cohort of Kramolowsky.[44–77] A study from the Uro-Oncology Research Group compared external beam radiation versus delayed hormonal therapy in a group of 77 patients with histologically documented prostate cancer.[45] In the group of 36 patients who were managed with delayed hormonal therapy, the median time to progression was 12.2 months, compared to 23.9 months in those men receiving radiation therapy ($p = .02$). Although significance was achieved for progression, survival was not significantly affected by radiation. It is highly likely that, due to the very small sample size of this study, any conclusions inferred are highly suspect.

A small study of 64 patients, 17 of whom were observed and 47 of whom received external beam radiotherapy, was reported by Smith.[46] At 5 years of follow-up, 17% of patients who received radiation were free of disease compared to 29% of patients who underwent delayed hormonal therapy. Similarly, death from prostate cancer at 5 years was reported in 40% of irradiated patients compared to 35% of patients who were observed. Notable, however, was the finding that local symptoms were reduced in patients who received radiation: from 65% to 51%. The aggregate of these data suggest that there may be a role for radiation therapy for nodal-positive disease but that the impact of such monotherapy may be quite small.

Radical Prostatectomy

While it has been a generally accepted notion that radical prostatectomy is most suitable for patients with disease limited to the prostate, because of a falling rate of positive lymph nodes, a known false-negative rate of frozen sections, and other factors, many patients are found to have positive nodes following the performance of radical prostatectomy. It is intriguing to note that a substantial number of these patients do quite well. In a group of 113 men from Johns Hopkins University who underwent radical prostatectomy and in whom hormonal therapy was deferred until disease progression, progression was noted relatively quickly: 80% of patients progressed by 5 years and 88% by 10 years of follow-up.[80] Despite such high progression rates, however, survival free of metastatic disease was observed in 66% of patients at 5 years and in 47% of patients at 10 years of follow-up. Further analysis of these data found that patients with metastases larger than 2 mm had a greater likelihood of early metastases. The greatest discriminator for outcome was whether the patient had any component of Gleason grade 8 or greater in the initial prostate needle biopsy. If such high-grade disease was present, 85% of patients had metastases at 5 years compared to only 18% of men with grades less than 8. The authors suggested that if prostatectomy is to be afforded to men with N+ disease, it should be reserved for those men with well-differentiated or moderately differentiated disease.

In a comprehensive review of the literature on the treatment of nodal-positive prostate cancer, Austenfeld and Davis acknowledged the inherent difficulties with comparing treatment results among series.[47] Nevertheless, in a summary of this review, the authors noted that by far the best disease-free survival rates were noted with radical prostatectomy, most often combined with early endocrine therapy. Employing radical prostatectomy and immediate hormonal therapy in a group of 162 patients with N+ disease, during a mean follow-up of 56.4 months Zincke noted 5- and 10-year disease-free survivals of 84 and 80%, respectively.[81] Further evidence of the potential efficacy of early hormonal therapy combined with radical prostatectomy was reported by deKernion and colleagues.[82] Of a total of 56 patients with N+ disease, 21 underwent early endocrine therapy, while the remainder did not. Despite the fact that those patients receiving early endocrine therapy had a worse prognosis (higher rate of seminal vesicle invasion, twice as many involved nodes), survival free of disease was significantly higher at 9 years of follow-up in those patients who received early endocrine therapy (67%) compared to those who did not (32%). While cause-specific survival was also improved (91 versus 71%), this difference did not achieve statistical significance.

Chemotherapy

Few series have employed adjuvant chemotherapy for nodal-positive prostate cancer. The reasons for this are many: the lack of demonstrated efficacy of chemotherapeutic agents, the high toxicity rates of such agents, the dramatic efficacy of hormonal therapy, and the often-prolonged survival of many patients with involved nodes.[83] Nevertheless, a small group (12) of patients from UCLA have been reported who received both radiation therapy and chemotherapy following radical prostatectomy and pelvic lymphadenectomy.[84] Actuarial 10-year disease-free survival of 92% was noted as well as a local and distant recurrence rate of 3 and 6%, respectively, at 5 years of follow-up. It remains to be determined what the marginal impact of chemotherapy was in this series as well as the identification of the optimal agent for use.

CONCLUSIONS

As can be quickly surmised from the discussions above, little is known about the relative efficacy of competing treatments for locally advanced prostate cancer. One ongoing clinical trial is addressing the issue of the need for adjuvant radiation therapy following radical prostatectomy for pT3 disease. Unfortunately, because of the "difficult randomization" in this trial (to be eligible, patients must be willing to be randomized to 6 weeks of adjuvant external beam radiation or to be enrolled in a program of observation alone), accrual has been slow and completion is expected in another 2 to 3 years. Nevertheless, it will be studies like this that will answer fundamental questions concerning optimal treatment of locally advanced prostate cancer. Until such trials are completed, it will remain the responsibility of the individual physician to provide as much information as possible regarding relative treatment efficacy and the distinct sets of complications and morbidity associated with individual treatments so as to allow patients to make informed choices, based upon their own sets of treatment goals.

REFERENCES

1. Schmidt JD, Mettlin CJ, Natarajan N, et al: Trends in patient care for prostate cancer, 1974–1983: results of surveys by the American College of Surgeons. J Urol 1986; 136: 416–421.
2. Mettlin CJ, Murphy GP, Lee F, et al: Characteristics of prostate cancer detected in the American Cancer Society–National Prostate Cancer Detection Project. J Urol 1994; 152:1737–1740.
3. Catalona WJ, Smith DS, Ratliff TL, Basler JW: Detection of organ-confined prostate cancer is increased through prostate-specific antigen screening. JAMA 1993; 270:948–954.
4. Corn BW, Hanks GE, Lee WR, Schultheiss T: Do the current subclassifications of stage T3 adenocarcinoma of the prostate have clinical relevance? Urology 1995; 45:484–490.
5. Petros JA, Catalona WJ: Lower incidence of unsuspected lymph node metastases in 521 consecutive patients with clinically localized prostate cancer. J Urol 1992; 147:1574–1575.
6. Bishoff JT, Reyes A, Thompson IM, et al: Pelvic lymphadenectomy can be omitted in selected patients with carcinoma of the prostate: development of a system of patient selection. Urology 1995; 45:270–274.
7. Wingo PA, Tong T, Bolden S: Cancer Statistics, 1995. CA Cancer J Clin 1995; 45:8–30.
8. Freeman JA, Esrig D, Grossfeld GD, et al: Incidence of occult lymph node metastases in pathologic stage C (pT3N0) prostate cancer. J Urol 1995; 154:474–478.
9. Gervasi LA, Mata J, Easley JD, et al: Prognostic significance of lymph nodal metastases in prostate cancer. J Urol 1989; 142:332.
10. Ohori M, Wheeler TM, Kattan MW, et al: Prognostic significance of positive surgical margins in radical prostatectomy specimens. J Urol 1995; 154:1818–1824.
11. Cheng WS, Frydenberg M, Bergstralh EJ, et al: Radical prostatectomy for pathologic stage C prostate cancer: influence of pathologic variables and adjuvant treatment on disease outcome. Urology 1993; 42:283–291.
12. Partin AW, Piantadosi S, Sanda MG, et al: Selection of men at high risk for disease recurrence for experimental adjuvant therapy following radical prostatectomy. Urology 1995; 45:831–838.
13. Boxer RJ, Kaufman JJ, Goodwin WE: Radical prostatec-

tomy for cancer of the prostate: 1951–1976. A review of 329 patients. J Urol 1977; 117:208–213.
14. Spaulding JT, Whitmore WF: Extended total excision of prostatic adenocarcinoma. J Urol 1978; 120:188–190.
15. Yamada AH, Lieskovsky G, Petrovich Z, et al: Results of radical prostatectomy and adjuvant therapy in the management of locally advanced, clinical stage TC, prostate cancer. Am J Clin Oncol (CCT) 1994; 17:277–285.
16. Van de Ouden VD, Davidson PJT, Hop W, Schroder FH: Radical prostatectomy as a monotherapy for locally advanced (stage T3) prostate cancer. J Urol 1994; 151:646–651.
17. Zagars G: Prostate specific antigen as an outcome variable for T1 and T2 prostate cancer treated by radiation therapy. J Urol 1994; 152:1786.
18. Van Poppel HV, deRidder D, Elgamal AA, et al: Neoadjuvant hormonal therapy before radical prostatectomy decreases the number of positive surgical margins in stage T2 prostate cancer: interim results of a prospective randomized trial. J Urol 1995; 154:429.
19. Cher ML, Shinohara K, Breslin S, et al: High failure rate associated with long-term followup of neoadjuvant androgen deprivation followed by radical prostatectomy for stage C prostatic cancer. Br J Urol 1995; 75:771–777.
20. Narayan P, Lowe BA, Carroll PR, Thompson IM: Neoadjuvant hormonal therapy and radical prostatectomy for clinical stage C carcinoma of the prostate. Br J Urol 1994; 73:544–548.
21. Partin AW, Yoo J, Carter HB, et al: The use of prostate specific antigen, clinical stage, and Gleason score to predict pathological stage in men with localized prostate cancer. J Urol 1993; 150:110–114.
22. Bluestein DL, Bostwick DG, Bergstralh EJ, Oesterling JE: Eliminating the need for bilateral pelvic lymphadenectomy in select patients with prostate cancer. J Urol 1994; 151: 1315.
23. Kavadi VS, Zagars GK, Pollack A: Serum prostate-specific antigen after radiation therapy for clinically localized prostate cancer: prognostic implications. Int J Radiat Oncol Biol Phys 1994; 30:279–287.
24. Rifkin HD, Zerhouni EA, Gatsonis CA, et al: Comparison of magnetic resonance imaging and ultrasonography in staging early prostate cancer. N Engl J Med 1990; 232: 621–626.
25. Chelsky MJ, Schnall MD, Seidmon EJ, et al: Use of endorectal surface coil magnetic resonance imaging for local staging of prostate cancer. J Urol 1993; 150:391–395.
26. Levran Z, Gonzalez JA, Diokno AC, et al: Are pelvic computerized tomography, bone scan, and pelvic lymphadenectomy necessary in the staging of prostate cancer? Br J Urol 1995; 75:778–781.
27. Wolf JS, Cher M, Dallera M, et al: The use and accuracy of cross-sectional imaging and fine needle aspiration cytology for detection of pelvic lymph node metastases before radical prostatectomy. J Urol 1995; 153:993–999.
28. Troxel S, Winfield HN: Comparative financial analysis of laparoscopic versus open pelvic lymph node dissection for men with cancer of the prostate. J Urol 1994; 151:675–680.
29. Byer DP: The Veterans Administration Cooperative Urological Research Group's studies of cancer of the prostate. Cancer 1973; 32:1126–1130.
30. Hanno PM: Carcinoma of the prostate—stage C. *In* Seidmon EJ, Hanno PM (eds): Current Urologic Therapy, 3rd edition, p 384. Philadelphia, WB Saunders Co, 1994.
31. Blackard CE: Re: Deferred treatment of low grade stage T3 prostate cancer without distant metastases (Letter; Comment). J Urol 1994; 151:436.
32. Adolfsson J: Deferred treatment of low grade, low stage T3 prostate cancer without distant metastases. J Urol 1993; 149:326–328.
33. Rana A, Chisholm GD, Khan M, et al: Conservative management with symptomatic treatment and delayed hormonal manipulation is justified in men with locally advanced carcinoma of the prostate. Br J Urol 1994; 74:637–641.
34. Aus G, Hugosson J, Norlen L: Long-term survival and mortality in prostate cancer treated with noncurative intent. J Urol 1995; 154:460–465.
35. Paulson DF, Moul JW, Walther PJ: Radical prostatectomy for clinical stage T1-2N0M0 prostatic adenocarcinoma: long-term results. J Urol 1990; 144:1180–1184.
36. Stein A, deKernion JB, Dorey F, et al: Adjuvant radiotherapy in patients post radical prostatectomy with tumor extending through capsule or positive seminal vesicles. Urology 1992; 39:59–62.
37. Eisbruch A, Perez CA, Roessler EH, Lockett MA: Adjuvant irradiation after prostatectomy for carcinoma of the prostate with positive surgical margins. Cancer 1994; 73:384–388.
38. Anscher MS, Prosnitz LR: Postoperative radiotherapy for patients with carcinoma of the prostate undergoing radical prostatectomy with positive surgical margins, seminal vesicle involvement and/or penetration through the capsule. J Urol 1987; 138:1407–1412.
39. Jacobson GM, Smith JA, Stewart JR: Postoperative radiation for pathologic stage C prostate cancer. Int J Radiat Oncol Biol Phys 1987; 13:1021–1024.
40. Shevlin BE, Mittal BB, Brand WN, Shety RM: The role of adjuvant irradiation following primary prostatectomy based on histopathologic extent of tumor. Int J Radiat Oncol Biol Phys 1989; 16:1425–1450.
41. Cheng WS, Frydenberg M, Bergstralh EJ, et al: Radical prostatectomy for pathologic stage C prostate cancer: influence of pathologic variables and adjuvant treatment on disease outcome. Urology 1993; 42:283.
42. Stamey TA, Villers AA, McNeal JE, et al: Positive surgical margins at radical prostatectomy: importance of the apical dissection. J Urol 1990; 143:1166.
43. Ohori M, Wheeler TM, Kattan KW, et al: Prognostic significance of positive surgical margins in radical prostatectomy specimens. J Urol 1995; 154:1818–1824.
44. Kramer SA, Cline WA, Farnham R, et al: Prognosis of patients with stage D1 prostatic adenocarcinoma. J Urol 1981; 126:817.
45. Paulson DF, Cline WA, Koefoot RB, et al: Extended field radiotherapy versus delayed hormonal therapy in node positive prostatic adenocarcinoma. J Urol 1982; 127: 935.
46. Smith JA, Haynes TH, Middleton RG: Impact of external irradiation on local symptoms and survival free of disease in patients with pelvic lymph node metastasis from adenocarcinoma of the prostate. J Urol 1984; 131:707.
47. Austenfeld MS, Davis BE: New concepts in the treatment of stage D1 adenocarcinoma of the prostate. Urol Clin North Am 1990; 17:867.
48. Thompson IM: Clinical stage C carcinoma of the prostate. AUA Update Series 1993; 11:82–87.
49. Lerner SE, Blute ML, Zincke H: Extended experience with radical prostatectomy for clinical stage T3 prostate cancer: outcome and contemporary morbidity. J Urol 1995; 154: 1447–1452.
50. Scott WW, Boyd HL: Combined hormone control therapy and radical prostatectomy in the treatment of selected cases of advanced carcinoma of the prostate: a retrospective study based upon 25 years of experience. J Urol 1969; 101:86.
51. Zagars GK, von Eschenback AC, Ayala AG: Prognostic factors in prostate cancer. Analysis of 874 patients treated with radiation therapy. Cancer 1993; 72:1709–1725.
52. Crook JM, Perry GA, Robertson S, Esche BA: Routine prostate biopsies following radiotherapy for prostate cancer: results for 226 patients. Urology 1995; 46:624.
53. Zietman AL, Coen JJ, Shipley WU, et al: Radical radiation therapy in the management of prostatic adenocarcinoma: the initial prostate specific antigen value as a predictor of treatment outcome. J Urol 1994; 151:640–646.
54. Leibel SA, Zelefsky MJ, Kutcher GJ, et al: The biological basis and clinical application of three-dimensional conformal external beam radiation therapy in carcinoma of the prostate. Semin Oncol 1994; 21:580–597.

55. Barendsen GW, Koot CJ, Van Kersen GR, et al: The effect of oxygen on impairment of the proliferative capacity of human cells in culture by ionizing radiations of different linear energy transfer. Int J Radiat Biol 1966; 10:317–327.
56. Russell KJ, Caplan RJ, Laramore GE, et al: Photon versus fast neutron external beam radiotherapy in the treatment of locally advanced prostate cancer: results of a randomized prospective trial. Int J Radiat Oncol Biol Phys 1993; 28:47–54.
57. Pilepich MV, Krall JM, Al-Sarraf M, et al: Androgen deprivation with radiation therapy compared with radiation therapy alone for locally advanced prostatic carcinoma: a randomized comparative trial of the Radiation Therapy Oncology Group. Urology 1995; 45:616–623.
58. Zelefsky MJ, Leibel SA, Burman CM, et al: Neoadjuvant hormonal therapy improves the therapeutic ratio in patients with bulky prostatic cancer treated with three-dimensional conformal radiation therapy. Int J Radiat Oncol Biol Phys 1994; 29:755–761.
59. Rozanski TA, Faerber GJ: Massive locally extensive prostate cancer. Urology 1994; 43:242–243.
60. Gonder MH, Soanes WA, Smith V: Experimental prostate cryosurgery. Invest Urol 1964; 1:610–618.
61. Lee F, Bahn DK, McHugh TA, et al: US-guided percutanous cryoablation of prostate cancer. Radiology 1994; 192: 769–776.
62. Miller RJ, Cohen JK, Merlotti LA: Percutaneous transperineal cryosurgical ablation of the prostate for the primary treatment of clinical stage C adenocarcinoma of the prostate. Urology 1994; 44:170–174.
63. Bahn DK, Lee F, Solomon MH, et al: Prostate cancer: US-guided percutaneous cryoablation. Radiology 1995; 194: 551–556.
64. Cox RL, Crawford ED: Complications of cryosurgical ablation of the prostate to treat localized adenocarcinoma of the prostate. Urology 1995; 45:932–935.
65. Bruchovsky N, Rennie PS, Coldman AJ, et al: Effects of androgen withdrawal on the stem cells composition of the Shionogi carcinoma. Cancer Res 1990; 50:2275–2282.
66. Akakura K, Bruchovsky N, Goldenberg SL, et al: Effects of intermittent androgen suppression on androgen-dependent tumors. Cancer 1993; 71:2782–2790.
67. Khan K, Thompson W, Bush S, et al: Transperineal percutaneous iridium-192 interstitial template implantation of the prostate: results and complications in 321 patients. Int J Radiat Oncol Biol Phys 1992; 22:935–939.
68. Holzman M, Carlton CE, Scardino PT: The frequency and morbidity of local tumor recurrence after definitive radiotherapy for stage C prostate cancer. J Urol 1991; 146: 1578–1582.
69. Zagars GK, von Eschenbach AC, Ayala AG, et al: The influence of local control on metastatic dissemination of prostate cancer treated by external beam megavoltage radiation therapy. Cancer 1991; 68:2370–2377.
70. McCarthy JF, Catalona WJ, Hudson MA: Effect of radiation therapy undetectable serum prostate specific antigen levels following radical prostatectomy: early versus delayed treatment. J Urol 1994; 161:1575–1578.
71. Thompson IM, Paradelo JC, Crawford ED, et al: An opportunity to determine optimal treatment of pT3 prostate cancer: the window may be closing. Urology 1994; 44: 804–811.
72. Veronesi U, Saccozzi R, Del Vechio M, et al: Comparing radical mastectomy with quandrantectomy, axillary dissection, and radiotherapy in patients with small cancers of the breast. N Engl J Med 1981; 305:6–11.
73. Fisher B, Redmond C, Poisson R, et al: Eight-year results of a randomized clinical trial comparing total mastectomy and lumpectomy with or without irradiation in the treatment of breast cancer. N Engl J Med 1989; 320:822–828.
74. Liljegren G, Holmberg L, Adami HO, et al: Sector resection with or without postoperative radiotherapy for stage I breast cancer. Five-year results of a randomized trial. J Natl Cancer Inst 1994; 86:717–722.
75. Thompson I, Crawford ED, Miller G, et al: Adjuvant radiotherapy following radical prostatectomy for pathologic stage C adenocarcinoma of the prostate: initial evaluation of toxicity. Proc Ann Meeting Am Soc Clin Oncol 1992; 11: 212.
76. Andriole G, Lieber M, Smith J, et al: Treatment with finasteride following radical prostatectomy for prostate cancer. Urology 1995; 45:491–497.
77. Kramolowsky EV: The value of testosterone deprivation in stage D1 carcinoma of the prostate. J Urol 1988; 139: 1242–1244.
78. Fleshner NE, Trachtenberg J: Combination finasteride and flutamide in advanced carcinoma of the prostate: effective therapy with minimal side effects. J Urol 1995; 154:642–646.
79. Lawton CA, Cox JD, Glisch C, et al: Is long-term survival possible with external beam irradiation for stage D1 adenocarcinoma of the prostate? Cancer 1992; 69:2761–2766.
80. Sgrignoli AR, Walsh PC, Stinberg GD, et al: Prognostic factors in men with stage D1 prostate cancer: identification of patients less likely to have prolonged survival after radical prostatectomy. J Urol 1994; 152:1077–1081.
81. Zincke H: Extended experience with surgical treatment of stage D1 adenocarcinoma of the prostate. Urology 1989; 33:27.
82. deKernion JB, Neuwirth H, Stein A, et al: Prognosis of patients with stage D1 prostate carcinoma following radical prostatectomy with and without early endocrine therapy. J Urol 1990; 144:700–703.
83. Eisenberger M, Simon R, O'Dwyer PJ, et al: A reevaluation of non-hormonal cytotoxic chemotherapy in the treatment of prostatic cancer. J Clin Oncol 1985; 3:827.
84. Carter GE, Lieskovsky G, Skinner DG, Petrovich Z: Results of local and/or systemic adjuvant therapy in the management of pathologic stage C or D1 prostate cancer following radical prostatectomy. J Urol 1989; 142:1266–1271.
85. Beahrs OH, Henson DE, Hutter RVP, Kennedy BJ: *In* Manual for Staging of Cancer, 4th edition, pp 487–512. Philadelphia, JB Lippincott Co, 1992.

28

METASTATIC ADENOCARCINOMA OF THE PROSTATE (TxNxM+): MANAGEMENT AND PROGNOSIS

STEVE WAXMAN, M.D. *and* E. DAVID CRAWFORD, M.D.

Adenocarcinoma of the prostate is the most common malignancy in men with an estimated 244,000 new cases being diagnosed in the United States in 1995.[1] The proportion of newly diagnosed stage D2 (M1) disease in most series is approximately 30%.[2] With approximately 70,000 new cases of metastatic adenocarcinoma of the prostate being newly diagnosed this year in the United States, a therapeutic dilemma exists as to the indications, selection, and timing of therapy. Treatment for metastatic prostate cancer was first begun following the discovery of the androgen dependence of prostatic cancer by Huggins and Hodges in the early 1940s.[3] They and others noted the symptomatic improvement and regression of disease in many patients treated with hormonal deprivation therapy. However, patients eventually progressed and died from their disease. Over 50 years have elapsed since the initial discovery of androgen sensitivity in prostate cancer, unfortunately without discovery of a cure for advanced prostate cancer. Many hormonal and nonhormonal therapies have been introduced during this time, some of which have increased the time to progression and improved survival. The management of metastatic prostate cancer continues to be a topic of controversy and ambiguity. This chapter will review the management and prognosis of metastatic adenocarcinoma of the prostate (TxNxM+).

DIAGNOSIS AND STAGING

The diagnosis of metastatic adenocarcinoma of the prostate has been addressed in an earlier chapter; however, several key points should be emphasized. The most common metastatic site for prostate cancer is bone, with the characteristic lesion being osteoblastic. Full-body bone scans with technetium-99m (^{99m}Tc) have been the mainstay for detecting and staging advanced prostate cancer for the past 20 years. The whole-body bone scan's sensitivity for detecting bone metastases from prostate cancer is superior to plain radiographs or serum markers.[4] Degenerative and arthritic disease, Paget's disease, and prior trauma can cause diagnostic confusion; however, correlation with plain radiographs will usually reliably differentiate metastatic disease from other processes. Prostate-specific antigen (PSA) can sometimes be helpful in predicting metastatic disease in patients with very high PSAs (>50 ng/ml). However, its greatest use in metastatic disease is in the monitoring of therapeutic intervention.

MANAGEMENT

The first treatment for metastatic adenocarcinoma of the prostate was bilateral orchiectomy, which was introduced by Huggins and Hodges in 1941.[1] While noting good initial symptomatic improvement and partial regression of disease, they found that patients eventually progressed and died from their disease. The discovery was crucial in establishing the androgen sensitivity of prostate cancer and led to the search for new forms of hormonal manipulation in this disease. Also in the early 1940s, it was realized that estrogen administration could achieve a "medical" castration through its negative feedback on the pituitary gland.[5] The endocrine axis and androgen production in humans has been very well characterized in the literature[6] (Fig. 28–1). The mechanism by which hormonal

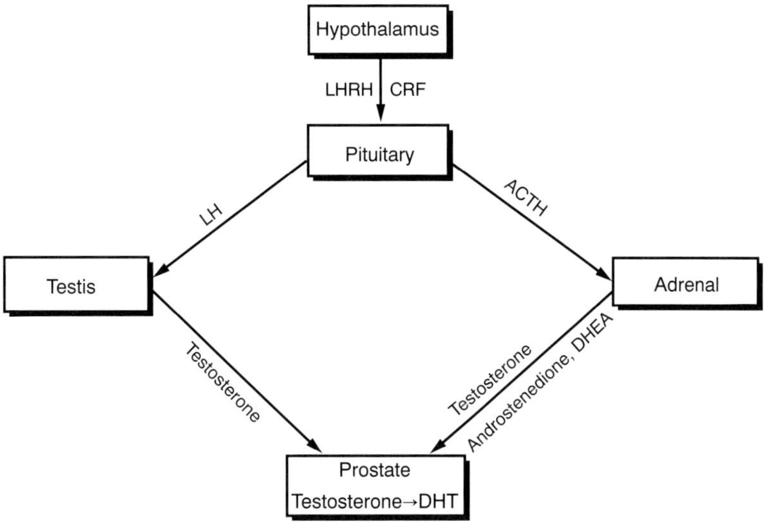
Hypothalamus
LHRH
CRF
Pituitary
LH
ACTH
Testis
Adrenal
Testosterone
Testosterone
Androstenedione, DHEA
Prostate
Testosterone→DHT

FIGURE 28–1. Mechanism of action of estrogens. Hypothalamus produces luteinizing hormone releasing hormone (LHRH), which stimulates release of luteinizing hormone (LH) from anterior pituitary. Luteinizing hormone stimulates production and release of testosterone by Leydig cells of testes. Testosterone and its metabolites are trophic hormones for benign and malignant prostatic tissue. Increased estrogen levels feed back on system to decrease luteinizing hormone release, thus decreasing testosterone levels in serum. Other mechanisms, including direct action on Leydig cells and direct toxicity to prostate cancer cells, are conjectured but not established with certainty. CRF, corticotropin-releasing factor; ACTH, adrenocorticotropic hormone; DHEA, dehydroepiandrosterone; DHT, dihydrotestosterone. (From Cox RL, Crawford ED: Estrogens in treatment of prostate cancer. J Urol 1995; 154:1991–1998, with permission.)

manipulation affects prostate cancer has also been described at length.[7] With the realization of the adrenal gland's ability to produce androgens and the eventual failure of orchiectomy to halt progress of metastatic prostate cancer, Huggins and Scott proposed bilateral adrenalectomy in patients whose prostate cancer was refractory to orchiectomy alone.[8] Unfortunately, replacement therapy in the mid 1940s was inadequate and these patients died of adrenal insufficiency, making it impossible to test the hypothesis of combined androgen blockade for many years to come. Over the past 50 years numerous medications have been developed and tested that achieve a medical castration (Table 28–1).

TABLE 28–1. ESTROGENS—DOSAGE, EFFICACY, AND TOXICITY*

Drug	Dose	Efficacy	Toxicity
Diethylstilbestrol	0.2 mg/day PO	Negligible	Negligible
	1 mg/day PO	Established	Mild
	3 mg/1 mg/day PO × 3	Established	Significant
	5 mg/day PO	Established	Excessive
Conjugated estrogens	2.5 mg/day PO	Established	Mild
Polyestradiol phosphate	80–160 mg/mo IM	Questionable	Mild
	240–320 mg/mo IM	Probable[†]	Mild or absent
Polyestradiol phosphate plus ethinyl estradiol	80 mg/mo IM plus 0.15 mg/day PO, respectively	Established	Significant
Estramustine phosphate	280 mg/day PO × 2	Established	Mild to significant
Ethinyl estradiol	0.05 mg/day PO × 3	Probable	Mild to significant
Stilbestrol diphosphate	100 mg/day PO × 3	Probable	Mild to significant
Chlorotrianisene	24–144 mg/day PO	Not established	Mild

*Modified from Cox RL, Crawford ED: Estrogens in treatment of prostate cancer. J Urol 1995; 154:1991–1998, with permission.

[†]Small studies.

The first and most commonly used estrogen for the hormonal treatment of prostate cancer was diethylstilbestrol (DES). The Veterans Administration Cooperative Urological Research Group (VACURG) studies of the 1960s demonstrated the effectiveness of DES in producing medical castration but also significant cardiovascular complications when used at a dose of 5 mg/day.[9] These cardiovascular complications were confirmed by several other studies.[10,11] Other estrogenic substances that have been used in the treatment of metastatic prostate cancer include Premarin, ethinyl estradiol, chlorotrianisene (TACE), and estramustine phosphate (EMCYT).[12–14] These estrogen preparations offer no advantage when compared to DES. Regardless of whether patients with metastatic prostate cancer underwent medical or surgical castration, patients with stage D2 disease had a median survival of only 30 months with a 5-year survival of 20%. Following initiation of hormonal ablation, progression to hormonal refractory disease usually occurred at 12 to 18 months.[15] Overall survival was not significantly changed from the 1940s through the 1980s with either therapy (medical or surgical castration). Once patients progressed on monotherapy, half died within 6 months of relapse.[16] In the 1980s, introduction of luteinizing hormone releasing hormone (LHRH) analogs provided patients with a relatively safe medical alternative to surgical castration. In randomized trials, leuprolide acetate was shown to be as effective as DES in producing medical castration without the cardiovascular complications and less gynecomastia when compared to estrogen.[17,18] The LHRH agonists cause pituitary desensitization by altering the normal pulsatile release of LHRH in the pituitary gland resulting in a greatly diminished luteinizing hormone. Testosterone supply falls to "castrate levels" (<50 ng/ml). Initially, LHRH agonists cause a transient stimulation of LH production (flare) that can potentially aggravate patient's symptoms; however, testosterone begins to fall within 1 to 2 weeks, with castrate levels being reached in approximately 1 month.[19] The "flare phenomenon," which occurs in 10% of patients, can have serious consequences; however, this can be cut with antiandrogen administration, which will be discussed later in this chapter.[20,21] While LHRH agonists have proven to be as effective as orchiectomy in producing castrate levels of testosterone, drawbacks include monthly parenteral administration and relatively high monetary cost. However, patient satisfaction and acceptance is much higher when compared to orchiectomy. Whether a patient undergoes bilateral orchiectomy, receives LHRH agonist, or DES therapy, approximately 60 to 80% of men with metastatic disease will respond to monotherapy with a mean duration of 20 to 24 months (subjective or objective response, disease stabilization). When these patients become hormone refractory, mean survival is only 6 to 9 months.

FORMS OF MONOTHERAPY IN THE TREATMENT OF METASTATIC PROSTATE CANCER

Progestational agents such as Megace and depostat have been used in metastatic prostate cancer due to their ability to suppress pituitary secretion of luteinizing hormone. They also directly inhibit steroidogenesis and weakly bind to androgen receptors in the prostate gland; however, escape eventually occurs with a gradual rise in plasma testosterone, thus requiring the combined administration of other agents such as DES.[22] Megace is also helpful in the treatment of hot flashes experienced by patients who have undergone monotherapy with orchiectomy or LHRH agonist therapy.

Prolactin antagonists (levodopa and bromocriptine) have demonstrated some efficacy in the relief of pain in patients who are hormone refractory. This is thought to be due to their ability to block pituitary-mediated androgen activity.[23]

ANTIANDROGENS

Androgens produced by the adrenal gland were thought to be contributory in the stimulation of prostate cancer as early as the 1940s. Bilateral adrenalectomy was unsuccessful mainly because of inadequate adrenal replacement at the time. "Medical adrenalectomy" was later begun using cortisone, aminoglutethimide, ketoconazole, and other agents. While adrenal androgens only account for 5 to 10% of the circulating androgen pool, 20 to 40% of total intraprostatic dihydrotestosterone is from the adrenal glands.[24] Furthermore, it was found that up to 50% of intraprostatic dihydrotestosterone (DHT) remains following medical or surgical castration.[25] The steroidal antiandrogens include cyproterone acetate (CPA) and Megace, which have both progestational and antiandrogenic properties. They block gonadotropin release from the pituitary and inhibit the formation of DHT-receptor complex in the prostate cells as well as the C21-19 decarboxylase enzyme, which is involved in the synthesis of adrenal androgens. Testosterone synthesis in the Leydig cells is also inhibited by CPA and Megace. Both drugs require the addition of low-dose DES to maintain castrate levels of testosterone.[26,27] Monotherapy with the steroidal antiandrogens show them to be no more effective than standard estrogen therapy.[28] The nonsteroidal antiandrogens were introduced in the 1980s and they are neither hormones nor hormone analogs. These compounds block the cellular action of androgens at the target organ by inhibiting nuclear uptake of DHT.[29] Nonsteroidal antiandrogens do not result in a decrease in serum testosterone, thus giving them the added benefit of potency preservation. There is no negative feedback on the hypothalamus, thus LHRH and LH levels are increased with a resultant in-

TABLE 28–2. AGENTS USED IN ANDROGEN BLOCKADE

Class	Mechanism of Action	Comments
LHRH analogues	Pituitary desensitization (↓ LH,* ↓ testosterone synthesis)	Transient flare of symptoms due to initial surge of LH secretion
Leuprolide		
Goserelin		
Steroidal antiandrogens	Primary: competitive inhibition of androgens at the receptor level	Require administration of DES, 0.1 mg/day, to ensure continued pituitary suppression
Megestrol acetate		
Cyproterone acetate	Secondary: progestational effect overrides the negative feedback of testosterone at the hypothalamus	
Nonsteroidal antiandrogens		
Flutamide	Competitive inhibitor of androgen binding at the target cell level	Short $T_{1/2}$, GI disturbances
Nilutamide	Same as flutamide	Reversible interstitial lung disease on 1% to 3% of patients; bothersome side effect of impaired adaptation to darkness
Casodex	Same as flutamide	Once-daily dosing
Other agents		
Aminoglutethimide	Inhibitor of adrenal steroidogenesis by blocking P-450–mediated hydroxylation	Requires the administration of hydrocortisone to suppress ACTH levels
Ketoconazole	Inhibitor of P-450 enzymes in testes and adrenals	Castrate levels achieved in <24 hr (useful with impending spinal cord compression)

*Modified from Mayer FJ, Crawford ED: Update on combined androgen blockade for metastatic prostate cancer. Adv Urol 1994; 7:93–107, with permission.

LHRH, luteinizing hormone releasing hormone; LH, luteinizing hormone; DES, diethylstilbestrol; $T_{1/2}$, half-life; ACTH, adrenocorticotropic hormone.

crease in serum testosterone. This high serum testosterone will overcome the blockade, thus prohibiting its use as monotherapy in metastatic prostate cancer. Nonsteroidal antiandrogens are not associated with cardiovascular toxicity or fluid retention; however, gynecomastia, diarrhea, flushing, and rarely liver function abnormalities may occur with its usage. The nonsteroidal antiandrogens have not been studied extensively as monotherapy and are mainly used in combination with orchiectomy or an LHRH analog. The three nonsteroidal antiandrogens used at this time are flutamide (Eulexin), nilutamide (Anandron), and bicalutamide (Casodex) (Table 28–2). The concept of metachronous combined androgen blockade was suggested by Huggins in the 1940s; however, it has only been safely and reliably achieved since the early 1980s. The first study of combined androgen blockade in the early 1980s by Labrie and associates was met with both enthusiasm and skepticism.[30] This first study lacked a control arm; however, the combination of LHRH agonist and an antiandrogen showed improved survival over historical control studies, thus stimulating further studies of maximal hormonal ablation. In 1989, the National Cancer Institute Intergroup Study (0036) reported increased survival in patients treated with LHRH agonist and antiandrogen when compared to LHRH agonist alone[31] (Fig. 28–2). Patients treated with combined androgen blockade had a 6-month increased survival overall. In a subset of men with good performance status and minimal bone disease a 19-month survival advantage was noted when compared to an equally matched cohort not receiving an antiandrogen (Fig. 28–3). Three other studies have confirmed a survival advantage in patients receiving combined androgen blockade when compared to orchiectomy or LHRH agonist alone.[32–34] Other trials, however, have not demonstrated any survival advantage with combined androgen blockade.[35,36] Criticism of these studies that do not show a survival advantage of combined androgen blockade is that they may be too immature or have too few patients to show statistical significance. This was, in fact, demonstrated in a later analysis of an initially negative study by the European Organization for Research and Treatment of Cancer (EORTC), which initially showed no advantage with combined androgen blockade but later reported a survival advantage after adequate time had elapsed to correctly assess the data (Table 28–3).

EARLY VERSUS LATE ENDOCRINE THERAPY

The timing of endocrine therapy in the treatment of metastatic prostate cancer has been debated for many decades. The VACURG study initially suggested no survival advantage of early hormonal therapy. However, in a recent update by Byar in the second VA study, 1 mg of DES had a beneficial effect on survival rate when compared to either placebo or 0.2 mg DES or 5 mg DES. It is possible that the cardiovascular complications associated with

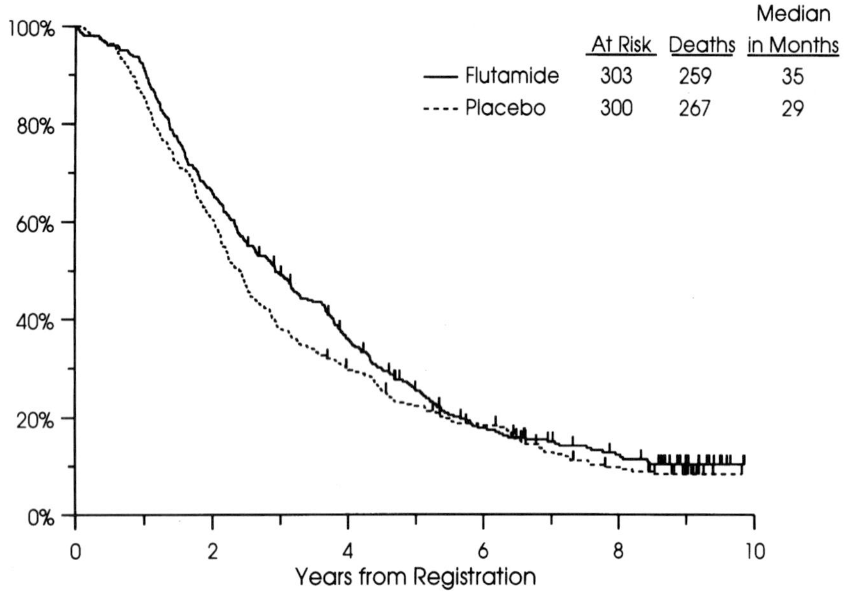
Median
At Risk Deaths in Months
Flutamide 303 259 35
Placebo 300 267 29
100%
80%
60%
40%
20%
0%
0 2 4 6 8 10
Years from Registration

FIGURE 28–2. National Cancer Institute intergroup protocol 0036. Leuprolide with flutamide or placebo. Overall survival, 21APR95.

the initial dose of 5 mg DES may have accounted for creating any survival advantage in the early hormonal treatment group.[9,37] While some studies have suggested a possible survival advantage with early hormonal therapy, no studies have any significant advantage with early as opposed to delayed endocrine treatment.

Regardless of what form or combination of hormonal therapy is used to treat metastatic adenocarcinoma of the prostate, the patient eventually develops a hormonal refractory state as evidenced by progression of disease. Typically, the PSA begins to rise and the bone scan may or may not indicate progressive metastatic disease. In patients who are on combined androgen blockade, several observations have been reported concerning the antiandrogen withdrawal syndrome. In those patients whose PSAs have begun to rise on combined androgen blockade, the withdrawal of antiandrogen (flutamide) resulted in a significant PSA decline as well as symptomatic relief.[38–41] Serum PSA decreased by greater than 80% in patients responding. It is hypothesized that the antiandrogen has a paradoxical effect on the androgen receptor, which undergoes mutation and recognizes the antiandrogen as an agonist. Other observations have included the possibility that patients may respond favorably to intermittent hormonal therapy for metastatic adenocarcinoma of the prostate. It is felt that once the patient shows a significant response to androgen deprivation therapy, the hormonal treatment may be stopped, thus allowing the androgen-sensitive

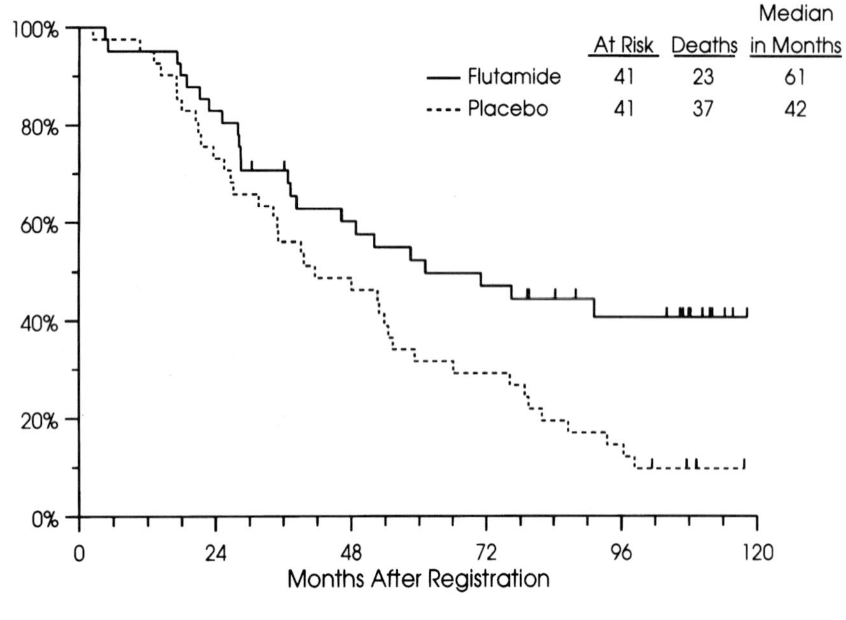
Median
At Risk Deaths in Months
Flutamide 41 23 61
Placebo 41 37 42
100%
80%
60%
40%
20%
0%
0 24 48 72 96 120
Months After Registration

FIGURE 28–3. National Cancer Institute intergroup protocol 0036. Leuprolide with flutamide or placebo. Overall survival, good prognosis subset, 21APR95.

TABLE 28–3. COMBINATION THERAPY WITH A PURE ANTIANDROGEN AND CASTRATION IN DOUBLE-BLIND, RANDOMIZED, PLACEBO-CONTROLLED AND PROSPECTIVE STUDIES OF STAGE D_2 DISEASE

Study	No. of Patients	Best Response	No Response	Pain Improvement	PSA or PAP Normalization	Duration of Response (Months)	Death Due to Cancer (Months)	Death from All Causes (Months)
Béland et al.[9,*]	194	46% vs. 20% $p < .01$	20% vs. 38% $p < .01$	$p < .05$	$p < .05$	Positive trend		24.3 vs. 18.9 (5.4) $p < .05$
National Cancer Institute[10,‡]	602	$p < .05$		$p < .05$	$p < .05$	16.9 vs. 13.8 (3.1) $p < .05$		35.6 vs. 28.3 (7.3) $p < .05$
Janknegt et al.[12,†§]	423	41% vs. 24% $p < .001$	22% vs. 36% $p < .002$	$p < .006$	$p < .05$	19.0 vs. 14.9 (4.1) $p = .006$	37.1 vs. 29.8 (7.3)	27.3 vs. 24.2 (4.1)
European Organization for Research and Treatment of Cancer[11,§]	327			$p < .05$	$p < .05$	30.7 vs. 19.6 (11.1) $p = .008$	43.9 vs. 29.9 (15.1) $p = .007$	34.4 vs. 27.1 (7.3) $p = .02$

*From Crawford ED, DeAntoni EP, Labrie E, et al: Endocrine therapy of prostate cancer: optimal form and appropriate timing. J Clin Endocrinol Metab 1995; 80:1062–1078, with permission.

†Nilutamide and orchiectomy versus orchiectomy as control.

‡Flutamide and luteinizing hormone releasing hormone (LHRH) agonist versus LHRH agonist as control.

§Flutamide and LHRH agonist versus orchiectomy as control.

NS, not significant; PAP, prostatic acid phosphatase; PSA, prostate-specific antigen.

cells to repopulate; then, hormonal therapy may be reinstituted, thus treating these cells and possibly delaying the progression of androgen-independent tumor cells.[42–44]

CHEMOTHERAPY AND RADIOTHERAPY

Eventually, patients with metastatic adenocarcinoma of the prostate on hormonal therapy will develop an androgen-refractory state that will lead to disease progression and eventual death. Cytotoxic chemotherapy has been attempted in patients with metastatic adenocarcinoma of the prostate, with and without hormone insensitivity.[45,46] Cytotoxic chemotherapeutic agents have also been tried in conjunction with endocrine therapy; however, no survival advantage has been demonstrated at this time.[47] The antiparasitic agent suramin has been tried in patients with hormone-refractory prostate cancer, with very little objective response in disease stabilization.[48] In patients with hormone-refractory prostate cancer with symptomatic bone metastases, palliation can be achieved with either selective external beam radiation therapy (XRT) to the metastases or with hemibody irradiation.[49,50] In patients with solitary symptomatic bone metastases, 20 to 40 Gy of XRT was able to improve symptoms in 80% of patients, with complete resolution of symptoms in 60%. Hemibody irradiation improved symptoms in 20 to 80% of patients depending on the extent of bone metastases. Another option for the treatment of symptomatic bone metastases involves the use of strontium-89 (^{89}Sr) administration. Strontium-89 is a pure β emitter that is taken up in the bones analogous to calcium. Studies have demonstrated a 20% complete symptomatic response, making it a useful adjunct in the treatment of patients with symptomatic bony metastases.[51–53]

PROGNOSIS

As stated earlier, patients with metastatic prostate cancer have a median survival of only 30 months. Following hormonal ablation therapy, a refractory state usually develops in 12 to 18 months after which approximately half of the patients die within 6 months of progression. The Veterans Administration Cooperative Urological Research Group, the National Prostatic Cancer Group, and the European Organization for Research on Treatment of Cancer Genitourinary Group (EORTC-GU), have all performed analyses to identify prognostic variables in patients with advanced prostate cancer. These studies have identified independent prognostic variables in newly diagnosed metastatic prostate cancer patients that may affect survival. Prognostic factors include elevated acid phosphates, upper tract obstruction, tumor grade, performance status, and other variables.[20,21,54] The introduction of PSA has provided clinicians with a much more sensitive tool for assessing initial response to treatment and assessing patient prognosis.[53,56–59] Patients whose PSAs dropped to a nadir of less than 4 mg/ml were found to have a significantly longer time to progression than those whose nadir remained elevated following treatment. Other prognostic indicators include the presence of aneuploidy of the tumor cells, nuclear and nucleolar morphology, neuroendocrine differentiation, androgen receptor status, serum tissue polypeptide antigen levels, and β-microseminal protein immunoreactivity. The degree of aneuploidy, however, parallels histologic grade and stage.[60,61]

SUMMARY

The incidence of adenocarcinoma of the prostate continues to rise, with a significant proportion of these men being newly diagnosed with metastatic disease. Many patients with advanced (T3) and nodal positive disease will also eventually progress to metastatic disease. It is thus imperative to develop more effective treatments for these patients so that not only time to progression but also overall survival is increased. Hormonal therapy has been practiced for over 50 years with only modest improvements in patient survival. It is hoped that with sound scientific research and judgment, effective therapies for androgen-independent tumor cells will be found. Once this is achieved, we may begin to realize potential cures rather than palliation in patients with metastatic disease.

REFERENCES

1. Wingo PA, Tong T, Boulden S: Cancer statistics, 1995. CA Cancer J Clin 1995; 35:8–30.
2. Mettlin C, Jones GW, Murphy GP: Trends in prostate cancer care in the United States, 1974–90: observations from the Patient Care Evaluation Studies of the American College of Surgeons Commission on Cancer. CA Cancer J Clin 1993; 43:83–91.
3. Huggins C, Hodges CV: Studies of prostatic cancer. I. Effect of castration, estrogen, and androgen injections on serum phosphatases in metastatic carcinoma of the prostate. Cancer Res 1941; 1:293–307.
4. Schaffer D, Pendergrass HP: Comparison of enzyme, clinical, radiographic, and radionuclide methods of detecting bone metastases from carcinoma of the prostate. Radiology 1976; 121:431–434.
5. Herbst WP: Effects of estradiol diproprionate and diethylstilbestrol on malignant prostatic tissue. Trans Am Assoc Genitourin Surg 1994; 34:195.
6. Daneshgari F, Crawford ED: Endocrine therapy of advanced carcinoma of the prostate. *In* Das S, Crawford ED (eds): Cancer of the Prostate, pp 333–354. New York, Marcel Dekker, Inc, 1993.
7. McConnell JD: Physiologic basis of endocrine therapy for prostatic cancer. Urol Clin North Am 1991; 18:1–13.
8. Huggins C, Scott WW: Bilateral adrenalectomy in prostatic cancer: clinical features and urinary excretion of 17-ketosteroids and estrogens. Ann Surg 1945; 122:1031.
9. VACURG: Treatment and survival of patients with cancer of the prostate. Surg Gynecol Obstet 1967; 124:1011–1017.
10. deVoogt HJ, Smith PH, Pavone-Macaluso M, et al: Cardiovascular side effects of diethylstilbestrol, cyproterone acetate, medroxyprogesterone acetate and estramustine phosphate used for the treatment of advanced prostatic cancer: results from European Organization for Research on Treatment of Cancer trials 30761 and 30762. J Urol 1986; 135:303–307.
11. Henriksson P, Edhag O: Orchiectomy versus oestrogen for prostatic cancer: cardiovascular effects. Br Med J 1986; 293: 413–415.
12. Resnik MI: Hormonal therapy in prostatic carcinoma. Urology 1984; 24(Suppl 5):18.
13. Foss SD, Miller A: Treatment of advanced carcinoma of the prostate with estramustine phosphate. J Urol 1976; 115: 406–408.
14. Benson RC, Wear JB, Gill GM: Treatment of stage D hormone resistant carcinoma of the prostate with estramustine phosphate. J Urol 1979; 121:452.
15. Blackard CE, Byar DP, Jordan WP Jr: Veterans Administration Cooperative Urological Research Group: orchiectomy for advanced carcinoma: a re-evaluation. Urology 1973; 1: 553.
16. Vest SA, Frazier TH: Survival following castration for prostatic cancer. J Urol 1946; 56:97.
17. Leuprolide Study Group: Leuprolide versus diethylstilbestrol for metastatic prostate cancer. N Engl J Med 1984; 311: 1281–1286.
18. Klioze SS, Miller MR, Spiro TP: A randomized, comparative study of buserelin with DES/orchiectomy in the treatment of stage D2 prostatic cancer patients. Am J Clin Oncol 1988; 2(Suppl):S5176–S5182.
19. Wenderoth UK, Jacobi GH: Gonadotropin-releasing hormone analogues for palliation of carcinoma of the prostate. World J Urol 1988; 1:40.
20. Kahan A, Delrieu F, Amor B, et al: Disease flare induced by D-Trp6-LHRH analogue in patients with metastatic prostatic cancer. Lancet 1984; 1:971–972.
21. Waxman J, Man A, Hendry WF, et al: Importance of early tumor exacerbation in patients treated with long-acting analogues of gonadotropin releasing hormone for advanced prostatic cancer. Br Med J 1985; 291:1387–1388.
22. Geller J, Albert J, Yen SSC, et al: Medical castration of males with megestrol acetate and small doses of diethylstilbestrol. J Clin Endocrinol Metab 1981; 52:576–580.
23. von Eschenbach AC: Cancer of the prostate. Curr Prob Cancer 1981; 5:12.
24. Harper ME, Pike A, Peeling WB, Griffiths KG: Steroids of adrenal origin metabolized by human prostatic tissue both in vivo and in vitro. J Endocrinol 1984; 60:117–125.
25. Labrie F, Luthy I, Veilleux R, et al: New concepts on the androgen sensitivity of prostate cancer. Prog Clin Biol Res 1987; 243A:145–172.
26. Bracci U: Antiandrogens in the treatment of prostatic cancer. Eur Urol 1979; 5:303.
27. Schroeder FH, et al: Metastatic cancer of the prostate managed with buserelin versus buserelin plus cyproterone acetate. J Urol 1987; 137:912.
28. Pavone-Macaluso M, deVoogt HJ, Viggiano G, et al: Comparison of diethylstilbestrol, cyproterone acetate and medroxyprogesterone acetate in the treatment of advanced prostatic cancer: final analysis of a randomized phase III trial of the European organization for research on Treatment of Cancer Urologic Group. J Urol 1986; 136:624–631.
29. Neri R, Kassem N: Biological and clinical properties of antiandrogens. *In* Bresciani F, King RJB, Lippman ME, et al (eds): Progress in Cancer Research and Therapy, pp 507–518. New York, Raven Press, 1984.
30. Labrie F, Dupont A, Belanger A, et al: New approach in the treatment of prostate cancer: complete instead of partial withdrawal of androgens. Prostate 1983; 4:579–594.
31. Crawford ED, Eisenberger MA, McLeod et al: A controlled trial of leuprolide with and without flutamide in prostatic carcinoma. N Engl J Med 1989; 321:419–424.
32. Crawford ED, Smith JA Jr, Soloway MS, et al: Treatment of stage D2 prostate cancer with leuprolide and anandron compared to leuprolide and placebo. Recent advances in urologic cancers: diagnosis and treatment. Atlanta, GA, American Cancer Society, June 1990.
33. Janknegt RA, Abbou CC, Bartoletti R, et al: Orchiectomy and nilutamide or placebo as treatment of metastatic prostate cancer in multinational double-blind randomized trial. J Urol 1993; 149:77–83.
34. Denis LJ, Whelan P, Carneiro JL, et al: Goserelin acetate and flutamide versus bilateral orchiectomy: a phase III EORTC trial. Urology 1993; 42:119–130.
35. Beland G, Elhilali M, Fradet Y, et al: Total androgen ablation: Canadian experience. Urol Clin North Am 1991; 18: 75–82.

36. Lunglmayr G: A multicenter trial comparing the luteinizing hormone releasing hormone analog Zoladex, with Zoladex plus flutamide in the treatment of advanced prostate cancer. The International Prostate Cancer Study Group. Eur Urol 1990; 18(Suppl):28–29.
37. Byar DP, Corle DK: Hormone therapy for prostate cancer: results of the Veterans Administration Cooperative Urological Research Group Studies. NCL Monogr 1988; 7:165–170.
38. Kelly K, Scher HI: Prostate specific antigen decline after antiandrogen withdrawal: the flutamide withdrawal syndrome. J Urol 1993; 149:607–609.
39. Scher HI, Kelly WK: Flutamide withdrawal syndrome: its impact on clinical trials in hormone-refractory prostate cancer. J Clin Oncol 1993; 11:1566–1572.
40. Dupont A, Gomez JL, Cusan L, et al: Response to flutamide withdrawal in advanced prostate cancer in progression under combination therapy. J Urol 1993; 150:908–913.
41. Sartor O, Cooper M, Weinberger M, et al: Surprising activity of flutamide withdrawal, when combined with aminoglutethimide, in treatment of "hormone-refractory" prostate cancer. J Natl Cancer Inst 1994; 86:222–227.
42. Akakura K, Bruchovsky N, Goldenberg SL, et al: Effects of intermittent androgen suppression of androgen-dependent tumors. Cancer 1993; 71:2782.
43. Klotz LH, Herr HW, Morse MJ, Whitmore WF Jr: Intermittent endocrine therapy for advanced prostate cancer. Cancer 1986; 58:2546.
44. Vahlensieck W, Wegner G, Lehmann HD, et al: Comparison between continuous and intermittent administration of extracyt in the treatment of carcinoma of the prostate. Urol Res 1985; 13:209.
45. Eisenberger MA: Chemotherapy in prostate cancer. *In* Crawford ED, Das S (eds): Current Genitourinary Cancer Surgery, pp 507–518. Philadelphia, Lea & Febiger, 1990.
46. Yagoda A, Petrylak D: Cytotoxic chemotherapy for advanced-resistant prostate cancer. Cancer 1993; 71:1098–1109.
47. Murphy GP, Beckely S, Brandy MF, et al: Treatment of newly diagnosed metastatic prostate cancer patients with chemotherapy agents in combination with hormones versus hormones alone. Cancer 1988; 51:1264–1272.
48. LaRocca RV, Cooper MR, Uhrich M, et al: Use of suramin in treatment of prostatic carcinoma refractory to conventional hormonal manipulation. Urol Clin North Am 1991; 18(1):123.
49. Tong D, Gillick L, Henrickson FR: The palliation of symptomatic osseous metastases: final results of the study by Radiation Therapy Oncology Group. Cancer 1982; 50:893–899.
50. Poulter CA, Cosmatos D, Rubin P, et al: A report of 8206: a phase III study of whether the addition of a single dose hemibody irradiation to standard fractionated local field irradiation is more effective than local field radiation alone in the treatment of symptomatic osseous metastases. Int J Radiat Oncol Biol Phys 1992; 23:207–214.
51. Breen SL, Powe JE, Porter AT: Dose estimation in strontium-89 radiotherapy of metastatic prostatic carcinoma. J Nucl Med 1992; 33:1316–1323.
52. Porter AT, McEwan AJB, Powe JE, et al: Results of a randomized phase III trial to evaluate the efficacy of strontium-89 adjuvant to local field external beam irradiation in the management of endocrine resistant metastatic prostate cancer. Int J Radiat Oncol Biol Phys 1993; 25:805–813.
53. Porter AT, Vaishampayan N: Strontium-89 in metastatic prostate cancer. Urol Symp 1994; 44:6A.
54. Sharife R, Soloway M, and the Leuprolide Study Group: Clinical study of leuprolide depot formulation in the treatment of advanced prostate cancer. J Urol 1990; 143: 68–71.
55. Cooper EH, Armitage TG, Robinson MRG, et al: Prostatic specific antigen and the prediction of prognosis in metastatic prostatic cancer. Cancer 1990; 20:749–756.
56. Petros JA, Andriole GL: Serum PSA after antiandrogen therapy. Urol Clin North Am 1993; 20:749–756.
57. Arai Y, Yoshiki T, Yoshida O: Prognostic significance of prostate specific antigen in endocrine treatment for prostatic cancer. J Urol 1990; 144:1415–1419.
58. Miller JI, Ahmann FR, Drach GW, et al: The clinical usefulness of serum prostate specific antigen after hormonal therapy of metastatic prostate cancer. J Urol 1992; 147: 956–961.
59. Mulders PFA, Del Moral PF, Theeuwes AGM, et al: Value of biochemical markers in the management of disseminated prostatic cancer. Eur Urol 1992; 21:2–5.
60. Benson MC, Ring K, Giella J: Flow cytometry in carcinoma of the prostate. Urol Clin North Am 1988; 17:885–891.
61. Winkler HZ, Rainwater LM, Myers RP, et al: Stage D1 prostatic adenocarcinoma: significance of nuclear DNA ploidy patterns studies by flow cytometry. Mayo Clin Proc 1988; 63:103–112.

29

BILATERAL PELVIC LYMPHADENECTOMY AND ANATOMICAL RADICAL RETROPUBIC PROSTATECTOMY

CHERYL T. LEE, M.D., JEROME P. RICHIE, M.D.,
and JOSEPH E. OESTERLING, M.D.

In 1996, an estimated 317,100 new cases of prostate cancer will be diagnosed in the United States.[1] This represents 41% of all newly diagnosed cancers in men. An estimated 41,400 patients with prostate cancer will die this year; only lung cancer has a higher mortality rate (~94,400).[1] At the age of 50 years, a man has a 42% chance of developing prostate cancer, and a 2.9% chance of dying from his disease.[2] Clearly, cancer of the prostate is an important disease process that deserves the attention of clinicians and researchers alike.

The treatment of prostate cancer continues to be controversial. Standard options for clinically localized disease include radical surgical therapy, radiation therapy, and watchful waiting. Over the past 15 years, advances in radical prostate surgery, most notably Walsh's[3] description of anatomic radical retropublic prostatectomy, have allowed the evolution of this procedure from a once feared and morbid treatment to a safe, cost-effective therapy with few untoward effects. In this chapter, the indications, surgical technique, and long-term results of bilateral pelvic lymphadenectomy and radical retropublic prostatectomy are discussed.

BILATERAL PELVIC LYMPHADENECTOMY

Accurate staging of prostate cancer has been difficult using physical examination, radiographic imaging, and/or biochemical studies. It is well established that lymphatic spread of prostate cancer occurs most commonly via the obturator lymph nodes, followed by the presacral, presciatic, and internal and external iliac nodes.[4] Since modern imaging techniques are poor detectors of pelvic lymph node metastases,[5,6] pelvic lymphadenectomy has been used for staging clinically localized prostate cancer via direct histologic evaluation of regional lymph nodes. As such, open pelvic lymph node dissection (PLND) is the standard by which all other studies must be judged. However, in 1996, with the aid of preoperative clinical variables, the practicing urologist can be selective in determining which patients should undergo a pelvic lymph node dissection.

Indications

Danella and coworkers[7] have found that the incidence of lymphatic metastases in patients with clinically localized prostate cancer is only 5.7%. Thus, Bluestein and colleagues[8] have established a reasonable means of predicting which patients are unlikely to have lymph node involvement and can avoid undergoing a staging bilateral pelvic lymphadenectomy. In a retrospective study, these researchers examined 1632 patients, aged 38 to 83 years (mean 66 years), who had localized prostate cancer and underwent a bilateral pelvic lymphadenectomy. None of these men had received preoperative radiation therapy or androgen-deprivation therapy. Univariate logistic regression models were used to predict the probability of positive pelvic lymph nodes as a function of patient age, prior transurethral resection of the prostate (TURP), serum prostate-specific antigen (PSA), primary Gleason grade, and local clinical stage. Neither patient age nor TURP was significant in predicting positive pelvic lymph nodes. Gleason grade, serum PSA level, and clinical stage all had a positive correlation with the presence of pelvic lymph node metastases ($p < .001$ for each).

Using multivariate logistic regression to analyze all three variables, Bluestein and coworkers were able to predict the probability of a patient having positive pelvic lymph nodes (Table 29–1) on the basis of serum PSA, primary Gleason grade, and local clinical stage. When the probability of positive pelvic lymph nodes is less than 3% according to serum PSA, stage, and grade, the authors suggest that a staging bilateral pelvic lymphadenectomy is not necessary. If this recommendation were applied to their patient population, 406 (25%) patients would not have undergone a bilateral pelvic lymphadenectomy. Among these 406 patients, 3 men actually had positive lymph nodes, representing a false-negative rate of less than 1%. These results suggest that 25% of patients with newly diagnosed prostate cancer may be spared a pelvic lymph node dissection when PSA is used in combination with tumor grade and clinical stage to predict lymph node involvement.

In support of these results, in a retrospective study of 945 men, Kleer and colleagues[9] found PSA to be the best single predictor of positive lymph node status. By including local clinical stage, as determined by digital rectal examination (DRE), and tumor grade, as determined from the biopsy specimen, there was a significant enhancement of the predictive power of PSA. Bishoff and colleagues[10] were also able to omit PLND in properly selected patients using PSA and clinical stage in combination with Gleason grade from the preoperative prostate biopsy. Likewise, Bangma and associates[11] used PSA in combination with the Anderson grade of the preoperative prostate biopsy to predict negative lymph node status with 95% certainty.

TABLE 29–1. COMBINATIONS OF LOCAL CLINICAL STAGE, PRIMARY GLEASON GRADE, AND SERUM PSA TO YIELD A FALSE-NEGATIVE RATE OF 3% FOR POSITIVE LYMPH NODES*

Local Clinical Stage	Primary Gleason Grade	Serum PSA† (ng/ml)
T1a–T2b	1 and 2	17.1
(A1–B1)	3	8.0
	4 and 5	4.2
T2c (B2)	1 and 2	4.1
	3	2.0
	4 and 5	1.0
T3a (C1)	1 and 2	1.4
	3	0.7
	4 and 5	0.3

*From Bluestein D, Bostwick D, Bergstralh E, Oesterling J: Eliminating the need for bilateral pelvic lymphadenectomy in select patients with prostate cancer. J Urol 1994; 151:1315–1320, with permission.

†Patients with lower serum PSA values have a false-negative rate of less than 3%.

The above studies support the concept of selective performance of PLND. Using preoperative clinical variables and accepting a 3% false-negative rate, Table 29–1 can be utilized to make specific recommendations to the practicing urologist. For a patient with a clinical stage T1a–T2b cancer, a PLND is not indicated if (1) the primary Gleason grade is 1 or 2 and the PSA is less than 17.1 ng/ml; (2) the primary Gleason grade is 3 and the PSA is less than 8 ng/ml; or (3) the primary Gleason grade is 4 or 5 and the PSA is less than 4.2 ng/ml. If the patient has a clinical stage T2c cancer, a PLND should not be performed if (1) the primary Gleason grade is 1 or 2 and the PSA is less than 4.0 ng/ml; (2) the primary Gleason grade is 3 and the PSA level is less than 2.0 ng/ml; or (3) the primary Gleason grade is 4 or 5 and the PSA is less than 1.0 ng/ml. If a patient is clinically suspected of having capsular penetration (clinical stage T3a), either by examination, transrectal ultrasound, or by prostatic biopsy, the PLND can be avoided if (1) the primary Gleason grade is 1 or 2 and the PSA is less than 1.4 ng/ml; (2) the primary Gleason grade is 3 and the PSA is less than 0.7 ng/ml; or (3) the primary Gleason grade is 4 or 5 and the PSA is less than 0.3 ng/ml. These data only apply to men who have not received adjuvant androgen deprivation therapy or radiation therapy. Nevertheless, the use of preoperative clinical variables to eliminate PLND has major implications in the prevention of patient morbidity from lymphadenectomy and in decreasing health care dollar expenditure; the mean total cost of an open pelvic lymphadenectomy is $8185 and that of a laparoscopic dissection is $9449.[12] Men not meeting the criteria stated above need to undergo a staging bilateral pelvic lymphadenectomy via one of three approaches: (1) open lymphadenectomy, (2) minilaparotomy, or (3) laparoscopic lymph node dissection.

Modified Pelvic Lymph Node Dissection

After making the decision to proceed with a PLND, the surgeon must decide which of three PLND techniques will be utilized. The surgeon and patient discuss the risks and benefits of each procedure and make a determination based on patient habitus, patient clinical situation, patient lifestyle, and the surgeon's familiarity and expertise with the different techniques.

Open Pelvic Lymph Node Dissection

Modified PLND has been shown[13] to be as effective in staging accuracy as complete pelvic lymphadenectomy and is associated with less morbidity. In addition, Paulson[14] has shown that an increase in lymph node dissection (beyond the modified borders) does not increase the rate of identifica-

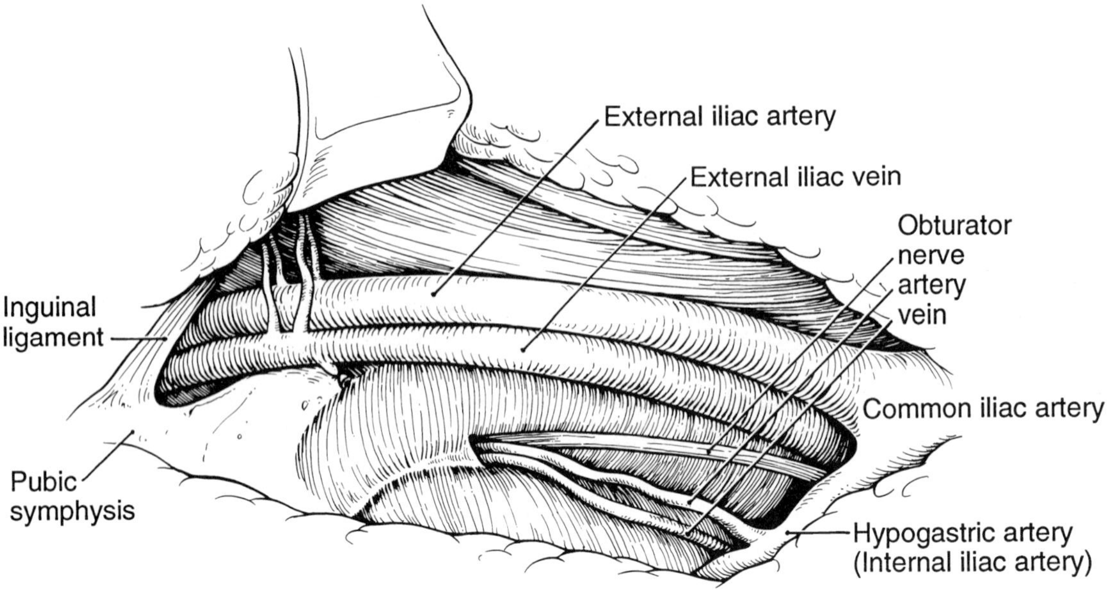
External iliac artery
External iliac vein
Obturator
nerve
artery
vein
Inguinal
ligament
Common iliac artery
Pubic
symphysis
Hypogastric artery
(Internal iliac artery)

FIGURE 29–1. View of the lateral pelvis. Borders of the modified template for pelvic lymphadenectomy.

tion of node-positive disease. The borders of the true modified template dissection, as discussed by Brendler et al.,[15] include the external iliac vein laterally, the hypogastric artery posteriorly, the inguinal ligament distally, and the bifurcation of the common iliac artery proximally (Fig. 29–1).

Technique

Prior to open PLND, careful physical examination of the patient's lower extremities is used to detect deep venous thrombosis/occlusion, phlebitis, and/or edema. The patient is placed in a supine position. The table is flexed and placed in 20 degrees of Trendelenburg position. The urethra is catheterized, and a vertical, midline abdominal incision is made from the infraumbilical area to the pubic symphysis. After separation of the rectus abdominis muscles in the midline and division of the transversalis fascia, blunt dissection is used to enter the prevesical space. The second and third digits are used to develop the perivesical space between the bladder and the iliac vessels.

A self-retaining retractor with a malleable blade (Balfour retractor) is used to retract the abdominal wall laterally and the peritoneal contents cephalad. An additional hand-held retractor may be necessary for medial bladder retraction. The fibrofatty tissue overlying the external iliac vein is sharply divided to skeletonize the vein. This dissection is continued caudally to the pelvic surface to allow resection of the medial retrocrural lymph node of Cloquet. The circumflex iliac vein is the true caudal limit. The external iliac vein is then skeletonized at its cephalad extent, where it enters the common iliac vein. The vein is skeletonized inferiorly, watching for aberrant veins. The nodal package is retracted medially, using blunt and sharp dissection. With this maneuver, the obturator nerve is exposed at the inferior aspect of the obturator fossa (Fig. 29–2). A ring or vascular forceps can be used to secure the obturator nodal tissue. The caudal attachments should be ligated (using clips or suture) and divided, again allowing resection of the node of Cloquet with the specimen.

The posterior dissection of the nodal package extends to the hypogastric artery, while subsequent cephalad extension is to the branching of the common iliac vessels. During this dissection, it may become necessary to ligate and divide the obturator artery and vein; usually, this can be avoided, as the structures reside inferior to the obturator nerve. All lymphatics should be clipped to avoid complicating lymphoceles. With progressive dissection cephalad to the iliac bifurcation, the nodal package will become progressively narrow and can be easily controlled with a surgical clip, divided, and removed (Fig. 29–3). The package is inspected for gross metastatic disease, and a Davol drain is placed within each obturator fossa and left in place until drainage is less than 75 ml for 24 hours.

Results and Complications

As reported by Bratt et al.,[16] complications of open PLND include wound infection (5.1%), hematoma or lymphocele (4.5%), venous thrombosis (1.9%), and myocardial infarction (0.6%). Their overall complication rate was 12%. McDowell et al.[17] reported a slightly higher overall complication rate of 19.4%, consisting of wound infection (5.1%), lymphocele (4.6%), prolonged ileus (3.7%), thromboembolic events (1.8%), pneumonia (0.9%), pelvic hematoma (0.9%), and lymphedema (0.5%). Others[18] have noted prolonged lymph leakage and a seven times greater formation of lymphoceles in

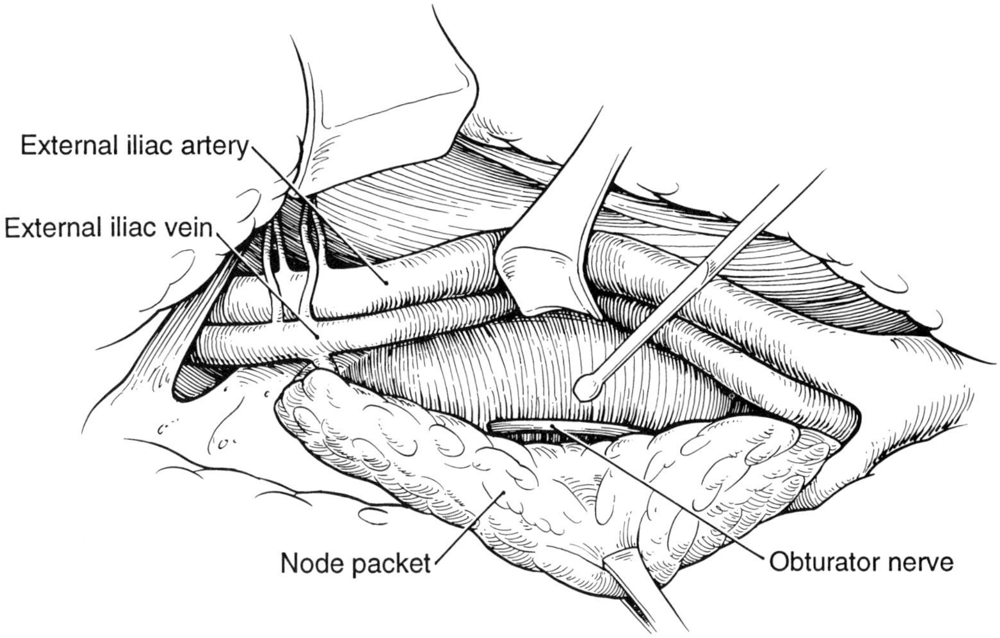
External iliac artery
External iliac vein
Node packet
Obturator nerve

FIGURE 29–2. View of the obturator fossa. Retraction of the obturator node packet, exposing the obturator nerve.

those patients undergoing staging PLND in conjunction with low-dose subcutaneous heparin sodium (5000 units every 12 hours for 7 days, starting 2 hours before surgery) for thromboembolic prophylaxis.

The Minilaparotomy for Pelvic Lymph Node Dissection

Indications

The minilaparotomy is indicated for most patients undergoing PLND, whether preceding a radical retropubic prostatectomy, a radical perineal prostatectomy, definitive radiation therapy, or cryosurgical ablation of the prostate. This procedure should be avoided in obese patients and in men with multiple previous pelvic surgeries.

Technique

The minilaparotomy staging pelvic lymphadenectomy (minilap) offers urologists a minimally invasive, open approach to the pelvic lymph nodes. This procedure, initially described by Steiner and Marshall,[19] is similar to the modified open pelvic lymphadenectomy in that it offers complete pelvic node excision under direct vision. However, it is performed through a 5- or 6-cm lower midline, abdominal incision (Fig. 29–4), instead of a 20-cm incision.

The procedure[19] begins with the patient placed in the supine position and the umbilicus centered over the kidney rest. The table is hyperextended to increase the space between the umbilicus and pubic symphysis. The urethra is catheterized as described above. A midline 5- or 6-cm incision is made 2 cm from the superior aspect of the pubic symphysis. Entrance is gained to the prevesical space as previously described. Richardson retractors are utilized to retract the incision laterally, and allow mobilization of the peritoneum off the external iliac vessels to the level of the common iliac arteries. In performing this maneuver, the surgeon may hook the vas deferens and mobilize it in a cephalad direction, providing improved visualization of the common iliac vessels. Steiner and Marshall utilize the Omni tract retractor to provide exposure of the obturator fossa. Alternatively, the surgeon may utilize a medium Richardson retractor for lateral retraction of the incision; a hand-held "sweetheart" retractor for medial retraction of the bladder; and a Deaver retractor for cephalad retraction of the vas deferens and peritoneum. Lateral table rotation facilitates further exposure and lymph node excision, as described above for the modified open pelvic lymphadenectomy.

Results

Like laparoscopic node excision, the minilap offers rapid postoperative recuperation and a shorter hospitalization because of the limited abdominal incision.[20] In addition, the minilap, like the modified open node dissection, requires less operative time, less disposable instrument usage, and less intraoperative cost than the laparoscopic PLND.[20] Mean operative time for the minilap procedure ranges from 32 to 90 minutes versus 150 to 190 minutes for the laparoscopic operation.[19,20] Perrotti et al.[20] reported mean numbers of lymph nodes retrieved from open PLND versus laparoscopic

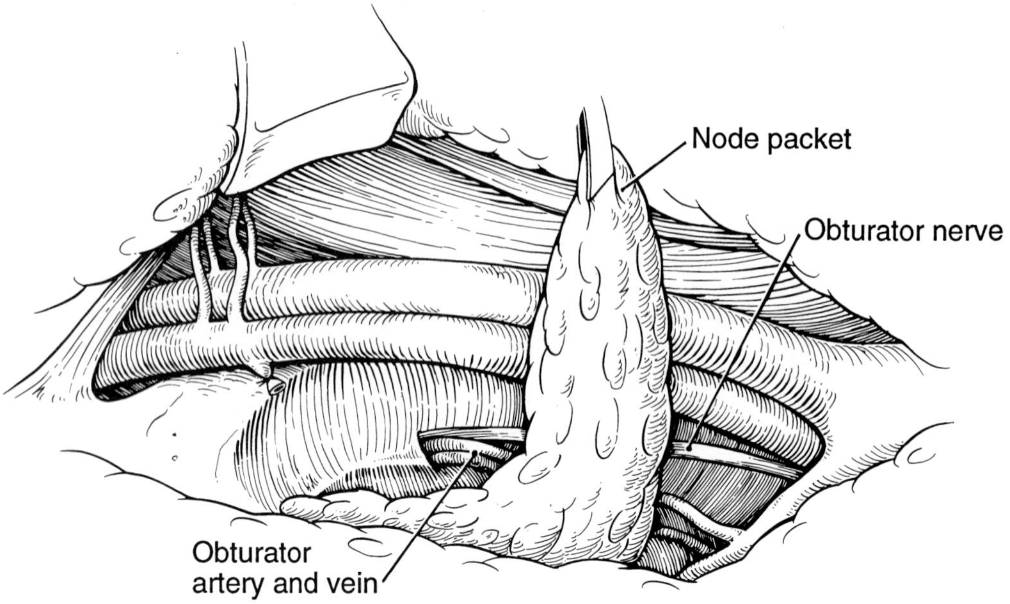
Node packet
Obturator nerve
Obturator
artery and vein

FIGURE 29–3. View of the obturator fossa. Removal of the obturator node packet.

PLND versus minilaparotomy to be 12, 9, and 9, respectively (the differences were not statistically significant).

Complications

Steiner[19] reported a 0% complication rate in those patients undergoing minilap solely. Perotti[20] reported two minilap complications. One patient had poorly characterized abdominal pain following the procedure, and another had a superficial skin separation after skin staple removal. This represented an overall 1% complication rate.

Cost Analysis

Perrotti et al.[20] provided a financial analysis of open PLND versus laparoscopic PLND versus minilaparotomy. Total costs for their institution were \$4262, \$4245, and \$2516, respectively. Factors that increased procedure costs were hospital stay (for modified open PLND) and intraoperative time (for laparoscopic PLND). This group demonstrated the minilap to be a cost-effective procedure with limited morbidity.

Laparoscopic Pelvic Lymph Node Dissection

Indications

Indications for laparoscopic (lap) PLND have not been clearly established. There is certainly utility in its use in staging prior to definitive radiation therapy. As well, its use has been reported after radiation therapy as a staging modality prior to salvage radical prostatectomy.[21] It is a reasonable option for lymph node sampling in the patient undergoing radical perineal prostatectomy. It also seems that it would be advantageous in patients with a high likelihood of nodal metastases (i.e., those with bulky tumor burden, poorly differentiated histology, and a markedly elevated serum PSA level). However, these latter indications are not well defined and require further study.

Certain patient characteristics increase the technical difficulty of laparoscopic surgery and therefore increase the risk of complications. As such, laparoscopic surgery should be avoided in the patient with obesity, previous pelvic or abdominal surgery, a large abdominal mass or aneurysm, or a history of hypercarbia (as in the patient with chronic ob-

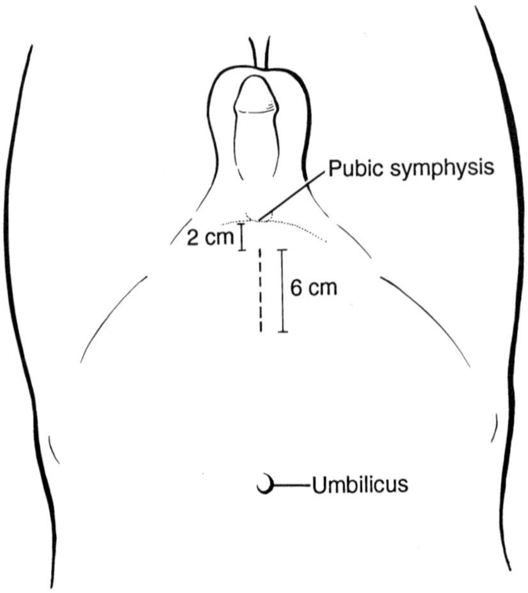
Pubic symphysis
2 cm
6 cm
Umbilicus

FIGURE 29–4. Surgical incision for the minilaparotomy pelvic lymph node dissection.

structive pulmonary disease). Other patient factors that preclude the performance of laparoscopic surgery include a history of peritonitis, hypotension, uncorrected coagulopathy, extensive adhesions, and dilated loops of intestine.

Technique

Laparoscopic PLND for prostate cancer staging has been performed since 1991,[22] and its popularity continues to grow. In performing this procedure, the patient should have a nasogastric tube and a urethral catheter placed to decompress the stomach and the bladder, respectively. The Trendelenburg position facilitates cephalad displacement of the intestines.

The technique of lap PLND[23] begins with a small umbilical incision, through which a Verres needle or Hasson cannula is placed. A pneumoperitoneum of 12 to 15 mm Hg is established using carbon dioxide. A trocar is introduced transumbilically, and a 10- or 11-mm port is established through which the camera lens is passed. The peritoneal cavity is inspected. Two additional trocars are then placed under direct visualization, one third the distance from the umbilicus to the iliac crest bilaterally (Fig. 29–5). Additional trocars can be placed if needed for introduction of supplementary scissors, cautery, suction, grasping, and dissecting instruments.

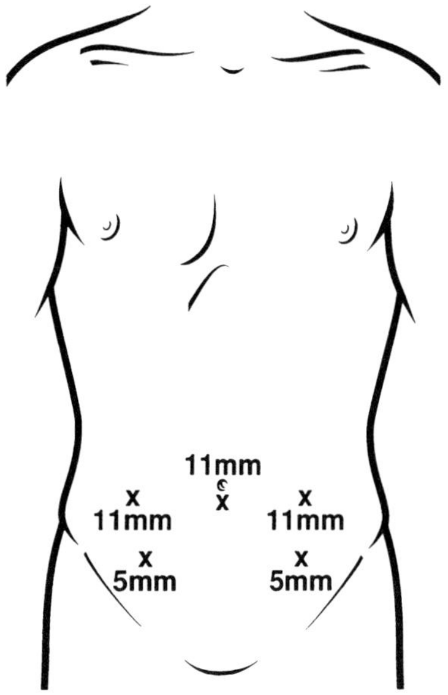
11mm
x
x
x
11mm
11mm
x
x
5mm
5mm

FIGURE 29–5. Schematic illustration of preferred trocar placement for laparoscopic PLND. (From Parro RD, Andrus CH, Boullier JA: Staging laparoscopic pelvic lymph node dissection: comparison of results with open pelvic lymphadenectomy. J Urol 1992; 147:875, with permission.)

After obtaining access, pertinent pelvic landmarks can be visualized, including the internal ring and the medial umbilical ligaments (Fig. 29–6). The external iliac vessels may be obscured by the overlying peritoneum but may be identified by their pulsations. Adhesions may require sharp incision. The pelvis is entered via a peritonectomy lateral to the umbilical ligament, and both medial and cephalad to the internal ring. The limits of dissection consist of the area delineated by the pubic rami distally, the bifurcation of the common iliac artery proximally, the external iliac artery laterally, and the umbilical ligament medially.

Blunt dissection is initiated at the pubis and is carried lateral and proximal to clear fibrofatty tissue overlying the external iliac veins. The dissection is continued proximally with node-bearing tissue (from the obturator fossa) removed using blunt and sharp maneuvers. This technique is performed

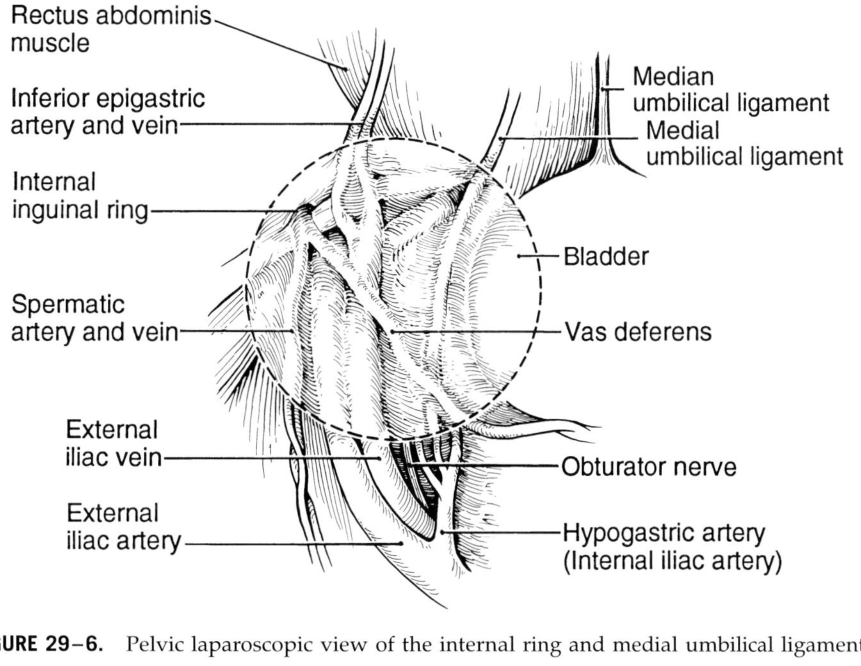
Rectus abdominis muscle
Inferior epigastric artery and vein
Internal inguinal ring
Spermatic artery and vein
External iliac vein
External iliac artery
Median umbilical ligament
Medial umbilical ligament
Bladder
Vas deferens
Obturator nerve
Hypogastric artery (Internal iliac artery)

FIGURE 29–6. Pelvic laparoscopic view of the internal ring and medial umbilical ligaments.

bilaterally. The specimens are removed using the corresponding 11-mm trocar. The areas of dissection are irrigated and examined for hemostasis, and the peritoneotomy is left open to reduce the occurrence of symptomatic lymphoceles. The pneumoperitoneum is then deflated, and the ports are removed.

There is a steep learning curve involved with the performance of laparoscopic PLND, as evidenced by the complication rates of Lang and colleagues.[24] They noted a 14% early complication rate in their first 50 patients undergoing laparoscopic PLND for genitourinary malignancy staging, in comparison to a 4% early complication rate in their next 50 patients.

Results

Laparoscopic lymphadenectomy is equivalent to the modified open PLND from a staging standpoint and offers the benefit of decreased morbidity and reduced hospital stay as well as a shorter convalescence period.[25] Additionally, the total number of lymph nodes retrieved by bilateral lap PLND is reported[25] to be 10 to 11.3, similar to open PLND. Indeed, its greatest utility is in sparing patients an open surgical procedure while accurately assessing lymph node involvement.

Complications

Complications of laparoscopic PLND are not inconsequential. Complications are noted to be 14 to 34% by laparoscopists, though these figures tend to improve with additional experience.[26–28] Kavoussi et al.[26] reported an overall 15% complication rate, with 3% related to vascular injury, 2% to viscus injury, 2.7% to genitourinary factors (bladder retention and scrotal swelling), 1.9% to intestinal obstruction, 1.3% to deep venous thrombosis, 1.3% to wound-related problems, 1.3% to lymphedema, 0.5% to anesthetic complications, and 0.5% to obturator nerve palsy. In another series, Chow et al.[27] described an overall 14% complication rate, with 2.4% related to small intestinal obstruction due to herniation of intestine through the trocar site in the abdominal wall, 2.4% to ureteral laceration, 4.7% to postoperative mesenteric edema, 1.2% to hematoma in the abdominal wall, 1.2% to infected retroperitoneal hematoma, 1.2% to sigmoid colon perforation, and 1.2% to lymphoceles. Others[28] have reported overall complication rates of 34%, predominantly involving intraoperative hypercarbia (16%), subcutaneous emphysema (12.5%), and shoulder tip pain (5.9%) related to incomplete deflation of pneumoperitoneum.

Cost Analysis

Troxel and Winfield[29] performed a financial analysis of open versus laparoscopic PLND. They found preoperative costs for both procedures to be similar. Intraoperative costs were significantly greater for laparoscopic dissection, primarily related to the prolonged operative time and use of disposable materials. Postoperative costs were significantly greater for the open technique, primarily related to prolonged hospital time. At their institution, the overall cost for laparoscopic PLND was $10,068 as opposed to $8723 for open PLND. This analysis did not take into account wages lost during the extended convalescent period associated with the open PLND. The authors felt the additional cost of laparoscopic dissection would likely be offset by this factor.

Accuracy of Frozen Lymph Node Pathologic Evaluation

Frozen section lymph node analysis in pelvic lymphadenectomy has been performed, often just prior to radical prostatectomy, in order to determine the patient's true nodal status. Epstein and colleagues[30] examined their experience with 310 pelvic lymphadenectomy specimens, comparing frozen and permanent sections. They showed false-negative rates of 27.5% for patients with grossly positive nodes and 32.3% for men with microscopic involvement of lymph nodes. Hermanson and Whitmore[31] reviewed six studies[30,32–36] directed at determining the accuracy of frozen section analysis. False-negative rates for this procedure ranged between 19 and 41%. Bearing these results in mind, the current authors do not perform frozen section analysis of all pelvic lymph node specimens. However, routine frozen section analysis is warranted in the patient at higher risk for lymph node metastases (men with serum PSA levels in excess of 20 ng/ml and Gleason scores of 8 to 10).

Summary

Bilateral pelvic lymph node dissection is the "gold standard" staging test for determining lymph node status in the patient with newly diagnosed prostate cancer. With the use of certain preoperative clinical variables, including serum PSA, clinical stage, and Gleason grade, lymph node status can be predicted accurately in many patients, thereby eliminating the morbidity and cost of lymph node excision. If a lymph node dissection is deemed necessary, there are three techniques to perform this procedure: open lymph node dissection, the minilaparotomy for open lymph node dissection, and laparoscopic lymph node dissection. All three procedures provide similar node retrieval, staging accuracy, and complication rates when performed by experienced surgeons. Open PLND has a shorter operative time than the laparoscopic approach, but a longer convalescent period. The minilap has a shorter operative time than the laparoscopic approach, and a similar hospital stay and convalescent period. The laparoscopic technique is more costly than the open procedures, but the shorter convalescent period and quicker return to work may offset these differences. Overall, the decision to proceed with one approach over the others must be made by the individual physician and patient working together as a team. This decision must take patient factors and physician skill into account.

ANATOMIC RADICAL RETROPUBIC PROSTATECTOMY

History of Prostatectomy

In 1904, Hugh Hampton Young first performed radical surgery of the prostate in an attempt at complete cancer cure. Billroth (1867), Leisrink (1882), Zuckerland (1889), Proust and Albaran (1901), and Goodfellow (1891) had all performed prostate surgery, but not in the sense of removal of the entire prostate (with its capsule and fascial coverings), a cuff of the bladder, and both seminal vesicles in one specimen, as reported by Young in 1905.[37] Since that time, other surgeons have made revisions of his technique, as outlined in the classic article on radical perineal prostatectomy for cancer control by Young.[38] Belt et al.[39] continued to improve this technique, as described in their article supporting an anatomic approach to perineal prostatectomy. The retropubic approach to prostatectomy came much later.

Retropubic prostatectomy was initially described by van Stockum in 1908.[40] Millin[41] later popularized this extravesical technique for prostatic obstruction in 1945, and, in collaboration with Memmelaar in 1949,[42] described the radical retropubic prostatectomy (RRP) for the treatment of cancer of the prostate. This technique was further refined approximately 15 years ago with the meticulous anatomic dissections of Walsh, delineating the autonomic innervation of the corpora cavernosa and the venous drainage of the penis in the area of the prostate gland.[3]

Prostate Anatomy

In performing radical prostatic surgery, the surgeon's knowledge of the prostate and pelvic floor anatomy is essential. The arterial supply (Fig. 29–7) of the prostate originates from the inferior vesical artery. This artery terminates into urethral and capsular branches, which supply the prostate directly. The capsular vessels travel in the lateral pelvic fascia along with the cavernous nerves to form the neurovascular bundle (NVB).

The venous drainage of the penis and prostate (Fig. 29–8) is highly variable, emptying into Santorini's plexus. In 1979, Walsh and Reiner[43] detailed the course of these veins. From their descriptions, it has been shown that a multitude of penile sinuses coalesce to form the deep dorsal vein, which exits the penile hilum anterior to the membranous urethra and the apex of the prostate. At this level it divides into a superficial branch, which travels between the puboprostatic ligaments, and right and

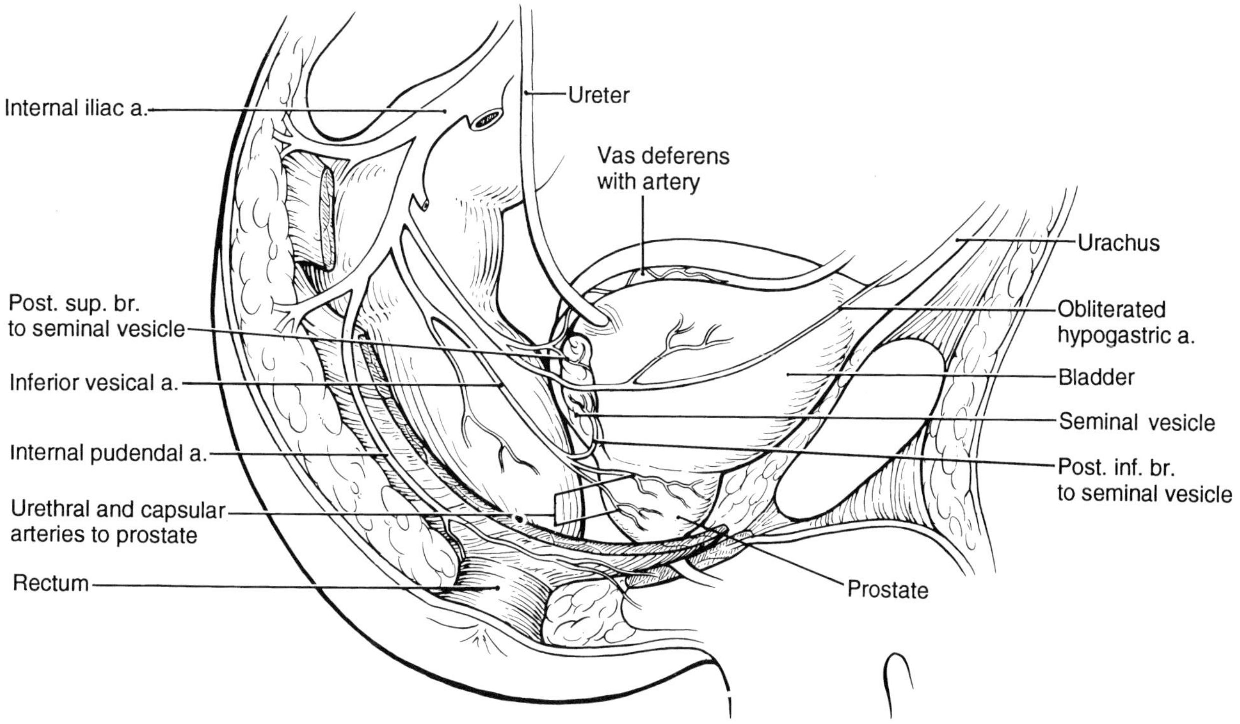
Internal iliac a.
Ureter
Vas deferens
with artery
Urachus
Post. sup. br.
to seminal vesicle
Obliterated
hypogastric a.
Inferior vesical a.
Bladder
Seminal vesicle
Internal pudendal a.
Post. inf. br.
to seminal vesicle
Urethral and capsular
arteries to prostate
Rectum
Prostate

FIGURE 29–7. Sagittal view of the pelvis demonstrating the arterial supply to the prostate.

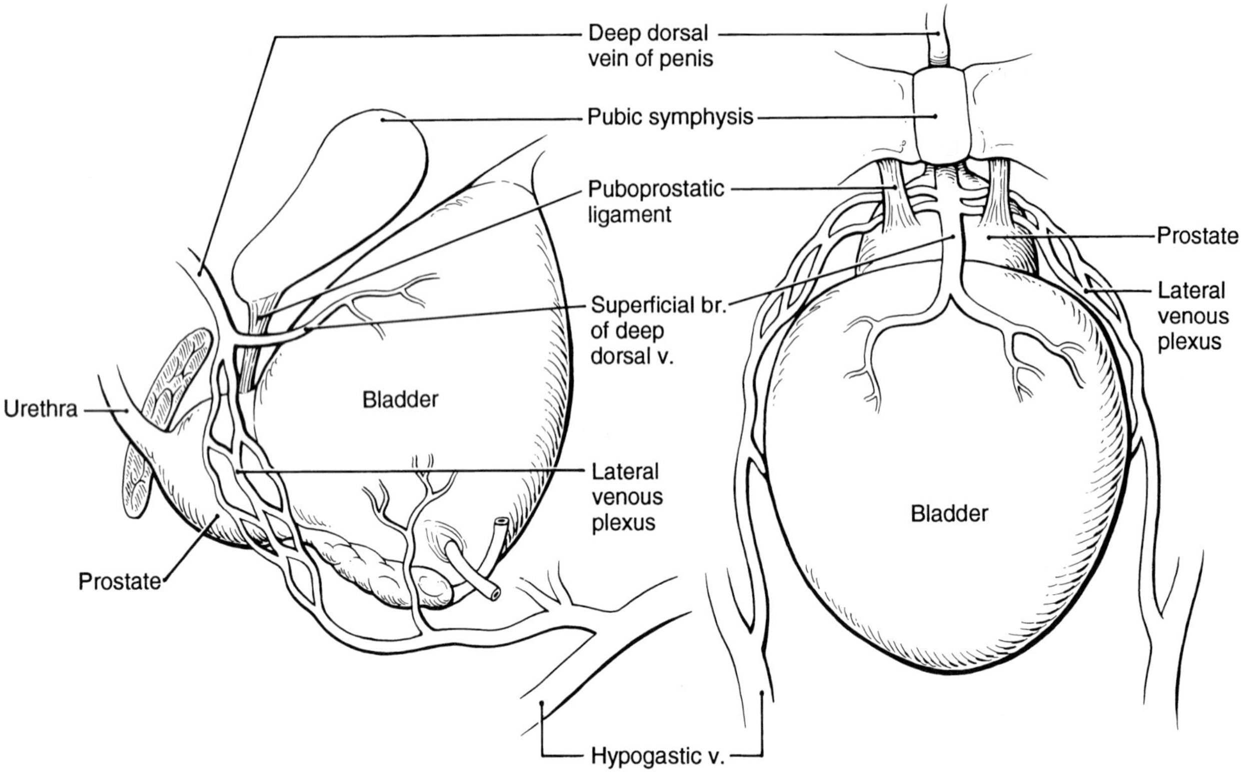
Deep dorsal vein of penis
Pubic symphysis
Puboprostatic ligament
Superficial br. of deep dorsal v.
Bladder
Urethra
Lateral venous plexus
Prostate
Hypogastic v.
Prostate
Lateral venous plexus
Bladder

FIGURE 29–8. Sagittal (*left*) and anterior (*right*) views of the pelvis demonstrating the venous drainage of the prostate.

left tributaries, which course posterolaterally draining into the internal iliac vein. Control of these veins is essential in obtaining the necessary bloodless exposure to perform an anatomic radical retropubic prostatectomy, while preserving urinary continence and erectile function.

The nerve supply to the prostate is outlined in Figure 29–9. Sympathetic nerve fibers from T11–L12 give rise to the sympathetic nerve chain forming the hypogastric nerve. Parasympathetic fibers from S2–S4 form the pelvic nerve, which innervates the prostate. The hypogastric and pelvic nerves enter the pelvic plexus and will give rise to the cavernous nerves, which are necessary for erectile function.[44]

Indications for Anatomic Radical Retropubic Prostatectomy

Radical prostate surgery is indicated in the patient with organ-confined prostate cancer, who has a life expectancy of 10 years or more. In determining which patients truly have organ-confined disease, the urologist can utilize preoperative local clinical stage, Gleason grade, and the serum PSA concentration. The use of nomograms that combine these three variables are extremely useful. Table 29–2 depicts one such nomogram for the prediction of final pathologic stage. There are no absolute values for Gleason grade or PSA that will preclude surgical therapy, as long as the patient is felt to have clinically localized disease. However, the urologist must confer with the patient and openly discuss the likelihood of having true organ-confined cancer. As the tumor grade and serum PSA concentration increase, the probability of having curable disease diminishes.

Preoperative Patient Preparation

Prior to surgery, the patient must undergo a thorough medical evaluation. If abnormal conditions are discovered, the patient is further evaluated by the appropriate subspecialist. After medical clearance has been obtained, the patient begins a process of thorough education regarding radical prostatectomy, the hospital stay, and expectations after discharge. The patient views a videotape describing (1) admission protocol, (2) anesthesia options, (3) operating room and recovery room practices, (4) routine inpatient care from nurses and physicians, and (5) the discharge protocol. In addition, the patient is instructed on incentive spirometry, which will reduce the risk of atelectasis and pneumonia postoperatively. In addition, the patient will begin perineal exercises to strengthen the external urinary sphincter. These exercises involve intermittent interruption of the urinary stream during micturition. These exercises are resumed 3 weeks postopera-

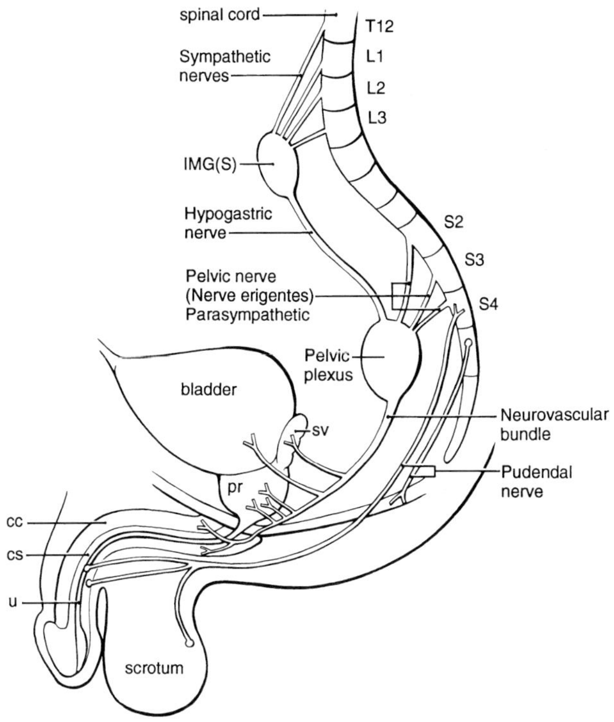
spinal cord
Sympathetic nerves
T12
L1
L2
L3
IMG(S)
Hypogastric nerve
S2
S3
Pelvic nerve (Nerve erigentes) Parasympathetic
S4
Pelvic plexus
bladder
sv
Neurovascular bundle
Pudendal nerve
pr
cc
cs
u
scrotum

FIGURE 29–9. Schematic illustration demonstrating autonomic innervation of the male lower urinary tract.

tively upon removal of the urethral catheter. Finally, the patient has the option to donate blood preoperatively, although he is not encouraged to do so, since the risk of a homologous blood transfusion is less than 5%.[45]

Surgical Technique

In 1996, preparation for an anatomic RRP includes abstinence from oral intake the night before surgery. Patients are admitted routinely the same day as the procedure.

The technique of anatomic RRP involves good positioning with adequate anesthesia. Some authors prefer epidural anesthesia, although the patient is given the option of general anesthesia as well. The procedure begins by placing the patient in the supine position. The table is hyperextended and placed in 20 degrees of Trendelenburg position. A 16-French urethral catheter is placed in the bladder, and 50 ml of water is placed in the balloon. A lower midline abdominal incision is made from 2 cm below the umbilicus to 1 cm above the pubic symphysis. Dissection is carried through transversalis fascia, and the peritoneal contents are swept cephalad with blunt dissection. A Balfour retractor is placed in the wound (Fig. 29–10), and the procedure is begun with a bilateral PLND if indicated. The anatomic limits of this dissection are noted above (Fig. 29–1). After completing the PLND, a midline malleable blade is used for cephalad retraction of the bladder, providing adequate exposure of the pelvis. The preprostatic adipose tissue is removed from the anterolateral surface of the prostate to expose the endopelvic fascia, which is a thin sheet of connective tissue that extends laterally from the pelvic sidewall onto the prostate and bladder medially. The puboprostatic ligaments are identified. These ligaments represent bands of condensed pelvic fascia that anchor the prostate to the distal third of the pubis close to the midline. The endopelvic fascia and the puboprostatic ligaments (Fig. 29–11) are incised and transected, respectively. When incising the endopelvic fascia, care is taken to preserve the levator ani musculature in its entirety. The levator ani musculature lies inferior and lateral to the endopelvic fascia. Additionally, care is taken to avoid violation of Santorini's plexus, which is located inferior and medial to the endopelvic fascia. At this point, the prostate gland can be palpated posterolaterally, and the surgeon can assess for any lateral extension of the tumor.

An angled Babcock clamp (Fig. 29–12) is used to bring the connective periprostatic tissue together on the anterior surface of the prostate (Fig. 29–13). Chromic sutures (2-0) are used to secure this tissue. A McDougal right-angle clamp (Fig. 29–14) is used to develop the plane between the urethra posteriorly and the dorsal vein complex (DVC) anteriorly. This dissection is performed distal to the apex of the prostate (Fig. 29–13, *inset*). The DVC represents the largest group of veins, providing a conduit for venous return from the deep dorsal vein of the penis, anteriorly, and the cavernosal veins, posteriorly. After isolating the DVC, it is ligated distally with a 0 Vicryl suture and transected with a No. 10 blade on a long handle. Alternatively, the DVC may be developed, transected, and oversewn using a running 2-0 Monocryl suture.

The striated urethral sphincter is intimately associated with the membranous urethra from the corpus spongiosum to the apex of the prostate. Examination of the male embryo reveals that this muscle invests the membranous urethra circumferentially; however, in the adult male, there is fibrous metaplasia of the posterior midline muscle fibers.[46] This results in a horseshoe-shaped striated urethral sphincter, which is most well developed anterior to the urethra just beneath the DVC. For this reason, when controlling hemorrhage from the DVC, care must be taken to avoid excessive posterior suture placement.

After transection of the DVC, the anterior membranous urethra is visualized and dissected in a most meticulous manner from the apical prostatic tissue. The anterior urethra is incised, the catheter is transected, and the posterior urethra is divided at the junction of the prostatomembranous urethra. Preservation of both membranous urethra and striated urethral sphincter demands a line of urethral transection that will provide an adequate surgical margin of resection, yet one that is as close to the

TABLE 29–2. NOMOGRAM FOR PREDICTION OF FINAL PATHOLOGICAL STAGE*

	PSA (ng/ml)																											
	0.0–4.0 Clinical Stage							4.1–10 Clinical Stage							10.1–20 Clinical Stage							>20 Clinical Stage						
Score	T1a	T1b	T1c	T2a	T2b	T2c	T3a	T1a	T1b	T1c	T2a	T2b	T2c	T3a	T1a	T1b	T1c	T2a	T2b	T2c	T3a	T1a	T1b	T1c	T2a	T2b	T2c	T3a
Prediction of organ-confined disease																												
2–4	100	85	92	88	76	82	—	100	78	82	83	67	71	—	100	—	—	61	52	—	—	—	—	33	20	7	—	—
5	100	78	81	81	67	73	—	100	70	71	73	56	64	43	100	49	55	58	43	37	26	—	—	24	32	—	3	—
6	100	68	69	72	54	60	42	100	53	59	62	44	48	33	—	36	41	44	28	37	19	—	—	22	14	11	4	5
7	—	54	55	61	41	46	—	100	39	43	51	32	37	26	—	24	24	36	19	24	14	—	—	7	18	4	5	3
8–10	—	—	—	48	31	—	—	—	32	31	39	22	25	12	—	11	—	29	14	15	9	—	—	3	3	1	2	2
Prediction of established capsular penetration																												
2–4	0	15	22	14	26	17	—	0	22	29	19	34	27	—	0	—	—	40	49	—	—	—	—	50	80	94	—	—
5	0	22	30	20	34	26	—	0	29	34	28	45	34	58	0	49	40	43	58	61	75	—	—	54	68	—	97	—
6	0	30	34	29	46	38	59	0	45	38	38	56	49	68	—	62	45	56	73	59	82	—	—	53	86	90	96	95
7	—	43	40	39	59	50	—	0	58	44	49	68	59	75	—	73	52	64	81	73	86	—	—	67	80	96	95	98
8–10	—	—	—	50	68	—	—	—	64	48	59	77	71	87	—	87	—	70	86	82	92	—	—	74	97	99	97	98
Prediction of seminal vesicle involvement																												
2–4	0	1	<1	1	2	2	—	0	2	<1	1	3	3	—	0	—	—	3	4	—	—	—	—	<1	12	30	—	—
5	0	3	<1	2	4	4	—	0	4	<1	3	6	6	5	0	7	<1	5	8	12	11	—	—	<1	11	—	29	—
6	0	6	1	5	9	9	8	0	9	1	6	11	12	11	—	15	1	11	19	17	18	—	—	2	35	40	53	31
7	—	12	4	9	17	17	—	0	18	5	12	22	23	18	—	28	6	19	33	33	31	—	—	9	31	73	62	55
8–10	—	—	—	17	29	—	—	—	29	23	22	38	40	40	—	55	—	29	50	53	49	—	—	81	81	93	73	65
Prediction of lymph nodal involvement																												
2–4	0	2	<1	1	2	4	—	0	2	1	1	2	5	—	0	—	—	1	3	—	—	—	—	6	2	7	—	—
5	0	4	1	2	4	8	—	0	4	1	2	5	10	8	0	5	3	2	6	13	11	—	—	9	3	—	29	—
6	0	8	2	3	9	17	15	0	9	2	4	11	19	16	—	11	4	5	13	22	20	—	—	8	9	18	53	31
7	—	15	2	7	18	31	—	0	18	3	8	20	34	28	—	21	7	9	24	39	35	—	—	24	11	44	62	55
8–10	—	—	—	13	32	—	—	—	30	5	15	35	53	50	—	41	—	17	40	59	54	—	—	41	35	76	73	65

*Numbers represent the percentage probability of the patient having a given pathologic stage based on a combined logistic regression analysis of clinical stage, Gleason grade, and serum PSA.

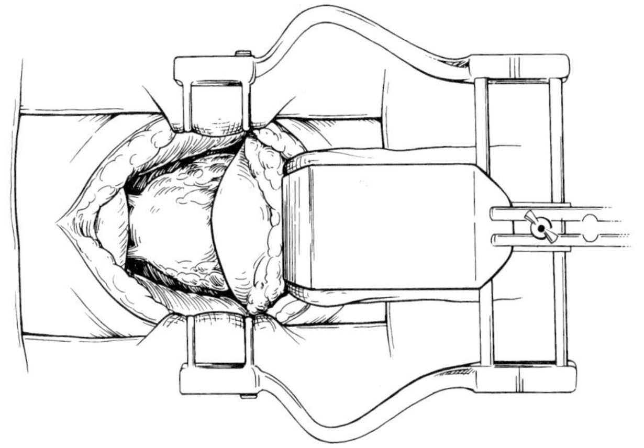

FIGURE 29–10. A lower midline abdominal incision is used for RRP. Balfour retraction allows for excellent exposure of the bladder and prostate.

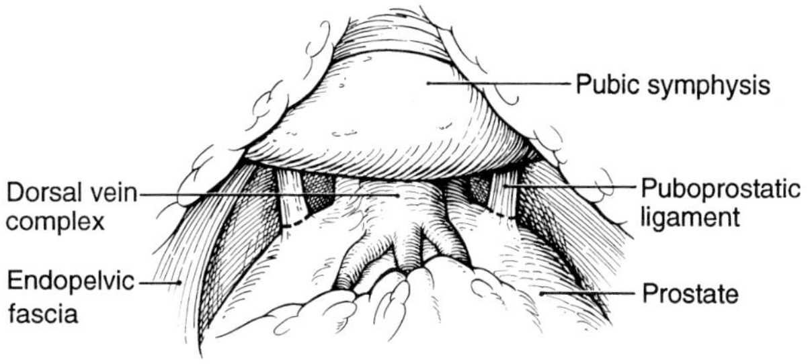
Pubic symphysis
Dorsal vein complex
Puboprostatic ligament
Endopelvic fascia
Prostate

FIGURE 29–11. View of the endopelvic fascia and puboprostatic ligaments.

apex of the prostate as possible. The more distal the transection, the shorter the residual continence zone and the greater the risk of long-term urinary incontinence. After posterior urethral transection, the urethral plate (rectourethralis muscle) comes into view. This structure can be sharply divided with a No. 10 blade on a long handle with the aid of a right-angle clamp.

Next, the lateral pelvic fascia (Fig. 29–15, *inset*), which is located on the posterolateral surface of the prostate, is meticulously incised at the 4-o'clock and 8-o'clock positions. This maneuver allows the neurovascular bundles to drop posteriorly and laterally, removing them from inadvertent injury. Using a fine-tip right angle (Fig. 29–16), the pedicles are carefully defined and divided in the space between the prostate capsule anteromedially and the neurovascular bundle posterolaterally. In order to avoid injury to the neurovascular bundle (see section on "Nerve-Sparing Indications and Technique"), the authors may or may not secure the pedicles with hemoclips or ligatures. If used, hemoclips are applied judiciously. Hemorrhage is typically minimal.

Once all the pedicles to the prostate gland are taken down, Denonvilliers' fascia is identified and incised in the midline. The vasa deferentia come into view and are dissected free of surrounding tissue down to the level of the tips of the seminal vesicles. A large hemoclip is placed across the vasa deferentia, and they are transected using a right-angle scissors. Using sharp dissection, the seminal vesicles are then dissected in their entirety (Fig. 29–17) from the posterior surface of the bladder and surrounding tissue. Before transecting, hemoclips are placed across the pedicle to the tip of the seminal vesicle.

The prostate can then be removed via sharp, circumferential vesical neck transection. When bladder neck reconstruction is required (see "Urethral-Sparing Indications and Technique"), interrupted 3-0 Monocryl sutures are used to reduce the vesical neck to 16 French (Fig. 29–18). The vesical mucosa is everted and secured to the neighboring seromuscular bladder wall using interrupted, 4-0 Monocryl sutures. This maneuver will ensure a mucosa-to-mucosa, watertight, urethrovesical anastomosis (Fig. 29–18, *inset*).

A 16-French catheter is placed in the urethra so that the tip of the catheter is visualized in the pelvis. The urethrovesical anastomosis is now performed by placing four to six, 3-0 Monocryl stitches (Fig. 29–19, *inset*) at the 12-, 1-, 4-, 6-, 8-, and 11-o'clock positions in the urethral stump emerging from the genitourinary diaphragm. Opposite ends of these urethral sutures are placed into corresponding positions on the bladder neck, using a French-eye needle. All sutures are placed from inside to outside, ensuring eversion of the mucosa, and therefore, accomplishing a mucosa-to-mucosa,

FIGURE 29–12. Angled Babcock clamp.

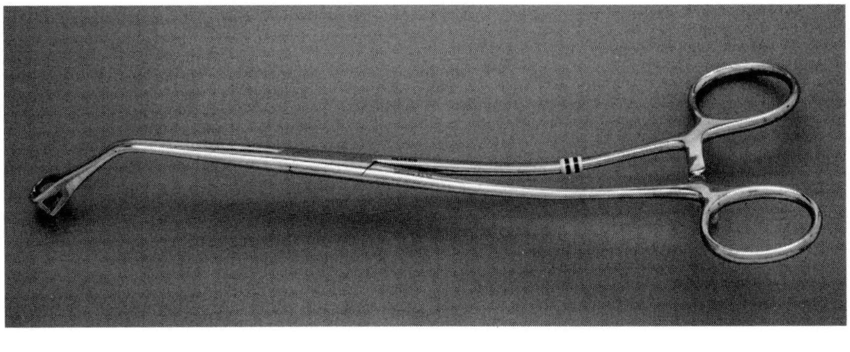

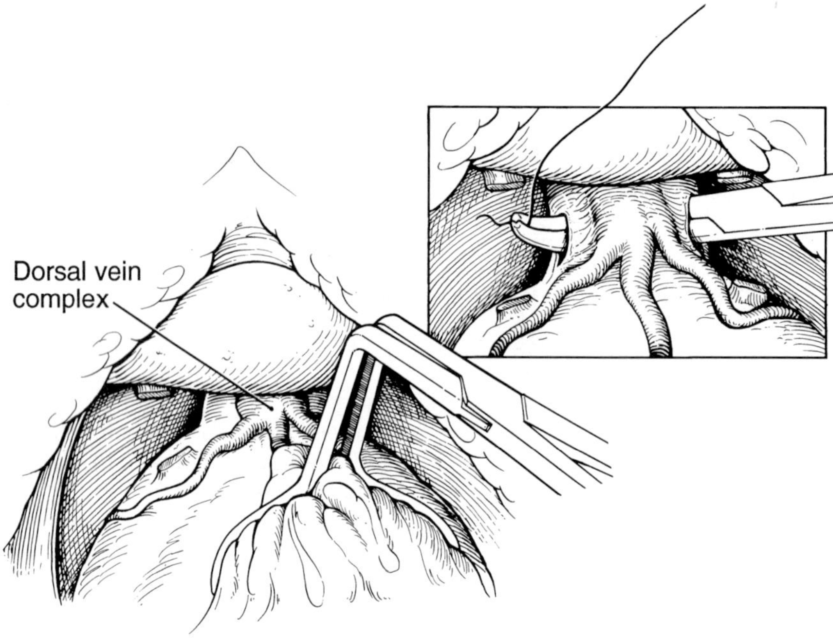
Dorsal vein complex

FIGURE 29–13. An angled Babcock clamp is utilized to secure bilateral edges of incised endopelvic fascia. Ligation of this tissue will prevent retrograde venous bleeding when the DVC is divided. *Inset,* The DVC is ligated.

watertight, urethrovesical anastomosis. After all sutures are placed, the 16-French urethral catheter is inserted into the bladder, and the sutures are tied (Fig. 29–19), apposing the vesicle neck and membranous urethra.

The wound is irrigated copiously. Bilateral Davol drains are positioned through separate stab incisions, so they enter percutaneously and exit the ipsilateral subcutaneous tissue. They are then situated between the rectus abdominis muscles in the midline before being placed into the ipsilateral obturator fossae. The drains are not tunneled through rectus fascia in order to reduce the risk of postoperative discomfort at the drain sites. The fascia is closed using a running No. 2 nylon suture, and the skin is apposed using a running, 4-0 Monocryl subcuticular suture. A 60-mg belladonna and opium (B&O) rectal suppository and a 30-mg intravenous infusion of ketorolac (Toradol) are given at the end of the procedure. The patient is then transferred to the recovery room and admitted to the hospital for a median stay of 2.8 days.

Nerve-Sparing Indications and Technique

In performing a "nerve-sparing" radical retropubic prostatectomy for select patients, the surgeon must be familiar with the location of the cavernous nerves, which originate from the pelvic plexus, cephalad and posterior to the tip of the seminal vesicles. They course posterolateral to the seminal vesicles and travel in the neurovascular bundle that continues along the posterolateral edge of the prostate, beneath the lateral pelvic fascia, and along the lateral edges of Denonvilliers' fascia.[46] Numerous cavernous nerves exist within each bundle. Branches to the membranous urethra and corpora cavernosa travel outside the prostatic capsule within the lateral pelvic fascia, in an inferior direction between the prostate and the rectum. At the level of prostatic apex and membranous urethra,

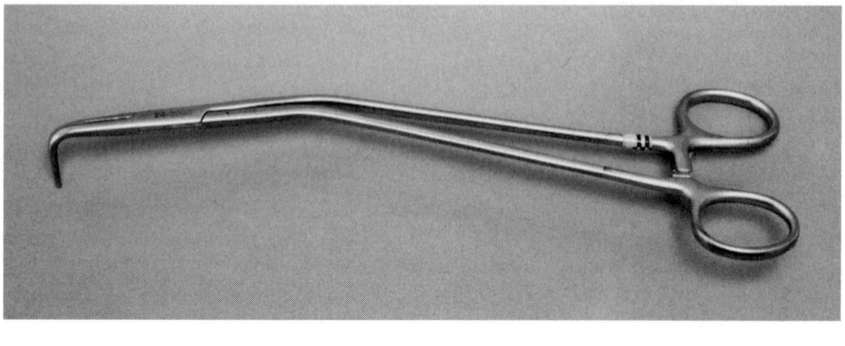

FIGURE 29–14. McDougal right-angle clamp.

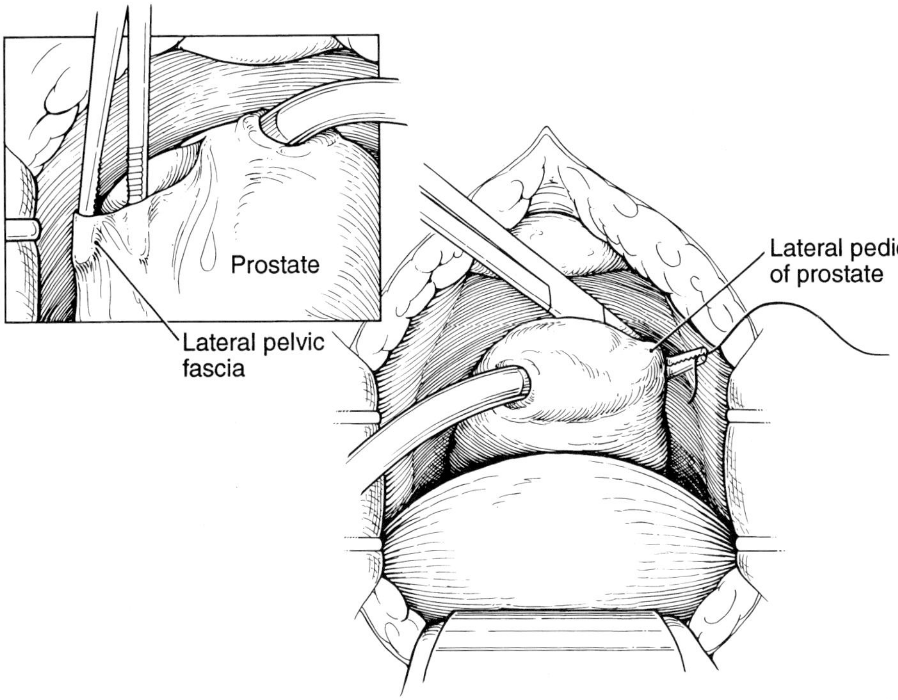
Prostate
Lateral pelvic fascia
Lateral pedicle of prostate

FIGURE 29–15. Lateral pedicles of the prostate are ligated and divided. *Inset,* The lateral pelvic fascia is incised.

the neurovascular bundles are located at the 5-o'clock and 7-o'clock positions with relation to the urethra.

Indications for nerve preservation include preoperative erectile function, organ-confined tumor, serum PSA concentration less than 10 ng/ml, and lack of induration or nodularity at the prostatic apex and posterolateral borders of the prostate. If induration or nodularity is noted ipsilaterally, the contralateral nerve bundle may be preserved, provided the patient has no other contraindication.

When performing a "nerve-sparing" RRP, the procedure is begun as described above. However, there are several maneuvers that must be performed throughout the procedure to preserve the autonomic innervation to the penis. During transection of the urethral plate, the NVBs are located slightly posterior and lateral to this structure. Aggressive dissection in this area could result in injury to one or both neurovascular bundles. Also, during the apical dissection, the urologist must not place excessive traction on the catheter. Pulling too hard on the catheter to manipulate the prostate can tear or traumatize the nerves traveling to the corpora cavernosa. When attention is turned to the lateral pelvic fascia, the incision should be performed at the 4- and 8-o'clock positions, allowing the NVBs to fall posteriorly and laterally. As the pedicles to the prostate are transected (Fig. 29–15), starting at the apex and continuing toward the base of the prostate, electrocautery must be avoided at all times. The electric current tends to travel along vascular and neural structures, and may compromise the cavernous nerves. Also, during seminal vesicle dissection, care must be taken to avoid injury to the pelvic nerve plexus, which is located in close proximity to the tip of the seminal vesicle. Lastly, with the aid of excellent exposure and a bloodless field, the surgeon should be able to visualize the NVBs within the pelvis (Fig. 29–20) prior to performing the urethrovesical anastomosis. This is important so that the anastomotic stitches are not placed through the tissue containing the cavernous nerves.

Urethral-Sparing Indications and Technique

A urethral-sparing radical retropubic prostatectomy may be performed in select patients. The authors feel that preservation of the vesical neck and

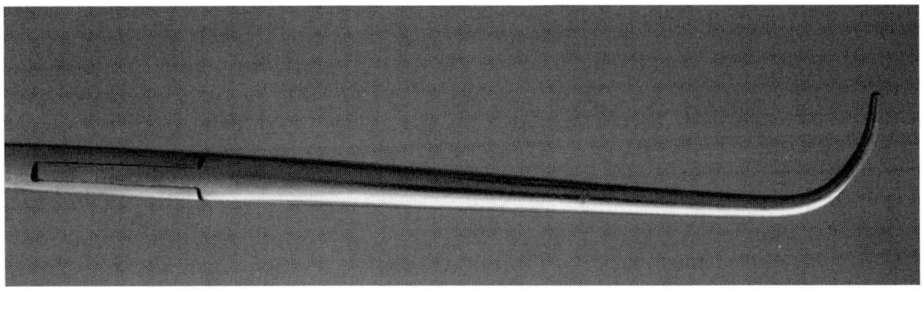

FIGURE 29–16. Fine-tip right-angle clamp.

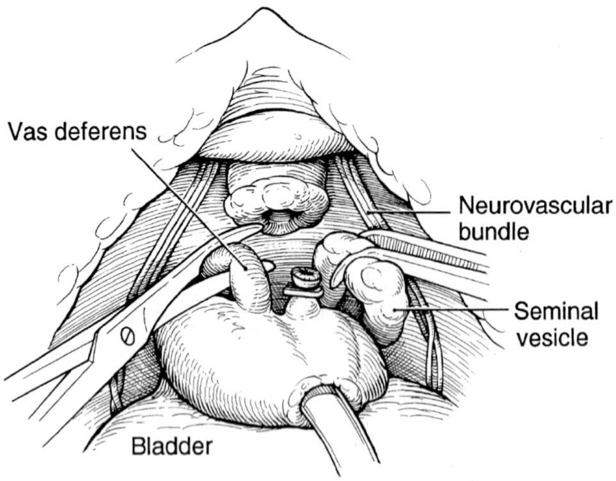
Vas deferens
Neurovascular bundle
Seminal vesicle
Bladder

FIGURE 29–17. Vas deferens and seminal vesicles are isolated and divided.

proximal prostatic urethra decreases the risk of a subsequent vesical neck contracture and may contribute to earlier return of urinary continence. This technique is indicated when the patient: (1) has no tumor in the transition zone of the prostate, (2) has no tumor at the base of the prostate, (3) has not had previous surgery involving the bladder neck (e.g., transurethral resection of the prostate), (4) does not have a significant median lobe, and (5) has a serum PSA level less than 10 ng/ml.

When performing a urethral-sparing technique, the prostatectomy procedure is begun as described above. After the seminal vesicles are freed from the posterior surface of the bladder, attention is turned to the prostatovesical junction. With the vasa deferentia and seminal vesicles dissected free, the plane between the prostate and the bladder comes into view. Using sharp dissection and a "posterior peel" approach, this plane can be further delineated, allowing the prostate to be freely dissected from the posterior base of the bladder. The dissection continues laterally and then anteriorly to free the prostate from the bladder circumferentially. Eventually, the prostate is only connected to the bladder at the vesical neck, where the proximal prostatic urethra begins. Continuation of sharp and blunt dissection, in combination with appropriate traction on the prostate gland, will allow complete dissection of the proximal prostatic urethra without violation of prostatic parenchyma (Fig. 29–21). With dissection of at least 1 cm of proximal prostatic urethra, a No. 15 blade is used to circumferentially transect the urethra. The prostate is removed, and 1.0 to 2.0 cm of proximal urethra remains on the vesical neck (Fig. 29–21, *inset*), resulting in urethral preservation without compromise of cancer eradication.

The urethrovesical anastomosis is performed by placing six urethral stitches, using 3-0 Monocryl (Fig. 29–19, *inset*), at the 12-, 1-, 4-, 6-, 8-, and 11-o'clock positions in the urethral stump emerging from the genitourinary diaphragm. Opposite ends of these urethral sutures are placed into corresponding positions on the proximal prostatic urethra, using a French-eye needle. All sutures are placed from inside to outside, ensuring eversion of the mucosa, and therefore, accomplishing a mucosa-to-mucosa, watertight, urethrourethral anastomosis. After the stiches are placed, the 16-French urethral catheter is then inserted into the bladder,

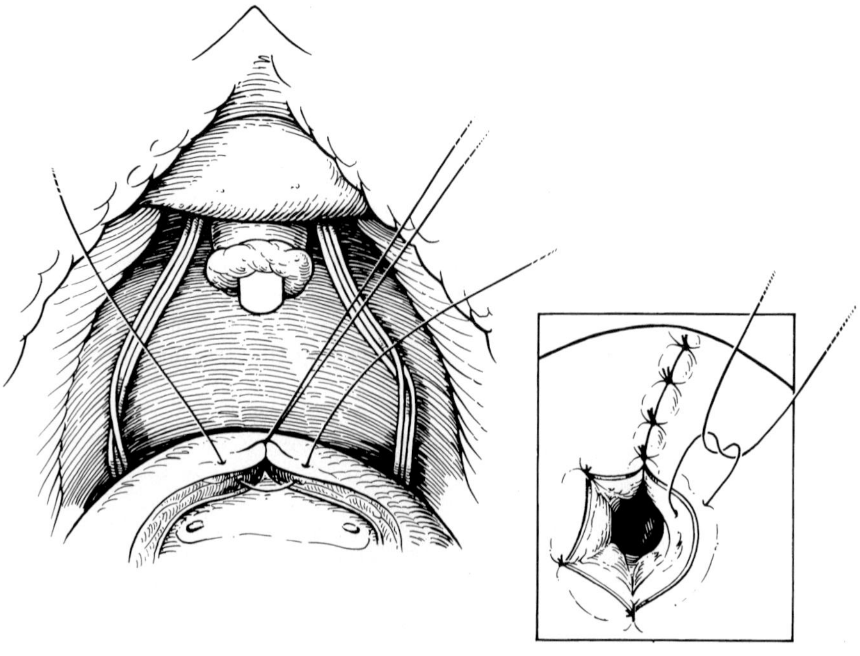

FIGURE 29–18. Bladder neck reconstruction.

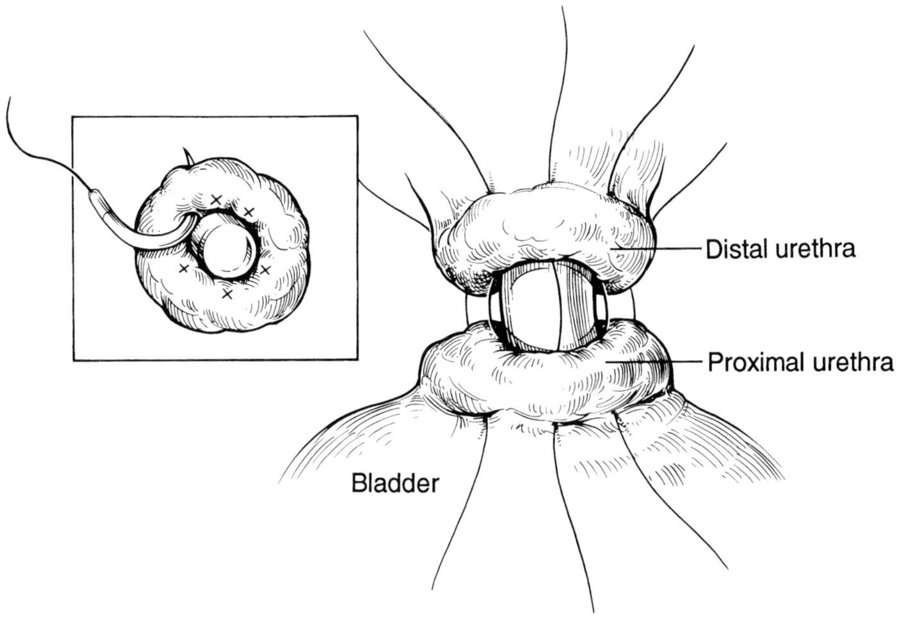
Distal urethra
Proximal urethra
Bladder

FIGURE 29–19. Urethral reconstruction.

and stitches are tied (Fig. 29–19), apposing the proximal prostatic urethra and membranous urethra. The remainder of the procedure is then performed as outlined above.

Postoperative Management

Equally important as performing an anatomically correct RRP is the postoperative care of the radical prostatectomy patient. The authors have developed a protocol involving aggressive pulmonary care, early ambulation and diet, and comprehensive patient education. This protocol for postoperative management is presented in Table 29–3. The patient is exposed to a liberal dietary program, which allows clear liquid intake on the operative day. The diet is then advanced as tolerated, with most patients enjoying solid food on the first postoperative day. Lower extremity exercise is stressed, beginning with dorsiflexion and plantarflexion on the operative day. Early ambulation is initiated on the first postoperative day with six walks, progressing in length. Patient education commences on the first postoperative day. Topics of instruction include urethral catheter care, postoperative activity restrictions, and signs and symptoms of postoperative complications, including thromboembolic events, wound infection, and catheter malfunction. Using this approach, the authors have been able to decrease the median hospital stay to 2.8 days, with many patients returning to the comfort of their home on the second postoperative day (J.E. Oesterling, personal communication, 1996).

Results of Anatomic Radical Retropubic Prostatectomy

Pathology

In evaluating the ability of RRP to provide adequate local cancer control, it is important to note the pathologic results after this procedure. Walsh and colleagues[47] analyzed the pathologic specimen of 955 men who underwent an RRP for clinically localized prostate cancer. The wide pathologic stages reflect the unfortunate inaccuracy of clinical staging for this disease. Organ-confined disease was noted in 37%, focal capsular penetration in 20.3%, established capsular penetration in 28.3%, seminal vesicle invasion in 7%, and positive pelvic lymph node involvement in 7.4%.

A similar pattern was seen in a series of 3170 consecutive patients who underwent RRP for clinically localized prostate cancer at the Mayo Clinic. Review of the pathologic specimens revealed organ-confined disease in 47%, capsular penetration and seminal vesicle involvement in 42%, and positive pelvic lymph nodes in 11%. Positive surgical margins were noted in 24% of the patients. The complete impact of a positive surgical margin is not known. In fact, Epstein,[49] in an intraoperative study, has shown that 40% of patients undergoing RRP diagnosed as having a positive margin after removal of the prostate actually have no residual tumor. This speculation helps to explain why many patients with positive margins will not have disease recurrence.

Survival

In a large series from a single institution, Zincke et al.[48] have noted overall 10- and 15-year survival

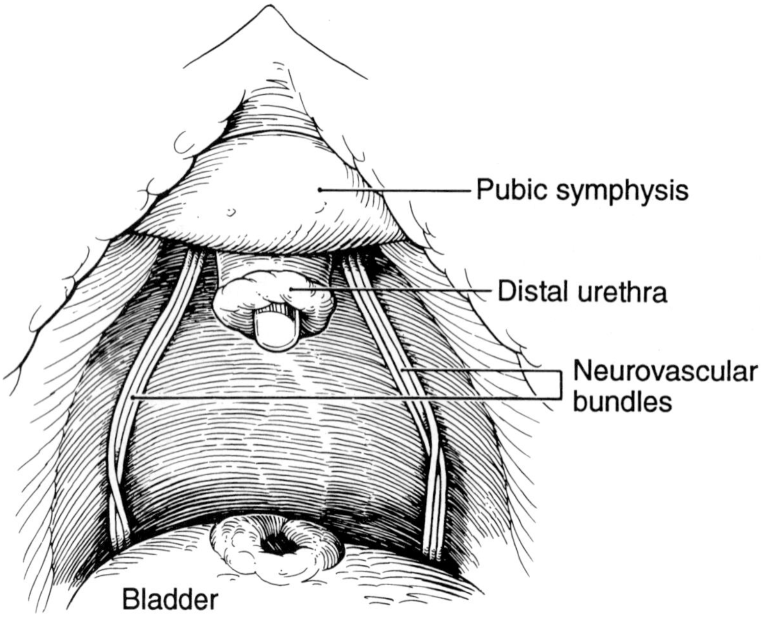
Pubic symphysis
Distal urethra
Neurovascular bundles
Bladder

FIGURE 29–20. The distal urethral edge (membranous urethra) and neurovascular bundles are visualized after prostatic removal.

rates after RRP to be 75 and 60%, respectively; cause-specific survival rates were 90 and 82%, respectively. Although clinical stage did not significantly affect survival, tumor grade did. The 10- and 15-year cause-specific survival rates for men with Gleason grades 3 or below were 95 and 93%, respectively; Gleason grades 4 to 6 were 90 and 82%, respectively; and Gleason grades 7 and above were 82 and 71%, respectively. The metastasis-free 10- and 15-year survival rates were 82 and 76%, respectively, and the local recurrence-free 10- and 15-year survival rates were 83 and 75%, respectively. Freedom from biochemical recurrence (undetectable serum PSA value) was 52 and 40% at these time intervals, respectively.

In evaluating biochemical recurrence as related to pathologic stage, Walsh and colleagues[47] noted freedom from biochemical recurrence (undetectable serum PSA value) 10 years after RRP for men with organ-confined disease to be 85%; for focal capsular penetration to be 82%; for low-grade (Gleason 2 to 6) established penetration to be 54%; for high-grade

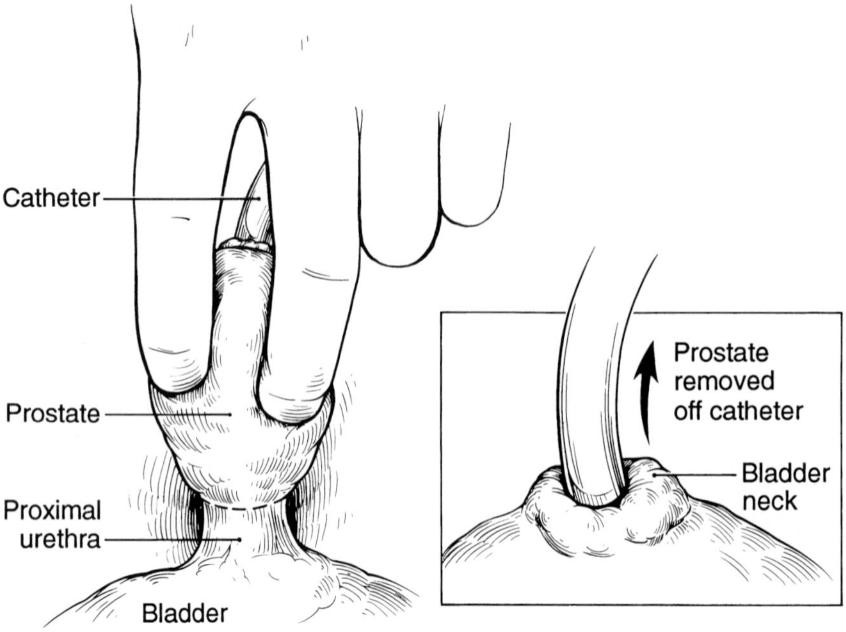
Catheter
Prostate
Proximal urethra
Bladder
Prostate removed off catheter
Bladder neck

FIGURE 29–21. The prostate is sharply dissected from the prostatic urethra, and then removed.

TABLE 29–3. POSTOPERATIVE MANAGEMENT OF RADICAL PROSTATECTOMY PATIENT

Operative Day

- Epidural catheter is removed in the postanesthesia care unit
- Pain control:
  - Patient-controlled anesthesia (PCA)
  - Ketoralac 15 mg IV every 6 hours for 48 hours
- Antibiotic therapy:
  - Cefotan 1000 mg IV every 12 hours for 48 hours
- Diet: clear liquids as tolerated
- Activity level:
  - Bedrest with scrotal elevation using a scrotal roll
  - Incentive spirometry 10 times per hour
- Deep venous thrombosis prophylaxis:
  - Sequential compression devices (SCD) while in bed or in a chair
  - Dorsiflexion/plantarflexion of feet 100 times per hour
- Hematocrit is obtained

Postoperative Day 1

- Diet: regular as tolerated
- Pain control:
  - PCA is discontinued
  - Oral narcotic such as hydrocodone/acetominophen is initiated (in combination with an oral stool softener)
- Activity:
  - Ambulation 6 times per day (SCD therapy is discontinued)
- Discharge instruction including Foley catheter care is begun
- Hematocrit is obtained

Postoperative Day 2

- Operative drains are removed if <75 ml/24 hours
- A Dulcolax suppository is provided as needed for constipation
- Discharge instructions are reinforced
- Iron supplementation is begun if the hematocrit is <30

Postoperative Day 3

- Discharge to home

(Gleason 7 to 10) established penetration to be 42%; for seminal vesicle involvement to be 43%; and for nodal-positive disease to be 0%. Clearly, pathologic stage impacts on the patient's ability to be free from biochemical recurrence, which appears to be an imminent predictor of clinical recurrence.

From these long-term results, it is clear that RRP is a most efficient treatment option for men with organ-confined prostate cancer. For men with capsular penetration and high-grade tumor, or involvement of the seminal vesicles, cure is less likely. Cure will not be achieved in the presence of node-positive disease.

Complications of Radical Retropubic Prostatectomy

Intraoperative and Perioperative Complications

HEMORRHAGE/BLOOD TRANSFUSION. Intraoperative and postoperative hemorrhage is always of concern to the surgeon. During RRP, large quantities of blood may be lost very rapidly. Because of the risk of hemorrhage and hemodynamic instability, most surgeons make provisions to have at least 2 units of blood available during the procedure. Many patients prefer to donate blood ahead of time in anticipation of receiving an autologous as opposed to homologous blood transfusion. Other centers perform acute normovolemic hemodilution (ANH) as an alternative to preoperative autologous blood donation.[50] Monk and colleagues[51] have shown transfusion costs for the autologous blood donation to be 73% higher than ANH. Additionally, the use of ANH does not significantly postpone the operative time and has demonstrated cost-effectiveness without compromise of postoperative outcome.

The mean blood loss during prostatectomy ranges from 600 ml[48] to 2266 ml.[52] Mean homologous transfusion rates range from 5 to 11.5%.[48,51,53] Many centers urge patients to donate blood preoperatively with the intention of avoiding homologous transfusion. Interestingly, Goad et al.[54] found autologous blood donation to be of limited benefit, as it increased the risk of homologous transfusion in their population. At the University of Michigan, the rate of homologous transfusion is reasonably low at 5%, and therefore patients are not encouraged to donate blood preoperatively.[45]

Postoperative hemorrhage was assessed by Hedican and Walsh.[55] In 1350 consecutive radical prostatectomy patients, only 7 (0.5%) had significant postoperative hemorrhage, requiring acute blood transfusion to support blood pressure. Four of the seven patients were managed with surgical reexploration, and three were managed expectantly. The cause of postoperative hemorrhage was attributed to unknown preoperative ingestion of anticoagulants, such as aspirin and nonsteroidal anti-inflammatory agents, unknown polycythemia vera, and technical factors relating to the surgery (nonligated or poorly ligated vessels). All patients in this series received 2 to 3 units of autologous blood and 0 to 27 units of homologous blood. The authors noted an increased incidence of vesical neck contracture rate in those patients who had postoperative hemorrhage but were managed expectantly. They postulated that this was most likely due to pelvic hematoma causing disruption of the vesicourethral anastomosis. As a result, they advocate exploration of patients who experience significant postoperative hemorrhage in order to completely evacuate the pelvic hematoma so there is no disruption of the vesicourethral anastomosis and later development of a vesical neck contracture and urinary incontinence.

RECTAL INJURY. Inadvertent rectal injury is a complication that can occur during radical prostatectomy because of the close proximity and intimate relationship of the prostate with the rectum. Reports of rectal injury had previously been as high as 8.2% in 1977.[56] With the introduction of the anatomic radical prostatectomy and improved guidelines for surgical therapy, contemporary series[57,58] now reveal a 1 to 1.2% incidence of rectal injury. In one series,[57] 27 of 2212 patients (1.2%) had rectal injuries. All but one of these injuries were identified immediately. Primary closure alone was performed in 21 of the 27 men, with 6 men requiring a temporary diverting colostomy. One patient died in the perioperative period due to sepsis from a rectourethral fistula. Other complications included three rectourethral fistulae and a fascial dehiscence. Predisposing factors for rectal injury included previous rectal surgery, previous pelvic radiation therapy, and previous transurethral resection of the prostate.

Another series[58] noted 10 rectal injuries in 1000 men who had undergone RRP. All injuries were in nonirradiated patients. Of the ten injuries, nine were recognized immediately, permitting primary closure. One patient required a temporary diverting colostomy. Within this series, no patient's postoperative course was complicated by wound infection, pelvic abscess, or urethrorectal fistula.

Rectal injuries are rare but serious complications of RRP. If recognized early, they can be repaired primarily, with minimal long-term morbidity to the patient.

Other. The incidence of other early complications of RRP include wound infection to 0.7 in 2.1%, urine leak due to anastomotic compromise in 2.9 to 5.2%, prolonged ileus in 0 to 2.6%, urinary tract infection/sepsis in 1.8%, pneumonia in 0.4%, cardiovascular events in 1.4 to 3.9%, and bladder retention in 0.4%. Aggressive preoperative medical evaluation and careful postoperative observation contribute to the relatively low rate of complications from this major surgical procedure.

Early Complications

Mortality. In contemporary series,[48,53,59,60] the mortality rate (death within 30 days of surgery) for RRP has ranged between 0.2 and 0.7%. However, when patients are stratified by age categories, elderly men may have a higher mortality rate. Kerr and Zincke[61] noted a 0% death rate in men less than 55 years of age, and a 1% rate for those older than 75 years of age. More striking results come from LuYao and colleagues[62]; men aged 65 to 75 years had a death rate of 1% or less versus men 80 years of age or older, who had a mortality rate of nearly 5%.

In modern times, RRP is a safe procedure for those men under age 75 years. Clearly, good clinical judgment must be used in selecting elderly candidates for this procedure. The authors do not recommend routine use of RRP as treatment for prostate cancer in the patient over 75 years of age. Exceptions may be made for the occasional elderly patient in excellent health, with extended family longevity, and high-grade prostate cancer.

Thromboembolic Events. Several groups[48,54,60,63] around the United States report a low incidence of deep venous thrombosis (DVT), from 1.2 to 1.8%. It follows that reports[48,53,60,61,63] of pulmonary embolus (PE) would similarly be low, ranging from 0 to 3.1%.

In the contemporary era of RRP, thromboembolic complications are rare, as reported by Cisek and Walsh.[64] One group of 784 men who were not managed with sequential compression device (SCD) prophylaxis had a 0.9% incidence of pulmonary embolism and 0.3% incidence of DVT. Those patients managed with SCD prophylaxis had a 1.7% incidence of PE and a 0.6% incidence of DVT. Of note is the fact that the men managed with SCDs had their complication a mean of 20 days after RRP as opposed to 11 days for those managed without SCDs. There was one fatality in each group. This study emphasized the need for patient education regarding signs and symptoms of thromboembolic phenomena, as the vast majority occur during outpatient status.

One wonders whether sequential compression devices are effective in preventing DVT and PE. The study cited above suggests there is no added benefit, although others have shown clear efficacy to SCD prophylaxis against deep venous thrombosis.[65–67] It is essential that the devices are functioning appropriately, are worn correctly, and are placed on the lower extremities prior to commencing surgery. In one study,[68] patients on routine nursing units had properly functioning devices only 48% of the time. Although the present authors utilize SCDs, our primary DVT prophylaxis involves early and aggressive ambulation as well as plantarflexion and dorsiflexion exercises while in bed.

Vesical Neck Contracture. Certainly, the evaluation of the patient with obstructive voiding symptoms or incontinence after RRP must include evaluation for vesical neck contracture. This complication of RRP has an incidence of 1.1 to 5.4%,[48,61,63] and tends to occur 6 to 12 weeks after the operation. The contracture may be the result of poor mucosal apposition of the bladder neck (or proximal prostatic urethra) to the membranous urethra. Flexible cystoscopy or placement of an 18-French urethral catheter will remove suspicion of a significant stricture. Strictures may be readily treated with vesical neck dilation or transurethral incision of the narrowing in association with selective injection of steroids into the contracture.

Late Complications

Urinary Incontinence. Walsh[47] recently reported his experience from the Johns Hopkins Hospital regarding stress urinary incontinence (SUI) following RRP. Upon reviewing his first 593 patients, 92% had complete continence, 6% had mild SUI (requiring 1 pad/day), 2% had moderate SUI (>1 pad/day), and 0.3% had severe SUI (requiring an artificial urinary sphincter) at 1-year follow-up. His subsequent 350 patients had similar results, with the exception that no one required an artificial urinary sphincter.

SUI is a complication of RRP that is difficult to assess, as there are no standard tests to gauge incontinence. The incidence of severe or total incontinence is reportedly 0.8 to 5%,[48,63] although elderly patients (>75 years of age) may have significant incontinence (>3 pads/day) as much as 16% of the time.[61] The incidence of mild to moderate incontinence varies greatly. When mail or telephone surveys are used to determine urinary incontinence, 30 to 50% of individuals are found to regularly wear pads, diapers, or clamps to stay dry.[69,70] Techniques involving careful apical dissection and preservation of the bladder neck and proximal prostatic urethra, when appropriate, may provide an improvement with regard to this untoward effect.

Erectile Dysfunction. Walsh[47,71] reported his experience from the Johns Hopkins Hospital regarding erectile dysfunction following RRP. In a review of 600 men, 503 (84%) were potent preoperatively and 68% were potent postoperatively. Potency was defined as the ability to achieve an erection sufficient for vaginal penetration. Patient age, stage of disease, and surgical technique served as factors correlating with return of sexual function. Sexual function was preserved in 91% of men less than 50 years old, 75% of those 50 to 60 years old, 58% of those 60 to 70 years old, and 25% of those over 70 years. Potency was achieved in men less than 50 years of age when either one or both neurovascular bundle(s) were preserved. In men older than 70 years of age, potency was better in those with bilateral bundle preservation. Also, the relative risk of impotency was two times greater (after age adjustment) when capsular penetration or seminal vesicle invasion was present.

In support of these findings, Catalona and Bigg[59] preserved sexual potency in 71 of 112 (63%) potent patients who had undergone bilateral nerve-sparing prostatectomy and 13 of 33 (39%) who had undergone a unilateral nerve-sparing procedure. They also noted a higher rate of potency preservation in younger men as well as in men with organ-confined tumor.

In general, erectile function can be preserved in two thirds of men undergoing nerve-sparing prostatectomy. Superior rates can be achieved when both neurovascular bundles are preserved, particularly in younger men with organ-confined disease. Patient selection is once again an extremely important factor. Additionally, potency may continue to improve at 12 to 18 months after surgery. This was demonstrated, in part, by Rossignol,[72] who reported potency rates of 33% at 6 months and 68.5% at 12 months following RRP.

Summary

Anatomic radical retropubic prostatectomy is clearly efficacious at long-term cancer control. In the modern era of anatomic prostate surgery,[3,44,73] blood loss is diminished, complications are few, and control of disease has been excellent. Several series[47,48,74] have reported cancer-specific survival rates following RRP of 85 to 90% at 10 years and 82% at 15 years. PSA-free recurrence has ranged from 78% at 5 years, to 42 to 85% at 10 years, and 41% at 15 years. Patients with lower Gleason grades have enjoyed even higher survival rates. Thus, it would seem that radical retropubic prostatectomy is an excellent treatment option for localized prostate cancer. Nevertheless, it should be reserved for those patients with organ-confined disease and a life expectancy that will allow benefit from the excellent cancer control. Patient selection is critical for true success with this therapeutic option.

REFERENCES

1. Parker SL, Tong T, Bolden S, Wingo PA: Cancer statistics, 1996. CA Cancer J Clin 1996; 46(1):5.
2. Scardino PT, Weaver R, Hudson MA: Early detection of prostate cancer. Hum Pathol 1992; 23:211.
3. Walsh PC, Lepor H, Eggleston JC: Radical prostatectomy with preservation of sexual function: anatomical and pathological considerations. Prostate 1983; 4:473.
4. Catalona WJ, Scott WW: Carcinoma of the prostate. *In* Walsh PC, Gittes RF, Perlmutter AD, Stamey TA (eds): Campbell's Urology, 5th edition, p 1463. Philadelphia, WB Saunders Co, 1986.
5. Rifkin MD, Zerhouni EA, Gatsonis CA, et al: Comparison of magnetic resonance imaging and ultrasonography in staging early prostate cancer. Results of a multi-institutional cooperative trial. N Engl J Med 1990; 323:621.
6. Walsh JW, Amendola MA, Konerding KR, et al: Computed tomographic detection of pelvic and inguinal lymph-node metastases from primary and recurrent pelvic malignant disease. Radiology 1980; 137:157.
7. Danella J, deKernion J, Smith R, Steckel J: The contemporary incidence of lymph node metastases in prostate cancer: implications for laparoscopic lymph node dissection. J Urol 1993; 149:1488–1491.
8. Bluestein D, Bostwick D, Bergstralh E, Osterling J: Eliminating the need for bilateral pelvic lymphadenectomy in select patients with prostate cancer. J Urol 1994; 151: 1315–1320.
9. Kleer E, Larson-Keller J, Zincke H, Oesterling J: Ability of preoperative serum prostate-specific antigen value to predict pathologic stage and DNA ploidy: influence of clinical stage and tumor grade. Urology 1993; 41(3):207–216.
10. Bishoff JT, Reyes A, Thompson IM, et al: Pelvic lymphadenectomy can be omitted in selected patients with carcinoma of the prostate: development of a system of patient selection. Urology 1995; 45(2):270–274.
11. Bangma CH, Hop WC, Schroder FH: Eliminating the need for peroperative frozen section analysis of pelvic lymph nodes during radical prostatectomy. Br J Urol 1995; 76: 595–599.
12. Winfield LH: Laparoscopy in urology. Urol Times 1993; 21:6.
13. Herr HW: Pelvic lymphadenectomy and iodine-125 implantation. *In* Johnson DE, Boileau MA (eds): Genitourinary Tumors: Fundamental Principles and Surgical Techniques, p 63. New York, Grune & Stratton, 1982.
14. Paulson DF: Staging lymphadenectomy should not be an antecedent to treatment in localized prostatic carcinoma. J Urol 1985; 25(2)S:7–14.
15. Brendler CB, Cleeve LK, Anderson EE, Paulson DF: Staging pelvic lymphadenectomy for carcinoma of the prostate: risk versus benefit. J Urol 1980; 124:849.

16. Bratt O, Elfving P, Flodgren P, Lundgren R: Morbidity of pelvic lymphadenectomy, radical retropubic prostatectomy and external radiotherapy in patients with localized prostatic cancer. Scand J Urol Nephrol 1994; 28:265–271.
17. McDowell GC, Johnson JW, Tenney DM, Johnson DE: Pelvic lymphadenectomy for staging clinically localized prostate cancer. Indications, complications, and results in 217 cases. Urology 1990; 35(6):476–482.
18. Tomic R, Granfors T, Sjodin JG, Ohberg L: Lymph leakage after staging pelvic lymphadenectomy for prostatic carcinoma with and without heparin prophylaxis. Scand J Urol Nephrol 1994; 28:273–274.
19. Steiner MS, Marshall FF: Mini-laparotomy staging pelvic lymphadenectomy (minilap): alternative to standard and laparoscopic pelvic lymphadenectomy. Urology 1993; 41(3):201.
20. Perrotti M, Gentle DL, Barada JH, et al: Mini-laparotomy pelvic lymph node dissection. J Urol 1996; 155:986.
21. Jarrard DF, Chodak GW: Prostate cancer staging after radiation utilizing laparoscopic pelvic lymphadenectomy. Urology 1995; 46(4):538–541.
22. Schuessler WW, Vancaillie TG, Reich H, Griffith DP: Transperitoneal endosurgical lymphadenectomy in patients with localized prostate cancer. J Urol 1991; 145:988.
23. Boullier JA, Hagood PG, Parra RO: Endocavitary (laparoscopic) pelvic lymphadenectomy with specific indications in urologic surgery. Urology 1993; 41(1):19–25.
24. Lang GS, Ruckle HC, Hadley HR, et al: One hundred consecutive laparoscopic pelvic lymph node dissections: comparing complications of the first 50 cases to the second 50 cases. Urology 1994; 44(2):221–225.
25. Parra RO, Andrus CH, Boullier JA: Staging laparoscopic pelvic lymph node dissection: comparison of results with open pelvic lymphadenectomy. J Urol 1992; 147:875.
26. Kavoussi LR, Sosa E, Chandhoke P, et al: Complications of laparoscopic pelvic lymph node dissection. J Urol 1993; 149:322.
27. Chow CC, Daly BD, Burney TL: Complications after laparoscopic pelvic lymphadenectomy: CT diagnosis. AJR 1994; 163:353.
28. Maffezzini M, Carmignani G, Perachino M: Benefits and complications of laparoscopic pelvic lymphadenectomy for detection of stage D1 prostate cancer: a multicenter experience. Eur Urol 1995; 27:135.
29. Troxel S, Winfield HN: Comparative financial analysis of laparoscopic versus open pelvic lymph node dissection for men with cancer of the prostate. J Urol 1994; 151:675–680.
30. Epstein JI, Oesterling JE, Eggleston JC, Walsh PC: Frozen section detection of lymph node metastases in prostatic carcinoma. Accuracy in grossly uninvolved pelvic lymphadenectomy specimens. J Urol 1986; 136:1234–1237.
31. Hermansen DK, Whitmore WF Jr: Frozen section lymph node analysis in pelvic lymphadenectomy for prostate cancer. J Urol 1988; 139(5):1073–1074.
32. McLaughlin AP, Saltzstein SL, McCullough DL, Gittes RF: Prostatic carcinoma: incidence and location of unsuspected lymphatic metastasis. J Urol 1976; 115:89.
33. Fowler JE, Torgerson L, McLeod DG, Stutzman RE: Radical prostatectomy with pelvic lymphadenectomy: observations on the accuracy of staging with lymph node frozen sections. J Urol 1981; 126:618.
34. Catalona WJ, Stein AJ: Accuracy of frozen section detection of lymph node metastases in prostatic carcinoma. J Urol 1982; 127:460.
35. Sadlowski RW, Donahue DJ, Richman AV, et al: Accuracy of frozen section diagnosis in pelvic lymph node staging biopsies for adenocarcinoma of the prostate. J Urol 1983; 129:324.
36. Kramolowsky EV, Narayana AS, Platz CE, Loening SA: The frozen section in lymphadenectomy for carcinoma of the prostate. J Urol 1984; 131:899.
37. Young HH: The early diagnosis and radical cure of carcinoma of the prostate. Bull Johns Hopkins Hosp 1905; 16(175):315.
38. Young HH: The cure of cancer of the prostate by radical perineal prostatectomy (prostato-seminal vesiculectomy): history, literature, and statistics of Young's operation. J Urol 1945; 53:188.
39. Belt E, Ebert C, Surber A Jr: A new anatomic approach in perineal prostatectomy. J Urol 1939; 41:482.
40. van Stockum WJ: Prostatectomia suprapubica extravesicalis. Zentralbelutt Für Chirurgie 1909; 30(2):41.
41. Millin T: Retropubic prostatectomy. A new extravesical technique. Lancet 1945; 2:693.
42. Memmelaar J: Total prostatovesiculectomy-retropubic approach. J Urol 1949; 62(3):340.
43. Reiner WG, Walsh PC: An anatomical approach to the surgical management of the dorsal vein and Santorini's plexus during radical retropubic surgery. J Urol 1979; 121:198.
44. Walsh PC, Donker PJ: Impotence following radical prostatectomy: insight into etiology and prevention. J Urol 1982; 128:492.
45. Goh M, Kleer CG, Wojno K, Oesterling JE: Autologous blood transfusion prior to anatomical radical retropubic prostatectomy: is it necessary? Urology 1996 (in press).
46. Myers RP: Practical pelvis anatomy pertinent to radical retropubic prostatectomy. AUA Update Series 1994; 13(4):26.
47. Walsh PC, Partin AW, Epstein JI: Cancer control and quality of life following anatomical radical retropubic prostatectomy: results at 10 years. J Urol 1994; 152:1831.
48. Zincke H, Oesterling JE, Blute ML, et al: Long-term (15 years) results after radical prostatectomy for clinically localized (stage T2c or lower) prostate cancer. J Urol 1994; 152:1850.
49. Epstein JI: Evaluation of radical prostatectomy capsular margins of resection. The significance of margins designated as negative, closely approaching, and positive. Am J Surg 1990; 14:626.
50. D'Ambra MN, Kaplan DK: Alternatives to allogeneic blood use in surgery: acute normovolemic hemodilution and preoperative autologous donation. Am J Surg 1995; 170(Suppl 6A):49S–52S.
51. Monk TG, Goodnough LT, Birkmeyer JD, et al: Acute normovolemic hemodilution is a cost-effective alternative to preoperative autologous blood donation by patients undergoing radical retropubic prostatectomy. Transfusion 1995; 35:559.
52. Oefelein MG, Colangelo LA, Rademaker AW, McVary KT: Intraoperative blood loss and prognosis in prostate cancer patients undergoing radical retropubic prostatectomy. J Urol 1995; 154:442.
53. Andriole GL, Smith DS, Rao G, et al: Early complications of contemporary anatomical radical retropubic prostatectomy. J Urol 1994; 152:1858.
54. Goad JR, Eastham JA, Fitzgerald KB, et al: Radical retropubic prostatectomy: limited benefit of autologous blood donation. J Urol 1995; 154:2103.
55. Hedican SP, Walsh PC: Postoperative bleeding following radical retropubic prostatectomy. J Urol 1994; 152:1181.
56. Veenema RJ, Gursel ED, Lattimer JK: Radical retropubic prostatectomy for cancer: a 20-year experience. J Urol 1977; 117:330–331.
57. McLaren RH, Barrett DM, Zincke H: Rectal injury occurring at radical retropubic prostatectomy for prostate cancer: etiology and treatment. Urology 1993; 42(4):401.
58. Borland RN, Walsh PC: The management of rectal injury during radical retropubic prostatectomy. J Urol 1992; 147:905.
59. Catalona WJ, Bigg SW: Nerve-sparing radical prostatectomy: evaluation of results after 250 patients. J Urol 1989; 143:538.
60. Licht MR, Klein EA: Early hospital discharge after radical retropubic prostatectomy: impact on cost and complication rate. Urology 1994; 44:700.
61. Kerr LA, Zincke H: Radical retropubic prostatectomy for prostate cancer in the elderly and the young: complications and prognosis. Eur Urol 1994; 25:305.

62. Lu-Yao GL, McLerran D, Wasson J, Wennberg JE: An assessment of radical prostatectomy: time trends, geographic variation and outcomes. JAMA 1993; 269(20):2633.
63. Igel TC, Barrett DM, Segura J, et al: Perioperative and postoperative complications from bilateral pelvic lymphadenectomy and radical retropubic prostatectomy. J Urol 1987; 137:1189.
64. Cisek LJ, Walsh PC: Thromboembolic complications following radical retropubic prostatectomy. Influence of external sequential pneumatic compression devices. Urology 1993; 42(4):406.
65. Baker WH, Mahler DK, Foldes MS, et al: Pneumatic compression devices for prophylaxis of deep venous thrombosis (DVT). Am Surg 1986; 52(7):371–373.
66. Chandhoke PS, Gooding GA, Narayan P: Prospective randomized trial of warfarin and intermittent pneumatic leg compression as prophylaxis for postoperative deep venous thrombosis in major urologic surgery. J Urol 1992; 147(4): 1056.
67. Haas SB, Insall JN, Scuderi GR, et al: Pneumatic sequential-compression boots compared with aspirin prophylaxis of deep-vein thrombosis after total knee arthroplasty. J Bone Joint Surg 1990; 72(1):27.
68. Comerota AJ, Katz ML, White JV: Why does prophylaxis with external pneumatic compression for deep vein thrombosis fail? Am J Surg 1992; 164(3):265.
69. Fowler FJ, Barry MJ, Lu-Yao G, et al: Patient-reported complications and follow-up treatment after radical prostatectomy. The National Medicare Experience: 1988–1990 (Updated June 1993). Urology 1993; 42(6):622.
70. Jonler M, Messing EM, Rhodes PR, Bruskewitz RC: Sequelae of radical prostatectomy. Br J Urol 1994; 74:352.
71. Quilan DM, Epstein JI, Carter BS, Walsh PC. Sexual function following radical prostatectomy: influence of preservation of neurovascular bundles. J Urol 1991; 145:998.
72. Rossignol G, Leandri P, Gautier JR, et al: Radical retropubic prostatectomy: complications and quality of life (429 cases, 1983–1989). Eur Urol 1991; 19:186.
73. Reimer WG, Walsh PC: An anatomical approach to the surgical management of the dorsal vein and Santorini's plexus during radical retropubic surgery. J Urol 1979; 121:198.
74. Catalona WJ, Smith DS: 5-year tumor recurrence rates after anatomical radical retropubic prostatectomy for prostate cancer. J Urol 1994; 152:1837.
75. Partin AW, Yoo J, Carter HB, et al: The use of prostate specific antigen, clinical stage and Gleason score to predict pathological stage in men with localized prostate cancer. J Urol 1993; 150:110.

30

RADICAL PERINEAL PROSTATECTOMY

DAVID F. PAULSON, M.D.

The perineum should be called the "gateway to the prostate." Radical perineal prostatectomy is a precise surgical exercise conducted under direct vision with excellent hemostatic control, identification and preservation of local anatomic structures and, ultimately, reconstruction of the urinary tract with preservation of continence. Radical perineal prostatectomy offers surgical control of prostatic malignancy equivalent to radical retropubic surgery, with certain advantages. Perineal prostatoseminal vesiculectomy has the advantage of providing a relatively avascular field, and excellent exposure for reconstruction of the urethrovesical junction and dependent postoperative drainage. The principal disadvantage of perineal prostatoseminal vesiculectomy is that this approach does not provide simultaneous exposure of the pelvic lymphatic drainage. Thus, two incisions are necessary if the patient elects radical perineal prostatectomy and requires a staging pelvic lymphadenectomy. However, the current practice of diagnosing prostatic carcinoma primarily on the basis of prostate-specific antigen (PSA) –driven biopsies, and the information that is available regarding the incidence of pelvic lymphatic spread as a function of Gleason grade of the biopsy specimen and the prebiopsy PSA, have reduced the necessity for staging pelvic lymphadenectomy. Potency-preserving surgery can be accomplished by the perineal route, although preservation of the periprostatic neurovascular plexus may be more difficult through the perineum than via the retropubic approach. Ankylosis of the hips or previous open prostatic surgery, which scars the bladder and prostate in the pelvis, complicating reconstruction at the urethrovesicle junction, may be a contraindication to perineal prostatectomy. The patient who is massively obese may have compromised diaphragmatic movement when placed in the exaggerated lithotomy position such that adequate ventilation cannot be maintained without excessively high pulmonary ventilation pressures.

PREOPERATIVE PREPARATION OF PATIENT

It is our current policy to use a GoLYTELY bowel preparation the day before surgery, combining this with oral antibiotics on the night before surgery. On the morning of surgery the patient receives an antibiotic enema several hours prior to entry into the operating room. No other preoperative preparation is necessary. The average patient loses approximately 5 to 8 pounds in fluid with the GoLYTELY preparation. This preparation can be conducted in-house or in an outpatient setting, depending upon the cardiovascular status of the patient and his ability to manage himself in the outpatient setting.

POSITIONING

Perineal prostatectomy is accomplished with the patient in an exaggerated lithotomy position. To achieve this, the sacrum is brought to the edge of the table, the buttocks extending several inches over the end of the operating table. The sacrum is elevated and placed on folded blankets or padding. The legs are then rotated towards the patient's head, lateral to the patient's torso. With the sacrum supported on appropriate soft padding, the weight of the patient is borne across the shoulder blades and the position is not supported by tension on the patient's extended lower extremities. With correct positioning, the perineum is parallel to the floor and optimum exposure is accomplished (Fig. 30–1).

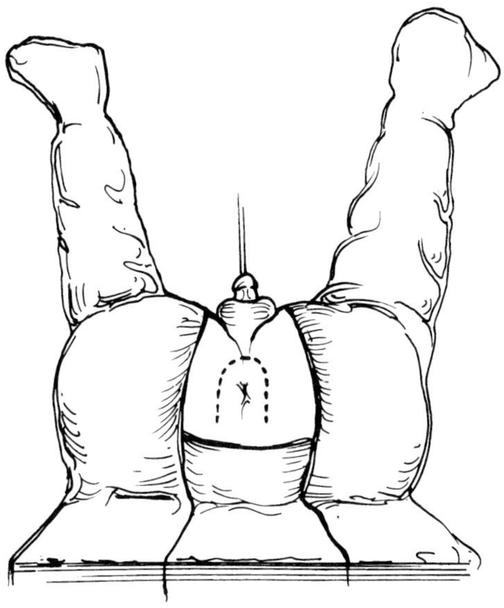

FIGURE 30–1. Exaggerated lithotomy position for radical perineal prostatectomy with line of incision indicated.

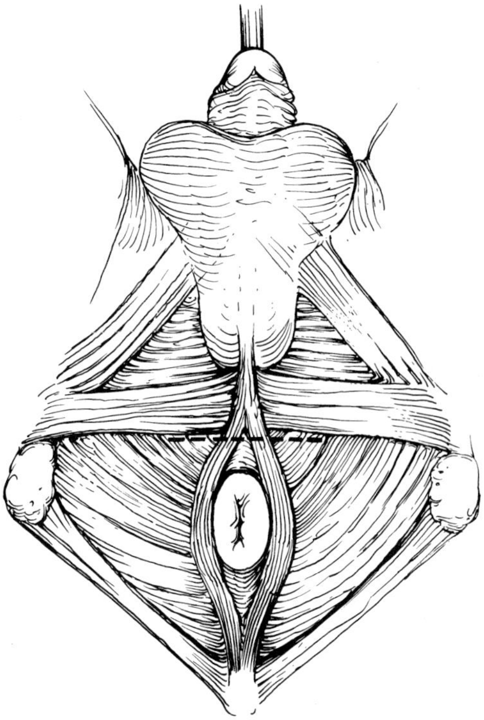

FIGURE 30–2. A *dotted line* drawn between the ischial tuberosities separates the anterior and posterior perineal triangles. The dissection carried out during radical perineal prostatectomy is conducted in the anterior urogenital triangle. A portion of the anterior urogenital triangle is filled by the urogenital diaphragm. The intent of the surgeon should be to approach the prostate beneath the posterior aspect of the urogenital diaphragm.

UNDERSTANDING PERINEAL ANATOMY

The perineum is defined as that area existing between the thighs and extending from the coccyx to the pubis. It is the external aspect of the pelvic outlet, the superior boundary being the levator ani. The lower, or perineal, surface of the levator ani forms the upper boundary of the perineum. Both the anal and the urogenital canal exit through the levator ani, presenting on the perineal surface. The surgeon may view the perineum as divisible into an anterior and posterior triangle, each segment divided by a transverse line that passes just anterior to the ischial tuberosities in front of the anal canal. The urologic surgeon is concerned only with the anterior perineal triangle, which is termed "the urogenital triangle" (Fig. 30–2). The anterior portion of the urogenital triangle contains a fibromuscular septum, the urogenital diaphragm, which extends across the anterior portion of the pelvic outlet below the levator ani. The prostate is approached posterior to the posterior edge of the urogenital diaphragm. If, during exposure of the prostate, the dissection is carried anteriorly into the urogenital diaphragm, the probability of damage to the external sphincteric mechanism, which accompanies the membranous urethra as it traverses the urogenital diaphragm, is high (Fig. 30–3). The urogenital diaphragm of the perineum shares, with the anal triangle, the levator ani, which forms its uppermost or cephalad boundary. Musculature that exists in the perineum below the levator ani has a common attachment in the midline between these two regions with the blending of two sets of muscles. The fibers that insert on the tip of the coccyx flow around the anus and insert on the perineal body, which represents the confluence of the central tendon and the transverse perineal musculature. When the "central tendon" is severed, the line of incision should be carried as close to the transverse perineal musculature as possible in order to preserve the fibers that flow around the anus and which are responsible for postoperative fecal continence. The appropriate line of incision is indicated by the dotted line in Figure 30–2. At the time of closure following completion of the radical perineal prostatectomy, these fibers are brought back to the central perineal body and fixed in place with multiple interrupted sutures. This is important in the preservation of rectal continence. Musculature that exists in the perineum below the levator ani has a common attachment in the midline between these two regions with the blending of the two sets of muscles, forming a fibromuscular mass referred to as the central tendon of the perineum. The central tendon is interposed between the anterior surface of the anal canal and the posterior surface of the urethra and must be sectioned in order to allow separation of the penile bulb from the anal canal. The ischial rectal fossa itself is a potential space that must be developed by the surgeon. It lies lateral to the anus, between the skin of the anal canal and the levator ani and posterior to the transverse perineal musculature, and is filled with fibrofatty tissue. Following incision of the skin overlying the

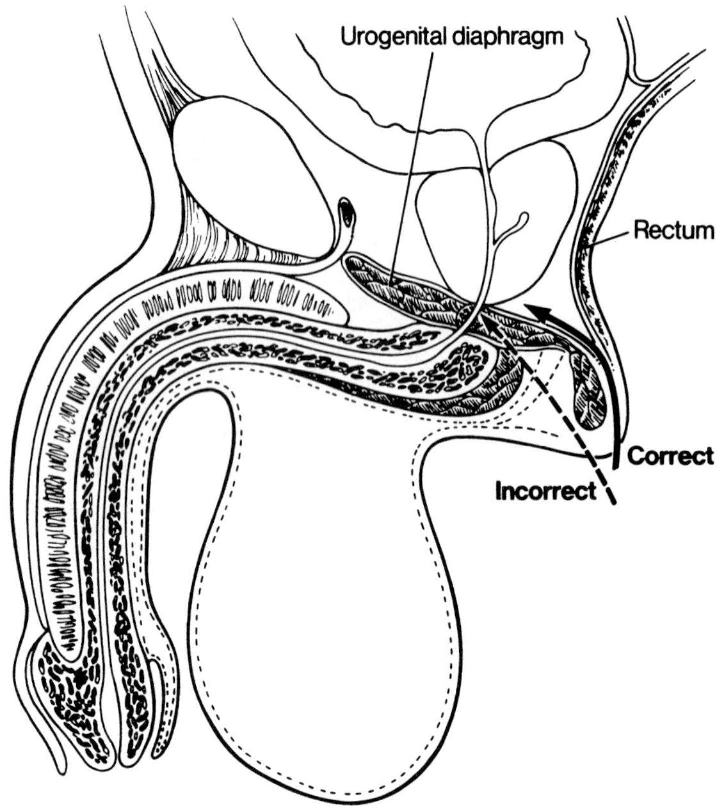
Urogenital diaphragm
Rectum
Correct
Incorrect

FIGURE 30–3. The *dotted line* indicates the incorrect line of dissection to the prostate. Note that the correct line of incision is beneath the anal sphincter and beneath the posterior margin of the urogenital diaphragm. Dissection through the urogenital diaphragm risks injury to the membranous urethra and the distal urethral sphincter. (From Paulson DF: Radical perineal prostatectomy. *In* Wein AJ, Malkowicz SB [eds]: Controversies in the Management of Prostate Cancer, pp 4–16. Philadelphia, CoMed Communications, 1992, with permission.)

perineum, the surgeon must make an incision through the outer condensation of fibrofatty tissue in order to enter this perineal space. This fibrofatty tissue is termed the superficial perineal fascia. After the surgical space has been created in the ischiorectal fossa, traction is placed on the anterior rectal wall. Palpating the taut rectal wall, the surgeon can identify a defect anterior to the rectal wall, beneath the central tendon, about 6 cm from the anal verge. A finger is placed through this defect and the central tendon severed with cautery as described above. This maneuver will expose the anterior rectal wall and the beginning of the rectourethralis.

Following the division of the central tendon, the surgeon should identify the anterior rectal fascia, as following this fascia on either side of the rectourethralis (Fig. 30–4) provides a secure highway through the perineum to the prostate with little risk of damage to the urogenital diaphragm or the rectum. The rectourethralis itself is a confluence of fibers with the levator ani that blend with the muscular walls of the rectum itself. Some of the longitudinal smooth muscle fibers from the anterior surface of the rectum leave the rectal wall to run upon the anterior surface of the levator ani where they pass forward to attach to the urethra, constituting the rectourethralis. When exposing the prostate, the rectourethralis must be either separated in the midline or divided completely in order to displace the rectum posteriorly. When exposing the prostate in the perineum, the surgeon should recognize the posterior aspect of the urogenital diaphragm, understanding that the correct approach to the apex of the prostate is cephalad to the transverse perineal musculature. Postprostatectomy uri-

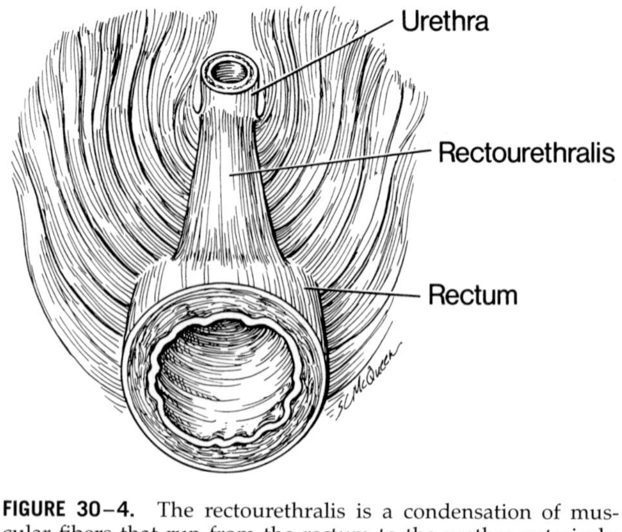
Urethra
Rectourethralis
Rectum

FIGURE 30–4. The rectourethralis is a condensation of muscular fibers that run from the rectum to the urethra anteriorly. It is variable in a cephalad caudad direction and is always in the midline. A surgical space may be created on each side of the rectourethralis, all the way to the prostate itself. (From Paulson DF: Radical perineal prostatectomy. *In* Wein AJ, Malkowicz SB [eds]: Controversies in the Management of Prostate Cancer, pp 4–16. Philadelphia, CoMed Communications, 1992, with permission.)

nary continence is dependent, in large portion, on the musculature of the membranous urethra as it exits through the urogenital diaphragm (or transverse perineal musculature). Improper perineal approach to the prostate may induce the surgeon to dissect within rather than cephalad to the urogenital diaphragm. In doing so, the membranous urethra may be fragmented, resulting in damage to a portion of the sphincteric mechanism, which is necessary for continence.

RADICAL PERINEAL PROSTATECTOMY

Exposure of Prostate

The surgeon who fully understands the perineal anatomy is prepared to perform a radical perineal prostatectomy. The patient is placed in an exaggerated lithotomy position. A Lowsley prostatic retractor is passed into the bladder through the urethra and the blades extended. If a Lowsley retractor cannot be passed into the bladder because of anatomic abnormalities of the bladder neck or because of false passage within the prostatic urethra, either a sound or the Lowsley retractor may be passed only to the apex of the prostate to identify the membranous urethra. It is not necessary to pass this instrument or sound into the bladder to expose the prostate through the perineum. After placement of the Lowsley retractor, the skin incision is made approximately 1 cm anterior to the anal verge and is curved posterolaterally within the medial borders of the ischial tuberosities (Fig. 30–5). The skin incision should be extended to the posterior anal margin. The superficial perineal fascia is incised

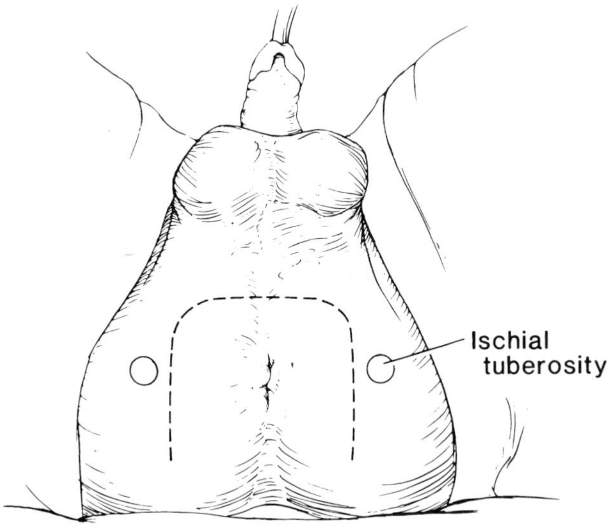
Ischial
tuberosity

FIGURE 30–5. Please note the placement of the skin incision. The skin incision is curved and carried behind the ischial tuberosities, behind the anus itself. This permits the rectum to be dropped far posteriorly and provides easy access to the prostate.

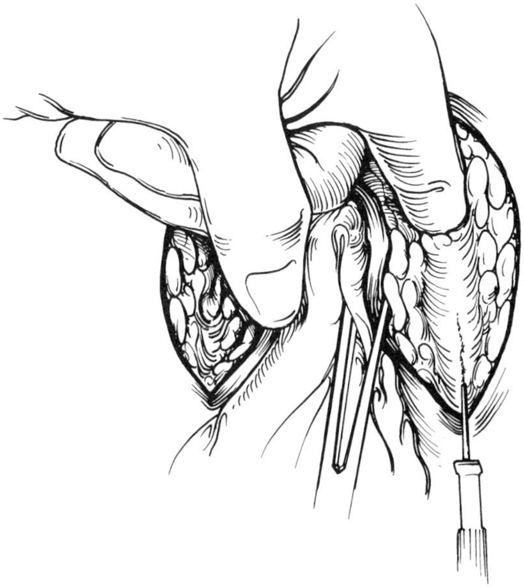

FIGURE 30–6. The surgical space and the ischial rectal fossa is developed by directing a finger directly towards the floor, pulling the finger towards the surgeon and cutting, with cutting cautery, down to the finger. This allows the rectum to be freed from its lateral fibrofatty attachments.

with cutting cautery and the surgical space within the ischial rectal fossa is developed. This is done by directing the finger directly to the floor beneath the patient, pulling the tissues toward the surgeon and cutting with cutting cautery (Fig. 30–6). After the ischial rectal space has been developed on either side, the surgeon may palpate the rectum in the midline and, by sliding his fingers anterior to the rectum, a defect can be created beneath the central tendon and anterior to the rectum. The central tendon and the associated muscular fibers, which are a portion of the superficial anal sphincter, are then incised at the margin of the skin incision (Fig. 30–7). This allows all of the muscles to remain intact and to be functional at the time of reconstruction following removal of the prostate.

At this time, an anterior retractor is put beneath the skin incision in the midline and the tissues retracted directly away from the floor of the operating room (Fig. 30–8). This places the rectourethralis and the rectum on tension, and the glistening fibers of the anterior rectal surface will be identified on either side of the rectourethralis. Using sharp dissection on both the right and left side, a space is created to either side of the midline, leaving the rectourethralis intact. This dissection is conducted by inverting the Metzenbaum scissors and creating a space just superior to the anterior surface of the rectum. At this time, a finger is placed into the rectum to pull the rectum posteriorly and digital blunt dissection is utilized to enlarge the potential space on the other side of the rectourethralis.

Although my previous publications have indicated that the rectourethralis is now to be divided, we have altered the procedure in such a way that

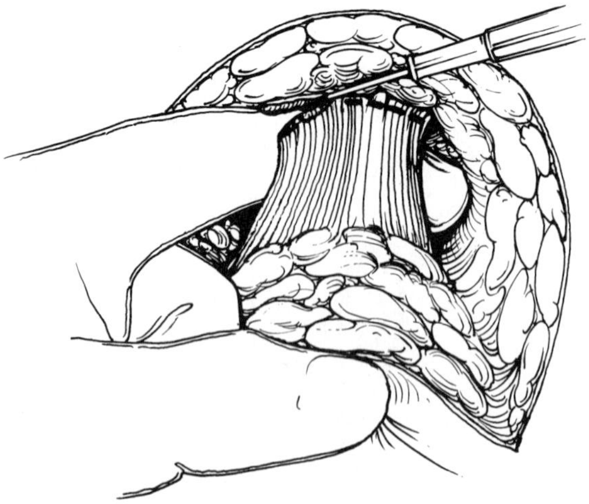

FIGURE 30–7. When the central tendon is incised, the margin of the transection should be at the skin margins rather than at the midportion of the central tendon. This allows the musculature of the central tendon to be reapproximated to the perineal body at the completion of the case.

only the very caudad fibers of the rectourethralis are divided. Then, using Metzenbaum scissors to spread the rectourethralis, a space is created in the midline between the rectourethralis fibers, which separate to the right and the left of the midline (Fig. 30–9). The tissues in the midportion of the rectourethralis are avascular and, by using the scissors for blunt dissection only, the curve of the rectum can be followed all the way to the level of the prostate.

At this point, the prostate is identified, the fibers overlying the prostate are incised and, with a bronchial dissector, a space is created lateral to the prostate and beneath the fibers of the rectourethralis, which merge with the fibers of the neurovascular fascia at the level of the prostate. These fibers are retracted to either side and this dissection then is carried to the reflection of the endopelvic fascia onto the prostate itself.

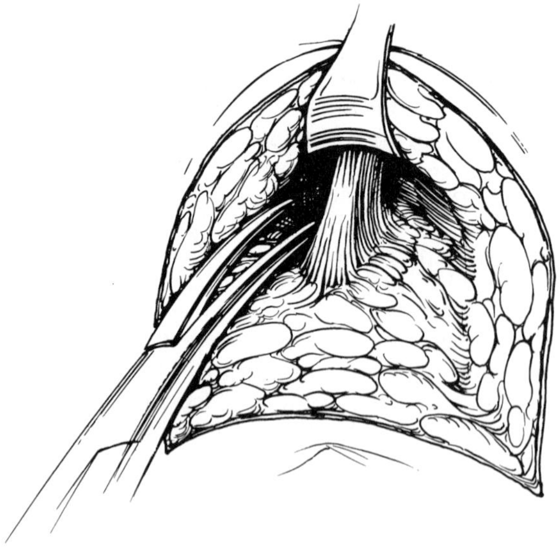

FIGURE 30–8. The rectourethralis may be placed on tension by pulling directly upwards with an anterior retractor and, placing a finger in the rectum, pulling the rectum posteriorly. The finger in the rectum is not used to identify the anterior rectal surface. The space on either side of the rectourethralis can be bluntly dissected to the level of the prostate. The anterior rectal surface will appear as a white glistening fascia.

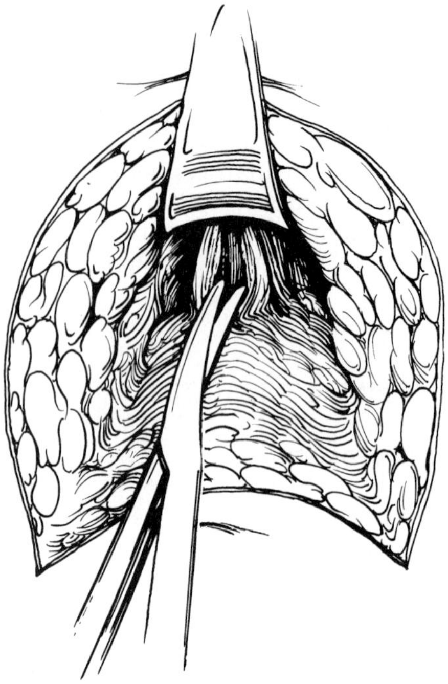

FIGURE 30–9. The rectourethralis is no longer totally divided but the rectourethralis fibers are split in the midline. Using curved Metzenbaum scissors, the rectourethralis can be separated all the way to the level of the prostate. This protects the anterior rectal surface and allows curved retractors to be placed beneath the rectourethralis, lateral to the prostate itself.

Baby Deaver retractors are utilized to separate the two leaves of the rectourethralis. If the rectourethralis and the associated neurovascular fascia do not dissect freely from the prostate, the rectourethralis and the associated neurovascular fibers are cut away and carried with the specimen. A weighted posterior retractor is then placed on top of the rectum and those rectal fibers that are attached to the fascia overlying the prostate are cut at the base of the prostate. This dissection is then carried on top of the anterior rectal fibers and outside Denonvilliers' fascia past the junction of the seminal vesicles and prostate.

Attention is now turned to the apex of the prostate. The fibromuscular fibers overlying the urethra at the apex of the prostate are sharply divided and, with blunt dissection, the apex of the prostate is displaced from the urethra. The vascular structures and lymphatics that egress from the apex of the prostate on either side of the urethra are separated from the urethra (Fig. 30–10). These structures then may be sharply divided or they may be controlled with cutting cautery prior to cutting. At this time,

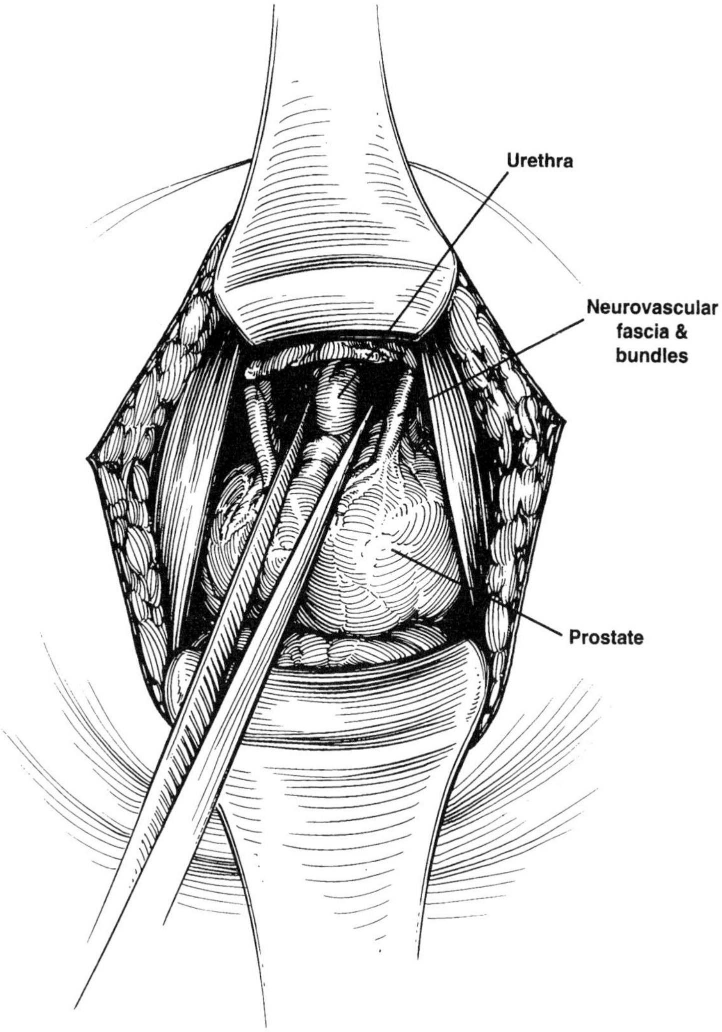
Urethra
Neurovascular fascia & bundles
Prostate

FIGURE 30–10. The urethra may be identified at its point of exit from the apex of the prostate. The lymphatics and vasculature, including the neurovascular fibers, may be separated at this point from the urethra itself. Approximately 1 cm or more of the urethra may be mobilized and the urethra may be safely transected at the level of the prostate. This tissue, when monitored by frozen section, has never proven to be positive. (From Paulson DF: Radical perineal prostatectomy. *In* Marshall FF [ed]: Textbook of Operative Urology. Philadelphia, WB Saunders Co, 1966, with permission.)

the surgeon may pass a finger on either side of the exposed urethra, curving the finger posteriorly as the dissection is carried beneath the dorsal venous complex to the level of the bladder anteriorly. Often this dissection can be enhanced by grasping the prostate at the apex following division of the urethra at the apex of the prostate and the prostate retracted away from the bladder neck.

With blunt digital dissection, the prostate can be separated from the detrusor fibers on either side of the midline. As the prostate is dissected from the anterior bladder neck, a "horse-collar" of bladder neck fibers at the level of bladder neck may be identified and preserved (Fig. 30–11). At this point the superior half of the urethra at the level of the bladder neck is severed. The Young tractor is then withdrawn and a Foley catheter or Penrose drain is passed through the prostatic urethra, being brought out superiorly between the line of incision at the level of the bladder neck and used for traction.

Before the prostate is completely cut away from the bladder neck, a tacking suture is placed in the bladder neck in order to ensure that it can be easily identified at the completion of the prostatectomy for reconstructive purposes.

Prior to complete division of the posterior portion of the urethra, using right-angle scissors, a plane is developed on either side of the posterior bladder neck between the prostate and the urethra. Right-angle scissors are then passed beneath the posterior bladder neck and the bladder neck divided. This allows the bladder to retract into the pelvis.

Following division of the posterior bladder neck, the glistening seminal vesicles should be evident beneath the posterior aspect of the bladder musculature. Should they not be readily apparent, with right-angle scissors, the surgeon should dissect in the midline until they are identified. Sharp dissection should allow the surgeon to expose the ampulla of the vas deferens. As the rectum has been previously separated from the posterior aspect of Denonvilliers' fascia behind the seminal vesicles, a finger may be placed in this surgical space to prevent damage to the rectum.

Once the seminal vesicles and ampulla of the vas deferens have been identified, using right-angle

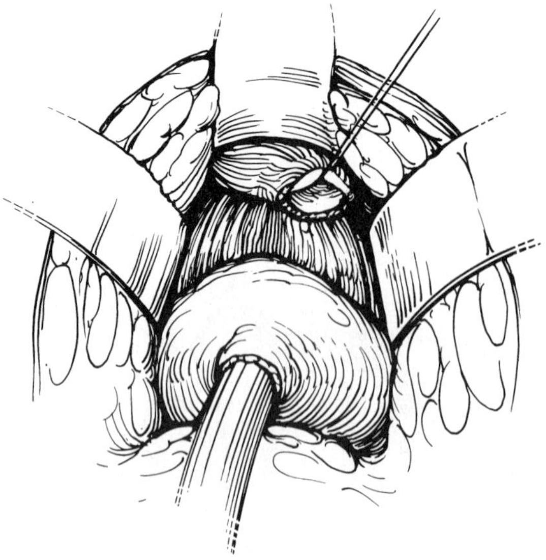

FIGURE 30–11. As the prostate is dissected from the urethra on both sides of the prostatovesical junction, a "horse-collar" of bladder neck fibers will be identified surrounding the egress of the urethra into the prostate. At this point the superior half of the urethra at the level of the bladder neck is transected, the bladder-side margin being tagged with 0 chromic catgut.

scissors, the fibromuscular tissue to the right and the left of the midline may be sharply cut away, bleeding points being controlled with electrocoagulation. At this point, the prostate is retained in place by the posterolateral extension of Denonvilliers' fascia behind the seminal vesicles, by the seminal vesicles themselves, and posterolaterally on the right and left side by the fibrovascular pedicles of the prostate itself (Fig. 30–12).

While protecting the rectum by a finger placed behind the prostate, a right-angle clamp is placed in the space between the seminal vesicles medially and the fibrovascular pedicle laterally. The pedicles may be controlled with surgical clips prior to division.

Following division of the vascular pedicles laterally, the specimen is attached only by the seminal vesicles and the posterior layer of Denonvilliers' fascia. The prostate may now be elevated within the perineum and the fascia overlying the seminal vesicles posteriorly incised transversely. The seminal vesicles are now removed with the specimen, using alternating sharp and blunt dissection. It is not necessary to remove the seminal vesicles in

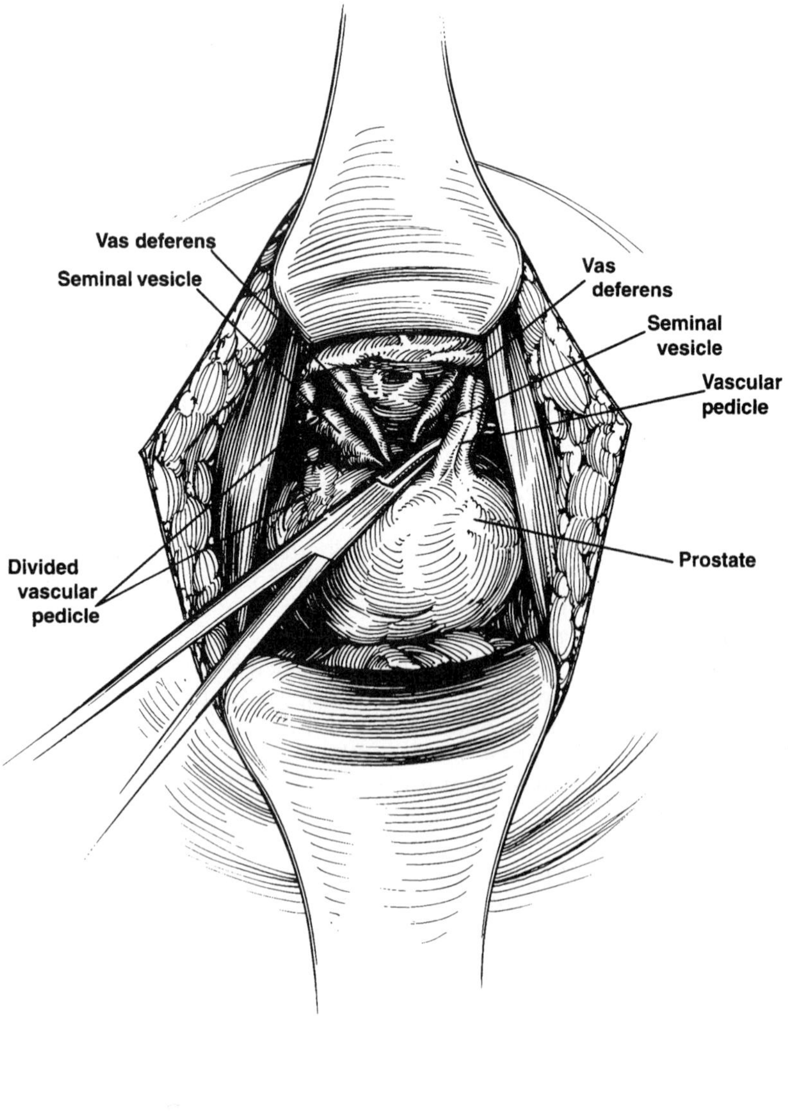
Vas deferens
Seminal vesicle
Vas deferens
Seminal vesicle
Vascular pedicle
Divided vascular pedicle
Prostate

FIGURE 30–12. By cutting directly posteriorly after the posterior urethra has been severed, the surgeon will encounter the seminal vesicles and vas deferens; these should be fully exposed in the midline. All tissues lateral to the seminal vesicles enclose portions of the vasculature to the prostate and may be controlled either by surgical clips or by electrocautery. (From Paulson DF: Radical perineal prostatectomy. *In* Marshall FF [ed]: Textbook of Operative Urology. Philadelphia, WB Saunders Co, 1966, with permission.)

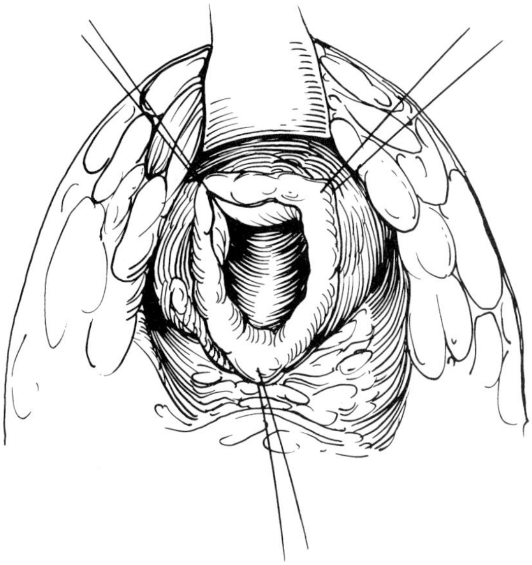

FIGURE 30–13. Sutures of 2-0 Monocryl are placed in the urethra at the 1-, 5-, 7-, and 11-o'clock positions; the sutures placed at the 5- and 7-o'clock positions are brought into the bladder neck at the 11- and 1-o'clock positions. The sutures placed in the urethra at the 11- and 12-o'clock positions are brought down and placed in the bladder neck at the 5- and 7-o'clock positions once the racket handle closure is completed.

their entirety, but they may be controlled after approximately 2 to 3 cm of seminal vesicular length has been identified. The patient side of the seminal vesicle may be controlled with surgical clips, the seminal vesicles and vas deferens divided, and the specimen removed.

After ascertaining that hemostasis is secure, continuity must be established between the reconstructed bladder neck and the membranous urethra. Bladder neck margins now are taken. An Allis clamp is placed on the bladder neck at the 6-o'clock position and the specimen pulled toward the perineal wound. Using right-angle scissors, a 0.5-cm margin of bladder neck is excised from the 6- to 12-o'clock position on both the left and the right side.

At this point, the mucosa of the bladder is brought up to the detrusor margin between the 9- to 12- to 3-o'clock positions using interlocking 0000 Monocryl suture material. At the 11:30 and 12:30 positions outside-in inside-out mattress sutures of 0 Monocryl are placed at the bladder neck and the tags left long. These will later be brought through the perineum to support the direct anastomosis. A Foley catheter now is passed through the urethra. Sutures of 00 Monocryl are placed posteriorly at the 5- and 7-o'clock positions in the urethra and brought down into the reconstructed bladder neck at the 11- and 1-o'clock positions. Sutures are then placed in the urethra at the 11- and 1-o'clock positions to be later placed in the reconstructed bladder neck (Fig. 30–13).

A racket handle closure then is conducted from the 6- to 12-o'clock positions with 0 Monocryl. The bladder neck is closed tightly around an 18-French Foley catheter. The last two stitches are left long to be brought through the perineum as vest sutures. The previously placed 2-0 Monocryl sutures placed into the urethra at the 11- and 1-o'clock positions now are brought into the reconstructed bladder neck on either side of the midline at the 6-o'clock position. The 2-0 sutures are then tied down to bring the urethra to the reconstructed bladder neck. Using a large surgeon's needle, the two anterior and two posterior vests are brought through the perineum on either side of the urethra and tied securely over the perineal body. The rectum is checked for defects. Drainage is established using a Penrose drain that is brought out the lateral aspect of the incision.

The previously transected muscular segment of the central tendon is brought to the perineal body in the midline and fixed with several interrupted sutures of 2-0 Monocryl. The perineum is closed with vertical mattress sutures of 2-0 chromic catgut.

The patient may be fed the next morning and mobilized within 12 hours of surgery. Discharge occurs 48 to 72 hours after surgery and after removal of the drain. The Foley catheter is left indwelling for 17 to 21 days depending on the day of discharge.

REFERENCES

1. Paulson DF: Radical perineal prostatectomy. Urol Clin North Am 1980; 7:847–854.
2. Paulson DF: Perineal prostatectomy. *In* Walsh PC, Retik AB, Stamey TA, Vaughan ED Jr (eds): Campbell's Urology, 6th edition, pp 2887–2897. Philadelphia, WB Saunders Co, 1992.
3. Paulson DF: Surgery for prostate: the perineal approach. *In* Droller MJ (ed): Genitourinary Surgery, pp 697–702, St Louis, CV Mosby, 1992.
4. Hollingshead WH: Anatomy for Surgeons, 2nd edition. New York, Harper & Row, 1971.
5. Frazier HA, Robertson JE, Paulson DF: Radical prostatectomy: the pros and cons of the perineal vs. retropubic approach. J Urol 1992; 147:888–890.
6. Paulson DF: Radical perineal prostatectomy. *In* Wein AJ, Malkowicz SF (eds): Controversies in the Management of Prostate Cancer, pp 4–16. Philadelphia, CoMed Communications, 1992.
7. Paulson DF, Frazier HA: Radical Prostatectomy. *In* Krane RJ, Siroky MB, Fitzpatrick JM (eds): Clinical Urology, pp 1020–1047. Philadelphia, JB Lippincott Co, 1994.
8. Paulson DF: Impact of radical prostatectomy in the management of clinically localized disease. J Urol 1994; 152: 1826–1830.
9. Paulson DF: Long term results of radical perineal prostatectomy. Eur Urol 1995; 27(Suppl 2):35–40.

31

SEMINAL VESICLES: DIAGNOSIS, STAGING, SURGERY, MANAGEMENT, AND PROGNOSIS

W. BEDFORD WATERS, M.D. *and* BRUCE W. LINDGREN, M.D.

The seminal vesicles are affected by disease processes ranging from congenital malformations to infections to neoplasms. Benign tumors of the seminal vesicles occur more frequently than malignancies and include papillary adenomas, cystadenomas, fibromas, and leiomyomas. Adenocarcinoma of the prostate is the most common malignant tumor to involve the seminal vesicles, although many others have been reported to involve the seminal vesicles secondarily. Although rare, primary malignancies of the seminal vesicles do occur. Carcinomas, sarcomas, and germ cell tumors have all been reported. Surgery for isolated seminal vesicle disease is uncommon and, when required, provides a technical challenge. Those disease processes that affect the seminal vesicles most commonly and are clinically most relevant are discussed in this chapter.

ANATOMY AND PHYSIOLOGY

The ureters each develop as a bud of the mesonephric duct in the fourth week of gestation. Arising as separate dorsolateral bulbous swellings of the distal mesonephric duct, the seminal vesicles appear at the twelfth to thirteenth week of gestation[1,2] (Fig. 31–1). Each seminal vesicle then joins the dilated ampulla of the vas deferens (mesonephric duct) to form the ejaculatory duct, which then courses through the prostate to empty into the prostatic urethra just lateral to the verumontanum. Anomalous connections between these structures occur as a result of their common origins. It has been reported that 50% of ectopic ureters in the male empty into the posterior urethra and another 30% drain into the ipsilateral seminal vesicle.[1]

The normal adult seminal vesicle is 5 to 10 cm long and 3 to 5 cm in diameter. The right seminal vesicle is larger than the left in roughly one third of men, and the size of both decreases with age.[1,2] The major arterial supply to the seminal vesicles arises as a branch of the vesiculodeferential artery, a branch of the umbilical artery that may also receive an accessory communicating vessel from the inferior vesicle artery. Lymphatic drainage is to the external and internal iliac nodes; the vesiculodeferential veins and inferior vesicle plexus receive venous drainage from the seminal vesicles. Innervation is via adrenergic fibers from the hypogastric nerve.[1,2]

The epithelial lining of the seminal vesicles consists of enfoldings of columnar and cuboidal epithelium, and three types of branching patterns of the ducts have been described. The muscularis consists of two layers: an outer longitudinal and an inner circular layer.[2]

An average of 2.5 ml of the ejaculate is produced by the seminal vesicles. Although the exact functional contribution of the seminal vesicles remains unknown, a number of components have been identified as having originated in the seminal vesicles, including fructose (and other carbohydrates); prostaglandins A, B, E, and F; and a coagulation factor.[2]

CYSTS OF THE SEMINAL VESICLES

Cysts of the seminal vesicles are rare. They may represent localized dilatations of one or several convolutions or generalized dilatation of the entire gland. They are usually unilocular, but the multilocular variety does occur. The cysts may or may

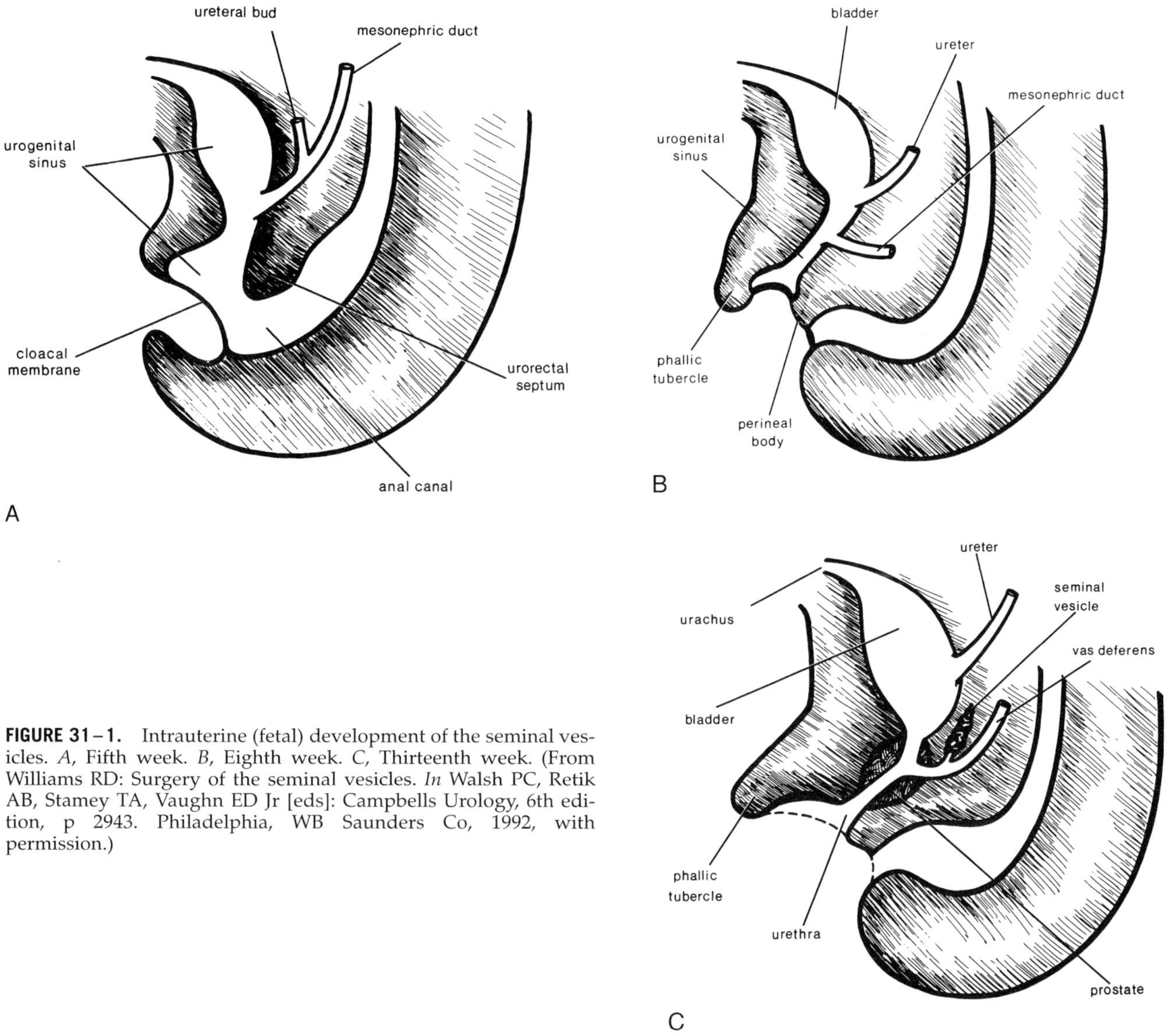
ureteral bud
mesonephric duct
urogenital sinus
cloacal membrane
urorectal septum
anal canal
A
bladder
ureter
mesonephric duct
urogenital sinus
phallic tubercle
perineal body
B
ureter
seminal vesicle
urachus
vas deferens
bladder
phallic tubercle
urethra
prostate
C

FIGURE 31–1. Intrauterine (fetal) development of the seminal vesicles. *A*, Fifth week. *B*, Eighth week. *C*, Thirteenth week. (From Williams RD: Surgery of the seminal vesicles. *In* Walsh PC, Retik AB, Stamey TA, Vaughn ED Jr [eds]: Campbells Urology, 6th edition, p 2943. Philadelphia, WB Saunders Co, 1992, with permission.)

not be infected. Seminal vesicle cysts are congenital or acquired. The congenital type has been associated with unilateral renal agenesis in many instances[3,4] (Figs. 31–2 and 31–3). Maldevelopment of the distal mesonephric duct causes atresia of the ejaculatory duct and seminal vesicle cyst formation as well as failure of development of the ureteral bud, which results in renal agenesis or dysgenesis. In one series, 12 of 13 patients with seminal vesicle cysts had ipsilateral renal anomalies, including agenesis, hypoplasia, complete duplication, and atrophy.[5] If the ureter buds too far cephalad, ectopic ureteral insertion into mesonephric duct derivatives (e.g., bladder neck, prostatic urethra, ejaculatory duct, seminal vesicle) can occur.[5] Cysts of the seminal vesicles may also be seen in patients with autosomal dominant polycystic kidney disease (Fig. 31–4). Seminal vesicle cysts are usually less than 5 cm in diameter but can be as large as 15 cm.[6] The ureter and trigone on the same side may be absent,[7,8] but a fibrous band[7,8] and a dilated blind-ending ureter have been found. The acquired type of cyst is probably the result of partial or complete obstruction of the ejaculatory duct.

Patients usually present at a time of peak sexual activity (second or third decade) with symptoms of dysuria, frequency of urination, difficult urination, perineal pain aggravated by defecation, and painful ejaculation, or they may be asymptomatic and present for evaluation of infertility. Hematospermia is rarely described.

Cystoscopically, the floor of the bladder may be elevated. The ureteral orifice on the affected side may be absent with unilateral trigone, or impossible to visualize. When associated with an absent ureteral orifice, ectopic ureteral insertion is suggested.[5] The lower ureter on the affected side may be deviated medially.[9]

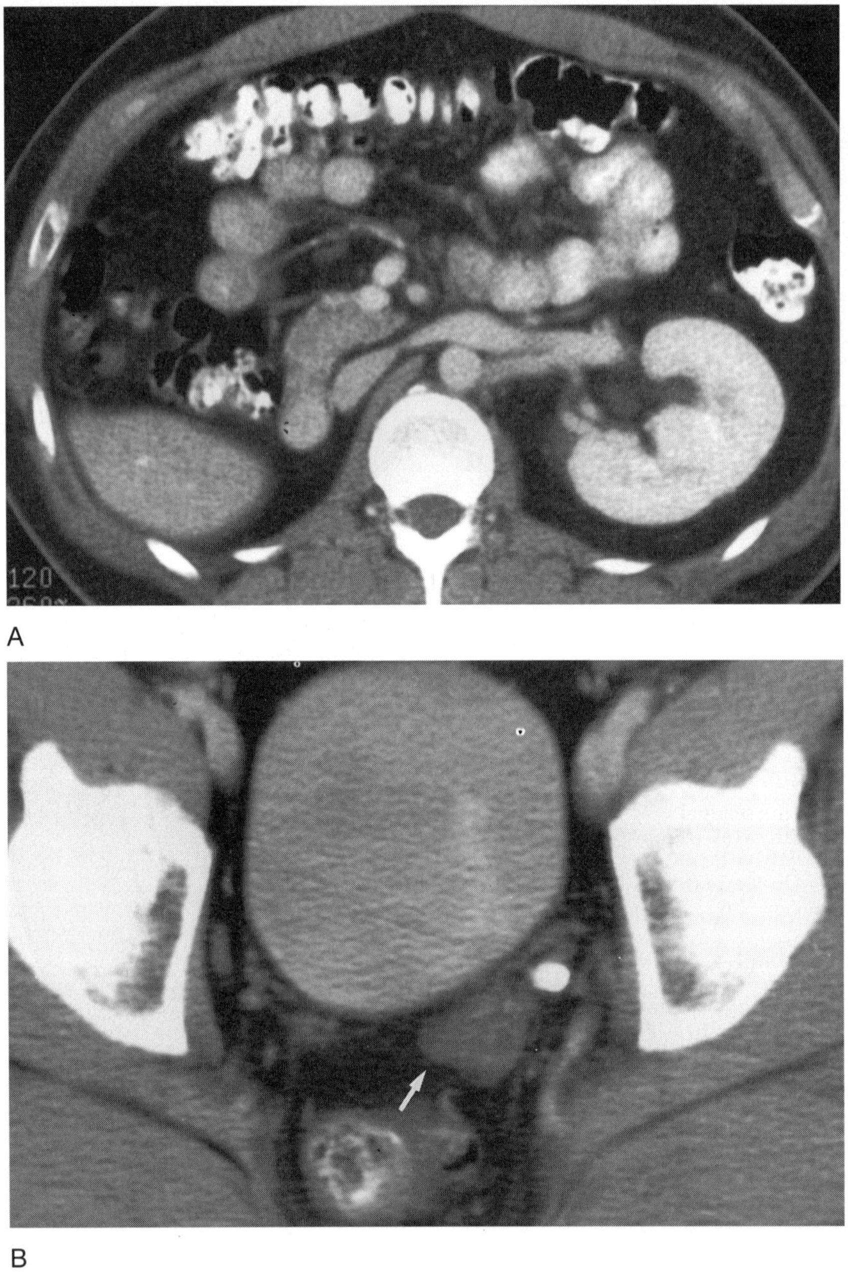
A
B

FIGURE 31–2. Agenesis of the kidney and ipsilateral seminal vesicle. *A*, CT image showing absence of the right kidney and hypertrophy of the left kidney. *B*, CT image showing a left seminal vesicle (arrow) but agenesis of the right seminal vesicle. (Courtesy of Terrance C. Demos, M.D., and Carl Kalbhen, M.D.)

BENIGN TUMORS OF THE SEMINAL VESICLES

Tumors of the seminal vesicles occur quite rarely, with benign tumors somewhat more common than malignant ones. Although symptoms such as hematuria, dysuria, urinary retention, and pain on defecation or micturition may occur, these tumors are diagnosed uncommonly because they are usually asymptomatic, are found on routine physical examination only as a supraprostatic or abdominal mass, and until recently were poorly delineated by available imaging studies.

Several histologic types of benign tumors have been reported to date. One of the most common consists of a cystic mass containing distinct epithelial and stromal components. It has been reported by different names, such as cystadenoma, benign mesenchymoma, and cystic epithelial-stromal tumor, but the term "cystadenoma" has been advocated by several authors.[10–12] Other histologic types of benign tumors include leiomyoma, papillary adenoma, fibroma, and amyloidosis.[1,13,14]

PRIMARY MALIGNANT TUMORS OF THE SEMINAL VESICLES

Primary malignancies of the seminal vesicles are rare, with a total of about 50 reported. A good deal of confusion exists in the literature with regard to primary tumors of the seminal vesicles. This is primarily due to the rarity of these tumors and the

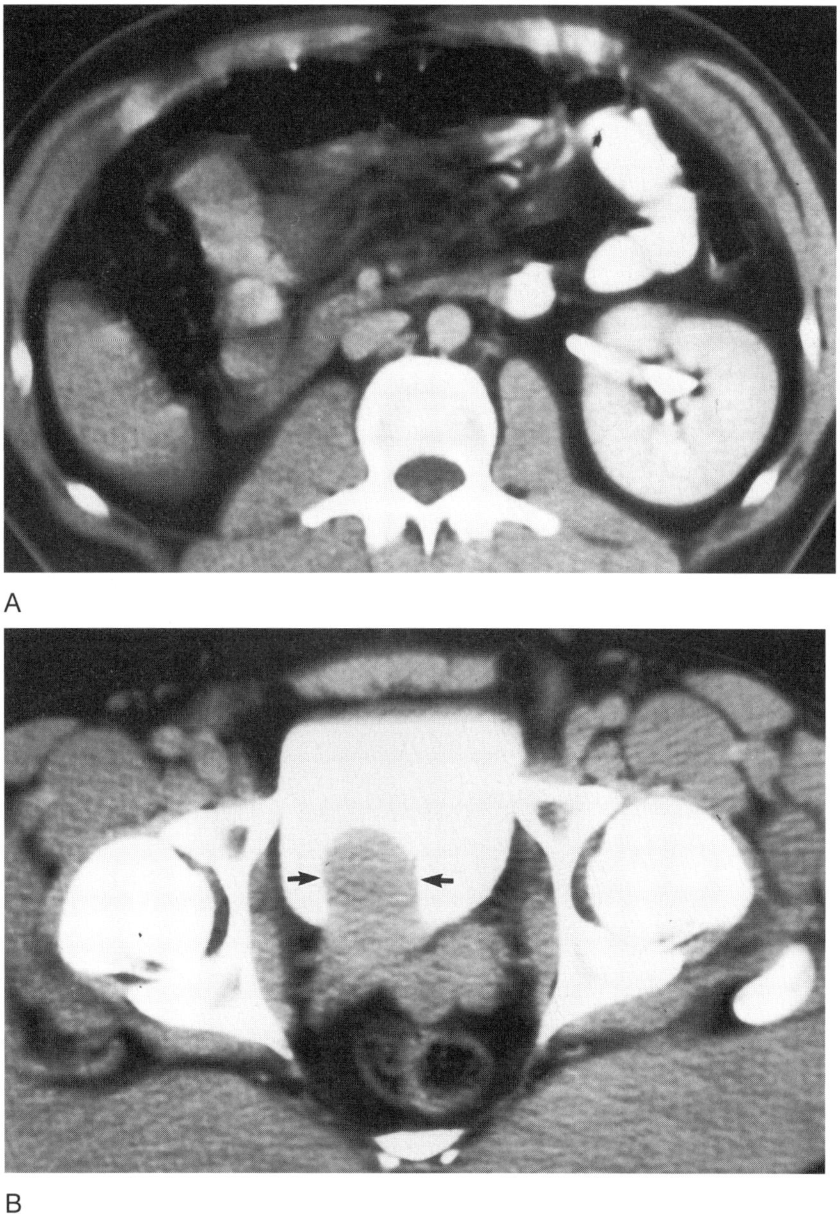
A
B

FIGURE 31–3. Agenesis of kidney and seminal vesicle cyst containing high-density fluid. *A*, CT image showing absence of the right kidney. *B*, CT image showing a high-attenuation seminal vesicle cyst (arrows) deforming the urinary bladder. (Courtesy of Terrance C. Demos, M.D., and Carl Kalbhen, M.D.)

lack of clear documentation in these reports. Adenocarcinomas are the more common malignant tumors arising in the seminal vesicles, with primary sarcomas of the seminal vesicles rare but documented. Many of the cases reported in the older literature either lack clear histologic descriptions or were characterized by large masses in the pelvis with gross involvement of contiguous organs, usually prostate. In light of these facts, Young and Davis believed that these tumors were best classified as "primary malignant tumors of the retrovesicle space."[15] In 1956, Lazarus presented a critical review of 20 previously reported cases, both carcinomas and sarcomas, and thought that only 7 qualified as true primary seminal vesicle tumors. He therefore agreed with Young and Davis that these tumors were best characterized as malignant tumors of the retrovesicle space.[16]

In 1956, Dalgaard and Giertsen reviewed previously reported cases of primary adenocarcinomas of the seminal vesicles and established the criteria that, to be considered an adenocarcinoma arising primarily in the seminal vesicle, the tumor must be a papillary or anaplastic carcinoma localized primarily to the seminal vesicle and must not involve the prostate, and there must be no other primary tumor demonstrated.[17] Benson et al. reviewed 12 cases of carcinoma of the seminal vesicle in the tissue registry at the Mayo Clinic and applied the above criteria. In addition, they required that cases, especially anaplastic carcinomas, show some degree of mucin production to differentiate them from anaplastic tumors of prostatic origin. Applying these criteria, this group concluded that only 2 of their 12 cases, and 35 of all previously reported cases, were indeed primary adenocarcinomas of the

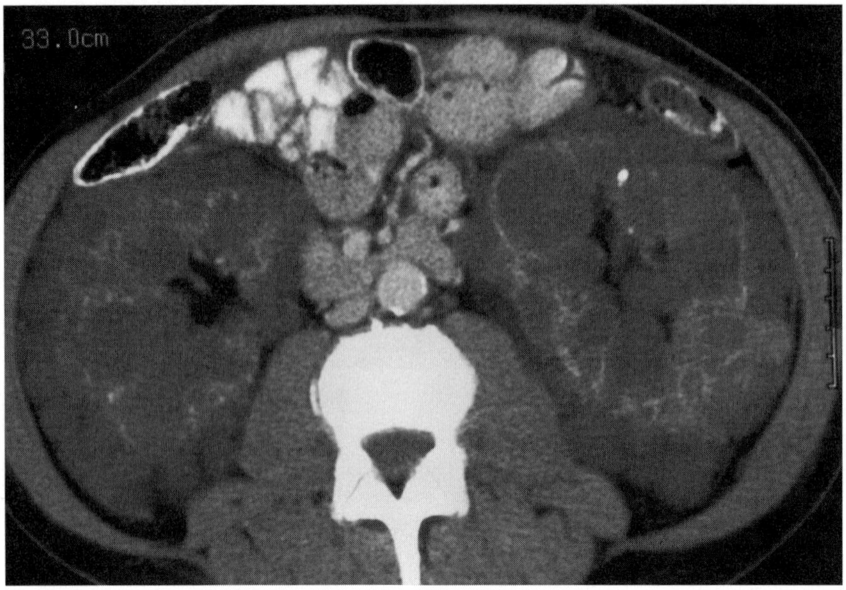
33.0cm

A

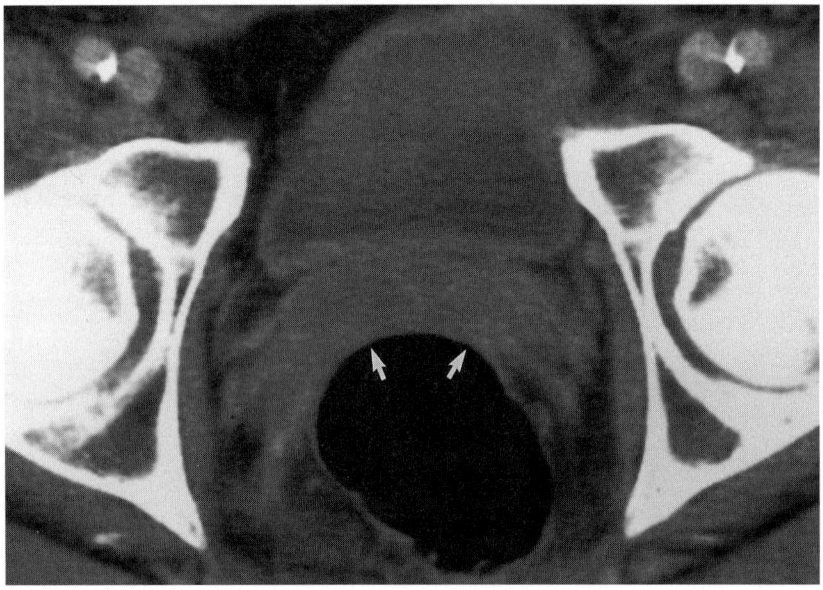

B

FIGURE 31–4. Polycystic kidneys and polycystic seminal vesicles. *A*, CT image showing markedly enlarged polycystic kidneys. *B*, CT image showing multiple large cysts in the seminal vesicles (arrows). (Courtesy of Terrance C. Demos, M.D., and Carl Kalbhen, M.D.)

seminal vesicles.[18] This group also recommended that tumors in question be stained for prostate-specific antigen (PSA) and prostatic acid phosphatase. Seminal vesicle tumors would not stain for either of these. A negative result, however, would not establish the diagnosis with certainty because poorly differentiated prostatic tumors may also be negative. Staining for carcinoembryonic antigen (CEA) was also suggested as potentially helpful. In their experience, normal seminal vesicle and gastrointestinal epithelium stain positively for CEA, whereas prostatic tumors do not. Therefore, positive staining for CEA would suggest a tumor of seminal vesicle or gastrointestinal origin.[18] Mazur and associates, however, reported that in their experience neither normal seminal vesicle epithelium nor adenocarcinoma of the seminal vesicles stained positively for CEA, and believed that this criterion was not helpful in differentiating these tumors from those of prostatic origin.[19]

Tumors of the seminal vesicles have been reported in men ranging in age from 17 to 87,[20,21] but most commonly occur in men over the age of 50. Many different presenting symptoms have been reported to date, including hematuria, hematospermia, dysuria, urethrorrhagia, urethralgia, obstructive voiding symptoms/urinary retention, and an abdominal mass.[20–24] These tumors may also present as incidental findings, either at the time of surgery or as a mass confluent with or adjacent to the prostate on routine digital rectal exam. Hemoptysis and shortness of breath secondary to pulmonary metastases from a seminal vesicle primary have also been reported as presenting complaints in one patient.[25] Physical examination of the patient with a seminal vesicle tumor is generally unremarkable with the exception of an abnormal digital rectal exam and/or an abdominal mass as stated previously. Evaluation of these patients with laboratory tests rarely gives insight into the etiology of the mass. Serum chemistry tests are usually normal; however, the rare patient with a primary seminal vesicle germ cell tumor may have an elevated β-human chorionic gonadotropin or α-fetoprotein level.[25] Serum PSA and acid phosphatase should be measured. An elevated level would raise the suspicion of prostatic adenocarcinoma rather than a primary seminal vesicle tumor. Elevation of CEA level has been reported in association with primary adenocarcinoma of the seminal vesicle.[21,26] Mild proteinuria or hematuria may be present on urinalysis.

RADIOLOGIC EVALUATION OF THE SEMINAL VESICLES

Before the availability of cross-sectional imaging modalities, the seminal vesicles could be directly imaged only by vasoseminal vesiculography (VSV). Abnormalities would occasionally be manifested indirectly on urography or cystourethrography. The introduction of ultrasonography, especially transrectal ultrasonography (TRUS), computed tomography (CT), and magnetic resonance imaging (MRI) now make it possible to image the normal and abnormal male seminal tract structures in a noninvasive fashion and with high resolution.[27]

The seminal vesicles are convoluted tubes that are obliquely oriented behind the bladder and above the prostate. They are usually oval in configuration, although they may be rounded or tubular.[28] They are widest in their midportions and then converge medially to join the vasa. Seminal vesicle symmetry is noted in only 67 to 78% of normal men on CT[28] or VSV.[29]

At autopsy, the normal seminal vesicle measures from 3.6 to 7.6 cm in length and from 1.2 to 2.4 cm in width. On CT, mean length has been given as 3.1 ± 0.5 cm and mean width as 1.5 ± 0.4 cm.[28] On TRUS, the combined length of the ampulla and the seminal vesicle exceeds 2.5 cm; the width varies from 0.7 to 1.5 cm.[30] The dimensions on VSV are slightly larger, probably because of the geometric magnification inherent in pelvic radiographs.[28]

The seminal vesicles are small in prepubertal boys. They are widest in the fifth and sixth decades, likely because of compression of the ejaculatory ducts by benign prostatic hyperplasia causing stasis and distention. They decrease in width and area (but not length) after 70 years of age.[28] There is no appreciable change in seminal vesicle dimensions following ejaculation.[31]

Imaging Modalities

The normal seminal vesicles have been imaged by the following techniques.

Vasoseminal Vesiculography

Vasoseminal vesiculography is also known as vasovesiculography. VSV is an invasive procedure that images structural changes in the seminal tract. It has lost most of its importance with the advent of ultrasound, TRUS, CT, and MRI and is mentioned for historical purposes only. The main indication for VSV currently is to confirm aplasia or occlusion of the vas and ejaculatory ducts in azoospermic men with normal spermatogenesis on testicular biopsy.[27]

Ultrasonography

Ultrasonography is a valuable imaging modality for diseases of the seminal vesicles. TRUS offers resolution superior to transabdominal ultrasonography and CT, but tissue penetration is limited with the high-frequency transducers employed.[27]

With TRUS, the patient is placed in a lateral decubitus position and the periprostatic seminal tract is imaged in axial and sagittal planes with transducers of 5.0 to 7.5 MHz. The normal seminal vesicles are symmetrically hypoechoic, have a few fine internal echoes or septations caused by their saccular convolutions, and are less echogenic than the prostate gland.[31]

The multiplanar capability of ultrasound often aids in determining the organ of origin of masses in the male pelvis; TRUS is particularly helpful in identifying and distinguishing seminal vesicle cysts from other masses (Fig. 31–5). TRUS also facilitates needle biopsy and drainage. The limitations of TRUS relate to the limited field of view of high-frequency transducers used for scanning and to its operator dependence.[31]

Computed Tomography

The seminal vesicles are easily identified in normal patients on CT as relatively symmetrical structures of soft tissue attenuation posterolateral to the urinary bladder and cephalad to the prostate, well delineated by surrounding periprostatic and perirectal fat. Although their orientation is somewhat related to distention of adjacent organs, they should be separated from the bladder by a triangular fat plane (seminal vesicle–bladder angle) with the patient in the supine position. This angle is obliterated with perivesicle extension of prostate or bladder tumors, but obliteration can occur if the patient is scanned in the prone position or if the rectum is overdistended.[27,32] Following abdominoperineal resection, the vesicles can shift posteriorly and simulate a presacral mass.

The only normal soft tissue densities that are imaged in the fat surrounding the seminal vesicles are the vasa, ureters, and pudendal veins. The latter

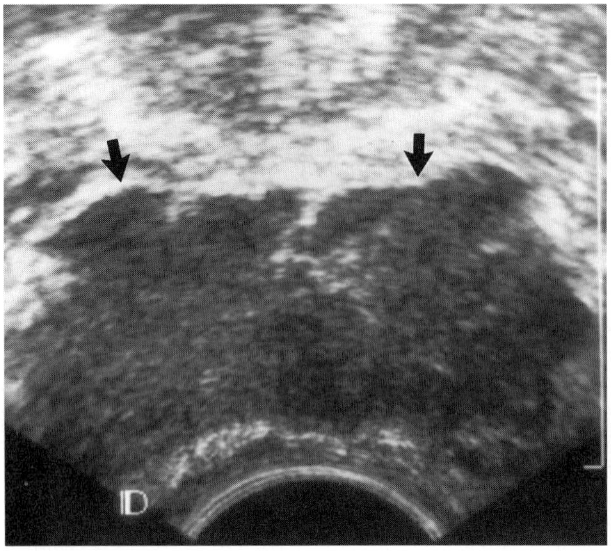

FIGURE 31–5. Prostate carcinoma with enlarged seminal vesicles (arrows) resulting from tumor invasion. Transrectal sonogram showing marked, symmetrical enlargement of both seminal vesicles, which are invaded by the prostate carcinoma. (Courtesy of Terrance C. Demos, M.D., and Carl Kalbhen, M.D.)

may be identified on the lateral aspects of the vesicles in the rectovesicle pouch.[27,28]

CT confirms the presence and size of the seminal vesicles and evaluates for cystic replacement or tumor invasion (Fig. 31–6). CT cannot depict internal vesicle morphology and is insensitive to early neoplastic involvement while contour and size are still normal. Imaging only transaxially may not be sufficient to determine the origin of a mass involving the seminal vesicles. In addition, CT imaging may be degraded by beam-hardening artifacts from the bony pelvis or a contrast-filled urinary bladder.[27]

Magnetic Resonance Imaging

The multiplanar capability of MRI and its high sensitivity to differences in tissue contrast make it superior to CT and TRUS in depicting the architecture of the seminal tract and delineating anatomic relations of pelvic organs.[33,34] Endorectal surface coil imaging further enhances spatial resolution.[33] Various pulse sequences facilitate tissue characterization and, in many instances, distinguish blood, fluid, fat, and tumor.[27]

On T1-weighted images (T1WI), the seminal vesicles exhibit an intermediate signal intensity (SI) equal to or greater than that of skeletal muscle and greater than that of urine. Both the convolutions of the vesicles and their low-intensity capsule are better imaged on T2-weighted images (T2WI), although contrast-enhanced vesicle walls may be seen on T1WI following gadolinium administration[27] (Fig. 31–7).

The SI of the seminal vesicles varies with age.[34] On T2WI it is less than that of fat or urine in prepubertal boys, greater than or similar to that of fat in men less than 70 years of age, and equal to or less than that of fat thereafter according to Secaf et al.,[34] who employed conventional body coil imaging. However, with the use of an endorectal coil and fast spin-echo T2WI techniques, the SI of seminal vesicle exceeds that of fat. The vas deferens and its ampulla, because they are thicker walled than the seminal vesicle, produce a low signal from the smooth muscle that can obscure the fact that these are basically hollow structures.[27]

Both radiation and endocrine therapy cause a decrease in size and change in appearance of the seminal vesicles. On T2WI, their SI becomes less than that of fat but remains higher than that of skeletal muscles.[27,34] Much of the imaging knowledge regarding the seminal tract derives from the intensive

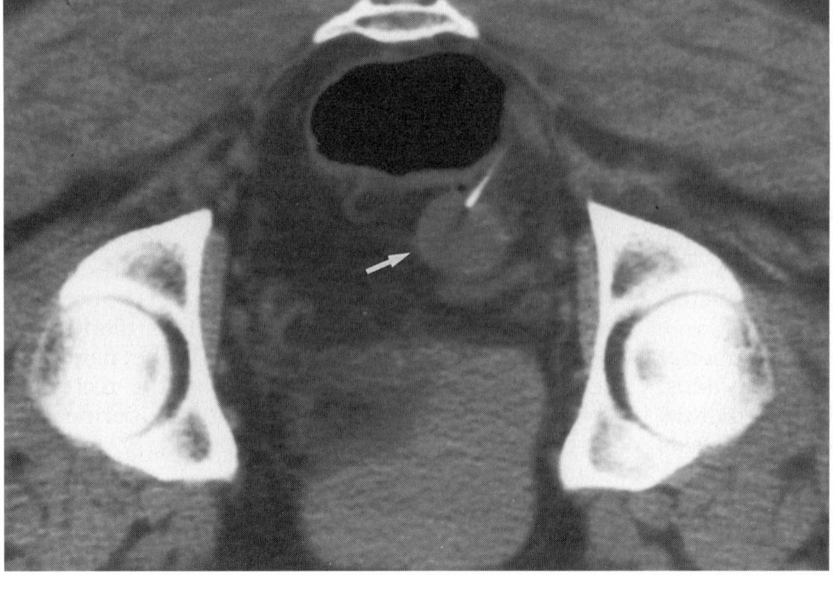

FIGURE 31–6. CT image showing a left seminal vesicle cyst (arrow) that was aspirated percutaneously. (Courtesy of Terrance C. Demos, M.D., and Carl Kalbhen, M.D.)

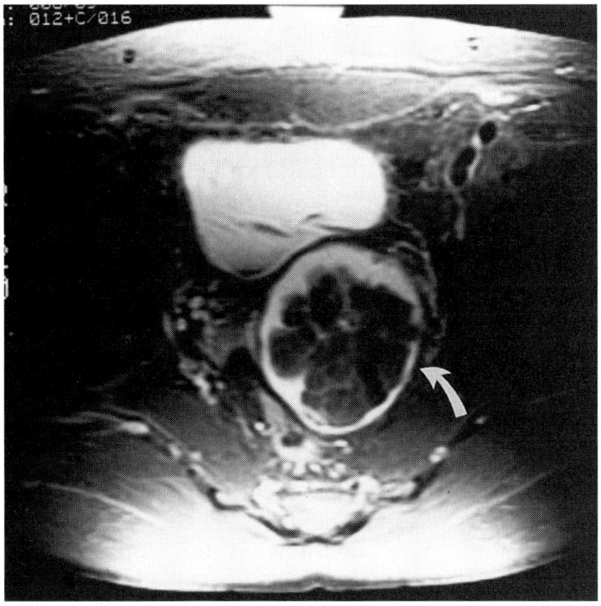
012+C/016

FIGURE 31–7. Seminal vesicle adenoma. T1-weighted MR image with fat suppression following gadolinium injection. There is a large lesion (arrow) of the left seminal vesicle that has an irregular enhancing wall and contains multiple low-signal, fluid-filled cystic areas with septae. (Courtesy of Paul Schellhammer, M.D.)

application of TRUS and MRI to the evaluation of prostate cancer (Fig. 31–8).

Imaging of Seminal Vesicle Pathology

Congenital anomalies and abnormalities and inflammatory diseases have been imaged on TRUS, CT, and MRI. These findings are not presented in this chapter. The reader is referred to two excellent articles on imaging of the seminal vesicles.[27,34]

Seminal Vesicle Cysts

Urography, ultrasound, CT, MRI, and VSV have all been used to diagnose seminal vesicle cysts. On urography, renal agenesis or duplication may be seen in association with an extrinsic bladder mass. Ultrasound is able to confirm the cystic nature of a pelvic mass and can usually localize the organ of origin, particularly with TRUS. Seminal vesicle cysts appear as typically cystic structures posterolateral to the bladder; internal echoes may be seen if the cyst is complicated by hemorrhage or infection. Seminal vesicle cysts may bulge the bladder wall or even intrude into its lumen.[27,35] TRUS can guide transrectal or transperineal puncture of pelvic cysts. Seminal vesicle cysts are usually filled with a viscous, brownish fluid that contains dead sperm at microscopy, unlike other pelvic cysts such

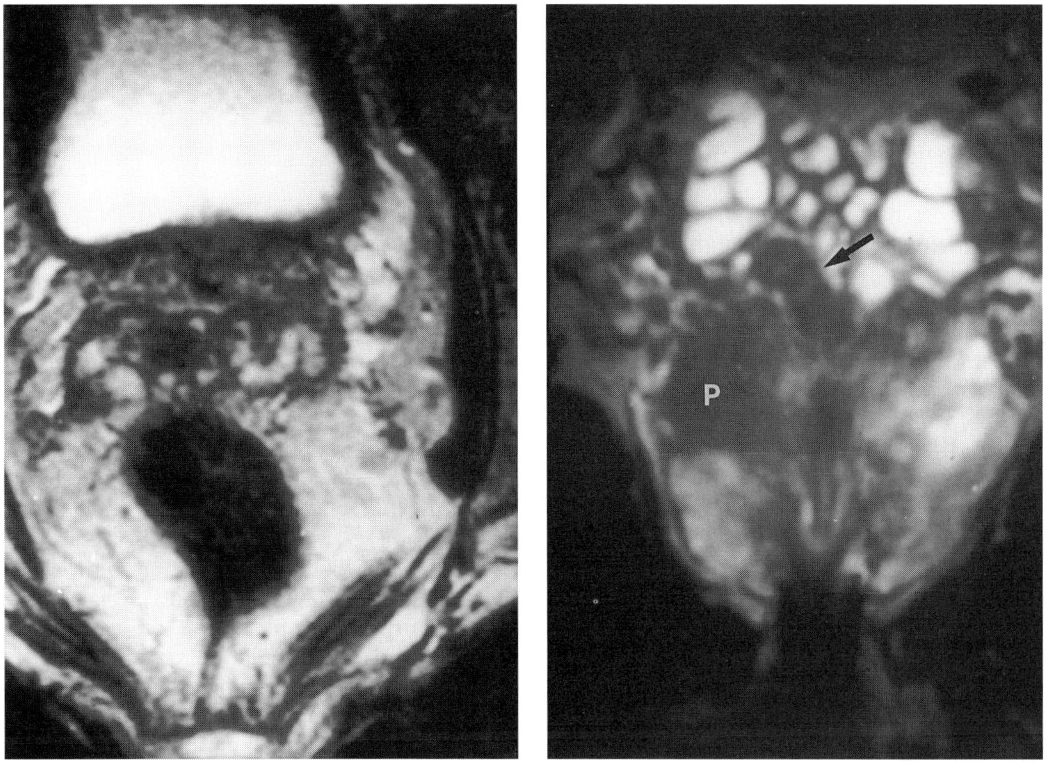
P

FIGURE 31–8. Prostate carcinoma invading the seminal vesicle. A T2-weighted MR image in the axial plane (left) does not show invasion clearly. The image in the coronal plane (right) clearly shows the prostate carcinoma (p) with extension (arrow) into the right seminal vesicle. (Courtesy of Terrance C. Demos, M.D., and Carl Kalbhen, M.D.)

as müllerian duct remnant cysts, dermoid cysts, and prostatic cysts.[27]

CT demonstrates a low-attenuation, unilocular cystic mass posterior to the bladder and cephalad to the prostate in the location of the expected seminal vesicle (Fig. 31–6). Associated renal anomalies and a dilated distal ureter that inserts ectopically somewhere near the seminal vesicle cyst may also be evident. Some of these cysts may be thick-walled, inhomogeneous, and of increased attenuation as a result of previous hemorrhage or infection.[36] The cyst wall may enhance following contrast administration, but the cyst contents should not. Cyst wall calcification is occasionally seen.[6]

On MRI, seminal vesicle cysts may appear as typically cystic structures (SI low on T1WI, high on T2WI) or may exhibit increased SI on both pulse sequences because of the presence of intracystic blood and/or proteinaceous material.[5,34] MRI can also demonstrate ectopic ureteral insertion into a dilated ejaculatory duct as well as the status of the ipsilateral kidney. Seminal vesicle cysts are unilocular; a multiloculated cystic mass involving the seminal vesicle is suggestive of a malignant cystosarcoma phylloides.[37]

Neoplasms

Primary Tumors. A variety of benign and malignant tumors occasionally arise in the seminal vesicles from either their epithelial or mesenchymal elements. Secondary involvement by tumors originating from the bladder, prostate, or rectum occurs more often.

Primary malignant tumors of the seminal vesicle include adenocarcinoma, a variety of sarcomas, and seminoma.[38,39] Adenocarcinomas can invade the urinary bladder and present as a bladder tumor.[30] Many benign tumors have been reported, including leiomyomas, fibromas, mesonephric hamartomas, cystadenomas (Fig. 31–7), and dermoid cysts. Fibromas and leiomyomas appear as soft tissue–density (solid) tumors without infiltrative growth characteristics; cystadenomas are multicystic lesions. Dermoids may contain fat and calcium.[27]

An irregularly enlarged seminal vesicle with an infiltrative growth pattern (pelvic wall, bladder, prostatic, or rectal involvement; streaky appearance of perivesical fat) and enlarged lymph nodes suggests a malignant nature of a seminal vesicle mass on CT, TRUS, or MRI. However, no specific features can reliably differentiate benign from malignant lesions or primary from metastatic tumors.[27]

Secondary Tumors. The seminal vesicles are most commonly affected by tumors occurring in adjacent organs. Seminal vesicle involvement by local spread of prostate cancer occurs in several ways: (1) tumor spread through the capsule to involve the seminal vesicles by contiguity; (2) invasion of the ejaculatory ducts with subsequent ascent of tumor in the periductal tissues to involve the seminal vesicles (seen in 40% of cases in Wheeler's series[40]); and (3) tumor ascent along the neurovascular bundles to involve the seminal vesicles[41] (seen in 30% of Wheeler's series[40]). In 30% of patients, Wheeler found focal tumor in the seminal vesicles without evidence of direct extension from the primary lesion; these were thought to represent metastatic disease rather than local spread.[40]

With endorectal coil MRI, one of the earliest indications of tumor involvement of the seminal vesicles is the thickening of tubules as the tumor spreads in the peritubular stroma. Low SI may also be seen, unilaterally or bilaterally, and is best demonstrated on axial T2WI. Often, the seminal vesicles may remain normal in size and architecture, despite extensive changes in the SI.[42]

Confirmatory sagittal or coronal images are important to obtain in cases in which there is apparent seminal vesicle involvement on the axial images to ensure that the appearance is not an artifact caused by partial volume averaging of an enlarged prostate with normal seminal vesicles.[41]

Less frequently, the seminal vesicles may be affected by either muscle-invasive or in situ transitional cell carcinoma of the bladder.[43,44]

Postoperative Appearance

The seminal vesicles are removed during radical prostatectomy. Postoperative CT and MRI scans may demonstrate structures that simulate residual normal seminal vesicles. There are several possible explanations for this: Postoperative reaction and scarring[45] or portions of the ampullae[46] may be mistaken for seminal vesicles. Alternatively, the tips of the seminal vesicles may have, in fact, been left behind.[27]

Hematospermia

In men under 40 years of age, hematospermia is usually caused by inflammation in the prostate, seminal vesicle, epididymis, or testicle. Occasionally, benign lesions such as seminal vesicle cysts or calculi, urethral hemangiomas, or, rarely, malignant tumors are responsible. In men over 40 years of age, carcinoma of the prostate, bladder, and seminal vesicles is more often etiologic, although benign causes still predominate. Overall, only 5 to 10% of hematospermia cases are related to underlying malignancy.[27]

Urologic evaluation is advised in men over 40 years of age with persistent hematospermia, coexistent hematuria, or associated ejaculatory or perineal pain.[47,48] Intravenous pyelography should be considered if there is coexistent hematuria. TRUS demonstrates abnormalities in 83% of patients and can guide biopsy of suspicious lesions.[49] However, the spatial resolution and high soft tissue contrast of MRI, particularly endorectal surface coil imaging, makes it the modality of choice to investigate the seminal vesicles and neighboring anatomy in patients with hematospermia.[33]

DIAGNOSIS

Although exploration with open biopsy was the mainstay of diagnosis reported in the early literature,[19,21,26,50,51] the more recent literature describes obtaining histologic confirmation of a suspected seminal vesicle tumor by needle biopsy.[52,53] Just as its use has become standard in conjunction with prostate needle biopsy, TRUS can greatly assist in directing the placement of the biopsy needle into a supraprostatic seminal vesicle mass.

Histologically, normal seminal vesicle tissue consists of many folds of columnar to cuboidal epithelium containing goblet cells.[1] There is a thin muscular wall arranged in two layers—an inner circular and an outer longitudinal.[2]

Benign tumors share the finding of a lack of mitotic activity.[10,54] Many histologic types have been described, as previously stated, and the specific histology of each is not discussed here. These tumors also tend to have a fibrous capsule surrounding them, and must be shown to arise from the seminal vesicle itself and not the prostate or other surrounding organs.

Primary adenocarcinoma of the seminal vesicle has a histologic pattern containing papillary architecture of tall, columnar or cuboidal cells in poorly formed glandular structures (Figs. 31–9 and 31–10). Abundant eosinophilic cytoplasm with intracytoplasmic or intracellular mucin is often present. Nuclei are usually located on the basal side of the cell, and are typically large, round or oval, and uniform in size, with one or two round, prominent, eosinophilic nucleoli.[18,22,38] The lipofuscin typically seen by light microscopy in normal seminal vesicle may not be easily seen in tumor cells, which is most likely explained by the electron microscopic finding of much smaller cytolysosomes reported in tumor cells as compared to normal seminal vesicle epithelium.[19]

Mesenchymal tumors of the seminal vesicles are quite rare, with only a handful of reported cases. Cell types reported in primary seminal vesicle sarcomas include hemangiosarcoma, leiomyosarcoma, fibrosarcoma, and cystosarcoma phylloides.[19,50–53,55] In general, histologic diagnosis is established as it would be for a sarcoma in any other location. These tumors most often exhibit local extension into surrounding tissues, but have also been reported to result in distant metastases.[19,51,55] A discussion of the histopathology of each of these sarcomas is beyond the scope of this chapter, and the interested reader is referred to the cited references for more detailed information.

Although extremely rare, the seminal vesicles have been reported as the primary site in two cases of extragonadal germ cell tumors. One well-documented case of seminoma reports no other site of origin. The tumor was excised entirely by radical cystoprostatectomy, and, although it was adherent to the prostate, the tumor was reportedly "clearly centered on and otherwise virtually confined to both seminal vesicles, except that it had infiltrated the left wall of the bladder and involved the left ureter."[56] Another patient presented with shortness of breath and was found to have choriocarcinoma

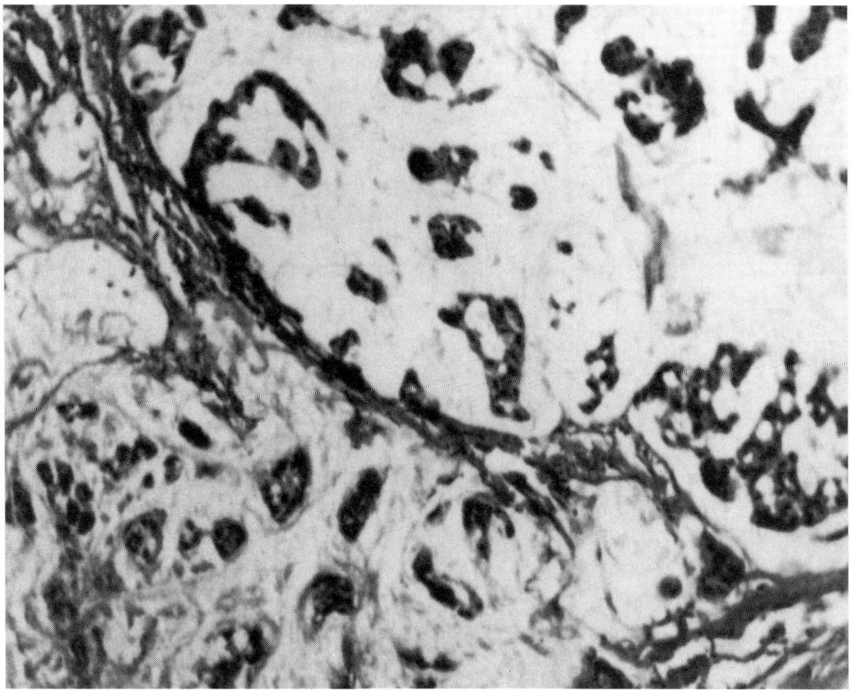

FIGURE 31–9. Adenocarcinoma of the seminal vesicle. Neoplastic epithelial cells in columns and poorly formed glandular structures are floating in mucus. H&E, reduced from ×160. (From Benson RC, Clark WR, Farrow GM: Carcinoma of the seminal vesicle. J Urol 1984; 132:484, with permission.)

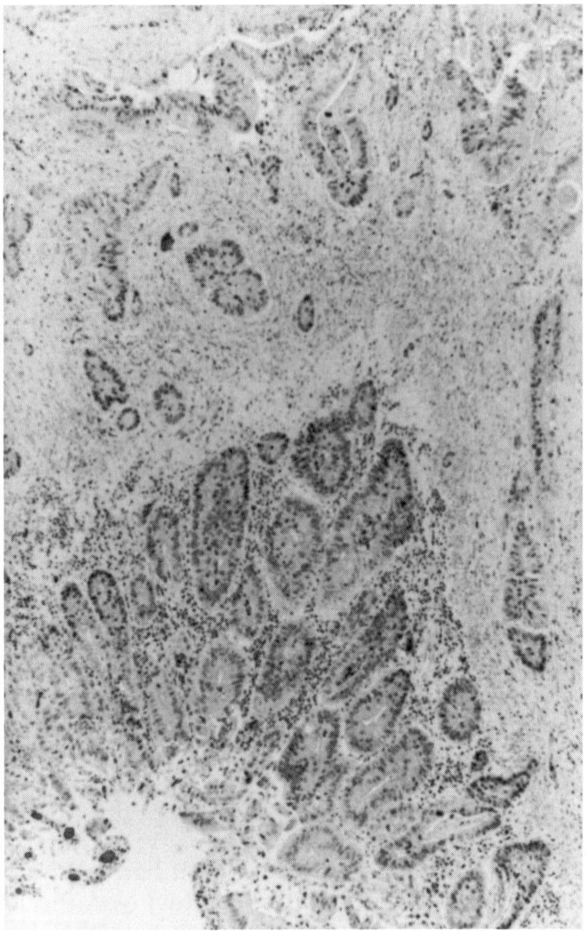

FIGURE 31-10. Adenocarcinoma in situ replacing seminal vesicle epithelium and lining. Its lumen (bottom) is associated with infiltrating adenocarcinoma (top). H&E, original magnification ×85. (From Davis NS, Merguerian PH, DiMarco PL, et al: Primary adenocarcinoma of seminal vesicle presenting as bladder tumor. Urology 1988; 32:467, with permission.)

with widespread metastases. Despite chemotherapy, he eventually succumbed to prolonged ventilatory dependence and sepsis. Autopsy confirmed a 12-cm mass in continuity with the seminal vesicles, and histologic examination of both testes failed to show any evidence of primary tumor.[25] The embryologic origin of these rare primary extragonadal germ cell tumors can be explained by the midline entrapment of primitive germ cells in the fetus. This is generally believed to result in extragonadal tumors found in the retroperitoneum or mediastinum or intracranially, but is also the most likely explanation for these primary germ cell tumors of the seminal vesicles.[56]

STAGING

There is no universally agreed upon staging system for malignancies of the seminal vesicles, likely because of the rarity of these tumors. Radiologic imaging studies help establish the diagnosis of a seminal vesicle tumor, as previously mentioned, and provide a good predictor of the local extent of disease. This information is useful in determining the likelihood of resectability. Because the commonly reported sites of metastases, other than local invasion, include the pelvic lymphatics, lungs, and bones, it seems reasonable that evaluation for the presence of metastases should include imaging studies of these tissues. This would most commonly include a chest radiograph, CT of the abdomen and pelvis, with or without chest CT, and a radionuclide bone scan. Intravenous urography (IVU) may also be considered to evaluate the location of the ureters, with particular reference to any degree of obstruction. Information gained from CT, however, may prove sufficient and make IVU unnecessary. Sarcomas reportedly have a greater likelihood of intracranial metastases, so a CT scan of the head should be considered in patients with primary seminal vesicle sarcomas.

SURGICAL MANAGEMENT

Surgical management of isolated seminal vesicle disease is uncommon. In the past, infection of the seminal vesicles was the most common reason for surgery; there are reports of up to 700 seminal vesiculectomies or vesiculotomies by a single surgeon for tuberculous disease.[57] In the current era, with the antibiotics available, surgical treatment of the seminal vesicles for infectious disease is rare. Surgical intervention is not necessarily required in the case of an asymptomatic mass that shows benign histology. Conservative management with repeat imaging may be all that is required in such a patient. When surgical intervention is required for either a malignant or a symptomatic benign mass, many surgical approaches have been described for excision of the seminal vesicles. Choices include the retrovesical, extraperitoneal, transperitoneal, transvesical, perineal, and posterior sacral/transcoccygeal approaches. The decision to choose one approach over another is in part due to the size and extent of the disease, but mostly depends on the expertise and comfort of the surgeon. Radical cystoprostatectomy including seminal vesiculectomy, the recommended treatment for malignant disease of the seminal vesicles, is the same as that routinely performed for bladder cancer and is not elaborated on here.

Preoperative preparation should include a full mechanical and routine antibiotic bowel preparation with oral erythromycin and neomycin. Antiembolic stockings and pneumatic compression boots are recommended to prevent deep venous thrombosis. A preoperative parenteral antibiotic, such as a first- or second-generation cephalosporin, is also recommended. Preoperative and postoperative incentive spirometry is emphasized.

Perineal Approach

The perineal approach to seminal vesiculectomy is similar to that for a perineal prostatectomy. Patient positioning, skin incision, and initial dissection are identical to those for perineal prostatectomy. The rectal wall must be dissected free higher than is usually necessary for a radical perineal prostatectomy. Once Denonvilliers' fascia has been incised, it is dissected off the seminal vesicles. If a nerve-sparing procedure is desired, one must take care not to injure the neurovascular bundles that run longitudinally in this area. Traction on the Lowsley retractor to lift the prostate may improve exposure during this portion of the procedure.

The extent of resection will depend in part on the seminal vesicle pathology in a particular patient. Benign lesions can be treated with unilateral excision of the seminal vesicle alone. Cancer may warrant a wider excision to include the vas deferens. Once the seminal vesicle has been carefully exposed, it is usually possible to place a clamp around its base and ligate the stump where the vascular pedicle is located (Fig. 31–11) using an absorbable suture. Just prior to dividing and removing the vesicle, the distal end where it enters the prostate can be secured with a clip or tie in order to prevent the secretions from obscuring the surgical field. The wound is then closed in layers and a Penrose drain is placed just as for a radical perineal prostatectomy.[1,58] The Foley catheter is removed on the first or second postoperative day, and the drain is removed when there is little or no drainage, usually the second or third postoperative day.

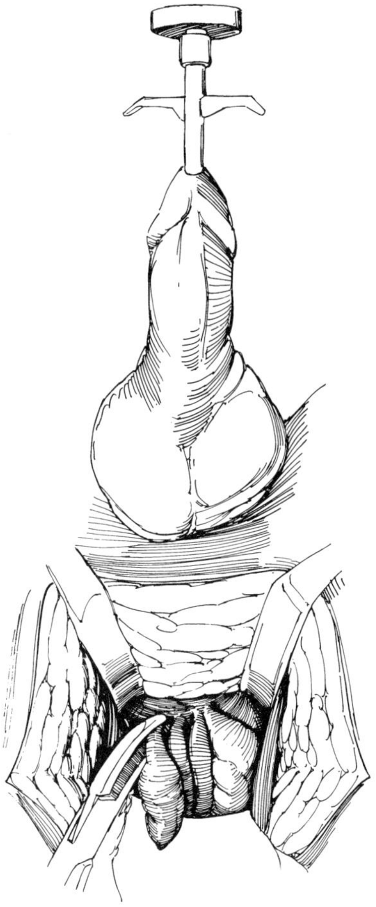

FIGURE 31–11. With upward traction on the Lowsley retractor to assist in visualization, the seminal vesicles and ampullae of the vas are identified from the perineal approach. (From Hinman F Jr: Atlas of Urologic Surgery, p 381. Philadelphia, WB Saunders Co, 1989, with permission.)

Transvesical Approach

The transvesical approach is probably the most direct route to the utricle,[58] and provides good visualization of the seminal vesicles as well. A midline incision from the pubic symphysis to the umbilicus or a Pfannenstiel incision is made, the rectus muscles are separated, and dissection is carried out to enter the space of Retzius. A Balfour or a Turner-Warwick self-retaining retractor is placed. The bladder is opened vertically for 7 to 10 cm, and stay sutures are placed on the bladder edge for retraction. Several moist 4 × 8 sponges are placed into the dome of the bladder, and a retractor blade is inserted into the bladder to place the dome on stretch. The ureteral orifices may be cannulated at this time to assist in identification of the location of the ureteral orifices and the subtrigonal ureter. A longitudinal trigonal incision of approximately 5 cm is preferred, but a transverse incision in the trigone just above the bladder neck can be performed (Fig. 31–12*A*).[1] Once the incision has been deepened through the entire thickness of bladder muscle, stay sutures can again be placed in the posterior bladder wall. The ampullae of the vas should then be visualized, and can either be dissected free and ligated or left intact as discussed earlier. The seminal vesicles should then be visualized just lateral to the ampullae of the vas (Fig. 31–12*B*). The seminal vesicle or vesicles can then be dissected out and the vascular pedicle either clipped or tied. The planes in this area may be difficult to delineate if there has been previous seminal vesiculitis. Should this be the case, the surgeon must pay particular attention to avoid entering the rectal wall; use of ureteral catheters as described previously is particularly helpful.[1]

The posterior bladder incision is then closed in two layers, with 2-0 absorbable suture in the muscle and running 4-0 absorbable suture in the mucosal layer. A 20-French urethral catheter is placed, and the ureteral catheters may either be removed or brought through the skin as stents. The anterior bladder wall is closed similar to the trigone, and a drain is placed in the perivesicle space. The drain is removed when the drainage is less than 50 to 60 ml/day, and the urethral catheter is removed in 7 to 10 days.[1,58]

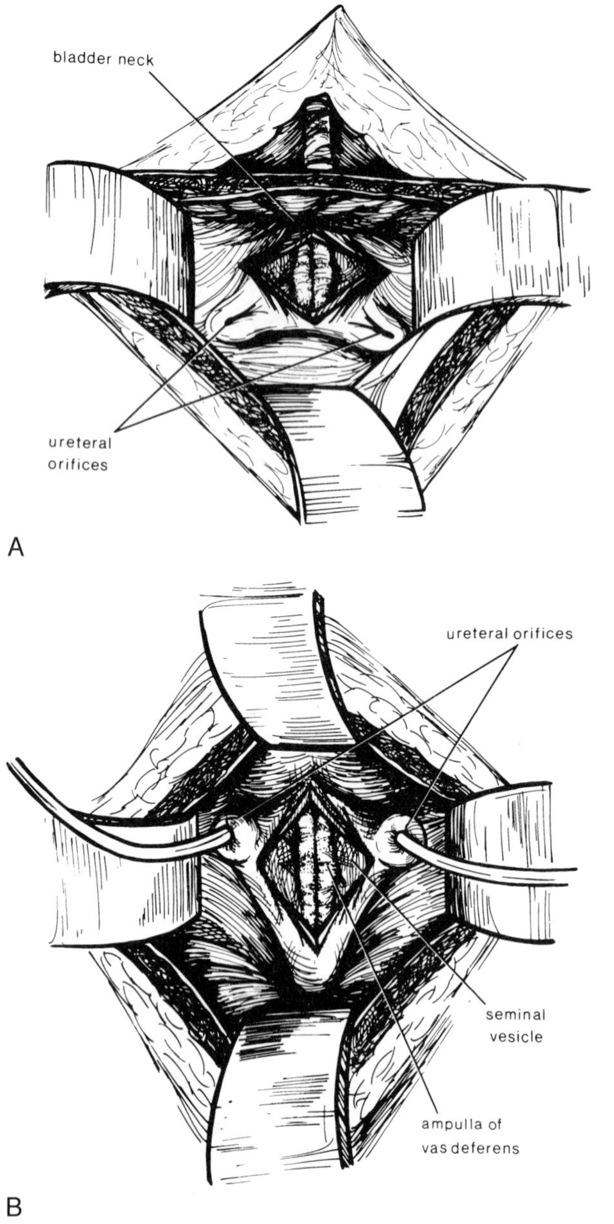
bladder neck
ureteral orifices
A
ureteral orifices
seminal vesicle
ampulla of vas deferens
B

FIGURE 31–12. Transvesical approach to seminal vesiculectomy. *A*, Transverse incision 2 cm superior to the bladder neck below the ureteral orifices. *B*, Vertical incision between the ureteral orifices. (From Williams RD: Surgery of the seminal vesicles. *In* Walsh PC, Retik AB, Stamey TA, Vaughn ED Jr [eds]: Campbells Urology, 6th edition, p 2951. Philadelphia, WB Saunders Co, 1992, with permission.)

Retrovesical Approach

In 1952, de Assis described the retrovesical approach to seminal vesiculectomy.[57] He advocated this as a method for extracapsular excision of cysts or benign (including infectious) masses, especially when bilateral excision is desired. Using a midline suprapubic incision from the symphysis pubis to just below the umbilicus, the rectus fascia is opened and the rectus abdominus muscles are split in the midline. Once access is gained to the perivesical space, the area of the peritoneal cul-de-sac is identified and the peritoneum is incised for a distance of 4 to 5 cm. The portion of peritoneum below its inferior region of adherence to the bladder is then identified and incised slightly longer than the previous peritoneal incision. These incisions should meet at their lateral aspects, and, once the inferior portion of peritoneum is freed from the loose connective tissue in the pelvis, the two edges of peritoneum are reapproximated, leaving a portion of peritoneum adherent to the posterior wall of the bladder. Alternatively, a transperitoneal, retrovesical approach can be performed by making the initial incision into the peritoneal cavity and then incising the cul-de-sac. A plane is then developed anterior to the rectum and posterior to the bladder and seminal vesicles (Fig. 31–13). The vasa should be visualized at this time, and care should be taken to identify the ureters where they cross the vasa to avoid injuring them. The vasa deferentia can then be isolated, ligated, and divided with absorbable sutures or clips. A clamp on the pelvic portion of the vas deferens can assist in retraction and aid in the dissection of the deeper, distal aspect of the seminal vesicles. Dissection of one or both seminal vesicles may also be performed while leaving the vasa intact. The superior and inferior vesical arteries may need to be sacrificed to improve visualization; this may be done without major concern because it will cause no harm to the overall vascular supply of the prostate and bladder.[1] The surgeon should take care to avoid dissection lateral to the seminal vesicle in an effort to preserve the neurovascular bundle.[1,58] When the distal aspect of the seminal vesicle has been identified where it enters the prostate, it is ligated and divided (Fig. 31–14).

A suction drain is placed into the retrovesical space and brought out through a separate stab incision, and the incision is closed. Again, the drain is removed when the output is less than 50 to 60 ml/day.

Transcoccygeal Approach

The transcoccygeal is an approach that is not particularly familiar to many urologists, and an uncommon choice for fear of rectal injury or impotence. It may be useful in patients whom it would be difficult to place in the supine or lithotomy positions, or who have had multiple previous perineal or retropubic operations.[1] The patient is placed prone in a jackknifed position, and the buttocks are retracted laterally with adhesive tape. Incision is made in an L shape, beginning in the midline from the midsacral level to the tip of the coccyx, then arcing along the gluteal cleft 3 cm from the anus on the side of the lesion. The coccyx is then exposed, dissected free from the underside of the rectum, and removed. The lateral wall of the rectum is then dissected free from surrounding tissue, including

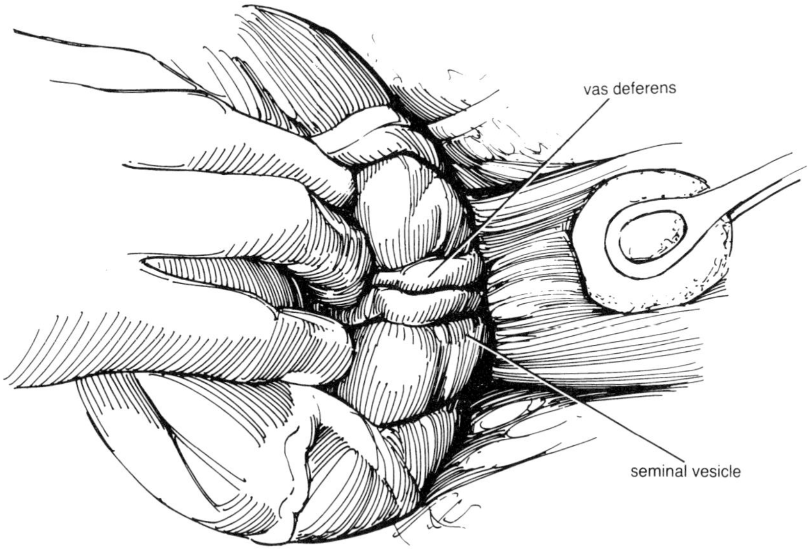
vas deferens
seminal vesicle

FIGURE 31-13. Retrovesical seminal vesiculectomy. A plane is developed between the posterior aspect of the bladder and seminal vesicles and the anterior rectal wall. Ureters, vas deferens, and seminal vesicles should be identified at this stage. (From Hinman F Jr: Atlas of Urologic Surgery, p 380. Philadelphia, WB Saunders Co, 1989, with permission.)

the levator ani muscles, until the prostate is encountered. When the prostate is identified, dissection is then performed superior to it until the ampullae of the vas are encountered. The seminal vesicles are located just lateral to the vas. Dissection and removal of the seminal vesicle or vesicles is as outlined previously. If difficulty is encountered in identifying the correct plane, a finger placed into

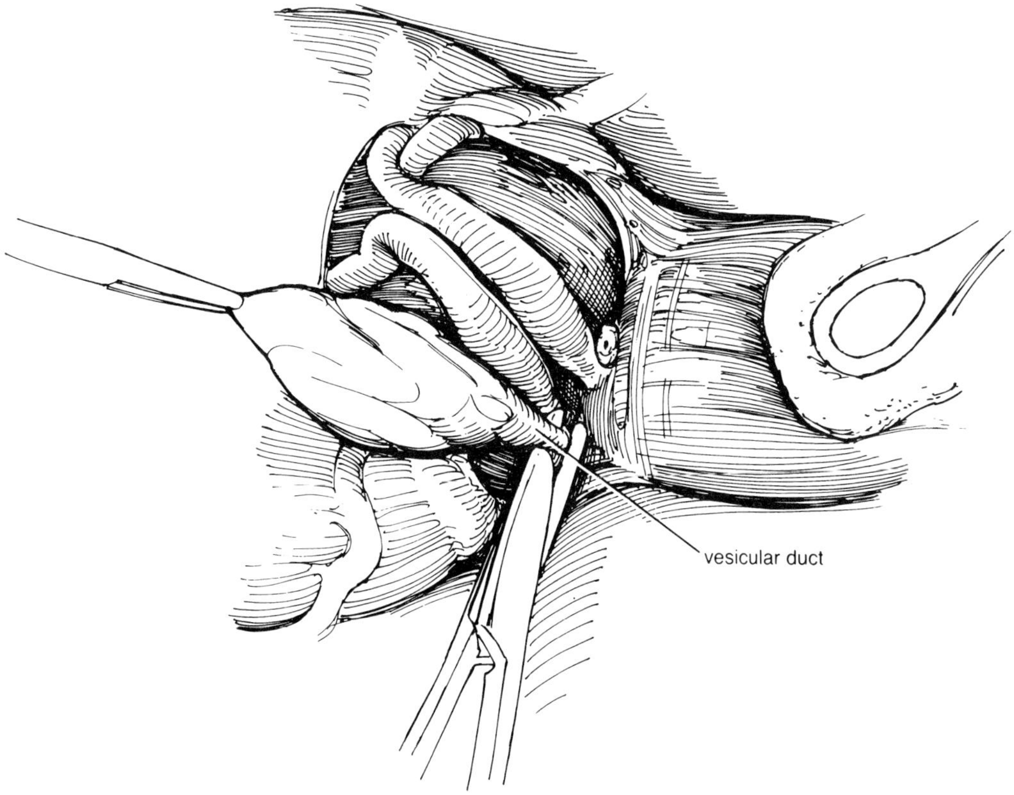
vesicular duct

FIGURE 31-14. Retrovesical seminal vesiculectomy. Once the seminal vesicle is dissected free and the vascular pedicle has been ligated, the distal end of the vesicle is ligated and divided and the specimen is removed. (From Hinman F Jr: Atlas of Urologic Surgery, p 380. Philadelphia, WB Saunders Co, 1989, with permission.)

the rectum via an O'Connor sheath may prove helpful. A Penrose drain is placed and brought out through a separate stab incision, and the wound is closed anatomically in layers. Postoperative recovery is usually uneventful, and the drain may be removed in 2 to 3 days if there is no drainage.[1]

Complications

As with any operative complication, the most important factor is careful inspection to identify the injury before the incision is closed. In particular, the rectum should be carefully scrutinized for any injury before the wound is closed.[1] Patients generally recover from rectal injuries uneventfully if they have had a full mechanical and antibiotic bowel preparation and if the laceration is closed in two layers at the time of the injury. Of note, however, is that, if a rectal injury occurs in conjunction with the retrovesical transperitoneal approach, consideration should be given to placing an omental patch over the repaired rectum and possibly performing a temporary diverting colostomy, because the rectal injury would be within the peritoneum and well above the levator ani muscles.[1]

Ureteral injuries are uncommon but can be managed with a stented primary repair. The stent should be left for 10 to 14 days postoperatively. Bladder injuries should likewise be repaired with a standard two-layer closure, and a urethral catheter left in place for 7 to 10 days postoperatively.[1] One should also consider obtaining a cystogram to rule out any extravasation prior to catheter removal.

Significant blood loss is uncommon. Nevertheless, because these cases are almost always performed on an elective basis, one should consider the possibility of autologous blood donation prior to surgery.

Impotence is of concern following seminal ve-

TABLE 31–1. PRIMARY CARCINOMAS OF THE SEMINAL VESICLES

Study	Patient Age	Diagnosis	Surgical Treatment	Other Treatment*	Follow-up
Okada et al.[20]	17	Well-differentiated papillary adenocarcinoma of seminal vesicle cyst	Excision of cyst (extraperitoneal)	—	Alive, NED† at 6 yr
Tanaka et al.[21]	87	Adenocarcinoma	Radical cystoprostatectomy with bilateral cutaneous ureterostomies	—	Died of cardiac disease at 6 mo; NED
Kawahara et al.[22]	19	Papillary adenocarcinoma 2 × 1.2 × 1.2 cm	Seminal vesiculectomy	—	4 yr, 2 mo NED
Benson et al.[18]	40	Papillary adenocarcinoma	Resection of both seminal vesicles and rectum; colostomy	Radium implant	Dead at 6 mo
	64	Adenocarcinoma (nodes positive)	Radical cystoprostatectomy with bilateral ureterosigmoidostomy	5FU + radiation	Symptoms at 10 mo; dead at 18 mo
Langham-Brown and Abercrombie[23]	21	Papillary carcinoma	—	Radiation—metastases at 1 yr, then chemotherapy (vincristine, 5FU, methotrexate, cyclophosphamide)	Dead at 3 yr
Kees[24]	60	Papillary adenocarcinoma	"Scooped out"	DES and bilateral orchiectomy at 9 mo for bone and pulmonary metastases	18 mo
Davis et al.[38]	43	Adenocarcinoma involving bladder, ureter, and seminal vesicle	Left nephroureterectomy and partial cystectomy with seminal vesiculectomy	Radiation	Unknown
Ewell[59]	62	Carcinoma with perineural and vascular invasion	Excision of mass	Estrogen × 8 yr	NED at 12 yr

*5FU, 5-fluorouracil; DES, diethylstilbestrol.
†NED, no evidence of disease.

siculectomy, particularly with either the transcoccygeal or perineal approach. Unilateral dissection may slightly reduce the risk of postoperative erectile dysfunction.

PROGNOSIS OF PRIMARY SEMINAL VESICLE TUMORS

Asymptomatic benign masses can be managed conservatively.[1] Repeat imaging studies should be obtained at regular intervals to evaluate for any increase in size that may warrant repeat biopsy to rule out a malignancy. Follow-up of patients with benign masses has been inconsistently reported in the literature, but in general these patients have an uneventful recovery. There have been reports of recurrent benign masses, mostly in the setting of cystadenoma of the seminal vesicle,[12] which raises the question of these lesions having a low malignant potential. As a result, patients who have undergone resection of a seminal vesicle tumor, either benign or malignant, should be followed regularly, with consideration given to either TRUS or CT to evaluate for the possibility of a recurrent mass.

Accurate statements with regard to the prognosis of patients with malignant seminal vesicle tumors are difficult to make as a result of the infrequent nature of these tumors, lack of uniform reporting (e.g., staging, histology, follow-up), and the absence of uniformity with regard to the surgical treatment employed. Tables 31–1 and 31–2 summarize the information available regarding primary seminal vesicle carcinomas and sarcomas, respectively. Because the majority of the case reports in the older literature[16,17] consisted of autopsy diagnoses, which would not contribute to a prediction of prognosis, they are not included in the tables.

There are cases in which local excision of the mass (seminal vesiculectomy) resulted in long-term survival[20,22,59]; however, other patients treated with radical excision died of their disease rather soon after surgery.[18] Although it would make intrinsic sense that small, low-grade malignant tumors have the potential to be cured by local excision, the lack of reported information with regard to size of tu-

TABLE 31–2. SEMINAL VESICLE SARCOMAS

Study	Patient Age	Diagnosis	Surgical Treatment	Other Treatment	Follow-up
Mazur et al.[19]	49	"Cystic epithelial stromal tumor" (cystosarcoma phylloides) 2 yr after excision of "teratoma"	Wide excision with partial cystectomy and excision of rectal wall; colostomy	—	18 mo "doing well"
Schned et al.[50]	60	Leiomyosarcoma of left seminal vesicle, 3.5 × 1.9 × 1.8 cm	Radical cystoprostatectomy with ileal loop	—	14 mo NED*
Buck and Shaw[51]	57	Fibrosarcoma, 14 × 6 cm	Excision of mass	—	6 mo NED
Lamont et al.[52]	52	Angiosarcoma (positive surgical margins)	Seminal vesiculectomy and pelvic lymphadenectomy	Radiation and chemotherapy for metastases	Dead at 3–4 mo with pulmonary and brain metastases
Amirkhan et al.[53]	68	Leiomyosarcoma	Radical cystoprostatectomy with orthotopic diversion	—	13 mo disease free
Chiou et al.[55]	63	Hemangiosarcoma	Radical cystoprostatectomy, urethrectomy, ileal loop	—	Died at 1 mo of "M.I.". Autopsy showed pulmonary, pleural, and peritoneal metastases
Fain et al.[60]	61	Cystosarcoma phylloides	Radical cystoprostatectomy, low anterior resection of sigmoid, ileal loop	Chemotherapy for pulmonary metastases at 4 yr postop	No recurrence 6 mo after chemotherapy
Tripathi and Dick[61]	?	Leiomyosarcoma	Seminal vesiculectomy	—	Alive at 1 yr

*NED, no evidence of disease.

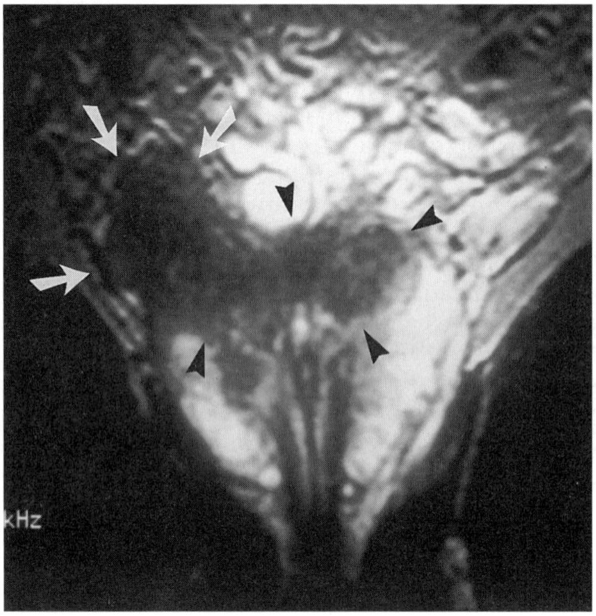
kHz

FIGURE 31–15. Prostate carcinoma invading the seminal vesicle. Coronal T2-weighted MR image showing tumor (arrowheads) at the base of the prostate with invasion (arrows) of the right seminal vesicle. (Courtesy of Terrance C. Demos, M.D., and Carl Kalbhen, M.D.)

mor, extent of local invasion, and "grade" of the tumor, and the lack of a defined staging system, do not permit such a recommendation. Radical cystoprostatectomy with seminal vesiculectomy and pelvic lymphadenectomy, therefore, seems to offer the best overall potential for cure, particularly because these tumors commonly spread by means of local invasion. Pelvic exenteration may be necessary if the rectal wall is involved with tumor as well.

In the reported germ cell tumors with a primary focus in the seminal vesicles, the patient with seminoma was treated with radical cystoprostatectomy and underwent postoperative radiation to the sacral region and para-aortic lymph nodes. He was reported to be free of disease at 8 months postoperatively.[56] The patient with metastatic choriocarcinoma died of his disease and complications of chemotherapy, which is consistent with the aggressive nature and high mortality rate of this tumor.[25]

Adjuvant therapy with external beam radiation,[23,38,52] interstitial radiation,[18] and chemotherapy[52,60] has been reported with both carcinomas and sarcomas. Although response to therapy has been shown in some patients, the paucity of data with regard to multimodal therapy does not allow generalized recommendations, and any adjuvant treatment should be undertaken on an individualized basis.

The use of androgen ablation therapy has also been advocated by some as an adjuvant to surgical excision.[24,59] The theoretical basis for this treatment stems from the embryologic origin from hormone-sensitive tissue and the functional dependence on testosterone of the glandular epithelium of the seminal vesicles.[59] In the case reported by Ewell, the patient underwent orchiectomy and received diethylstilbestrol (DES) for 8 years after development of bony metastases, and then survived another 4 years after DES was discontinued.[59] Ewell's report lacks detailed histologic description of the tumor, however, and no special stains on the specimen were reported that might allow differentiation from a high-grade adenocarcinoma of the prostate. Furthermore, the infrequent occurrence of seminal vesicle tumors, in contradistinction to the very prevalent prostatic carcinoma, decreases the theoretical validity of significant contribution of androgens to the development and progression of seminal vesicle tumors, because both the prostate and the seminal vesicles are exposed to essentially the same androgen milieu.

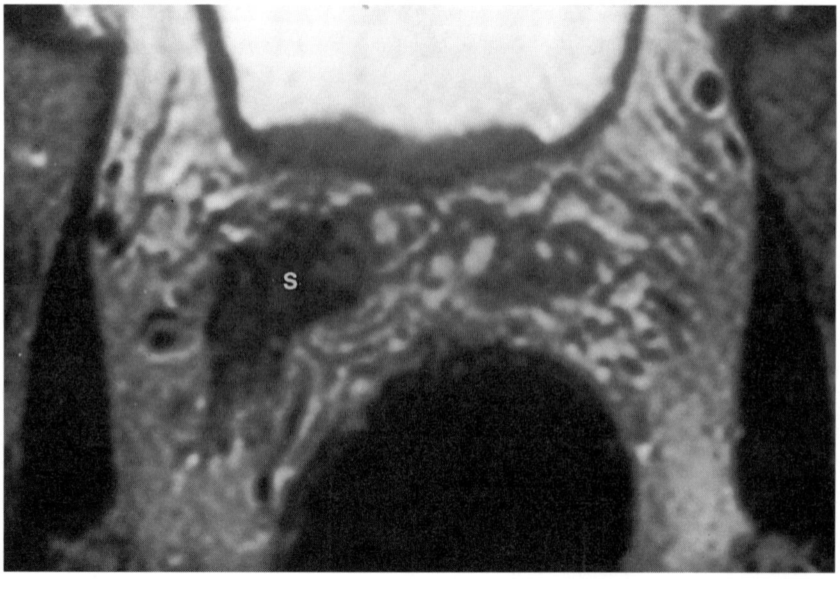
S

FIGURE 31–16. Prostate carcinoma invading and enlarging the seminal vesicle. Axial T2-weighted MR image showing an enlarged right seminal vesicle that has low signal as a result of invasion by a prostate carcinoma. (Courtesy of Terrance C. Demos, M.D., and Carl Kalbhen, M.D.)

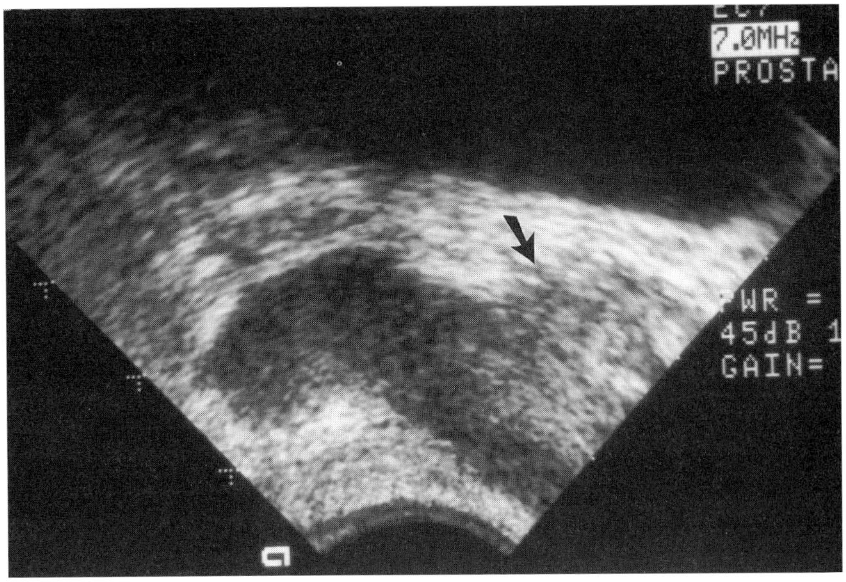
7.0MHz
PROSTA
PWR =
45dB
GAIN=

FIGURE 31–17. Prostate carcinoma invading a seminal vesicle. Sagittal transrectal sonogram showing invasion of the seminal vesicle (arrow) causing loss of the normal beak configuration of the prostate and adjacent seminal vesicle. (Courtesy of Terrance C. Demos, M.D., and Carl Kalbhen, M.D.)

SEMINAL VESICLES AND PROSTATE CANCER

The seminal vesicles are most commonly affected by prostate cancer (Figs. 31–15 through 31–17). Invasion of the seminal vesicles by prostate cancer is one of the most important prognostic indicators in this disease and is defined as involvement of the muscularis layer (not simply the fat adjacent to the seminal vesicles) by tumor.[62,63] Most commonly, prostate cancer involves the seminal vesicles by extension up the loose connective tissue of the ejaculatory ducts (type I). The second most common mechanisms of involvement are from across the base of the prostate directly into the seminal vesicles (type IIA) or retrograde extension of tumor into the seminal vesicles along nerves in the periprostatic fat (type IIB). Many tumors are large enough to involve the seminal vesicles by more than one mechanism (type I + II). Both types I and II are the result of spread of tumor in direct contiguity to tumor in the prostate. Rarely, tumor may appear in the seminal vesicles as isolated deposits (type III). This type is considered to represent metastases, or, perhaps, regression of tumor between the prostatic primary site and the focus in the seminal vesicles (Fig. 31–18).[64]

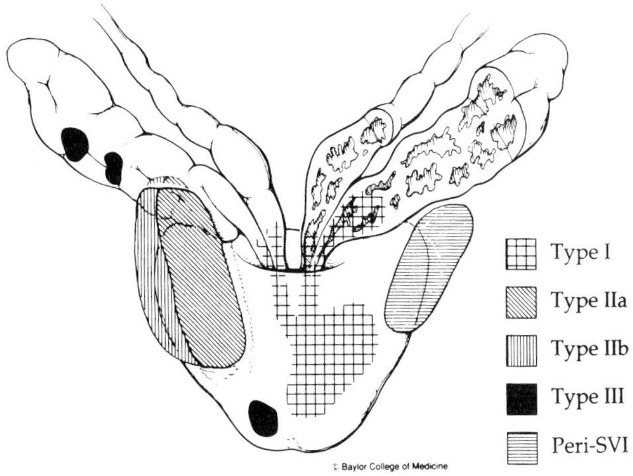
Type I
Type IIa
Type IIb
Type III
Peri-SVI
© Baylor College of Medicine

FIGURE 31–18. Diagrammatic representation of the three patterns of seminal vesicle involvement (SVI) and peri-SVI. The combination of types I and II is categorized as type I + II. (From Ohori M, Scardino PT, Lapin SL, et al: The mechanisms and prognostic significance of seminal vesicle involvement by prostate cancer. Am J Surg Pathol 1993; 17:1253, with permission.)

There are controversies regarding the definition of seminal vesicle invasion. Some studies define tumor in the periseminal vesicle soft tissue as seminal vesicle invasion.[65–69] Others define seminal vesicle invasion as tumor invading the muscular wall of the seminal vesicle.[65,70–72] Most studies do not provide a definition of seminal vesicle invasion. There are also controversies regarding the prognostic significance of seminal vesicle invasion. Most studies have reported the presence of seminal vesicle invasion to be associated with a worse prognosis than capsular penetration[65,73–76]; however, other studies have reported conflicting results.[65,77] Epstein et al. evaluated 115 cases of established capsular penetration, 16 of periseminal vesicle invasion, and 45 of seminal vesicle invasion in patients without lymph node metastases.[65] Patients with seminal vesicle invasion had a significantly worse prognosis than those with capsular penetration; periseminal vesicle invasion was associated with an intermediate risk of progression. Gleason grade, surgical margins, and seminal vesicle invasion were all independent predictors of progression in a multivariate analysis, whereas tumor volume was not. In patients with seminal vesicle invasion, there was a trend for surgical margins and Gleason grade to predict progression; with tumor volume there was none.[65] The clarification of the definition of seminal vesicle invasion in prostate cancer will allow more accurate stratification of patients with prostate cancer for the assessment of new predictors of tumor progression as well as in future adjuvant treatment protocols.[65]

Acknowledgment. The authors wish to thank Dr. Terrence C. Demos, Professor of Radiology, Loyola University Medical Center, for his help in the preparation of this chapter.

REFERENCES

1. Williams RD: Surgery of the seminal vesicles. *In* Walsh PC, Retik AB, Stamey TA, Vaughn ED Jr (eds): Campbells Urology, 6th edition, pp 2942–2956. Philadelphia, WB Saunders Co, 1992.
2. Redman JF: Anatomy of the genitourinary system. *In* Gillenwater JY, Grayhack JT, Howards SS, Duckett JW (eds): Adult and Pediatric Urology, 2nd edition, pp 3–62. St. Louis, Mosby–Year Book, 1987.
3. Greenbaum E, Pearman RO: Vasovesiculography: cyst of the seminal vesicle associated with cyst agenesis of ipsilateral kidney. Radiology 1971; 98:362.
4. Hot SA, Petersen NE: Ectopia of seminal vesicle associated with agenesis of ipsilateral kidney. Urology 1974; 4:322–324.
5. King BF, Hattery RR, Lieber MM, et al: Congenital cystic disease of the seminal vesicle. Radiology 1991; 178:207–211.
6. Heaney JA, Pfister RC, Meares EM: Giant cyst of the seminal vesicle with renal agenesis. AJR 1987; 149:139–140.
7. Hart JB: A case of cyst of the seminal vesicle. J Urol 1966; 96:247–249.
8. Linhares-Furtado AJ: Three cases of cystic seminal vesicle associated with unilateral renal agenesis. Br J Urol 1973; 45:536–540.
9. Klotz PG: Congenital cystic abnormality of the seminal vesicle associated with ipsilateral renal agenesis: report of a case. Can J Surg 1967; 10:471–473.
10. Mazucchelli L, Studer UE, Zimmermann A: Cystadenoma of the seminal vesicle: case report and literature review. J Urol 1992; 147:1621–1624.
11. Lundhus E, Bundgaard N, Sorensen FB: Cystadenoma of the seminal vesicle: a case report. Scand J Urol Nephrol 1984; 18:341–342.
12. Bullock KN: Cystadenoma of the seminal vesicle. J R Soc Med 1988; 81:294–295.
13. Ramchandani P, Schnall MD, LiVolsi VA, et al: Senile amyloidosis of the seminal vesicles mimicking metastatic spread of prostatic carcinoma on MR images. AJR 1993; 161:99–100.
14. Carris CK, McLaughlin AP III, Gittes RF: Amyloidosis of the lower genitourinary tract. J Urol 1976; 115:423–426.
15. Young HH, Davis DM: Young's Practice of Urology, Volume 1, pp 558–559. Philadelphia, WB Saunders Co, 1926.
16. Lazarus JA: Primary malignant tumors of the retrovesical region with special reference to malignant tumors of the seminal vesicles: report of a case of retrovesical sarcoma. Acta Pathol Microbiol Scand 1956; 39:255–267.
17. Dalgaard JB, Giertsen JC: Primary carcinoma of the seminal vesicle: case and survey. Acta Pathol Microbiol Scand 1956; 39:255–267.
18. Benson RC, Clark WR, Farrow GM: Carcinoma of the seminal vesicle. J Urol 1984; 132:483–485.
19. Mazur MT, Myers JL, Maddos WA: Cystic epithelial-stromal tumor of the seminal vesicle. Am J Surg Pathol 1987; 11:210–217.
20. Okada Y, Tanaka H, Takeuchi H, et al: Papillary adenocarcinoma in a seminal vesicle cyst associated with ipsilateral renal agenesis: a case report. J Urol 1992; 148:1543–1545.
21. Tanaka T, Takeuchi T, Oguchi K, et al: Primary adenocarcinoma of the seminal vesicle. Hum Pathol 1987; 18:200–202.
22. Kawahara M, Matsuhashi M, Tajima M, et al: Primary carcinoma of the seminal vesicle. Urology 1988; 32:269–272.
23. Langham-Brown JJ, Abercrombie GF: Carcinoma of the seminal vesicle. Br J Urol 1986; 58:339–340.
24. Kees OSR: Clinical improvement following estrogenic therapy in a case of primary adenocarcinoma of the seminal vesicle. J Urol 1964; 91(6):665–670.
25. Fairey AE, Mead GM, Murphy D, et al: Primary seminal vesicle choriocarcinoma. Br J Urol 1993; 71:756–757.
26. Gohji K, Kamidono S, Okada S: Primary adenocarcinoma of the seminal vesicle. Br J Urol 1993; 72:514–515.
27. Ramchandani P, Banner MP, Pollack HM: Imaging of the seminal vesicles. Semin Roentgenol 1993; 27:83–91.
28. Silverman PM, Dunnick NR, Ford KK: Computed tomography of the normal seminal vesicles. Comput Radiol 1985; 9:379–385.
29. Banner MP, Hassler R: The normal seminal vesiculogram. Radiology 1978; 128:339–344.
30. Carter SS, Shinohara K, Lipshulz LI: Transrectal ultrasonography in disorders of the seminal vesicles and ejaculatory ducts. Urol Clin North Am 1989; 16:773–790.
31. Hernandez AD, Urry RL, Smith JA: Ultrasonographic characteristics of the seminal vesicles after ejaculation. J Urol 1990; 144:1380–1382.
32. Lee JKT, Marx MV: Pelvis. *In* Lee JKT, Sagel SS, Stanley RJ (eds): Computed Body Tomography with MRI Correlation, pp 852–853. New York, Raven, 1989.
33. Schnall MD, Pollack HM, Van Arsdalen K, et al: The seminal tract in patients with ejaculatory dysfunction: MR imaging with an endorectal surface coil. AJR 1992; 159:337–341.
34. Secaf E, Nuruddin RN, Hricak H, et al: MR imaging of the seminal vesicles. AJR 1991; 156:989–994.
35. Sheih CP, Hung CS, Wei CF: Cystic dilatations within the pelvis in patients with ipsilateral renal agenesis or dysplasia. J Urol 1990; 144:324–327.
36. Kenney PJ, Leeson MD: Congenital abnormalities of the seminal vesicles: spectrum of computed tomographic findings. Radiology 1983; 149:247–251.
37. Genevois PA, VanSinor ML, Sintzoff SA, et al: Cysts of the prostate and seminal vesicles: MR imaging findings in 11 cases. AJR 1990; 155:1021–1024.
38. Davis NS, Merguerian PA, DiMarco PL, et al: Primary adenocarcinoma of the seminal vesicle presenting as a bladder tumor. Urology 1988; 32:466–468.
39. Murphy WM, Gaeta JF: Diseases of the prostate gland and seminal vesicles. *In* Murphy WM (ed): Urological Pathology, pp 210–218. Philadelphia, WB Saunders Co, 1989.
40. Wheeler T: Anatomic considerations in carcinoma of the prostate. Urol Clin North Am 1989; 16:623–634.
41. Ramchandani P, Schnall MD: Magnetic resonance imaging of the prostate. Semin Roentgenol 1993; 28:74–82.
42. Schnall MD, Bezzi M, Pollack HM, et al: Magnetic resonance imaging of the prostate. Magn Reson Q 1990; 6:1–16.
43. Jaske G, Putz A, Hofstadter F: Carcinoma in situ of the bladder extending into the seminal vesicles. J Urol 1987; 137:44–45.
44. Ro JY, Ayala AG, el-Naggar A, et al: Seminal vesicle involvement by in situ and invasive transitional cell carcinoma of the bladder. Am J Surg Pathol 1987; 11:951–958.
45. Summers RM, Korobkin MT, Ellis JH, et al: Pelvic CT findings after radical prostatectomy. Radiology 1991; 181(p)(Suppl): 243.
46. Ramchandani P, Kressel HY, Pollack HM, et al: Endorectal surface coil imaging for suspected recurrence of prostate cancer after radical prostatectomy. Radiology 1991; 181(p)(Suppl):262.
47. Ganabathi K, Chadwick D, Feneley RCL, et al: Hemospermia. Br J Urol 1992; 69:225–230.
48. Littrup PJ, Lee F, McLeary RD, et al: Transrectal US of the seminal vesicles and ejaculatory ducts: clinical correlation. Radiology 1988; 168:625–628.
49. Etherington RJ, Clements R, Griffiths GJ, et al: Transrectal

ultrasound in the management of hemospermia. Clin Radiol 1990; 41:175–177.
50. Schned AR, Ledbetter JS, Selikowitz SM: Primary leiomyosarcoma of the seminal vesicle. Cancer 1986; 57:2202–2206.
51. Buck AC, Shaw RE: Primary tumours of the retro-vesical region with special reference to mesenchymal tumors of the seminal vesicles. Br J Urol 1972; 44:47–50.
52. Lamont JS, Hesketh PJ, de las Morenas A, et al: Primary angiosarcoma of the seminal vesicle. J Urol 1991; 146: 165–167.
53. Amirkhan RH, Molberg KH, Wiley EL, et al: Primary leiomyosarcoma of the seminal vesicle. Urology 1994; 44: 132–135.
54. Gentile AT, Moseley HS, Quinn SF, et al: Leiomyoma of the seminal vesicle. J Urol 1994; 151:1027–1029.
55. Chiou R-K, Limas C, Lange PH: Hemangiosarcoma of the seminal vesicle: case report and literature review. J Urol 1985; 134:371–373.
56. Adachi Y, Rokujyo M, Kojima H, et al: Primary seminoma of the seminal vesicle: report of a case. J Urol 1991; 146: 857–859.
57. de Assis JS: Seminal vesiculectomy. J Urol 1952; 68:747–753.
58. Hinman F Jr: Section 7—Prostate: Excision. *In* Atlas of Urologic Surgery, pp 315–388. Philadelphia, WB Saunders Co, 1989.
59. Ewell GH: Seminal vesicle carcinoma. J Urol 1963; 89: 908–912.
60. Fain JS, Cosnow I, King BF, et al: Cystosarcoma phyllodes of the seminal vesicle. Cancer 1993; 71:2055–2061.
61. Tripathi VNP, Dick VS: Primary sarcoma of the urogenital system in adults. J Urol 1969; 101:898–904.
62. Villers AA, McNeal JE, Redwine EA: Pathogenesis and biological significance of seminal vesicle invasion in prostatic adenocarcinoma. J Urol 1990; 143:1183–1187.
63. Ohori M, Scardino PT, Lapin SL, et al: The mechanisms and prognostic significance of seminal vesicle involvement by prostate cancer. Am J Surg Pathol 1993; 17:1252–1261.
64. Wheeler TM: Anatomy of the prostate and the pathology of prostate cancer. *In* Vogelzang NJ, Scardino PT, Shipley WU, Coffey DS (eds): Comprehensive Textbook of Genitourinary Oncology, pp 621–639. Baltimore, Williams & Wilkins, 1996.
65. Epstein JI, Carmichael M, Walsh PC: Adenocarcinoma of the prostate invading the seminal vesicle: definition and relation of tumor volume, grade, and margins of resection to prognosis. J Urol 1993; 149:1040–1045.
66. Jewett HJ: Radical perineal prostatectomy for cancer of the prostate: an analysis of 190 cases. J Urol 1949; 61:277–280.
67. Jewett HJ: Radical perineal prostatectomy for carcinoma: an analysis of cases at Johns Hopkins Hospital, 1904–1954. JAMA 1954; 156:1039–104.
68. Jewett HJ, Eggleston JC, Yawn DH: Radical prostatectomy in the management of carcinoma of the prostate: probable causes of some therapeutic failures. J Urol 1972; 107: 1034–1040.
69. Catalona WJ, Bigg SW: Nerve-sparing radical prostatectomy: evaluation of results after 250 patients. J Urol 1990; 143:538.
70. Jones EC: Resection margins status in radical retropubic prostatectomy specimens: relationship to type of operation, tumor size, tumor grade and local tumor extension. J Urol 1990; 144:89–93.
71. Partin AW, Epstein JI, Cho KR, et al: Morphometric measurement of tumor volume and per cent of gland involvement as predictors of pathological stage in clinical stage B prostate cancer. J Urol 1989; 141:341–345.
72. Christensen WN, Partin AW, Walsh PC, et al: Pathologic findings in clinical stage A2 prostate cancer: relation of tumor volume, grade, and location to pathologic stage. Cancer 1990; 65:1021–102.
73. Fowler JE Jr, Mills SE: Operable prostatic carcinoma: correlations among clinical stage, pathological stage, Gleason histological score and early disease-free survival. J Urol 1985; 133:49–52.
74. Middleton RG, Smith JA Jr, Melzer RB, et al: Patient survival and local recurrence rate following radical prostatectomy for prostatic carcinoma. J Urol 1986; 136:422–424.
75. Paulson DF, Moul JW, Walther PJ: Radical prostatectomy for clinical stage T1–2N0M0 prostatic adenocarcinoma: long-term results. J Urol 1990; 144:1180–1184.
76. Schellhammer PF: Radical prostatectomy: patterns of local failure and survival in 67 patients. Urology 1988; 31:191–197.
77. Zincle H, Utz DC, Benson RC Jr, et al: Bilateral pelvic lymphadenectomy and radical retropubic prostatectomy for stage C adenocarcinoma of prostate. Urology 1984; 24: 532–539.

VII

TESTIS AND OTHER SCROTAL TUMORS

32

TESTIS TUMORS: DIAGNOSIS AND STAGING

CHRISTOPHER L. COOGAN, M.D. *and*
RANDALL G. ROWLAND, M.D., PH.D

Testicular cancer is the most common malignancy in men ages 15 to 35 years.[1] This tumor grows rapidly, with a doubling time of 20 to 30 days, has a high risk of metastatic spread, and affects predominately young men.[2] In 1970, the mortality rate for testicular cancer was approximately 90% compared to less than 10% in 1990.[1] Testicular cancer represents a paradigm for the multimodal treatment of tumors. The discoveries of accurate tumor markers, improved multiagent chemotherapy, and modification in surgical techniques have led to improved survival in patients with testicular cancer.

INCIDENCE

Testicular cancer accounts for 6600 new cases per year, with a lifetime probability of developing testis cancer of 0.2%.[3] Testicular cancer may appear at any age, but tends to occur in three distinct age groups: infants and children (0 to 10 years), young adults (15 to 40 years), and older adults (over 60 years).[4] The majority of cases occur in men ages 15 to 35, making it the most common malignancy in this age group.[1] Different histologies tend to occur at different ages. The median age range at diagnosis for a nonseminomatous germ cell tumor (25 to 29 years) is about 10 years earlier compared to that for seminoma (35 to 39 years).[5,6] Yolk sac tumors are the most common testicular malignancy in children; germ cell tumors of children are discussed in Chapter 48.

Dixon and Moore cited an incidence of 2.88 cases per year per 100,000 men in the U.S. Army between 1940 and 1947.[7] The incidence in England during a similar time period was 2.3 cases per year per 100,000 population.[8] In 1995, the incidence of testicular cancer in white males in the United States had increased to approximately 4.5 cases per year per 100,000 population.[9] In England, Scotland, the Nordic countries, Australia, and New Zealand, the incidence of testicular cancer has also increased since the turn of the century.[6] Only cancers of the mouth and skin and non-Hodgkin's lymphoma have increased at a rate faster than testicular cancer.[6] U.S. blacks, however, are one of the few groups in which there has been no increase in the incidence of testicular cancer.[9,10] Forman and Moller compared the incidence rate between 1970 and 1985 in several countries' tumor registries and found an increase in the incidence of testicular cancer ranging from 1.9% to 6.6%, with a median of 2.7% per annum.[6] In Switzerland, which has an extremely high incidence of testis cancer, the rate has not increased between 1974 and 1987, indicating that, in certain high-risk populations, a steady state may be reached.[11] The increasing incidence of testicular cancer appears to be due to more than just increasing patient awareness and cancer registries, but the exact etiology is uncertain.

The incidence of testicular cancer varies among different geographical regions and races. Denmark has one of the highest recorded incidences of testicular cancer.[12] White males in the United States and Western Europe have a high incidence of testis cancer, whereas Asians, Africans, Puerto Ricans, and North American blacks have a low rate of testis cancer.[13] The age-adjusted incidence between 1986 and 1990 for whites in the United States (5.1: 100,000) is over seven times that of blacks in the United States (0.7:100,000).[9] Although some have stated that the low incidence of testis tumors in blacks is attributable to a decreased incidence of nonseminomatous germ cell tumors, others have shown no significant difference in the distribution of tumor types in blacks compared to the general population.[10] An increased incidence has been noted in patients living in rural populations.[14] Testicular tumors occur more commonly on the right side, which is probably related to the increased incidence of cryptorchidism on the right.

ETIOLOGY

Many etiologic agents have been associated with the development of testicular tumors. Up to 10% of testicular cancer patients have a history of cryptorchidism.[13] The incidence of cryptorchidism may be as high as 20% in the premature male, but is slightly less than 1% at 1 year of age.[15] The location of the testis may play a role in the development of testicular cancer. Martin found an increased incidence of testicular tumors in patients with testes located in the abdomen compared to those located in the inguinal region.[16] Patients with cryptorchidism have a 3- to 46-fold increased incidence of testicular tumors.[16] Patients with cryptorchidism should undergo orchiopexy after the age of 1, because some testicles may descend properly up to 1 year of age. The exact timing of orchiopexy, however, remains controversial. Patients with cryptorchidism and their parents should be counseled on the necessity of scrotal examination because both testicles have an elevated risk of developing testicular cancer.[16] A second important risk factor in the development of testicular tumors is the presence of a contralateral tumor. Up to 5% of patients with testicular cancer will develop a contralateral testis tumor, most often metachronously.[17]

Trauma has also been considered an etiologic agent in the development of testicular cancer, but there are few data to support this.[18] It is more likely that the traumatic event causes the patient to seek medical attention, allowing the diagnosis to be made. Recent literature has also implicated minor inguinoscrotal traumatic events, such as a hydrocele, testis injury, hernia, or vasectomy, in the etiology of testicular cancer.[18–20] Although many controlled studies have shown no significant increase in testicular tumors in patients undergoing vasectomy, there may be an increased incidence of testicular tumors in patients with complications after vasectomy.[21]

Gilbert initially suggested that atrophy may have an etiologic role in testicular tumors when he noted that 80 of 5500 patients with testicular cancer (1.5%) had an atrophic testis prior to developing a tumor.[22] In addition, Beard et al. found testis tumors in 2 of 132 cases of mumps-associated atrophied testes (1.5%), significantly higher than the 0.2% noted in the general population.[23] Although the exact mechanism is unclear, nonspecific or mumps-associated atrophy is associated with a higher likelihood of developing testicular cancer. Possibly an altered hormonal milieu or viral agent causes the development of tumors in atrophied testes. Atrophied testes must be followed closely for the development of possible tumor. Anecdotal reports have associated the development of acquired immunodeficiency syndrome with subsequent testicular cancer.[24]

Hormonal factors have been associated with the development of testis tumors. There are conflicting studies on the role of maternal exposure to diethylstilbestrol in the development of testis cancer in male offspring. Cosgrove et al.'s study showed a possible increased incidence,[25] whereas Brown et al.'s study showed no significant difference.[26] Other prenatal factors, such as maternal severe nausea, unusual bleeding during pregnancy, low birth rate, or early birth order, have all been associated with excess risk of developing testicular tumors.[26] Those whose occupations are associated with the highest risk of tumor formation are paper and printing workers, administrators, and professionals.[27]

Genetic factors may also play a role in the etiology of testicular tumors. Cooper and associates described three brothers with testicular cancer.[28] They suggest a multistep etiology in the development of testicular tumors in patients with a genetic predisposition. Patients with a history of testicular tumors have up to a 5% chance of developing a contralateral testicular tumor,[17] suggesting a genetic predisposition to developing testicular cancer. Nicholson and Harland have implicated a genetic etiology in up to one third of cases of testicular cancer.[29] The decreased incidence of testicular cancer in blacks further supports the genetic basis in the etiology of testis cancer. Finally, isochromosomal deletions on the short arm of chromosome 12 have been found in many patients with both seminoma and nonseminomatous germ cell tumors,[2] supporting a genetic role in the development of testis cancer.

PATHOLOGY

The American classification of testicular tumors is shown in Table 32–1. Tumors purely of germ cell origin comprise approximately 90 to 95% of testicular neoplasms.[3] (Testicular tumors of non–germ cell origin are discussed in Chapter 35.) Intratubular germ cell neoplasia is considered a precursor lesion and is defined as the presence of atypical germ cells in the seminiferous epithelium. The true incidence of intratubular germ cell neoplasia is unknown, but Giwercman et al. did not find any patients with intratubular germ cell neoplasia on postmortem testis biopsies among 396 men between the ages of 18 and 50.[30] In subfertile men, however, the incidence has been reported to be as high as 1.1%.[31] Intratubular germ cell neoplasia is a precursor lesion that may precede both seminoma and nonseminomatous germ cell tumors.[32] The incidence of intratubular germ cell neoplasia in patients with contralateral cancer of the testis is over 5%.[33,34] Germ cell tumors of testicular origin are classically divided into seminoma and nonsemi-

TABLE 32–1. CLASSIFICATION OF TESTICULAR GERM CELL TUMORS

Precursor Lesion
- Intratubular germ cell neoplasia (unclassified type equivalent to "carcinoma in situ")

Tumors of One Histologic Type
- Seminoma
  - Variant: seminoma with syncytiotrophoblast cells
- Spermatocytic seminoma
  - Variant: spermatocytic seminoma with a sarcomatous component
- Embryonal cell carcinoma
- Yolk sac tumor (endodermal sinus tumor)
- Choriocarcinoma
- Teratoma
  - Mature teratoma
  - Immature teratoma
  - Teratoma with an overtly malignant component
  - Monodermal variants
    - Carcinoid (pure and with teratomatous elements)
    - Primitive neuroectodermal tumor

Tumors of More than One Histologic Type
- Mixed germ cell tumors (specify individual components)
- Polyembryoma and diffuse embryoma

noma. The incidences of each type of germ cell tumor are shown in Table 32–2.

Seminoma remains the most common germ cell tumor, followed by embryonal cell carcinoma and teratocarcinoma. Classically, seminoma was divided into typical, anaplastic, and spermatocytic. Spermatocytic seminoma occurs at a later age and is unlikely to metastasize. Today, however, the prognostic differences between the histologic types of seminoma are debatable.[5] Nonseminomatous germ cell tumors include embryonal cell carcinoma, yolk sac carcinoma, choriocarcinoma, and teratoma. Approximately 25% of testicular germ cell tumors are composed of multiple cell types, with embryonal cell carcinoma and teratoma being the most common.[5]

CLINICAL MANIFESTATIONS

The most common presentation of testicular cancer is painless swelling of one testis. Patients may also complain of fullness, dull ache, pain, or infertility. Bosl and associates cited a median time from onset of symptoms to first physician visit of 36 days, followed by an additional 10 days before histologic diagnosis.[35] Moul reviewed almost 5000 cases of testicular cancer and found a mean duration of 26 weeks from onset of symptoms to surgical diagnosis.[36] Although patients with higher stage disease present with a longer delay in diagnosis,[35] conflicting data exist on whether this affects overall survival.[37] Any hard mass in the scrotum should be considered a germ cell tumor until proven otherwise. Testicular tumors may be confused with epididymitis, orchitis, torsion, hydrocele, spermatocele, varicocele, or hernia. The key to managing young males with a presumed diagnosis of epididymitis is to perform careful follow-up examinations to ensure the mass has resolved with proper therapy.

TABLE 32–2. PRIMARY CELL TYPES OF GERM CELL TUMORS IN 2562 CASES FROM NINE SERIES*

Cell Type	Average Incidence (%)	Range (%)
Seminoma	42	34–55
Embryonal cell carcinoma	26	23–34
Teratocarcinoma	26	9–32
Teratoma	5	1–6
Choriocarcinoma	1	1–4

*Tabulated from Johnson DE: Epidemiology. *In* Johnson DE (ed): Testicular Tumors, 2nd ed, p 37. Flushing, NY, Medical Examination Publishing Co, 1976.

Forty to 50% of patients will have metastatic disease at presentation.[38] Approximately 10% of patients will present with manifestations of metastatic disease,[35] such as a neck mass from supraclavicular adenopathy, hemoptysis from lung metastasis, abdominal mass, back pain from retroperitoneal adenopathy, bone pain from metastasis, gynecomastia secondary to elevated serum human chorionic gonadotropin level,[39] or gastrointestinal disturbances from direct or indirect involvement.[40] A high index of suspicion, proper scrotal examination, and radiologic imaging are necessary to make the diagnosis in these patients.

The normal testis is oval, firm, and smooth, with a posteriorly attached epididymis. The testes are best palpated using warm hands, beginning with the unaffected testis. The tips of the thumb and opposing fingertips are placed on opposite sides of testis or the fingertips of opposite hands are placed on each side and the testis is gently palpated. The uninvolved testis is examined first, allowing the patient to relax and giving the examiner a good baseline. A normal testicle is smooth in consistency, freely mobile, and able to be differentiated from the posteriorly placed epididymis. The suspicious testis is examined in a similar fashion. Any solid mass within the tunica albuginea should be considered malignant until proven otherwise. Transillumination of the testis is useful to differentiate between a solid and a cystic structure. Ultrasound examination aids in localizing and determining the consistency of the mass (Fig. 32–1).

TUMOR MARKERS

Up to 90% of patients with testis cancer will have an elevated α-fetoprotein (AFP) or β-human chorionic gonadotropin (β-hCG) level.[41] Tumor markers are useful in diagnosis, initial staging, assessing the response to therapy, and early detection of relapse. The development of tumor markers in testis cancer has, in part, accounted for the improved sur-

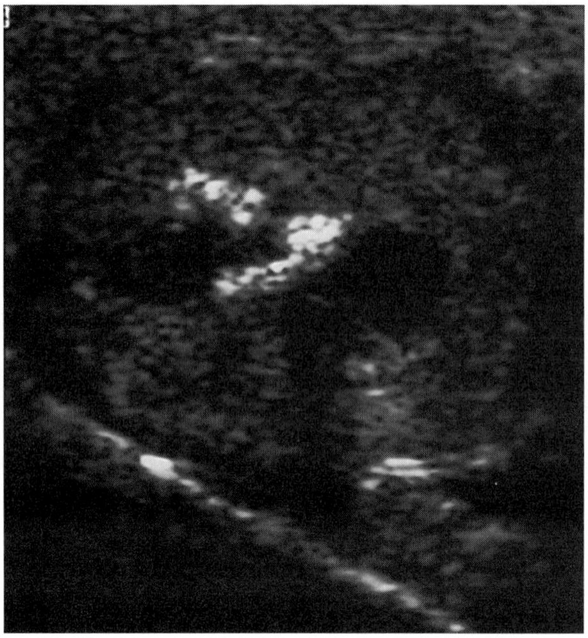

FIGURE 32–1. Ultrasound of the testicle. Note the mixed echogenicity of the mass within the testicle. Radical orchiectomy revealed a mixed germ cell tumor.

vival seen in patients with testis cancer. Accurate tumor markers have allowed patients with relapse to be detected at an earlier stage, resulting in improved survival. The presence of elevated levels of tumor markers is useful; however, normal serum tumor marker levels do not eliminate the diagnosis of testis cancer.

hCG is a glycoprotein with a molecular weight of 38,000 and is normally made by the syncytiotrophoblast of placenta. The serum half-life of β-hCG ranges between 24 and 36 hours. hCG is a polypeptide consisting of two subunits designated α and β. The α subunit has homology with other hormones, including follicle-stimulating hormone, thyroid-stimulating hormone, and luteinizing hormone. The β subunit is antigenically distinct, and immunoassays have been developed to this subunit. Forty to 60% of nonseminomatous germ cell tumors and up to 30% of pure seminomas have an elevated hCG level.[38] Choriocarcinoma is characterized by a markedly elevated hCG level, but an elevated level of hCG may also be seen with other nonseminomatous germ cell tumors and in patients with seminoma. Elevated hCG levels may also be seen in other carcinomas, including stomach, pancreas, colon, bladder, small intestine, bronchus, and breast, and in Hodgkin's disease, non-Hodgkin's lymphoma, myeloma, leukemia, retroperitoneal sarcoma, melanoma, and insulinomas.[42]

AFP is an embryonic glycoprotein with a molecular weight of 70,000 produced by the yolk sac, and subsequently by the fetal liver. Serum AFP levels fall dramatically at birth and become undetectable by 1 year of age.[42] The serum half-life of AFP ranges from 5 to 7 days. An elevated AFP level is seen in approximately 70% of yolk sac and embryonal germ cell tumors.[38] An elevated serum AFP level should always indicate the presence of nonseminomatous germ cell tumor. If the histologic diagnosis is seminoma and the AFP level is elevated, the surgical specimen must be re-examined by the pathologist. AFP can also be elevated by liver damage or metastasis, gastrointestinal carcinoma, or hepatocellular carcinoma. In addition, ataxia-telangiectasia, hereditary tyrosinemia, and hereditary persistence of AFP may all cause an elevated AFP level.[42,43]

Other tumor markers for testicular cancer have also been investigated. Although AFP and hCG are excellent tumor markers, additional tumor markers are necessary not only for additional prognostic and survival data, but also for evaluation of "marker-negative" patients. The level of placental-like alkaline phosphatase (PLAP) is elevated in 40 to 100% of seminomas and is useful in following the course of disease.[42] It is less useful in patients with nonseminomatous germ cell tumors. Unfortunately, the PLAP level is also elevated in up to 35% of normal patients, many of whom smoke.[42] The level of serum lactate dehydrogenase (LDH), particularly the isoenzyme fraction, LDH-1, is elevated in up to 60% of nonseminomatous germ cell tumors.[38] LDH levels may also be elevated in patients with liver disease, myocardial damage, or hemolysis.[42] Serum LDH levels have been shown to correlate with the extent of disease.[44] A number of additional markers are available, including placental proteins 5, 10, and 15, neuron-specific enolase, γ-glutamyl transpeptidase, ferritin, prolactin, estradiol, and the oncogene c-*myc*.[42]

As stated previously, serum tumor markers are useful in diagnosis, staging, assessing response to therapy, and early detection of relapse. The most useful role of AFP and hCG is monitoring the response to therapy in patients with metastatic disease. Marker levels often initially rise following the onset of chemotherapy—the "surge phenomenon." Patients should have an approximate 1-log reduction in their marker levels with each course of chemotherapy.[1] Failure to decline at the normal rate may indicate the necessity to change chemotherapy.[45]

IMAGING EVALUATION

Accurate imaging examinations are useful in both the initial diagnosis and staging of testis cancer patients. The improved overall survival enjoyed by patients with testicular cancer is, in part, due to technological advances and improved accuracy in imaging. An algorithm for the diagnosis and staging of testis cancer is presented in Figure 32–2. After the diagnosis is established by radical orchiectomy, patients are staged by appropriate imaging and, in selected patients, subsequent pathologic

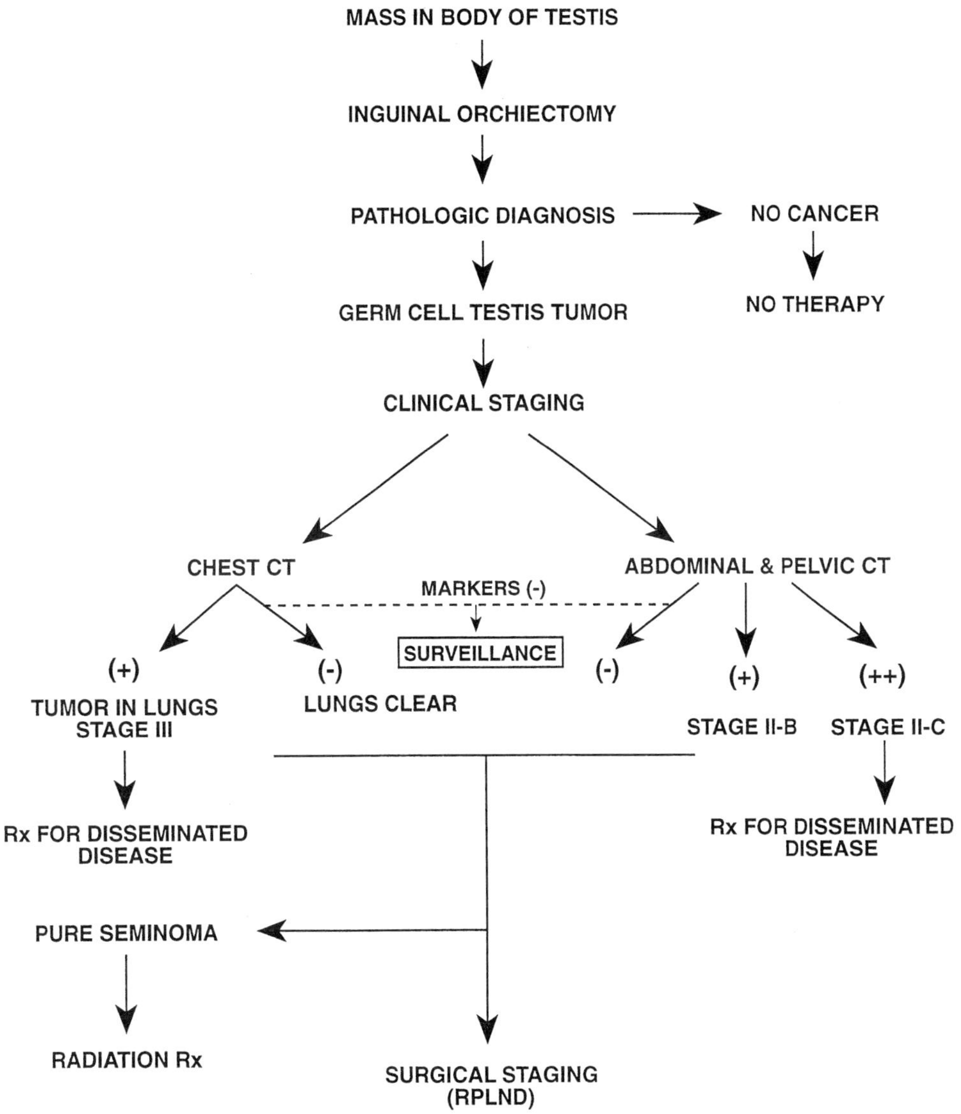
MASS IN BODY OF TESTIS
INGUINAL ORCHIECTOMY
PATHOLOGIC DIAGNOSIS
NO CANCER
NO THERAPY
GERM CELL TESTIS TUMOR
CLINICAL STAGING
CHEST CT
ABDOMINAL & PELVIC CT
MARKERS (-)
SURVEILLANCE
(+)
TUMOR IN LUNGS
STAGE III
(-)
LUNGS CLEAR
(-)
(+)
(++)
STAGE II-B
STAGE II-C
Rx FOR DISSEMINATED DISEASE
Rx FOR DISSEMINATED DISEASE
PURE SEMINOMA
RADIATION Rx
SURGICAL STAGING (RPLND)

FIGURE 32–2. Algorithm for the diagnosis of staging of testis cancer. The staging system specified is detailed in Table 32–3. RPLND, retroperitoneal lymph node dissection.

staging based on retroperitoneal lymph node dissection (RPLND).

Historically, lymphangiography was utilized in the staging of patients with testis cancer. Following injection of contrast into lymphatic vessels, the lymph nodes became opacified and metastases appeared as filling defects. Metastases may then be visualized in patients with "normal-size" lymph nodes.[46] However, lymphangiography is extremely difficult and painful to perform and only opacifies nodes up to the first or second lumbar vertebrae, and the overall predictive accuracy is only 62%.[46,47] In addition, lymphangiograms have been associated with pulmonary embolism and impaired pulmonary diffusion capacity, and RPLND is more difficult to perform after a lymphangiogram.[48] Intravenous urography was often carried out at the time of lymphangiography to delineate tumor extent and the anatomy of the kidneys and ureters.

Ultrasound examination is useful in the visualization of the testicles and retroperitoneum. Scrotal palpation remains the primary method of diagnosis in testis cancer. However, it is often difficult to palpate a tumor because of its small size or a large or tense hydrocele. In these patients, scrotal ultrasound is mandatory. Scrotal ultrasound is noninvasive, radiation free, and highly accurate in the diagnosis of testicular cancer.[49] Ultrasound is able to differentiate between an intratesticular mass and a mass that lies outside the tunica albuginea. Figure 32–1 shows a scrotal ultrasound that displays a typical testicular tumor. Seminoma is classically a hypoechoic lesion, whereas a nonseminomatous germ cell tumor may show a mixed echogenicity. Color Doppler has been utilized in the evaluation of testicular tumors with limited advantage over traditional gray-scale ultrasound.[50] Ultrasound examination of the retroperitoneum is limited secondary to excessive adipose tissue and overlying bowel gas. Rowland and associates found an overall accuracy of 53% utilizing ultrasound in the examination of the retroperitoneum in 64 patients with testis cancer.[51] In select patients with a small amount of retroperitoneal fat, especially children, ultrasound may be superior to computed tomography (CT).

CT is the primary modality in the evaluation of the retroperitoneal lymph nodes. It is noninvasive, easy to reproduce, and accurate and allows visualization of adjacent organs. Figures 32–3 and 32–4 display representative CT scans of patients with clinical B2 and B3 disease, respectively. The diagnosis of metastasis on CT is based on the size of the lymph nodes. The exact cutoff between a normal and an enlarged lymph node is controversial and ranges between 5 and 15 mm.[46] As one changes the size criterion for a normal lymph node, the accuracy of CT will change. Previous studies using a diameter of 10 to 15 mm as the criterion for metastatic disease found a false-negative rate ranging between 23 and 44%.[48,51] Leibovitch et al. were able to lower the false-negative rate to less than 10% by changing the threshold to 3 mm in the predicted landing zone and 10 mm out of the predicted landing zone.[52] CT has also been associated with an approximately 25% rate of false-positive tests.[53] Work using third- and fourth-generation CT scanners still yields a 33% false-negative rate.[54] The pattern of metastatic spread has been well documented by Donohue et al.[55] and should aid in the interpretation of retroperitoneal CT in patients with testis cancer. Fernandez et al. stated that any number of nodes in the primary landing zone, regardless of size, is suspicious for occult disease.[54]

CT scanning of the chest is the most sensitive method of identifying pulmonary metastasis.[46] The improved sensitivity, however, allows visualization of many small lesions that are usually of benign etiology. It is hoped that continued improvement in

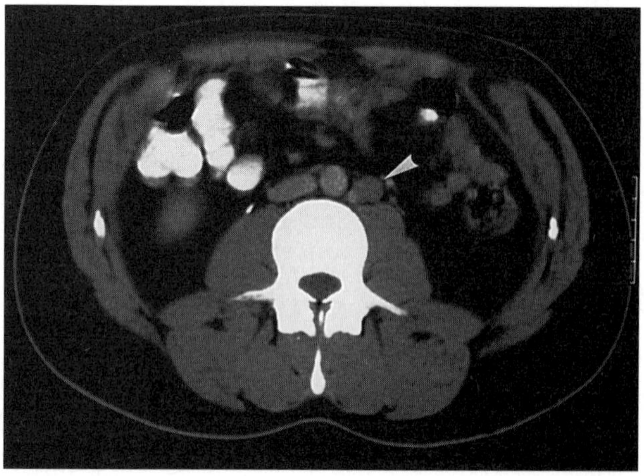

FIGURE 32–3. CT scan of the abdomen displaying a patient with clinical stage B2 disease. Arrow marks a mass in the periaortic area measuring 2.5 × 1.7 cm.

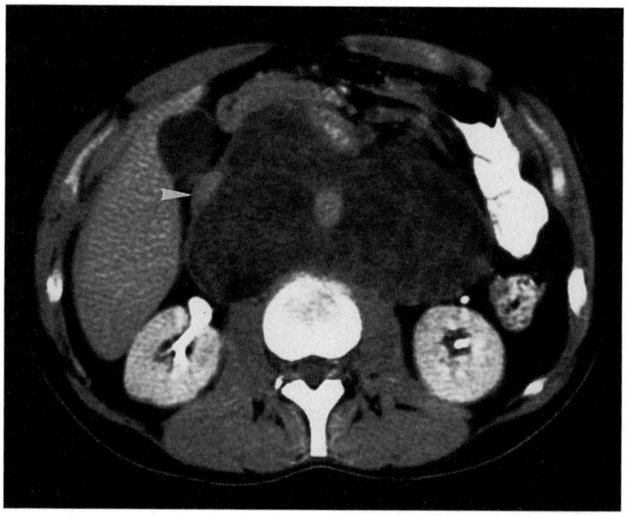

FIGURE 32–4. CT scan of the abdomen in a patient with clinical stage B3 disease. Note that the mass has completely surrounded the aorta and displaced the inferior vena cava (arrow).

CT, including the use of spiral CT in both the retroperitoneum and chest, will decrease both the false-positive and false-negative rates. Until a more accurate staging system exists, however, RPLND is the primary modality utilized by the authors in patients with low-stage disease. Improved markers and accuracy of clinical staging may better define patients in whom surveillance is a better alternative.

Magnetic resonance imaging (MRI) has been utilized in the evaluation of scrotal masses[56] and the retroperitoneum. MRI was utilized in the evaluation of 205 patients with scrotal pathology, and a 100% sensitivity was found in the diagnosis of testicular cancer.[56] Ultrasound, however, will likely remain the test of choice because it is 98.5% sensitive, universally available, and less costly and has a shorter exam time.[56] CT scanning of the abdomen and pelvis is currently the test of choice to examine the retroperitoneum for evidence of metastatic spread. Unlike CT, retroperitoneal MRI is able to obtain images in many planes, does not require injection of contrast, and allows a more accurate visualization of vasculature. Although it was hoped that MRI would be useful in distinguishing between malignant and benign processes on T1- and T2-weighted images, to date this is not possible.[46]

STAGING

The staging of testicular cancer patients is based on both their clinical and pathologic findings. Patients must be accurately classified and the extent of disease determined for proper therapeutic decisions. Clinical staging is used to determine whether patients are best suited for surveillance, RPLND, or induction chemotherapy. Once the diagnosis of an intratesticular mass is made, serum is drawn to

TABLE 32–3. CLINICAL STAGING OF TESTIS CANCER

Stage	Description
A or I	Tumor limited to the testis alone
B1 or IIA	Tumor of the testis and retroperitoneal lymph nodes (<2 cm)
B2 or IIB	Tumor of the retroperitoneal lymph nodes 2–6 cm in greatest dimension by CT
B3 or IIC	Tumor of retroperitoneal lymph nodes >6 cm in greatest dimension by CT
C or III	Tumor above the diaphragm or involving abdominal solid organ

measure tumor markers and radical orchiectomy is performed (the technique for radical orchiectomy is described elsewhere). Repeat serum samples are drawn after the orchiectomy to determine if the rate of decay of tumor markers is in accord with the expected half-life of each tumor marker. The rate of decay is critical in establishing the treatment necessary for a given patient.

Clinical staging is based on the radiographic findings. The clinical staging system utilized at Indiana University is shown in Table 32–3. All testis cancer patients require a CT scan of their abdomen and pelvis and a chest x-ray to determine if there is any evidence of metastatic spread. We routinely utilize CT scanning of the chest in all patients with testis cancer. Testis cancer primarily spreads via the lymphatics to the retroperitoneum. Donohue et al. determined that the distribution of lymphatic metastasis is predictable and occurs along defined pathways.[55] Right testicular tumors spread first to the interaortocaval area, whereas left testis tumors spread initially to the left paraortic area. The crossover of metastatic spread is greater from right to left than from left to right. The ability to accurately predict where a tumor will spread should be reflected during the interpretation of the CT scan, allowing a more accurate clinical staging. The 30% false-negative rate of CT, however, precludes more accurate clinical staging.

TABLE 32–4. TNM STAGING SYSTEM FOR TESTICULAR CANCER

T0—No apparent primary
T1—Testis only (excludes rete testis)
T2—Beyond the tunica albuginea
T3—Rete testis or epididymal involvement
T4—Spermatic cord
  a—spermatic cord
  b—scrotum

N0—No nodal involvement
N1—Ipsilateral regional nodal involvement
N2—Contralateral or bilateral abdominal or groin nodes
N3—Palpable abdominal nodes or fixed groin nodes
N4—Juxtaregional nodes

M0—No distant metastases
M1—Distant metastases present

TABLE 32–5. INDIANA UNIVERSITY CLASSIFICATION OF EXTENT OF DISEASE*

Minimal
1. Elevated hCG or AFP only
2. Cervical nodes (+/− nonpalpable retroperitoneal nodes)
3. Unresectable, but nonpalpable, retroperitoneal disease
4. Minimal pulmonary metastases—less than five per lung field and the largest <2 cm (+/− nonpalpable abdominal disease)

Moderate
5. Palpable abdominal mass as only anatomic disease
6. Moderate pulmonary metastases—5 to 10 pulmonary metastases per lung field and the largest <3 cm; *or* a mediastinal mass <50% of the intrathoracic diameter; *or* a solitary pulmonary metastasis any size >2 cm (+/− nonpalpable abdominal disease)

Advanced
7. Advanced pulmonary metastases—mediastinal mass >50% of the intrathoracic diameter; *or* greater than 10 pulmonary metastases per lung field; *or* multiple pulmonary metastases >3 cm (+/− nonpalpable abdominal disease)
8. Palpable abdominal disease plus pulmonary metastases
   8.1—minimal pulmonary
   8.2—moderate pulmonary
   8.3—advanced pulmonary
9. Hepatic, osseous, or central nervous system metastases

*From Birch R, Williams SD, Cohn A, et al: Prognostic factors for a favorable outcome in disseminated germ cell tumors. J Clin Oncol 1986; 4:400, with permission.

Surgical staging allows a more accurate staging and is therapeutic in about two thirds of the patients.[53] Patients are classified on the basis of the orchiectomy specimen and nodal status after RPLND (Table 32–4). Patients are classified into high versus low risk based on the findings of the orchiectomy. Patients with vascular invasion, presence of embryonal or undifferentiated cells, or absence of yolk sac are considered to be at a high risk of metastatic disease.[57–59] The histologic findings combined with DNA analysis have also been utilized to predict the likelihood of recurrence.[60] These findings enable a physician to more accurately define a given patient's probability of distant metastasis. The volume and region of nodal disease directly affect the probability of recurrence after RPLND.[53]

Patients with metastatic testicular cancer are classified on the basis of various prognostic factors. Birch and associates classified patients into three groups (minimal, moderate, and advanced) based on the extent of disease (Table 32–5).[61] Patients with minimal or moderate disease have a 99% and 90% response rate, respectively,[61] whereas patients with advanced disease have only a 58% chance of response with standard therapy. The extent of disease based on the Indiana University classification system and the number of elevated markers have been shown to be statistically significant predictors of response to therapy.[38,61] Other staging classifications for patients with high-risk disease have been formulated based on serum tumor markers and response, specific metastatic sites, size and number of lung metastasis, and histology that attempt to predict a given patient's response to therapy. Continued emphasis on redefining the classification system as well as developing new prognostic indicators, such as new tumor markers or genetic markers, will continue to improve survival in patients with testis cancer.

Awareness of the necessity for testicular self-exam, as well as careful examinations or imaging of all testicular masses by physicians, will allow testicular cancer to be diagnosed in a timely fashion. Exact clinical and pathologic staging will allow proper therapy and treatment outcomes of patients with testicular cancer. Continued research efforts should increase survival, especially in "poor-risk" patients.

REFERENCES

1. Einhorn LH, Richie JP, Shipley WU: Cancer of the testis. *In* De Vita VT, Hellman S, Rosenburg SA (eds): Cancer: Principles and Practice of Oncology, 4th edition, p 1126. Philadelphia, JB Lippincott Co, 1993.
2. Sagalowsky AI: Current consideration in the diagnosis and initial treatment of testicular cancer. Compr Ther 1994; 20: 688–694.
3. Richie JP: Detection and treatment of testicular cancer. CA Cancer J Clin 1993; 43:151–175.
4. Richie JP: Neoplasm of the testis. *In* Walsh PC, Retik AB, Stamey TA, Vaughan ED Jr (eds): Campbell's Urology, 6th edition, p 1222. Philadelphia, WB Saunders Co, 1992.
5. Rowland RG, Foster RS, Donohue JP: Scrotum and testis. *In* Gillenwater JY, Grayhack JT, Howards SS, Duckett JW (eds): Adult and Pediatric Urology, 3rd edition, p 1917. St. Louis, Mosby–Year Book 1996.
6. Forman D, Moller H: Testicular cancer. *In* Doll R, Fraumeni JF, Muir CS (eds): Cancer Surveys Volume 19/20: Trends in Cancer Incidence and Mortality, p 323. Cold Spring Harbor, NY, Cold Spring Harbor Laboratory Press, 1994.
7. Dixon FJ, Moore RA: Tumors of the male sex organs. *In* Atlas of Tumor Pathology, Section VIII, Fascicles 31b and 32, p 127. Washington, DC, Armed Forces Institute of Pathology, 1952.
8. Collins DH, Pugh RCB: Classification and frequency of testicular tumors. Br J Urol 1972; 36(Suppl):1.
9. Feuer EJ, Brown LM, Kaplan RS: Testis. *In* Miller BA, Gloeckler LA, Hankey BF, et al (eds): SEER Cancer Statistics Review 1973–1990. Bethesda, MD, National Institutes of Health, 1993.
10. Moul JW, Schanne FJ, Thompson IM, et al: Testicular cancer in blacks. Cancer 1994; 73:388.
11. Levi F, Te VC, La Vecchia C: Testicular cancer trends in the canton of Vaud, Switzerland, 1974–1987. Br J Cancer 1990; 62:871.
12. Osterlind A: Diverging trends in incidence and mortality of testicular cancer in Denmark, 1943–1982. Br J Cancer 1986; 53:501.
13. Schottenfeld D, Warshauer ME, Sherlock S, et al: The epidemiology of testicular cancer in young adults. Am J Epidemiol 1980; 112(2):232.
14. Sharma KC, Gaeta JF, Bross ID, et al: Testicular tumors: histologic and epidemiologic assessment. NY State J Med 1972; 72:2421.
15. Walker RD: Diagnosis and management of the nonpalpable undescended testicle. AUA Updates, Lesson 20 (XI). Houston, American Urological Association, 1992.
16. Martin DC: Malignancy in the cryptorchid testis. Urol Clin North Am 1982; 9:371–376.
17. Dieckmann K, Boeckmann W, Brosig W, et al: Bilateral testicular germ cell tumors: report of nine cases and review of the literature. Cancer 1986; 57:1254.
18. Swerdlow AJ, Huttly SRA, Smith PG: Is the incidence of testis cancer related to trauma or temperature? Br J Urol 1988; 61:518.
19. Strader CH, Weiss NS, Daling JR: Vasectomy and the incidence of testis cancer. Am J Epidemidol 1988; 128:56.
20. Pike MC, Chilvers C, Peckham MJ: Effect of age at orchiopexy on risk of testis cancer. Lancet 1986; 1:1246.
21. Oliver RTD: Clinical relevance of modern understanding of testis cancer epidemiology and etiology. *In* Moul JW (ed): Problems in Urology, Volume 8(1), p 12. Philadelphia, JB Lippincott Co, 1994.
22. Gilbert JB: Tumors of the testis following mumps orchitis: case report and review of 24 cases. J Urol 1944; 51:296.
23. Beard CM, Benson RC, Kelalis PP, et al: The incidence and outcome of mumps orchitis in Rochester, Minnesota, 1935 to 1974. Mayo Clin Proc 1977; 52:3.
24. Tessler AR, Catanese A: AIDS and germ cell tumors of testis. Urology 1987; 30:203.
25. Cosgrove MD, Benton B, Henderson BE: Male genitourinary abnormalities and maternal diethylstilbestrol. J Urol 1977; 117:220.
26. Brown LM, Pottern LM, Hoover RN: Prenatal and perinatal risk factors for testicular cancer. Cancer Res 1986; 46: 4812.
27. Swerdlow AJ, Douglas AJ, Huttly SRA, et al: Cancer of the testis, socioeconomic status and occupation. Br J Ind Med 1991; 48:670.
28. Cooper MA, Fellows J, Einhorn LH: Familial occurrence of testicular cancer. J Urol 1994; 151:1022.
29. Nicholson PW, Harland SJ: Inheritance and testicular cancer. Br J Cancer 1995; 71:421.
30. Giwercman A, Muller J, Skakkebaek NE: Prevalence of carcinoma in situ and other histopathological abnormalities in testis from 399 men who died suddenly and unexpectedly. J Urol 1991; 145:77.
31. Skakkebaek NE: Carcinoma in situ of the testis: frequency and relationship to invasive germ cell tumours in infertile men. Histopathology 1978; 2:157.
32. Berthelsen JG, Skakkebaek NE, Giwercman A: Carcinoma in situ of testis: a precursor of germ cell tumors. *In* Moul JW (ed): Problems in Urology, Volume 8(1), p 46. Philadelphia, JB Lippincott Co, 1994.
33. von der Maase H, Rorth M, Walbom-Jorgensen S, et al: Carcinoma in situ of contralateral testis in patients with testicular germ cell cancer: study of 27 cases in 500 patients. BMJ 1986; 293:1398.
34. Berthelsen JG, Skakkebaek NE, von der Maase H, et al: Screening for carcinoma in situ of the contralateral testis in patients with germinal testicular cancer. BMJ 1982; 285: 1683.
35. Bosl GJ, Vogelzang NJ, Goldman A, et al: Impact of delay in diagnosis on clinical stage of testicular cancer. Lancet 1981; 2:970.
36. Moul JW: Early and accurate diagnosis of testicular cancer. *In* Moul JW (ed): Problems in Urology, Volume 8(1), p 58. Philadelphia, JB Lippincott Co, 1994.
37. Horwich A: Testicular germ cell tumors: an introductory overview. *In* Horwich A (ed): Testicular Cancer: Investigation and Management, p 1. London, Chapman and Hall Medical, 1991.
38. Sarosdy M: Testicular cancer: an overview. *In* Crawford ED, Das S (eds): Current Genitourinary Cancer Surgery, p 306. Philadelphia, Lea & Febiger, 1990.
39. Flood JG, Lighman SL, Francis N: Unusual presentation of a testicular tumor. Br J Urol 1991; 68:549.
40. Miller TT, Mendelson DS, Wu L, et al: Seminoma of the testis presenting as an ulcerating mass of the duodenum. Clin Imag 1992; 16:201.
41. Scardino PT, Cox HD, Waldman TA, et al: The value of serum tumor markers in the staging and prognosis of germ cell tumors of the testis. J Urol 1977; 118:994.
42. Mason MD: Tumour markers. *In* Horwich A (ed): Testic-

ular Cancer: Investigation and Management, p 33. London, Chapman and Hall Medical, 1991.
43. McVey JH, Michaelides K, Hansen LP, et al: A G to A substitution in an HNF 1 binding site in the human alphafetoprotein gene is associated with hereditary persistence of alpha-fetoprotein. Hum Mol Genet 1993; 2:379.
44. Bosl GJ, Geller NL, Cirrincione C, et al: Multivariate analysis of prognostic variables in patients with metastatic disease. Cancer Res 1983; 43:3403.
45. Lange PH, Raghavan D: Clinical applications of tumor markers in testicular cancer. *In* Donohue JP (ed): International Perspectives in Urology, Volume 7: Testis Tumors, p 112. Baltimore, Williams & Wilkins, 1983.
46. Husband J: Advances in tumor imaging. *In* Horwich A (ed): Testicular Cancer: Investigation and Management, p 15. London, Chapman and Hall Medical, 1991.
47. Storm PB, Kern A, Loening SA, et al: Evaluation of pedal lymphangiography in staging nonseminomatous testicular carcinoma. J Urol 1977; 118:1000.
48. Richie JP, Garnick MB, Finberg H: Computerized tomography: how accurate for abdominal staging of testis tumors? J Urol 1982; 127:715.
49. Richie JP, Birnholz J, Garnick MB: Ultrasonography as a diagnostic adjunct for the evaluation of masses in the scrotum. Surg Gynecol Obstet 1982; 154:695.
50. Horstman WG, Melson GL, Middleton WD, et al: Testicular tumors: findings with color Doppler US. Radiology 1992; 185:733.
51. Rowland RG, Weisman D, Williams SD, et al: Accuracy of preoperative staging in stages A and B nonseminomatous germ cell testis tumors. J Urol 1982; 127:718.
52. Leibovitch I, Foster RS, Kopecky KK, et al: Improved accuracy of computerized tomography based clinical staging in low stage nonseminomatous germ cell cancer using size criteria of retroperitoneal lymph nodes. J Urol 1995; 154:1759.
53. Donohue JP, Thornhill JA, Foster RS, et al: The role of retroperitoneal lymphadenectomy in clinical stage B testis cancer: the Indiana University experience (1965 to 1989). J Urol 1995; 153:85.
54. Fernandez EB, Moul JW, Foley JP, et al: Retroperitoneal imaging with third and fourth generation computed axial tomography in clinical stage 1 nonseminomatous germ cell tumors. Urology 1994; 44:548.
55. Donohue JP, Zachary JM, Maynard BR: Distribution of nodal metastases in nonseminomatous testis cancer. J Urol 1982; 128:315.
56. Schultz-Lampel D, Bogaert G, Thuroff JW, et al: MRI for evaluation of scrotal pathology. Urol Res 1991; 19:289.
57. Freedman LS, Parkinson MC, Jones WG, et al: Histopathology in the prediction of relapse with stage 1 testicular teratoma treated by orchiectomy alone. Lancet 1987; 2:294.
58. Read G, Stenning SP, Cullen MH, et al: Medical Research Council prospective study of surveillance for stage 1 testicular teratoma. J Clin Oncol 1992; 10:1762.
59. Moul JW, McCarthy WF, Fernandez EB, et al: Percentage of embryonal carcinoma and of vascular invasion predicts pathological stage in clinical stage I nonseminomatous testicular cancer. Cancer Res 1994; 54:362.
60. Albers P, DeRiese WT, Ulbright TM, et al: Prognostic factors in patients with pathological stage 1 non-seminomatous testicular germ cell tumors and tumor recurrence during follow-up. Urol Res 1995; 23:211.
61. Birch R, Williams SD, Cohn A, et al: Prognostic factors for a favorable outcome in disseminated germ cell tumors. J Clin Oncol 1986; 4:400.

33

SEMINOMA: MANAGEMENT AND PROGNOSIS

MICHAEL A. S. JEWETT, M.D., F.R.C.S.(C),
GHOLAMREZA KHAKPOUR, M.D., *and*
MARY K. GOSPODAROWICZ, M.D., F.R.C.P.(C)

More than 95% of testicular cancer is of germ cell origin, and approximately 50% of these are seminoma[1]. Seminoma typically occurs in younger men with a mean age of 35 years, which is approximately 7 years older than nonseminoma patients. The incidence of testicular cancer is rising in Canada and the United States as well as Europe, but the reasons are unclear.[2–4] The current incidence of testicular cancer in the white U.S. population is 6:100,000 males per year, and that in Canada is 4:100,000.[5,6] Treatment results have been good for many years because of the relatively low metastatic rate and high radiosensitivity. More recent advances in chemotherapy have improved the cure rate to greater than 95% overall. More accurate staging has resulted in a potential for decreased treatment and the attendant morbidity.

DIAGNOSIS AND STAGING

Painless swelling in one testis is the most common presenting complaint in at least 65% of patients.[7] Approximately 20 to 30% have pain or a heaviness in the affected side. Less common presentations include loss of libido, infertility with an incidental mass detected, acute symptoms resembling torsion, hematospermia, associated varicocele, and thrombosis of the pampiniform plexus. Nipple tenderness or swelling has been reported in up to 5% of patients. Very rarely, symptoms including back pain may develop as a result of metastatic lesions. The duration of symptoms has not clearly been shown to correlate with increased stage.[8]

Any history of cryptorchidism and previous inguinal or scrotal surgery, including orchiopexy, should be noted. The latter may alter the pattern of metastasis and therefore be important for future treatment. It is important, in patients who may undergo radiotherapy, to note any history of inflammatory bowel disease, previous abdominal or pelvic surgery or other intra-abdominal disease.

On physical examination, the diagnosis is usually suspected by palpation of an intratesticular mass or a hard mass replacing the entire testicle. The mass cannot be transilluminated. The differential diagnosis includes many of the causes of scrotal mass. Ultrasonography has assumed an important role in diagnosis. Hypoechoic lesions that are frequently homogeneous are characteristic for seminoma (with sharp demarcation from the surrounding testicular tissue). Patchy necrosis may produce a heterogeneous appearance that is more characteristic of the nonseminoma tumors. Echoes from bone or cartilage present in teratocarcinoma are not seen in seminoma; however, all would be treated similarly by orchiectomy to definitively establish the diagnosis.

Radical inguinal orchiectomy establishes the diagnosis and is definitive treatment for the primary tumor. Transcrotal needle biopsy has been reported in special cases.[9] There may be a role for partial orchiectomy in a solitary testis (see later). Routine examination of pathologic sections stained with hematoxylin and eosin reveals the characteristic seminoma morphology. A baseline ultrasound of the contralateral testicle should be obtained in all cases, and biopsy may be indicated at the time of orchiectomy to detect carcinoma in situ if risk factors, such as small size, soft texture, and poor semen quality, are present.

Testicular self-examination has been promoted as a means of early detection of testicular tumors. There is some controversy about this because of a lack of a clear-cut correlation between stage at presentation and duration of symptoms. In addition there are many benign lesions of the genitalia that will be detected by testicular self-examination and may require further assessment.

There is limited information regarding the safety, sensitivity, and specificity of percutaneous needle biopsy of testis tumors.[9] Scrotal violation by any means has been discouraged because of a perceived risk of tumor implantation and change in the pattern of spread.

Serum tumor markers, including the β-subunit of human chorionic gonadotropin (β-hCG) and α-fetoprotein (AFP), should be measured immediately before and after orchiectomy. The levels of these markers are of considerable significance in terms of treatment and prognosis. Their half-lives are less than 24 hours and 5 days, respectively, so that a persistent elevation after orchiectomy indicates metastatic disease unless the level is low.

β-hCG is a glycoprotein synthesized by the syncytiotrophoblastic giant cells. The immunohistochemistry of the primary tumor will identify these cells. Care must be taken to exclude nonseminomatous elements. Whenever pure seminoma with isolated elevation of β-hCG is diagnosed, histologic work-up of the entire primary tumor site must be done to exclude the presence of teratoid structures, especially chorioepithelial cells. An elevation of AFP indicates a nonseminomatous tumor, and the patient should be treated as having that type of tumor, not as having a seminoma. Low-level β-hCG elevation occurs in 8 to 40% of pure seminoma.[10] A level above 200 ng/ml is usually associated with metastases, and nonseminoma elements are often eventually detected. Lactate dehydrogenase is a nonspecific enzyme that has some usefulness as a marker in seminoma.[11] Patients with advanced disease have elevated levels that may be useful in monitoring their therapy. Placental leukocyte alkaline phosphatase has not been found useful in the management of seminoma to date because of a lack of specificity.[12,13] Repeated marker determinations may be necessary until they become normal or they plateau at an above-normal level.

All patients require a chest x-ray and a computed tomography (CT) scan of the abdomen and pelvis to document the presence, location, and size of any abnormal retroperitoneal lymph nodes.[14] If lymph nodes greater than 1 cm in diameter are considered abnormal, the overall accuracy of CT scans to detect lymph node metastases has been reported to be approximately 70%.[15,16] CT is also useful in demonstrating the position of normal kidneys and in identifying renal abnormalities such as horseshoe or pelvic kidney for radiation treatment planning. Lymphangiography has been recommended for those patients with negative CT scans and in patients for surveillance, but its value has been questioned.[14] Although the concept that lymphangiography could improve on the accuracy of CT is appealing, experience in nonseminomatous germ cell testis tumors (NSGCTTs) has been disappointing.[17]

Routine magnetic resonance imaging appears to have little advantage over CT.[18] CT of the thorax is not required for patients with a normal CT scan of the abdomen and pelvis. However, CT of the thorax should be performed in the presence of abdominal disease.[19]

Sperm banking should be offered if the patient is going to have radiation therapy or chemotherapy.[20]

The current International Union Against Cancer TNM and American Joint Committee on Cancer (AJCC) staging classifications for testicular cancer have not been universally adopted, and a new classification from AJCC is being proposed[21,22] (Table 33–1). Other staging classifications have been favored by some, and the designations of stage II and its substages differ considerably between systems.[23]

PATHOLOGY

There are three histologic subtypes of seminoma: classical (70 to 85%), anaplastic (10 to 30%), and spermatocytic (2 to 12%).[1,23] *Classical seminoma* occurs most commonly in the fourth decade. These tumors are composed of sheets of relatively large cells with clear cytoplasm and densely staining nuclei. Syncytiotrophoblastic elements occur in 10 to 15% and lymphocytic infiltration occurs in 20%. There is a correlation between the incidence of syncytiotrophoblastic cells and elevation of β-hCG.

Anaplastic seminoma occurs in patients at an age similar to that for the classical type. It has a worse prognosis than classical seminoma, and 30% of patients dying with seminoma have this type. Characteristics include increased mitotic activity, with three or more mitoses per high power field; a greater incidence of microinvasion; a higher rate of β-hCG production (36%); and an increased incidence of metastasis. Histologically, there is also more nuclear pleomorphism and cellular anaplasia. There may be some histologic similarity to histiocytic lymphoma and embryonal carcinoma. Up to 46% of patients have extragonadal extension of the primary tumor, 25% present with stage II disease, and 36% have an elevated β-hCG.

Spermatocytic seminoma tends to occur in older patients, with the average age in the sixth decade, and does not occur in extragonadal locations. Most cases appear as large, multinodular, fleshy, gelatinous, and hemorrhagic tumors. On microscopic examination, solid sheets of cells may be interrupted by pseudoglandular patterns. Nests of cells may occur in an edematous stroma. Unlike classical seminoma, lymphocytes are usually but not invariably absent and a granulomatous reaction does not occur. Intratubular spermatocytic seminoma is commonly identified. Periodic acid–Schiff stains and placental alkaline phosphatase (PALP) immunostains are usually negative in spermatocytic semi-

TABLE 33–1. PROPOSED UICC/AJCC STAGING CLASSIFICATION FOR TESTIS TUMORS

Definition of TNM

Primary Tumor (T)
- pTx Primary tumor cannot be assessed (if no radical orchiectomy has been performed, Tx is used)
- pT0 No evidence of primary tumor (e.g., histologic scar in testis)
- pTis Intratubular germ cell neoplasia (carcinoma in situ)
- pT1 Tumor limited to the testis and epididymis and no vascular/lymphatic invasion
- pT2 Tumor limited to the testis and epididymis with vascular/lymphatic invasion; or tumor extending through the tunica albuginea with involvement of tunica vaginalis
- pT3 Tumor invades the spermatic cord with or without vascular/lymphatic invasion
- pT4 Tumor invades the scrotum with or without vascular/lymphatic invasion

Regional Lymph Nodes (N)

Clinical
- Nx Regional lymph nodes cannot be assessed
- N0 No regional lymph node metastases
- N1 Lymph node mass 2 cm or less in greatest dimension; or multiple lymph nodes, none more than 2 cm in greatest dimension
- N2 Lymph node mass, more than 2 cm but not more than 5 cm in greatest dimension; or multiple lymph nodes, any one mass greater than 2 cm but not more than 5 cm in greatest dimension
- N3 Lymph node mass more than 5 cm in greatest dimension

Pathologic
- pN0 No evidence of tumor in lymph nodes
- pN1 Lymph node mass, 2 cm or less in greatest dimension and <5 nodes positive, none >2 cm in greatest dimension
- pN2 Lymph node mass, more than 2 cm but not more than 5 cm in greatest dimension; more than 5 nodes positive, none >5 cm; evidence of extranodal extension of tumor
- pN3 Lymph node mass more than 5 cm in greatest dimension

Distant Metastases (M)
- M0 No evidence of distant metastases
- M1a Nonregional nodal or pulmonary metastases
- M1b Nonpulmonary visceral metastases
- Mx Presence of distant metastases cannot be assessed

Serum Tumor Markers (S)

	LDH* (units)	hCG (mIu/ml)	AFP (ng/ml)
S0	≤N	≤N	≤N
S1	<1.5 × N	<5000	<1000
S2	1.5–10 × N	5000–50,000	1000–10,000
S3	>10 × N	>50,000	>10,000

Stage Grouping

Stage	T	N	M	S
0	pTis	N0	M0	S0
1	T1–4	N0	M0	Sx†
1A	T1	N0	M0	S0
1B	T2	N0	M0	S0
	T3	N0	M0	S0
	T4	N0	M0	S0
IS	any T	N0	M0	S1–3
II	any T	N1–3	M0	Sx
IIA	any T	N1	M0	S0
	any T	N0	M0	S1
IIB	any T	N2	M0	S0
	any T	N2	M0	S1
IIC	any T	N3	M0	S0
	any T	N3	M0	S1
III	any T	any N	M1	Sx
IIIA	any T	any N	M1a	S0
	any T	any N	M1a	S1
IIIB	any T	N1–3	M0	S2
	any T	any N	M1a	S2
IIIC	any T	any N	M1a	S3
	any T	any N	M1b	any S

*N indicates the upper limit of normal for the lactate dehydrogenase (LDH) assay.

†Sx, serum tumor markers cannot be assessed.

noma, in contrast to classical seminoma. Spermatocytic seminoma never metastasizes, and therefore orchiectomy alone is usually adequate treatment.

ETIOLOGY

Cryptorchidism is the only clear-cut risk factor with a well-established association.[24] Pure seminoma accounts for a large proportion of testicular germ cell tumors occurring in cryptorchid testes. Undescended testis is the most common disorder of sexual differentiation and occurs in 3.4% of full-term male infants; however, 75 to 80% of these testes will descend in the first year of life, leaving 0.7 to 0.8% of 1-year-olds with true cryptorchid testis. The reason that cryptorchidism increases the risk of tumor is unknown, but the cause of the cryptorchidism may also be the cause of the neoplasia. The location of the cryptorchid testis is important; those patients with intra-abdominal or high inguinal testes are substantially more likely to develop tumors. Early reports suggested that seminoma presenting in an undescended testis was associated with an adverse prognosis, but more recent data do not support this finding.[25] A painful groin mass or abdominal pain is the presenting symptom in more than half of these patients. The size of the primary tumor is larger in pelvic than in inguinal seminoma. An impalpable testis may be detected by ultrasound or CT scan. The accuracy of tumor detection is 91% for ultrasound and 96% for CT, which is more accurate for intra-abdominal testes. Probably as a result of a length of time bias, there is a higher incidence of metastatic involvement (62%) with tumors arising in an intra-abdominal testis than in seminoma presenting in a scrotal testis (25%). In addition, the pattern of nodal metastases is different, with a much higher incidence of pelvic lymph node involvement.

There is a racial variation; black Americans have an incidence 1/10th that of the white population.

Epidemiologic studies have demonstrated a correlation between incidence and socioeconomic conditions. There is an association with human leukocyte antigen typing (BW41). Molecular genetic changes are now being defined.[26–28]

MANAGEMENT

Stage I Disease

When the diagnosis is suspected, the initial management is radical inguinal orchiectomy. This permits high division of the spermatic cord with complete removal of adnexa. Following orchiectomy, patients have routinely received prophylactic abdominal radiation because of a probable high rate of retroperitoneal metastases undetectable prior to CT scanning. Over the past 15 years, improved staging techniques and combination platinum-based chemotherapy have permitted more precise stratification of these patients for therapy and have permitted surveillance as a treatment option. Single-agent chemotherapy is being studied in trial settings as a further option.

Radiation Therapy

Considerable experience in treating stage I seminoma with retroperitoneal radiation has been accumulated[29–55] (Table 33–2). With the use of moderate-dose radiation (25 to 35 Gy), in-field disease control has been observed in 92 to 98% of patients.

The lymphatic drainage of the testis is directly to the para-aortic lymph nodes. There are documented differences in the distribution of metastases from left and right nonseminomatous testis tumors that presumably apply to seminomas as well.[56] The left testicular vein drains to the left renal vein and the lymphatic drainage is primarily to the lymph nodes in the para-aortic area directly below left renal hilum. There is no direct crossover to the right unless there are extensive metastases. On the right side, the testicular vein drains directly to the inferior vena cava below the level of the renal vein, and therefore paracaval and interaortocaval nodes are usually the first ones to be involved. Left-sided nodes may also be involved. Pelvic and inguinal lymph node involvement is very rare. Factors predisposing to inguinal lymph node involvement and inguinal relapse are well established and include past history of scrotal or inguinal surgery, seminoma involving a cryptorchid testis, scrotal orchiectomy with incision of the tunica albuginea, and tumor invasion of the tunica vaginalis or lower third of the epididymis.[42,43] Disruption of lymphatic vessels in the spermatic cord during inguinal surgery has been shown to induce anastomosis between testicular lymphatic vessels and regional lymphatics destined for inguinal or pelvic lymph nodes. In an occasional patient, a connection with the contralateral inguinal lymph nodes may be established, but this is uncommon. In a small proportion of patients with inguinal relapse, no predisposing factors may be apparent.[29,30]

Standard postorchiectomy radiation therapy in

TABLE 33–2. RESULTS OF RETROPERITONEAL RADIATION THERAPY IN STAGE I SEMINOMA

Series	No. of Cases	Survival Rate (%)	Relapse Rate (%)
Allhoff et al.[55]	64	100	3.1
Bayens et al.[42*]	132	99	5
Brunt and Scoble[33]	25	100	4
Duncan et al.[130]	103	96	5
Dosmann and Zagers[52]	282	97[†]	3
Epstein et al.[131]	42	100	2
Fosså et al.[34]	365	99	4
Germa Lluch et al.[58]	36	100	0.3
Giacchetti et al.[132]	184	96	2
Gospodarowicz et al.[44]	194	100	5
Hannum et al.[133]	48	97	4
Kellokumpu and Halme[46]	129	95	6
Lai et al.[47]	95	97	2
Lindeman et al.[134]	73	90	2
Read and Johnson[29‡]	94	98	1
Singhal et al.[30]	56	96	7
Sommer et al.[135]	133	100	0
Stein et al.[136]	64	94	9.3
Thomas[38]	150	99	1.3
Tongaonkar et al.[39]	71	100	7.4
Willan and McGowan[40]	149	98	7
Yeoh et al.[137]	69	96	1.4

*Para-aortic radiation therapy alone; 17 patients.
†Disease-free survival.
‡Para-aortic radiation therapy; 94 patients.

stage I seminoma is directed to the para-aortic and ipsilateral pelvic lymph nodes. At the Princess Margaret Hospital (PMH), parallel opposed anteroposterior fields are treated with 6- to 18-MV linear accelerator photons. The treatment volume includes the para-aortic and ipsilateral pelvic lymph nodes and is based on the information obtained from CT of the abdomen and pelvis to avoid excessive irradiation of renal parenchyma. This plan is called "hockey stick" in North America and "dog leg" in the United Kingdom and Europe.[31] The contralateral testis is placed in a scrotal shield to protect fertility and hormonal function. A dose of 25 Gy is prescribed at the midplane and delivered in 20 daily fractions over 4 weeks. Inguinal lymph nodes are not routinely treated, but the radiation field is extended to cover the inguinal area in patients with risk factors for inguinal lymph node involvement. Scrotal irradiation is avoided, including in patients with scrotal violation unless the presence of gross contamination is suspected. Meta-analysis of the literature suggests that local therapy is unnecessary in patients who experienced scrotal violation because they have a very low recurrence rate of 2.9% that does not appear to change with local treatment.[32]

The low incidence of pelvic lymph node involvement in stage I seminoma has led to the suggestion to limit the radiation volume to the para-aortic lymph nodes alone. Occasional reports of patients treated in such a manner have consistently showed excellent results with no pelvic failures.[29,33] The Medical Research Council Testicular Study Group in the United Kingdom has conducted a prospective randomized trial of the traditional para-aortic and pelvic radiation versus para-aortic radiation alone.[34] In patients with stage I seminoma and with undisturbed lymph node drainage, adjuvant radiation to the para-aortic nodes is associated with a higher risk of pelvic recurrence but reduced morbidity, although recurrence rates overall are low.

The in-field control rate following retroperitoneal radiation therapy is close to 100%, and there were no in-field failures seen in a cohort of 194 stage I seminoma patients treated at the PMH between 1981 and 1991.[23,25,35–48] The minimum dose of radiation required to control occult retroperitoneal disease has not been defined. Published reports include radiation doses ranging from 2500 to 4000 cGy.[43,49] Isolated local failures have been reported at 1500 and 2100 cGy.[49,50] Recently, Read et al. described 91 patients who received radiation to the para-aortic nodes only with a dose of 2000 cGy in eight fractions, treating alternate fields daily.[29] With a median follow-up of 34 months, no local failures have been reported.

Approximately 5% of patients are expected to relapse outside the treatment volume (Table 33–2). Relapse is most common in the first 18 months following diagnosis of primary seminoma, but late relapses have been reported.[30,44] A small proportion of patients, usually with predisposing factors, relapse in the inguinal lymph nodes. The pattern of relapse has been well documented, with the majority of relapses occurring in the supraclavicular lymph nodes, mediastinum, lung, or bone. Uncommon sites of isolated metastases, such as brain, bone, and tonsil, have also been noted.[51–54]

The cause-specific survival rate in stage I seminoma approaches 100%.[41–43,45–48] However, the overall survival rate ranges between 92 and 99% at 5 to 10 years. Most deaths are due to intercurrent illness, but there is concern that premature deaths may be occurring from radiation-induced cancers. With such excellent treatment results, the prognostic factors for relapse are often not apparent. However, up to 1 in 20 patients treated with postorchiectomy radiation therapy will develop disease recurrence. Factors that predispose to distant relapse include anaplastic histology and locally extensive tumor with invasion of the tunica albuginea, epididymis, or spermatic cord, but their predictive value is low.[45,57] Recognition of factors strongly predictive for early disease dissemination beyond the retroperitoneal lymph nodes would help to identify those patients who may better be treated with initial chemotherapy.

Surveillance

Although adjuvant retroperitoneal radiation therapy continues as the standard management of stage I seminoma, there has been increasing interest over the past 10 years in surveillance, reserving treatment for those who relapse. The reasons for considering surveillance include the possibility of reducing overall treatment morbidity, the availability of CT to both more accurately stage and follow patients, and the development of curative chemotherapy regimens. Several prospective nonrandomized studies of surveillance have been conducted over the past decade (Table 33–3).[55,57–63] The largest reported experience with surveillance is from the Danish Testicular Carcinoma Study Group.[48,64] With a median follow-up of 48 months, the crude relapse rate in 261 patients was 19%. Other studies with adequate follow-up (>36 months) have reported similar relapse rates.[44,52,59] The predominant site of relapse in all studies was in the para-aortic lymph nodes—41 of 49 relapses (82%) in the Danish study and 90% in the PMH series.[61,62,65] The median time to relapse ranged from 12 to 18 months, but late relapses (>4 years) have also been reported. In the PMH series, late relapse occurred in 8 of 31 patients who relapsed (26%). Only 2 of the 727 patients in the surveillance series died of disease, with an additional 2 patients dying of the results of chemotherapy-induced neutropenia.[61] Prognostic factors for relapse have been studied in the three large surveillance studies.[59,61,62] In the Danish study, with univariate analysis, tumor size, histologic subtype, necrosis, and invasion of the rete testis predicted relapse.[61] On multivariate analysis, tumor size was

TABLE 33–3. RESULTS OF SURVEILLANCE IN 727 CASES OF STAGE I SEMINOMA

Series	No. of Patients	Median Follow-up (mo)	Relapse (No. of pts.)	Survival—CSS (%)
Allhoff et al.[55]	33	—	3	100
Charig et al.[57]	15	31	5	100
Germa Lluch et al.[58]	45	34	5	100
Horwich et al.[59]	103	62	17	100
Oliver[138]	26	18	4	100
Ramakrishnan et al.[60]	72	44	13	100
von der Masse et al.[61]	261	46	49	98.9
Warde et al.[62]	172	50	27	99

the only significant factor. The cumulative risk of relapse after 4 years was 6% in patients with tumors less than 3 cm in diameter, 18% in those with tumors 3 to less than 6 cm, and 36% in those with tumors 6 cm or larger. In the PMH series, age at diagnosis and tumor size were the factors predictive for relapse on univariate analysis.[62,66] The risk of progression at 5 years was 21% in patients less than 34 years old, in contrast to a 9% risk in those over 34 years of age. With tumors of 6 cm or less, risk of progression was 12%, and with tumors larger than 6 cm it was 33%. Age was not a significant factor in the Danish study. The only significant factor in the Royal Marsden Hospital study was the presence of lymphatic and/or vascular invasion (9 vs. 17% relapse rate). At relapse, most patients have been treated with retroperitoneal radiation therapy. One of the concerns about surveillance is the potential for more patients to require chemotherapy, which involves a prolonged and more toxic course of treatment. This concern is difficult to address because, in some centers, chemotherapy was used electively at relapse.[58,67]

Chemotherapy

Carboplatin in the adjuvant setting produces minimal morbidity and appears effective in pilot studies.[68] Myelosuppression and gonadal toxicity are reported to be mild. A randomized trial comparing radiotherapy and carboplatin has been initiated by the British Medical Research Council.

Stage II Disease

Stage II seminoma includes a wide spectrum of disease extent. Currently, staging is based on the transverse diameter of the largest retroperitoneal lymph node mass (Table 33–1). The definition of stage II seminoma and its substages has varied over time, and the literature must be interpreted with caution. The most common presentation is with stage IIA disease. The frequency of stage IIA depends on the staging investigations performed, and it is more commonly seen when stage allocation is based on lymphangiography alone. Presentations with stage IIB disease are very rare, and only retrospective studies are available to study patterns of failure and treatment outcome in this group of patients. The traditional approach to the management of stage II seminoma is radiation therapy to the para-aortic and pelvic lymph nodes. With this approach, excellent local disease control can be expected, but there is an increasing risk of distant relapse with increasing bulk of retroperitoneal metastases.

Radiation Therapy

The technique of radiation therapy in stage II seminoma is similar to that used in stage I disease. In patients with small (<2 cm) and solitary para-aortic lymph node metastases, no alterations in the radiation dose or technique are required. With more extensive metastases, the radiation field is extended to cover the common iliac lymph nodes bilaterally. A dose of 25 Gy is usually delivered to the entire treatment volume and is followed by a boost of 10 Gy to the involved lymph nodes. The planning process ideally includes a CT-based plan and distribution to ensure appropriate coverage of the disease, without excessive irradiation of the kidneys. The question of including the inguinal lymph nodes and/or scrotum in the radiation volume is analogous to the problem in stage I seminoma, but bulky (>5 cm) para-aortic lymph nodes have been associated with an increased risk of inguinal lymph node involvement.[69]

Until the early 1980s with the exception of some U.K. and Canadian centers, most patients with stage II seminoma received elective mediastinal and supraclavicular irradiation.[70–72] The rationale for this policy was based on the recognition of the orderly spread of seminoma from the abdominal to the supraclavicular and mediastinal lymph nodes. Such treatment reduced the supradiaphragmatic failure rate.[52] However, in the last decade, this practice has been completely abandoned because supradiaphragmatic irradiation does not affect the risk of hematogenous metastases to the lung or bone and effective salvage chemotherapy is available for supradiaphragmatic relapse. Mediastinal irradiation has also been shown to be associated with an increased risk of premature cardiac death.

In stage IIA disease, complete regression of retroperitoneal adenopathy is commonly seen toward the end of the course of radiation, but, in patients with bulky disease, a residual mass may be noted for 12 to 18 months following treatment. Follow-up CT of the abdomen should be continued until complete response has been documented.

The ultimate local control rates with radiation therapy in stage II seminoma have not been well described. Most reports include patients diagnosed and treated without the benefit of CT evaluation of disease extent. Prior to the availability of CT, the extent of abdominal disease was poorly defined and relapse inadequately documented. Even with CT, the difficulties in estimating local control are compounded by the occasional persistence of a residual mass following treatment of bulky retroperitoneal disease.[70,73,74] Data from other contemporary series of patients with stage II seminoma include only an occasional in-field recurrence.[34,42,46–48,52,74–77] The presence of nonseminomatous tumor in metastatic lymph nodes, or at relapse, in patients with pure seminoma has been documented in several series.[44,52,76] Therefore, failure to achieve complete regression in the retroperitoneal lymph nodes in patient with pure seminoma should alert the clinician to the possible presence of nonseminomatous tumor. If the residual mass is small and continues to regress, observation is recommended. On occasion, regression is minimal and a persistent mass may be observed for a number of years. The management of such cases has been controversial, and there are few data on the risk of continuing observation rather than intervention. The need for retroperitoneal lymphadenectomy (RPL) in patients with a residual mass following chemotherapy of seminoma has been questioned, and the indications for surgery have been revised to include only a residual mass greater than 3 cm in diameter, rather than resecting smaller masses or diffuse fibrotic changes.[70,78] An elective resection of a persistent mass is useful to include the presence of teratoma and to obviate the need for continuous monitoring of the abdomen.

The majority of relapses occur outside the irradiated area. The main risk factor predictive for distant relapse is the extent of retroperitoneal lymph node disease. The failure rate for patients with stage IIA and IIB seminoma is 10 to 20%,[79] that for stage IIC seminoma between 20 and 50%, and that for stage IID in excess of 50%. In 99 stage II seminoma patients treated with retroperitoneal radiation at the PMH, the size of retroperitoneal lymph nodes was the most important predictor of relapse and survival.[80] Eight of 69 stage IIA and IIB patients relapsed, but relapse was outside the irradiated area in all but 2, and 1 of these was embryonal carcinoma.

Chemotherapy

Chemotherapy has been used with success in the management of advanced stage II seminoma, with local control rates comparable to those obtained with radiation therapy, bearing in mind the difficulties in evaluating the presence of viable residual disease. The toxicity of chemotherapy, however, should not be ignored. RPL is an alternative strategy for stage IIA–IIB seminoma, especially in patients with limited retroperitoneal involvement and contraindications to the use of radiation therapy. The toxicity of RPL compares favorably with that of chemotherapy in stage IIA–IIB disease.

Our experience supports the use of chemotherapy in all patients with stage IIC–IIB disease, and it is possible that some patients with lymph nodes 3 to 4 cm in diameter, but multiple, may also be better treated with chemotherapy.[44] Unfortunately, the total burden of infradiaphragmatic disease has not been analyzed as a possible prognostic factor for distant relapse, and our own data are not sufficient to answer this question. Chemotherapy results are discussed in the section on stage III disease.

Retroperitoneal Lymphadenectomy

This rarely indicated option is reserved for the rare patient who has a contraindication to radiotherapy (e.g., inflammatory bowel disease, a second contralateral seminoma after abdominal irradiation, or uncertain histology). Modern chemotherapy has reduced the indications for RPL. The procedure is similar to that done for nonseminoma, according to the surgeon's preference.

Stage III Disease

The development of highly effective cisplatin-based chemotherapy for seminoma has dramatically improved survival in stage II and stage III seminoma and offered a curative option to a few patients with stage I disease who recur following radiotherapy. Although no phase III trials specifically address the efficacy of different chemotherapy regimens for seminoma, the results with a combination of etoposide and cisplatin offer response rates and survival in excess of 90%.

In the 1980s, the chemotherapy regimens of weekly cisplatin and cyclophosphamide pioneered at the M.D. Anderson Cancer Center produced 85% response rates. The Royal Marsden Hospital studies with single-agent carboplatin produced 75% response rates, with a high proportion of failures successfully salvaged using cisplatin-based regimens.

A recent report of the Memorial Sloan-Kettering Cancer Center experience with chemotherapy in 140 patients with advanced seminoma documented an overall durable response in 86% with a median follow-up of 3.5 years.[81] The highest proportion of patients were alive and event free following treatment with etoposide and cisplatin (97% alive and 94% event free). The adverse prognostic factors for response to chemotherapy include elevated pretreatment lactate dehydrogenase levels and high β-hCG levels.

In summary, cisplatin-based chemotherapy is a highly effective treatment for patients with advanced seminoma. Four cycles of cisplatin and etoposide are highly effective and form the standard therapy at PMH and other centers.

Relapse

The management of recurrent disease depends on the previous therapy, extent of disease, and histology at relapse. Patients who develop disease progression on surveillance, and who have not had previous retroperitoneal radiation, are managed similarly to new patients with seminoma. Depending on the extent of disease, they receive either radiation therapy alone (for those with retroperitoneal or inguinal relapse <5 cm in diameter) or chemotherapy (for those with >5-cm metastases or distant disease). Patients who are not candidates for radiation therapy may be treated with retroperitoneal lymph node dissection. The management of recurrent disease following treatment depends on the previous therapy, extent of disease, and histology at relapse. Patients who relapse following radiation therapy are usually managed with chemotherapy. The exception to this is isolated inguinal relapse, which may be effectively treated with local irradiation or surgical excision. The choice of chemotherapy depends on the histology of recurrent disease. In patients with unknown histology at relapse, consideration should be given to the use of chemotherapy appropriate for NSGCTT, rather than relying on the two-drug combination of etoposide and cisplatin. Most recurrences are detected on follow-up visits.

Management of Carcinoma in Situ

Carcinoma in situ (CIS) is a premalignant lesion. Germ cell transformation to CIS or testicular intraepithelial neoplasia appears to be a precursor to most germ cell tumors and may occur during early fetal life.[36] Proliferation with subsequent invasion usually occurs after puberty and may be hormonally induced. Deteriorating semen quality in the population may reflect abnormalities that predispose to these events and explain the increasing incidence of these tumors. Patients at relative risk for CIS include those with a history of cryptorchidism, contralateral tumor, infertility, extragonadal germ cell tumor, and sexual ambiguity.[37] Poor semen quality and decreased testicular size may be associated. Testicular biopsy should be considered in these patients because CIS is multifocal and can usually be detected on random sampling. Needle biopsy percutaneously with local anesthesia is feasible and may be as sensitive as open biopsy.[82] Modest-dose reduction radiotherapy to the affected testis will eradicate the CIS, prevent the development of invasive disease, and usually preserve testosterone production, leaving Sertoli cells only in the tubules. Sperm banking should be offered, but semen quality is usually poor. The burden of lifelong testosterone replacement has focused interest on detection of contralateral disease at the time of orchiectomy for clinically unilateral disease. However, the risk for CIS is low (less than 5%) and not all pathologists recognize CIS. Therefore routine biopsy has not been adopted, at least in North America. Nevertheless, it is increasingly evident that virtually all men with CIS on biopsy will progress to develop clinically invasive tumor. Cytologic (with immunochemistry) or biochemical screening of seminal fluid for markers of CIS in at-risk patients may be useful in the future. The subsequent occurrence of a contralateral invasive tumor has traditionally resulted in orchiectomy, although there is recent experience with enucleation or partial orchiectomy, which may be an alternative.[83]

EFFECTS OF TREATMENT

Complications of Radiation—Acute and Chronic

The radiation doses employed in treatment of seminoma are lower than those used for other malignancies, and the acute complications have been assumed to be of minor importance. However, the morbidity of abdominal radiation has not been well documented. A minor degree of nausea occurs in most patients, but less than 50% develop vomiting. Approximately 10% of patients develop severe nausea and vomiting requiring regular antiemetics and are unable to complete normal daily tasks. Antiemetic drugs control nausea in most patients, and the availability of ondansetron has improved symptom control in patients with severe nausea and vomiting. Diarrhea develops in a minority of patients. Significant depression of white blood cells and platelets is uncommon and almost never requires treatment interruption. In spite of the outpatient therapy, many patients are unable to continue full employment or study while receiving radiation therapy. Weakness and lassitude requiring additional rest develops in many patients.

Reports in the literature describe isolated cases of bowel obstruction; however, this only occurred with higher radiation doses.[84] Late radiation complications following radiation treatment for seminoma are uncommon. Only major complications are usually recorded, and the incidence of severe hepatic, renal, bladder, and bowel damage is reported to be less than 1%.[85] Indeed no severe complications are expected unless the patient has an underlying medical problem, or a technical error occurs. The only documented complication is an increased incidence of peptic ulceration in patients treated with a 30- to 45-Gy radiation dose.[85] This was observed in a retrospective study, and other reports did not make the same observation. The results of another study showed that treatment of seminoma with abdominal irradiation is frequently associated with long-term effects on gastrointestinal function; stool frequency was above the control range and gastric emptying was faster, but there were no significant effects on vitamin B_{12}, bile acid, lactose, or fat absorption.[85] However, with the demonstration that a policy of close surveillance following orchidectomy produces a long-term survival equivalent to that for immediate postoperative radiation therapy for stage I seminoma of the testis,[86] the morbidity of treatment, even if relatively minor, assumes a new significance.

Effects on Reproduction

Testicular germinal epithelium is exquisitely sensitive to ionizing radiation. Although the contralateral testis is not in the radiation field, the scatter dose can be significant and may cause profound depression of spermatogenesis and compromise future fertility. A radiation dose between 20 and 50 cGy may produce temporary aspermia, and doses greater than 50 cGy may preclude recovery of spermatogenesis. The use of scrotal shielding reduces the scattered radiation dose but cannot assure protection of spermatogenesis in all patients. The use of sperm banking is recommended for patients who wish to optimize their chances for future fertility and who are to be treated with radiation therapy. In men who recover spermatogenesis after radiation therapy for seminoma, there is no evidence of an increased incidence of genetic abnormalities among their subsequent offspring.[87] Increasing use of radiation therapy to the para-aortic and common iliac nodes alone will also eliminate radiation to the remaining testicle.

Psychological Problems after Treatment

Most studies of the psychosocial well-being of patients after treatment for testicular cancer have analyzed patients without considering the different treatment modalities used. The majority of the studies show that most patients do not have any serious psychological sequelae from their diagnosis or treatment.[88–90] Indeed, some patients report an improved outlook on life compared to their premorbid state and also compared to control groups.[88–91] It is certainly true that some patients do experience severe psychological symptoms, mainly in the areas of sexual activity, infertility, distress, and social upheaval.[92,93] They frequently have had previous emotional problems and they should be referred for therapy.[93] Schover et al. reported that 19% of 84 patients who were treated for seminoma had low rates of subsequent sexual activity.[94] Fifteen per cent had erectile dysfunction and 10% had difficulty reaching orgasm. Data on the psychological morbidity associated with surveillance programs are sparse, but the evidence suggests that these patients may have fewer sexual problems than those who undergo treatment.[91] However, they may have other significant problems with anxiety regarding relapse, and social or work-related problems associated with the follow-up necessary in surveillance programs. Open discussions with clinicians, active participation in treatment decisions, and continuous support after therapy has been completed are helpful in alleviating anxiety regarding therapy, its effects, and outcome.

MANAGEMENT OF RESIDUAL RETROPERITONEAL MASSES

Residual masses may persist after both radiation and chemotherapy. Their management is controversial to some degree. After radiation, most masses will slowly shrink and appear as scars on imaging with CT. A persistent mass after chemotherapy is more common. Two significant features distinguish seminoma from NSGCTT in this clinical setting. First, teratoma in the residual specimen is rare. Second, a complete RPL is technically difficult because tissue planes may be obliterated secondary to the severe scirrhous reaction of these tumors to chemotherapy.[78] The perioperative morbidity with seminoma has been reported to be significantly higher than that for NSGCTT.[70]

There are two clinical presentations of the residual mass. First, the tumor ''implodes'' around the great vessels and obliterates radiographic planes. Residual disease merges with the great vessels, the psoas muscles, and other retroperitoneal structures and resembles the clinical findings seen with retroperitoneal fibrosis; it is ill defined and usually represents fibrosis. Patients with these radiographic findings do not benefit from surgery because the pathologic findings do not justify the high morbidity. In contrast, some masses are well delineated and distinct from surrounding structures. These masses are usually easily resectable. This operation can be accomplished with low morbidity and is effective in excluding residual viable tumor or teratoma. If the postchemotherapy CT scan is normal or the residual mass is smaller than 3 cm, most investigators suggest observation. Controversy exists for the 20 to 30% of patients in whom a residual mass is 3 cm or larger. Although both radiation therapy to the area of residual disease and careful observation have been recommended, our bias is to resect residual mass. This protocol is based on the greater than 40% incidence of seminoma in this subset of patients, the rare occurrence of NSGCTT or teratoma, and the low morbidity of the approach with modern surgical techniques and perioperative care.

The Memorial Sloan-Kettering Cancer Center experience has been updated with a report of 104 patients. Patients with residual masses less than 3 cm in diameter rarely have residual active tumor (3%), whereas 27% of those with masses of 3 cm or larger have residual tumor.[95] Given this high proportion of persistent malignancy, they have recommended resection or biopsy of masses of 3 cm or larger to be followed by additional therapy for those with viable cancer. Options also include further chemotherapy or observation. The time from completion of therapy to surgery is not reported but may be important because masses tend to regress slowly over many months. The EORTC trials have reported that masses can regress over as long as a year and that many can persist for a year or more without relapse.[96] Therefore, patients with a residual mass less than 3 cm or complete remission in response to chemotherapy should be observed.

Several studies have evaluated the management of residual masses in patients receiving chemotherapy for advanced seminoma.[78,95,97] Freidman et al.[97] reported on 20 patients with residual radiographic abnormalities after PVB therapy; 14 who had no prior residual mass were observed, and all remained disease free. Six patients received additional radiation therapy to residual sites of disease, and all remained disease free for a median follow-up of 17 months. Three patients had resection of residual disease, with two postoperative deaths, which were in part related to bleomycin-associated pulmonary toxicity; the third patient was alive without evidence of disease. The authors concluded that patients with a postchemotherapy residual mass did not require surgery in view of the excellent overall prognosis and the significant surgical morbidity.

Loehrer et al. examined 62 patients who received cisplatin-based chemotherapy for seminoma.[98] Thirteen underwent attempted surgical exision of residual disease, among whom three (23%) had evidence of residual malignancy. Fosså et al. reported on 39 patients with advanced seminoma, 15 of whom had received prior radiation therapy.[70] Twelve patients underwent exploration for residual disease, three of whom proved to have viable seminoma. One postoperative death from pulmonary toxicity was observed. The conclusion of both groups of investigators was to observe patients with residual disease because of the excessive surgical morbidity involved in detecting persistent tumor.

OTHER ISSUES AND MANAGEMENT OF UNUSUAL CASES

Seminoma with High Levels of β-Human Chorionic Gonadotropin

Gonadotropins can be secreted by most types of testicular tumors, including pure seminoma. Histologic studies have shown that β-hCG is secreted by syncytiotrophoblastic giant cells. In pure seminoma, the frequency of β-hCG production measured in peripheral blood has been reported to be 8 to 13%,[99–101] and in some reports it was even higher (39 to 68%).[102,103] Mumperow and Hartmann reported a much higher incidence of β-hCG secretion by pure seminoma, by measuring β-hCG levels in blood from the testicular vein and the antecubital fossa.[104] They found elevated β-hCG levels in the cubital vein in 26% of patients and in the testicular vein in 80% of patients. Syncytiotrophoblastic cells were found in only 39% of patients with elevated serum β-hCG (cubital and/or testicular).

The question is whether β-hCG–secreting seminomas have a prognosis inferior to that of tumors not secreting β-hCG. The interpretation of the literature is confounded by the lack of attention to the decay of β-hCG levels following orchiectomy. Reports of seminoma treated in the 1960s and 1970s have claimed a worse prognosis.[41,105,106] It is possible that these reports may have included tumors with NSGCTT components, or have failed to confirm an elevated β-hCG level in the context of known disease extent. More recent reports, taking disease extent into account, failed to confirm worse outcome in patients with β-hCG–secreting seminomas.[101,107,108] Weissbach and Busser-Maatz, in a large prospective study of seminoma, found 31% of patients with β-hCG–secreting tumors were more likely to have metastases in retroperitoneal lymph nodes.[109] However, stage by stage, there was no difference in their risk of later relapse. These results imply that the detection of β-hCG is an indicator of tumor burden rather than a sign of tumor aggressiveness. There are few reports of pure seminoma with very high postorchiectomy β-hCG levels without evidence of metastases. If the level of β-hCG reflects tumor burden, and imaging of the retroperitoneal lymph nodes does not reveal metastases, the possibility of occult disease outside the retroperitoneum must be considered. In such cases chemotherapy, rather than retroperitoneal radiation therapy, may be the preferred treatment approach, although it is likely that these patients can be successfully treated with radiation therapy.

Bilateral Tumors

There is an increased risk of developing a tumor in the contralateral testis in patients with testicular tumors.[110,111] The risk of developing a second contralateral testicular tumor is 1 to 4% and appears to be increasing as a result of improved survival of patients of all stages. The second tumor may be synchronous or metachronous. The interval to a synchronous tumor may be long, but 30% appear within 2 years and 50% by 5 years. The relative risk (as compared to the general population) in 1909 patients with testicular cancer diagnosed in the Netherlands with a median follow-up of 7.7 years was 35.7.[112] This increased risk was confined to those patients treated with radiation therapy or with surgery alone. The cumulative risk of developing a second testicular tumor at 25 years of follow-up was reported to be as high as 5.2% by Osterlind et al. in 1991.[113] They reported on the follow-up of 2850 patients with testicular tumors in Denmark diagnosed between 1960 and 1984 and found the risk of developing a second testicular primary to be 9.4% in 224 patients treated with surgery alone, 4.7% in 1994 patients treated with radiation therapy, and 4.3% in 582 patients given chemotherapy. The risk was greater in patients with nonseminomatous tumors (8.4%) as compared to seminomas (3.6%). Interestingly, no second testicular tumors were observed in Manchester, England, where routine prophylactic radiation therapy was given to the contralateral testis.[114]

Patients with second testis cancers resulting in bilateral orchiectomy have an unsatisfactory quality of life because of hormonal imbalance. Bilateral orchidectomy produces infertility and impotence requiring hormonal replacement, which may be a major burden.

When tumor in the contralateral testis is diagnosed, an orchiectomy is usually performed. The two tumors have the same histology 50% of the time, and 80% of bilateral tumors are seminomas. The postorchiectomy management depends on the extent of disease and treatments used for the first tumor. For patients with stage I previously treated with radiation therapy, surveillance or RPL may be used. In stage II disease, the choice of RPL or chemotherapy depends upon the extent of disease and prior treatment.

Because of the morbidity of bilateral orchidectomy, partial orchidectomy of the remaining testis or enucleation has been described.[83,115,116] Percutaneous needly biopsy of the second tumor with radiotherapy to the testis has also been reported.[9] Some experience is being obtained with high-energy focused ultrasound and other high-energy treatments.

Seminoma in Patients with Horseshoe or Pelvic Ectopic Kidney

Horseshoe kidney occurs in approximately 1 in 400 of the general population.[117] There is also an association between renal fusion abnormalities and cryptorchidism, which in turn is associated with an increased incidence of testicular neoplasms.

The association of horseshoe kidney and testicular tumors may occur more commonly because it represents another abnormality in the development of the urogenital ridge.[118] Because of this anomaly, variation in the normal pathways of lymphatic spread might be expected. There are two main problems in the management of seminoma associated with horseshoe kidney or pelvic kidney. In a number of cases of horseshoe kidney, a large part of the renal parenchyma directly overlies the regional lymph nodes, thus lying within the standard radiation volume, and a standard radiation dose would lead to an unacceptable risk of radiation nephritis. Furthermore, the possible abnormalities in lymphatic drainage of the testis lead to an increased risk of relapse with the standard radiation fields. Unusual patterns of relapse have been observed in patients managed by surveillance, confirming concerns regarding abnormal lymphatic pathways.[119] For these reasons, surveillance in stage I and chemotherapy in stage II patients have usually been the treatments of choice. However, a retroperitoneal lymph node dissection is another option for patients unwilling to follow the surveillance program. Reports in the literature suggest that RPL was both safe and effective in the selected cases in which it was performed.[120]

Seminoma in Immunosuppressed Patients

A number of cases of seminoma have been reported following renal transplantation.[121,122] Dieckmann et al. reported a case of stage I seminoma in a renal transplant patient receiving cyclosporin.[123] The patient was managed with routine postoperative radiation therapy and remained well 2 years after therapy. Villalona-Calero et al. reported two stage 1 cases, one managed with radiation therapy and the other with surveillance, with no recurrence at up to 2 years.[121] Stage I and II seminoma in renal transplant patients has usually been treated with postoperative radiation therapy. However, concerns regarding potential damage to the transplanted kidney may dictate surveillance. Short-term follow-up of these patients does not suggest a higher risk of relapse, but available data are limited.

Several reports have documented the presentation and course of testis tumors in human immunodeficiency virus (HIV)-positive patients.[124,125] Moyle et al. found 3 patients with seminoma among 2205 known HIV-positive patients (136 per 100,000), which is 68 times the expected incidence.[126] Testis tumors in HIV-positive patients are most commonly NSGCTT. Some reports suggested that the pattern of presentation in HIV-associated seminoma is similar to that of non–HIV-related seminoma, but there are also reports of an increased frequency of bilateral tumors.[127] Staging of testis tumors in HIV-positive patients may be difficult, especially in those with normal tumor markers and retroperitoneal adenopathy, because the enlarged retroperitoneal lymph nodes may be benign. Most patients with stage I and II HIV-related seminoma and a good performance status were treated with the usual radiation therapy, although surveillance was also employed in this population. Retroperitoneal radiation therapy has been shown to result in a prolonged decrease in the CD4 count. The concern that wide-field irradiation and chemotherapy both worsen immunosuppression and may precipitate HIV-related infection has led to a recommendation for surveillance in stage I seminoma. However, the risk of early tumor dissemination may be greater in HIV-positive than HIV-negative patients. In patients without severe infections, chemotherapy may be well tolerated without risk of activation of HIV-related infections. In some series, the stage I patients managed with surveillance progressed in the retroperitoneal lymph nodes and required treatment soon after diagnosis. However, to date there are few data on the therapy, pattern of relapse, and survival of patients with HIV and seminoma. As in other malignancies, the prognosis is related more to the severity of AIDS and its complications.[128] Further information regarding the tolerance and response of these patients to radiation therapy and chemotherapy will be helpful in determining the optimal treatment strategy.

Management of Noncompliant Patients

As the cure rate for patients with stage I and II seminoma approaches 100%, problems with patient compliance with treatment or follow-up recommendations may affect the outcome more than choice of therapy. Every large cancer center has experience with a patient who refuses conventional therapy, or fails to attend for follow-up and eventually dies of disease. Little attention has been given to this problem, and it is important to examine factors contributing to lack of compliance. Patient education regarding the diagnosis, available treatment options, and outcome in testis tumors, and the need for regular evaluation, should be given high priority.

Management of Seminoma in the Cryptorchid Testis

The postorchiectomy management of seminoma presenting in cryptorchid testis depends on the location of the primary tumor and the extent of disease. Stage I and II disease, other than in patients with large nodal metastases (>5 cm), is treated with radiation therapy. Comparable survival can be achieved by giving similar doses of radiation and adjusting the size of the para-aortic and pelvic radiation fields to cover the known extent of disease.[129] In patients with pelvic lymph node involvement, irradiation of the whole pelvis is recommended. The prognosis of patients with seminoma arising from cryptorchid testis depends more on the stage and extent of disease than the tumor origin in a cryptorchid testis.

FINAL COMMENTS

The survival of patients with seminoma is excellent and the overall risk of relapse is low. These results have been achieved by more accurate staging, knowledge of risk factors, better understanding of the patterns of spread of germinal tumors, and more effective chemotherapy as well as careful diligence in treatment delivery. Continuous vigilance regarding treatment results and failures as well as late effects is required to optimize the survival and quality of life of patients with this disease.

REFERENCES

1. Ulbright TM: Germ cell neoplasms of the testis. Am J Surg Pathol 1993; 17:1075.
2. Zheng T, Holford TR, Ma Z, et al: Continuing increase in incidence of germ-cell testis cancer in young adults: experience from Connecticut, USA, 1935–1992. Int J Cancer 1996; 65:723.
3. Hoff Wanderas E, Tretli S, Fossa S: Trends in incidence of testicular cancer in Norway 1955–1992. Eur J Cancer 1995; 31:2044.
4. Brown LM, Potter LM, Hoover RN, et al: Testicular cancer in the United States: trends in incidence and mortality. Int J Epidemiol 1986; 15:164.
5. Muir C, Waterhouse J, Mack T, et al: Cancer Incidence in Five Continents. Lyon, International Agency for Research on Cancer, Vol 5, 1987.
6. Kwiatkowska K: Cancer in Ontario 1993–1994. Toronto, Canada, Ontario Cancer Treatment and Research Foundation, 1994.
7. Kennedy B, Schmidt J, Winchester D, et al: National survey of patterns of care for testis cancer. Cancer 1987; 60:1921.
8. Moul JD, Paulson DF, Dodge RK, Walther PJ: Delay in diagnosis and survival in testicular cancer: impact of effective therapy and changes during 18 years. J Urol 1990; 143:520.
9. Bos SD, Ypma AF: Synchronous bilateral seminoma of testis treated with unilateral orchiectomy and contralateral irradiation: a therapeutic option. Case report. Scand J Urol Nephrol 1993; 27:559.
10. Fosså A, Fosså SD: Serum lactic dehydrogenase and human choriogonadotropin in seminoma. Br J Urol 1991; 63:408.
11. Edler Von Eyben F, Lindegaard Madsen E, Blaabjerg O, Hyltoft Petersen P: Serum lactate dehydrogenase isoenzyme 1: an early indicator of relapse in patients with testicular germ cell tumors. Acta Oncol 1995; 34:925.
12. Nielsen OS, Munro AJ, Duncan W, et al: Is placental alkaline phosphatase (PLAP) a useful marker for seminoma? Eur J Cancer 1990; 26:1049.
13. Munro AJ, Nielsen OS, Duncan W, et al: An assessment of combined tumour markers in patients with seminoma: placental alkaline phosphatase (PLAP), lactate dehydrogenase (LDH) and beta human chorionic gonadotropin (beta HCG). Br J Cancer 1991; 64:537.
14. MacVicar D: Staging of testicular germ cell tumours [Review]. Clin Radiol 1993; 47:147.
15. Lien HH, Stenwig SE, Ous S, Fosså SD: Influence of different criteria for abnormal lymph node size on reliability of computed tomography in patients with non-seminomatous testicular tumor. Acta Radiol Diagn 1986; 27:199.
16. Stomper PC, Fung CY, Socinski MA, et al: Detection of retroperitoneal metastases in early-stage non-seminomatous testicular cancer: analysis of different CT criteria. Am J Roentgenol 1987; 149:1187.

17. Pizzocaro G, Nicolai N, Salvioni R, et al: Comparision between clinical and pathological staging in low stage nonseminomatous germ cell testicular tumors. J Urol 1992; 148:76.
18. Hogeboom WR, Hoekstra HJ, Mooyaart EL, et al: The role of magnetic resonance imaging and computed tomography in the treatment evaluation of retroperitoneal lymphnode metastases of non-seminomatous testicular tumors. Eur J Radiol 1991; 13:31.
19. See WA, Hoxie L: Chest staging in testis cancer patients: imaging modality selection based upon risk assessment as determined by abdominal (CT) results. J Urol 1993; 150:874.
20. Agarwal A, Tolentino MVJ, Sidhu RS, et al: Effect of cryopreservation on semen quality in patients with testicular cancer. Urology 1995; 46:382.
21. Beahrs OH, Henson DE, Hutter RV, Kennedy BJ: American Joint Committee on Cancer: Manual for Staging of Cancer. 4. Philadelphia, JB Lippincott, 1992.
22. Hermanek P, Sobin LH, UICC International Union Against Cancer, TNM Classification of Malignant Tumors. Berlin, Springer-Verlag, 1992.
23. Mostofi FK: Testicular tumors: epidemiologic, etiologic and pathologic features. Cancer 1973; 32:1186.
24. Batata MA, Whitmore JWF, Chu RCH, et al: Cryptorchidism and testicular cancer. J Urol 1980; 124:382.
25. Gauwitz MD, Zagars GK: Treatment of seminoma arising in cryptorchid testis. Int J Radiat Oncol Biol Phys 1992; 24:153.
26. Lothe RA, Peltomaki P, Tommerup N, et al: Molecular genetic changes in human male germ cell tumors. Lab Invest 1995; 73:606.
27. Al-Jehani RMA, Povey S, Delhanty JDA, Parrington JM: Loss of heterozygosity on chromosome arms 5q, 11p, 1q, and 16p in human testicular germ cell tumors. Genes Chromosom Cancer 1995; 13:249.
28. Peng H-Q, Bailey D, Bronson D, et al: Loss of heterozygosity of tumor suppressor genes in testis cancer. Cancer Res 1995; 55:2871.
29. Read G, Johnston R: Short duration radiotherapy in stage I seminoma of the testis: preliminary results of a prospective study. J Clin Oncol 1993; 5:364.
30. Singhal S, Dixit S, Vyas R, et al: Post-orchiectomy management in stage I testicular seminoma: elective irradiation or surveillance? Australas Radiol 1993; 37:205.
31. Dobbs J, Barrett A, Ash D: Practical Radiotherapy Planning. London, Edward Arnold, 1992.
32. Capelouto CC, Clark PE, Ransil BJ, Loughlin KR: A review of scrotal violation in testicular cancer: is adjuvant local therapy necessary? J Urol 1995; 153:981.
33. Brunt AM, Scoble JE: Para-aortic nodal irradiation for early stage testicular seminoma. Clin Oncol 1992; 4:165.
34. Fosså SD, Horwich A, Russell JM, et al: Optimal field size in adjuvant radiotherapy (XRT) on stage I seminoma—a randomized trial. J Clin Oncol 1996; 15:239.
35. Floyd C, Ayala A, Logothetis C, et al: Spermatocytic seminoma with associated sarcoma of the testis. Cancer 1988; 61:409.
36. Giwercman A, von der Maase H, Skakkebæk NE: Epidemiological and clinical aspects of carcinoma in situ of the testis. Eur Urol 1993; 23:104.
37. von der Maase H: Clinical aspects of carcinoma in situ of the testis: concluding remarks. Eur Urol 1993; 23:251.
38. Thomas G: Controversies in the management of testicular seminoma. Cancer 1985; 55:2296.
39. Tongaonkar H, Dalal A, Kelkar D, et al: Stage I testicular tumours: the TATA Memorial Hospital experience. J Surg Oncol 1993; 54:114.
40. Willan BD, McGowan DG: Seminoma of the testis: a 22 year experience with radiation therapy. Int J Radiat Oncol Biol Phys 1985; 11:1769.
41. Babaian R, Zagers G: Testicular seminoma: the MD Anderson experience. An analysis of pathological characteristics and treatment recommendations. J Urol 1988; 139: 311.
42. Bayens YC, Helle PA, Van PW, Mali SP: Orchidectomy followed by radiotherapy in 176 stage I and II testicular seminoma patients: benefits of a 10-years follow up study. Radiother Oncol 1992; 25:97.
43. Fosså S, Aass N, Kaalhus O: Radiotherapy for testicular seminoma stage I: treatment results and long-term post-irradiation morbidity in 365 patients. Int J Radiat Oncol Biol Phys 1989; 16:383.
44. Gospodarowicz MK, Warde PR, Panzarella T, et al: The Princess Margaret Hospital Experience in the management of stage I and II seminoma 1981–1991. Adv Biosci 1994; 91:177.
45. Hamilton C, Horwich A, Easton D, Peckham M: Radiotherapy for stage I seminoma testis: results of treatment and complications. Radiother Oncol 1986; 6:115.
46. Kellokumpu L, Halme A: Results in irradiated testicular seminoma patients. Radiother Oncol 1990; 18:1.
47. Lai PP, Bernstein MJ, Kim H, et al: Radiation therapy for stage I and IIA testicular seminoma. Int J Radiat Oncol Biol Phys 1994; 28:373.
48. Zagars GK: Stage I testicular seminoma following orchidectomy—to treat or not to treat? Eur J Cancer 1993; 14:1923.
49. Dosoretz D, Shipley W, Blitzer P, Gilbert S, et al: Megavoltage irradiation for pure testicular seminoma: results and patterns of failure. Cancer 1981; 48:2184.
50. Lester S, Morphis J, Hornback N: Testicular seminoma: analysis of treatment results and failures. Int J Radiat Oncol Biol Phys 1986; 12:353.
51. Abdeen N, Souhami L, Freeman C, Yassa M, et al: Radiation therapy of testicular seminoma: a 15-year survey. Am J Clin Oncol 1992; 15:87.
52. Dosmann MA, Zagers G: Post-orchiectomy radiotherapy for stages I and II testicular seminoma [see comments]. Int J Radiat Oncol Biol Phys 1993; 26:381.
53. Raina V, Singh SP, Kamble N, et al: Brain metastasis as the site of relapse in germ cell tumor of testis. Cancer 1993; 72:2182.
54. Rathmell AJ, Mapstone NP, Jones WG: Testicular seminoma metastasizing to palatine tonsil. Clin Oncol 1993; 5: 185.
55. Allhoff EP, Liedke S, de Riese W, et al: Stage I seminoma of the testis: adjuvant radiotherapy or surveillance? Br J Urol 1991; 68:190.
56. Donohue JP, Maynard B, Zachary M: The distribution of nodal metastases in the retroperitoneum from nonseminomatous testis cancer. J Urol 1982; 128:315.
57. Charig MJ, Hindley AC, Lloyd K, Golding SJ: "Watch policy" in patients with suspected stage I testicular seminoma: CT as a sole staging and surveillance technique. Clin Radiol 1990; 42:40.
58. Germa Lluch JR, Climent M, Villavicencio H, et al: Treatment of stage I testicular tumours. Br J Urol 1993; 71:473.
59. Horwich A, Alsanjari N, A'Hern R, Nicholls J, et al: Surveillance following orchidectomy for stage I testicular seminoma. Br J Cancer 1992; 65:775.
60. Ramakrishnan S, Champion A, Dorreen M, et al: Stage I seminoma of the testis: is post-orchidectomy surveillance a safe alternative to routine postoperative radiotherapy? Clin Oncol 1992; 4:284.
61. von der Maase H, Specht L, Jacobson GK, et al: Surveillance following orchidectomy for stage I seminoma of the testis. Eur J Cancer 1993; 29A:1931.
62. Warde PR, Gospodarowicz MK, Goodman PJ, Catton CN: Results of a policy of surveillance in stage I testicular seminoma. Int J Radiat Oncol Biol Phys 1993; 27:11.
63. Warde PR, Gospodarowicz MK, Panzarella T, et al: Stage I testicular seminoma: results of adjuvant irradiation and surveillance. J Clin Oncol 1995; 13:2255.
64. von der Maase H, Specht L, Jacobsen GK, et al: Surveillance following orchidectomy for stage I seminoma of the testis. Eur J Cancer 1993; 14:1931.
65. Toner GC, Gabrilove JL, Gordon M, et al: Phase I trial of intravenous and intraperitoneal administration of gran-

ulocyte-macrophage colony-stimulating factor. J Immunother 1994; 15:59.
66. Warde PG, Gospodarowicz MK, Panzarella T, et al: Prognostic factors in stage I testicular seminoma managed by surveillance. J Urol 1996; 155(5 Suppl):326a.
67. Oliver R, Edmonds P, Ong J, et al: Pilot studies of 2 and 1 course carboplatin as adjuvant for stage I seminoma: should it be tested in a randomized trial against radiotherapy? Int J Radiat Oncol Biol Phys 1994; 29:3.
68. Dieckmann K-P, Drain J, Kuster J, Bruggeboes B: Adjuvant carboplatin treatment for seminoma clinical stage I. J Cancer Res Clin Oncol 1996; 122:63.
69. Mason MD, Featherston T, Olliff J, Horwich A: Inguinal and iliac lymph node involvement in germ cell tumours of the testis. J Clin Oncol 1991; 3:147.
70. Fosså SD, Borge L, Aass N, et al: The treatment of advanced metastatic seminoma: experience in 55 cases. J Clin Oncol 1987; 5:1071.
71. Hanks G, Herring D, Kramer S: Patterns of care outcome studies; results of the national practice in seminoma of the testis. Int J Radiat Oncol Biol Phys 1981; 7:1413.
72. Thomas G, Rider W, Dembo A, et al: Seminoma of the testis: results of treatment and patterns of failure after radiation therapy. Int J Radiat Oncol Biol Phys 1982; 8: 165.
73. Gregory C, Peckham M: Results of radiotherapy for stage II testicular seminoma. Radiother Oncol 1986; 6:285.
74. Lindeman G, Tiver K: Management of testicular seminoma at Westmead Hospital from 1980 to 87. Aust N Z J Surg 1991; 61:211.
75. Epstein BE, Order S, Zinreich E: Staging, treatment, and results in testicular seminoma: a 12-year report. Cancer 1990; 65:405.
76. Evensen J, Fosså S, Kjellevold K, et al: Testicular seminoma: analysis of treatment and failure for stage II disease. Radiother Oncol 1985; 4:55.
77. Smalley S, Earle J, Evans R, et al: Modern radiotherapy results with bulky stages II and III seminoma. J Urol 1990; 144:685.
78. Herr HW, Bosl G: Residual mass after chemotherapy for seminoma: changing concepts of management. J Urol 1987; 137:1234.
79. Evensen J, Fosså S, Kjellevold K, et al: Testicular seminoma: histological findings and their prognostic significance for stage II disease. J Surg Oncol 1987; 36:166.
80. Warde PR, Gospodarowicz M, Panzarella T, et al: Management of stage II seminoma. J Clin Oncol 1966; 15:242.
81. Mencel PJ, Motzer RJ, Mazumdar M, et al: Advanced seminoma: treatment results, survival, and prognostic factors in 142 patients. J Clin Oncol 1994; 12:120.
82. Heikkila R, Heilo A, Stenwig AE, Fosså SD: Testicular ultrasonography and 18G biopsy for clinically undetected cancer or carcinoma in situ in patients with germ cell tumours. Br J Urol 1993; 71:214.
83. Heidenreich A, Bonfig R, Derschum W, et al: A conservative approach to bilateral testicular germ cell tumors. J Urol 1995; 153:10.
84. Sommer K, Brockmann W, Hubener K: Treatment results and acute and late toxicity of radiation therapy for testicular seminoma [Review]. Cancer 1990; 66:259.
85. Hamilton C, Horwich A, Bliss J, et al: Gastrointestinal morbidity of adjuvant radiotherapy in stage I malignant teratoma of the testis. Radiother Oncol 1987; 10:85.
86. Peckham M, Hamilton C, Horwich A, et al: Surveillance after orchidectomy for stage I seminoma of the testis. Br J Urol 1987; 59:343.
87. Senturia Y, Peckham C, Peckham M: Children fathered by men treated for testicular cancer. Lancet 1985; 2:766.
88. Cassileth B, Steinfeld A: Psychological preparation of the patient and family. Cancer 1987; 60:547.
89. Fosså S, Aass N, Kaalhus O: Testicular cancer in young Norwegians [Review]. J Surg Oncol 1988; 39:1091.
90. Kassa S, Aass N, Mastekassa A: Psychological well-being in testicular cancer patients. Eur J Cancer 1991; 27: 1091.
91. Tinker S, Howard G, Kerr G: Sexual morbidity following radiotherapy for germ cell tumours of the testis. Radiother Oncol 1992; 25:1091.
92. Moynihan C: Psychosocial assessments and counselling of the patient with testicular cancer. *In* Horwich A (ed): Testicular Cancer: Investigation and Management, p 353. London, Chapman and Hall Medical, 1991.
93. Rieker PP: How should a man with testicular cancer be counseled and what information is available? Semin Urol Oncol 1996; 14:17.
94. Schover LR, Gonzales M, von Eschenbach A: Sexual and marital relationships after radiotherapy for seminoma. Urology 1986; 27:117.
95. Puc HS, Heelan R, Mazumdar M, et al: Management of residual mass in advanced seminoma: results and recommendations from the Memorial Sloan-Kettering Cancer Center. J Clin Oncol 1996; 14:454.
96. Fosså SD, Droz JP, Stoter G, et al: Cisplatin, vincristine, and ifosphamide combination chemotherapy of metastatic seminoma: results of EORTC trial 30874. Br J Cancer 1995; 71:619.
97. Freidman EL, Garnick MB, Stomper PC, et al: Therapeutic guidelines and results in advanced seminoma. J Clin Oncol 1985; 3:1325.
98. Loehrer PJ, Birch R, Williams SD, et al: Chemotherapy of metastatic seminoma: the Southeastern Cancer Study Group experience. J Clin Oncol 1987; 5:1212.
99. Mann K, Siddle K: Evidence for free beta-subunit secretion in so-called human chorionic gonadotropin-positive seminoma. Cancer 1988; 62:2378.
100. Mirimanoff R, Shipley W, Dosoretz D, et al: Pure seminoma of the testis: the results of radiation therapy in patients with elevated human chorionic gonadotropin titers. J Urol 1985; 134:17.
101. Mirimanoff R, Sinzig M, Kruger M, et al: Prognosis of human chorionic gonadotropin-producing seminoma treated by postoperative radiotherapy. Int J Radiat Oncol Biol Phys 1993; 27:17.
102. Paus E, Fosså SD, Risberg T, Nustad K: The diagnostic value of human chorionic gonadotrophin in patients with testicular seminoma. Br J Urol 1987; 59:572.
103. Swartz D, Johnson D, Hussey D: Should an elevated human chorionic gonadotropin titer alter therapy for seminoma? J Urol 1984; 131:63.
104. Mumperow E, Hartmann M: Spermatic cord beta-human chorionic gonadotropin levels in seminoma and their clinical implications. J Urol 1992; 147:1041.
105. Morgan D, Caillaud J, Bellet D, et al: Gonadotropin-producing seminoma: a distinct category of germ cell neoplasm. Clin Radiol 1982; 33:149.
106. Norgaard P, Scultz H, Arends J, et al: Tumour markers in testicular germ cell tumours: five year experience from the DATECA Study 1976–1980. Acta Radiol (Oncol) 1984; 23:287.
107. Diekmann K, Due W, Bauer H: Seminoma testis with elevated serum beta-HCG—a category of germ-cell cancer between seminoma and nonseminoma [Review]. Int Urol Nephrol 1989; 21:175.
108. Mauch P, Weichselbaum R, Botnik K: The significance of positive chorionic gonadotropins in apparently pure seminoma of the testis. Int J Radiat Oncol Biol Phys 1979; 5: 887.
109. Weissbach L, Busser-Maatz R: HCG-positive seminoma. Eur Urol 1993; 2:229.
110. Bokemeyer C, Schmoll H, Schoffski P, et al: Bilateral testicular tumours: prevalence and clinical implications. Eur J Cancer 1993; 6:874.
111. Ondrus D, Matoska J, Hornak M: Bilateral germ cell tumors of the testis. Neoplasma 1993; 40:329.
112. van Leeuwan F, Stiggelbout A, van den Belt-Dusebout A, et al: A follow-up study of 1,909 patients. J Clin Oncol 1993; 11:415.
113. Osterlind A, Berthelsen J, Abildgaard N, et al: Risk of bilateral testicular germ cell cancer in Denmark: 1960–1984. J Natl Cancer Inst 1991; 83:1391.

114. Read G, Robertson A, Blair V: Radiotherapy in seminoma of the testis. Clin Radiol 1983; 34:469.
115. Weissbach L: Organ preserving surgery of malignant germ cell tumors. J Urol 1995; 153:90.
116. Robertson GSM: Radical orchidectomy and benign testicular conditions. Br J Surg 1995; 82:342.
117. Bauer S, Perlmutter A, Retik A: Anomalies of the upper urinary tract. *In* Walsh PC, Retik AB, Stamey TA, Vaughan ED Jr (eds): Campbell's Urology, 6th edition, p 1357. Philadelphia, WB Saunders Co, 1992.
118. Li F, Fraumeni J: Testicular cancers in children: epidemiologic characteristics. J Natl Cancer Inst 1972; 48:1575.
119. Elyan S, Reed D, Ostrawski M, et al: Problems in the management of testicular seminoma associated with a horseshoe kidney. Clin Oncol 1990; 2:163.
120. Key D, Moyad R, Grossman H: Seminoma associated with crossed fused renal ectopia. J Urol 1990; 143:1015.
121. Villalona CM, Ducker T, Holasek M, et al: Management of testicular seminoma following organ transplantation. Med Pediatr Oncol 1992; 20:338.
122. Leibovitch I, Baniel J, Rowland RG, et al: Malignant testicular neoplasms in immunosuppressed patients. Journal d'Urologie 1996; 155:1938.
123. Dieckmann KP, Due W, Offermann G: Testicular seminoma in an immunosuppressed renal transplant recipient. Br J Urol 1989; 63:549.
124. Hentrich MU, Brack NG, Schmid P, et al: Testicular germ cell tumors in patients with human immunodeficiency virus infection. Cancer 1996; 77:2109.
125. Bernardi D, Salvioni R, Vaccher E, et al: Testicular germ cell tumors and human immunodeficiency virus infection: a report of 26 cases. J Clin Oncol 1995; 13: 2705.
126. Moyle G, Hawkins DA, Gazzard BG: Seminoma and HIV infections. Int J STD AIDS 1991; 2:293.
127. Roehrborn CG, Worrell JT, Wiley EL: Bilateral synchronous testis tumors of different histology in a patient with the acquired immunodeficiency syndrome related complex. J Urol 1990; 144:353.
128. Timmerman JM, Northfelt DW, Small EJ: Malignant germ cell tumors in men infected with the human immunodeficiency virus: natural history and results of therapy. J Clin Oncol 1995; 13:1391.
129. Sham JS, Choy D, Chan KW, Choi PH: Seminoma of normally descended and cryptorchid testis. Eur J Surg Oncol 1992; 16:33.

34

NONSEMINOMATOUS GERM CELL TUMORS: MANAGEMENT AND PROGNOSIS

JEROME P. RICHIE, M.D.

Testicular cancer is relatively rare, with an incidence of approximately 3.5 per 100,000 men per year. In 1996, there will be an estimated 7400 new cases but only 370 deaths.[1] Nonetheless, testicular cancer represents the most common malignancy in men from the ages of 15 to 35 and the second most common malignancy from age 35–39. Occurring in a crucial evolutionary period of a young man's career (family planning, etc.), testicular cancer has a major emotional impact on this population. Testicular cancer evokes widespread interest for a variety of reasons. First and foremost, testicular cancer has become one of the most curable solid neoplasms in 1996 and can serve as a paradigm for the multimodal treatment of solid malignancies. Dramatic improvements in survival, with almost a total reversal from a 10% survival in the 1970s to a 90% survival in the 1990s, has resulted from the combination of effective diagnostic techniques, improvement in serum tumor markers, effective multidrug chemotherapeutic regimens, and modifications of surgical technique. All of these advances have led to a decline in morbidity and mortality. In 1996, overall survival for all stages of testicular cancer should be well above 80% and should approach 100% for patients with low-stage disease. For all stages of disease, 5-year survival exceeds that for any other malignancy.

Survival advances have resulted from better understanding of accurate serum tumor markers, which allow careful follow-up with intervention earlier in the course of disease, as well as additional characteristics of testicular tumors that favor successful therapy. These characteristics include origin from germ cells, which in general are more sensitive to radiation therapy and a wide variety of chemotherapeutic agents, as well as capacity for differentiation, rapid rate of growth, predictable and systematic patterns of spread, and occurrence in young individuals without comorbid disease.

MOLECULAR BIOLOGY

The burgeoning field of molecular biology holds promise for the identification of intracellular changes that will alter the kinetics of growth of normal testicular cells. In the 1980s cell surface antigens and morphologic characteristics could be evaluated; in the 1990s, the potential for better understanding and possible elucidation of the etiology of testicular cancer, based upon molecular factors, may well be achieved. Germ cell tumors may manifest a variety of chromosomal abnormalities. Most frequent abnormalities involve chromosomes 1 and 12. Abnormalities have been noted with rearrangements in both the short and long arm of chromosome 1.[2] Chromosome 12 abnormalities may either be polysomy or monosomy. Utilizing the technique of fluorescent in situ hybridization, many germ cell tumors will have multiple copies of chromosome 12. Thus, significant attention is being focused on chromosome 12 for possible tumor suppressor genetic abnormalities.[3]

Carcinoma In Situ

Preneoplastic changes in the testis, so-called carcinoma-in-situ, have been described by a variety of investigators. Controversy exists, however, concerning the premalignant alteration of intratubular germ cell neoplasia with the development of frank malignancy. Skakkebaek and associates have described the occurrence of intratubular germ cell clusters that are atypical when seen on testicular biopsies in men who presented with infertility.[4] Precancerous changes have been described in adjacent uninvolved areas of the testis in patients with germinal tumors.[5] Skakkebaek and associates have reported that 50% of men harboring carcinoma in situ will progress to develop "invasive" growth during the next 5 years.[6] Radiation therapy has been recommended as the treatment for carcinoma in situ, consisting of 1600 to 2000 cGy given in ten equal daily fractions.[7] These findings raise the difficult question of how to deal with the opposite gonad, particularly since there is a known tendency for patients to develop contralateral tumor in approximately 1% of cases. The rate of intratubular germ cell neoplasia has been well defined. The problem that remains in the 1990s is how to deal with this intratubular germ cell neoplasia, and in what percentage of patients will clinically apparent testicular tumors develop?

Frequency of Histologic Types

Seminoma is the most common single germinal cell tumor, accounting for 40%, with embryonal carcinoma 20 to 25%, teratocarcinoma 25 to 30%, teratoma 5 to 10%, and pure choriocarcinoma 1%. When combined histologic patterns are considered as a separate entity, the frequency approximates seminoma 30%, embryonal carcinoma 30%, teratoma 10%, teratocarcinoma 25%, choriocarcinoma 1%, and other combined patterns 15%.[8]

EPIDEMIOLOGY

Estimates of lifetime probability for American white males of developing testicular cancer are approximately 0.2%.[1] The average age-adjusted rate for American males from 1969 to 1971 was 3.7 per 100,000, nearly twice the rate of 2.0 per 100,000 seen in the 1930s. Amongst American black males, the rate is 0.9 per 100,000, unchanged in the past 40 years. Similar trends have been noted in Denmark with an increased but almost doubled age-adjusted incidence between 1945 and 1970.[9]

Peak incidence of testicular tumor occurs from 20 to 40 years and again in late adulthood over 60 years of age. Seminoma is rare below the age of 10 and above the age of 60, but is the most common histologic type overall. Approximately 2 to 3% of testicular cancers are bilateral, occurring either simultaneously or successively. A history of cryptorchidism in nearly half the men with bilateral tumors is consistent with observations that bilateral dysgenesis occurs frequently even in patients with unilateral maldescent.

Cryptorchidism

LeComete in 1851 is credited with the initial observation of a relationship between cryptorchidism and subsequent tumor formation.[10] Approximately 10% of patients with testicular tumors will have a prior history of cryptorchidism. Gilbert and Hamilton in 1940, based upon the observed incidence of cryptorchidism in military inductees, calculated estimated risks of tumorigenesis in a man with a history of cryptorchidism to be 48 times that of men with normally descended testes.[11] More recent studies have reported the relative risk to be lower, some 3 to 14 times normal expected incidence.[12] Approximately 5 to 10% of patients with a history of cryptorchidism will develop malignancy in the contralateral normally descended gonad. This observation may be representative of carcinoma in situ or some hormonal dysfunction in patients predisposing to the development of subsequent malignancy.

NATURAL HISTORY

Once a palpable nodule exists within the testicular substance, local involvement or metastases either via the lymphatic or hematogenous route may occur. Approximately half the patients with nonseminomatous tumor will present with disseminated disease. Involvement of the epididymis or cord may lead to pelvic and/or inguinal lymph node metastases, although most tumors confined to the testis proper will spread primarily to the retroperitoneal lymph nodes. Hematogenous spread to lung, bone, or liver may occur as a result of direct tumor invasion.

The tunica albuginea functions as a natural barrier to expansile local growth. Local involvement of the epididymis or spermatic cord is seen in 10 to 15% of patients.

Lymphatic metastasis is common to all forms of germinal testis tumors. The lymphatics generally tend to follow the spermatic vessels to primary landing sites in the retroperitoneum. The primary drainage to the right testis is located in the interaortal caval group of nodes at the region of L2. The first echelon of nodes draining the left testis is located in the left para-aortic region, just below the left renal hilum. Subsequent drainage cephalad may be to the cisterna chyli, thoracic duct, and supraclavicular nodes. Extranodal metastases may result from direct vascular invasion or from lymphatic metastases with subsequent vascular invasion.

In general, growth rate among germ cell tumors tends to be high. Doubling rates have been calculated from between 10 to 30 days.

CLINICAL STAGING

Once the diagnosis of germ cell neoplasm has been established by radical inguinal orchiectomy, with early clamping of the cord, clinical staging is necessary in order to further define treatment modalities. Staging should take into account the pathologic examination of the primary specimen, history and physical findings, as well as a variety of other diagnostic modalities. Clinical staging attempts to define the extent of disease at the time of diagnosis. The accuracy of clinical assessment is imperative if the physician is to be able to make a logical decision as to therapy. Importance of clinical staging cannot be overemphasized; such knowledge allows the orderly decision of algorithms for appropriate treatment as well as reasonable expectations for prognosis. With the advent of alternative treatment protocols (surveillance) for patients with clinical low-stage testicular cancer, the impact of staging and its accuracy assumes ever greater import.

Sites of Metastases

The majority of testicular cancer spreads through lymphatics in an orderly fashion, although vascular dissemination may occur early in some tumors. Primary lymphatic drainage from the right testicle is through interaortal caval lymph nodes with subsequent drainage to precaval, preaortic, and paracaval lymph nodes. There tends to be spread from right to left into the left para-aortic area. Primary drainage of the left testis is to the left para-aortic nodes just below the level of the renal hilum. Cross metastases occur more commonly in patients with right-sided tumors. The lymphatics tend to follow the aorta below the crus of the diaphragm into the retrocrural space. Landing sites from minimal, moderate, or extensive disease have been accurately reported by Donohue and associates.[13]

Distant metastases occur most commonly to the pulmonary region with intraparenchymal involvement. Subsequent spread may be noted to liver, viscera, brain, or bone. In general, bony metastases are encountered late in the course of disease. Central nervous system metastases may be understaged.

Staging Systems

The predictable mode of metastases along with advances in imaging and biochemical markers have improved the accuracy of initial clinical evaluations, although they remain far from perfect. A variety of clinical staging systems has been advocated.

For seminoma, the system proposed by Boden and Gibb in 1951 has remained the mainstay of clinical staging[14] (Table 34–1). These investigators separated extent of disease into three stages: stage I, tumor limited to the testis with no spread through capsule or spermatic cord; stage II, with clinical or radiologic evidence of tumor extension beyond testicle but contained within the regional lymph nodes; and stage III, disseminated disease above the diaphragm or visceral disease.

TABLE 34–1. CLINICAL STAGING SYSTEMS FOR SEMINOMA

Boden/Gibb Stage	MSKCC	AJCC
A (I) Tumor confined to testis	A	I (A) Negative II (B) Positive N1 Microscopic involvement
B (II) Spread to regional nodes	B1 <5 cm	N2 Nodes grossly involved A (B1) <5 nodes involved with none >2 cm diameter
	B2 >5 cm	B (B2) >5 nodes involved and/or nodes >2 cm diameter N3 Extranodal extension (gross or microscopic), resectable
	B3 >10 cm ("bulky")	N4 (B3) Incompletely resected/unresectable disease
C (III) Spread beyond retroperitoneal nodes	CIII	

MSKCC, Memorial Sloan-Kettering Cancer Center; AJCC, American Joint Committee on Cancer.

The system of Boden and Gibb has been modified through the years as clinical staging procedures have become more precise. The Memorial Sloan-Kettering Cancer Center (MSKCC) group has subdivided stage B patients into B1 (<5 cm in diameter), B2 (>5 cm in diameter), and B3 (bulky retroperitoneal disease). The American Joint Committee on Cancer (AJCC) has described the TNM system. All of these systems are detailed in Table 34–1.

For nonseminomatous germ cell tumors, accurate clinical staging is desirable. The principal differences between staging systems for seminomas and nonseminomas relate to the roles of surgical lymph node sampling and serum tumor markers. Pathologic staging systems for nonseminomatous germ cell tumors are detailed in Table 34–2, including the USC system, the Walter Reed system, and the TNM system.[15,16]

Clinical Staging Accuracy

Following orchiectomy, persistent elevation of one or both tumor markers suggests residual tumor. Rapid normalization of previously elevated markers conceivably represents elimination of tumor, although this is not necessarily the case. In

TABLE 34–2. PATHOLOGIC STAGING SYSTEMS FOR NONSEMINOMATOUS GERM CELL TUMORS

Skinner*	Walter Reed†	TNM
A—confined to testis	I	N0
B—Spread to retroperitoneum		
B1	IA	N1
<6 positive nodes		N2a
No node >2 cm		
No extranodal extension		
B2	IIB	N2b
>6 positive nodes		
Any node >2 cm		
B3	IIC	N3
Massive retroperitoneal disease		
C—Metastatic	III	M+

*Data from Skinner (1976).[15]
†Data from Maier and Sulak (1973).[16]

patients with disease clinically confined to the testis, approximately 30% will develop metastatic disease while under surveillance despite negative tumor markers immediately following orchiectomy. Tumor markers, when elevated, are very helpful in predicting residual disease. The converse, however, is not necessarily true. Approximately 40% of patients with documented disease in the retroperitoneum will have negative tumor markers.

Abdominal computed tomography (CT) scans remain the most effective means to identify retroperitoneal lymph node involvement. CT scanning has replaced intravenous urography and pedal lymphangiography. Abdominal CT scans, especially with third- and fourth-generation scanners, can identify lymph node deposits less than 2 cm in diameter in the upper para-aortic regions. CT scanning generally provides three-dimensional estimate of tumor size as well as involvement of soft tissue structures. CT scanning, however, has significant limitations. In thin patients, with absence of intraperitoneal versus retroperitoneal fat planes, retroperitoneal metastases may often be missed even when 2 to 3 cm in diameter. CT scanning is not sufficiently accurate to distinguish fibrosis, teratoma, or malignancy. There is an estimated 25% underestimation of regional nodal involvement with negative CT scans.[17] Thus, a positive CT scan is likely to accurately identify metastatic disease. The converse, however, is not necessarily true. As many as an estimated 25 to 30% of patients with documented retroperitoneal metastases will have apparently negative CT scans.

TREATMENT

Seminoma (Fig. 34–1)

Treatment strategies for patients with germ cell tumor have evolved from understanding of tumor natural history, clinical staging, as well as effectiveness of treatment. Multimodal therapy has been largely credited with recent treatment success, but the current accuracy of clinical staging, ability to recognize failure early, and high probability of successful treatment of failures have prompted investigations aimed at reducing morbidity associated with treatment.

Seminoma is the most common histologic testis tumor in adults and accounts for approximately 60% of all germ cell tumors of the testis. Established treatment for low-stage seminoma has been inguinal orchiectomy followed by therapeutic or adjuvant radiation therapy. This treatment represents a highly effective method of treating low-stage disease with minimal morbidity; with the advent of multidrug chemotherapy for cure of patients with more disseminated disease, the overall cure rate for all stages should exceed 90%.

The natural history and radiosensitivity of seminoma favor megavoltage irradiation in relatively modest amounts as the treatment of choice in the vast majority of patients following inguinal orchiectomy. Since the staging error may be 15 to 25% for stage I seminoma, any treatment (or lack of it) should produce a cure in 75% of patients, or better. The overall effectiveness of radiation therapy is confirmed, however, in that 2500 to 3500 cGy delivered over a 3-week period to the periaortic and ipsilateral inguinopelvic lymph nodes results in 5-year survival rates of 90 to 95%. In stage II disease, 5-year survival rates of roughly 80 per cent are anticipated following therapeutic retroperitoneal irradiation. Deposits in supradiaphragmatic nodes or distant sites and bulky abdominal disease respond less favorably to primary radiation therapy, which by itself yields survival rates as low as 20 to 30%. Evidence indicates that seminoma is exquisitely sensitive to various chemotherapy regimens, particularly platinum-based ones, with response rates of 60 to 100% being reported.

Nonseminomatous Germ Cell Tumors
(Fig. 34–2)

Stage 1

Removal of the testis via an inguinal approach, the so-called radical orchiectomy, remains the definitive procedure for pathologic diagnosis as well as local treatment of testicular neoplasms. Morbidity is minimal and mortality should be virtually zero while allowing 100% local control. Transcrotal biopsy is to be condemned. The inguinal approach permits early control of the vascular and lymphatic supply as well as en bloc removal of the testis with all its tunics.

In patients with nonseminomatous germ cell tumor, following inguinal orchiectomy, the accuracy of clinical staging is critical as a determinant for further treatment selection. Because of the inexactitude of clinical staging accuracy, retroperitoneal

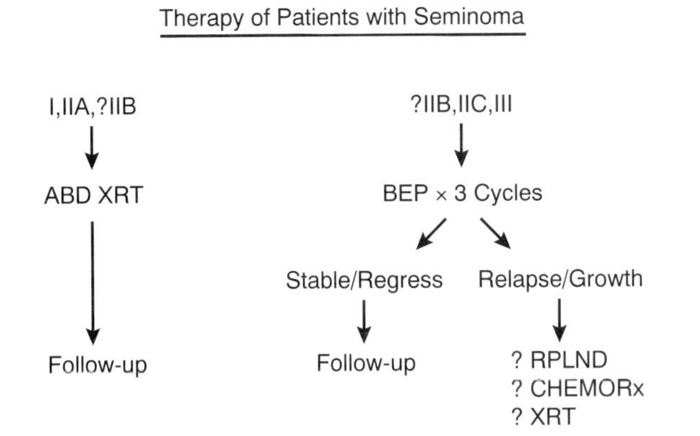
Therapy of Patients with Seminoma
I,IIA,?IIB
ABD XRT
Follow-up
?IIB,IIC,III
BEP × 3 Cycles
Stable/Regress
Relapse/Growth
Follow-up
? RPLND
? CHEMORx
? XRT

FIGURE 34–1. Treatment plan for patients with pure seminoma. BEP, bleomycin, etoposide, and cis-platinum.

lymphadenectomy remains the mainstay of surgical therapy in patients with nonseminomatous germ cell tumors (Table 34–3). These tumors generally spread to the retroperitoneal lymph nodes before further dissemination, and the primary landing sites are well identified. After spread to the retroperitoneum, the next most common site of metastasis is to the lungs which can be identified early with plain radiographs. Furthermore, these tumors often produce beta-human chorionic gonadotropin (β-hCG) or alpha-fetoprotein (AFP), both of which are measurable in the serum at nanogram levels.

Historical Perspectives

Anatomic studies at the turn of the century by Most[23] and Cuneo[24] as well as later work by Jamieson and Dobson[25] and Rouviere[26] demonstrated the lymphatic drainage of the testis with the primary echelon of drainage for right-sided tumors to be interaortal caval and for left-sided tumors to be left para-aortic and preaortic nodes. There exists some crossover, especially from right to left. These anatomic studies provided the basis for regional control after establishing local control by orchiectomy. The first site of metastasis in patients with nonseminomatous tumors is generally the retroperitoneal lymph nodes (90%). In approximately 10% of patients the first site of metastasis will be outside the borders of a standard retroperitoneal lymph node dissection. Thorough excision of the retroperitoneal lymph nodes remains the epitome or "gold standard" of staging. Although noninvasive staging techniques are somewhat accurate, 20 to 25% of patients with clinical stage I disease are understaged by all available modalities of nonsurgical staging. The cure rate for patients with pathologically confirmed stage I disease is 99.6% with surgery alone (Table 34–3). The 5 to 10% of patients who may relapse following negative retroperitoneal lymph node dissection for stage I disease have a high cure rate with salvage chemotherapy.

The 5 to 10% of patients who relapse will generally do so within the first 2 years after diagnosis. Thus, careful follow up is necessary for the first 2 years, generally with monthly chest x-rays and tumor markers for the first year and every other month for the second year. Because relapse beyond 2 years is rare, these patients can be followed annually for the next several years. Patients who relapse generally do so in the lungs, suggesting hematogenous spread that preceded lymphatic dissemination. Recurrences in the retroperitoneum have been recognized rarely in patients who previously had a negative lymph node dissection.

Retroperitoneal lymph node dissection was established as a primary therapy for nonseminomatous germ cell tumors by Lewis in 1948.[27] Kimbrough and Cook fostered inguinal orchiectomy plus retroperitoneal lymphadenectomy as the preferred local regional treatment for patients with testis tumors.[28] In Europe, conversely, radiation therapy was utilized as a primary means for sterilizing nodal deposits. Lewis reported a 46%

TABLE 34–3. SURVIVAL AFTER ORCHIECTOMY AND RPLND IN CLINICAL STAGE I NONSEMINOMATOUS GERM CELL TUMORS

Series	No. of Patients	No. Relapsed (%)	No. Dead
Fraley et al. (1979)[18]	28	0	0
Pizzocaro (1986)[19]	36	4 (11%)	0
Richie (1990)[20]	85	7 (8%)	0
Donohue et al. (1993)[21]	266	31 (12%)	2
Sosnowski et al. (1994)[22]	52	4* (2%)	0
Total	467	46 (10%)	2 (0.4%)

*Adjuvant chemotherapy—15 patients with pathologic stage II.

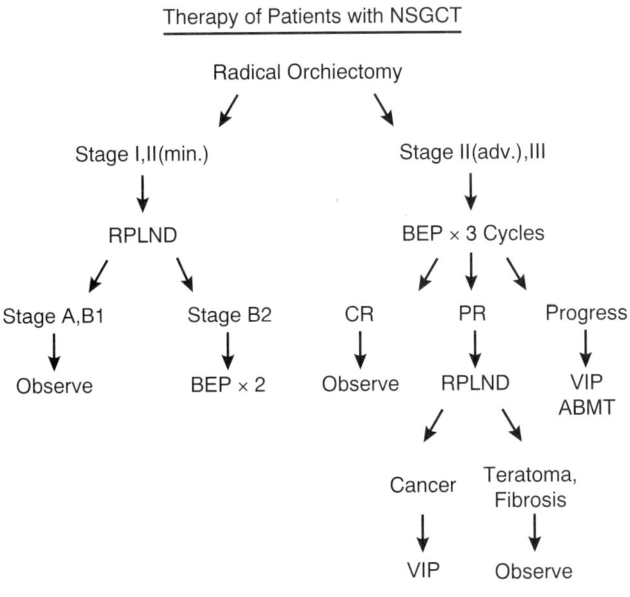
Therapy of Patients with NSGCT
Radical Orchiectomy
Stage I,II(min.)
Stage II(adv.),III
RPLND
BEP × 3 Cycles
Stage A,B1
Stage B2
CR
PR
Progress
Observe
BEP × 2
Observe
RPLND
VIP
ABMT
Cancer
Teratoma,
Fibrosis
VIP
Observe

FIGURE 34–2. Treatment algorithm for patients with nonseminomatous germ cell testicular tumors. RPLND, retroperitoneal lymph node dissection; BEP, bleomycin, etoposide, and cis-platinum; VIP, vinblastine, ifosfamide, and cis-platinum; ABMT, autologous bone marrow transplantation.

5-year survival among 28 patients treated with lymphadenectomy and/or radiation therapy after orchiectomy.[27]

A variety of surgical approaches has been advocated for retroperitoneal lymphadenectomy. Cooper and associates popularized the transthoracic approach in 1950.[29] Staubitz et al.[30] and Whitmore[31] utilized the transabdominal approach. The question of bilateral suprahilar dissection was invoked by Donohue and associates,[13] leading to important mapping studies for the distribution of retroperitoneal lymph node metastases in patients with minimal, moderate, or advanced retroperitoneal disease. These studies have allowed tailoring of the surgical procedure to the amount of retroperitoneal adenopathy that is present.

Retroperitoneal lymph node dissection, via a transabdominal or thoracoabdominal approach, is a generally well-tolerated, 3- to 4-hour procedure with negligible mortality and minimal morbidity. The mortality rate is less than 1%. Morbidity ranges from 5 to 25%, usually related to atelectasis, pneumonitis, ileus, lymphocele, or pancreatitis.[32]

Fertility After Retroperitoneal Lymph Node Dissection

Semen quality as an indicator of potential fertility has been studied by many investigators before, during, and after various treatments for testicular cancer. Approximately 50 to 60% of males are reportedly subfertile at the time of diagnosis of a nonseminomatous germ cell tumor. Controversy exists as to whether spermatogenesis is impaired prior to the clinical manifestation of testicular cancer or whether semen quality is impaired as a result of diagnosis and/or initial therapy. Nonetheless, in a large proportion of patients, spermatogenesis impairment may be reversible.

Emission and Ejaculation

Prior to 1980, a high incidence of infertility was noted following retroperitoneal lymph node dissection in patients with testicular cancer. This infertility was largely due to either failure of seminal emission or retrograde ejaculation secondary to damage to the sympathetic nerve fibers involved in ejaculation.

Early descriptions of retroperitoneal lymphadenectomy included a complete bilateral dissection from above the renal hilar area bilaterally, encompassing both ureters down to where each ureter crossed the common iliac artery. Retroperitoneal tissue was removed both anterior to and posterior to the great vessels in order to completely remove all nodal-bearing tissue. Thorough removal of all lymphatic tissue was considered essential because of the lack of effective alternative therapies. Indeed, retroperitoneal lymph node dissection using the above template has been curative in patients with minimal nodal involvement, even without the use of adjunctive chemotherapy. With the development of effective combination platinum-based chemotherapy, testicular cancer has become one of the most curable of all genitourinary tumors. As survival rates have improved, the long-term effects of infertility resulting from retroperitoneal lymph node dissection have assumed greater import. A major impetus for close observation or surveillance therapy has been the long-term effect of ejaculatory compromise and infertility in patients with low-stage testicular cancer.

Modified Retroperitoneal Lymph Node Dissection

In the early 1980s, Narayan and associates published an important paper concerning ejaculation after extended retroperitoneal lymph node dissection.[33] This paper showed that modification of surgical boundaries could allow return of ejaculation in approximately half of patients with low-stage testicular cancer following retroperitoneal lymph node dissection. Even with more extensive dissections for stage B2 or B3 retroperitoneal involvement, ejaculatory capability returned in approximately one third of patients.

Richie reported a prospective study of modified lymph node dissection in 85 patients with clinical stage I nonseminomatous germ cell tumor of the testis.[20] The dissection is bilateral above the level of the inferior mesenteric artery but unilateral below the inferior mesenteric artery. The technique involves a thoracoabdominal approach through the ipsilateral side with mobilization of the peritoneal envelope completely as previously described. Once the peritoneum is peeled from the posterior rectus fascia, an incision is made in the peritoneum and palpation carried out to be certain there is no bulk disease or more extensive disease, which would preclude retroperitoneal rather than transperitoneal lymphadenectomy. By peeling the peritoneal envelope and remaining in a retroperitoneal fashion, along with preservation of the inferior mesenteric artery, injury to the contralateral side of the aorta and great vessels below the inferior mesenteric artery is avoided (Figs. 34–3 and 34–4).

Thus, for a right-sided tumor, the dissection would encompass the renal hilar area bilaterally to the level of the left ureter or gonadal vein. On the left side, dissection is carried down to the level of the inferior mesenteric artery, then across to the right side and down the right side of the aorta encompassing the right common iliac artery. All nodal-bearing tissue in the interaortal caval area is removed, and posteriorly the margin is the anterior spinous ligament. Both sympathetic chains are preserved. On the right side, the dissection is carried along the right renal hilar area to the level of the right ureter and down to where the ureter crosses the common iliac artery. The ipsilateral spermatic vessels are removed to the level of the deep inguinal ring and the previously ligated stump of the cord (Fig. 34–3).

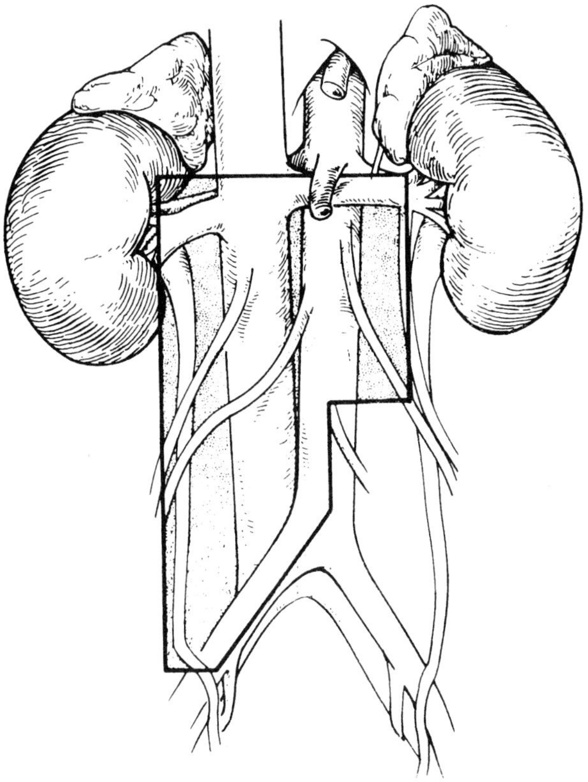

FIGURE 34–3. Modified right-sided retroperitoneal lymph node dissection template. The dissection is complete above the level of the inferior mesenteric artery, but limited to the unilateral/ipsilateral side below the level of the inferior mesenteric artery.

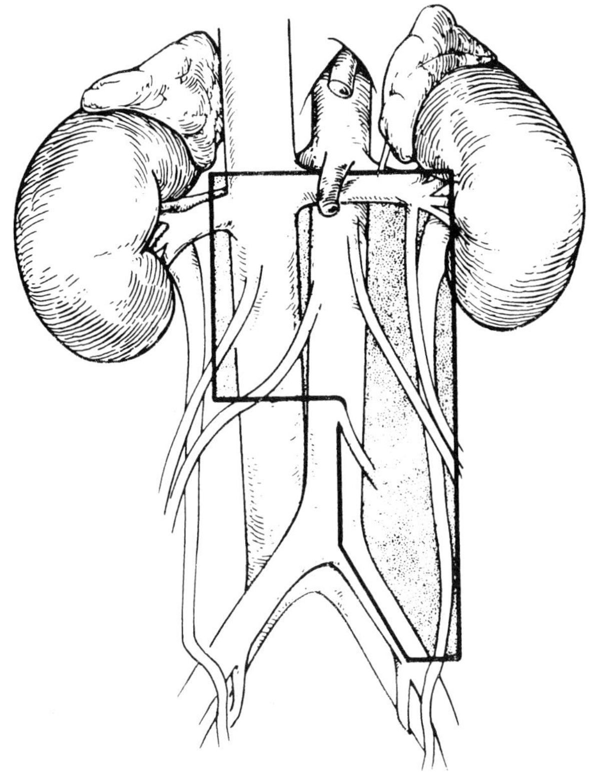

FIGURE 34–4. Template for modified left-sided retroperitoneal lymph node dissection. The right-sided border is near the right margin of the inferior vena cava.

For left-sided dissection, a similar dissection is performed with the exception of the right lateral margin (Fig. 34–4). Since nodal spread tends to be from right to left, dissection is only carried to the lateral margin of the inferior vena cava rather than all the way over to the right ureter. This dissection is bilateral above the inferior mesenteric artery and unilateral below the inferior mesenteric artery.

The final pathology report of the 85 patients who underwent modified retroperitoneal lymph node dissection was stage A in 64 patients and stage B1 in 21 patients. Patients have been followed from 12 to 84 months with a median of 38 months. Seven patients have relapsed, all with pulmonary metastases. All patients have been salvaged with chemotherapy and remain free of disease. There have been no retroperitoneal recurrences other than one retrocrural recurrence.

With respect to preservation of ejaculatory function, 75 of 85 patients have reported spontaneous return of antegrade ejaculation, usually within 1 month postoperatively. An additional five patients have been converted to antegrade ejaculation with imipramine (Tofranil). Thus, 80 of 85 patients (94%) have recovered antegrade ejaculation, either spontaneously or with medication. Five patients remain with retrograde ejaculation, as documented by sperm in the urine following ejaculation. Sperm counts have been obtained in 65 patients. The counts range from a low of 2×10^6/ml to a high of 120×10^6/ml. Volume has ranged from 0.5 to 4.5 ml. Most patients report that post–node dissection ejaculate volume is approximately one half that of pre–node dissection ejaculate volume. There have been 11 pregnancies in this group of patients.

The template or boundary method of retroperitoneal lymph node dissection has significant advantages. By utilization of this technique, a complete bilateral dissection can be performed in the area most likely to be involved with retroperitoneal nodal disease, yet modification in a less likely area can spare some of the ejaculatory consequences. This type of procedure is universally transferable to surgeons with some experience in performance of retroperitoneal lymph node dissection and requires no additional new skills or techniques of identification. The above techniques represent a therapeutically and diagnostically sound technique for treatment of patients with pathologic stage A and B1 disease, with preservation of ejaculation in more than 90% of patients.

Various centers have described modifications of retroperitoneal lymph node dissection with a variety of techniques to preserve ejaculation. Donohue reported modifications with preservation of ejaculation in two thirds of patients with right-sided tumors and one third of those with left-sided tumors.[34] Pizzocaro reported on unilateral retroperitoneal lymph node dissection with excellent preservation of ejaculation. Nineteen per cent of patients with stage A and B1 testicular cancer had preservation of ejaculation, whereas only 23% of patients with stage B2 had preservation of ejaculation.[34]

Attempts have been made to identify individual retroperitoneal sympathetic nerves responsible for antegrade ejaculation. Jewett and Torbey describe early experience with nerve-sparing techniques with excellent return of ejaculation.[35] Likewise, Donohue and associates have performed a similar procedure with excellent return of ejaculation.[34] These techniques involve removal of nodal-bearing tissue from around the postganglionic fibers. The techniques are somewhat more time consuming and may require a steeper learning curve as well. Nonetheless, ejaculation can be preserved in 100% of patients and fertility noted in 75% of patients using these techniques.[36]

Laparoscopy to perform retroperitoneal lymph node dissection has been described but has a very steep learning curve and may not completely remove all the retroperitoneal nodal tissue.[37]

Radiation Therapy

Megavoltage irradiation has been available since the 1950s and in common use since the 1960s, by which time retroperitoneal lymph node dissection had already become established, especially in the United States. Radiation therapy of the retroperitoneum in patients with clinical stage I nonseminomatous germ cell tumor remains accepted practice in many treatment centers outside North America. The main objections to the use of retroperitoneal lymph node irradiation have been the inaccuracy of clinical staging of the retroperitoneal lymph nodes; the resultant lack of survival data that could be reasonably compared with surgical data; and the concern that, in the event of postirradiation relapse, the prior irradiation might preclude adequate chemotherapy or surgical excision. Modern staging techniques have reduced the falsely negative staging error in clinical stage I to approximately 20%. In patients with clinical stage I disease subjected to retroperitoneal lymph node dissection, 10 to 15% will harbor undetected nodal metastasis and another 5 to 10% will relapse following surgery, almost always in extranodal sites. The tumoricidal dose for nonseminomatous germ cell tumor ranges between 4000 and 5000 cGy, far in excess of that required to sterilize seminoma. A dose of 4000 to 4500 cGy delivered in 4 to 5 weeks to the para-aortic and ipsilateral pelvic lymph nodes is the recommended radiation standard in clinical stage I nonseminomatous germ cell tumor. The long-term complications of para-aortic irradiation include radiation enteritis, bowel obstruction, and bone marrow suppression, with a reported frequency of between 5 and 10%. Secondary malignancy has been reported following abdominal radiation therapy for Hodgkin's disease, but such reports following treatment for testis tumors are anecdotal.

The overall success rate of radiation therapy in the treatment of clinical stage I nonseminomatous germ cell tumor in terms of 5-year survival is between 80 and 95% when chemotherapy is used to treat relapses. Relapse rates following radiation therapy for clinical stage I are as high as 24 per cent (14 of 59), 3% within the irradiated volume, and 21% outside.[38]

SURVEILLANCE

If staging modalities were sufficiently accurate to identify patients whose disease is truly confined to the testis, orchiectomy alone should yield survival results equal to therapeutic strategies that incorporate treatment of the regional lymph nodes. With the inaccuracies of staging, however, retroperitoneal lymph node dissection remains the only modality that can accurately delineate pathologic stage I from pathologic stage II testicular cancer. Clinical understaging approximates 25% even in the best of series. Nonetheless, approximately 70% of patients who undergo retroperitoneal lymph node dissection are found to have pathologic stage I disease and, therefore, receive no therapeutic benefit from the operation. Additionally, 5 to 10% of patients will relapse outside of the field of the retroperitoneal node dissection.

With the advent of effective chemotherapy, coupled with concerns about the need for retroperitoneal lymph node dissection in all patients with clinical stage I testicular cancer as well as the complications of loss of ejaculation and infertility, postorchiectomy observation or surveillance has a certain appeal. Several large surveillance programs have been undertaken throughout the world. In several of the largest series, detailed in Table 34–4, the relapse rate is approximately 30%. Unfortunately, the death rate in those patients who relapse has been 7%, or 2% of the entire series. Even with monitoring, 80% of relapses are noted at more advanced stage compared to those patients who undergo retroperitoneal lymph node dissection and who tend to relapse with pulmonary metastases at a lower stage of advanced disease.[50] Considering that the majority of these patients have very favorable factors in order to enter a surveillance protocol, death rates should be exceedingly rare in this subset of patients.

A further concern about surveillance protocols is the extraordinary period of time necessary to follow patients as well as concerns about patients becoming lost to follow-up. There have been at least two reports of late relapses, 6 and 9 years, respectively, for patients with nonseminomatous germ cell tumor on surveillance protocols.[51,52] In addition to the potential problems of long and detailed

TABLE 34–4. SURVEILLANCE STUDIES IN PATIENTS WITH CLINICAL STAGE I NONSEMINOMATOUS GERM CELL TUMOR

Series	No. of Patients	No. Relapsed (%)	No. Dead
Johnson et al. (1984)[39]	36	12 (33)	2
Freedman et al. (1987)[40]	259	70 (27)	3
Rorth et al. (1987)[41]	79	24 (30)	2
Raghavan et al. (1988)[42]	46	13 (8)	2
Sogoni et al. (1988)[43]	45	10 (22)	2
Thompson et al. (1988)[44]	36	12 (33)	2
Read et al. (1992)[45]	373	93 (25)	5
Sturgeon et al. (1992)[46]	105	37 (35)	1
Colls et al. (1995)[47]	115	34 (30)	2
Gels et al. (1995)[48]	154	42 (27)	2
Nicolai-Pizzocaro (1995)[49]	85	25 (29)	3
Total	1333	362 (27%)	26 (2%)

follow-up, difficulties obtaining adequate imaging studies, and a higher mortality rate with relapse, one must factor in the increased cost and labor for longer surveillance.[53] As more experience has been generated, patient selection should identify those individuals at low risk for metastases in whom close observation could be elected. These patients require meticulous evaluation prior to entering a well-designed and well-managed surveillance protocol. Staging should be carried out compulsively in selected patients with no evidence of suspicious nodes or pulmonary masses.

Several series have evaluated prognostic factors associated with relapse.[54–56] Patients with a significant percentage of embryonal carcinoma in the primary are felt to be at high risk of relapse.[56] The local T stage or extent of involvement of the tumor is also an important prognostic factor. Patients with invasion of the epididymis or tunica albuginea (T2 or greater) have a higher rate of relapse. Finally and most importantly, the presence of vascular or lymphatic invasion is significantly associated with relapse.

In patients in whom surveillance therapy is elected, this should be considered an active form of treatment with careful follow-up being mandatory. Physical examination, chest x-rays, and tumor markers are performed monthly for the first year, every 2 months for the second year, and every 3 to 6 months thereafter. Because of the difficulty with assessment of the retroperitoneum, CT scan should be performed approximately every 2 to 3 months for the first 2 years and at least every 6 months thereafter. Surveillance is necessary for a minimum of 5 years and possibly 10 years following orchiectomy.

TREATMENT OF STAGE II (SPREAD TO RETROPERITONEAL LYMPH NODES)

Surgical Treatment

Stage II

The potential advantages of retroperitoneal lymph node dissection for testicular cancer stem from the fact that retroperitoneal deposits are usually the first and often the only evidence of spread beyond the testis. Therefore, retroperitoneal lymph node dissection should be capable of eradicating all disease in over half of patients with stage II tumors. A variety of surgical approaches has been utilized, including the thoracoabdominal or midline transperitoneal exposure. Clinical experience has shown that surgical exploration alone is more than 90% accurate in assessing presence or absence of lymph node metastases. When suspicious lymph nodes are encountered at operation, a complete bilateral retroperitoneal lymphadenectomy is recommended. Suprarenal nodal metastases occur infrequently in the absence of advanced infrarenal disease. Retrocrural metastases must be evaluated carefully.

Retroperitoneal lymph node dissection is certainly capable of controlling regional nodal metastases in select patients.[57] In my experience, in patients with metastases greater than 3 cm in diameter, chemotherapy will often be necessary and these patients are generally recommended for primary chemotherapy. In patients with clinical metastases less than 3 cm in diameter, retroperitoneal lymph node dissection often will suffice without the need for additional chemotherapy.

Chemotherapy

The high relapse and unresectability rates for patients with bulky retroperitoneal disease, combined with effectiveness of multidrug regimens incorporating cis-platinum for treatment of disseminated cancer, have prompted the use of chemotherapy as initial therapy for patients with advanced nodal or pulmonary metastases during the mid-1970s. Because chemotherapy was so effective in treating disseminated disease, the role of surgery has been redefined in an era of potential primary chemotherapy. In patients with masses in the retroperitoneum and rising tumor markers, chemotherapy is preferable to surgical approach. In patients with disease greater than 3 cm in diameter, and certainly greater than 5 cm in diameter, chemotherapy is the initial treatment of choice followed by retroperitoneal lymph node dissection if necessary for residual disease.

The recognition of teratoma within excised residual masses following combination chemotherapy is a relatively recent phenomenon. Mature or immature teratoma should be removed because preoperative studies cannot exclude the possibility of residual malignancy, expansion of benign solid and cystic teratomatous elements may compromise vital organ function, and teratoma may degenerate into a malignant sarcomatous form. Approximately 10 to 25% of patients with advanced nonseminomatous germ cell tumors with normal serum tumor markers following preoperative cytoreductive chemotherapy will still have a malignant component within the excised tissues. Because untreated disease may possess a lethal potential, surgical resection of residual masses following chemocytoreduction is mandatory.

Adjuvant Chemotherapy

Surgical excision has been the standard treatment for patients with clinical stage I or low stage II nonseminomatous germ cell tumors. At issue is whether adjuvant chemotherapy is necessary in patients with disease in the retroperitoneum that has been resected completely. Two-year disease-free survival rate for such patients is 60 to 80%, indicating that 20 to 40% of these patients will recur, usually in the lungs. These patients can be salvaged with three or four cycles of combination chemotherapy.

A national intergroup study published by Williams and associates reported a 48% relapse rate for patients with any positive nodes who were observed following retroperitoneal lymphadenectomy.[58] This relapse rate was compared to a 2% relapse rate in patients who received two cycles of adjuvant chemotherapy, either VAB-VI or PVB (platinum, vinblastine, bleomycin), postoperatively. This study included all patients with positive retroperitoneal lymph nodes dissected, from stage N1 to N3. There was no difference in relapse rate among patients with nodal stages—40% for N1, 53% for N2a, and 60% for N2b.

In a review of 39 patients who underwent retroperitoneal lymph node dissection at the Brigham and Women's Hospital for pathologic stage B1 disease, with less than six positive nodes and no node greater than 2 cm, only 3 of 39 patients have relapsed with a median follow-up of 3.5 years.[59] Thus, for patients with minimal retroperitoneal disease, resected completely, careful follow-up is recommended. For patients with more extensive disease, adjuvant chemotherapy with two cycles can be initiated relatively shortly after retroperitoneal lymph node dissection. The other alternative is careful follow-up with three or four cycles of chemotherapy to be used at the time of relapse. Two cycles of cis-platinum–based adjuvant chemotherapy will almost always prevent relapse.

STAGE III

Prior to the 1970s, advanced stages of testicular cancer were treated with chemotherapy but with only modest response rates. Li and associates described so-called triple therapy consisting of chlorambucil, methotrexate, and actinomycin D in 1960.[60] They reported a 50% objective response rate and a 5 to 10% complete response rate. Subsequently, actinomycin D was shown to be the most effective agent. The concept of combination of vinblastine with bleomycin was initially described by Samuels and associates at M.D. Anderson Cancer Center.[61] Cis-platinum, the most active single agent in the treatment of testicular cancer, was identified initially on studies of agents that inhibit bacterial replication.[62] Einhorn added cis-platinum to the standard two-drug regimen of vinblastine and bleomycin beginning in 1974.[63] Originally, this consisted of cis-platinum 20 mg/m^2 every 3 weeks, vinblastine 0.2 mg/kg on day 1 and 2 every 3 weeks, and bleomycin 30 units IV push. This cycle was repeated four times. Saline hydration was utilized to prevent nephrotoxicity. In their early trial, complete response was achieved in 70% and virtually 100% objective response rate was noted.

Because of toxicity with high-dose vinblastine, specifically myalgias, neuropathy, and ileus, a second randomized prospective trial was introduced to study the standard PVB regimen with a lower dose of vinblastine (0.3 mg/kg). Maintenance vinblastine was used for 2 years after achievement of response. In this trial there was no significant difference in efficacy with the lower vinblastine dosage with or without the addition of Adriamycin.[64] Thus, the lower dose of vinblastine, 0.3 mg/kg, was shown to be equally effective with long-term, durable response rates.

Beginning in 1978, a third-generation study was performed in a randomized prospective fashion comparing four cycles of PVB chemotherapy versus four cycles with maintenance vinblastine. This study confirmed the fact that cure rates could be achieved with four cycles of chemotherapy without the need for maintenance.[65] Overall, 80% of patients on this study were alive and disease-free with follow-up greater than 5 years. Etoposide (VP-16) has single-agent activity in patients with testicular cancer. Because of the toxicity, especially neuromuscular, with vinblastine, VP-16 was studied in a randomized prospective trial under the auspices of the Southeastern Cancer Study Group.[66] In this multi-institutional trial, 121 patients were treated with PVB with a 61% complete response (CR) rate. One hundred twenty-three patients were treated with bleomycin, platinum, and VP-16 with a 60% CR rate. Including patients rendered free of disease after resection of teratoma, 74% were disease-free in the PVB group versus 83% in the platinum, bleomycin, VP-16 group. Toxicity was similar in both arms. Thus, BEP (bleomycin, etoposide, platinum) would seem to be a superior combination chemotherapy and has become the standard treatment for patients with disseminated germ cell tumor.

Randomized studies have compared three cycles versus four cycles of BEP. The response rate is equivalent in both groups. Thus, for patients without adverse risk factors (vide infra), three cycles of BEP chemotherapy should suffice. Three cycles of EP is inferior to three cycles of BEP.[67]

Cis-platinum combination chemotherapy will effect cure rates in approximately 70% of patients with disseminated germ cell tumors. In patients in whom serum markers have normalized after three cycles of chemotherapy, residual masses should be resected surgically. The operative procedures for surgical resection are more extensive. Surgeons should be aware of potential bleomycin-related complications, especially with pulmonary fibrosis.[68] Barneveld and colleagues[69] reported 8 of 93 patients with evidence of bleomycin pneumonitis, 1 of whom died from bleomycin toxicity. Bleomycin toxicity can be minimized by careful monitoring intra- and postoperatively, reduction in the forced inspiratory oxygen (<0.25), and restriction of free water intraoperatively and immediately postoperatively.

Cytoreductive Surgery After Chemotherapy

Primary chemotherapy has been accepted as the initial treatment for patients with advanced or disseminated testicular cancer. In patients with bulk abdominal disease on CT scan, or evidence of pulmonary metastases, as well as those with rising tumor markers, platinum-based chemotherapy is the initial treatment of choice. On occasion, a patient will undergo abdominal exploration and biopsy of a mass confirming the histologic diagnosis of a germ cell tumor. In such instances, the primary in the testis may remain in place.

In patients with extensive retroperitoneal disease (stage B3), or disease above the diaphragm (stage C), primary chemotherapy has resulted in complete remissions in approximately 70% of patients. A combination of chemotherapy and surgery is advocated for those patients who do not achieve a complete response. Although changes in the treatment of low-stage disease have centered around reduction in the extent of surgical treatment, with preservation of ejaculation, changes in the treatment of advanced disease have focused on finding less toxic but equally efficacious chemotherapeutic regimens. Chemotherapeutic toxicity has been reduced by decreasing the amount of vinblastine in the PVB regimen. Another advance was the recognition that maintenance vinblastine was not helpful. Further reduction in toxicity has resulted from the substitution of etoposide (VP-16) for vinblastine (BEP).

In patients who have completed chemotherapy and have evidence of residual disease, a full bilateral retroperitoneal lymph node dissection is required. This procedure is based upon the findings of the distribution of tumor at the time of retroperitoneal lymph node dissection. Even though a large residual mass may remain, much of this mass may represent fibrosis with the possibility of tumor in other areas of the retroperitoneum. Because the nodal spread in bulk disease cannot be accurately predicted, a complete bilateral retroperitoneal lymph node dissection is essential and biopsy alone is to be condemned.

Retroperitoneal lymph node dissection yields important factors in determining the patient's subsequent course of treatment. If the patient has residual cancer at the time of surgery, then additional treatment with primary or secondary chemotherapy may be indicated. If only scar tissue or teratoma remain, then observation is appropriate as long as the margins remain negative.

The surgical approach for extensive retroperitoneal disease following chemotherapy should be a left thoracoabdominal approach with the patient placed in a torqued position. The larger the mass, the higher incision should be in the thoracic cavity, carried down as a paramedian incision. The peritoneal cavity is entered and the bowel mobilized completely based on the superior mesenteric artery (Fig. 34–5). The descending colonic mesentery should be divided near the tumor mass with sacrifice of the inferior mesenteric artery. The colon should be mobilized from the lateral peritoneal reflection allowing full mobility. The large fibrotic mass usually covers the aorta and often the vena cava as well (Fig. 34–6). The right ureter should be identified and carefully dissected free of the fibrotic mass. The vena cava should next be identified and dissected free with control above and below. The lumbar veins should be ligated as identified. It is important during this dissection to carefully identify and preserve the renal arteries. The aorta is next extricated from the mass with division of lumbar

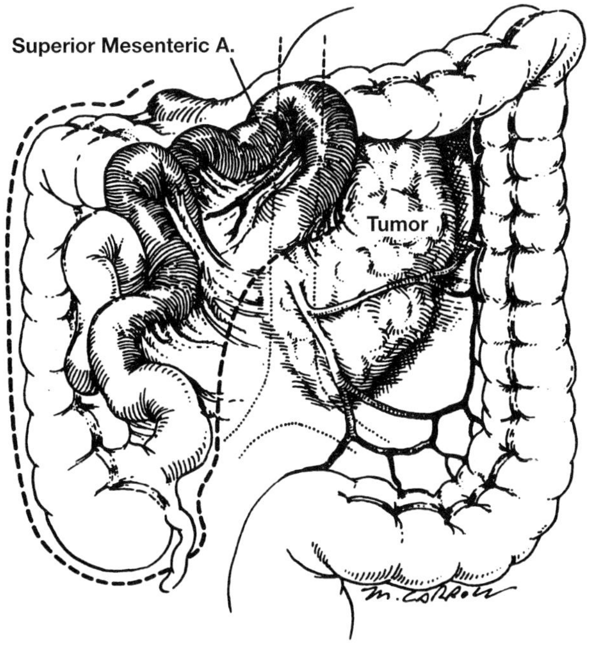
Superior Mesenteric A.
Tumor

FIGURE 34–5. Incision along the root of the mesentery to mobilize small bowel based upon the pedicle of the superior mesenteric artery. The bowel may be packed in a plastic bag and placed on upper abdomen to ensure adequate exposure. (From Waters WB: Retroperitoneal lymph node dissection for tumors of the testis. *In* Nyhus LM, Barker RJ [eds]: Mastery of Surgery, 2nd edition, p 1144. Boston, Little, Brown & Co, 1992, with permission.)

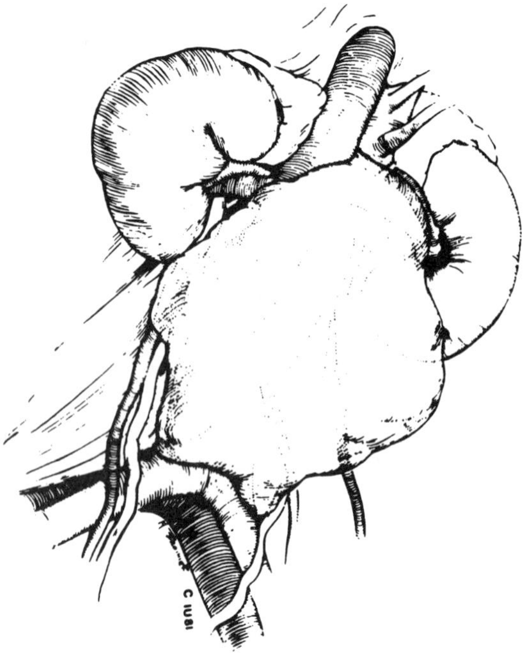
C IUBI

FIGURE 34–6. Typical tumor mass overlying the great vessels following completion of platinum-based chemotherapy. Bowel and mesenteric incisions have been made as described previously to allow exposure. (From Donohue JP: Transabdominal lymphadenectomy. *In* Donohue JP [ed]: Testis Tumors, p 190. Baltimore, Williams & Wilkins, 1983, with permission.)

arteries, carefully protecting the renal arteries and superior mesenteric artery. The mass can then be removed from the left kidney and left ureter. Occasionally, with a large mass the left kidney must be sacrificed en bloc along with the mass. It is essential to explore the retrocrural space, especially in patients with bulk disease.

In patients with residual cancer that has been resected after chemotherapy, or more commonly in patients who don't respond to the traditional courses of induction therapy, salvage therapy with different agents is available and should be considered (Fig. 34–2). In patients who show evidence of progression during cis-platinum combination chemotherapy, salvage chemotherapy with cis-platinum should not be utilized. In patients who progress after having received cis-platinum, cis-platinum may still be useful and should be considered in salvage regimens.

Ifosfamide is an active agent in patients with testicular cancer with a 22% single-agent response rate.[70] Ifosfamide in combination with vinblastine and cis-platinum (VIP regimen) has achieved an approximate 30% disease-free status in patients who have failed initial chemotherapy regimens.[71] In patients who receive ifosfamide, Mesna should be utilized prior to starting ifosfamide to prevent the complication of hemorrhagic cystitis. In patients who have initially received vinblastine, VP-16 should be used in the VIP regimen. In patients who receive VP-16, vinblastine should be used.

Third-line chemotherapy for patients who have failed first- and second-line therapy includes autologous bone marrow transplantation with high-dose chemotherapy regimens.[72] Carboplatin, an agent with activity similar to cis-platinum, has myelosuppression as its dose-limiting toxicity. Therefore, carboplatin can be used in lieu of cis-platin in patients who are undergoing autologous bone marrow transplantation.[73]

Management of High-Risk Testicular Cancer Patients

Patients with stage C nonseminomatous testicular cancer can be subdivided into patients who will respond to standard chemotherapy versus more aggressive chemotherapy. The Indiana University staging system detailed in Table 34–5 has proven to be a workable model with therapeutic advantages. Patients with minimal or moderate disease will do well with standard chemotherapy, with response rates in the 91 to 95% category.[74] Patients with advanced disease, however, had only a 53% therapeutic response. Therefore, more aggressive chemotherapy should be utilized in patients with advanced-extent disease according to this category.

Testicular cancer represents one of the real success stories in modern oncology. Testicular cancer has become one of the most curable solid neoplasms. Attention is now being turned to fine tuning aspects of the disease, attempting to reduce morbidity from chemotherapy as well as modified surgical approaches. A challenge for the 1990s will be to maintain effective response rates while reducing morbidity and better identification of risk fac-

TABLE 34–5. INDIANA UNIVERSITY STAGING SYSTEM FOR DISSEMINATED TESTICULAR CANCER*

Minimal Extent
1. Elevated markers only
2. Cervical nodes (± nonpalpable retroperitoneal nodes)
3. Unresectable nonpalpable retroperitoneal disease
4. Fewer than five pulmonary metastases per lung field *and* largest <2 cm (± nonpalpable retroperitoneal nodes)

Moderate Extent
1. Palpable abdominal mass only (no supradiaphragmatic disease)
2. Moderate pulmonary metastases: 5–10 metastases per lung field and largest <3 cm *or* solitary pulmonary metastasis of any size <2 cm (± nonpalpable retroperitoneal disease)

Advanced Extent
1. Advanced pulmonary metastases: primary mediastinal nonseminomatous germ cell tumor *or* >10 pulmonary metastases per lung field, *or* multiple pulmonary metastases
2. Palpable abdominal mass plus supradiaphragmatic disease
3. Liver, bone, or CNS metastases

tors in order to select appropriate therapy for individual patients.

EXTRAGONADAL TUMORS

Primary tumors of extragonadal origin are rare, with fewer than 1000 cases described in the literature. Distinction between a primary extragonadal germ cell tumor and metastatic disease from an undetected testis primary tumor may be difficult but has obviously important clinical implications. Surgical and autopsy series have confirmed the absence of a "burned-out" testicular primary lesion in a number of cases, laying to rest some of the skepticism surrounding the diagnosis of extragonadal germ cell tumor in the past.[75] More recently, testicular ultrasonography has emerged as a sensitive technique for the detection of tiny neoplasms a few millimeters in size within the clinically "normal" testis. Although the exact incidence of extragonadal germ cell tumors is unknown, clinical data suggest that roughly 3 to 5% of all germ cell tumors are of extragonadal origin.

The most common sites of origin are, in decreasing order of frequency, the mediastinum, retroperitoneum, sacrococcygeal region, and pineal gland, although many unusual sources have also been reported. Two schools of thought exist as to the origin of these neoplasms: (1) displacement of primitive germ cells during early embryonic migration from the yolk sac entoderm; and (2) persistence of pluripotential cells in sequestered primitive rests during early somatic development. The theory of misplaced germ cells holds that during ontogeny, migration through the retroperitoneum is misdirected cephalad to the mediastinum and pineal gland or caudad to the sacrococcygeal region, rather than to the genital ridges. The alternative hypothesis maintains that primitive pluripotential cells may be dislocated during early embryogenesis (blastema or morula phase). A germ cell rest in the third brachial cleft, for example, could result in a mediastinal tumor, which, interestingly, often resembles a thymoma histologically.

Males are predominantly affected, although a female predominance has been noted with sacrococcygeal lesions. With the exception of sacrococcygeal tumors in the newborn, these tumors generally lack encapsulation, unlike their testicular counterparts, and tend to invade or envelope contiguous structures. The majority of adults with extragonadal germ cell tumors present with advanced local disease and distant metastases. These tumors most commonly spread to regional lymph nodes, lung, liver, and bone. Histologically, all germ cell types are represented, with pure seminoma accounting for roughly half the tumors in the mediastinum and retroperitoneum. In general, sacrococcygeal tumors of the newborn and young adult are functionally and histologically benign, whereas tumors discovered during infancy prove malignant in about half the cases.

Extragonadal germ cell tumors may reach a large size with no or relatively few symptoms. Diagnosis of mediastinal extragonadal germ cell tumor is most commonly established during the third decade, with or without signs and symptoms of chest pain, cough, or dyspnea. Patients with primary retroperitoneal tumors may present with abdominal or back pain, a palpable mass, vascular obstruction, or other vague constitutional symptoms. Sacrococcygeal tumors are most often diagnosed in the neonate (1 in 40,000 births) and less frequently during infancy or adulthood, with findings of a palpable mass, skin discoloration or hairy nevus, or bowel or urinary obstruction. Tumors of the pineal gland occur in children and young adults, producing symptoms of increased intracranial pressure (headache, visual impairment), oculomotor dysfunction (diplopia, ptosis), hearing loss, hypopituitarism (abnormal menses), and hypothalamic disturbances (diabetes insipidus).

Complete local excision of mediastinal or retroperitoneal tumors is rarely feasible because of frequent local extension and high rates of metastatic disease. In reviewing 30 cases of primary mediastinal tumors, Martini et al. found only 4 of 30 patients who presented with no metastasis.[76] Three of these four had pure seminoma. In the ten patients with pure seminoma, only four were long-term survivors following surgery or radiotherapy. Of 20 patients with elements of embryonal carcinoma, only 1 was alive at 20 months following surgery, radiotherapy, and chemotherapy. Sterchi and Cordell reviewed 108 patients with mediastinal seminoma, finding a 5-year survival rate of 58% following primary radiation therapy or surgery.[77] The recent MSKCC experience with 21 cases of extragonadal seminoma was reviewed with primary cisplatinum–based chemotherapy; only one died of metastatic disease, with the remainder disease-free at 19+ to 46+ months' follow-up. Patients with primary retroperitoneal seminoma appear equally responsive to intensive chemotherapy regimens.[78] In contrast, patients with nonseminomatous extragonadal germ cell tumor have done poorly despite surgery, radiotherapy, and chemotherapy.[79,80] Disappointingly, only 2 of 18 patients treated at MSKCC with successive VAB protocols have achieved CR. While Garnick et al.[81] reported similar results, those of Hainsworth et al.,[82] using the PVB regimen, were superior. The reason for this apparent discrepancy remains unclear.

Wide local excision is the treatment of choice for sacrococcygeal tumors, in that the majority are benign. Limited experience renders uncertain the advisability of adjunctive irradiation or chemotherapy for malignant tumors. Radical excisions for pineal tumors have been disappointing from the standpoints of local control and operative morbidity. Such procedures have been largely abandoned in favor of primary radiation therapy, although a cerebrospinal fluid shunt may be required.[83]

REFERENCES

1. Parker SL, Tong T, Bolden S, Wingo PA: Cancer Statistics, 1996. CA Cancer Clin J 1996; 65:5.
2. Chagantirsk R, Rodriquez E, Bosl GJ: Cytogenetics of male germ cell tumors. Urol Clin North Am 1993; 20:55–66.
3. Suijkerbuijk RF, Looijenga L, DeJong B, et al: Verification of isochromosome 12p and identification of other chromosome 12 aberrations in gonadal and extagonadal human germ cell tumors by bicolor double fluorescence in situ hybridization. Cancer Genet Cytogenet 1992; 63:8–16.
4. Skakkebaek NE: Possible carcinoma in situ of the testis. Lancet 1972; 2:516.
5. Skakkebaek NE: Atypical germ cells in the adjacent "normal" tissue of testicular tumors. Acta Pathol Microbiol Scand 1975; 84:127.
6. Skakkebaek NE, Berthelsen JG, Muller J: Carcinoma in situ of the undescended testis. Urol Clin North Am 1982; 9: 377–385.
7. Giwereman A, von der Maase H, Berthelsen JG, et al: Localized irradiation of testis with carcinoma in situ: effects on Leydig cell function and irradiation of malignant germ cells in 20 patients. J Clin Endocrinol Metab 1991; 73:596–603.
8. Mostofi FK: Testicular tumors. Epidemiologic, etiologic and pathologic features. Cancer 1973; 32:1186.
9. Clemmesen J: Statistical studies in malignancy. Microbiol Scand 1974; 247:1.
10. LeComete (1851): Quoted by Grove JS. The cryptorchid problem. J Urol 1954; 71:735.
11. Gilbert JB, Hamilton JB: Studies in malignant testis tumors; incidence and nature of tumors in ectopic testis. Surg Gynecol Obstet 1940; 71:731.
12. Farrer JH, Walker AH, Rajfer J: Management of the postpubertal cryptorchid testis: a statistical review. J Urol 1985; 134:1071.
13. Donohue JP, Zachary JM, Maynard BR: Distribution of nodal metastases in nonseminomatous testis cancer. J Urol 1982; 128:315.
14. Boden JP, Gibb R: Radiotherapy and testicular neoplasms. Lancet 1951; 2:119.
15. Skinner DG: Non-seminomatous testis tumors: a plan of management based on 96 patients to improve survival in all stages by combined therapeutic modalities. J Urol 1976; 115:65.
16. Maier JG, Sulak MH: Radiation therapy in malignant testis tumors. Part II: nonseminoma. Cancer 1973; 32:1212.
17. Stomper PC, Kalish LA, Garnick MB, et al: CT and pathologic predictive features of residual mass histologic findings after chemotherapy for nonseminomatous germ cell tumors: can residual malignancy or teratoma be excluded. Radiology 1991; 180:711–714.
18. Fraley E, Lange PH, Kennedy BJ: Germ-cell testicular cancer in adults. N Engl J Med 1979; 301:1370, 1420.
19. Pizzocaro G: Retroperitoneal lymphadenectomy in clinical stage I nonseminomatous germinal testis cancer. Eur J Surg Oncol 1986; 12:25–33.
20. Richie JP: Clinical stage I testicular cancer: the role of modified retroperitoneal lymphadenectomy. J Urol 1990; 144: 1160–1163.
21. Donohue JP, Thornhill JA, Foster RS, et al: Retroperitoneal lymphadenectomy for clinical stage A testis cancer (1965–1989): modifications of technique and impact on ejaculation. J Urol 1993; 149:237–243.
22. Sosnowski M, Jeromin L, Pluzanska A, Puzanska A: Is modified retroperitoneal lymph node dissection still feasible in the treatment of patients with clinical stage I nonseminomatous testicular cancer? Int Urol Nephrol 1994; 26: 471–477.
23. Most H: Uber malique loden ges chwulste und ihremetastasin. Arch Pathol Anat 1898; 54:235.
24. Cuneo B: Note sur les lymphatiques du testicle. Bull Soc Anat (Paris) 1901; 76:105.
25. Jamieson JK, Dobson JF: The lymphatics of the testicle. Lancet 1910; 1:493.
26. Rouviere H: Anatomy of the Human Lymphatic System (Translated by MJ Tobias). Ann Arbor, Edward Bros, 1938.
27. Lewis LG: Testis tumor: report on 250 cases. J Urol 1948; 59:763.
28. Kimbrough JC, Cook FE Jr: Carcinoma of the testis. JAMA 1953; 153:1436.
29. Cooper JF, Leadbetter WF, Chute R: The thoracoabdominal approach for retroperitoneal gland dissection: its application to testis tumors. Surg Gynecol Obstet 1950; 90:46.
30. Staubitz WJ, Early KS, Magoss IV, Murphy GP: Surgical management of testis tumors. J Urol 1974; 111:205.
31. Whitmore WF Jr: Germinal tumors of the testis. *In* Proceedings of the Sixth National Cancer Conference, pp 219–221. Philadelphia, JB Lippincott Co, 1970.
32. Baniel J, Foster RS, Rowland RG, et al: Complications of primary retroperitoneal lymph node dissection. J Urol 1994; 152:424–427.
33. Narayan P, Lange PH, Fraley EE: Ejaculation and fertility after extended retroperitoneal lymph node dissection for testicular cancer. J Urol 1982; 127:685.
34. Donohue JP, Foster RS, Rowland RG, et al: Nerve-sparing retroperitoneal lymphadenectomy with preservation of ejaculation. J Urol 1990; 144:287.
35. Jewett MAS, Torbey C: Nerve-sparing techniques in retroperitoneal lymphadenectomy in patients with low-stage testicular cancer. Semin Urol 1988; 6:233.
36. Foster RS, McNulty A, Rubin LR: The fertility of patients with clinical stage I testis cancer managed by nerve sparing retroperitoneal lymph node dissection. J Urol 1994; 152:1139.
37. Gerber GS, Bissada NK, Hulbert JC: Laparoscopic retroperitoneal lymphadenectomy: multi-institutional analysis. J Urol 1994; 152:1188.
38. Raghavan D, Peckham MJ, Heyderman E, et al: Prognostic factors in clinical stage I non-seminomatous germ-cell tumours of the testis. Br J Cancer 1982; 45:167.
39. Johnson DE, Lo RK, von Eschenbach AC, et al: Surveillance alone for patients with clinical stage I nonseminomatous germ cell tumors of the testis. Preliminary results. J Urol 1984; 131:491.
40. Freedman LS, Jones WG, Peckham MJ, et al: Histopathology in the prediction of relapse of patients with stage I testicular teratoma treated by orchidectomy alone. Lancet 1987; 2:294.
41. Rørth M, von der Maase H, Nielsen ES, et al: Orchidectomy alone versus orchidectomy plus radiotherapy in stage I nonseminomatous testicular cancer: A randomized study by the Danish Carcinoma Study Group. Int J Androl 1987; 10:255.
42. Raghavan D, Colls B, Levi J, et al: Surveillance for stage I nonseminomatous germ cell tumors of the testis: the optimal protocol has not yet been defined. Br J Urol 1988; 61: 522.
43. Sogani PC, Whitmore WF Jr, Herr HW, et al: Long-term experience with orchiectomy alone in treatment of clinical stage I non-seminomatous germ cell tumor of the testis. J Urol 1988; 133:246A.
44. Thompson PI, Nixon J, Harvey VJ: Disease relapse in patients with stage I non-seminomatous germ cell tumor of the testis on active surveillance. J Clin Oncol 1988; 6:1597.
45. Read G, Stenning SP, Cullen MH, et al: Medical Research Council prospective study of surveillance for stage I testicular teratoma. Medical Research Council Testicular Tumors Working Party. J Clin Oncol 1992; 10:1762–1768.
46. Sturgeon JF, Jewett MA, Alison RE, et al: Surveillance after orchiectomy for patients with clinical stage I nonseminomatous testis tumors. J Clin Oncol 1992; 10:564–568.
47. Colls BM, Harvey VJ, Skelton L, et al: Results of the surveillance policy of stage I nonseminomatous germ cell testicular tumours. Br J Urol 1992; 70:423–428.
48. Gels ME, Hoekstra HJ, Sleijfer DT, et al: Detection and recurrence in patients with clinical stage I nonseminomatous testicular germ cell tumors and consequences for further follow-up: a single-center 10-year experience. J Clin Oncol 1995; 13:1188–1194.

49. Nicolai N, Pizzocaro G: A surveillance study of clinical stage I nonseminomatous germ cell tumors of the testis: 10-year followup. J Urol 1995; 154:1054–1059.
50. Rowland RG, Weisman D, Williams S, et al: Accuracy of preoperative staging in stage A and B non-seminomatous germ cell testis tumors. J Urol 1982; 127:718.
51. McCrystal MR, Zwi LJ, Harvey VJ: Late seminomatous relapse of a mixed germ cell tumor of the testis on intensive surveillance. J Urol 1995; 153:1057.
52. Hurley LJ, Libertino JA: Recurrence of a nonseminomatous germ cell tumor 9 years postoperatively: is surveillance alone acceptable? J Urol 1995; 153:1060.
53. Donohue JP, Thornhill JA, Foster RS, et al: Stage I nonseminomatous germ cell testicular cancer—management options and risk benefit considerations. World J Urol 1994; 12:170–177.
54. Fung CY, Kalish LA, Brodsky GL, et al: Stage I nonseminomatous germ cell testicular tumor: prediction of metastatic potential by primary histology. J Clin Oncol 1988; 6: 1467.
55. Dunphy CH, Ayala AG, Swanson DA, et al: Clinical stage I nonseminomatous and mixed germ cell tumors of the testis. A clinicopathologic study of 93 patients on a surveillance protocol after orchiectomy alone. Lancet 1988; 62: 1202.
56. Moul JW, McCarthy WF, Fernandez EB, Sesterhenn IA: Percentage of embryonal carcinoma and of vascular invasion predicts pathological stage in clinical stage I nonseminomatous testicular cancer. Cancer Res 1994; 54:362–364.
57. Donohue JP, Thornhill JA, Foster RS: The role of retroperitoneal lymphadenectomy in clinical stage B testis cancer: the Indiana University experience (1965–1989). J Urol 1995; 153:85.
58. Williams SD, Stablain DM, Einhorn LH, et al: Immediate adjuvant chemotherapy versus observation with treatment at relapse in pathologic stage II testicular cancer. N Engl J Med 1987; 317:1433.
59. Richie JP, Kantoff P: Is adjuvant chemotherapy necessary for patients with stage B_1 testicular cancer? J Clin Oncol 1991; 9:1393–1396.
60. Li MC, Whitmore WF Jr, Golbey R, Grabstald H: Effects of combined drug therapy on metastatic cancer of the testis. JAMA 1960; 174:1291.
61. Samuels ML, Johnson DE, Holoye PY: Continuous intravenous bleomycin therapy with vinblastine in stage III testicular neoplasia. Cancer Chemother Rep 1975; 59:563.
62. Rosenberg B, VanCamp L, Krigas T: Inhibition of cell division in *E. coli* by electrolysis products from a platinum electrode. Nature 1965; 205:678.
63. Einhorn LH, Donohue JP: Cis-diamminedichloroplatinum, vinblastine and bleomycin combination chemotherapy in disseminated testicular cancer. Ann Intern Med 1977; 87: 293.
64. Einhorn LH, Williams SD: Chemotherapy of disseminated testicular cancer. Cancer 1980; 46:1339.
65. Einhorn LH, Williams SD, Troner M, et al: The role of maintenance therapy in disseminated testicular cancer. N Engl J Med 1981; 305:727.
66. Williams SD, Birch R, Einhorn LH, et al: Treatment of disseminated germ cell tumors with cis-platinum, bleomycin and either vinblastine and etoposide. N Engl J Med 1987; 316:1435.
67. Loehrer PJ Sr, Johnson D, Elson P, et al: Importance of bleomycin in favorable-prognosis disseminated germ cell tumors: an Eastern Cooperative Oncology Group trial. J Clin Oncol 1995; 13:470–476.
68. Sleijfer S, Van der Mark TW, Schrafford T, et al: Decrease in pulmonary function during bleomycin-containing combination chemotherapy for testicular cancer: not only a bleomycin effect. Br J Cancer 1995; 71:120–123.
69. Barneveld PW, Sleijfer DT, Van der Mark TW, et al: Natural course of bleomycin-induced pneumonitis. Am Rev Respir Dis 1987; 135:48.
70. Wheeler BM, Loehrer PJ, Williams SD, Einhorn LH: Ifosfamide and refractory germ cell tumors. J Clin Oncol 1986; 4:28.
71. Lauer RL, Roth B, Loehrer PJ, et al: Cis-platinum plus ifosfamide plus either VP-16 or vinblastine as third-line therapy for metastatic testicular cancer. Proc Am Soc Clin Oncol 1987; 6:99.
72. Siegert W, Beyer J, Strohscheer I, et al: High-dose treatment with carboplatin, etoposide, and ifosfamide followed by autologous stem-cell transplantation in relapsed or refractory germ cell cancer: a phase I/II study. J Clin Oncol 1994; 12:1223–1231.
73. Lotz JP, Andre T, Donsimoni R, et al: High dose chemotherapy with ifosfamide, carboplatin, and etoposide combined with autologous bone marrow transplantation for the treatment of poor-prognosis germ cell tumors and metastatic trophoblastic disease in adults. Cancer 1995; 75: 874–885.
74. Birch R, Williams SD, Cohn A, et al: Prognostic factors for a favorable outcome in disseminated germ cell tumors. J Clin Oncol 1986; 4:400.
75. Luna MA, Valenzuela-Tamariz J: Germ cell tumors of the mediastinum: post-mortem findings. Am J Clin Pathol 1976; 65:450.
76. Martini N, Golbey RB, Hajdu SI, et al: Primary mediastinal germ cell tumors. Cancer 1974; 33:763.
77. Sterchi M, Cordell AR: Seminoma of the anterior mediastinum. Ann Thorac Surg 1975; 19:371.
78. Stanton GF, Bosl GJ, Vugrin D, et al: Treatment of patients with advanced seminoma with cyclophosphamide, bleomycin, actinomycin D, vinblastine and cis-platin (VAB-6). Proc Am Soc Clin Oncol 1983; 2:1.
79. Recondo J, Libshitz HI: Mediastinal extragonadal germ cell tumors. Urology 1978; 11:369.
80. Reynolds TF, Tagoda A, Vugrin D, Golbey RB: Chemotherapy of mediastinal germ cell tumors. Semin Oncol 1978; 6:113.
81. Garnick MB, Canellos GP, Richie JP: Treatment and surgical staging of testicular and primary extragonadal germ cell cancer. JAMA 1983; 250:1733–1741.
82. Hainsworth JD, Einhorn LH, Williams SD, et al: Advanced extragonadal germ cell tumors. Successful treatment with combination chemotherapy. Ann Intern Med 1982; 97:7.
83. Cole H: Tumours in the region of the pineal. Clin Radiol 1971; 22:110.

35

NON–GERM CELL TUMORS OF THE TESTIS

ERIC A. KLEIN, M.D. *and* HOWARD S. LEVIN, M.D.

Non–germ cell tumors of the testis comprise a heterogeneous group of benign and malignant neoplasms that may be primary or metastatic. As a group they account for only 5 to 6% of all testicular neoplasms, the remaining testicular tumors being of germ cell origin (Fig. 35–1). The most commonly occurring primary tumors of non–germ cell origin are classified as sex cord/stromal tumors or tumors of specialized gonadal stroma. These tumors may be associated with somatic or constitutional chromosomal syndromes. Other less commonly encountered primary tumors include mesenchymal tumors from nonspecialized stroma such as blood vessels or smooth muscle, tumors arising from hematopoietic cells, and a multitude of other benign tumors that mimic malignant lesions. In addition, a number of malignancies from other sites may rarely present initially or as a late sign of more diffuse disease. Cases of malignant lymphoma and malignant germ cell tumors in patients with acquired immunodeficiency syndrome (AIDS) have also been reported.[1] A useful practical classification of non–germ cell testicular tumors is presented in Table 35–1.

Most primary tumors of non–germ cell origin are biologically benign. The clinical presentation of these tumors is similar to and often indistinguishable from those of germ cell origin. Common presenting symptoms include testicular pain and enlargement that may be of prolonged duration. Breast tenderness or enlargement may also be present. Physical examination typically confirms the presence of testicular swelling or intratesticular mass. Most primary non–germ cell tumors will appear as discrete hypoechoic lesions on ultrasonography, whereas leukemic or lymphomatous infiltration will demonstrate enlargement with multiple focal or diffuse areas of decreased echogenicity. The presence of diffuse unilateral or bilateral testicular enlargement rather than a discrete mass on physical exam or scrotal ultrasonography suggests a secondary rather than primary neoplasm. Peripheral lymphadenopathy is rare with primary non–germ cell tumors and should prompt a search to exclude a primary tumor from another site, notably lymphoma. Gynecomastia, loss of libido, or other signs of feminization may be present in some tumors (notably Leydig or Sertoli cell tumors) as a result of active secretion of estrogens or alterations in serum estrogen/testosterone ratios or peripheral aromatization of testosterone.[2] Serum levels of human chorionic gonadotropin (hCG) and α-fetoprotein (AFP) will be normal. All of these clinical features may also be present with primary germ cell tumors, and histologic examination of the affected testicle is the sine qua non for distinguishing these tumor types and determining the need for further evaluation and treatment. In adults with a palpably normal opposite testis, inguinal orchiectomy without frozen section is considered standard therapy. Occasionally a non–germ cell tumor or other benign process may be strongly suspected based on presenting signs and symptoms and/or the ultrasonographic appearance of the lesion, and inguinal exploration and excisional biopsy with the intent of sparing the uninvolved ipsilateral testis may be considered. In such instances, frozen section examination of the excised tumor is necessary to exclude the presence of malignancy. In all such cases, the clinical aspects and topography of the mass should be shared with the pathologist. In cases with equivocal findings on frozen section, inguinal orchiectomy should be performed in patients with a normal contralateral testis. Frozen section is useful in identifying malignant lymphomas so that fresh tissue can be used for tumor phenotyping.

A description of individual tumor types with characteristic clinical and pathologic features and recommendations for management follows.

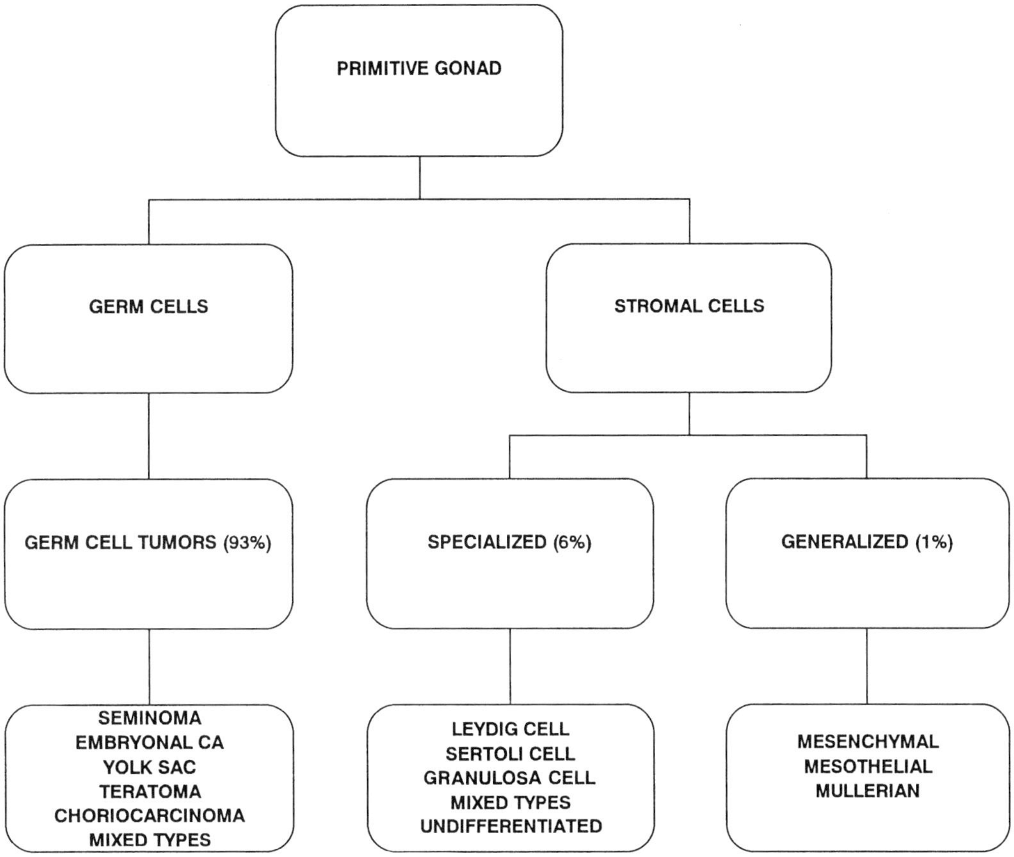
PRIMITIVE GONAD
GERM CELLS
STROMAL CELLS
GERM CELL TUMORS (93%)
SPECIALIZED (6%)
GENERALIZED (1%)
SEMINOMA
EMBRYONAL CA
YOLK SAC
TERATOMA
CHORIOCARCINOMA
MIXED TYPES
LEYDIG CELL
SERTOLI CELL
GRANULOSA CELL
MIXED TYPES
UNDIFFERENTIATED
MESENCHYMAL
MESOTHELIAL
MULLERIAN

FIGURE 35–1. Embryologic origin of testis tumors.

PRIMARY TUMORS OF SEX CORD/ STROMAL ORIGIN

Leydig Cell Tumors

Clinical Presentation

Leydig cell tumors (LCTs) comprise approximately 1 to 3% of testicular tumors. They occur in males of all ages, with predominance in children older than 4 and adults in their 20s to 50s. In prepubertal boys, they produce isosexual precocity with penile enlargement, sexual hair growth, increased bone growth, deepened voice, and aggressive behavior as a consequence of increased testosterone production by the neoplasm. Clinical signs and symptoms are usually manifest before the discovery of the neoplasm. In postpubertal males, LCTs usually present with a unilateral painless testicular mass or incidentally as a mass discovered during physical examination. Only 30% have signs of increased hormonal function and, in contrast to the prepubertal group, affected adults exhibit feminization with unilateral or bilateral gynecomastia, impotence, and hair loss.[2] LCTs have been reported in cryptorchid testes before and after orchiopexy, in the contralateral testis of a 40-year-old 7 years after orchiectomy for a mixed malignant germ cell tumor, and in association with Klinefelter's syndrome and tuberous sclerosis.[3,4]

TABLE 35–1. CLASSIFICATION OF NON–GERM CELL TESTICULAR TUMORS

Tumors of Specialized Stroma	Tumors of Generalized Stroma	Hematologic Tumors	Miscellaneous Tumors
Leydig cell tumor	Vascular tumors	Lymphoma	Carcinoid
Sertoli cell tumor	Smooth and skeletal muscle tumors	Leukemia	Epidermoid cyst
Granulosa cell tumor	Adenomatoid tumor	Plasmacytoma	Adenocarcinoma of the rete testis
Mixed tumor	Mesothelioma		Metastatic tumors
Incompletely differentiated tumors			Ovarian surface epithelial–type tumors

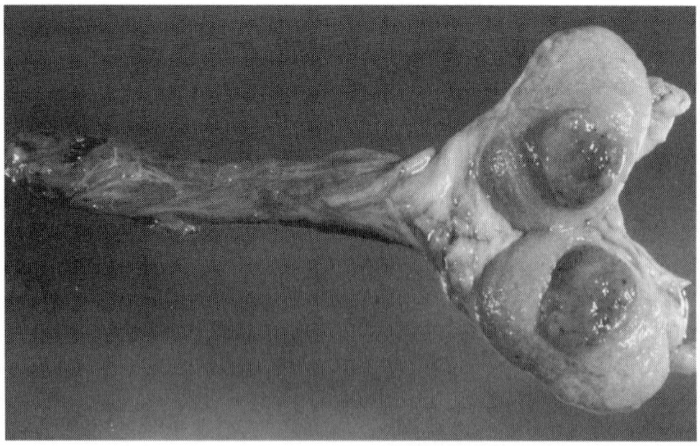

FIGURE 35–2. Benign Leydig cell tumor. Discrete unencapsulated, soft, tan 2.2-cm mass in bivalved testis in a 29-year-old man with left testicular mass and bilateral gynecomastia.

Pathologic Characteristics

The gross appearance of LCTs is characteristically mahogany or yellow-brown in color, rubbery, discrete, nonencapsulated, and nonnecrotic. LCTs vary considerably in size, ranging from nonpalpable to more than 10 cm in diameter (Fig. 35–2). The microscopic appearance is variable, with a spectrum of cell shapes extending from polygonal to spindled. Leydig cell nuclei are generally round with a small, single nucleolus, but binucleate, multinucleate, and giant cells with giant nuclei may be present (Fig. 35–3). Mitotic figures are generally sparse. Cell cytoplasm is usually eosinophilic and sometimes ground glass in appearance, but may be vacuolated depending on the amount of intracytoplasmic lipid. Approximately 40% of LCTs contain intracytoplasmic Reinke's crystals.[5] Lipochrome pigment may also be present in varying amounts. The tumor cells may grow in sheets, cords, and tubular formations. Capillaries are abundant between aggregates of epithelial cells. The stroma may be loose or dense and hyaline. The ultrastructural appearance resembles that of other steroid hormone–producing cells. LCTs stain positively for lipid. In tumors of prepubertal males, seminiferous tubules adjacent to the neoplasm have shown response to local androgen manifested as proliferative activity of germinal epithelium with development to the spermatid stage.[6] Seminiferous tubules in the contralateral testis and distant from the tumor in the ipsilateral testis typically retain prepubertal morphology. Conversely, in postpubertal men, seminiferous tubules adjacent to feminizing LCTs show reduced spermatogenesis and thickening of the tunica propria.

Approximately 10% of LCTs are malignant, and over 30 such cases have been reported. Malignant LCTs are larger than benign LCTS, have no clinical endocrine hyperfunction, and have a shorter clinical duration prior to orchiectomy.[7] Collins and Cameron debated the malignancy of some of these cases on the basis of unproven metastases and the nonperformance of autopsies.[8] The absolute criterion for malignancy of a LCT is metastasis, but other morphologic features that strongly suggest malignancy include large tumors, marked cellular anaplasia, frequent or atypical mitoses, infiltrating margin, and necrosis[7] (Fig. 35–4). Invasion of lymphatics and/or blood vessels is suggestive of malignancy (Fig. 35–5). Metastases usually occur within months to years after the original diagnosis, but initial metastasis has been recorded as late as 9 years after orchiectomy. Initial metastasis is usually to retroperitoneal lymph nodes, but subsequent metastases involve remote lymph nodes and possibly viscera. Benign LCTs generally have diploid DNA content, whereas malignant LCTs generally have aneuploid DNA by flow cytometry.[9]

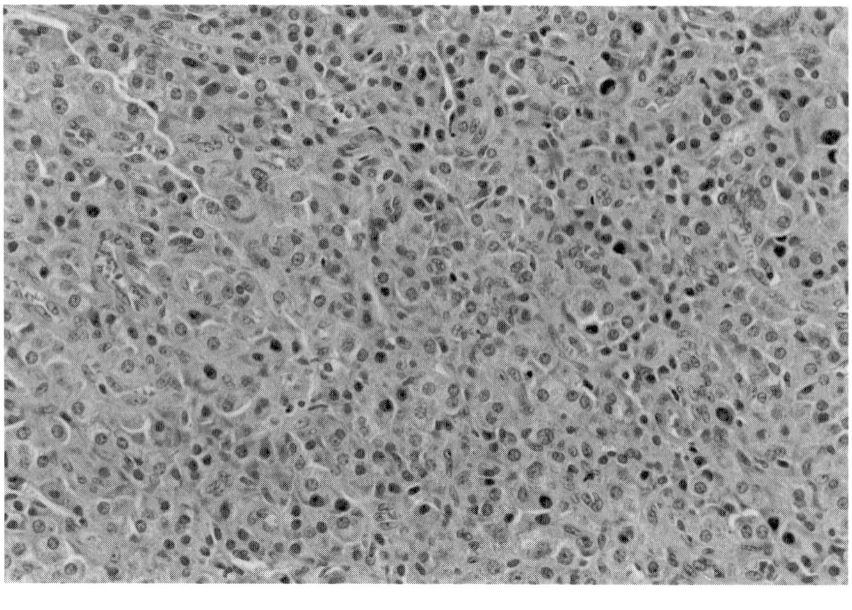

FIGURE 35–3. Leydig cell tumor in a 20-year-old with an enlarged testis. The testicular parenchyma was substantially replaced by a yellow-brown mass. The Leydig cells contain round uniform nuclei and eosinophilic granular cytoplasm. H&E, ×31.2.

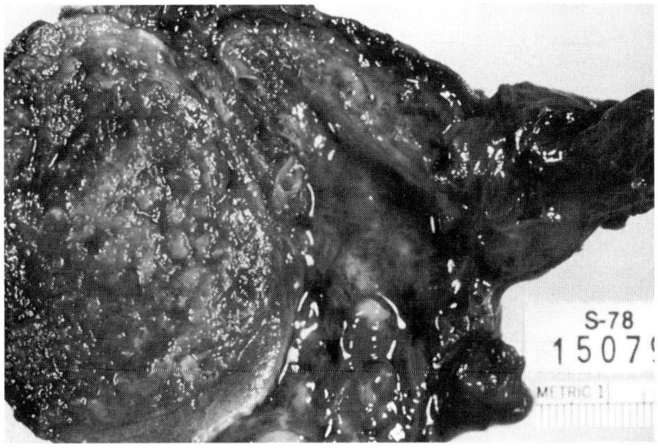

FIGURE 35–4. Malignant Leydig cell tumor in a 63-year-old man who noted enlargement and soreness of the testis for 4 to 5 weeks. The testis measured 6 × 7 × 7 cm and was almost totally replaced by a bulging light tan to dark brown variegated mass with multiple apparent septae. (Courtesy of the California Tumor Tissue Registry.)

Tumors in Males with Congenital Adrenal Hyperplasia

An important distinction must be made between LCTs and the testicular masses in the salt-losing form of congenital adrenal hyperplasia (CAH). Males with CAH from the neonatal period to adulthood may develop bilateral testicular or peritesticular masses that are histologically similar to LCT[10] (Figs. 35–6 and 35–7). The cells of these masses do not contain Reinke's crystals but do contain abundant lipochrome pigment, which gives the gross tumors a brown or black appearance. These masses resemble those in patients with Nelson's syndrome. The fact that the masses often disappear after corticosteroid therapy and are sensitive to corticotropin stimulation suggests they are of adrenocortical origin. Davis et al. described the only instance of a malignant LCT in a patient with CAH.[11] In order to avoid inappropriate orchiectomy in patients with CAH, and because of their response to corticosteroid therapy and the risk of adrenal insufficiency if these patients are not treated with corticosteroids after orchiectomy, it is important to distinguish true LCT from CAH with testicular masses.

Evaluation and Management

In children presenting with precocious puberty, biochemical evaluation is necessary to distinguish primary LCT from Leydig cell hyperplasia secondary to CAH. The presence of a unilateral tumor with normal serum or urinary levels of dehydroepiandrosterone, androstenedione, and 17-hydroxyprogesterone strongly favors the diagnosis of primary LCT, whereas bilateral tumors or those associated with abnormalities of steroid biosynthesis favor CAH. In either instance, serum testosterone levels may be elevated. Corticotropin stimulation and dexamethasone suppression tests are occasionally necessary to establish tumor origin. Gabrilove et al. reviewed 37 cases of feminizing LCTs of the testis, 5 of which were in prepubertal boys.[2] In 20 patients in whom estrogens were measured, 13 had high urinary titers. Serum estrogen levels may also be elevated, with a concomitant reduction in serum testosterone. Gonadotropin levels will vary with associated levels of serum androgens and estrogens.

The treatment of LCT is surgical excision. In cases in which the diagnosis of LCT is not suspected preoperatively, inguinal orchiectomy is the procedure of choice. In children and adults in whom the diagnosis is suspected, a testis-sparing enucleation or excisional biopsy is acceptable provided that histologic confirmation of the lesion is obtained by frozen section. Following tumor excision, the endocrinologic manifestations of the tumor typically disappear in adults. In children with

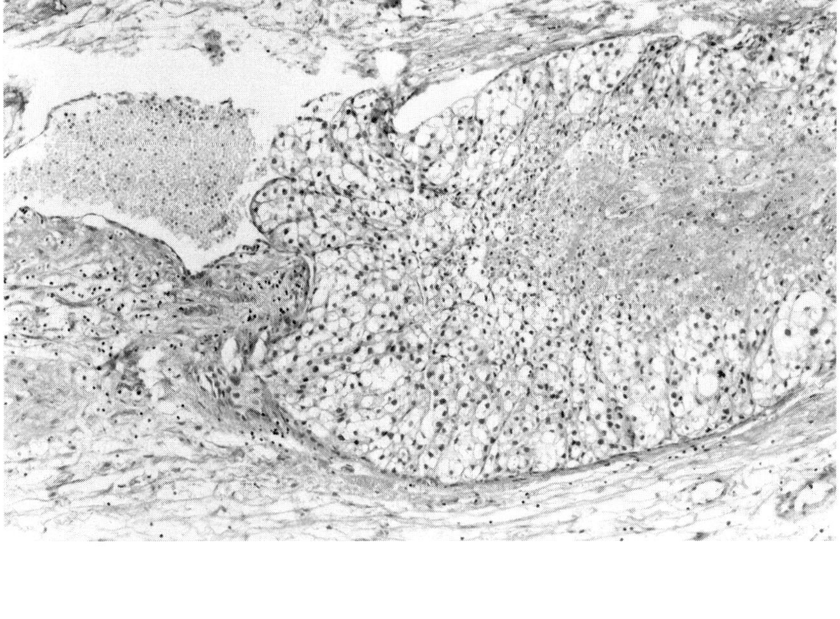

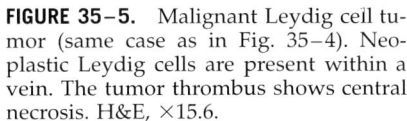

FIGURE 35–5. Malignant Leydig cell tumor (same case as in Fig. 35–4). Neoplastic Leydig cells are present within a vein. The tumor thrombus shows central necrosis. H&E, ×15.6.

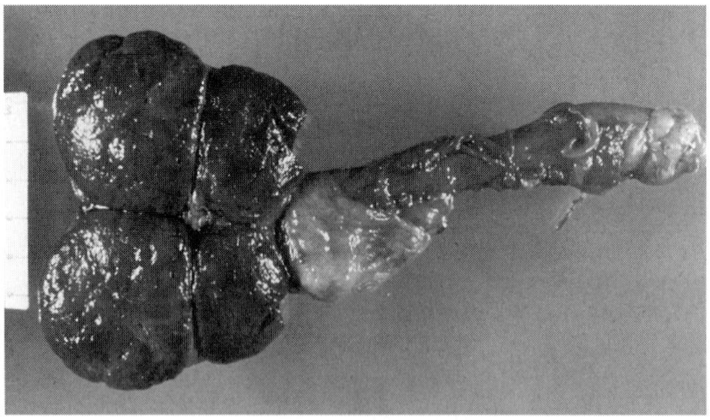

FIGURE 35–6. Probable congenital adrenal hyperplasia in a 29-year-old man who has had right testicular enlargement for 2 years. Left testis was removed 4 years earlier and demonstrated a similar mass. Bivalved testis demonstrates a dark mahogany-colored, bilobed 6.8-cm mass replacing testicular parenchyma.

symptoms of short duration, the signs of masculinization generally abate and puberty will proceed normally. However, in some children with long-standing symptoms, the signs of precocious puberty will persist.

Virtually all LCTs in children and 90% of LCTs in adults are benign, have a good prognosis, and require no therapy other than excision. Patients with malignant tumors have a poor prognosis and usually die within 2 years after the discovery of metastatic disease. Patients in whom a malignant tumor is suspected on histopathology should undergo a metastatic evaluation, including chest x-ray, abdominal and pelvic computed tomography scan, and biochemical evaluation in the hopes of identifying a usable tumor marker. The optimum management of patients with malignant LCT following excision of the primary lesion is unknown. There are no available data to evaluate the benefit of prophylactic retroperitoneal lymphadenectomy versus observation in patients with disease clinically localized to the testis. In a review of the management of 32 patients with established metastatic LCT, Bertram et al. reported no objective responses to radiation therapy, minimal or no benefit from various combinations of chemotherapy (including platinum-based regimens), and only isolated reports of benefit from resection of low-volume or solitary metastatic deposits.[12] Several cases of complete response to mitotane have been reported, but in all instances the patients ultimately relapsed and died of progressive disease.

Sertoli Cell Tumor

Clinical Presentation

A variety of Sertoli cell tumors (SCTs) have been described, which together comprise only 1% of testicular tumors. The principal cell types are classic SCT, sclerosing SCT, large-cell calcifying SCT, and Sertoli cell adenoma (SCA) associated with androgen insensitivity syndrome (AIS). All but the last of these variants typically present with painless testicular enlargement and occur in males of any age. SCA in AIS occurs in phenotypic females. Gynecomastia is present in about 20% of cases of SCT and is a typical feature of malignant SCTs. These tumors must be distinguished from microscopic or barely grossly visible masses of persistent immature tubules that have been termed Pick's adenomas or androblastomas, which are seen in cryptorchid testes and have no malignant potential.

Pathologic Characteristics

Classic SCT. On gross inspection, classic SCTs are generally circumscribed and yellow, tan, or

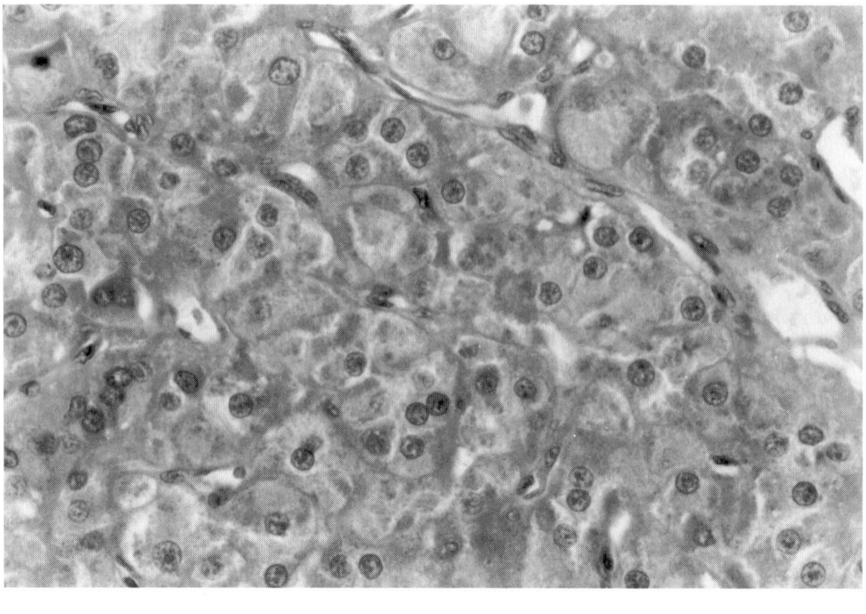

FIGURE 35–7. Probable congenital adrenal hyperplasia mimicking Leydig cell tumor (same case as Fig. 35–6). Uniform cells contain similar-appearing round nuclei and granular cytoplasm containing fine brown pigment. H&E, ×128.

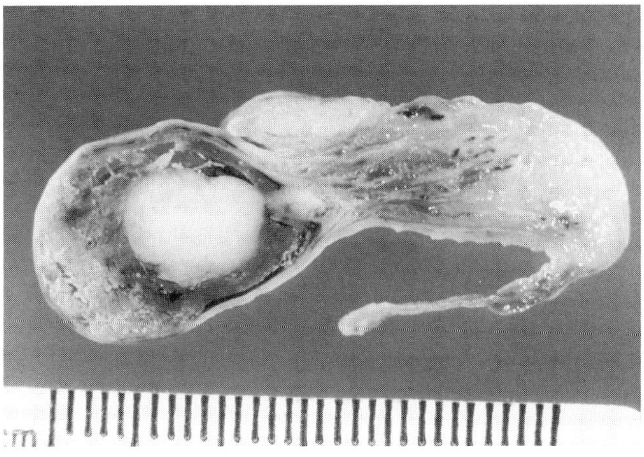

FIGURE 35–8. Sertoli cell tumor. The tumor is a discrete 8-mm nonencapsulated, nonnecrotic, firm mass in a 44-year-man.

white and may be hemorrhagic (Fig. 35–8). Microscopically, they grow in tubules, cords, sheets, aggregates, and occasional retiform configurations separated by fibrovascular septae (Fig. 35–9). Nuclei are round to ovoid and may contain nucleoli. Tumor cell cytoplasm may be pale or eosinophilic and may contain lipid vacuoles. The latter finding in a tumor with a diffuse growth pattern may be confused with the appearance of a LCT. The stroma of a classic SCT may be scant or abundant and hyalinized. Most recognizable classic SCTs behave in a benign fashion, but up to 30% may be malignant, as evidenced by the presence of local invasion and metastases.

SCLEROSING SCT. Sclerosing SCT is a newly described entity. Zukerberg et al. described 10 patients aged 18 to 80 years (median 30) with sclerosing SCT.[13] The tumors generally presented as a painless mass, with one arising in a cryptorchid testis and another in a testis that had undergone orchiopexy. All tumors were unilateral and ranged from 0.4 to 4.0 cm in diameter. Eight of 10 tumors were 1.5 cm or less. The tumors were well demarcated, hard, and yellow-white to tan. Microscopically, 9 of 10 tumors were discrete; the tenth tumor invaded the rete testis, epididymis, and blood vessels. The tumors contained simple and anastomosing tubules, large cellular aggregates, and cords of epithelial cells. The cells were medium sized with rounded vesicular to dark nuclei. The epithelial elements proliferated in a dense hyaline stroma within which were entrapped nonneoplastic seminiferous tubules lined by immature Sertoli cells. No patient showed evidence of malignant behavior, including the 80-year-old man with histologic evidence of invasion.

LARGE-CELL CALCIFYING SCT. Proppe and Scully in 1980 characterized unusual and distinctive tumors of the testis in 10 patients as large-cell calcifying SCTs.[14] Since then, at least 21 additional such SCTs have been reported.[15,16] Age at presentation ranges from 5 to 48 years, with the majority less than age 20. As of 1995, only two reported cases were deemed malignant.[17] The tumor has been associated with a variety of somatic syndromes, including Carney's syndrome, Peutz-Jeghers syndrome, adrenal cortical hyperplasia, and primary pigmented adrenal cortical disease and with LCTs of the testis, cardiac myxomas, mucocutaneous pigmentation, acromegaly, pituitary gigantism, Cushing's syndrome, acidophilic adenoma of the pituitary gland, gynecomastia, isosexual precocity, and AIS.[15,16,18] The neoplasms may involve the entire testis, but in general are 4 cm or less in maximum dimension. They are frequently multifocal, are bilateral in approximately 40%, and are well circumscribed. On cross section the masses are yellow-tan, sometimes with calcific foci. Microscopically, the tumor grows both within

FIGURE 35–9. Sertoli cell tumor. The tumor contains solid and tubular structures with round to oval nuclei and prominent nucleoli. The tubules are surrounded by basement membrane. Elsewhere, similar-appearing cells lack lumens and grow in more solid configurations. H&E, ×62.2.

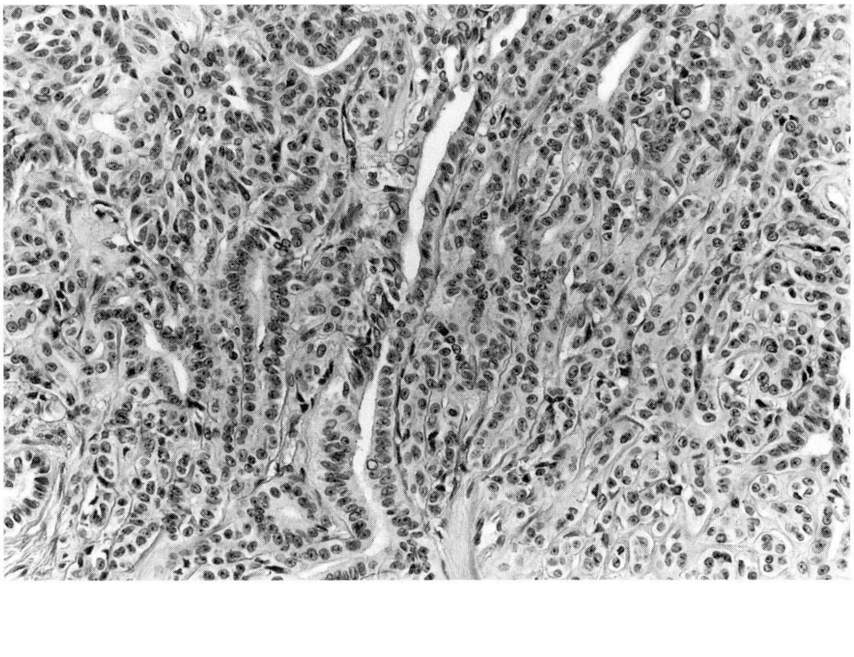

seminiferous tubules and within the interstitium. Within tubules the neoplastic cells are large, with abundant pink cytoplasm, and expand the tubules. Some tubules have a markedly thickened tunica propria that extends into tubular lumens as eosinophilic spherules. The interstitial tumor is composed of cords, nests, and trabeculae. The tumor cells range from 12 to 25 μ in diameter and have ground glass or finely granular cytoplasm. Transitions between intratubular and interstitial growth may be seen. Calcific rounded nodules, plaques, and masses may be present as intratubular and extratubular aggregates.

Sertoli Cell Adenoma Associated with Androgen Insensitivity Syndrome. AIS is caused by defective or absent cellular androgen receptors. As a result, patients with complete AIS are phenotypic females with a shallow vagina and absent wolffian duct derivatives. The patients have 46,XY karyotypes and bilateral intra-abdominal testes that frequently contain nodular masses comprised of multiple tubules lined almost exclusively by Sertoli cells (Fig. 35–10). Hamartomas contain small solid tubules lined by immature Sertoli cells and may have hyperplastic Leydig cells and ovarian-type stroma. Young and Scully[19] and Rutgers and Scully[20] distinguish between hamartomas and pure SCA, which is comprised exclusively of tubules lined by Sertoli cells (Fig. 35–11). Although the SCA may be a monomorphic manifestation of a hamartoma, some SCAs achieve a size up to 25 cm in diameter. SCAs and hamartomas are completely benign. Rarely, other types of sex cord/stromal tumors have been reported in AIS, including a few malignant tumors. Although the SCAs and hamartomas are benign, it is well to remember that these masses are occurring in cryptorchid testes, and malignant germ cell tumors, principally malignant intratubular germ cell neoplasia and seminomas, may develop concomitantly. Approximately 30% of patients with complete AIS will develop malignant germ cell tumors by age 50.[19]

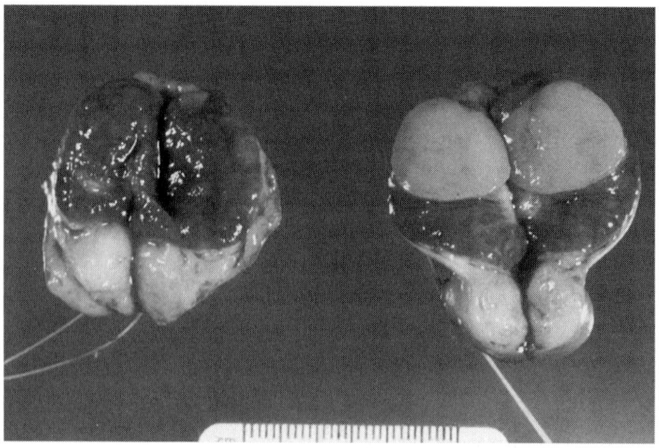

FIGURE 35–10. Sertoli cell adenoma of right testis in patient with androgen insensitivity syndrome. The patient was a 17-year-old virilized phenotypic female. In the right orchiectomy specimen is a firm, 1.6-cm unencapsulated tan nodule. The white firm areas at the bottom of the photographs of the testes are smooth muscle masses at the medial portion of the testes and are of probable müllerian duct origin.

Evaluation and Management

Most SCTs are not suspected preoperatively and are diagnosed only at the time of orchiectomy performed for a testicular mass. In the context of a known associated syndrome, the presence of the large-cell calcifying SCT variant may be suspected preoperatively by the presence of testicular calcifications on scrotal ultrasound, but this finding is not specific to large-cell calcifying SCT. When suspected, a testis-sparing surgical approach as described for LCT may be considered, remembering that rare large-cell calcifying SCTs may be malig-

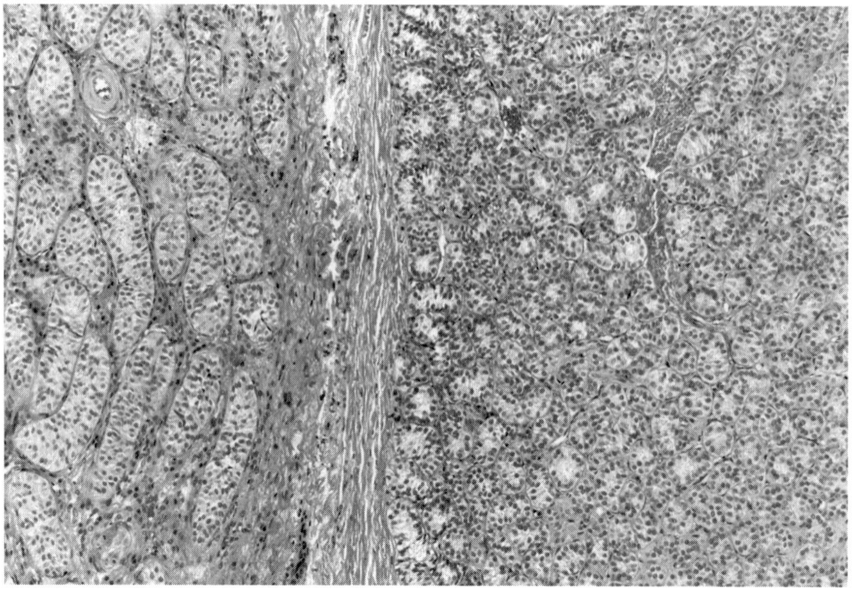

FIGURE 35–11. Sertoli cell adenoma (same patient as in Fig. 35–10). The Sertoli cell adenoma is on the right and is composed of discrete uniform tubules lined by Sertoli cells. The larger tubules on the left are of the nonadenomatous testis and are separated by prominent Leydig cells. H&E ×31.2.

nant and that some may be multifocal. Histologically benign tumors require no further therapy, although long-term follow-up may be indicated because the occurrence of metastatic disease has been reported as long as 15 years after initial diagnosis. For metastatic lesions, involvement of the retroperitoneal nodes is frequent, and there are several case reports of long-term complete remission following retroperitoneal lymphadenectomy. Experience with chemotherapy for malignant SCTs is limited, and the response rate is undefined. Several cases of complete responses to chemotherapy with platinum, etoposide, and ifosfamide have been reported in men with mixed gonadal stromal tumors with prominent Sertoli cell elements.[26,28]

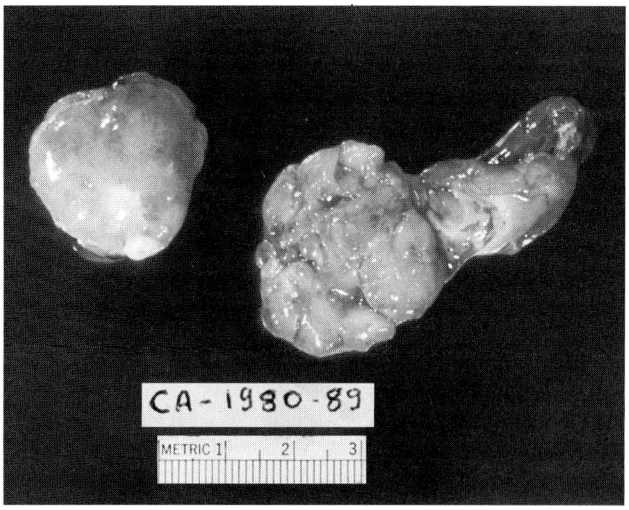
CA-1980-89
METRIC 1
2
3

FIGURE 35–12. Juvenile granulosa cell tumor in a 1-month-old boy with left testicular mass. The testis measured 3 × 2.5 × 1.5 cm. The surface was smooth and red-tan. On cut section, there was a variegated red to yellow lobulated parenchyma with cystic areas up to 5 mm in diameter. (Courtesy of the California Tumor Tissue Registry.)

Granulosa Cell Tumors

Clinical Presentation

Two forms of granulosa cell tumors have been described in males, adult and juvenile. Nineteen cases of adult granulosa cell tumor (GCT) of the testis have been reported in the English literature, although additional sex cord/stromal tumors with granulosa cell differentiation have been reported.[21] The majority have presented as scrotal masses with testicular enlargement ranging from 2 months to 15 years in the described cases. The patient with a mass of 15 years' duration had delayed testicular descent, and two other patients had been cryptorchid. Five tumors have had associated estrogenic clinical manifestations. Four of these patients had lymph node or visceral metastases, and two patients died of their disease. One patient developed metastases 121 months after diagnosis and died of disease 13 months later.

Juvenile GCTs rarely arise in infants over 6 months old and in all probability arise in utero. They have been associated with 45/XO/46,XY and 45,XO/46/XY,iso(Yq) karyotypes and other forms of mosaicism.[22] The tumors are generally found in descended testes, although they have been discovered in undescended and torsed testes. The tumor is not associated with isosexual precocity. The testis harboring this tumor is usually enlarged, solid, and/or cystic (Fig. 35–12).

Pathologic Characteristics

The reported adult GCTs ranged in size from four microscopic lobules to 13 cm and were well circumscribed.[21] They have been described as brownish, white, yellow, and pink and either solid or cystic. Two of Jiminez-Quintero et al.'s patients with me-

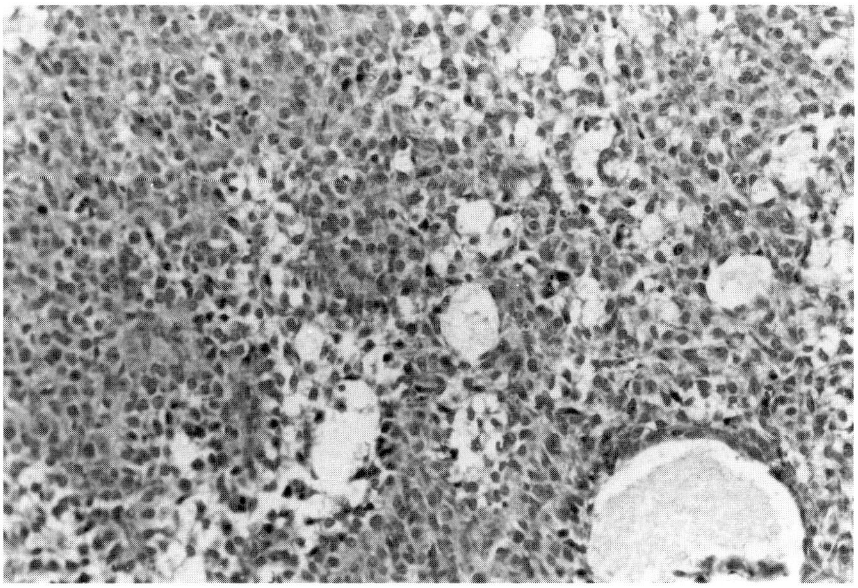

FIGURE 35–13. Juvenile granulosa cell tumor (same patient as in Fig. 35–12). Multiple small cysts and areas of solid polyhedral to rounded cells comprise the tumor. Elsewhere, larger follicles were present. H&E, ×31.2.

tastases had hemorrhagic or friable and necrotic foci in their tumors.[21] Their microscopic appearance has resembled that of ovarian granulosa cell tumor with solid, cystic, insular, gyriform, and trabecular patterns. Individual granulosa cells have been described as fairly uniform with scanty cytoplasm, indistinct cell borders, and longitudinal nuclear grooves in elongate cells. Jiminez-Quintero et al. record up to 26 mitotic figures in 50 high-power microscopic fields. Tumor cells have been described as positive for vimentin and negative for keratin or epithelial membrane antigen (EMA). Juvenile GCTs are grossly multicystic and contain follicular structures of varying size lined by one to multiple layers of cells, and contain pale eosinophilic or basophilic intraluminal material (Figs. 35–12 and 35–13). The stroma is fibrous and may contain groups of cells that resemble theca cells and granulosa cells that do not resemble the cells of adult GCT. Lawrence et al. found only a few grooved cells in a minority of tumors.[22] In the juvenile GCTs, the granulosa cells have round to oval nuclei and pale to eosinophilic cytoplasm. Tumor granulosa cells stain positively for vimentin, and some cells stain positively for keratin and S-100 protein with immunoperoxidase stains.[23] The cells that resemble theca cells have been demonstrated to stain positively for muscle-specific actin, vimentin, and focally for desmin with immunoperoxidase stains. Mitoses may be numerous. Tumor cells may be present in relationship to seminiferous tubules and have even been described within a seminiferous tubule. The differential diagnosis of juvenile GCT of the testis consists of those tumors developing in the neonatal period. Probably most congenital testicular tumors and those discovered in the first 4 months of life are juvenile GCTs rather than yolk sac tumors. Yolk sac tumors may be solid and/or cystic and may have macrocystic or microcystic areas. However, definitive areas diagnostic for yolk sac tumor, including Schiller-Duval bodies and immunoperoxidase staining for AFP, are absent in juvenile GCT. Levels of serum AFP are elevated in the neonate relative to adult values, so serum AFP levels are of no value in the diagnosis of this tumor.

Evaluation and Management

The diagnosis of adult GCT is not usually established until the time of orchiectomy, and surgical excision is usually curative. There is insufficient experience with malignant forms of this tumor to comment on therapy. Juvenile GCT can be suspected on the basis of patient age and karyotype. These tumors are invariably benign and are cured by excision, although follow-up in many cases is still limited.

Mixed Sex Cord/Gonadal Stromal Tumors and Incompletely Differentiated Tumors

Tumors of mixed histology occasionally occur and may consist of some areas with recognizable elements mixed with incompletely differentiated cells resembling ovarian stroma (Fig. 35–14). A recently described transgenic mouse model suggests that at least some of these neoplasms may arise from tumors that begin as Sertoli cell tumors.[24] Like pure forms, tumors of mixed histology and incompletely differentiated tumors present as an isolated testicular mass, usually without endocrinologic signs or symptoms, and are diagnosed at the time of orchiectomy (Fig. 35–15). Most are biologically benign, but some metastatic tumors have been described.[25,26] Treatment is by inguinal orchiectomy. Retroperitoneal lymph node dissection may have value in some cases with metastasis.[27] Good re-

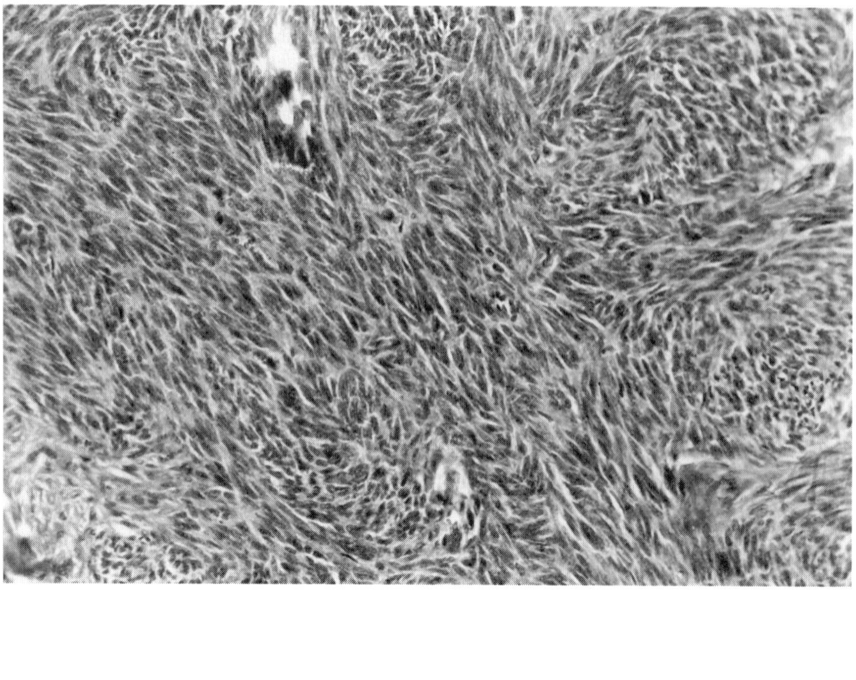

FIGURE 35–14. Incompletely differentiated gonadal stromal tumor presenting as a testicular mass in a 46-year-old. Interlacing fascicles of basophilic spindled cells with large uniform nuclei resemble cells of ovarian stroma. H&E, ×62.2.

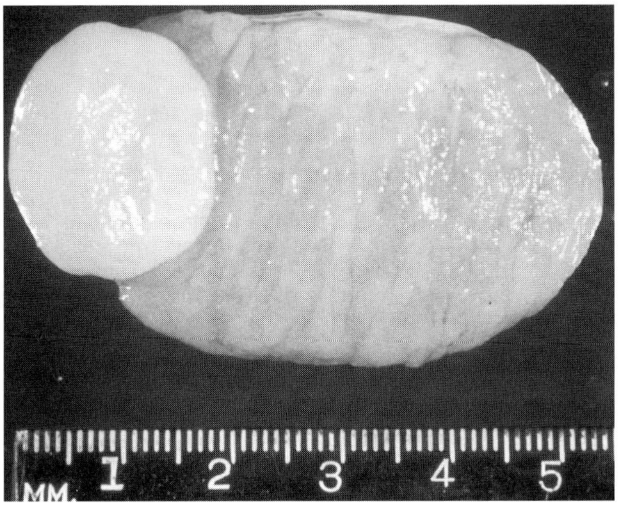
MM 1 2 3 4 5

FIGURE 35–15. Incompletely differentiated gonadal stromal tumor (same patient as in Fig. 35–14). The tumor is a firm, 2.2-cm nonencapsulated subcapsular mass.

sponses to platinum-based chemotherapy have been described for metastatic disease.[28]

MISCELLANEOUS TUMORS

Epidermoid Cysts

Epidermoid cysts are benign lesions that typically present as a painless testicular mass and are frequently noted incidentally on physical examination. They occur slightly more commonly on the right side and rarely are much larger than 2 to 3 cm. Grossly they appear as a usually solitary cyst containing laminated keratinaceous material (Fig. 35–16). Histologically, they are composed of a squamous lining and filled with keratin.[29] Treatment has historically been by orchiectomy, but there are several reports in the literature describing a characteristic appearance of this lesion on ultrasound that may allow diagnosis preoperatively. In such cases, inguinal exploration and excisional biopsy seem reasonable, especially in children or patients with a solitary testicle.[30] Epidermoid cysts have rarely been reported in a patient with Klinefelter's syndrome[31]; we have seen another such patient (Fig. 35–17).

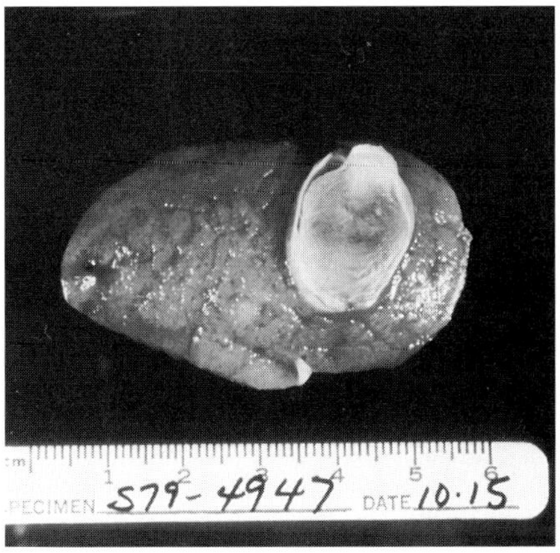
S79-4947
DATE 10·15

FIGURE 35–16. Epidermoid cyst in an 18-year-old with a 3-month history of a nontender mass of the left testis. The testis contains a well-circumscribed 2-cm cyst with a 1-mm-thick gray wall filled with yellow-white, friable, cheesy material.

RETE TESTIS CARCINOMA

Clinical Presentation

Orozco and Murphy reported one case and reviewed 43 cases of rete testis carcinoma (RTC) that have been recorded in the English literature through 1992.[32] The patients have ranged in age from 17 to 91 years, with a mean age of 50. The clinical onset may or may not be associated with pain. Testicular enlargement averaged about 2 years in duration but had been present for 5 years in four instances. Serum tumor marker levels were not elevated. All patients were treated by orchiectomy and some were also treated with radiotherapy, chemotherapy, and retroperitoneal lymphadenectomy. Of the reviewed patients, 33% died of RTC, 75% within a year of diagnosis. Twenty patients were alive at the time of the report, with 80% free of disease at a maximum 2-year follow-up.

Pathologic Characteristics

RTCs are poorly circumscribed gray nodules at the hilus of the testis. Most tumors are single, but multiple masses have been reported. The tumors range in size from 1 to 15 cm. Histologically, RTCs are adenocarcinomas. The predominant growth pattern is papillary, with solid, spindled, and cystic areas less common (Figs. 35–18 and 35–19). Tumor cells are columnar to cuboidal with acidophilic to amphophilic cytoplasm. Nuclei are enlarged, pleomorphic, and round to oval, with coarsely granular chromatin and sometimes prominent nucleoli. Mitoses may be frequent. The tumors stain negative for mucin, occasionally positive for carcinoembryonic antigen (CEA), and positive for vimentin, EMA, and keratin with immunoperoxidase stains. Immunoperoxidase stains are negative for AFP, hCG, and prostate-specific antigen. The diagnosis of RTC should be made in cases where the tumor is present in the hilus of the testis, where there is a transition from histologically normal rete testis to RTC, where primary testicular tumors of germ cell and non–germ cell origin and mesothelioma can be excluded, and where extratesticular origin can be reasonably excluded on a histologic and clinical basis. The distinction between a RTC and adenoma or hyperplasia of the rete testis should not be difficult.

Evaluation and Management

RTCs are usually found incidentally by palpation or at the time of orchiectomy for a testicular mass.

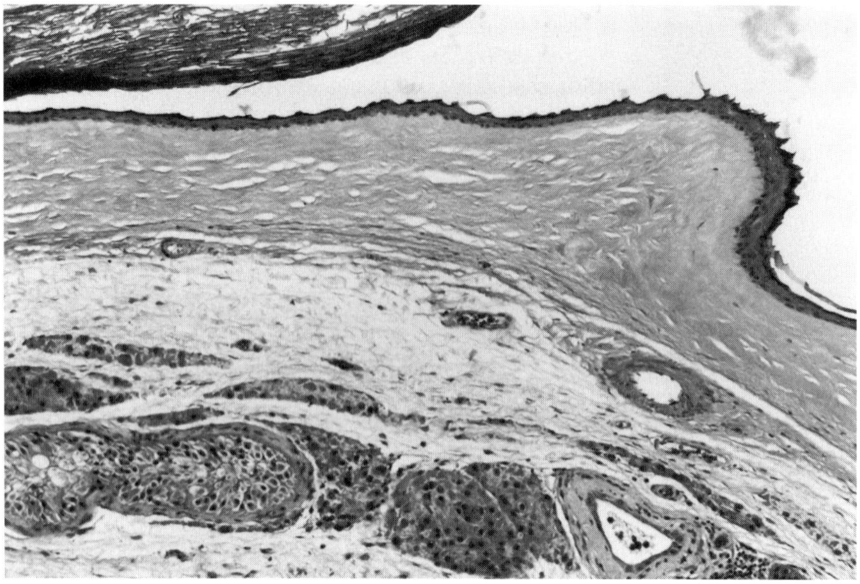

FIGURE 35–17. Epidermoid cyst in a 16-year-old with a cystic testicular mass. The cyst is lined by flattened squamous epithelium. Laminated keratin is present in the left upper corner. Mostly flattened seminiferous tubules lined by Sertoli cells are present beneath the cyst. Leydig cells are prominent. The patient was subsequently found to have Kleinfelter's syndrome. H&E, ×31.2.

They may be suspected on preoperative exam or ultrasound by a hilar location or involvement of the epididymis. Initial therapy is by orchiectomy, followed by a staging evaluation for distant disease.[33] One long-term complete remission has been reported following retroperitoneal lymphadenectomy for micrometastatic disease. Chemotherapy for disseminated disease has generally been unsuccessful.[33]

Malignant Mesothelioma of the Tunica Vaginalis

Clinical Presentation

Malignant mesothelioma (MM) is a rare lesion. The literature consists of 64 cases, with the largest series reported by Jones et al. in 1995.[34] The age range is 7 to 80 years, with a mean of 53.5. Two thirds of patients were over 50 years at the time of diagnosis. Most patients presented with a benign-appearing hydrocele with or without an inguinal or scrotal mass. Of those patients who were asked about asbestos exposure, 41% had some degree of occupational exposure. The large majority of patients had a hydrocele sac studded with papillary excrescences ranging in size from several millimeters to several centimeters (Fig. 35–20). In some cases a mass involved the spermatic cord, other paratesticular structures, or, rarely, the testis proper. MM that extended beyond the confines of the hydrocele invaded local structures, including spermatic cord, epididymis, testis, and penile, scrotal, and lower abdominal wall skin. Twenty-five

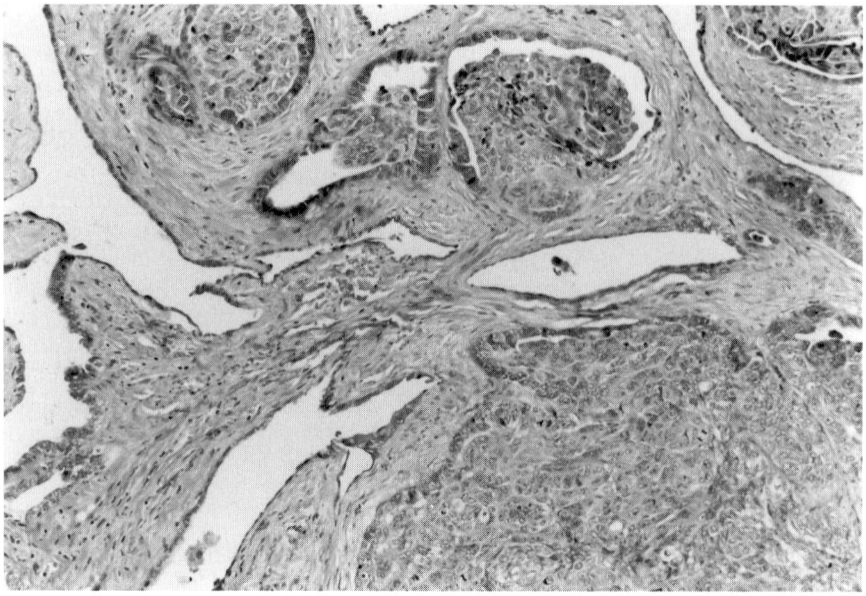

FIGURE 35–18. Rete testis carcinoma in a 47-year-old with recurrent hydrocele and a firm, nontender mass at the superior pole of the right testis. Orchiectomy specimen contained numerous irregular, firm, 1- to 4-cm nodules with involvement of the epididymis. Papillary and solid neoplasm involves the rete testis, surrounding and projecting into rete testis lumens. H&E, ×31.2.

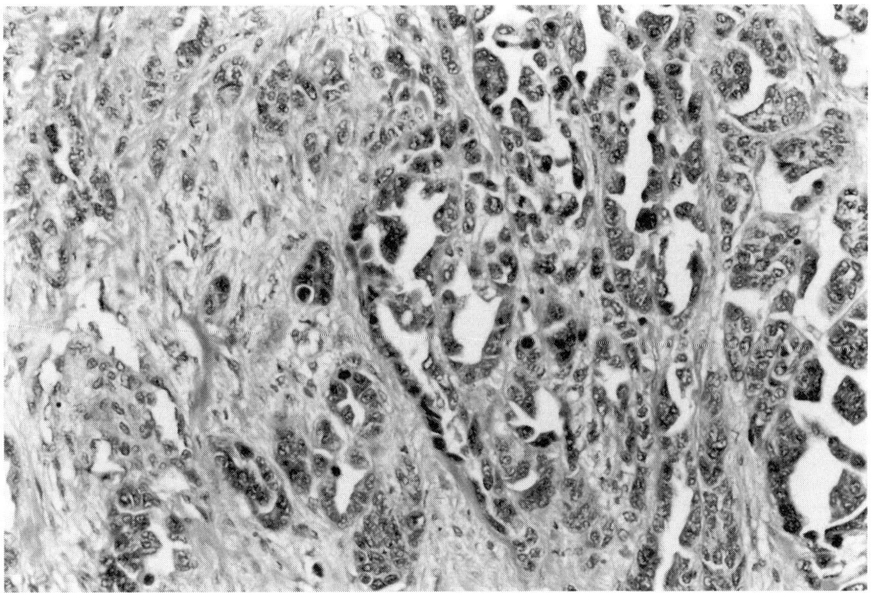

FIGURE 35–19. Rete testis carcinoma (same case as in Fig. 35–18). Glandular spaces are lined by epithelial cells with round to oval, pleomorphic, enlarged nuclei with prominent nucleoli. Glands are infiltrating connective tissue. H&E, ×62.2.

of 62 patients had distant metastases. The principal sites of metastases were retroperitoneal and inguinal lymph nodes, other lymph nodes, and lung. Retroperitoneal and inguinal lymph node involvement was sometimes present at the time of diagnosis. Of 52 patients with follow-up data, 44% died of disease, 17% were alive with disease, and 38% had no evidence of disease. The latter figure should be considered with caution because late recurrence of well-differentiated epithelial MM has been observed.

Pathologic Characteristics

Seventy-five per cent of the tumors described by Jones et al. were epithelial and 25% were biphasic.[34] Epithelial tumors grew in a tubular and/or papillary growth pattern (Fig. 35–21). Cellular anaplasia was variable, with some tumors composed of bland cells without mitotic activity growing in a papillary pattern on fibrous stalks and others containing large eosinophilic cells with hyperchromatic irregular nuclei, prominent nucleoli, and frequent mitoses growing in an infiltrating tubular pattern. Tumor stroma was usually dense. Psammoma bodies were occasionally present. The majority of tumors, even the best differentiated, showed some degree of stromal invasion. MMs with a biphasic pattern had a sarcomatous component with spindled cells of variable differentiation, sometimes containing numerous mitotic figures.

MM must be distinguished from a number of benign and malignant lesions. Mesothelial cell hyperplasia, although prominent in a hernia sac, is rarely present in a hydrocele and does not contain the fibrous stalks characteristic of the papillary MM. Adenomatoid tumor is a benign tumor derived from mesothelial cells, but has a characteristic gland-like architecture and cytology that distinguishes it from MM. It is far more difficult to distinguish MM from serous borderline tumors of müllerian origin (ovarian surface epithelial type) that resemble ovarian tumors of borderline malignancy that may involve the testis or paratesticular tissue, metastatic adenocarcinoma, and RTC.[35] Borderline serous tumors generally have broad papillae with stratified epithelial cells, some of which are ciliated, having a more columnar appearance. Immunohistochemical stains may be useful in distinguishing between these two tumors because serous tumors are frequently positive for Leu-M1, B72.3, CEA, and CA125, whereas MMs are negative for these antigens.[35] RTC may be associated with a hydrocele and focally may have a histologic resemblance to MM, but if the criteria of diagnosis enumerated earlier are adhered to, there should be no problem distinguishing the two entities. Electron microscopy may also help distinguish the entities because me-

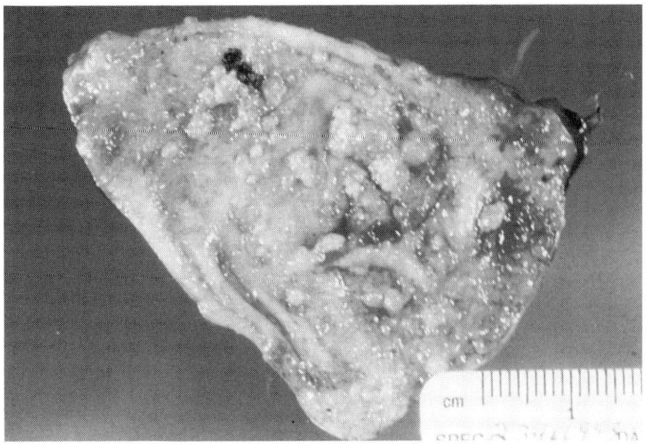

FIGURE 35–20. Papillary mesothelioma in a 53-year-old man with recurrent left hydrocele. The tunica vaginalis is studded with yellow-tan excrescences from 0.2 to 1.0 cm in maximum dimension.

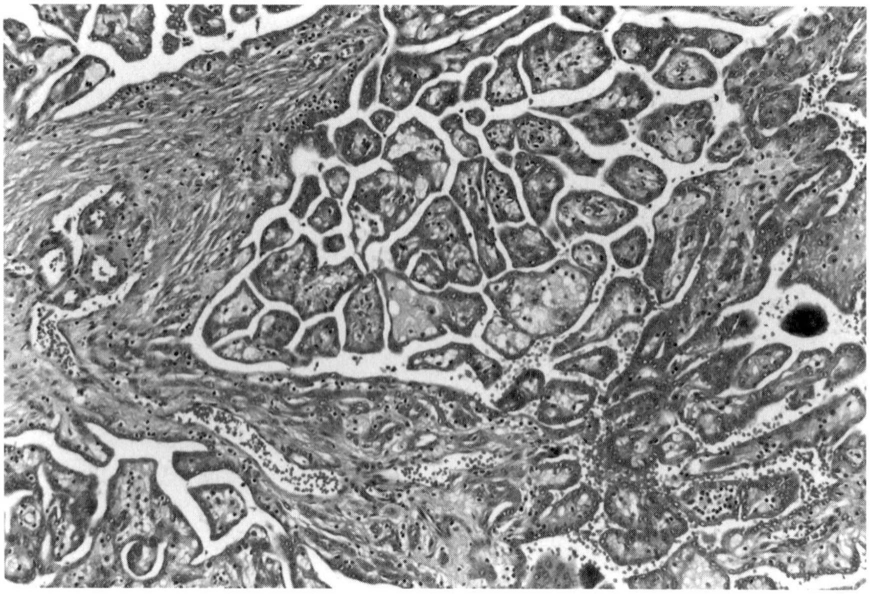

FIGURE 35–21. Papillary mesothelioma (same case as in Fig. 35–20). The tumor is multifocal and comprised of a complex papillary growth lined by a single layer of mesothelial cells with oval, prominently nucleolated nuclei growing on fibrous stalks. H&E, ×31.2.

sothelial cells have long, thin, bushy microvilli, and epithelial cells of rete testis origin do not. As in the pleura and peritoneum, there may rarely be a problem distinguishing MM from metastatic adenocarcinoma. The same immunohistochemical stains used to distinguish müllerian papillary serous tumors are useful in distinguishing metastatic adenocarcinomas from MM. Adenocarcinomas, which may be of gastrointestinal origin, should stain positively for Leu-Ml, B72.3, and CEA and may contain intracytoplasmic mucin.

Evaluation and Management

MM is usually not suspected preoperatively and may occasionally be encountered incidentally during hydrocelectomy. When the initial presentation is a scrotal mass, inguinal orchiectomy should be performed with en bloc excision of involved adjacent structures. If the tumor is incidentally discovered during a transscrotal procedure, frozen section should be performed and inguinal orchiectomy completed at the same sitting or soon thereafter after consultation with the patient. A metastatic evaluation is appropriate, but there is little experience in the literature to address the issues of surveillance, adjuvant chemotherapy, or prophylactic retroperitoneal or inguinal lymphadenectomy.

Metastatic Tumors

Symptomatic metastatic nonhematologic tumors of the testis occur only rarely. Price and Mostofi identified only 38 metastatic carcinomas involving the testis suitable for study at a time when the Armed Forces Institute of Pathology had 1600 primary testicular tumors.[36] Four of the patients had bilateral tumors. Only six tumors were clinically symptomatic, generally as a result of testicular enlargement. The majority of tumors in their report were discovered at autopsy. Of the 38 tumors, 14 were from the lung and 12 were from the prostate gland. Tiltman found metastases in six of 248 autopsies in males with metastatic carcinoma.[37] Testicular metastases occurred in 2 of 12 cases of prostate carcinoma, two of nine cases of malignant melanoma, one of four cases of malignant pleural mesothelioma, and 1 of 89 cases of carcinoma of the lung. Haupt et al. reviewed the literature through 1982 and found that the most common tumors metastasizing to the testes were (in descending order) carcinomas of the prostate and lung, malignant melanoma, and carcinomas of the kidney, stomach, and pancreas.[38] These findings emphasize the relative rarity of metastases to the testis and the fact that in most patients testicular involvement will be discovered incidentally despite a known history of cancer. Only 24 cases of testicular enlargement as the primary manifestation of a tumor metastasis have been reported. These included primary tumors of the prostate, kidney, and gastrointestinal tract, some of which were initially thought to represent primary testicular tumors even after histologic examination. Grossly metastatic tumors are generally multinodular (Fig. 35–22). Microscopically, the tumor grows in the interstitium and may be within endothelial-lined spaces. The morphology of the tumor may be characteristic of the primary tumor (Fig. 35–23). Treatment for tumors metastatic to the testis is directed at the underlying malignancy.

Carcinoid Tumors

Carcinoid tumor involving the testis and testicular adnexa represents a special problem inasmuch as both primary and metastatic tumors may have

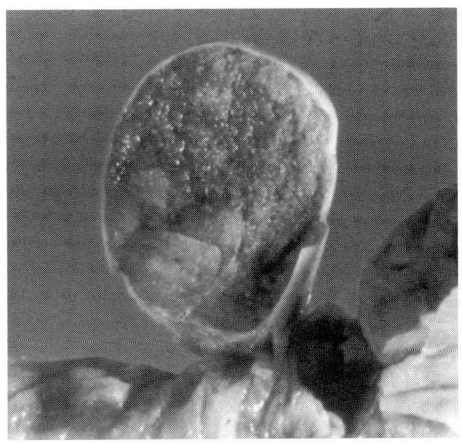

FIGURE 35–22. Metastatic undifferentiated carcinoma, small-cell type, of the lung in a 76-year-old man with a left testicular mass and previous history of undifferentiated small-cell carcinoma of lung. Metastatic confluent nodules of neoplasm are present in the lower left portion of the testis.

similar morphology. The nests of tumor grow in an insular pattern with groups of uniform, centrally nucleated cells having fine nuclear chromatin and granular eosinophilic cytoplasm (Fig. 35–24). The majority of carcinoid tumors stain positively with argentaffin and argyrophil stains and for chromogranin, neuron-specific enolase, and other polypeptides with immunoperoxidase stains. Zavala-Pompa et al. indicated that 9 of 62 testicular carcinoid tumors reported through 1992 were metastatic.[39] The largest of the metastatic carcinoid tumors on which data were recorded was 2.5 cm, and three patients had symptoms of the carcinoid syndrome. Most patients with metastatic carcinoid tumors died within a year, although one patient survived for 12 years. Factors that favor a metastatic origin for a carcinoid tumor are bilaterality, involvement of peritesticular structures, absence of a teratomatous component, and the presence of carcinoid syndrome symptomatology. Most primary testicular carcinoids are cured with inguinal orchiectomy. However, all patients should have a metastatic evaluation and retroperitoneal lymphadenectomy should be considered in those tumors associated with teratoma. Carcinoid tumors are generally considered to be of germ cell origin.

Other Miscellaneous Tumors

A variety of other uncommon and usually benign lesions may mimic more aggressive testicular tumors. *Simple cysts* have been described in 17 patients of all ages, ranging in size from 1 to several centimeters in diameter, and are probably more common than noted.[40] Histologically they are lined by flat or cuboidal epithelium and have a benign appearance. Cysts may be suspected preoperatively by a smooth-walled, anechoic appearance on ultrasound. *Adenomatoid tumors* are benign mesenchymal proliferations that usually arise from the epididymis but may also arise from the tunica albuginea and may infiltrate testicular parenchyma. Only a single report of a true intratesticular adenomatoid tumor has been published. These tumors present as painless enlargement and are firm or hard to palpation (Figs. 35–25 and 35–26). *Fibromas* and *fibrous pseudotumors* of the testicular tunics presenting as hard, painful or incidentally discovered masses have also been reported. *Granulomatous orchitis* and *malakoplakia* are benign inflammatory conditions usually diagnosed following orchiectomy. They have characteristic histologic appearances that are pathognomonic. All of these lesions are cured by orchiectomy or simple excision and are important mostly to be differentiated from malignant testicular tumors and, in the case of mal-

FIGURE 35–23. Metastatic prostatic adenocarcinoma in a 58-year-old man with bilateral orchiectomy for prostate cancer. One testis contained a firm, tan, irregular mass. Solid aggregates of tumor and neoplastic glands expand the interstitium adjacent to a seminiferous tubule. H&E, ×31.2.

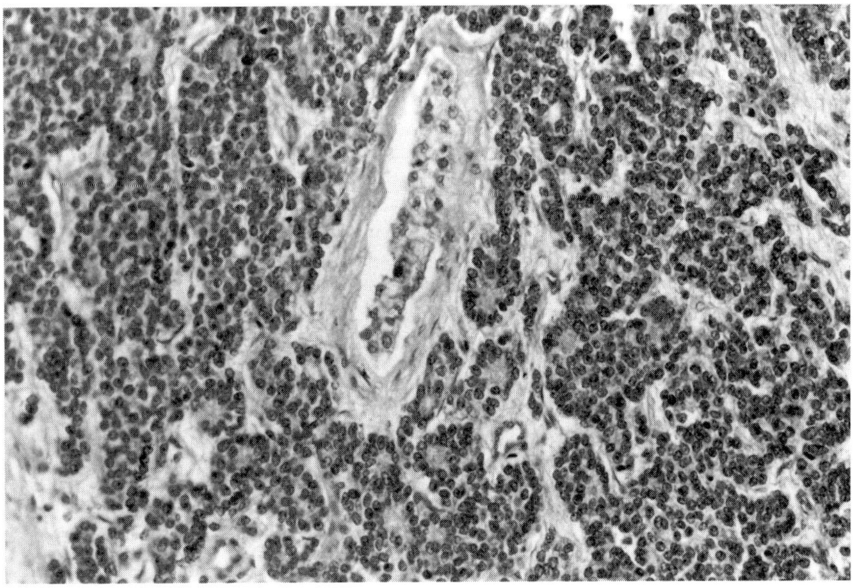

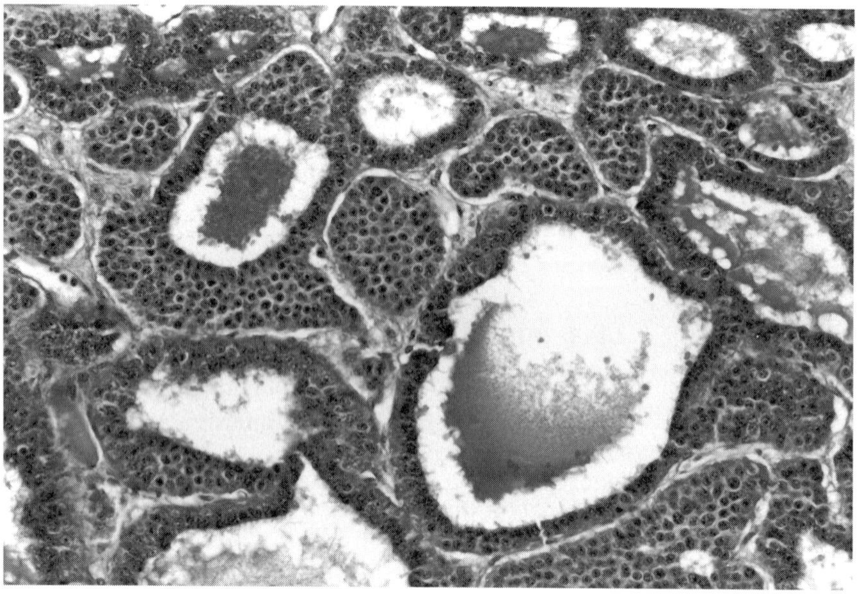

FIGURE 35–24. Carcinoid tumor in a 42-year-old male with enlarged right testis and epididymis containing a 3.5-cm yellow to red, firm to fibrous mass. The tumor is comprised of solid nests and cysts growing in an insular pattern. Tumor cells contain uniform, centrally nucleated cells with fine nuclear chromatin and granular eosinophilic cytoplasm. H&E, ×31.2. (Courtesy of the California Tumor Tissue Registry.)

acoplakia and granulomatous orchitis, from malignant lymphoma.

HEMATOLOGIC TUMORS

Malignant Lymphoma

Clinical Presentation

Although malignant lymphomas (MLs) comprise only a small percentage of testicular tumors, they account for more than 50% of testicular tumors in men over age 65. About 80% of testicular MLs occur in men over age 50. The neoplasm generally presents as a unilateral, painless, intrascrotal mass. About 5% of men present with bilateral synchronous involvement, and approximately 20% with a unilateral presentation will develop lymphomatous involvement of the opposite testis. Generally, the diagnosis of ML is first made at the time of orchiectomy. Only a small percentage of patients have a history of antecedent lymphoma. Of 127 men with ML of the testis, Gowing reported only 8 with antecedent ML and 13 with active lymphoma at the time of orchiectomy.[41]

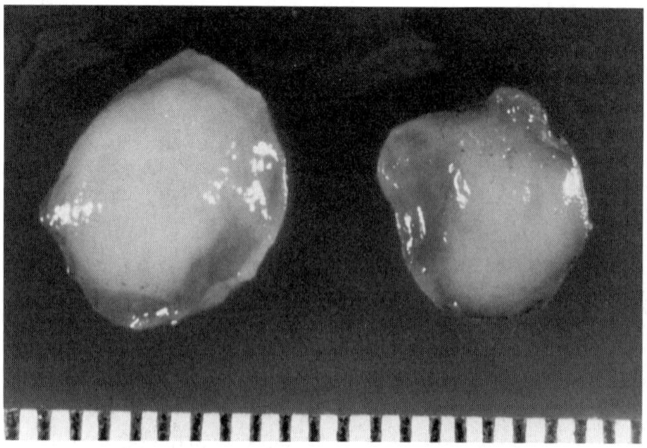

FIGURE 35–25. Adenomatoid tumor of epididymis. The epididymal specimen consists of a discrete white, uniform, rubbery, 0.9-cm nodule in a 44-year-old man.

Pathologic Characteristics

The neoplasm mainly involves the testis but often extends into the epididymis or spermatic cord. The testis is enlarged, sometimes massively, and on cut section is partially or extensively replaced by an ill-defined tan-grey mass. The tumor merges imperceptibly with testicular parenchyma. Tumor consistency is more rubbery than hard, and necrosis may be present. The large majority of testicular lymphomas are of the diffuse non-Hodgkin's type. Gowing indicated that 41% of the British Testicular Tumor Panel cases were poorly differentiated lymphocytic lymphomas and 59% were large-cell lymphomas (undifferentiated "stem cell reticulum cell type").[41] They had no cases of Hodgkin's disease among their 127 cases. Virtually all types of ML other than Hodgkin's disease occur in the testis. Ferry et al. in 1994 reported 64 MLs that presented primarily in the testis.[42] Of these, 53 had diffuse large-cell lymphoma of which 27 were of the noncleaved type in the Working Formulation, 10 were immunoblastic, 6 were small noncleaved, and 6 were not otherwise specified. Of those tumors that were immunophenotyped, 33 were of B-cell lineage, 1 was of T-cell lineage, and 5 were of indeterminate lineage. Irrespective of cell type, the pattern of infiltration is similar. Tumor cells proliferate in the interstitium, separating seminiferous tubules, infiltrating their tunica propria and blood vessel walls, and eventually obliterating many tubules and vessels (Fig. 35–27). Sections may contain no

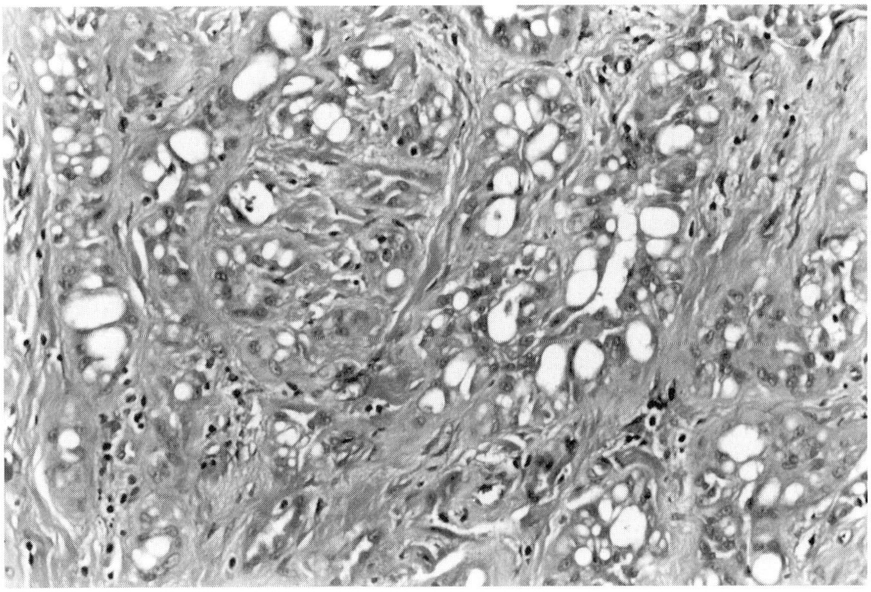

FIGURE 35–26. Adenomatoid tumor of the epididymis (same patient as in Fig. 35–25). Gland-like structures lined by flattened cells infiltrate collagenous tissue. Numerous intraluminal and intracytoplasmic vacuoles of varying size are present, creating a spiderweb appearance in some areas. H&E, ×31.2.

recognizable testicular parenchyma. Tumor cells may extend into the rete testis, epididymis, tunica albuginea, or peritesticular soft tissue.

Evaluation and Management

The prognosis of men with ML of the testis has been poor. Gowing et al. indicated 62% of their patients died of disseminated ML.[41] Only 12 of 124 patients (10%) survived 5 years after orchiectomy. In a more recent study, Ferry et al. found 20 of 55 patients (36%) to be free of disease a median of 49 months after orchiectomy, 6 (11%) were alive with disease, and 29 (53%) died of ML.[42] With careful staging of ML, it is apparent that prognosis is related to the stage of the disease at the time of orchiectomy. Turner et al. reported 60% disease-free survival in stage I ML, contrasted with a 17% disease-free survival for stages II, III, and IV.[43] Turner et al.'s cases were classified according to the Rapaport system and the Working Classification of Non-Hodgkin's Lymphomas. In the latter classification, the large-cell noncleaved, large-cell cleaved, and diffuse mixed lymphomas were designated intermediate-grade lymphomas, and immunoblastic lymphoma, Burkitt's lymphoma, and diffuse undifferentiated lymphomas were designated as high-grade lymphomas. Eight of 17 men with intermediate-grade ML were alive and well with an average follow-up of 24 months. There were no survivors among six men in the high-grade group, whose average survival was 13 months. Thus grade appears to be another prognostic variable. Stage I

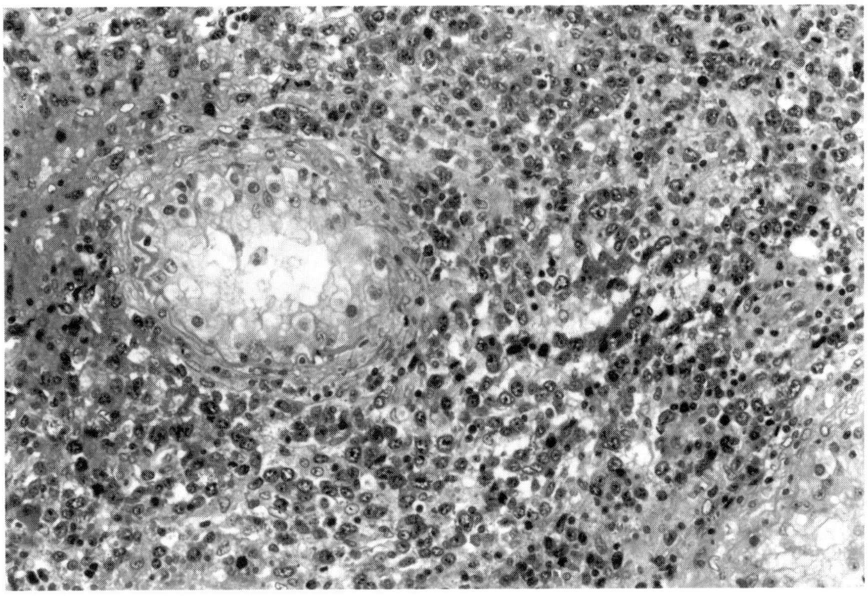

FIGURE 35–27. Malignant lymphoma, diffuse large-cell type. A 225-g, 9.5-cm in maximum dimension testis was subtotally replaced by a dark tan, focally hemorrhagic, focally necrotic, ill-defined mass. An extensive cellular infiltrate greatly expands the interstitium and compresses seminiferous tubules. The individual cells contain large, variably shaped, prominently nucleolated nuclei with sparse cytoplasm. H&E, ×62.2.

disease, unilateral right-sided ML, and microscopic sclerosis were associated with an improved prognosis in Ferry et al.'s study.[42]

It is clear that some cases of ML originate in the testis. Although rare survivals have been reported following orchiectomy alone, this is certainly insufficient therapy because the large majority of men ultimately develop extratesticular ML. Extratesticular involvement tends to occur in several areas, including Waldeyer's ring and the central nervous system. Turner et al.'s series also suggests that MLs at these sites may have been present at the time of orchiectomy.[43] Ferry et al.'s data indicate that MLs that relapsed in the testis tended to be extranodal, and that ML presenting in the testis tended to have lymphoma in extranodal sites, notably bone, central nervous system, skin, orbit, paranasal sinuses, stomach, nose, thyroid, and larynx.[42] Treatment should be based on stage and histologic type of lymphoma.

Plasmacytoma

Plasma cell neoplasms involving the testis are rare and have the same implications as ML. The tumors are bilateral and sequential in about 20% of men. Tumors are generally manifest as painless enlargement and are part of a systemic process sometimes identified prior to orchiectomy. All patients with sufficient follow-up reviewed by Levin and Mostofi, and all seven in the literature until that time, succumbed to systemic disease.[44] In 1991 there had been 38 reported cases, only 6 of which had no documented systemic myeloma. The mean age at the time of diagnosis was 55 years, with only eight patients under 50 and the youngest age 26. The gross and microscopic appearances of plasmacytoma are similar to those of ML, the only difference being the cell type, which is a neoplastic plasma cell of variable morphology (Fig. 35–28).

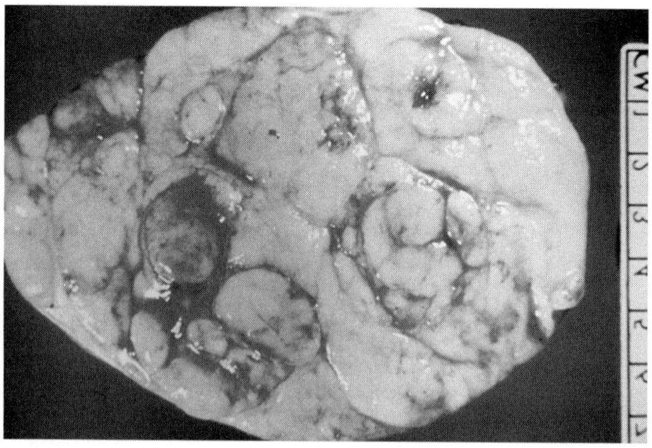

FIGURE 35–28. Plasmacytoma. Massive enlargement and complete replacement of testicular parenchyma by a lobulated, gray-yellow, 11-cm mass in a 42-year-old man.

Leukemia

Leukemic involvement of the testis is common. In an autopsy study, Givler found that 63% of 140 males with acute leukemia and 22% of 76 males with chronic leukemia had testicular involvement.[45] All varieties of acute leukemia were represented. It is recognized that children with acute lymphoblastic leukemia (ALL) in bone marrow remission may have recurrence first demonstrated in the testis. In Givler's study, eight children with ALL developed testicular masses while receiving chemotherapy. Five of the children were in hematologic remission, and the testicular masses were either the sole evidence of leukemia or associated with other extramedullary leukemic masses. Hematologic relapse followed in all cases. In five of eight cases testicular involvement was bilateral. Following completion of chemotherapy in cases of ALL, biopsy of the testes to rule out occult leukemic involvement is part of some current protocols. Neither palpation nor studies such as ultrasound or magnetic resonance imaging are sufficiently sensitive to the presence of leukemic infiltrates to obviate the need for biopsy. Buchanan et al. reported that one third of patients with overt testicular recurrence of ALL treated with an intense treatment protocol exhibited prolonged second remissions with the potential for cure.[46] Only a small percentage of patients will develop testicular recurrence following a negative biopsy. The interstitial pattern of testicular involvement in ALL is similar to that of ML. Occasionally ALL involvement of the testis produces a massive enlargement (Fig. 35–29).

TUMORS OF GENERALIZED STROMA

Tumors of generalized stroma (blood vessels, smooth muscle, and other supporting stroma), also known as mesenchymal tumors, rarely occur in the testis. Petersen reported a total of 26 such tumors described in the literature, most of which (62%) were malignant.[47] The histologies of the benign tumors included five hemangiomas, three hemangioendotheliomas, one leiomyoma, and one myxoid neurofibroma.[47] The malignancies included 14 rhabdomyosarcomas, 1 osteosarcoma, and 1 leiomyosarcoma. The microscopic appearance of these tumors is similar to that of those occurring at more typical sites. Most of these patients presented with testicular enlargement and underwent inguinal orchiectomy, with the diagnosis of a mesenchymal tumor made only after surgical excision of the testis. Benign tumors found in this manner do not require further evaluation or treatment. Rhabdomyosarcomas of the testis proper occur less frequently than in paratesticular locations but should be similarly treated with retroperitoneal lymphadenectomy, chemotherapy, and radiation, depending on stage.

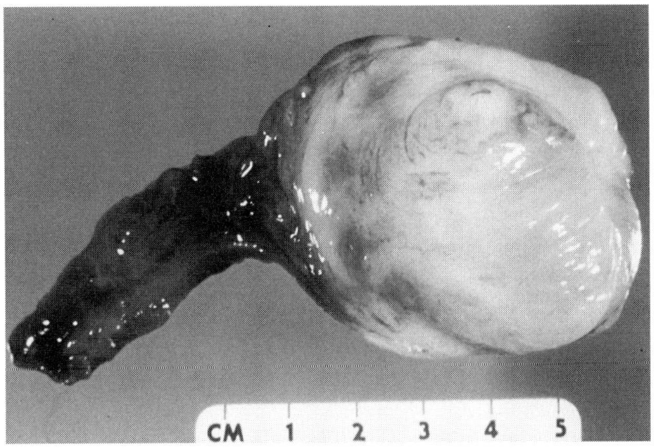
CM 1 2 3 4 5

FIGURE 35–29. Acute lymphocytic leukemia. Massive replacement of right testis by a cream-colored, focally hemorrhagic, ill-defined mass in a 10-year-old with an 8-year history of treated ALL.

TESTIS TUMORS IN AIDS

Patients infected with human immunodeficiency virus (HIV) or with full-blown AIDS appear to be at a higher risk of developing primary or secondary testis tumors. The first two cases of germ cell tumors of the testis in AIDS patients were reported in 1985.[48] Wilson et al. reported 5 of 3015 HIV-positive men presenting with testicular tumors over a 5-year period, an incidence of 0.2%, more than 50 times the incidence of testis tumors in the general population.[48] There have been additional cases in the urologic literature of testis tumors described in the AIDS population, including seminoma and mixed nonseminomatous germ cell tumors, Kaposi's sarcoma, and ML. Some of the cases of non–germ cell tumors presented with testicular swelling as the initial and primary manifestation of HIV infection, and some of these patients presented with symptoms of acute prostatitis or epididymo-orchitis and were initially treated with antibiotics before returning with complaints of progressive testicular enlargement. Reported cases were ultimately managed by inguinal orchiectomy and additional therapy based on tumor histology and status of the patient's immune system. These reports highlight the need for a high index of suspicion for testicular tumors in men at risk for HIV who present with testicular enlargement.

TESTICULAR AND PARATESTICULAR TUMORS OF OVARIAN SURFACE EPITHELIAL TYPE

Prior to 1995, 17 cases had been reported of testicular and paratesticular tumors of ovarian surface epithelial type, when Jones et al. reported an additional 5 cases of paratesticular serous carcinoma.[49,50] These occurred in an age range of 11 to 68 years, with a median of 47 years, in Young and Scully's series of testicular and paratesticular tumors[49] and in a range of 16 to 42 years, with a mean of 31 years, in Jones et al.'s series of paratesticular serous carcinoma.[50] The majority of tumors of ovarian surface epithelial origin are paratesticular, but at least seven principally involved testicular parenchyma. Other areas of involvement included the tunica vaginalis and the testiculoepididymal groove at the upper pole of the testis. The majority of cases have been of serous borderline type, but serous papillary carcinoma, mucinous cystadenoma and cystadenocarcinoma, endometroid adenoacanthoma, clear cell carcinoma, and Brenner tumors have been reported.[49,50] These tumors may be derived from müllerian duct remnants, the tunica vaginalis, or both. Most borderline serous tumors behave in a benign fashion if completely excised, but the clear cell adenocarcinoma and two cases of papillary serous carcinoma behaved in a malignant fashion, one causing metastasis and death and another having extensive abdominal recurrence.[50] A third patient without demonstrable recurrence had persistent elevation of serum CA125.[50] It is important to recognize the müllerian nature of these neoplasms and to accurately distinguish between borderline and frankly malignant variants.

The differential diagnosis of müllerian surface epithelial tumors includes germ cell tumors, rete testis adenocarcinoma, mesothelioma of the tunica vaginalis, and metastatic adenocarcinoma. Germ cell tumors, because they are the most frequent tumor in this region, must be considered in the differential diagnosis, but only teratomas with mucinous glandular differentiation or transitional cell foci might remotely be considered in the differential diagnosis of mucinous or Brenner variants of müllerian tumors. As described earlier, rete testis adenocarcinomas have a combination of diagnostic features that must be recognized for a correct diagnosis. Paratesticular and tunica vaginalis MM may closely resemble paratesticular and tunica vaginalis borderline serous müllerian tumors. MMs are about three times more frequent. Müllerian tumors stain positively for keratin and frequently for CEA, B72.3, BER-EP4, EMA, Leu-M1, S-100 protein, and placental-like alkaline phosphatase, whereas MMs stain positively for keratin and EMA.[44] Although borderline serous tumors and epithelial MMs may have similar papillary configurations, borderline serous tumors generally have stratified nuclei and may be ciliated, whereas MMs are lined by a single cell layer. Metastatic carcinomas to the testis, tunica vaginalis, and paratesticular tissues are rare but should be considered in the differential diagnosis.

REFERENCES

1. Buzelin F, Karam G, Moreau A, et al: Testicular tumor and the acquired immunodeficiency syndrome. Eur Urol 1994; 26:71–76.
2. Gabrilove JL, Nicolis GL, Mitty HA, Sohval AR: Feminizing interstitial cell tumor of the testis: personal obser-

vations and a review of the literature. Cancer 1975; 35: 1184–1202.
3. Dieckmann K, Loy V: Metachronous germ cell and Leydig cell tumors of the testis: do testicular germ cell tumors and Leydig cell tumors share common etiologic factors? Cancer 1993; 72:1305–1307.
4. Poster RB, Katz DS: Leydig cell tumor of the testis in Klinefelter syndrome: MR detection. J Comput Assist Tumogr 1993; 17:480–481.
5. Sohval AR, Churg J, Gabrilove JL: Ultrastructure of feminizing testicular Leydig cell tumors. Ultrastruct Pathol 1982; 3:335–345.
6. Gittes RF, Smith G, Conn CA, Smith F: Local androgenic effect of interstitial cell tumor of the testis. J Urol 1970; 104: 774–777.
7. Kim F, Young RH, Scully RE: Leydig cell tumors of the testis: a clinicopathologic analysis of 40 cases and review of the literature. Am J Surg Pathol 1985; 9:177.
8. Collins DH, Cameron KM: Interstitial-cell tumor. Br J Urol 1964; 36(Suppl):62–69.
9. Palazzo JP, Petersen RO, Young RH, Scully RE: Deoxyribonucleic acid flow cytometry of testicular Leydig cell tumors. J Urol 1994; 152:415–417.
10. Kirkland RT, Kirkland JL, Keenan BS, et al: Bilateral testicular tumors in congenital adrenal hyperplasia. J Clin Endocrinol Metab 1977; 44:369–378.
11. Davis JM, Woodroof J, Sadasivan R, Stephens R: Case report: congenital adrenal hyperplasia and malignant Leydig cell tumor. Am J Med Sci 1995; 309:63–65.
12. Bertram KA, Bratloff B, Hodges GF, Davidson H: Treatment of malignant Leydig cell tumor. Cancer 1991; 68: 2324–2329.
13. Zukerberg LR, Young RH, Scully RE: Sclerosing Sertoli cell tumor of the testis: a report of 10 cases. Am J Surg Pathol 1991; 15:829–834.
14. Proppe KH, Scully RE: Large-cell calcifying Sertoli cell tumor of the testis. Am J Clin Pathol 1980; 74:607–619.
15. Proppe KH, Dickerson GHL: Large-cell calcifying Sertoli cell tumor of the testis. Hum Pathol 1982; 13:1109–1114.
16. Tetu B, Ro JY, Ayala AG: Large cell calcifying Sertoli cell tumor of the testis: a clinicopathologic, immunohistochemical and ultrastructural study of two cases. Am J Clin Pathol 1991; 96:717–722.
17. Nogales FF, Andujar M, Zuluaga A, Garcia-Puche JL: Malignant large cell calcifying Sertoli cell tumor of the testis. J Urol 1995; 153:1935–1937.
18. Dryer L, Jacyk WK, du Plessis DJ. Bilateral large-cell calcifying Sertoli cell tumor of the testes with Peutz-Jeghers syndrome: a case report. Pediatr Dermatol 1994; 11:335–337.
19. Young RH, Scully RE (eds): Tumors and tumorlike lesions in intersexual disorders. *In* Testicular Tumors, pp 140–150. Chicago, ASCP Press, 1990.
20. Rutgers JL, Scully RE: Pathology of the testis in intersex syndromes. Semin Diagn Pathol 1987; 4:275–291.
21. Jimenez-Quintero LP, Ro JY, Zavala-Pompa A, et al: Granulosa cell tumor of the adult testis: a clinicopathologic study of seven cases and a review of the literature. Hum Pathol 1993; 24:1120–1126.
22. Lawrence WD, Young RH, Scully RE: Juvenile granulosa cell tumor of the infantile testis. Am J Surg Pathol 1985; 9: 87–84.
23. Tanaka Y, Sasaki Y, Tachibana K, et al: Testicular juvenile granulosa cell tumor in an infant with X/XY mosaicism clinically diagnosed as true hermaphroditism. Am J Surg Pathol 1994; 18:316–322.
24. Paquis-Flucklinger V, Rassoulzadegan M, Michiels J-F: Experimental Sertoli cell tumors in the mouse and their progression into a mixed germ cell-sex cord proliferation. Am J Pathol 1994; 144:454–459.
25. Lawrence WD, Young RH, Scully RE: Sex cord-stromal tumors. *In* Talerman A, Roth LM (eds): Contemporary Issues in Surgical Pathology: Pathology of the Testis and Its Adnexa, Vol 7, pp 67–92. New York, Churchill Livingstone, 1986.
26. Dieckmann K-P, Loy V: Response of metastasized sex cord gonadal stromal tumor of the testis to cisplatin-based chemotherapy. J Urol 1994; 151:1024–1026.
27. Gohji K, Higuchi A, Fujii A, Kizaki T: Malignant gonadal stromal tumor. Urology 1994; 43:244–247.
28. Stewart DA, Stewart DJ, Mai KT: Active chemotherapy for metastatic stromal cell tumor of the testis. Urology 1993; 42:732–734.
29. Price EB Jr: Epidermoid cysts of the testis: a clinical and pathologic analysis of 69 cases from the testicular tumor registry. J Urol 1969; 102:708–731.
30. Ross JH, Kay R, Elder J: Testis sparing surgery for pediatric epidermoid cysts of the testis. J Urol 1993; 149:353–56.
31. Baniel J, Perez JM, Foster RS: Benign testicular tumor associated with Klinefelter's syndrome. J Urol 1994; 151: 157–158.
32. Orozco RE, Murphy WM: Carcinoma of the rete testis: case report and review of the literature. J Urol 1993; 150:974–977.
33. Stein JP, Freeman JA, Esrig D, et al: Papillary adenocarcinoma of the rete testis: a case report and review of the literature. Urology 1994; 44:588–594.
34. Jones MA, Young RH, Scully RE: Malignant mesothelioma of the tunica vaginalis: a clinicopathologic analysis of 11 cases with review of the literature. Am J Surg Pathol 1995; 19:815–825.
35. De Nictolis M, Tommasoni S, Fabris G, Prat J: Intratesticular serous cystadenoma of borderline malignancy: a pathological, histochemical and DNA content study of a case with long-term follow-up. Virchows Arch A Pathol Anat 1993; 423:221–225.
36. Price EB Jr, Mostofi FK: Secondary carcinoma of the testis. Cancer 1957; 10:592–595.
37. Tiltman AJ: Metastatic tumors of the testis. Histopathology 1979; 3:31–37.
38. Haupt HM, Mann RB, Trump DL, Abeloff MD: Metastatic carcinoma involving the testis: clinical and pathologic distinction from primary testicular neoplasms. Cancer 1984; 54:709–714.
39. Zavala-Pompa A, Ro JY, el-Naggar A, et al: Primary carcinoid tumor of testis: immunohistochemical, ultrastructural and DNA flow cytometric study of three cases with a review of the literature. Cancer 1993; 72:1726–1732.
40. Peterson RO: Urologic Pathology, 2nd edition, p 451. Philadelphia, JB Lippincott Co, 1992.
41. Gowing NFC: Malignant lymphoma of the testis. *In* Pugh RCB (ed): Pathology of the testis, pp 334–355. Oxford, England, Blackwell Scientific Publications, 1976.
42. Ferry JA, Harris NL, Young RH, et al: Malignant lymphoma of the testis, epididymis and spermatic cord: a clinicopathologic study of 69 cases with immunophenotypic analysis. Am J Surg Pathol 1994; 18:376–390.
43. Turner RR, Colby TV, MacKintosh FR: Testicular lymphomas: a clinicopathologic study of 35 cases. Cancer 1981; 48: 2095–2102.
44. Levin HS, Mostofi FK: Symptomatic plasmacytoma of the testis. Cancer 1970; 25:1193–1203.
45. Givler RL: Testicular involvement in leukemia and lymphoma. Cancer 1969; 23:1290–1295.
46. Buchanan GR, Boyett JM, Pollock BH, et al: Improved treatment results in boys with overt testicular relapse during or shortly after initial therapy for acute lymphoblastic leukemia: a Pediatric Oncology Group study. Cancer 1991; 68:48–55.
47. Petersen RO: Urologic Pathology, 2nd edition, p 496. Philadelphia, JB Lippincott Co, 1992.
48. Wilson WT, Frenkel E, Vuitch F, Sagalowsky AI: Testicular tumors in men with human immunodeficiency virus. J Urol 1992; 147:1038–1040.
49. Young RH, Scully RE: Testicular and paratesticular tumors and tumor-like lesions of ovarian common epithelial and Mullerian types. Am J Clin Pathol 1986; 86:146–152.
50. Jones MA, Young RH, Srigley JR, Scully RE: Paratesticular serous papillary carcinoma: a report of six cases. Am J Surg Pathol 1995; 19:1359–1365.

36

RADICAL ORCHIECTOMY AND RETROPERITONEAL LYMPH NODE DISSECTION

JOHN P. DONOHUE, M.D.

PHYSICAL DIAGNOSIS OF TESTIS TUMORS AND RADICAL ORCHIECTOMY

Any mass within the body of the testicle itself must be considered a germ cell tumor until proven otherwise. Once the index of suspicion for a testis tumor is aroused, it is advisable to have the patient examined by a trained urologist. The urologist should be able to help differentiate the physical findings between epididymitis, spermatocele, varicocele, hydrocele, and testicular cancer. One of the most important aspects of physical examination is determining the location of the mass in question. The examiner should use two hands (Fig. 36–1). One hand steadies the testicle and the other grasps the testicle using the fingertips and the tip of the thumb to try to differentiate between a mass located in the body of the testicle versus a mass located in the epididymis. Transillumination is helpful to detect solid versus fluid-filled masses. Ultrasonography has been extremely helpful in differentiating between solid versus cystic lesions and also helping to pinpoint the location of the lesion. Ultrasound is also extremely helpful in illustrating the status of the underlying testicle in a patient who has a hydrocele that is too tense to allow adequate examination. The sensitivity of ultrasound in diagnosing testis tumors (i.e., in placing the lesion within the testis proper) is 98 to 99%.

If a mass in or adjacent to the body of the testis cannot be satisfactorily diagnosed with physical examination, transillumination, and ultrasonography, then the burden of proof is upon the urologist to further examine the mass through a surgical exploration. Because the lymphatics of the testis flow along the cord structures, it is important to explore the testicle through an inguinal incision to avoid contamination of the superficial inguinal and scrotal lymphatics by the testicular lymphatics in the event of tumor spillage. After the incision is made, the external oblique aponeurosis is incised in the line of its fibers and the cord structures are mobilized. The easiest way to get around the cord structures is to sweep from lateral to medial at the level of the pubic tubercle. One should take care to make certain the vas deferens as well as the testicular vessels are included in this bundle of tissue. Once the cord structures are isolated, they can be dissected more proximally and a noncrushing clamp can be placed on the cord structures to help prevent any theoretical spread by lymphatics or any bloodborne metastasis during the remainder of the surgical procedure. At this point the testicle can be delivered into the incision by placing traction on the cord structures. Loose connective tissue and cremasteric fibers must often be mobilized from the cord structures to allow delivery of the testicle. The testicle will still be attached to the dependent portion of the scrotum by the gubernaculum of the testis.

At this point direct examination of the testis should be accomplished. If the mass is clearly within the body of the testicle and is solid, an orchiectomy should be performed by ligating the cord structures at the level of the internal inguinal ring. During this part of the procedure, one should take care to separate the vas deferens from the vasculature. These two structures should be tied separately and should be mobilized to allow their separation. This aspect is important because, if the patient comes to retroperitoneal lymph node dissection at a future time, separating these structures at the time of orchiectomy facilitates the dissection of the gonadal vessels in the retroperitoneum.

If at the time of exploration the location and con-

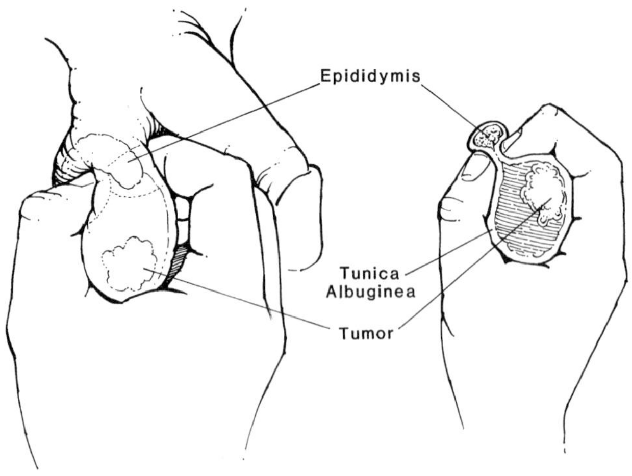
Epididymis
Tunica Albuginea
Tumor

FIGURE 36–1. Scrotal examination emphasizing the digital separation of the testis from the epididymis with the thumb and forefinger. By sliding these fingers across the testis, one can appreciate an intratesticular (tumor) mass. Any mass lesion within the tunica albuginea by definition has arisen from testicular tubules and is malignant at the 97th percentile in adolescents and adults.

sistency of the mass is not obvious (a very rare event), the tunica vaginalis can be incised to expose the tunica albuginea of the testis. If with this level of observation and testicular palpation it is still not possible to confirm an intratesticular mass in question, a biopsy can be performed. However, this should be an extremely rare scenario. Prior to performing a biopsy, however, it is recommended that the testicle be walled off with dry laparotomy pads to avoid any potential spill into the wound. If there is any doubt at the time of biopsy and frozen section, the testicle should be removed. It is an error of much greater significance if a testis with a tumor is left in place than if a testis without a malignant neoplasm is removed. Intratesticular mass lesions in adolescents and adults are malignant at the 97th percentile. If the mass is shown to be benign at biopsy, however, the tunica albuginea of the testis can be reapproximated with an absorbable suture and the testis can be returned to the scrotum. Because noncrushing clamps were used, the blood supply of the testis should not be jeopardized.

Levels of the serum markers β-human chorionic gonadotropin (β-hCG) and α-fetoprotein (AFP) should be obtained prior to surgical exploration in anyone suspected of having a testis tumor. This will be helpful at a later time in terms of monitoring the level of markers as an indication of response to therapy.

When a non–germ cell paratesticular tumor is encountered, the same inguinal orchiectomy with high ligation of the cord is also indicated. Oftentimes simple surgical excision of these tumors is satisfactory treatment. However, because one cannot be certain ahead of time of the precise diagnosis of the tumor, it is advisable to treat it in the same manner as one would a potential germ cell tumor.

In the case of either a suspected germ cell tumor or a suspected non–germ cell tumor, the mass should not be approached through the scrotum by open biopsy or by fine-needle aspiration. The inguinal approach is definitely recommended to avoid potential cross-contamination of different lymphatic drainage systems.

In dealing with germ cell neoplasms, one must differentiate between clinical and pathologic staging. Table 36–1 shows the definitions of the clinical stages of testis tumors (Fig. 36–2) and Table 36–2 shows the pathologic stages of testis tumor. The following sections of this chapter explain in detail the procedures involved in clinical and pathologic staging. Modifications of the staging classification for

TABLE 36–1. CLINICAL STAGES OF TESTIS TUMORS

Stage		Description
A		Tumor limited to the testis alone
B		Tumor of the testis and retroperitoneal lymph nodes
	B-2	Tumor of retroperitoneal lymph nodes 2–6 cm in greatest dimension by CT
	B-3	Tumor of retroperitoneal lymph nodes >6 cm in greatest dimension by CT
C		Tumor above the diaphragm or involving abdominal solid organs

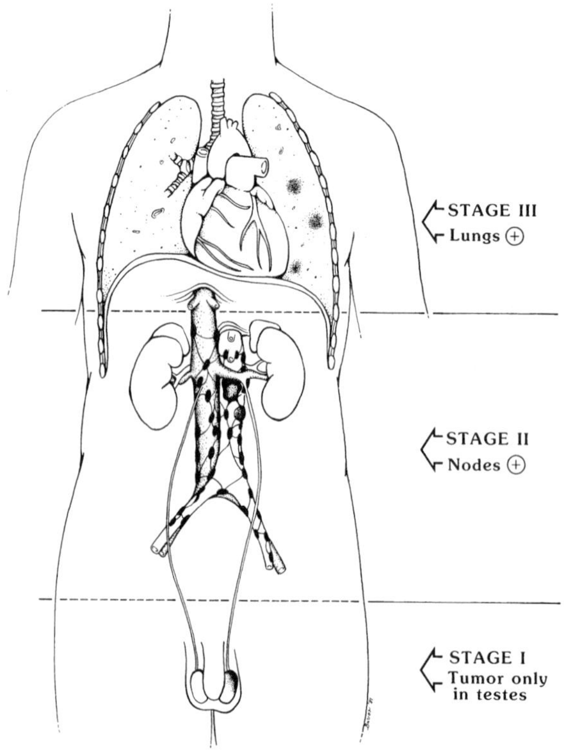
STAGE III
Lungs ⊕
STAGE II
Nodes ⊕
STAGE I
Tumor only in testes

FIGURE 36–2. Staging template for testis cancer. Both clinical and pathologic staging are based on the principle of disease. *A*, Confined to the testis; *B*, metastatic to the regional (i.e., retroperitoneal) nodes but not above the diaphragm; *C*, tumor involving chest (mediastinum, lungs, or other viscera).

TABLE 36–2. PATHOLOGIC STAGES OF TESTIS TUMORS

Stage	Description
A	Tumor limited to the testis and paratesticular structure
B-1	Microscopic metastases to retroperitoneal lymph nodes (1–5 nodes)
B-2	Microscopic metastases to retroperitoneal lymph nodes (>5 nodes) or gross nodal involvement (2–6 cm)
B-3	Gross tumor of retroperitoneal lymph nodes (>6 cm)
C	Metastases above the diaphragm or to abdominal solid organs

advanced disease are being examined by many investigators to try to develop groupings that allow more precise divisions into specific treatment groups and also allow one to assess the prognosis of the patient more accurately.

RETROPERITONEAL LYMPH NODE DISSECTION: INTRODUCTION AND HISTORICAL BACKGROUND

Traditionally, full bilateral retroperitoneal lymph node dissection (RPLND) for low-stage nonseminomatous testis cancer has offered two benefits. First, it enabled precise pathologic staging to occur early in the course of the disease. With the advent of computed tomography (CT) scanning, clinical staging has improved, although current clinical staging techniques are unable to identify the 30% of patients who indeed are pathologic stage B. Pathologic staging early in the course of the disease enables therapeutic options and prognosis to be defined.

The second benefit of RPLND has been the therapeutic aspect of the procedure. For the 30% of patients who are pathologic stage B, RPLND offers a 70% chance of long-term care without subjecting the patient to platinum-based chemotherapy. Therefore, the staging and therapeutic aspects of RPLND in low-stage nonseminomatous testis cancer are well recognized as benefits of the procedure. The traditional objection to RPLND has involved the morbidity side of the equation, specifically related to the almost universal loss of emission and ejaculation after full bilateral RPLND. The development of the nerve-sparing RPLND, with its attendant preservation of emission/ejaculation, has eliminated this source of morbidity without impacting on the staging and therapeutic aspects of the procedure. Therefore, nerve-sparing RPLND remains an excellent method of managing patients with low-stage nonseminomatous testis cancer.

Proponents of the surveillance scheme for patients with clinical stage A nonseminomatous testis cancer maintain that surveillance will have comparable long-term cure rates but will spare patients with pathologic stage A disease the morbidity of a laparotomy. Certainly correctly classifying clinical stage A patients as pathologic stage A without the necessity of a laparotomy is an admirable goal. Work is in progress at several centers attempting to improve clinical staging. However, currently clinical staging is not highly accurate, and current surveillance management methods must be judged based on long-term cure rates, compliance of patients in the community setting, cost, and ultimate morbidity for the patient who requires full-dose platinum-based chemotherapy and subsequent postchemotherapy RPLND.

We believe the results attained using nerve-sparing RPLND must be the standard by which surveillance is ultimately judged. Additionally, we believe patient care should be individualized; the patient presenting with clinical stage A nonseminomatous testis cancer at the current time must be apprised of the facts and allowed to choose his method of management.

NERVE-SPARING RETROPERITONEAL LYMPH NODE DISSECTION

Development of the Nerve-Sparing Procedure

The traditional full bilateral suprahilar RPLND involved removal of all lymphatic tissue from the suprahilar areas to the bifurcation of the common iliac, from ureter to ureter. This was by intent a radical procedure because chemotherapy rescue was not available at the time of development of full bilateral RPLND. All sympathetic efferent fibers were sacrificed and lymphatic tissue was removed en bloc. Therefore, these patients suffered from anejaculation postoperatively.

With the advent of CT scanning, it became apparent that the pathway of lymphatic channels from the abdomen to the chest was posterior, through the crus of the diaphragm, and not anterior to the suprahilar zones. Therefore, the suprahilar aspect of the full bilateral RPLND was eliminated. Because no modification of the surgical resection template below the renal vessels occurred during the full bilateral dissection, anejaculation again was the rule postoperatively.

The next development in the evolution of RPLND involved the use of mapping studies to modify the surgical resection templates.[1–3] These studies identified sites of retroperitoneal disease for both right- and left-sided primary testicular tumors for patients with low- and high-volume retroperitoneal disease. It became apparent that patients with low-volume retroperitoneal disease had metastatic disease in predictable sites, depending on whether or not the primary was right or left sided. From this information, templates were derived for

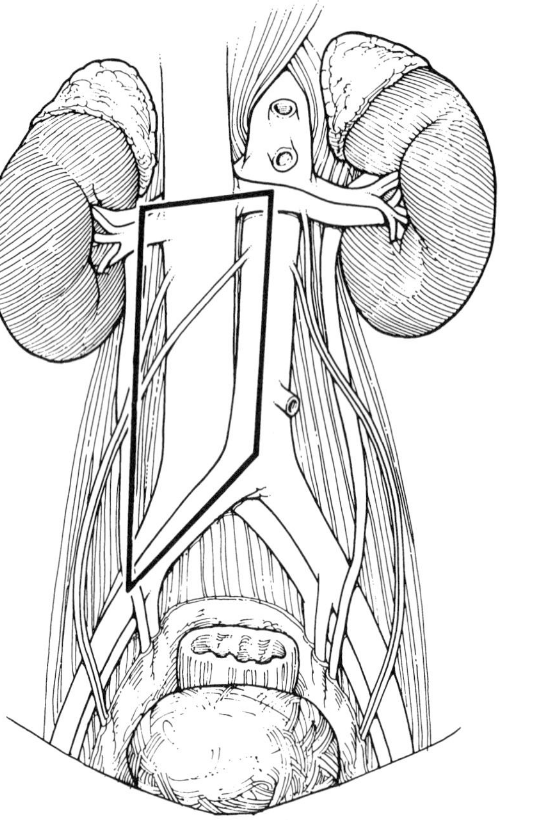

FIGURE 36–3. Template for modified right unilateral RPLND. (After Whitmore.)

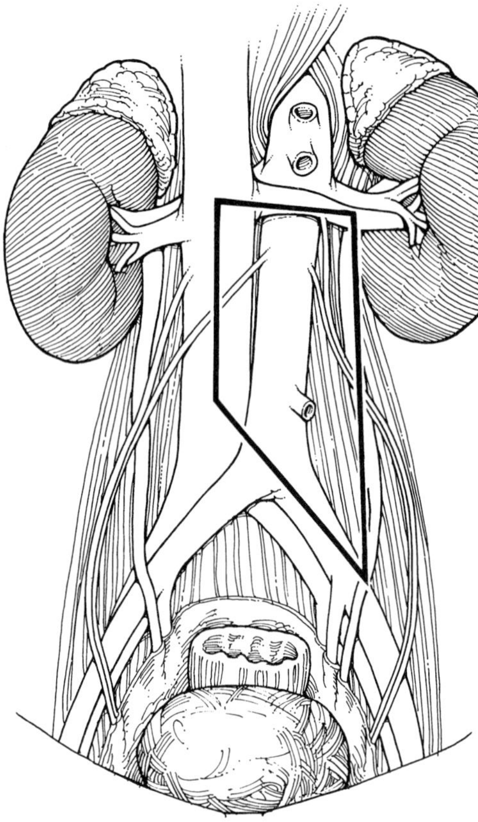

FIGURE 36–4. Template for modified left unilateral RPLND. (After Whitmore.)

both right- and left-sided dissections (Figs. 36–3 and 36–4) that would remove lymphatic tissue at high risk for harboring metastatic disease, with preservation of other retroperitoneal lymphatic tissue at low risk for containing metastasis. Additionally, these templates saved some retroperitoneal efferent sympathetic fibers because the dissections were basically unilateral and these fibers exist bilaterally. Therefore, these so-called modified dissections were capable of preserving emission/ejaculation roughly 50 to 70% of the time.[4–6]

The nerve-sparing RPLND was developed because experienced retroperitoneal surgeons realized that these efferent sympathetic fibers, although quite small in some patients, were able to be identified and dissected prospectively prior to the removal of retroperitoneal lymphatic tissue. The nerve-sparing dissection therefore prospectively identifies and dissects retroperitoneal efferent sympathetic fibers prior to removing lymphatic tissue according to templates similar to the templates used for the modified dissection (Figs. 36–5 through 36–8). By preserving these efferent fibers, emission/ejaculation is reliably preserved.[6–9]

Technique of Nerve-Sparing Dissection

Although we use a transperitoneal midline approach to the retroperitoneum for nerve-sparing

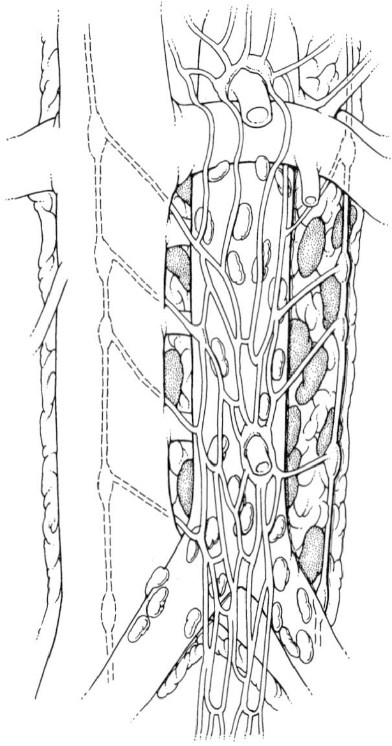

FIGURE 36–5. Schematic of retroperitoneal sympathetic nervous system.

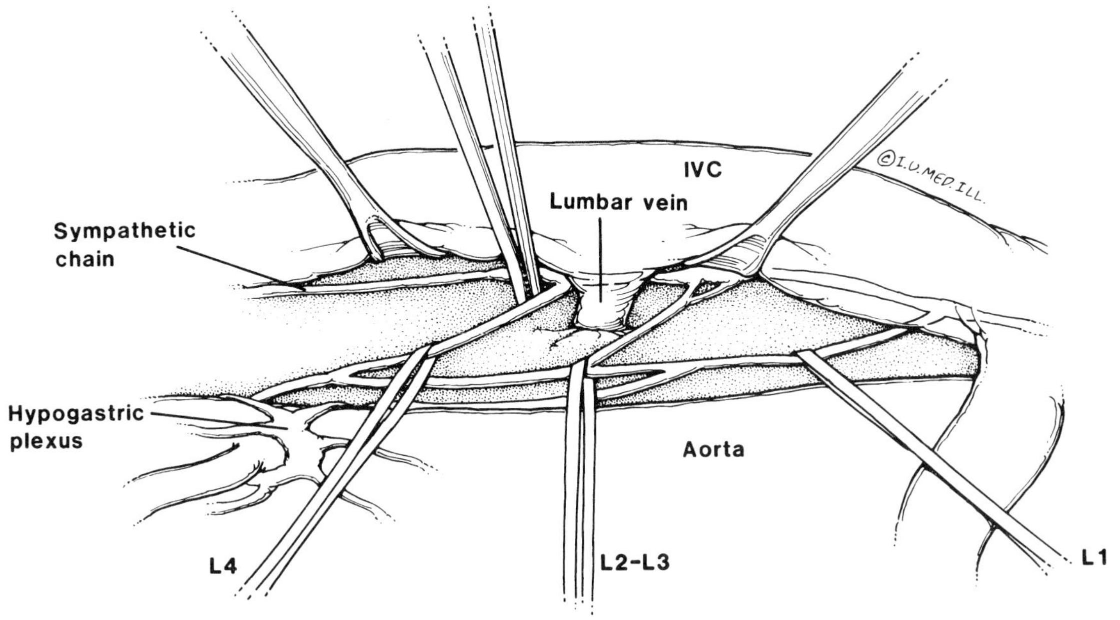
IVC
Lumbar vein
Sympathetic chain
Hypogastric plexus
Aorta
L4
L2-L3
L1
©I.U. MED. ILL.

FIGURE 36–6. Relationships of right postganglionic fibers and right sympathetic chain to the inferior vena cava.

RPLND, a thoracoabdominal extraperitoneal approach certainly is acceptable. After the midline transperitoneal incision is performed, a self-retaining retractor is used. The posterior peritoneal incision varies dependent on whether or not the patient had a right testicular primary or left testicular primary.

Right-Sided Dissection

For a right-sided primary the posterior peritoneal incision is performed from the cecum superiorly along the inferior aspect of the duodenum to the ligament of Treitz. The duodenum is then reflected using blunt and sharp dissection off the anterior surface of the vena cava, taking care to reflect the root of the small bowel anteriorly, leaving the right gonadal vein posteriorly with the remaining retroperitoneal tissue. Self-retaining retractors are placed, giving good exposure of the interaortocaval, precaval, and paracaval zones. The anterior split of lymphatic tissue is then carried out over the anterior surface of the aorta and the vena cava. The caval split extends from the origin of the renal veins to the bifurcation; the aortic split extends from the left renal vein to the origin of the inferior mesenteric artery. Care must be taken to identify any precaval right lower pole renal arteries. The hypogastric plexus is identified at the bifurcation of the aorta. Lymphatic tissue is then rolled medially off the side of the vena cava, at which time lumbar veins are identified coursing from the posterior body wall to the posterior vena cava. Efferent sympathetic fibers are characteristically seen passing around these lumbars from the sympathetic chain

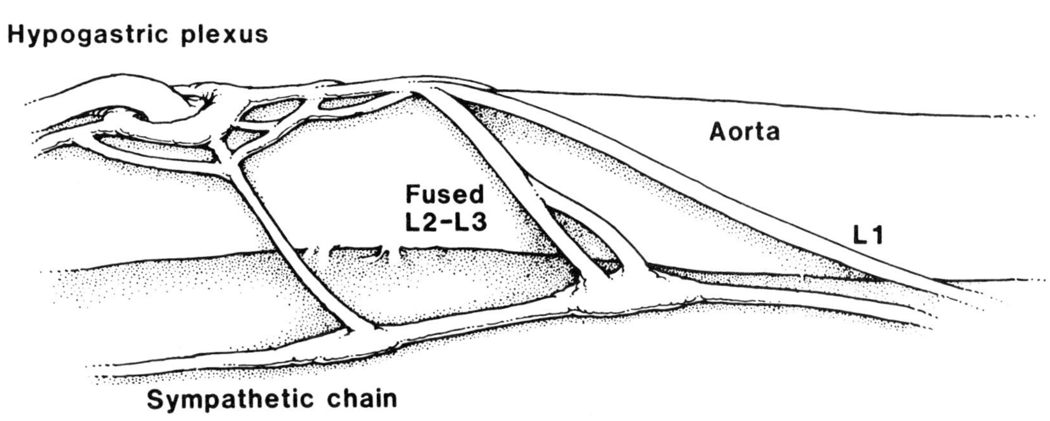
Hypogastric plexus
Aorta
Fused L2-L3
L1
Sympathetic chain

FIGURE 36–7. Relationship of left postganglionic fibers and left sympathetic chain to the abdominal aorta.

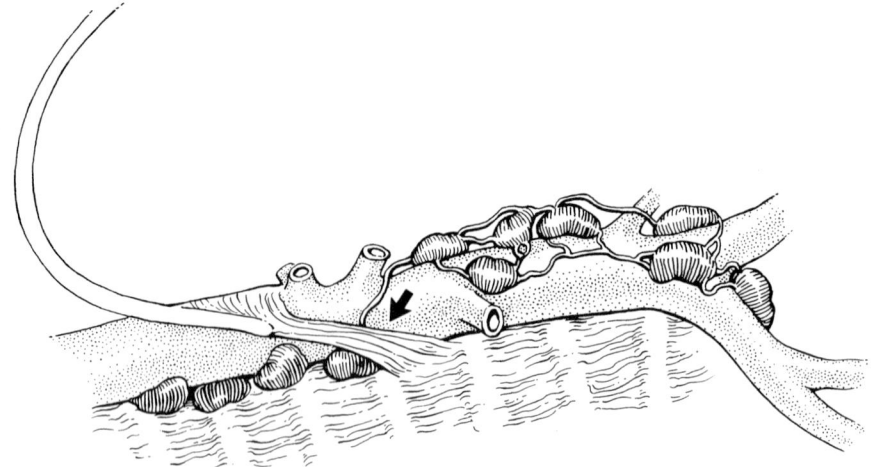

FIGURE 36–8. Lymphatic flow from the retroperitoneum to the chest passes through the aortic hiatus of the diaphragm posterolaterally. Nodes in this area are called retrocrural because of their location posterior to the right and left crura of the diaphragm.

to the preaortic plexus. The lumbar veins are divided between silk ties, after which the sympathetic fibers are dissected free of remaining retroperitoneal tissue and placed in vessel loops.

Next, the "roll" of lymphatic tissue medially off the right side of the aorta is carried out, thus setting up the interaortocaval package. Lumbar arteries are divided only as needed and not on a routine basis as is done for full bilateral RPLND. Looped sympathetic fibers are retracted to the right as lymphatic tissue is removed en bloc off the posterior body wall, taking care to clip any lumbar veins or arteries as they penetrate the posterior body wall. The right renal artery is identified superiorly near the crus of the diaphragm and lymphatic tissue is dissected from the artery. Clips are used at the point where the interaortocaval package penetrates the crus of the diaphragm and the interaortocaval package is excised and passed off. Next, the "roll" of tissue off the right side of the cava is performed, after which the precaval and right paracaval packages are harvested, taking care not to injure the right ureter. Finally, the right gonadal vein and artery are dissected distally to the internal ring, at which time the ligatures from the orchiectomy are seen. The vas deferens is divided, and the gonadal vessels are passed off as specimen. Irrigation is then carried out, after which the posterior peritoneum is closed using a running absorbable suture.

Left-Sided Dissection

One of two posterior peritoneal incisions may be performed for a left-sided dissection. An incision may be performed lateral to the left colon, similar to the incision performed for a transperitoneal nephrectomy. The splenocolic ligament is divided and the bowel and its mesocolon are reflected medially. Sympathetic fibers are visualized in the left periaortic zone distally as they cross the left common iliac artery. This represents the preaortic plexus. They are dissected proximally until they have been freed from left periaortic retroperitoneal tissue. Next, the left sympathetic chain is identified by dissecting along the psoas, lateral to the nodal package. Efferent fibers from the chain are freed by splitting overlying lymphatic tissue. Hence, sympathetic fibers are dissected proximally from the hypogastric plexus, and distally from the sympathetic chain. The net result is the complete dissection of left-sided sympathetic fibers. The split of lymphatic tissue over the aorta from the left renal vein to the inferior mesenteric artery is carried out, after which lymphatic tissue is rolled laterally, taking care to not injure any sympathetic fibers. The gonadal vein is divided between silk ties and is dissected distally to the left internal ring, at which time the vas is ligated and the stump from the previous left orchiectomy is identified. Gonadal vessels are then passed off as specimen. The left periaortic package is then harvested, with the distal margin being the bifurcation of the left common iliac. Superiorly, the left renal artery is identified and dissected free of lymphatic tissue, taking care to not injure any efferent sympathetic fibers. The tissue is then removed, taking care to clip lymphatics as they pierce the left crus of the diaphragm. The upper interaortocaval package is then harvested using the same technique as was used for a right-sided dissection. Only the superior-most aspect of the interaortocaval zone is taken for a left-sided dissection because mapping studies have shown that the lower interaortocaval zone is rarely involved in low-volume retroperitoneal disease from a left primary (Figs. 36–6 and 36–7).

An alternative posterior peritoneal incision for a left-sided dissection involves access to the upper left periaortic and interaortocaval zones via an incision along the inferior aspect of the duodenum, with reflection of the duodenum superiorly and to the right. After completion of the upper portion of the dissection, the sigmoid colon is mobilized medially after a posterior peritoneal incision lateral to the sigmoid has been made. This yields good access to the lower left periaortic zone and to the gonadal vessels. These two incisions are necessary because the inferior mesenteric artery is not divided.

TABLE 36–3. RESULTS OF PRIMARY RPLND IN NONSEMINOMATOUS GERM CELL TESTIS CANCER—CLINICAL STAGE A (1965–1989)

Disease Extent (Pathologic Stage)	Patients N	Patients %	Relapse N	Relapse %	Survival (%)	Deaths
A						
1965–1978	57	66	6	11	100	0
1979–1989	267	71	29	11	99.2	2*
Cumulative	324	70	35	11	99.1	2
B, no adjuvant						
1965–1978	9	11	4	44	100	0
1979–1989	65	17	21	32	98.5	1†
Cumulative	74	16	25	34	98.6	1†
B, plus adjuvant‡						
1965–1978	20	23	3	15	95	1§
1979–1989	46	12	0	0	100	0
Cumulative	66	14	63	14	98.5	1†
All cases						
1965–1978	86		13	15	98.8	1
1979–1989	378		50	13	99.2	3
Cumulative	464		63	14	99.1	4

*One cancer death, one postoperative death.
†One cancer death.
‡Non–platinum-based chemotherapy.
§One death from testis cancer.

After completion of the left-sided dissection, the posterior peritoneum is routinely closed using a running absorbable suture. Abdominal closure is performed using a running nonabsorbable monofilament suture. Most patients do not have a significant ileus after nerve-sparing RPLND for low-volume disease. Although we have used nasogastric decompression for 2 to 3 days in the past, our current technique is to omit nasogastric tube decompression and restrict the patient to no oral intake for 1 to 2 days. Hospitalization ranges from 4 to 7 days. Transfusions are not necessary, and our patients are not cross matched. The only significant morbidity involves small bowel obstruction secondary to adhesions, which occurs in approximately 1% of patients.

Results with Nerve-Sparing Dissection

Primary Results

Our initial experience with nerve-sparing RPLND has already been described.[9] We have now performed this procedure in over 225 patients. The therapeutic aspect of the procedure has been maintained because roughly 70% of our patients who

TABLE 36–4. RESULTS OF PRIMARY RPLND IN NONSEMINOMATOUS GERM CELL TESTIS CANCER—CLINICAL STAGE B

Disease Extent (Pathologic Stage)	Patients N	Patients %	Relapse N	Relapse %	Survival (%)	Deaths
A						
1979–1989	32	23	2	6	100	0
1965–1989	41	24	2	5	100	0
B, no adjuvant						
1979–1989	49	35	18	37	96	2
1965–1989	54	31	19	35	96.2	2
B with adjuvant*						
1979–1989	59	42	0	0	98.3	1
1965–1989	79	45	11	14	93.6	5
All cases						
1979–1989	140		20	14	98	3†
1965–1989	174		32	18	95.9	7‡

*Adjuvant = cis-platinum, vinblastine, bleomycin (PVB × 2): 1979–1989.
†One cancer death, one postoperative death, one chemotherapy.
‡Five cancer deaths, one postoperative death, one chemotherapy.

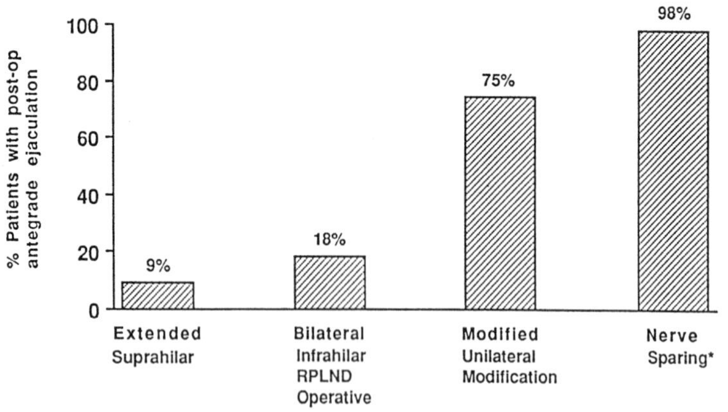
% Patients with post-op antegrade ejaculation
100
80
60
40
20
0
9%
18%
75%
98%
Extended Suprahilar
Bilateral Infrahilar
RPLND Operative
Modified Unilateral Modification
Nerve Sparing*

FIGURE 36–9. Influence of modifications of operative technique on the incidence of postoperative antegrade ejaculation after primary RPLND in clinical stage A nonseminomatous germ cell testis cancer. *, Of these cases, 89% had nerve-sparing modified unilateral RPLND.

were pathologic stage B and who elected not to have adjuvant chemotherapy have been cured as a result of nerve-sparing RPLND. Local recurrence occasionally occurs in pathologic stage B patients, although it is extremely rare in our experience (less than 1%; Tables 36–3 and 36–4). Almost all patients subjected to nerve-sparing RPLND ejaculate (Fig. 36–9).

Postchemotherapy Results

Between March of 1988 and November of 1991, a total of 40 patients underwent some form of nerve-sparing RPLND at Indiana University after receiving primary chemotherapy for either bulky retroperitoneal or clinical stage C testicular carcinoma at presentation. A minimum of 12 months' follow-up is available for 38 of these patients.

DISSECTION PROCEDURES. Thirty-one of the 38 patients underwent full bilateral dissections, including one patient who had a left suprahilar dissection as well. The other seven patients had unilateral procedures, with three having left template dissections, two having right template procedures, and two having right-sided dissections modified according to the location and volume of disease. Two patients were approached through thoracoabdominal transperitoneal incisions, and the remaining 36 patients were explored through midline laparotomies. Two patients had concomitant pulmonary resections for residual pulmonary disease, and two patients required nephrectomies for complete excision of their disease.

LUMBAR ROOTS SPARED. Three patients were noted on dictated operative summaries to have had all postganglionic lumbar sympathetic roots dissected and preserved during their RPLNDs. Twelve patients had all right-sided roots preserved and eight patients had all left-sided roots spared. One patient had all left-sided roots and three right-sided roots spared, one patient had all right-sided roots (L2 and L3) spared, and one patient had three right-sided roots (L1, L2, and L3) and one left-sided root (L1) preserved. Ten patients had from one to three roots on either side spared during their RPLNDs.

SPECIMEN PATHOLOGY. Twenty-three patients (60%) had teratoma in their RPLND specimen, including the patient with elevation of β-hCG preoperatively, and 12 patients (32%) had necrosis. Two patients (5%) had choriocarcinoma present in their specimen, and one patient (3%) had ganglioneuroma as the predominant histology from his RPLND. One patient from the teratoma group also had a small area of atypical myelomyoma present in his specimen.

FOLLOW-UP DATA. All 38 patients are alive with no evidence of disease at their most recent visit to our office or that of their local physician. The mean follow-up period is 34 months, with a range of 12 to 57 months. One patient had a pulmonary relapse treated with salvage chemotherapy and subsequent pulmonary resection with pathology of the lung specimen showing necrosis only. One patient had a marker-normal mediastinal relapse treated with surgical resection, with the pathology showing teratoma. One patient developed a new contralateral left testis mass that was treated with radical orchiectomy; the pathology of the testis showed embryonal cell carcinoma. Although the postorchiectomy markers were normal, an abdominal CT obtained at the local hospital was read as showing a small retroperitoneal mass in the interaortocaval area. He received two courses of platinum/VP-16–ifosfamide. Retrospective interpretation of this CT scan by radiologists at our facility concluded that the tissue believed to be interaortocaval tumor was actually unopacified bowel lying in the region of his previous resection. This patient has since had a repeat CT scan at our facility that was normal. Two patients, 26 and 47 months after RPLND with normal markers, are being followed for small areas of residual pulmonary densities that have been stable on serial chest radiographs and are presumed to be areas of necrosis.

POSTOPERATIVE COMPLICATIONS. One patient had a superficial wound infection with fascial dehiscence of a portion of his incision during the first week postoperatively, requiring exploration and closure. Two patients developed partial small bowel obstructions months after discharge and underwent exploration and adhesiolysis procedures.

TABLE 36–5. SEMEN ANALYSES

Patient	Specimen Sampling Time*	Volume (ml)	Count (million/ml)
1	28	1.8	0
2	21	1.7	0
3	18	3.0	93
4	21	5.0	93
5	33	2.0	78.2
6	24	2.5	45.4
7	21	4.0	142
8	23	1.0	29
9	37	8.0	0.7

*Number of months after surgery that specimen was obtained.

Two patients developed symptomatic lymphoceles postoperatively that were treated with percutaneous drainage procedures. One patient experienced transient partial left femoral neurapraxia that was thought to be related to the self-retaining retractor used during surgery.

Status of Ejaculation. Thirty-four of the 38 patients report normal ejaculation after their RPLNDs, with one patient experiencing a delay of 21 months prior to return. Of the four patients reporting absence of ejaculatory function postoperatively, one had all roots spared, two had all right-sided roots spared, and one had only a single root (right L3) preserved during RPLND. One of the three patients with all right-sided roots spared received an intraoperative injury to the right sympathetic chain during the procedure.

Fertility. Nine of the 34 ejaculatory patients report 10 pregnancies in their partners, with six partners completing uneventful term pregnancies and giving birth to seven healthy children without complication. There have been four miscarriages reported in three patients' partners, one attributed to cervical incompetence in the patient's wife. Post-RPLND semen analysis data are available in nine patients (Table 36–5). Mean ejaculate volume is 3.2 ml, and three of the nine analyses, obtained 21, 28, and 37 months postoperatively, show persistent azoospermia.

Impact on Treatment Methods. The method of surgical treatment of testicular carcinoma continues to evolve in an effort to improve efficacy and reduce morbidity. Initial studies of patterns of nodal metastasis from nonseminomatous germ cell tumors (NSGCTs) of the testes led to limitations of standard bilateral and suprahilar retroperitoneal dissections to template procedures without sacrificing efficacy of treatment.[10] These modifications in dissection borders limited but did not eliminate postoperative ejaculatory dysfunction (Fig. 36–8). Recent advances and review of previous findings in anatomic knowledge and surgical technique have led to the ability to define and surgically preserve ejaculation.[4–6,10–14] At our institution, patients with clinical stage A nonseminomatous testicular carcinoma who undergo RPLND routinely have procedures that spare the postganglionic lumbar sympathetic roots. Postoperative ejaculatory dysfunction has been virtually eliminated in these patients. In light of the success of these nerve-sparing procedures in patients with low-stage disease, we have begun applying nerve-sparing techniques to selected patients with relatively small volumes of residual retroperitoneal disease after receiving primary chemotherapy for metastatic disease.

It should be stressed that the patients in this series represent a select group among the many patients treated at our facility for residual disease after chemotherapy. In the 44-month period of this series, a total of 256 patients underwent full bilateral postchemotherapy RPLND without the use of nerve-sparing technique. Our 40 patients therefore represent only 13.5% of the total population of postchemotherapy RPLND patients during the period of our initial experience. These 40 patients were chosen on the basis of the relatively small and predominantly unilateral distribution of their initial retroperitoneal adenopathy and residual disease after chemotherapy. The fact that only 2 (5%) of the 40 patients had persistent germ cell elements in their RPLND specimens also reflects the selection bias in the series.

Thirty-four of 38 patients report normal ejaculatory function postoperatively. Although other authors have noted delay in return of ejaculation after RPLND,[6,7] only one patient in our series reported a delay of 21 months prior to return. Of the four anejaculatory patients, one had only a single root spared and one had an intraoperative sympathetic chain injury that might explain anejaculation. All four patients in our series who report absence of ejaculation postoperatively initially presented with left-sided primaries and eventually underwent full bilateral dissections. This observation raises the possibility that patients undergoing a full left-sided cleanout are more prone to "downstream" sympathetic fiber injury in the preaortic area below the inferior mesenteric artery or in the hypogastric plexus, despite adequate preservation of right-sided lumbar roots in the interaortocaval region.

All of our patients were requested to obtain semen analyses at our expense, but only nine complied. Three patients are persistently azoospermic, two who received salvage chemotherapy and one who underwent high-dose carboplatinum therapy with autologous bone marrow transplantation. The adverse effects of testicular carcinoma and chemotherapy on semen parameters are well documented,[15] and must be considered when discussing fertility in patients who have undergone post-chemotherapy RPLNDs.

We are encouraged that, despite a mean follow-up period of almost 3 years, we have not seen an abdominal relapse in these patients, and we believe that our efforts to preserve their ejaculatory function have not compromised the efficacy of their procedures. The fact that six of our patients have been

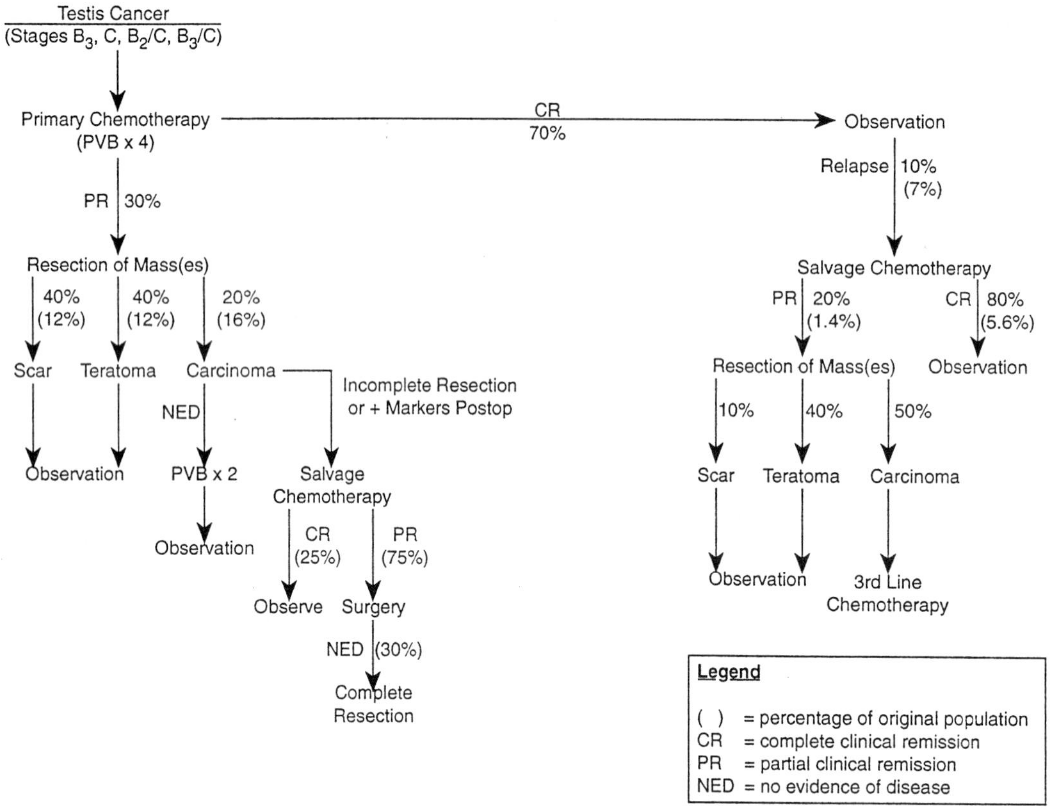
Testis Cancer
(Stages B_3, C, B_2/C, B_3/C)
Primary Chemotherapy
(PVB x 4)
CR
70%
Observation
Relapse 10%
(7%)
PR 30%
Resection of Mass(es)
40%
(12%)
40%
(12%)
20%
(16%)
Scar
Teratoma
Carcinoma
Incomplete Resection
or + Markers Postop
NED
Observation
PVB x 2
Salvage
Chemotherapy
Observation
CR
(25%)
PR
(75%)
Observe
Surgery
NED (30%)
Complete
Resection
Salvage Chemotherapy
PR 20%
(1.4%)
CR 80%
(5.6%)
Resection of Mass(es)
Observation
10%
40%
50%
Scar
Teratoma
Carcinoma
Observation
3rd Line
Chemotherapy
Legend
( ) = percentage of original population
CR = complete clinical remission
PR = partial clinical remission
NED = no evidence of disease

FIGURE 36–10. Treatment scheme for disseminated testis cancer at Indiana University.

able to father seven healthy children gives us additional encouragement and strengthens our belief that the careful application of nerve-sparing techniques to patients undergoing RPLND after receiving primary chemotherapy for metastatic disease improves the means of surgical treatment of testicular carcinoma by further reducing its morbidity.

DISSECTION AFTER CHEMOTHERAPY FOR ADVANCED TESTIS CANCER

Figure 36–10 outlines the treatment scheme for advanced testis cancer relative to the timing of surgical intervention. Advanced testicular cancer is best treated with combination platinum-based chemotherapy as primary therapy. Those with more bulky tumor who obtain a partial remission should then have residual tumor completely resected by surgery. This effectively restages the patient, provides therapeutic benefit to many, and determines the need for additional chemotherapy. If carcinoma is found in the resected specimen, further "salvage" chemotherapy is a possible additional option. If the resection is grossly complete, even this group can obtain survival with or without salvage chemotherapy.[16]

Clinical experience and long-term follow-up (>5 years) with over 700 such cases permits several other observations. Some patients who achieve a partial remission can still be observed. Those with pure seminoma in the primary specimen who still have a radiographic abnormality after treatment for bulky metastatic disease usually have necrotic tumor if resected. Therefore, several groups have demonstrated a successful conservative approach in the partial responders. We have noted another group who can be observed after a partial remis-

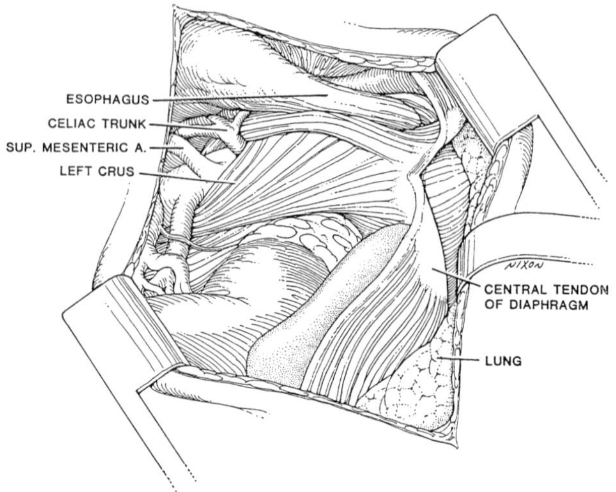
ESOPHAGUS
CELIAC TRUNK
SUP. MESENTERIC A.
LEFT CRUS
NIXON
CENTRAL TENDON
OF DIAPHRAGM
LUNG

FIGURE 36–11. Exposure of the left crus of the diaphragm through a left thoracoabdominal incision, as an approach to left retrocrural tumor.

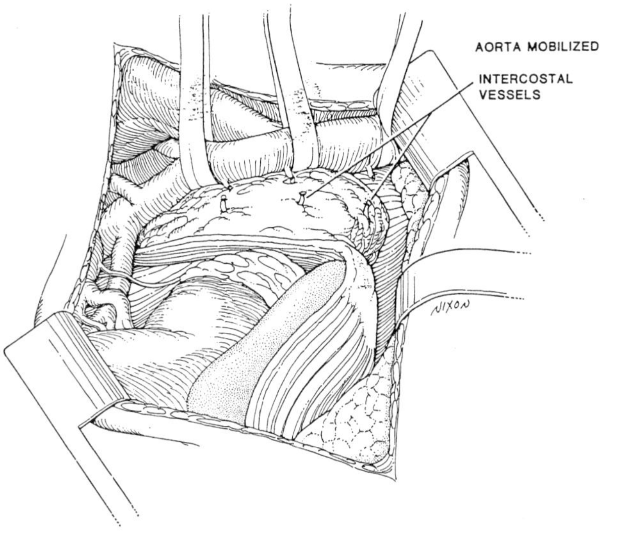
AORTA MOBILIZED
INTERCOSTAL VESSELS

FIGURE 36–12. Left crus divided longitudinally, aorta mobilized, intercostals ligated and divided (L1 through T9), and retrocrural tumor exposed in posterior inferior mediastinal space.

sion: those who had pure embryonal cancer in the primary tumor and who had a 90% or greater reduction in measured tumor volume. All of these patients had necrosis in the resected specimens.[17] Also, we have noted that the relapse potential is related to three major variables: site of the disease (e.g., mediastinal vs. retroperitoneal), histology (sarcomatous elements vs. none), and bulk of disease (massive vs. moderate vs. small).[18]

Two different groups of patients must be considered for postchemotherapy RPLND. The first group are those who have had a partial remission with primary therapy. The second group are those who once had a complete remission after primary chemotherapy, but who relapse and then achieve a partial remission after salvage chemotherapy.

The first group, who do not have complete resolution of findings on abdominal CT scan or abdominal ultrasound after chemotherapy, are considered as candidates for radical RPLND. If the residual mass is high in the abdomen and extends into the retrocrural area, or apparently involves the diaphragm and has extension into the chest, a combined abdominal and thoracic approach is indicated. Depending upon the circumstances of the individual case, either a thoracoabdominal incision or a median sternotomy in combination with a midline abdominal incision is used. When patients have residual unilateral chest disease, either in the parenchyma or the mediastinum, a thoracotomy incision alone is sufficient, assuming the abdominal findings have completely normalized or were normal initially. If bilateral chest disease is present, particularly in the posterior mediastinum, separate thoracotomy incisions may be indicated. If the bilateral chest disease is in any other location, adequate exposure can frequently be obtained through a median sternotomy. Any of these approaches can be used in combination with a midline abdominal incision if there is residual disease in the abdomen (Figs. 36–11 through 36–13).

If any patient in this group, having undergone primary cytoreductive chemotherapy, has persistently elevated serum markers (AFP or β-hCG), he is treated with salvage chemotherapy rather than surgical resection based upon the knowledge that there is still active disease present.

The second set of patients are those who have undergone salvage chemotherapy. The same indications for surgery are used in this set of patients; that is, they would have evidence of only a partial remission. Again, in general, if the patient had an elevated AFP or β-hCG level, he would be a candidate for further chemotherapy rather than surgical treatment. There are occasional exceptions to

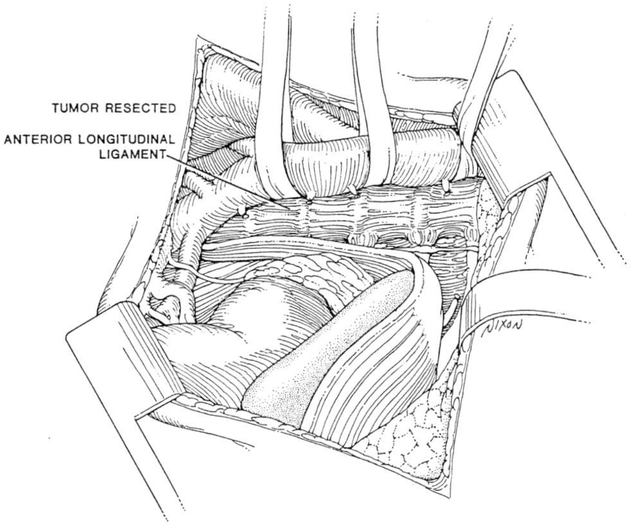
TUMOR RESECTED
ANTERIOR LONGITUDINAL LIGAMENT

FIGURE 36–13. Retrocrural tumor removed from posterior inferior mediastinal space after securing distal intercostal vessels at foramina L1 through T9.

TABLE 36–6. INDICATIONS FOR SURGERY AFTER CHEMOTHERAPY

	Indicated Surgery		
Finding	RPLND	Thoracotomy	Median Sternotomy
Residual abdominal mass on CT or ultrasound	+		
Retrocrural mass on CT	+	+/0	+/0
Unilateral parenchymal mass on WLT*		+	
Unilateral mediastinal mass on WLT		+	
Bilateral parenchymal or mediastinal masses			+
Elevated serum AFP	0	0	0
Elevated serum β-hCG	0	0	0

*WLT, whole lung tomogram; CT, computed axial tomogram.

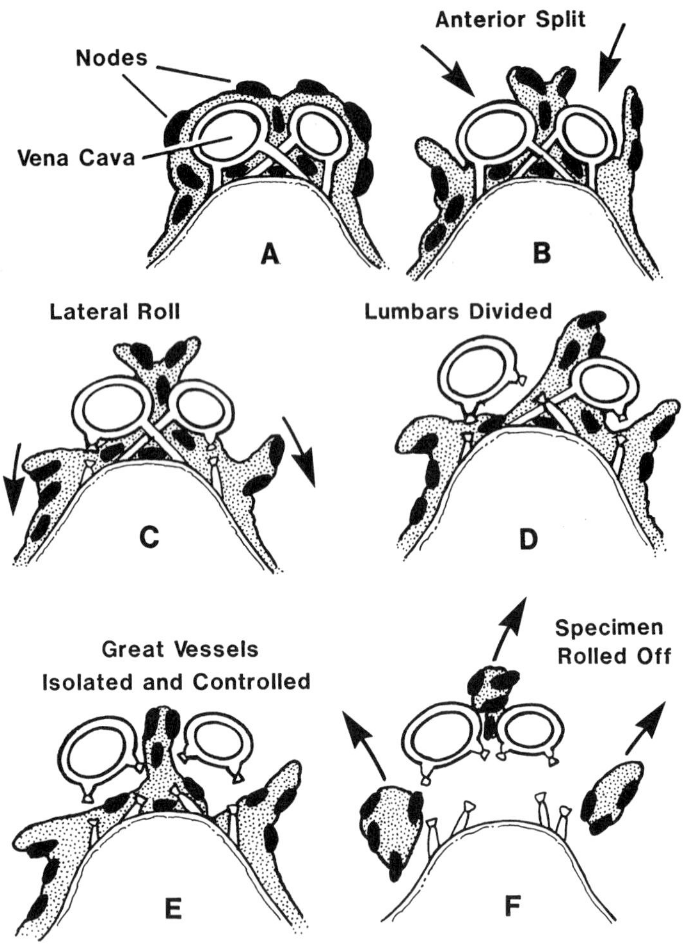
Anterior Split
Nodes
Vena Cava
A
B
Lateral Roll
Lumbars Divided
C
D
Great Vessels
Isolated and Controlled
Specimen
Rolled Off
E
F

FIGURE 36–14. Original description of the "split and roll" technique using axial view of great vessels. *A*, Before split. *B*, Anterior split at 12 o'clock on both inferior vena cava and aorta. *C*, Lateral "roll" of each lymphatic package to better expose lumbar vessel. *D*, Medial "roll" off each vessel permits completion of each lumbar vessel division. *E*, Once the lumbar vessels are divided, both great vessels are easily mobilized. *F*, Then, with great vessels isolated and free, the associated lymphatic packages are removed—"subtracted"—from the anterior spinous ligaments and lumbar foramina.

this rule: if the patient has exhausted all chemotherapeutic regimens that have any likelihood of success and has a limited focus of disease deemed resectable (Table 36–6).

The technical portions of the RPLND have been thoroughly described by Donohue et al.[19–21] (Figs. 36–14 through 36–17). A full bilateral RPLND is indicated in most cases. Tissue analysis from full RPLND specimens confirms the diverse nature of histologic change in these patients who have had widespread metastatic disease.[22] Therefore, a simple "lumpectomy" is a dangerous practice because it risks missing tumor elsewhere in the retroperitoneum. The "split and roll" technique in postchemotherapy dissections is essentially a vascular isolation (analogous to radiographic "subtraction" technique) and mobilization, permitting safe, complete, and reproducible postchemotherapy RPLND.

Results at Indiana University

Patients with either partial remission after primary chemotherapy or who had relapsed after primary therapy and had a partial response to salvage chemotherapy were present in all groups. There was roughly a two fifths/two fifths/one fifth division in the reported series among the findings of fibrotic-cystic-necrotic tissue (two fifths of cases), teratoma (two fifths), and carcinoma (one fifth).[23] This varies according to initial patient response (Table 36–7).

In general, the patients who have only necrotic or fibrocystic tissue at the time of exploration do well postoperatively. Table 36–8 outlines the outcomes of postchemotherapy surgery according to the histology of the tumor resected. Clearly, the necrosis group does best and the teratoma group does well. Those with persistent cancer (NSGCT) or sarcoma do less well, although many are still curable with a complete tumor resection.[16,24]

Technical Considerations in Postchemotherapy Dissection

Dissection of Bulky Nodal Disease

The requirements of retroperitoneal dissection sometimes extend to nodal disease that is para-aortic, retrocrural, and posterior mediastinal; such is the extension of the lymphatic drainage from the abdomen into the chest. Precrural tissues below the diaphragm consist largely of splenic lymphatic ganglia and nerves from the superior mesenteric

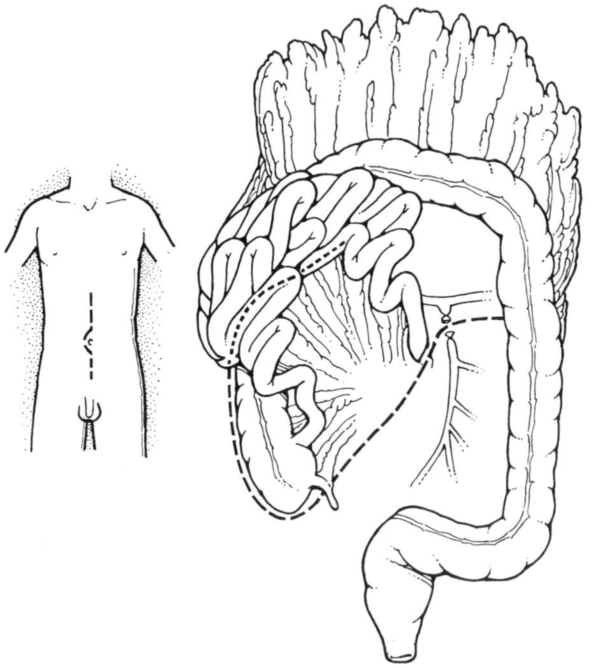

FIGURE 36–15. Mesenteric attachments of right colon and root of the small bowel can be divided to the ligament of Treitz. Dividing the inferior mesenteric vein facilitates mobilization of pancreas and cephalad retraction.

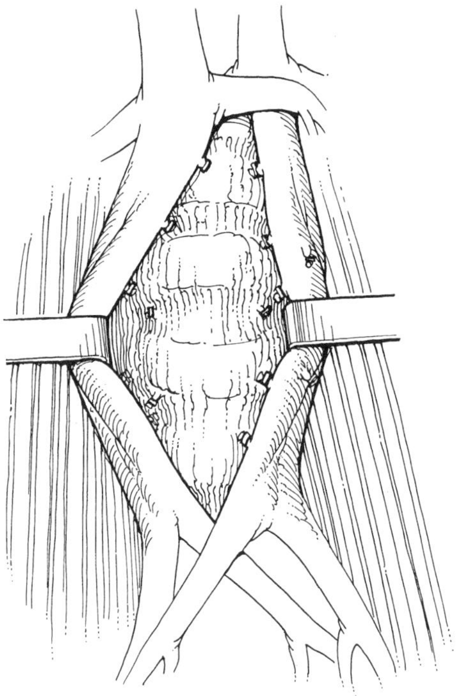

FIGURE 36–17. Original anterior view of completely mobilized great vessels, with lumbar vessels divided, retracted to show anterior spinous ligaments. The lymphatic package ± tumor has been "subtracted" from the retroperitoneal space.

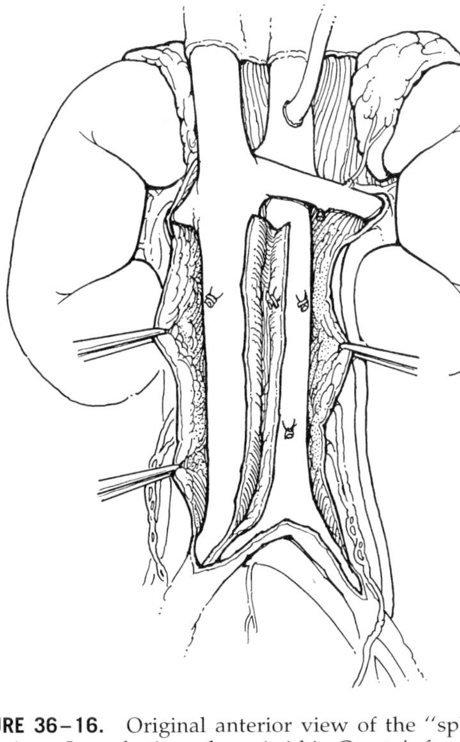

FIGURE 36–16. Original anterior view of the "split and roll" technique. Lymphatic package (within Gerota's fascia extending across vessels) is divided longitudinally at 12 o'clock over both great vessels. In this view the inferior mesenteric artery is also divided.

and celiac axes. Para-aortic tumor below the renal arteries for the most part will drain into the posterior mediastinum at the level of the renal arteries and through the aortic hiatus in the diaphragm. This hiatus is created by the right and left crus of the diaphragm, which insert on the anterior spinous ligaments around the aorta. The diaphragmatic fibers decussate superior to the celiac axis, and the aortic hiatus is thus created in something of an inverted U shape. The lymphatics course lateral and posterior to the aorta as it passes the diaphragm. Positive nodes in this area are quite reliably demonstrated by upper abdominal and chest CT scans. We reserve dissection there for only those patients who have demonstrated tumor following chemotherapy. It is inappropriate and unnecessary to dissect these retrocrural para-aortic nodes in low-stage disease.

The technique of this dissection is based upon the volume of disease. Those patients with bulky nodal disease require a thoracoabdominal approach. The choice of a right or left approach is dependent upon the distribution of nodes as viewed on the CT scan. All things being equal, the left thoracoabdominal approach through an eighth, ninth, or tenth interspace incision is usually adequate. For extremely large retrocrural or posterior mediastinal disease, we may resort to a thoracotomy several interspaces higher.

Figures 36–11 through 36–13 demonstrate the principles of dissection in this area, which are much

TABLE 36–7. HISTOLOGIC FINDINGS IN SURGERY AFTER CHEMOTHERAPY

Treatment	Fibrosis/ Necrosis	Teratoma	Cancer
Primary chemotherapy only	44%	44%	12%
Salvage chemotherapy (multiple courses for refractory disease)	10%	40%	50%

the same as the principles in the abdomen. First, the parietal pleura must be incised as well as the overlying fibers of the diaphragm as they condense to form the crus. This would then expose the lateral aspect of the aorta and the posterolateral nodal tissue, which can sometimes be fairly bulky. The parietal pleural incision is carried cephalad to the pulmonary hilum if necessary. Then the so-called split and roll technique is used to mobilize the aorta in the chest. We are mindful of the fact that the anterior spinal artery arises from the thoracic aorta cephalad to T8. Nonetheless, we have often divided the intercostals from this level through T12 bilaterally without any untoward effect on the spinal cord function. The point of these remarks is that the intercostal vessels must be prospectively identified and secured between ligatures and clips and then divided if the aorta is to be appropriately mobilized and elevated in the mediastinum. It is crucial to approach this posterolaterally. Only in this manner can the aorta be well visualized together with its intercostal posterior branches. An anterior sternal splitting incision is a very difficult and inappropriate approach to posterior mediastinal dissection, particularly in the inferior portion of the mediastinum. It is far better to approach this structure with a lateral thoracotomy combined with midline transperitoneal approach as needed.

If each intercostal segment can be secured with clips and ligatures, then the aorta can be elevated away from the posterior spinous ligament in Penrose drains, for example. This then will permit clearance of the posterior mediastinal nodal tissue, with attendant preservation of the aorta, esophagus, and contralateral crus, which can be visualized as the nodes are stripped off the anterior spinous ligaments. Occasionally, posterior passage of the vessels through the foramina T8–T12 requires electrocautery and/or suture ligation for control.

If the dissection is extensive, we then make no effort to reconstruct the pleura and simply close the chest in the traditional manner with insertion of a chest tube, which usually remains in place for several days depending upon the amount of chest drainage.

Several principles apply in the management of these patients postoperatively. Our treatment options are based upon the histopathology of the resected tissue. If there are still active malignant elements present in the tumor, two courses of salvage chemotherapy are indicated. If only teratoma or necrosis and scar tissue are found, we would then recommend close follow-up with interval CT scans of the chest at least semiannually, together with more frequent serum markers and chest films, usually on an every-2-months schedule.

Resection of the Great Vessels During Extensive Dissection

Although it is infrequently necessary, nonetheless extensive vascular repair and/or resection is sometimes required in the course of extended postchemotherapy testis tumor dissections. In most cases the tumor can be dissected from the great vessels with the usual "split and roll" technique; however, there are some occasions when the tumor actually involves the wall of the great vessel or, in the case of the venous system, actually invades the vessel as a tumor thrombus.

In approximately 500 postchemotherapy RPLNDs, we have had to resect the infrarenal vena cava 45

TABLE 36–8. OUTCOMES OF POSTCHEMOTHERAPY SURGERY BY TUMOR TYPE, 1975–1990

		Current Status*											
		NED		LWD		Unknown		DOD		DOp		DOC	
Tumor Type	Total Cases	N	%	N	%	N	%	N	%	N	%	N	%
Fibrosis-necrosis	150	139	92.7	2	1.3			8	5.3	1	0.7	0	
Teratoma	274	244	89.1	11	4	1	0.4	12	4.4	3	1.1	3†	1.1
Nonseminomatous germ cell tumor	121	63	52.1	11	9.1	1	0.8	41	33.9	5	4.1	0	
Non–germ cell tumor	13	5	38.5	1	0.8	4	30.7	3	23	0	0	0	0
TOTALS	558	451		25		6		64		9		3	

Overall survival: $\frac{\text{(NED + LWD)}}{\text{Total cases}} = \frac{476}{558} = 85\%$

Disease-free survival: $\frac{\text{NED}}{\text{Total cases}} = \frac{451}{558} = 81\%$

*NED, no evidence of disease; LWD, living with disease; DOD, died of disease; DOp, died of operative complications; DOC, died of other causes.
†Two testis-negative patients (0.7%) died of unrelated causes and one patient (0.4%) died of another malignancy.

times. In most of these cases the cava was directly involved with tumor thrombus. In the early years we resected several cavae with active tumor thrombus from extensive retroperitoneal tumor prior to chemotherapy. In more recent years this problem has been largely eliminated with prior chemotherapy for extensive bulky disease, which has a marked cytoreductive effect. Occasionally, however, we still have tumor thrombus in the cava in the form of necrotic tumor covered by fibrous thrombus and/or teratoma. In fact, on two occasions, despite salvage chemotherapy for relapsing advanced disease, active tumor with malignant elements has been found as intracaval tumor thrombus.

Caval resection should not be undertaken lightly because there is significant morbidity with this procedure. The morbidity referred to is not only immediate venous congestion of the lower extremities, but also continued extravasation of lymphatic tissue into a third space (i.e., retroperitoneum). In analyzing our postoperative complications, we have noted a greater frequency of abdominal ascites in patients who have had their cavae resected. Therefore, abdominal ascites is an added risk factor in any patient who has the cava resected.[25,26]

The technique of caval resection is relatively simple. The vena cava is mobilized by dividing the various lumbar tributaries and mobilizing it as completely as possible in the infrarenal area. Usually there are several major lumbar vessels just below the level of the renal vessels, and these need to be secured in order to obtain a good 360-degree clearance. Normally we use the vascular staple clamp for this, but these vessels can also be oversewn with any vascular suture material in a continuous suture while controlled in vascular clamps.

The distal extent of the caval resection should be as limited as possible. When possible, it is preferable to leave the iliac veins intact. This is not always possible, however, and on occasion we have resected the venous structure below the hypogastric venous entry (i.e., at the external iliac level). This simply compounds the felony of lower extremity venous stasis and lymphedema, which gradually reverse. The major morbidity once again is the risk of transient abdominal ascites in these patients, presumably secondary to massive alternate lymphatic drainage along the body wall with leakage into a large third space created by the dissection. The absence of venous connections for lymphatic drainage is probably the culprit in such cases.

In this same cohort of postchemotherapy RPLND patients, we have had to use interposition aortic or tube grafts or bifurcated aortoiliac grafts in nine patients. One of these was done on an emergent basis in a patient who ruptured his aorta while in the recovery room after an extended subadventitial dissection hours earlier. Fortunately, he was rescued and had a remarkably smooth postoperative course. The other four were done in a planned manner because of evident aortic involvement with tumor during the RPLND procedure itself. In each of these remaining four cases, it was apparent that the aortic wall was so heavily involved and so damaged by the tumor dissection that it would be best replaced. The decision can be made more easily if the dissection is clearly required in the subadventitial plane and the aortic wall is pale, "cheesy," and poorly controlled with suture ligature. In such patients, it is safer to simply resect the involved segment and replace it with an interposition Dacron tube graft. In each of the five cases, the patients did very well postoperatively.

The technique is essentially the same as in aortic aneurysm repair. Care is taken to develop a safe cuff below the renal arteries, which is virtually always possible in testis tumor cases. In none of the five cases was a shunt necessary for aortic involvement in the suprarenal area. Usually we use a running 4-0 Prolene suture to anastomose the tube graft, which has been sized and preclotted. Of course, the distal limb of the dissection must also be prepared at the time of the interposition graft so as to minimize the distal ischemic time. Once again, 360-degree continuous 4-0 Prolene suture is suitable for the distal anastomosis. Care is taken to backflush the graft by removal of the distal clamps first and then, under low-pressure conditions, to review the integrity of the graft itself and the connections. Following this, the cephalad clamp is removed and additional hemostasis can then be obtained at the suture line. Normally this is unnecessary, and simple digital occlusion and time are all that is needed for hemostasis. Depending on the extent of the time required, heparinization is used and then reversed with protamine. Normally we use 1 mg/kg heparin and reverse it with about two thirds that dose of protamine. In the event of a patch graft or a relative brief clamping, no heparinization at all is required.

Based on these experiences, it is prudent to attempt the dissection in the extra-adventitial plane whenever possible. This should obviate the need for grafting.

Review of the Role of Postchemotherapy Surgery

Figure 36–10 provides an algorithm of the progress of a patient who presents with advanced stage III or advanced abdominal disease. Normally platinum-based consolidation chemotherapy is given to reduce or eliminate the tumor burden and then the patient is reevaluated. If the tumor burden has been eliminated to the extent that a complete remission is obtained, then fewer patients will relapse. Furthermore, they tend to relapse in the chest, and therefore retroperitoneal lymphadenectomy is unnecessary in someone who has a truly negative clinical CT scan of the abdomen *after* completion of chemotherapy. Among our relapses in this group, only one in four patients actually relapsed in the belly. Therefore, retroperitoneal lymphadenectomy in this group is unwarranted *if* they have a solid, complete remission after chemotherapy. Unfortunately, approximately 30% of the patients do not obtain complete remission. These are the patients who require postchemotherapy surgery. Whether the tumor is in the chest or belly, any residual mass lesion following chemotherapy should be excised for both histologic assessment and assignment of further therapy in the event of persistent malignant elements. The approach to patients with advanced disease after chemotherapy has been extensively described.[20,21]

Those patients with bulky teratomatous tumors remain difficult problems, particularly if their tumor is massive and even more so if it contains abundant immature elements. The significance of this resected teratoma and its relapse potential are the subjects of much interest and current study. Regression analysis studies reveal that site, tumor burden, and histology of the surgical specimen are the primary factors in postchemotherapy relapse in teratoma patients.[18] There is also a significant difference between small versus moderate versus massive disease resected postchemotherapy. Those patients with the most massive disease relapse most commonly. Usually relapse is outside the field of resection, but it is also not uncommon to have relapse occur within the dissected field, particularly related to posterior body wall foramina, gastrointestinal viscera, or deep pelvic or mediastinal nodes.

Finally, patients with cancer in the histology of the surgical specimen represent a more difficult group because they have not responded as well to prior chemotherapy. If the resecton is complete, they still have a fair chance of cure with the addition of salvage chemotherapy. One of the most difficult subsets in this histologic analysis are those patients with sarcomatous elements in the resected surgical specimen. Analysis reveals these patients to be at particularly high risk for relapse. Ulbright et al.[27] have described such non–germ cell elements as adenocarcinoma and embryonal rhabdomyosarcoma in these tumors. Of interest is the fact that in most cases these non–germ cell elements were found in the primary tumors. Of 10 cases, 7 were found to have foci of non-germ cell elements coexistent with the primary testicular.

The heterogeneity among germ cell tumors in the testis is becoming well recognized.[28] New insights are provided by study of tumors resected following chemotherapy. In reviewing 269 cases of teratoma

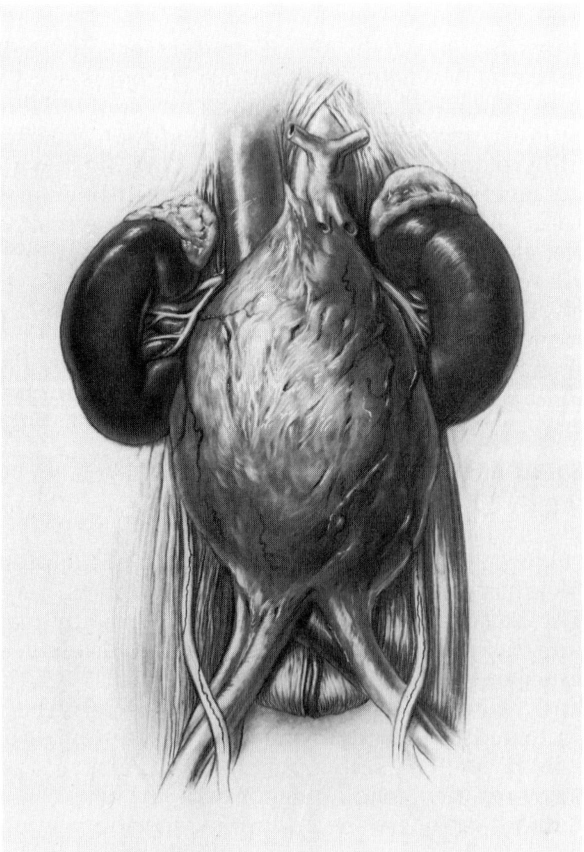

FIGURE 36–18. Anterior view of bulky residual tumor in a postchemotherapy patient; note its relationships, enveloping the great vessels.

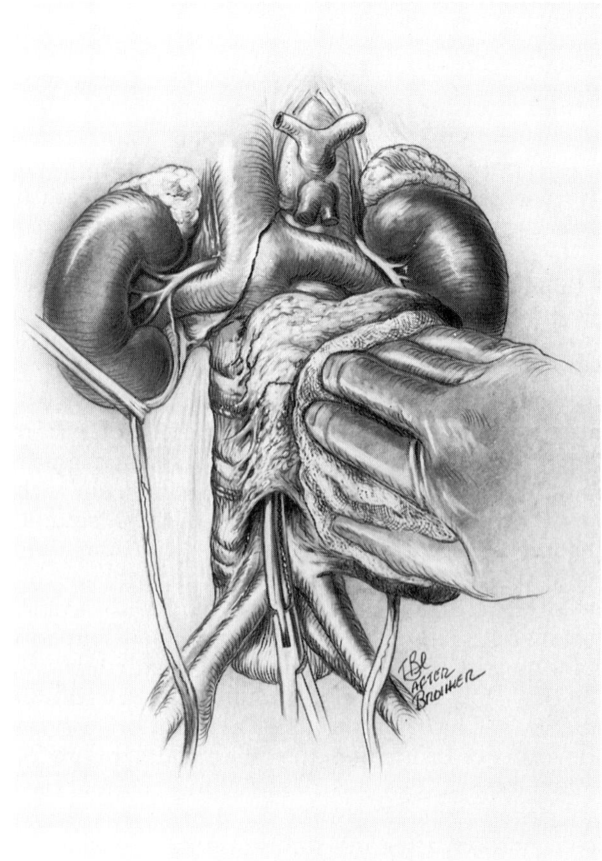

FIGURE 36–19. A clamp is introduced in the adventitial space around the vena cava. By splitting tissue (e.g., with electrocautery), the tumor can be rolled off the vessel and lumbar vessels exposed, ligated, and divided.

seen at Indiana University Medical Center from 1974 to 1982, 11 patients with NSGCT were found to have elements of non–germ cell malignancies as noted previously. Apparently platinum-based combination chemotherapy eliminated the more sensitive germ cell elements in these metastatic tumors, unmasking the remaining non–germ cell elements, which persisted following chemotherapy.

The technique of resecting the retroperitoneum following chemotherapy is also well described in earlier publications.[20,21] Figures 36–18 through 36–21 show the basic strategy of postchemotherapy RPLND for residual bulk disease. Not only should the tumor itself be excised, but tissues within the original retroperitoneal template of nodal drainage from the testis should be removed as well. Normally the exposure is the same as that described for low-stage disease. In most cases, not only is the root of the small bowel mesentery incised, but also the posterior attachments to the cecum and the mesocolon of the right side are divided and bowel is mobilized up and away from the anterior aspect of Gerota's fascia and placed on the chest in a bowel bag. Also, it is common to need additional exposure in such cases. Therefore, we usually divide the inferior mesenteric vein between silk ligatures and then mobilize the left colonic mesentery. We also usually divide the inferior mesenteric artery so as to complete this mobilization of the left colonic mesentery and retract this away from the tumor and the retroperitoneal nodes. Of course, most of these patients will have their lumbar postganglionic fibers dissected in the preaortic dissection in this area and will not be able to ejaculate if they have a very complete dissection in the lower periaortic zone. (This is quite the opposite from current nerve-sparing techniques in low-stage disease, wherein ejaculation is preserved.)

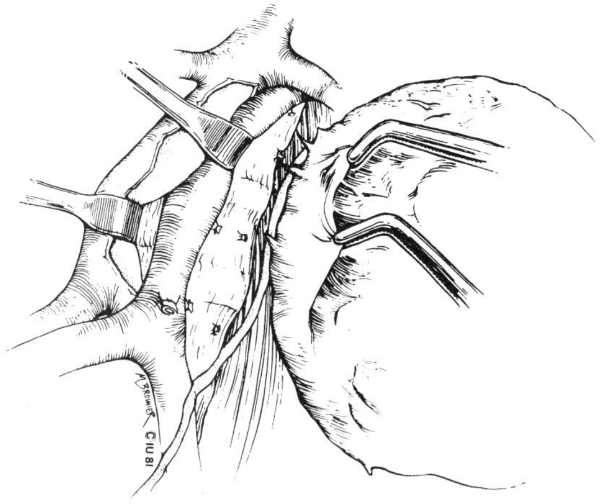

FIGURE 36–21. The tumor has been freed from both great vessels. Now it must be swept off the anterior spinous ligaments, the lumbar foramina must be secured, and the ipsilateral ureter dissected free from the tumor.

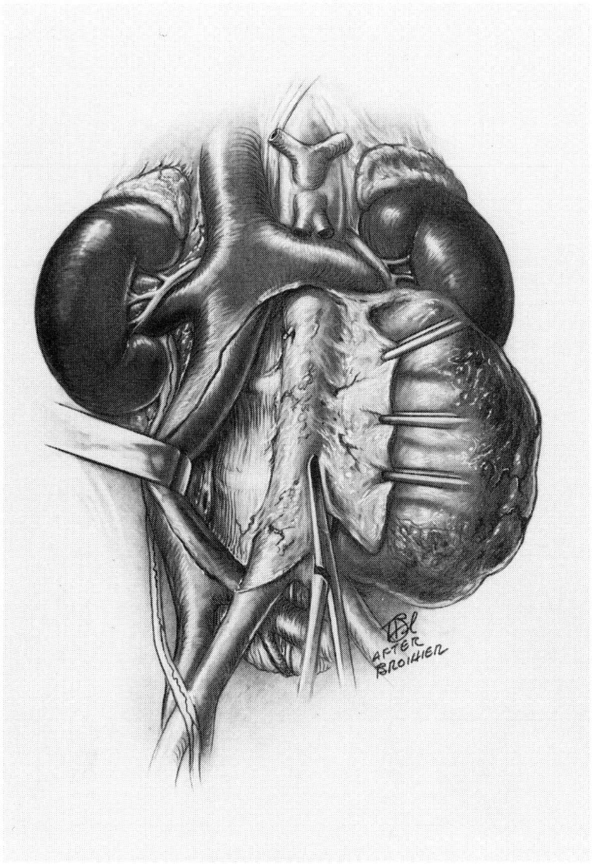
AFTER BROIHIER

FIGURE 36–20. Similarly, the aorta can be mobilized using this "split and roll" technique throughout its length. Note division of inferior mesenteric artery, which is often necessary when dissecting bulky para-aortic tumors.

A basic strategy is to begin anterior to the great vessels, again either in the iliac or left renal venous area. The longitudinal split is made over the great vessels, sometimes with the need to retract tumor laterally as one does so. It is usually helpful to divide the lumbar vessels so as to better retract the great vessels off and away from the tumor. At length, if all the lumbar vessels are divided and the vessels elevated from the tumor, the tumor can then be resected from the posterior body wall. At this point the lumbar vessels are controlled at the foramina with clips and/or suture ligatures. Bovie cautery using an extender if necessary is usually helpful in these postchemotherapy dissections. Figures 36–14 through 36–21 illustrate this.

Another special consideration is the presence of suprahilar disease. This can take two forms. Direct extension from a massive infrahilar tumor may project into the suprahilar zone. In this case, it is usually precrural and can be rolled down and away from the great vessels. Occasionally it must be removed en bloc, with one kidney or the other being basically inseparable from the renal hilum. The usual lymph flow into the chest from the retroperitoneum is periaortic and posterior. CT scans have shown that the majority of suprahilar positive-scan disease is in the retrocrural zone. As this becomes larger, it becomes more expedient to do a thoracoabdominal approach. This reflects the essential nature of a posterior mediastinal fixed tumor. However, with early and low-bulk involvement, this part of the dissection can still be done well through the anterior approach even if it requires splitting the crus for a few centimeters. This can always be repaired by direct suture reapproximation of the crura and the posterior ligamentous attachments of the spine. The cysterna chyli is based anywhere from L1 to T10 in the posterior periaortic retrocrural space, together with the azygos and hemiazygos venous systems, and can usually be recognized as such. It must be handled with great care and suture ligated and/or clipped at its base so as to avoid leakage and subsequent ascites. About 1% of advanced cases will develop postoperative ascites, which can usually be managed conservatively with hyperalimentation and then oral feedings with a medium- and short-chain triglyceride diet. Surgical intervention with peritoneal venous shunting, for example, is a rarely needed alternative to conservative management.

Concerning high-stage disease, the selection of cases for surgery depends on clinical studies. One could argue that CT scan is much too insensitive in these postchemotherapy patients. In fact, its analysis suggests there would be only two abdominal relapses out of every 100 patients with clinically positive retroperitoneal tumor who have actually achieved a complete remission with chemotherapy.[29] These patients can be detected in due course with close follow-up and repeat CT scans. This is quite different from the clinical stage I patients who have not had chemotherapy; in the best of hands, 30% of this group will have positive nodes. Furthermore, without prior chemotherapy, the relapse in this group tends to be rapid and fulminating. Relapse in the postchemotherapy group is usually represented by a slower presentation if the relapse is in the retroperitoneum. Therefore, our own practice is to permit clinical staging in postchemotherapy patients to direct selection of patients for surgery. Those with a radiographic lesion in the retroperitoneum are scheduled for full bilateral retroperitoneal lymphadenectomy. Those stage III patients who become completely negative are followed with interval CT scans (about every 3 months in the first year postchemotherapy, every 4 to 6 months in the second year, and yearly thereafter for those enjoying a continuous complete remission). The same is true for chest disease.[17] We resect persistent radiographic lesions and give salvage chemotherapy for those with any residual malignancy in the resected specimen.[30] If there is scar, necrosis, or simple teratoma in the resected specimen, we believe that salvage chemotherapy can be withheld. At the present time it is unclear to us whether those patients with abundant immature elements in their resected teratoma should have further or salvage chemotherapy. To this point we have chosen to withhold further chemotherapy and treat those who do relapse with chemotherapy or surgery at that time. Teratoma seems to be a surgical problem rather than a medical one.[16,24,31]

All things considered, postchemotherapy surgery for metastatic testis cancer represents a great surgical challenge. This is never more true than when the surgeon is presented with extended abdominal and chest disease. Demands for safe and thorough tumor removal are both great and exacting.

Complications of Postchemotherapy Dissection

Two reports in the literature have discussed the complications of postchemotherapy lymph node dissections in sizable groups of patients.[32,33] The rate of complications seems to be proportionately related to the bulk of disease present. This is evidenced by an overall combined complication rate of 12% in patients undergoing primary retroperitoneal lymph node dissection for stage A, B1, or B2 disease versus an overall complication rate of 25% in those patients initially presenting with stage B or C disease who have undergone postchemotherapy RPLND. The death rate in the low-stage disease patients was 0.3%, whereas the death rate in the high-stage postchemotherapy node dissection patients was 3%. Of the complications, approximately one half were minor and one half were major. Although there were major complications, only a small percentage of these required reoperation. Virtually all of the deaths in the postchemotherapy node dissection group were related to complications of the previous chemotherapy, notably compromise in pulmonary function.[34] This finding of compromised pulmonary function with a decrease in the diffusion capacity and a restrictive defect as well has been noted by others.[24] In the more recent cases at the author's institution, there have been no pulmonary-related deaths in the last 3 years.

Although there is a significant complication rate and a mortality rate now of less than 3%, the ben-

TABLE 36–9. PRIMARY RPLND COMPLICATIONS, 1982–1992 (478 PATIENTS)

Complication	Total	Minor	Major
Wound infection	23	11	12
Small bowel obstruction	11	1	10
Atelectasis/pneumonitis	10	1	9
Urinary tract infection	3	1	2
Ascites (chylous)	1	—	1
Lymphocele	1	—	1
Pancreatitis	1	—	1
Other			
Rectus sheath hematoma	1	1	—
Scrotal hematoma	1	—	1
Ureteral injury	1	1	—
Ventral postoperative hernia	1	—	1

TABLE 36–10. COMPLICATIONS: 1982–1986 VERSUS 1987–1992

	1982–1986 (164 Patients)			1987–1992 (314 Patients)			
	Minor	Major	Total	Minor	Major	Total	
Wound infection	6	6	12 (8%)	5	6	11 (3.5%)	$p<0.004$
Small bowel obstruction	—	8	8 (4.8%)	1	2	3 (0.9%)	$p<0.007$
Atelectasis/pneumonitis	1	5	6 (3.2%)	—	4	4 (1.2%)	$p<0.08$
Urinary tract infection	3	—	3	—	—	—	
Ascites	—	1	1	—	—	—	
Lymphocele	—	1	1	—	—	—	
Pancreatitis	—	1	1	—	—	—	
Other	—	1	1	2	1	3	

efit gained from reassessment of the patient after four courses of chemotherapy far outweighs the risks. The reassessment of the patient's pathologic status at that point allows appropriate follow-up or additional treatment for the patient.

We have reviewed the surgical complications of RPLND for low-stage (I and II) disease to update our prior report of 1981[32] (Table 36–9). There is a significant reduction in the incidence over the course of time related to experience (Table 36–10) and also related to the extent of the procedure done (Table 36–11). Cost-benefit and risk-benefit analyses become possible with this detailed information.

Usually all patients who have had a primary RPLND are seen back at the Medical Center by a urologist and medical oncologist approximately 3 to 4 weeks after surgery. Beginning with this first checkup, chest x-rays and serum marker measurements are obtained monthly for the first year. A physical examination with particular emphasis on recurrent abdominal masses and inguinal, axillary, or cervical adenopathy is performed on an every-other-month basis. After the first year has passed, the testing and physical examination can be decreased in frequency. During this second year, the chest x-rays and serum marker measurements are performed every other month and physical examinations every 3 to 4 months. At the end of 2 years the patient can be followed on a semiannual or annual basis. The one exception to this is the patient who has had teratoma in a specimen obtained at surgery after chemotherapy. In this group of patients there seems to be a subset that are prone to having late relapses, as long as 5 or more years after surgery. For these patients prolonged follow-up is recommended. Because the recurrence of teratoma is often at the margins of resection in the retroperitoneum, a CT scan on an annual basis is recommended for at least the first 5 postoperative years. Axial imaging is an important part of the follow-up in postchemotherapy patients. The frequency of these scans depends on the clinical situation.

CURRENT PROBLEMS AND FUTURE PROSPECTS

Although great progress has been made in the management of germ cell cancer, there are a number of issues that remain difficult and not completely resolved. These are discussed here in the order of clinical stage.

Clinical Stage I

The management of the patient with nonseminomatous germ cell tumor postorchiectomy has been generally a "local option" according to the

TABLE 36–11. COMPLICATIONS: FULL BILATERAL DISSECTION VERSUS MODIFIED TEMPLATE ± NERVE-SPARING DISSECTION

	Full Bilateral (62 Patients)			Modified Template (416 Patients)		
	Minor	Major	Total	Minor	Major	Total
Wound infection	1	4	5 (8%)	10	8	18 (4.3%)
Small bowel obstruction	—	3	3 (4.8%)	1	7	8 (2%)
Atelectasis/pneumonitis	—	2	2 (3.2%)	1	7	8 (2%)
Urinary tract infection	1	—	1	2	—	2
Ascites	—	—	—	—	1	1
Lymphocele	—	—	—	—	1	1
Pancreatitis	—	1	1	—	—	—
Other	—	1	1	2	1	3

customs and experience of the region. For example, in the United Kingdom, radiotherapy for low-stage disease was abandoned in favor of surveillance in the 1980s. In the United States, RPLND was practiced as both a staging and a therapeutic maneuver, the therapeutic aspects being confined to those patients with pathologic stage II disease.

Our current problem with clinical stage I disease is the assignment of primary management relative to risk of relapse. A major contribution was the study from the MRC Group in the United Kingdom, clearly relating risk factors based on the primary histology of the testis tumor.[35,36] This has now led to the pre-emptive use of chemotherapy in the high-risk clinical stage I group, recognizing, of course, that virtually half or more of the patients will never relapse (thus such management constitutes overtreatment and needless toxicity for that cohort destined not to relapse). Those at very low risk for relapse are followed with surveillance, and there is general agreement on this. In the United States, the most common approach is to do a modified or nerve-sparing RPLND in clinical stage I patients, recognizing that it becomes merely a staging procedure in the 70% of patients who indeed turn out to be pathologic stage I also. Therefore, the unsolved problem in clinical stage I relates to the insensitivity (30%) and nonspecificity (about 20%) of clinical staging. The issue of nonspecificity is particularly worrisome. Nearly one fifth of patients with suspicious CTs or lymphography will indeed be pathologic stage I. Pre-emptive chemotherapy on the basis of clinical risk is particularly unfortunate in this group. The answers shall be forthcoming as ongoing development of statistical models of cost-benefit and risk-benefit is completed.

Clinical Stage II

Again, the initial management of clinical stage II remains somewhat imperfect and controversial. In areas wedded to the primary chemotherapy approach, the survival data are excellent, but the total toxicity of treatment and ultimate requirement for surgical treatment as well in about 20 to 30% of patients remain cause for concern. Conversely, modified RPLND will provide accurate retroperitoneal staging, but the requirement for double therapy in about 30% of patients is a concern. This was the subject of a prospective randomized study[29] that supports the view that a patient with clinical stage BII is at relatively high risk for relapse (50%), whereas a patient with clinical stage BI is at much less risk of relapse (15 to 30%). Thus the question of management of these pathologic stage II patients post-RPLND is not perfectly solved. It is fair enough to say that adjuvant chemotherapy is not a requirement but, if elected, a relapse can be reliably prevented. The issue of relating the decision to the nodal histology is not perfectly resolved. Generally, those patients with tumors with undifferentiated elements that were embryonal or seminomatous are more amenable than those with primary teratoma.

Another continuing question is "How big is big?" Again, this is a function of local decision making and experience. In many areas in the United States, tumors above 3 cm are considered to be stage BII and, therefore, suitable for primary chemotherapy, particularly in those patients with basically embryonal or seminomatous components in the primary. Those patients with basically teratomatous components in the primary should probably proceed to RPLND in settings where this is available.

Clinical Stage III

Definition of risk status and segregation of high-risk patients into a more aggressive primary chemotherapy regimen remain unsolved problems. The choice of the drug delivery schedules and selections remains a subject of debate. Also, the corollary of this issue is being actively studied: What is the minimal chemotherapy for good-risk patients? Although there is general agreement that more aggressive primary chemotherapy schedules are indicated for high-risk patients, the role of autologous bone marrow transplant is most difficult to determine, and this procedure is also a very expensive proposition. Another unsolved problem is the definition of a "safe" partial remission versus an "unsafe" partial remission. Many experienced clinicians believe there are some predictive criteria related to response rate and primary histology that allow clinical speculation as to who may be safely followed with clinical studies as opposed to operated for resection of a partial remission. Also, the management of refractory disease (i.e., persistent serologic positive) is undergoing re-evaluation. A number of centers have noticed that surgical excision of a locally persistent refractory tumor may provide better and more immediate results than continued chemotherapy, with the provision that the disease be localized enough to be surgically resectable.[24]

The management of the histologic cancer subset following postchemotherapy RPLND is being distinguished more carefully. Those patients who have completed only primary chemotherapy are apparently benefited by salvage chemotherapy postoperatively. However, those who have already received salvage chemotherapy and who still have cancer in their resected specimen may well be managed expectantly postoperatively as opposed to undergoing still more "salvage" chemotherapy. Our own experience would suggest that the cancer subset in the postchemotherapy setting dose indeed require a distinction between those who have had only primary chemotherapy versus those who have already had extensive salvage chemotherapy.[24] Although some of the latter may be curable with surgery, it appears that additional salvage in this subset may be of little avail. Another concern is the timing and extent of postchemotherapy surgery. There seems to be a limited role for nerve-sparing techniques in those patients with low-volume, lateralized disease. Also, our own retrospective analysis of risk factors suggests that volume, sites, and histologic non–germ cell elements are major factors in prediction of relapse.[18]

Of great concern and as yet unsolved is the management of extragonadal germ cell tumors, which are biologically more difficult and less responsive to chemotherapy. At this point, the patient's best hope for a cure is a simple complete surgical resection.

The management of carcinoma in situ remains a difficult clinical and social question. Although there is general agreement about the "high-risk" contralateral testis (soft, small, undescended, and hypofertile), the management of a contralateral testis that is not apparently a high risk remains controversial relative to the requirement for initial testicular biopsy. Because the progression rate is 2 to 3% for a second testicular solid tumor, and because the disease-specific death rate from these second tumors is extremely low, there has been a general expectant attitude in the clinical management of NSGCT in the normal-risk patient. Emphasis has been placed on self-examination in such cases. Nevertheless, it remains very well demonstrated that those patients destined to develop a second testis primary are to be found among the 5% of patients with contralateral carcinoma in situ. Should they be biopsied and treated initially? How? The intriguing question remains: "What happens to the 2 to 3% of patients with carcinoma in situ that never progresses to a phenotypic solid tumor?"

REFERENCES

1. Donohue JP, Zachary JM, Maynard SD: Distribution of nodal metastases in nonseminomatous testicular cancer. J Urol 1982; 128:315.
2. Ray B, Hajdu SI, Whitmore WF Jr: Distribution of retroperitoneal lymph node metastases in testicular germinal tumors. Cancer 1974; 33:340.
3. Weisbach L, Boedefield E: Localization of solitary and multiple metastases in stage II nonseminomatous testis tumor as a basis for a modified staging lymph node dissection in stage I. J Urol 1982; 138:77.
4. Pizzocaro G, Salvioni R, Zononi F: Unilateral lymphadenectomy in intraoperative stage I nonseminomatous germinal testis cancer. J Urol 1985; 134:485.
5. Richie JP: Clinical stage I testicular cancer: the role of modified retroperitoneal lymphadenectomy. J Urol 1990; 144: 1160.
6. Jewett MA, Kong YP, Goldberg SD, et al: Retroperitoneal lymphadenectomy for testicular tumor with nerve-sparing for ejaculation. J Urol 1988; 139:1220.
7. Narayan P, Lang P, Fraley EE: Ejaculation and fertility after extended retroperitoneal lymph node dissection for testicular cancer. World J Urol 1982; 127:685.
8. Colleselli K, Poisel S, Schachtner W, et al: Nerve-preserving bilateral retroperitoneal lymphadenectomy: anatomical study and operative approach. J Urol 1990; 144:293.
9. Donohue JP, Foster RS, Rowland RG, et al: Nerve-sparing retroperitoneal lymphadenectomy with preservation of ejaculation. J Urol 1988; 139:206A; J Urol 1990; 144:287.
10. Foster RS, Donohue JP: Surgical treatment of clinical stage A nonseminomatous testis cancer. Semin Oncol 1992; 19: 166.
11. Whitelaw GP, Smithwick RH: Some secondary effects of sympathectomy with particular reference to the disturbance of sexual function. N Engl J Med 1951; 245:121.
12. Jones DR, Norman AR, Horwich A, Hendry WF: Ejaculatory dysfunction after retroperitoneal lymphadenectomy. Eur Urol 1993; 23:169.
13. Leiter E, Brendler H: Loss of ejaculation following bilateral retroperitoneal lymphadenectomy. J Urol 1967; 98:375.
14. Brenner J, Vurgin D, Whitmore WF Jr: Effect of treatment on fertility and sexual function in males with metastatic nonseminomatous germ cell tumors of testis. Am J Clin Oncol 1985; 8:178.
15. Drasga RE, Einhorn LE, Williams SD, et al: Fertility after chemotherapy for testicular cancer. J Clin Oncol 1983; 1: 179.
16. Murphy BR, Breeden ES, Donohue JP, et al: Surgical salvage of chemorefractory germ cell tumors. J Clin Oncol 1993; 11:324.
17. Donohue JP, Rowland RG, Kopecky KK, et al: Correlation of computerized tomographic changes and histologic findings in eighty patients having radical retroperitoneal lymph node dissection after chemotherapy for testis cancer. J Urol 1987; 137:1176.
18. Loehrer PJ, Williams SD, Clark SA, et al: Teratoma following chemotherapy for nonseminomatous germ cell tumor (NSGCT): a clinicopathologic correlation. J Urol 1986; 135: 1183.
19. Donohue JP, Einhorn LH, Williams SD: Cytoreductive surgery for metastatic testis cancer: considerations of timing and extent. J Urol 1980; 123:876.
20. Donohue JP: Surgical management of testis cancer. *In* Einhorn LE (ed): Testicular Tumors—Management and Treatment, p 29–46. New York, Masson Publishing, 1980.
21. Donohue JP, Rowland RG, Bihrle R: Transabdominal retroperitoneal lymph node dissection. *In* Skinner DG, Leiskovsky G (eds): Diagnosis and Management of Genitourinary Cancer, p 802. Philadelphia, WB Saunders Co, 1988.
22. Donohue JP, Roth LM, Zachary JM, et al: Cytoreductive surgery for metastatic testis cancer: tissue analysis of retroperitoneal masses after chemotherapy. J Urol 1982; 127: 1111.
23. Donohue JP, Rowland RG: The role of surgery in advanced testicular cancer. Cancer 1984; 54:2716.
24. Fox EP, Weathers TD, Williams SD, et al: Outcome analysis for patients with persistent non-teratomatous germ cell tumor in post chemotherapy retroperitoneal lymph node dissections. J Clin Oncol 1993; 11:1294.
25. Donohue JB, Thornhill J, Foster R, et al: Resection of the inferior vena cava or intraluminal thrombectomy during retroperitoneal lymph node disection for metastatic germ cell cancer: indications and results. J Urol 1991; 146:346.
26. Baniel J, Foster R, Rowland R, et al: Complications of post chemotherapy retroperitoneal lymph node dissection. J Urol 1995: 153:976.
27. Ulbright TM, Loehrer PJ, Roth LM, et al: The development of non-germ cell malignancies within germ cell tumors: a clinicopathologic study of 11 cases. Cancer 1984; 54:1824.
28. Loehrer PJ, Sledge GW, Einhorn LH: Heterogeneity among germ cell tumors of the testis. Semin Oncol 1985; 12:304.
29. Williams S, Stablien D, Einhorn L, et al: Immediate adjuvant chemotherapy versus observation with treatment of relapse in pathological stage II testicular cancer. N Engl J Med 1987; 317:1433.
30. Mandelbaum I, Williams SD, Einhorn LH: Aggressive surgical management of testicular carcinoma metastatic to lungs and mediastinum. Ann Thorac Surg 1980; 30:224.

31. Einhorn LH, Williams SD: The management of disseminated testicular cancer. *In* Einhorn LH (ed): Testicular Tumors—Management and Treatment, pp 117–149. New York, Masson Publishing, 1980.
32. Donohue JP, Rowland RG: Complications of retroperitoneal lymph node dissection. J Urol 1981; 125:338.
33. Skinner GD, Melamed A, Lieskovsky G: Complications of thoracoabdominal retroperitoneal lymph node dissection. J Urol 1982; 127:1107.
34. Rowland RG, Moorthy SS, Donohue JP: Anesthetic considerations for post chemotherapy radical retroperitoneal lymph node dissection. Paper presented at the North Central Section American Urological Association meeting, Marco Island, FL, 1982.
35. Freedman LS, Jones WG, Peckham MJ, et al: Histopathology in the prediction of relapse of patients with stage I testicular teratoma treated by orchidectomy alone. Lancet 1987; 2:294.
36. Hosking P, Dilly S, Easton D, et al: Prognostic factors in stage I nonseminomatous germ cell testicular tumors managed by orchidectomy and surveillance: implications for adjuvant chemotherapy. J Clin Oncol 1986; 4:1031.

VIII

RETROPERITONEUM

37

RETROPERITONEAL TUMORS: DIAGNOSIS, STAGING, SURGERY, MANAGEMENT, AND PROGNOSIS

S. BRUCE MALKOWICZ, M.D.

Retroperitoneal tumors (primarily sarcomas) in the adult are rare and account for less than 0.5 to 1.0% of adult malignancies. Sarcomas of distinct urinary tract origin are even less common. These lesions, although uncommon, tend to be dramatic in their clinical presentation and repeatedly raise questions regarding their appropriate evaluation and treatment. Unlike rare lesions, which are studied in a systematic fashion, primary retroperitoneal tumors of soft tissue and urologic origin are generally reported in small- to moderate-size clinical series that extend over an appreciable period of time. Furthermore, such lesions are often lumped together with soft tissue sarcomas of the extremities when data are presented.

The pooled data from multiple series have provided some insight into the major determinants of the clinical behavior of primary retroperitoneal sarcomas, and the collective surgical experience with these lesions allows for a rational approach to the clinical assessment and technical treatment of these tumors. Surgery remains the foundation for the treatment of primary soft tissue retroperitoneal sarcomas, and total extirpation of the tumor with negative surgical margins is the ideal goal. At the present time, the completeness of the surgical resection and low tumor grade remain the primary determinants of successful long-term outcome. Although the urologic oncologist will not encounter such lesions frequently, it is important to be well versed in the general pathology, clinical assessment, and surgical approach to these soft tissue sarcomas.

The roles of radiation therapy and chemotherapy have been better defined in the treatment of extremity soft tissue sarcomas, yet their place in the treatment of retroperitoneal tumors in either the neoadjuvant, adjuvant, or advanced disease setting has yet to be established. Recent chemotherapy and radiation series have defined the toxicity and therapeutic efficacy of these treatment modalities in retroperitoneal sarcomas.

Although genitourinary sarcomas are exceedingly rare, their incidence patterns, modes of presentation and clinical responsiveness can be demonstrated by the available data. While radical extirpation is the general rule for therapy, in some instances, particularly urinary bladder sarcoma, other therapeutic options do exist. A general assessment of the effectiveness of secondary therapy on these sarcomas can also be made.

PRIMARY RETROPERITONEAL SARCOMA

Incidence and Etiology

Retroperitoneal sarcomas are rare tumors that account for only 0.1 to 0.2% of all malignant tumors and approximately 10 to 20% of all soft tissue sarcomas.[1] Less than one half of all retroperitoneal tumors are retroperitoneal sarcomas. Generally 15 to 20% of retroperitoneal tumors are benign (e.g., lipoma). The remainder are composed of lymphomas or primary urologic tumors.[2] Approximately 500 to 1000 new cases of retroperitoneal sarcoma are diagnosed each year. Incidence figures on specific genitourinary sarcomas are difficult to establish because of the rarity of such lesions.[2,3] Retroperitoneal sarcomas arise most commonly in the fifth and sixth decades of life, but age incidence may span from the second to eighth decades.[3,4]

There is a slight male predominance but no distinct ethnic or racial distribution. Although any histologic pattern may be seen at any age, rhabdomyosarcoma generally clusters in younger patients, even excluding the pediatric population, and malignant fibrous histiocytoma is usually seen in older age groups. Generally, these lesions are not associated with other conditions, and a pattern of familial transmission has not been demonstrated. However, rare patients with neurofibromatosis may develop malignant schwannomas at some anatomic site.[5]

There is little known with regard to the etiology of retroperitoneal sarcomas. Radiation injury, prior trauma, and environmental exposure to agents such as dioxin and asbestos have been implicated.[6,7] Radiation may predispose patients to the development of sarcomas. Approximately 0.1% of patients treated with radiation therapy who survive greater than 5 years may develop a sarcoma at that site.[8] To qualify as a postradiation sarcoma, a lesion must meet specific established criteria.[6] In these cases, the sarcoma must develop within the irradiated field and prior documentation that the area was normal must be established. Additionally, histologic confirmation of the diagnosis is necessary, and a latency of at least 3 years is required. There appears to be no difference in the incidence of radiation-induced disease between those patients treated with orthovoltage and megavoltage. The most common postradiation tumor is the malignant fibrous histiocytoma, followed by osteosarcoma and fibrosarcoma. Most of these radiation-induced lesions appear to be of high grade and generally have poorer survival.[8]

Earlier epidemiologic studies reported that exposure to herbicides such as dioxin and wood preservatives may contribute to the development of retroperitoneal sarcomas.[9] In a more recent case-referent occupational study, several occupations (gardeners, forestry workers, construction workers) involved with exposure to phenoxy herbicides and/or chlorophenols (a component of herbicides and wood impregnating agents) displayed a significant odds ratio (4.1:1.7) of developing soft tissue sarcomas.[10] In studies of Vietnam era soldiers exposed to Agent Orange, no significant association was found between the development of sarcomas and exposure in case-control studies.[11] In some industrial studies, an association was noted between dioxin exposure and the development of sarcomas if the exposure was prolonged (greater than 1 year) and the latency period significant (over 20 years).[12] No distinct viral or immunologic etiologies have been proposed for the development of retroperitoneal sarcomas.

Pathology

Retroperitoneal sarcomas arise primarily from soft tissues of fibrous and adipose origin as well as muscle, nerve, and lymphatic tissue. These tissues are derived from primitive mesenchyme from the mesoderm, with some contribution from neuroectoderm.[13] Their location allows for a rather long, indolent preclinical course, during which time the tumor can grow to significant proportions. This growth may result in local areas of necrosis or liquefaction as the tumor outstrips its vascular supply.

In classic reviews of these lesions the common tissue distribution, in descending order, is liposarcoma, leiomyosarcoma, and fibrosarcoma, followed by other histologies.[4,14–26] Malignant fibrous histiocytoma (MFH) figures much more prominently in contemporary series; however, owing to intensive pathologic interest in defining this disorder, many tumors previously described as variants of fibrosarcoma or liposarcoma have been reclassified as MFH.[27,28] Therefore fibrosarcoma has been replaced in frequency order by this condition.

Although a well-developed understanding of the fundamental pathology of these lesions has not yet emerged, evaluation of the cytogenetic alterations in many sarcomas is beginning to suggest a common molecular theme. Several of these tumors display specific chromosomal translocations. Although the translocations appear unique for specific tumors (t[12;16][q13;p11] in myxoid liposarcoma), nearly all of these translocations result in the production of novel, tumor-specific, chimeric transcription factors. These factors interact with the upstream regulatory component of a gene and can significantly affect the expression of that gene at the messenger RNA level. The nucleic acid binding domain of the chimeric transcription factor confers target specificity within the tissue genome, whereas the transcription factor portion of this novel protein determines the transactivation potential and expression level of the target gene.[29,30] Novel insights into sarcoma pathology such as this unique transcription factor motif may provide the foundation for future therapeutic strategies directed at these lesions.

Benign Lesions (Table 37–1)

Lipomas. Lipomas consist almost entirely of mature fat and are uncommonly found in the retroperitoneum. They are probably the most common soft tissue tumor in humans. Most of these lesions occur superficially, but they may occur in other areas such as the retroperitoneum. Deep lipomas within the retroperitoneum are usually not as well circumscribed as their superficial counterparts and can conform to irregular spaces in this body space.[31,32] The adipocytes are normal or slightly

TABLE 37–1. BENIGN LESIONS OF THE RETROPERITONEUM

Lipoma
Pelvic lipomatosis
Myelolipoma
Leiomyoma
Ganglioneuroma
Hemangiopericytoma
Schwannoma

larger in appearance and have a well-developed vascular network. There is very little in the way of nuclear irregularity. Differing levels of fibrous connective tissue can be found in these lesions. The rim of the lipocyte is reactive for S-100 protein. Although the majority of these masses are idiopathic in nature, they can occasionally be a manifestation of steroid lipomatosis.

Pelvic Lipomatosis. Pelvic lipomatosis, although not a distinct tumor per se, was first described in 1959 as an overgrowth of fat in the perivesical and perirectal area. It is a hyperplastic rather neoplastic entity that can create a space-occupying lesion. Approximately two thirds of patients are African American, and women are rarely affected.[33] The growth is diffuse rather than nodular, and oftentimes it is difficult to distinguish it from normal adipose tissue. The condition may be associated with cystitis glandularis.[34] The general clinical course is slowly progressive and may result in the need for urinary diversion.[35]

Myelolipoma. This is a tumor-like growth of mature fat and bone marrow elements. Although it usually occurs in the adrenal gland, it can be seen as an isolated pelvic lesion.[36,37] It is distinct from extramedullary hematopoietic tumors, which are usually multiple and generally associated with mild proliferative diseases and skeletal disorders. Myelolipomas generally occur in patients older than 40 years of age and are rarely greater than 5 cm in size.[38] They are usually found as incidental imaging findings. The adrenal lesion can create inferior renal displacement seen as a radiolucent mass. Pathologically, it may display the features of a lipoma or have a darker appearance if myeloid elements predominate. Adrenal myelolipoma development may be secondary to prolonged stress and excessive stimulation with adrenocorticotropic hormones.[36]

Retroperitoneal Xanthogranuloma. This is an older classification of retroperitoneal tumors noted to consist of xanthoma and inflammatory cells. An impression that these lesions were benign was misleading, and with close follow-up it could be shown that many patients died of their disease. This diagnosis is rare, and the majority of similar lesions discovered contemporarily are now generally subclassified under the greater category of MFH tumors.[39]

Leiomyoma. These generally rare lesions are seen in a distribution that represents smooth muscle tissue in the body. They occur overwhelmingly in the female genital tract but have also been reported in the urinary bladder. There are occasional reports of these tumors in the retroperitoneum, where they can grow asymptomatically to a considerable size. They may have some calcifications. Leiomyomas stain positive for desmin, which separates them from their malignant counterpart. Extension of these lesions from the uterus into the vascular system can create tumor thrombi not unlike those seen with renal lesions.[40,41]

Ganglioneuroma. These lesions are fully differentiated tumors of neuroectodermal origin that are usually seen in patients over the age of 10. They can occur in the posterior mediastinum and the retroperitoneum. The retroperitoneal masses may grow quite large, yet they are grossly well circumscribed and have a uniform microscopic appearance. Some calcification may be present, and in some cases vasoactive intestinal peptide may be secreted, resulting in a diarrhea-like syndrome.[42,43]

Malignant Lesions (Table 37–2)

Liposarcoma. Liposarcomas, among the most common of primary retroperitoneal tumors, are distinguished by their often large dimensions and range of subtypes. These lesions have a peak incidence between ages 40 and 60.[44] Approximately 20% of these lesions arise in the retroperitoneum. One unfortunate clinical feature of these lesions is their great tendency to recur, often within the first 6 months after surgery. The principal tissue type is usually recapitulated at the time of recurrence. The rate of metastasis depends on the degree of tumor differentiation, with nearly 90% of poorly differentiated tumors metastasizing.[45,46]

Unlike benign lipomas, liposarcomas may bear little resemblance to classic fat-filled structures. The gross lesion is usually described as having a "fish flesh" appearance and, although generally encapsulated, it can often display invasive characteristics. Besides the retroperitoneum, these lesions arise in the deep soft tissues of the proximal extremities. They generally present as very large lesions when originating from the retroperitoneum. Histologi-

TABLE 37–2. MALIGNANT LESIONS OF THE RETROPERITONEUM AND HISTOLOGIC SUBCLASSIFICATIONS

Liposarcoma
Myxoid liposarcoma
Well differentiated
Lipoma-like
Inflammatory
Sclerosing
Differentiated
Round cell
Pleomorphic
Leiomyosarcoma
Malignant fibrous histiocytoma (MFH)
Storiform-pleomorphic
Myxoid MFH
MFH–giant cell type
Inflammatory MFH
Fibrosarcoma
Rhabdomyosarcoma
Embryonal
Botryoid
Alveolar
Pleomorphic
Spindle cell
Malignant hemangiopericytoma
Malignant peripheral nerve sheath tumors (malignant schwannoma)
Synovial sarcoma
Angiosarcoma

cally these lesions are subclassified as myxoid, well-differentiated, round cell, and pleomorphic variants.[47]

Myxoid liposarcoma is the most common liposarcoma and represents approximately 45% of this category of retroperitoneal lesions. It displays a background of stellate mesenchymal cells and a prominent capillary pattern often described as "chicken wire" (Fig. 37–1). The distinct cell is the lipoblast, which is similar to the fetal adipocyte. These cells are characterized by a lipid vacuole that scallops the nucleus. This creates the lipoma-like appearance of these lesions (Fig. 37–2).

Well-differentiated liposarcomas most resemble lipomas and are usually designated as low grade. Subvariants include the lipoma-like, inflammatory, sclerosing, and differentiated. The first three variants are often confused with benign processes such as scarring or inflammation, whereas the differentiated subtype is often noted in longstanding retroperitoneal lesions and considered higher grade.

The *round cell subtype* is also referred to as a lipoblastic variant and is distinguished by sheets of round cells with lipoblastic differentiation.

Pleomorphic liposarcoma is defined as a high-grade malignant variant with very bizarre nuclei and huge lipoblasts.

Leiomyosarcoma. This tumor accounts for less than 10% of all soft tissue sarcomas yet comprises a significant percentage of retroperitoneal sarcomas. It has a 2:1 female-to-male presentation. Low-grade leiomyosarcoma can be difficult to distinguish from leiomyomas, but higher grade lesions display a more infiltrative flesh-like appearance.[48] Low-grade lesions are often distinguished from leiomyomas by their chromatin pattern and the number of mitoses (greater than five mitoses per high-power field) present in the specimen. The characteristic findings in leiomyosarcoma are malignant spindle cells with cigar-shaped nuclei. The muscle fascicles interweave. These tumors immunohistochemically stain for vimentin, actin, and less often desmin; they stain negative for S-100. Ultrastructural features include bundles of thin cytofilaments, which can help distinguish leiomyosarcomas from other lesions.

A rare retroperitoneal variant of these tumors are leiomyosarcomas that originate from the great vessels.[49] These occur predominantly in women. Tumors of the iliac vessels usually present with lower extremity edema, whereas those of the inferior vena cava can display findings consistent with Budd-Chiari syndrome.[50] Resection of these lesions is recommended when anatomically feasible. However, survival is usually less than 2 years and many inferior vena caval lesions are unresectable because of their intrahepatic locations.

Malignant Fibrous Histiocytoma. MFH was originally described in 1963 and has come to be the predominant histologic diagnosis for contemporarily reported soft tissue sarcomas.[51] It is defined as a sarcoma of primary histiocytic origin. Many pleomorphic variants of fibrosarcoma, liposarcoma, and rhabdomyosarcoma have been reclassified in to this category. With the thorough evaluation of a tumor specimen, distinct regions of

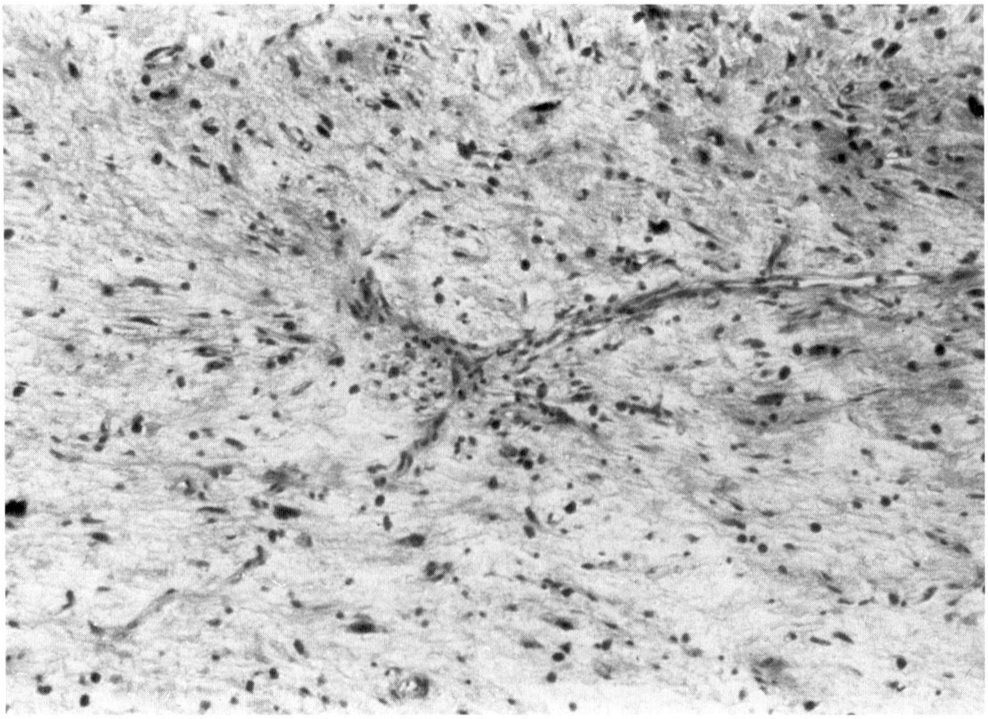

FIGURE 37–1. Myxoid liposarcoma displaying myxoid vascular pattern and minimal lipoblasts. Hematoxylin & eosin stain, ×250.

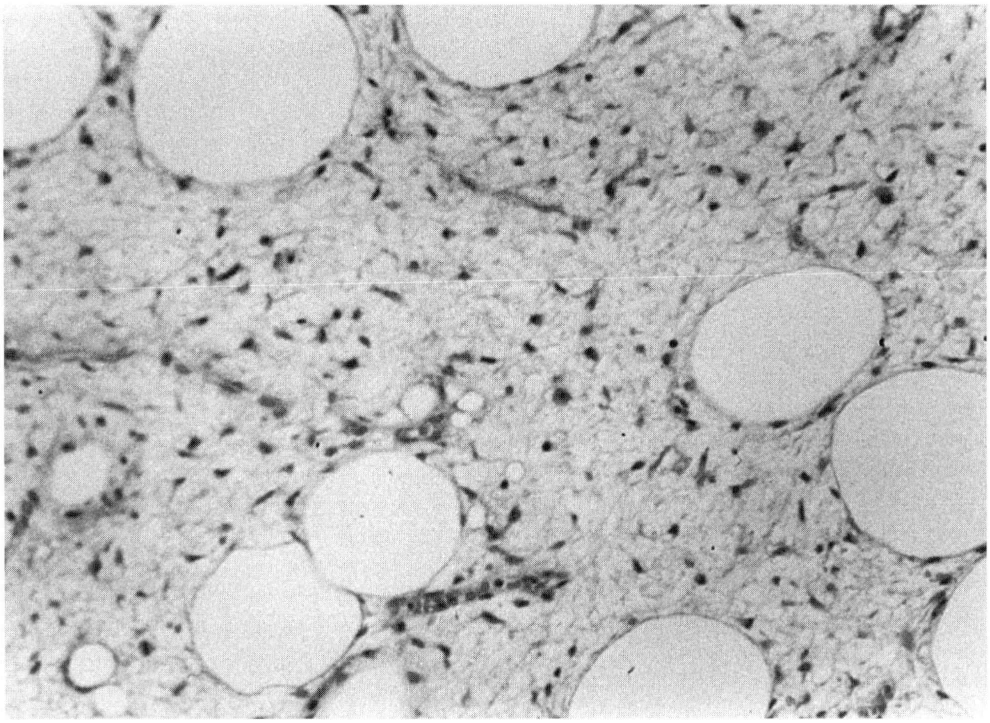

FIGURE 37–2. Myxoid liposarcoma displaying lipoblasts and myxoid matrix. ×250.

leiomyosarcoma, liposarcoma, and other soft tissue sarcomas may be identified. In such cases the tumor may be defined by those findings and the mention of associated MFH pattern.[52] There are four subtypes of MFH that may coexist in a particular lesion: storiform-pleomorphic, myxoid, giant cell, and inflammatory. The angiomatoid variant is seen almost exclusively in the extremities and trunk.[53]

The *storiform-pleomorphic variant* has a distinct but not pathognomonic pinwheel pattern caused by the collagen pattern of curling fascicles of cells (Fig. 37–3). It is the most common variant, usually comprising 40 to 60% of most series. Although this pattern may predominate, it may not be present throughout the lesion in question. Areas of collagen or foamy cells may also be encountered. The nuclei tend to be irregular and large, with discernible mitoses. Additionally, inflammatory cells and cellular phagocytosis may be detected (Fig. 37–4). The constellation of tissue histology and nuclear irregularities in addition to the inflammatory components differentiate this lesion from benign entities.

Myxoid MFH makes up 25% of this overall tumor type. It is often difficult to distinguish it from liposarcoma, yet the mixoid MFH has little neutral fat but is rich in mucopolysaccharide residing in intracytoplasmic vacuoles.

MFH–giant cell type is distinguished by large, benign-appearing osteoclasts. Multinucleated giant cells and the stroma comprise the malignant components of this lesion. If cartilage or osteoid is detected, these lesions are classified as soft tissue osteosarcomas, which usually have a poorer prognosis than MFH.

Inflammatory MFH is rare and often difficult to distinguish from benign processes such as nodular fasciitis when the presentation is truncal or extremity. A neutrophilic infiltrate is generally noted, with a matrix of reticular cells. Often an exact diagnosis is not made until a recurrence is biopsied.

FIBROSARCOMA. Fibrosarcomas are malignant tumors of fibroblast origin. They have a range of gradation and grossly display a classic "fish flesh" pattern, with hemorrhage and necrosis. Low-grade lesions can display a herringbone–spindle-shaped histologic pattern. On retrospective review, these lesions are often reclassified as MFH or as a desmoid lesion (aggressive fibromatosis). Therefore, these lesions represent a smaller proportion of primary retroperitoneal tumors than previously reported. There is a greater incidence of blood-borne metastases with this tumor to the lung and bones.[54]

RHABDOMYOSARCOMA. Rhabdomyosarcoma comprises a minor percentage of reported retroperitoneal sarcomas, yet is a significant lesion in pediatric oncology as well as pediatric tumors associated with the genitourinary system. (This topic is dealt with extensively in Chapter 47.) These lesions are generally classified as embryonal, botryoid, alveolar, or pleomorphic, with spindle cell more recently described as a subtype of the embryonal form.[55,56]

Embryonal rhabdomyosarcoma comprises more than half of all rhabdomyosarcomas and has a large array of anatomic locations, including the genitourinary tract and retroperitoneum. It can range from very well to poorly differentiated lesions and can express the multiple stages of muscle development.

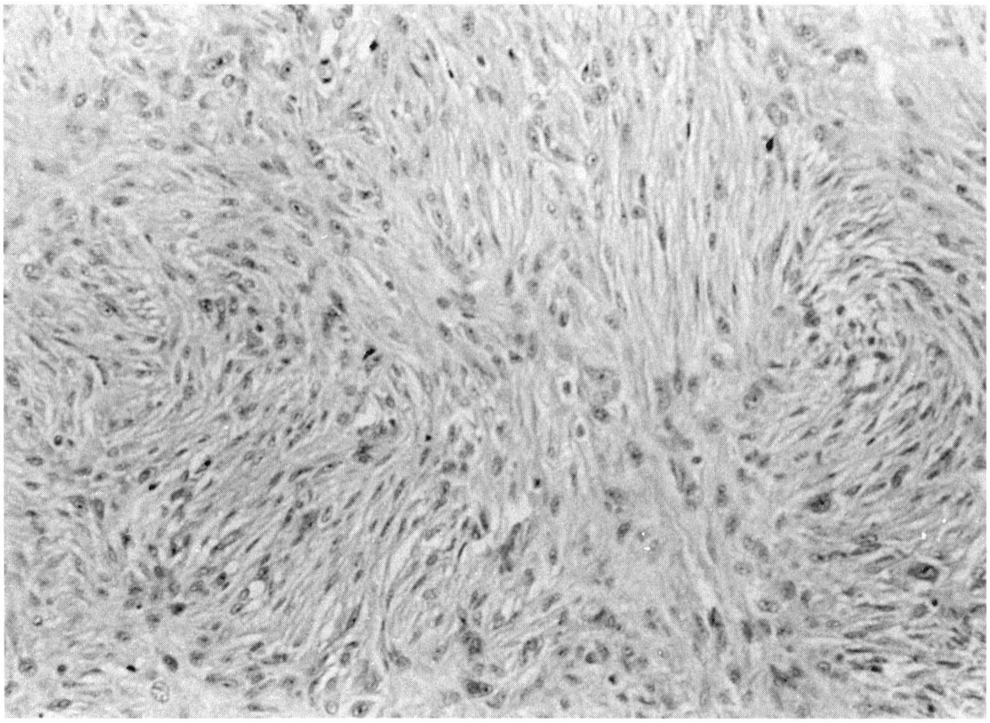

FIGURE 37–3. Storiform pattern of malignant fibrous histiocytoma. ×250.

Botryoid lesions are an anatomic variant of the embryonal type and generally are seen in hollow viscera. The *spindle cell subtype* is noted for its favorable clinical behavior.

Alveolar rhabdomyosarcoma accounts for approximately 20% of rhabdomyosarcomas and tends to occur more frequently in the extremities. The tumor is arranged in aggregates of round or oval cells that create irregular spaces reminiscent of alveoli. These tissues may be surrounded by fibrous septae, and areas of necrosis are not uncommon.

Pleomorphic rhabdomyosarcoma comprises 5% of

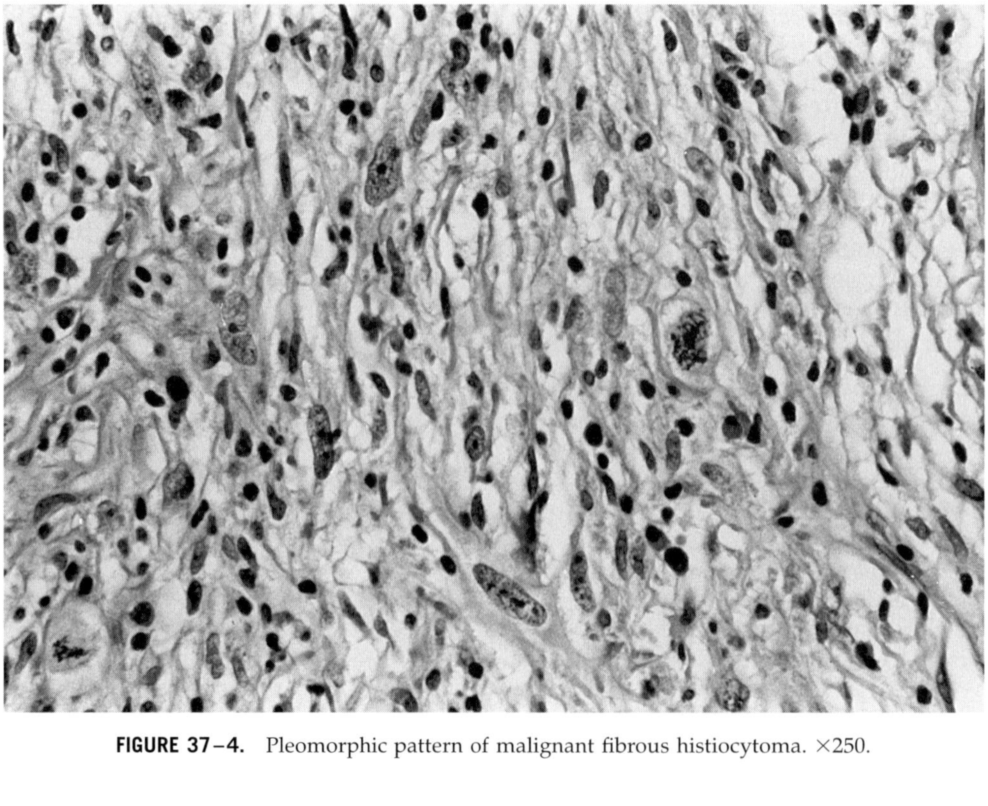

FIGURE 37–4. Pleomorphic pattern of malignant fibrous histiocytoma. ×250.

adult rhabdomyosarcomas and generally occurs in older patients. It generally occurs in the extremities and is not unlike MFH in its appearance. The absence of cross-striations makes diagnosis difficult. With all rhabdomyosarcomas, immunostaining for desmin, myoglobin, and muscle-specific actin is useful.

MALIGNANT HEMANGIOPERICYTOMA. These rare lesions originate from pericytes, which are unique cells that arborize about small vessels and capillaries. Their contractile properties allow them to control microvascular flow and permeability. Less than 200 of these lesions have been described, yet 25% of them have occurred in the retroperitoneum or pelvis.[57] They are usually well circumscribed, and if possible complete surgical excision is warranted. Hemangiopericytomas display a rich vascular pattern and stain positive for factor VIIIa; they are negative for desmin and actin. The clinical behavior of these lesions is difficult to predict, but metastases may develop in 20 to 50% of cases. Those lesions with greater than four mitoses per 10 high-power fields have a worse prognosis.[58,59]

MALIGNANT PERIPHERAL NERVE SHEATH TUMOR (MALIGNANT SCHWANNOMA). Those lesions generally referred to as malignant schwannomas are now referred to by this more general classification because it accounts for lesions of nerve, neurofibroma, and lesions showing nerve sheath differentiation. The majority of these lesions arise in the extremities, yet they can occasionally be seen in the pelvis, originating from the sciatic nerve or sacral plexus. These lesions are associated with neurofibromatosis type I.[60]

SYNOVIAL CELL SARCOMA. These lesions are usually associated with the extremities and articular surfaces, but occasionally are reported in series of retroperitoneal lesions because of their origination from the lumbar joint areas. They may resemble malignant neural sheath tumors. It is clinically important to realize the anatomic origin of this lesion because complete resection would be unlikely with the usual approach to retroperitoneal tumor extirpation.[61,62] Vanishingly rare as retroperitoneal tumor, it is almost always an extremity lesion.

Diagnosis

Because of their slow growth and anatomic location, retroperitoneal tumors (usually sarcomas) tend to grow to a large size before they are detected. In a series of MFH cases, the average size at diagnosis for extremity lesions was 5 cm, whereas retroperitoneal lesions were 16.5 cm in size[27]; thus such lesions can often be enormous by usual pathologic standards. Although the age at presentation is distributed across a large spectrum, the majority of patients are diagnosed with retroperitoneal tumors in the sixth decade of life. Because the progression of symptoms is slow, there is usually a lag time of 5 months from initial symptoms to diagnosis. The principal clinical finding is abdominal mass and abdominal pain (60 to 80% of cases)[11]; many patients also experience nausea-vomiting and weight loss (20 to 30%). Neurologic findings are noted in 30% of patients.[64] Lower extremity edema is seen in 17 to 20% of patients, but urinary symptoms are surprisingly rare, seen in only 3 to 5% of patients in most series. In very rare cases hypoglycemia has been reported as a presenting symptom secondary to the secretion of insulin-like substances.[1]

Physical examination will generally demonstrate a protuberant abdomen that may be accompanied by an appearance of extremity wasting. Peripheral or inguinal adenopathy may be present although lymphadenopathy is not usually associated with these tumors (<5%).[65] Lower extremity edema and/or increased abdominal wall venous markings suggest the presence of vena caval compression or obstruction.

Diagnostic imaging is imperative to delineate the anatomic limits of the lesion and assess the integrity and function of adjacent organs. This is most appropriately demonstrated with computed tomography (CT).[66,67] Important issues to address with this modality are bilateral renal function, the presence or absence of visceral metastases, and lymphadenopathy. Attention should also be given to the axial skeleton. Tumor involvement of neural foramina suggests unresectability of the lesion. Germ cell tumors, which should be suspected in young men and diagnosed through a thorough physical examination and testicular ultrasound, are usually distinguished on CT scan from other primary retroperitoneal lesions. This is also generally true for lymphomas. However, the CT scan is not particularly diagnostic for the multiple tumor histologies of primary retroperitoneal tumors besides a liposarcoma with high fat content. Even the classic findings of fat density and tissue septa are not a tissue signature for this disease (Fig. 37–5).

Earlier literature attests to the value of intravenous urography, upper and lower gastrointestinal tract series, and angiography in defining displacement and delineating function (Fig. 37–6). Given the vascularity of many of these lesions and the technical difficulty they may present at surgery, angiography was considered the principal study before undertaking a therapeutic resection. Although it may clearly augment a CT study, it is now thought that angiography should not be used as the sole criterion for unresectability because it may not accurately display the degree of vascular encasement. The superiority of magnetic resonance imaging (MRI) over conventional CT scanning has not been definitely demonstrated in retroperitoneal sarcomas, yet the apparent refinement in delineating tissue boundaries and the multiplanar imaging provided by MRI make it a valuable adjunctive study when dealing with a large, generally uncommon

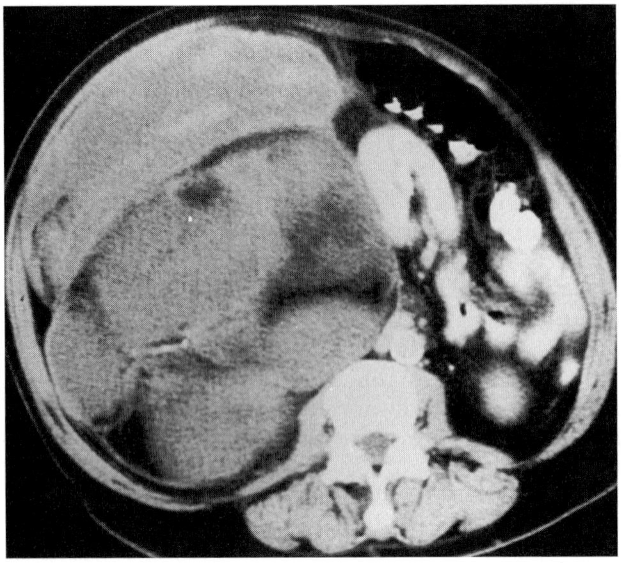

FIGURE 37–5. CT image demonstrating massive right-sided liposarcoma with suggestion of internal fibrous bands displacing the liver and right-sided retroperitoneal structures.

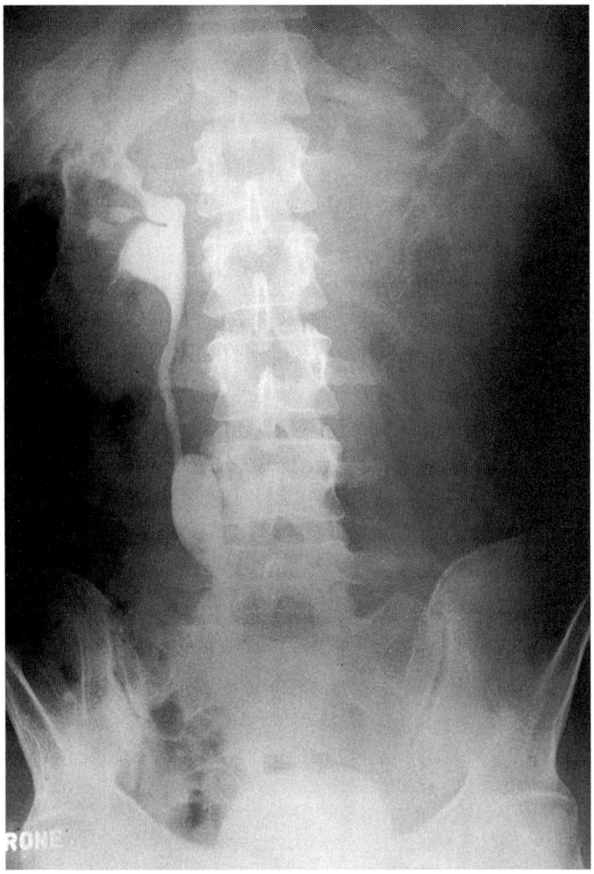

FIGURE 37–6. Intravenous urogram (prone position) demonstrating displacement of right renal unit by massive liposarcoma.

tumor. There is strong evidence to suggest that it may better delineate tissue planes in extremity lesions.[68,69] From a practical standpoint, the two imaging modalities may be complementary rather than redundant in certain cases, and MRI should be employed as needed. The role for magnetic resonance angiography in the diagnosis and staging of these lesions is yet to be determined.

In some cases imaging will not provide a reasonable diagnosis; these patients may require a biopsy prior to definitive resection. Classic references suggest that percutaneous needle biopsies of these retroperitoneal masses are generally unsatisfactory even when aided with imaging techniques such as ultrasound or CT.[21] More recent sources indicate that diagnosis may be a function of experience with these lesions and that percutaneous biopsy or even needle aspiration may be adequate.[70] As a result of the uncommon nature of these lesions at most centers, it would seem appropriate to obtain a correct tissue diagnosis with a reasonable tissue sample when the diagnosis is in question.

In specific cases an intraoperative biopsy may be indicated to diagnose the lesion or differentiate it from a lymphoma or germ cell tumor. In those instances care must be taken to obtain the sample from a solid part of the lesion and employ meticulous technique to avoid any tumor spillage. This is accomplished through appropriate draping of the operative field, excellent hemostastis, and meticulous closure with covering of the wound.[21] Laparoscopic sampling, although possible, would probably not be feasible in most of these patients. Tumor specimens should be sent for frozen section and touch preparations prepared to establish a diagnosis. In the appropriate patient, levels of the serum tumor markers for germ cell tumors (β-human chorionic gonadotropin and α-fetoprotein) should be obtained preoperatively. There are no specific serum tumor markers for primary retroperitoneal sarcomas, although levels of vanillylmandelic acid may be elevated in the rare case of ganglioneuroma or extra-adrenal pheochromocytoma.

With a greater appreciation for the multitude of histologic subtypes of retroperitoneal tumors, many diagnoses can be made on the basis of hematoxylin-eosin staining alone. However, immunostaining for intermediate filaments and muscle or nerve components may aid in cases in which a diagnosis is in doubt[63] (Table 37–3).

Staging

The primary determinant of staging for primary retroperitoneal tumors is the tumor grade. The grading is based on a 1 through 3 or 4 scale, and stage grouping is done through the TNM system. Because of the impact of tumor grade, this is often referred to as a GTNM system (Table 37–4).[71]

Tumor grading is determined by several factors, including atypical mitosis, cytoplasmic and nuclear pleomorphism, and necrosis.[72,73] Grade 1 lesions are

TABLE 37–3. IMMUNOHISTOCHEMICAL SPECIFICITY OF SOME COMMON PRIMARY RETROPERITONEAL SARCOMAS

	Immunohistochemical Staining Results						
Tumor Histology	S-100	Vimentin	Desmin	Actin	Cytokeratin	Factor XIIa	Fibroblast Antigen
Leiomyosarcoma	—	+	+/—	+	Rare		
Liposarcoma	+	+					
Rhabdomyosarcoma			+	+			
Hemangiopericytoma		+	—	—		+	
Mixed nerve sheath tumor	+						
Synovial sarcoma	—						
MFH							+

denoted by few mitoses, acellularity, minimal alterations of the nucleus, and absent or few nucleoli. Scoring often takes into consideration other factors, such as tumor size and patient age. Grade 2 lesions display small to moderate-size nucleoli, moderate nuclear pleomorphism, irregular chromatin distribution, and a moderate amount of mitoses. Areas of necrosis may be noted in the microscopic field. Grade 3 lesions are characterized by numerous mitoses, gross chromatin clumping, moderate or considerable necrosis, and variation in nuclear morphology. The distinction between T1 and T2 lesions is made at 5 cm.

Clinical staging beyond physical exam should also include a bone scan and a dedicated chest CT as well as an abdominal/retroperitoneal CT scan with attention to the liver. Bilateral renal function must be determined preoperatively. In experienced hands, CT scanning alone may provide enough local staging information. Because these lesions are rare, however, any question regarding the extent of contiguous organ involvement should be answered by the appropriate confirmatory imaging test (e.g., upper gastrointestinal tract series). Laboratory tests may provide some diagnostic discrimination, yet generally add little to a staging evaluation.

TABLE 37–4. AMERICAN JOINT COMMITTEE ON CANCER GTNM CLASSIFICATION AND STAGE GROUPING OF SOFT TISSUE SARCOMAS

G: Tumor Grade
G1—well differentiated
G2—moderately well differentiated
G3—poorly differentiated
T: Primary Tumor
T1—tumor ≤5 cm in greatest diameter
T2—tumor >5 cm in greatest diameter
N: Regional Lymph Node Involvement
N0—no known metastases to lymph nodes
N1—verified metastases to lymph nodes
M: Distant Metastasis
M0—no known distant metastasis
M1—known distant metastasis
Stage Grouping

IA	G1	T1	N0	M0
IB	G1	T2	N0	M0
IIA	G2	T1	N0	M0
IIB	G2	T2	N0	M0
IIIA	G3	T1	N0	M0
IIIB	G3	T2	N0	M0
IVA	Any G	Any T	N1	M0
IVB	Any G	Any T	Any N	M1

Surgery

Extirpative surgery is the principal and most effective form of therapy for primary retroperitoneal tumors. Preoperative planning to assess the extent of the disease is essential because successful surgery is defined by complete excision of the mass with adequate margins of normal tissue. A complete resection rate between 38 and 78% (average, 55%) is reported in many large series[14–26,74–76] (Table 37–5). In several large series of retroperitoneal sarcomas, univariate and multivariate analysis of independent treatment variables has been performed. In over 280 patients, completeness of resection was the single most important positive predictive feature.[77] Intermediate or high tumor grade is a strong negative feature.[20,77–79] In most reported series, intermediate- and high-grade lesions comprise 55 to 70% of the tumors described. Tumor histology, tumor size, and patient age were not significant factors in survival. Therefore, carefully planned and skillfully executed surgical therapy is critical for any chance at long-term success.

Operative Technique

The classic approach for surgery on these lesions is through long midline incisions or chevron incisions. The tumors are usually right or left sided, however, with few actually arising from the midline. A full flank approach, such as that employed for renal stone surgery, is discouraged because it can limit exposure to the full retroperitoneum or abdomen.[1,21] Because these lesions are not compartmentalized by the retroperitoneum, they can cross many anatomic boundaries. It is important, therefore, to determine the potential for resectability, beyond that presupposed through imaging. This is first accomplished by developing a subadventitial plane along the lateral borders of the great vessels extending dorsally between the spine and the psoas and quadratis muscles (Fig. 37–7). In this manner one can determine if the tumor has spread along a

TABLE 37–5. POOLED DATA ON COMPLETE VERSUS PARTIAL RESECTION*

Series	No. of Patients	Resection (No./%)		Mean Survival (Months)		Complete Resection 5-yr Survival (%)
		Complete	Partial	Complete	Partial	
Dalton et al.[19]	116	63/54	25/21	72	13	54
Jacques et al.[20]	86	43/50	34/39.5	65	28	74
McGrath et al.[18]	47	18/38	18/38	120	24	70
Glenn et al.[22]	50	37/74	8/16	40	—	38
Karakouis et al.[24]	68	27/40	7/10	84	48	64
Kilkeny et al.[26]	63	49/78	10/16	41	9	48
Zornig et al.[23]	51	30/59	21/41	60	—	35
TOTAL	481	267/55.5	123/25.6	70.3	24.4	54.7

*Biopsy-only patients excluded.

spinal nerve route and into the spinal foramina or even farther into the spinal cord. If this is the case, the tumor is generally considered unresectable. It has also been suggested that a lateral incision of the peritoneum into the deep body wall is important to explore on a level posterior to the spinous processes (Fig. 37–7). If the operator's fingers can be bimanually palpated, this sarcoma is considered resectable.

It is imperative in the preoperative period that both the patient and the surgeon realize the potential need for en bloc resection of affected organs. This can include vascular structures as well as the kidney and portions of the diaphragm, liver, stomach, gallbladder, spleen, pancreas, and gut. In a review of several series, up to 68% of operations required resection of an adjacent organ to ensure adequate negative margins. The most frequently resected organs are listed in decreasing order in Table 37–6. Although a Dacron graft is necessary to replace a portion of resected aorta, there is debate among surgeons with regard to the need for venous reconstruction. Many believe that the venous collaterals that develop secondary to vena caval compression are adequate to allow for appropriate drainage from otherwise vascularly compromised organs. When bowel viability is questionable, the bowel portion should be resected if possible. Although many visceral organs can be resected, unresectability is usually denoted by sarcomatosis, nerve root involvement, pelvic sidewall involvement, malignant ascites, or the presence of distant metastasis.[1,21]

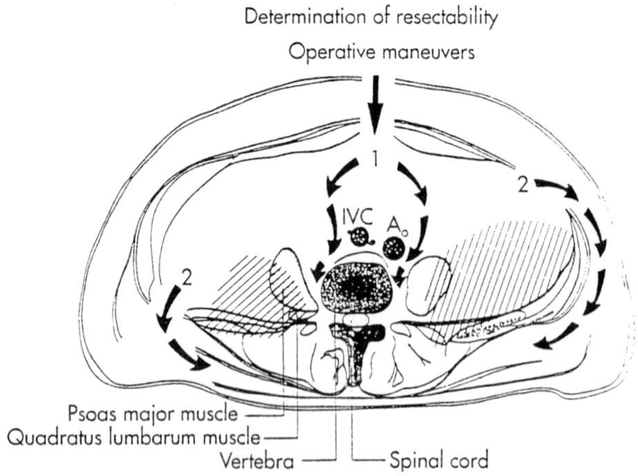
Determination of resectability
Operative maneuvers
1
2
2
IVC
Ao
Psoas major muscle
Quadratus lumborum muscle
Vertebra
Spinal cord

FIGURE 37–7. Transabdominal approach to determine resectability of a primary retroperitoneal sarcoma. Pertinent maneuvers consist of intra-abdominal assessment of visceral and vascular contents and retroperitoneal assessment of attachment to musculoskeletal and spinous structures. (From Storm FK, Mahvi DM: Diagnosis and management of retroperitoneal soft-tissue sarcoma. Ann Surg 1991; 214:2, with permission.)

When defining the operative field, it is often necessary to release multiple intra-abdominal adhesions. This must be performed meticulously because an enterotomy and subsequent fistula formation can cause major morbidity. Tactile as well as visual perceptions aid in avoiding violation of the bowel. In addition, the use of sharp curved Mayo scissors rather than Metzenbaum scissors may aid in avoiding this complication. During the dissection of a large tumor mass, it is often necessary to shift the location of the dissection when one particular area becomes difficult because of concerns of a clear margin or the potential for vascular damage. A centripetal dissection allows one to dissect those areas that are amenable to dissection and whose release in turn may free up a previously more constrained area of the operative field.[80] Morbidity and mortality rates for contemporary surgical series are acceptable. An operative mortality of 2 to 7% with morbidity rates of 6 to 25% are the norm. Hemorrhage, intra-abdominal abscess, and enterocutaneous fistula are the most commonly described complications.

TABLE 37–6. ORGANS SACRIFICED DURING COMPLETE RESECTION OF SARCOMA

Organ	Frequency of Resection (%)
Kidney	32–46
Colon	25
Adrenal gland	18
Pancreas	15
Spleen	10

Another surgical technique is the modified thoracoabdominal approach, which has been developed and popularized by Skinner. Those familiar with the technique believe that it allows maximum exposure to the posterior retroperitoneum, which is often a difficult area to assess through a midline incision. Additionally, it provides access and control to the ipsilateral great vessels above the diaphragm. Whether a left- or right-sided procedure is performed, excellent exposure can be developed in the contralateral retroperitoneal region without difficulty. The technique described here is a summary of Skinner's approach.[81]

With the thoracoabdominal approach, patient positioning is critical. The patient is not placed in a "pure flank" position, similar to that used in stone surgery. Rather, a modified flank position is employed (Fig. 37–8). The contralateral leg is flexed 90 degrees and the hip is flexed approximately 30 degrees. The ipsilateral shoulder and chest are placed 20 degrees off the horizontal, with the arm brought across the chest and placed in an adjustable arm rest. The pelvis is at most rotated 10 degrees off the horizontal, and this position is maintained with a roll sheet. The table is fully hyperextended, with the break located above the iliac crest. The patient is secured with wide adhesive tape and the ipsilateral leg is supported on a pillow.

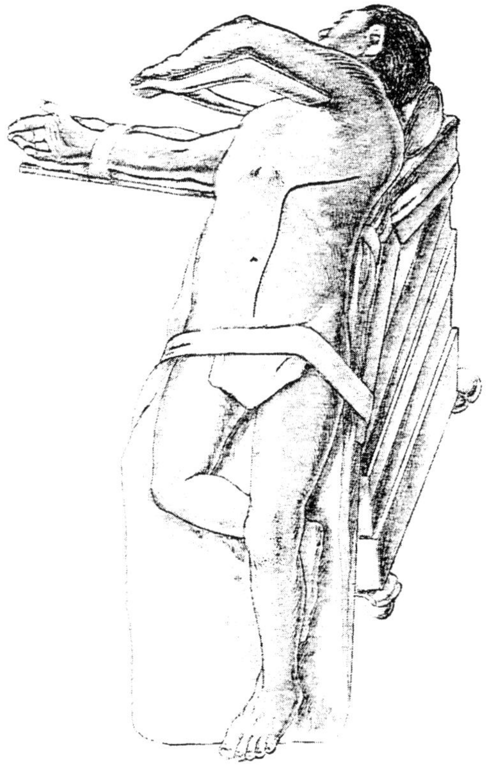

FIGURE 37–8. Patient positioning and modified thoracoabdominal approach to primary retroperitoneal tumor. (From Skinner DG: Considerations for management of large retroperitoneal tumors: use of the modified thoracoabdominal approach. J Urol 1977; 117:605, with permission.)

A midaxillary incision is carried in the midaxillary line from the eighth, ninth, or tenth rib. The height of this incision is based on the size of the primary lesion. It extends over the rib and costochondral junction into the epigastrium, and then proceeds inferiorly as a midline incision into the pelvis. The rib is resected subperiosteally and the costochondral junction is divided. The rectus muscle is divided and retracted laterally. In most instances, the peritoneum will be opened and the bowel contents mobilized superiorly. This mobilization is based on the superior mesenteric artery pedicle. It is important that this artery be identified initially, and care be taken not to traumatize it. In many instances, the inferior mesenteric artery may have to be resected. Most care should be taken to maintain the marginal artery. In most instances a large bowel section will be avoided, yet, if there is a question of viability at the end of the case, any suspect area of bowel should be resected. Vena cava obstruction may be associated with any right-sided lesions; if this is the case, it is usually best to resect the vena cava en bloc with removal of the tumor. Often, a right nephrectomy may also be required. If this maneuver is performed, it is best to maintain vascular connection between the vena cava and left renal vein to decrease the possibility of acute or long-term renal insufficiency.

In general, the aorta can be dissected free of large retroperitoneal tumors, but rarely may require replacement with a Dacron graft. During dissection or mobilization of the great vessels, care must be taken to control the lumbar vessels with ligation and division to avoid problematic bleeding. Whereas the distal vessels may be controlled with hemoclips, it is appropriate to ligate lumbar vessels at their origin on the great vessel. In the case of significant bleeding, the vessel tear can be controlled with the use of a Judd or Allis clamp. Although the possibility of spinal devascularization exists, it is very uncommon because of the significant collateral blood supply to the spine from the artery of Adamkiewicz. In younger patients the potential for ejaculatory dysfunction is significant.

Postoperative Monitoring

There is no set protocol for the postoperative monitoring of patients with primary retroperitoneal sarcoma, but recommendations can be made given the rapidity of recurrence, the advantage of complete tumor re-resection, and the lethality of this condition. It would be appropriate to perform an abdominal CT scan, chest x-ray, and biochemistry profile with complete blood count every 6 months. A lengthening of this follow-up interval should be considered only after 5 years.

Surgical Outcome

The overall survival for patients presenting with retroperitoneal sarcomas is poor. In a multi-institutional review the 2-, 5-, and 10-year mean survival rates for patients with this disease were 56%, 34%, and 18%, respectively.[21] The effective surgical management of retroperitoneal tumors has been limited by their size at presentation, which often results in secondary organ involvement. This has a poor impact on the ability to achieve negative surgical margins even with the resection of adjacent organs. Historically, a complete surgical resection with negative margins was achieved in 50 to 60% of patients. The more recent series demonstrate complete resection rates in the 60 to 80% range, which may be due to improvements in imaging, preoperative planning, and surgical technique.

Those patients in whom a complete resection is achieved display superior survival to those patients with incomplete resection of their tumors (Table 37–5). On average, the 5-year survival of patients with completely resected tumors is 54% compared to 17% for incomplete resections; at 10 years this difference is 45% to 17%. Thus a nearly 40% survival advantage is seen at 5 to 10 years in those patients with complete surgical resection of their lesion (Fig. 37–9). Tumor recurrence after complete surgical resection is significant, however. There is a 72% chance of local recurrence at 5 years and a 90% chance of recurrence at 10 years in most series. These data imply very poor survival at 15 years.[21]

Reoperative surgery for the treatment of recurrent retroperitoneal sarcoma can be of value. In one series, 30 patients with a previous complete resection of the primary lesion experienced local tumor recurrence at a mean interval of 23 months. Sixty per cent of these patients were rendered free of disease after reoperative surgery. To accomplish this, 33% required the resection of adjacent viscera. Those patients in whom a complete resection was achieved with a second operation had a 33-month median survival, compared to a 14-month median survival in those patients who did not experience a second complete resection.[82]

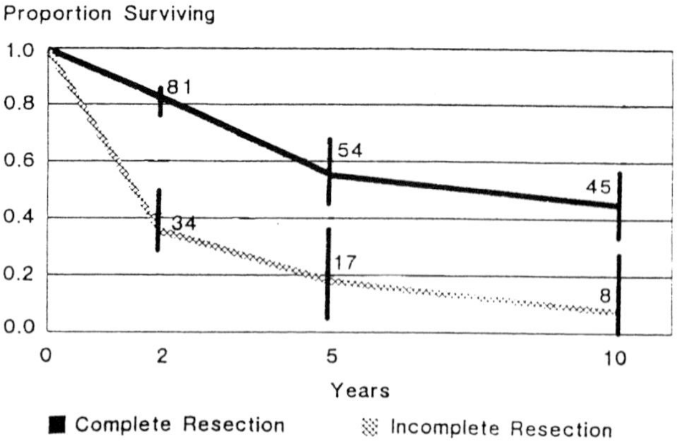
Proportion Surviving
1.0
0.8
0.6
0.4
0.2
0.0
0
2
5
10
Years
81
54
45
34
17
8
Complete Resection
Incomplete Resection

FIGURE 37–9. Patient survival as a function of completeness of the surgical resection. The data represent *x* complete resections and *y* incomplete resections from collected series. (From Storm FK, Mahvi DM: Diagnosis and management of retroperitoneal soft-tissue sarcoma. Ann Surg 1991; 214:2, with permission.)

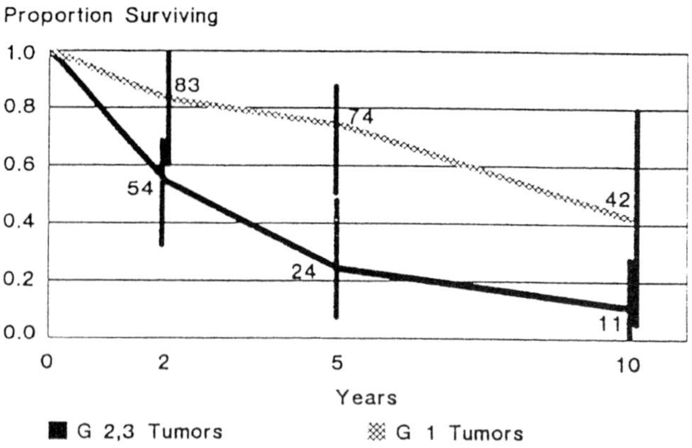
Proportion Surviving
1.0
0.8
0.6
0.4
0.2
0.0
0
2
5
10
Years
83
74
54
42
24
11
G 2,3 Tumors
G 1 Tumors

FIGURE 37–10. Patient survival as a function of tumor grade in cases of primary retroperitoneal sarcoma. The data represent 50 low-grade and 80 high-grade tumors from collected series. (From Storm FK, Mahvi DM: Diagnosis and management of retroperitoneal soft-tissue sarcoma. Ann Surg 1991; 214:2, with permission.)

The role of subtotal resection has never been clearly established, yet some data suggest that this may have some positive value compared to palliative or debulking surgery. In one report, 22 patients with complete resection of tumor displayed a median survival similar to that of 15 patients with subtotal resection (median survival >120 months), compared to those only having a partial palliative resection or exploration (12 to 20 months).[83] An aggressive surgical approach in cases in which near-complete resection can be obtained has also been advocated by others.[24]

The effect of tumor grade on patient survival cannot be underestimated. Low-grade lesions display a 50% survival advantage over intermediate- and high-grade lesions at 5 years (74 versus 24%) and a 30% survival advantage at 10 years (42 versus 11%) (Fig. 37–10). This is demonstrated even in the face of total surgical resection. Although aggressive surgical resection of retroperitoneal sarcoma serves as the foundation of therapy for this condition, the high local recurrence rate and eventual mortality from this disease have prompted the exploration of adjuvant therapeutic modalities.

Adjuvant Therapy

Radiation Therapy

The treatment of extremity sarcomas has been significantly advanced by the addition of preoperative radiation therapy to the affected site. Maintenance of function and decreased local recurrence can be achieved through the use of this modality in the adjuvant and neoadjuvant setting. Doses of 60 to 65 Gy are generally administered in the treatment of soft tissue extremity sarcoma.[84] Unfortunately, the low tolerance of the bowel and associated abdominal organs for radiation has limited the application of such therapy for the treatment of ret-

TABLE 37–7. RESULTS IN FOUR SERIES OF IORT VERSUS EXTERNAL BEAM RADIATION THERAPY (XRT) FOR RETROPERITONEAL SARCOMA RESECTION PATIENTS

Series	No. of Patients	IORT (Gy)	Total XRT (Gy)	Local Failure (%)	Follow-Up (Months)
Sindelar et al.[89]	15/35	20	50–55	40	96
Willett et al.[90]	10	10–20	40–50	10	60
Gunderson et al.[87]	20	10–20	45–60	15	30
Kiel et al.[88]	12	12.5–20	45–54	17	18

roperitoneal lesions. Both external beam therapy and the application of intraoperative radiation therapy (IORT) have been studied in these tumors, yet no marked advances have been made.

Local control of the retroperitoneal sarcoma site in a dose-dependent fashion has been suggested in several radiation therapy series.[85,86] Increased toxicity can accompany this, however, thus negating any potential beneficial effect. In older series in which external beam therapy alone was administered, the dose-limiting effects of radiation enteritis were significant.[22] This prompted the application of IORT combined with additional external beam treatment to provide dose escalation at lower toxicity.

The results of four such series employing this strategy are reported in Table 37–7.[87–90] The National Cancer Institute trial, which was a prospective randomized series of 35 patients, is representative of this effort. These patients underwent resection of their lesions and 20 Gy of intraoperative radiation in combination with 35 to 40 Gy of postoperative radiation versus 50 to 55 Gy of external beam radiation therapy alone. Fifteen of these patients received chemotherapy. An interim analysis suggested no significant differences in survival in either treatment group, and this was supported in the final results.[89,91] Although median survival times were similar in each group (45 months in IORT patients versus 52 months in controls), there was a significantly lower number of local recurrences (6 of 15 IORT patients versus 16 of 20 controls) and less radiation enteritis (2 of 15 IORT patients versus 10 of 20 controls) with the use of IORT. Unfortunately those patients receiving IORT had more radiation-related peripheral neuropathy (9 of 15) than did control patients (1 of 20). The use of brachytherapy in the treatment of soft tissue sarcomas is also being explored as an alternative to conventional IORT.[86]

The use of neoadjuvant radiation therapy has also been explored employing novel therapies to lessen preoperative gastrointestinal morbidity. Dynamic three-dimensional conformal pion radiotherapy was administered to 21 patients deemed to have unresectable retroperitoneal sarcomas. Treatment morbidity was tolerable, and nine patients later underwent surgery. Three patients experienced a complete surgical resection. Five-year actuarial local control in all lesions was 60% with a 33% 5-year actuarial survival.[92]

Radiosensitizers such as iododeoxyuridine (IdUrd) have also been tested in the presurgical radiation treatment of retroperitoneal sarcomas. In one phase I/II trial, IdUrd was administered in a dose-escalated fashion (1000 to 1600 mg/m^2/day) to 16 patients. Up to 65 Gy of external beam and intraoperative radiation were administered. Toxicity in these patients was minimal. Eleven patients underwent resection, and negative margins were present in four of these patients. In several cases significant preoperative tumor shrinkage was noted.[93,94]

Retroperitoneal sarcomas are radioresponsive lesions, but the ability to provide a therapeutic advantage, even locally, with radiation therapy is offset by competing morbidity. Improved delivery techniques and novel radiation therapy approaches may define a minimally toxic, therapeutic role for radiation therapy in the treatment of retroperitoneal sarcoma in the future.

Chemotherapy

The role of chemotherapy for retroperitoneal sarcoma, especially in the adjuvant setting, is poorly defined. When one considers soft tissue sarcomas as a group, the risk of distant disease and subsequent death is still significant even with adequate local control. Although this makes a compelling argument for adjuvant chemotherapy, there is no large-scale prospective randomized trial that supports this proposition. The adjuvant chemotherapy trials reported for these lesions are generally small and treat a heterogeneic group of lesions with multiple drug combinations. They are therefore of insufficient power from which to draw any conclusions. It generally requires several hundred patients in each arm of an adjuvant trial to appropriately demonstrate a 10 to 15% improvement in outcome with adjuvant therapy.[95]

The results of several studies evaluating adjuvant multiagent doxorubicin-based chemotherapy in extremity soft tissue sarcoma have been conflicting. Some studies display a survival advantage and others do not.[96,97] A meta-analysis of the pooled data, however, suggests that adjuvant therapy significantly decreases the risk of recurrence and death in patients with high-grade extremity sarcomas.[98] Unfortunately, these data cannot be extrapolated to patients with retroperitoneal tumors.

Adjuvant single-agent or multiagent doxorubicin-based combinations that include methotrexate and cyclophosphamide have not proven useful in retroperitoneal tumors or tumors in other nonextremity sites. When taken as a whole, the adjuvant chemotherapy data on nonextremity sarcoma suggest significant toxicity and do not support the use of adjuvant therapy in retroperitoneal sarcomas on a routine basis.[96]

Metastatic Disease

Approximately one fifth of patients with soft tissue retroperitoneal sarcoma will present with metastatic disease. After definitive treatment for local disease, recurrence at multiple sites is the predominant pattern (47%) of metastasis. This is followed by isolated local recurrences (30%), isolated lung metastases (17%), and findings at other isolated sites (6%).[99,100] Generally all local and distant disease presents itself by 60 months. When technically feasible, local recurrence should be resected as discussed previously. Aggressive resection of isolated lesions at other sites is indicated, especially in the case of isolated pulmonary metastases. The demonstration of pulmonary metastases in the presence of extrapulmonary disease does not merit an attempt at pulmonary control. In the case of isolated pulmonary disease, however, those patients undergoing complete resection can experience a 38% 3-year actuarial survival.[101]

Doxorubicin serves as the foundation of chemotherapy for advanced disease in soft tissue sarcoma.[102,103] Initial studies reported a soft tissue sarcoma response rate of 20 to 25%, yet sustained complete responses with this agent are rare. Other agents that display activity are dacarbazine and ifosfamide.[104] Methotrexate and cyclophosphamide have also been classic constituents of doxorubicin-based chemotherapy.[105] Some early data on combination therapy including ifosfamide or dacarbazine suggested increased tumor responsiveness; thus several phase III trials were conducted to test these combinations against doxorubicin or doxorubicin plus carbazine control arms.[106,107] None of these studies demonstrated improved survival.

This sobering trend was confirmed by a recent phase III three-arm European Organization for Research and Treatment of Cancer report comparing doxorubicin alone to doxorubicin and ifosfamide and to cyclophosphamide, vincristine, doxorubicin, and dacarbazine (CYVADIC).[108] Thirty-five cancer centers treated 648 patients at multiple sites for metastatic soft tissue sarcoma. The overall response rate was 24%, and no significant difference was detected among the three study arms. The duration of remission ranged from 44 to 48 weeks and median survival was 51 to 55 weeks. Increased cardiotoxicity and myelosuppression were noted in the doxorubicin plus ifosfamide arm. Response rates related to site of tumor origin were not reported. These data confirm single-agent doxorubicin as the standard therapy for metastatic retroperitoneal soft tissue sarcoma.

Data on investigational therapy for advanced disease are sparse, yet one area of interest is the use of granulocyte-macrophage colony-stimulating factor (GM-CSF) to enhance immune recognition and tumor destruction in these lesions. Data on advanced sarcoma patients treated with exogenous GM-CSF as part of a standard chemotherapy protocol revealed a complete remission in one third (5 of 15) of the patients.[109] The further use of GM-CSF as an exogenous adjuvant agent or as part of a GM-CSF autologous tumor-based vaccine program may provide a qualitative improvement in the treatment of advanced soft tissue retroperitoneal sarcoma.[110,111]

ADULT URINARY TRACT SARCOMA

Primary sarcomas arising from the genitourinary system are extremely rare lesions overall and comprise only 1 to 2% of urologic tumors in adults. Only 800 to 1000 such tumors have been described from multiple genitourinary sites; thus practice principles in the diagnosis and treatment of these tumors must be derived from anecdotal pooled data.[112,113] General treatment principles are also extrapolated and applied from the clinical experience with primary retroperitoneal sarcomas. These lesions behave differently from pediatric genitourinary sarcomas, notably pediatric rhabdomyosarcoma (see Chapter 47). Thus treatment strategies, especially for advanced disease, tend to be empirical.

Despite the rarity of these tumors, the collective data regarding sarcomas of the genitourinary tract provide significant information with regard to clinical presentation and clinical outcome, which provides a rough guideline for treatment when these uncommon lesions are encountered. The most common sarcomatous lesions of the urinary system originate in the spermatic cord and paratesticular structures, which are not strictly speaking retroperitoneal. In decreasing order of incidence, sarcomas of the kidney, the bladder, and the prostate are encountered (Table 37–8).

Renal Sarcoma

Approximately 1 to 2% of kidney tumors are renal sarcomas. This excludes the spindle cell variant of renal cell carcinoma. The most frequent histologic subtypes of sarcoma encountered in the kidney are listed in Table 37–8. Leiomyosarcoma is the most common renal sarcoma comprising 30 to 40%

TABLE 37–8. MOST COMMON GENITOURINARY SARCOMAS (DECREASING ORDER OF FREQUENCY)

Renal
Leiomyosarcoma
Liposarcoma
MFH
Hemangiopericytoma
Rhabdomyosarcoma
Osteogenic sarcoma
Bladder
Leiomyosarcoma
Rhabdomyosarcoma
Osteogenic sarcoma
Liposarcoma
MFH
Fibrosarcoma
Prostate
Leiomyosarcoma
Rhabdomyosarcoma
Fibrosarcoma
Spindle cell sarcoma
Spermatic Cord, Testis, Paratestis
Leiomyosarcoma
Rhabdomyosarcoma
Liposarcoma
Fibrosarcoma
MFH

of most reported series. Liposarcoma and MFH are encountered in near-equal frequency because many fibrosarcomas have been reclassified under the general heading of MFH. Other major reported lesions include rhabdomyosarcoma, osteosarcoma, and hemangiopericytoma.[114–117] Renal sarcoma usually presents at a slightly younger age than in the average patient with renal cell carcinoma, with pain and flank mass as the common symptoms. Hematuria is seen less frequently with classic renal cell carcinoma. Renal sarcomas have no distinguishing imaging characteristics but tend to be hypervascular. When small, they are hard to distinguish from renal cell carcinoma, but hypovascularity combined with contiguous tumor spread may suggest one of these lesions.

Treatment for renal sarcoma is similar to that for renal cell carcinoma, namely, wide surgical excision. The principles for a standard radical nephrectomy conform to those for sarcoma surgery, and the modified thoracoabdominal approach is particularly suited to these lesions. As is the case in all soft tissue sarcomas, tumor size, reflected in complete resectability, and grade are the major determinants of clinical outcome. There are no data to support chemotherapy or radiation in the adjuvant setting, and it is unlikely that these modalities will confer a survival benefit for patients with advanced disease. The overall 5-year survival for these patients is approximately 30%. Those individuals with liposarcoma or hemangiopericytoma perform much better than patients with leiomyosarcoma. The survival rate at 5 years is in the 80 to 90% range for liposarcoma yet less than 50% for leiomyosarcoma. This is more than likely a reflection of tumor grade at presentation.[112,113,116]

Patients with renal sarcoma should adhere to close postoperative follow-up, including more frequent evaluation of the renal bed because local recurrence is the rule rather than the exception with sarcomas. Therapy for advanced disease usually consists of single-agent doxorubicin or multiagent doxorubicin-based chemotherapy. Although responses may be seen, sustained complete responses are not reported.

Urinary Bladder Sarcoma

In the adult, primary urinary bladder sarcomas are very rare, with less than 200 cases reported in the medical literature.[112,113] They comprise approximately 0.1 to 0.2% of all primary bladder tumors, yet present in a manner similar to typical bladder tumors. Most patients display hematuria, dysuria, or urinary frequency as the presenting signs and symptoms of their lesions. Imaging studies can display upper urinary tract obstruction or filling defects of the bladder.[116,118–121] The diagnosis can usually be made by transurethral resection of the bladder tumor. Pelvic and abdominal imaging with CT or MRI is useful in perioperative staging. The most common tumor histology in adult bladder sarcoma is leiomyosarcoma, followed by rhabdomyosarcoma. These lesions of muscle origin comprise 70 to 80% of all adult bladder sarcomas. Liposarcoma, MFH, and osteosarcoma account for less than 5% each of bladder sarcomas.[122,123] The development of some bladder sarcomas has been attributed to the secondary effects of radiation or chemotherapy exposure.[124,125]

The treatment of bladder sarcoma results in exceptionally good outcomes for a tumor type generally expected to perform poorly. In one series of patients with leiomyosarcoma treated with cystectomy and diversion, six of seven patients were alive at 35 to 95 months, with the other patient lost to follow-up. These patients underwent combinations of presurgical and postsurgical chemotherapy and/or radiation therapy.[121] Significant long-term disease-free survival rates have also been achieved with less aggressive surgery. In an earlier series from Memorial Sloan-Kettering Cancer Center, 14 of 15 patients with resectable bladder tumors displayed no evidence of disease 1 to 9 years after surgery; this included four patients who underwent partial cystectomy.[112] In a more recent series from the same institution, 7 of 10 patients with bladder sarcoma are alive without evidence of disease with over 5 years of follow-up, including 2 patients treated only with transurethral resection of 2-cm leiomyosarcomas of the bladder.[116] These data suggest that bladder preservation is a reasonable option in the treatment of this disease, especially in the case of leiomyosarcoma. Partial cystectomy is a reasonable option if wide (3- to 4-cm) margins can be obtained. Involvement of the trigone or more distal structures, however, would suggest total cystectomy and continent reconstruction as an appropriate option. Although the data are anecdotal, the use of chemotherapy and external beam radiation may be appropriate in patients with bladder sarcoma at high risk for local or distant recurrence. Overall 5-year survival for patients with bladder sarcomas is 60%. Those patients with adult rhabdomyosarcoma of the bladder have a poorer prognosis than their pediatric counterparts and adults with leiomyosarcoma. The 5-year survival for patients with adult rhabdomyosarcoma is approximately 30%.[126]

Prostate Sarcoma

There are fewer than 150 reported cases of primary sarcoma of the prostate.[112,113,121,127,128] Given the estimated yearly incidence of prostate cancer (over 300,000 cases), these lesions comprise well less than 0.1% of primary prostate tumors. The majority of prostate sarcomas are either leiomyosarcoma (50%) or rhabdomyosarcoma (30%); the remainder are distributed over multiple tissue types. In general, patients with prostate sarcoma tend to present somewhat younger than the typical patient with adenocarcinoma of the prostate. The most common presenting symptoms are bladder outlet obstruction and dysuria. A combination of symptoms and a palpable mass (often smooth) on physical examination lead to endoscopic evaluation and needle biopsy diagnosis. The majority of patients present with regional or local disease; 10 to 20% of patients may have metastases.

Cystoprostatectomy has generally been the treatment of choice for these tumors because most are large at the time of diagnosis, and because usually defined tissue planes may be obliterated by these tumors. In the case of extensive retroperitoneal disease, it may be preferable to perform a total pelvic exenteration to achieve complete local control. Because the potential for total continent reconstruction of both the urinary and lower gastrointestinal tract exists, this aggressive approach is a more favorable option than double ostomies or palliative therapy.[129] As in the case of bladder sarcoma, a pelvic lymph node dissection should accompany the exenterative procedure because nodal involvement, especially in rhabdomyosarcoma, can exist.

In general, patients with prostate sarcoma have an unfavorable outcome. The average 5-year survival is approximately 25%. Patients with leiomyosarcoma have a 40% 5-year survival rate and those with rhabdomyosarcoma have a 0 to 10% 5-year survival rate. It is difficult to assess the value of combined adjuvant therapy but, in the case of high-grade or extensive disease, a doxorubicin-based protocol and the addition of external beam radiation would be appropriate.

Paratesticular Tumors

The most common primary genitourinary sarcomas are those of the paratestis, spermatic cord, and testis proper.[112,113,116] Almost 300 cases of such lesions have been reported. The majority of these lesions are of muscle origin and are either rhabdomyosarcoma or leiomyosarcoma (50% of tumors). Liposarcomas and fibrosarcomas are commonly seen, along with a distribution of other rare lesions (Table 37–8). The most common benign tumor of the spermatic cord, however, is a lipoma, and the most common benign lesion of the paratesticular region is an adenomatoid tumor.

These lesions segregate into adolescent–early adult and older age (over 50) groups, with the majority of rhabdomyosarcomas concentrated in the younger patients. Rhabdomyosarcomas also have a greater predilection for occurring in an intrascrotal area. Liposarcoma and leiomyosarcoma can occur anywhere along the inguinal to paratesticular region and are often found in the inguinal region. It is unusual to have a sarcoma in the testicular parenchyma.

Patients with paratesticular sarcomas have a firm palpable mass in the scrotum or the spermatic cord. Any lesions of the scrotal contents should be evaluated with ultrasound, and all solid lesions should be classically treated with inguinal exploration biopsy and radical orchiectomy if indicated. Transcrotal exploration should not be performed. Further therapy for these tumors is dictated by tissue histology.

Rhabdomyosarcoma and leiomyosarcoma generally perform poorly. It is necessary to assess these patients for the presence of metastatic disease, particularly retroperitoneal lymph node involvement. In the absence of gross disease, a retroperitoneal lymph node dissection is appropriate, especially in the case of rhabdomyosarcoma, where the incidence of positive retroperitoneal nodes may be greater than 50%.[130,131] If gross nodal or distant metastatic disease is detected, doxorubicin-based chemotherapy is the classic treatment for advanced disease and is generally employed in the presence of microscopic metastasis. Those patients with liposarcoma generally show nearly complete cure through local excision.[132] Ninety per cent of patients may be treated in this fashion, but local recurrences have been reported and can result in fatalities.

Carcinosarcoma is a very rare lesion that can affect the genitourinary system. It is a malignant mixed tumor with sarcomatous and carcinomatous components. There are less than 100 reported cases, and the majority of these affected the urinary bladder.[133,134] Carcinosarcoma also has been reported in the prostate and kidney. Patient outcomes are uniformly poor, and treatment for this disease is anecdotal beyond radical surgery.

Summary

Genitourinary sarcomas are exceedingly rare lesions that are not amenable to controlled clinical trials. Precise standards for clinical care are therefore difficult to establish. Although the management of renal sarcomas differs little from the classic management of renal tumors, it is interesting to note that bladder sarcoma is a very treatable disease in which cure may be obtained in many cases without the loss of function. Prostate sarcomas are best treated with very aggressive surgery, and the outcome of paratesticular sarcoma is very much affected by primary histology. In urologic sarcomas there appears to be a role for lymph node dissection in conjunction with primary therapy, which is different than the clinical recommendations for primary retroperitoneal sarcomas. Adult rhabdomyosarcoma generally responds less well than its pediatric counterpart even when successful pediatric therapeutic protocols are employed. In all instances of genitourinary sarcoma, the overall lack of sustained responses to doxorubicin-based therapy suggests that patients with advanced disease should be enrolled in novel protocols.

REFERENCES

1. McGrath PC: Retroperitoneal sarcomas. Semin Surg Oncol 1994; 10:364.
2. Wingo PA, Tong T, Bolden S: Cancer statistics, 1995. CA Cancer J Clin 1995; 45:8.
3. Mack TM: Sarcomas and other malignancies of soft tissue, retroperitoneum, peritoneum, pleura, heart, mediastinum, and spleen. Cancer 1995; 75:211.
4. Pack GT, Tabah EJ: Primary retroperitoneal tumors: a study of 120 cases [International Abstracts of Surgery]. Surg Gynecol Obstet 1954; 99:209–231, 313–341.
5. Woodruff JM: Peripheral nerve tumors showing glandular differentiation (glandular schwannoma). Cancer 1976; 32:2399.
6. Arlen M, Higinbotham NL, Huvos AG, et al: Radiation-induced sarcoma of bone. Cancer 1971; 28:1087.
7. Bailar JC: How dangerous is dioxin? N Engl J Med 1991; 324:260.
8. Laskin WB, Silverman TA, Enzinger FM: Postradiation soft tissue sarcomas: an analysis of 53 cases. Cancer 1988; 62:2330.
9. Hardell L, Sandstrom A: Case-control study: soft tissue sarcoma and exposure to phenoxyacetic acids or chlorophenols. Br J Cancer 1979; 39:711.
10. Wingren G, Fredrikson M, Brage HN, et al: Soft tissue sarcoma and occupational exposures. Cancer 1990; 66:806.
11. Greenwald P, Kovasznay B, Collins DN, et al: Sarcomas of soft tissues after Vietnam service. J Natl Cancer Inst 1984; 73:1107.
12. Suruda AJ, Ward EM, Fingerhut MA: Identification of soft tissue sarcoma deaths in cohorts exposed to dioxin and to chlorinated naphthalenes. Epidemiology 1993; 4:14.
13. Economou JS, Sondak VK, Eilber FR: General considerations. *In* Eilber FR (ed): The Soft Tissue Sarcomas, Vol 2, pp 3–31. Orlando, FL, Grune & Stratton, 1987.
14. Bose B: Primary malignant retroperitoneal tumors: analysis of 30 cases. Can J Surg 1979; 22:215.
15. Armstrong JR, Cohn I Jr: Primary malignant retroperitoneal tumors. Am J Surg 1965; 110:937.
16. Coran AG, Crocker DW, Wilson RE: A twenty-five year experience with soft tissue sarcomas. Am J Surg 1970; 119: 288.
17. Oriana S, Bonardi P, Preda F: Primary retroperitoneal tumors. Tumori 1977; 63:397.
18. McGrath PC, Neifeld JP, Lawrence W Jr, et al: Improved survival following complete excision of retroperitoneal sarcomas. Ann Surg 1984; 200:200.
19. Dalton RR, Donohue JH, Mucha P, et al: Management of retroperitoneal sarcomas. Surgery 1989; 106:725.
20. Jacques DP, Coit DG, Hajdu SI, Brennan MF: Management of primary and recurrent soft-tissue sarcoma of the retroperitoneum. Ann Surg 1990; 212:51.
21. Storm FK, Mahvi DM: Diagnosis and management of retroperitoneal soft-tissue sarcoma. Ann Surg 1991; 214:2.
22. Glenn J, Sindelar WF, Kinsella T, et al: Results of multimodality therapy of resectable soft-tissue sarcomas of the retroperitoneum. Surgery 1985; 97:316.
23. Zornig C, Weh HJ, Krull A, et al: Retroperitoneal sarcoma in a series of 51 adults. Eur J Surg Oncol 1992; 18:475.
24. Karakousis CP, Velez AF, Emrich LJ: Management of retroperitoneal sarcomas and patient survival. Am J Surg 1985; 150:376.
25. Rossi CR, Nitti M, Foletto S, et al: Management of primary sarcomas of the retroperitoneum. Eur J Surg Oncol 1993; 19:355.
26. Kilkenny JW III, Bland KI, Copeland EM, et al: Retroperitoneal sarcoma: the University of Florida experience. J Am Coll Surg 1996; 182:329.
27. Rooser B, Willen H, Gustafson P, et al: Malignant fibrous histiocytoma of soft tissue. A population-based epidemiologic and prognostic study of 137 patients. Cancer 1991; 67:499.
28. Pezzi CM, Rawlings MS, Esgro JJ, et al: Prognostic factors in 227 patients with malignant fibrous histiocytoma. Cancer 1992; 69:2098.
29. Crozat A, Aman P, Mandahl N, Ron D: Fusion of CHOP to a novel RNA-binding protein in human myxoid liposarcoma. Nature 1993; 363:640.
30. Ladanyi M: The emerging molecular genetics of sarcoma translocations. Diagn Mol Pathol 1995; 4(3):162.
31. DeWeerd JH, Dockerty MB: Lipomatous retroperitoneal tumors. Am J Surg 1952; 84:397.
32. Mowat AP, Clark CG: Presacral lipomata. Br J Surg 1961; 49:230.
33. Heyns CF: Pelvic lipomatosis: a review of its diagnosis and management. J Urol 1991; 146:267.
34. Yalla SV, Ivker M, Burros HM, et al: Cystitis glandularis with perivesical lipomatosis: frequent association of two unusual proliferative conditions. Urology 1975; 5:383.
35. Klein FA, Vernon-Smith MJ, Kasenetz I, et al: Pelvic lipomatosis: 35 year experience. J Urol 1988; 139:998.
36. Sanders R, Nabil B, Curry N, et al: Clinical spectrum of adrenal myelolipoma: analysis of 8 tumors in 7 patients. J Urol 1995; 153:1791.
37. Chen KT, Felix EL, Flam MS: Extraadrenal myelolipoma. Am J Clin Pathol 1982; 78:386.
38. Fowler MR, Williams RB, Alba JM, et al: Extra-adrenal myelolipomas compared with extramedullary hematopoietic tumors: a case of pre-sacral myelolipoma. Am J Surg Pathol 1992; 6:363.
39. Kyriakos M, Kempson RL: Inflammatory fibrous histiocytoma: an aggressive and lethal lesion. Cancer 1976; 37: 1584.
40. Clement PH: Intravenous leiomyomatosis of the uterus. Pathol Annu 1988; 23:153.
41. Scurry JP, Carey MP, Targett CS, et al: Soft tissue lipoleiomyoma. Pathology 1991; 23:360.
42. Moriwaki Y, Miyake M, Yamamoto T, et al: Retroperitoneal ganglioneuroma: a case report and review of the Japanese literature. Int Med 1992; 31:82.

43. Mendelsohn G, Eggleston JC, Olson JL, et al: Vasoactive intestinal peptide and its relationship to ganglion cell differentiation in neuroblastic tumors. Lab Invest 1979; 41: 144.
44. Kindblom LG, Angervall L, Svendsen P: Liposarcoma: a clinicopathologic, radiographic and prognostic study. Acta Pathol Microbiol Scand 1975; 253:1.
45. Spittle MF, Newton KA, Mackenzie DH: Liposarcoma: a review of 60 cases. Br J Cancer 1971; 24:696.
46. Weiss SW, Rao VK: Well differentiated liposarcoma (atypical lipoma) of deep soft tissue of the extremities, retroperitoneum and miscellaneous sites: a follow-up study of 92 cases with analysis of the incidence of "dedifferentiation." Am J Surg Pathol 1992; 16:1051.
47. Enterline HT, Culberson JD, Rochlin DB, et al: Liposarcoma: a clinical pathological study of 53 cases. Cancer 1960; 13:932–950.
48. Shmookler BM, Lauer DH: Retroperitoneal leiomyosarcoma: a clinicopathologic analysis of 36 cases. Am J Surg Pathol 1983; 7:269.
49. Demers ML, Curley SA, Romsdahl MM: Inferior vena cava leiomyosarcoma. J Surg Oncol 1992; 51:89.
50. Cardell BS, McGill DAF, Williams F: Leiomyosarcoma of inferior vena cava producing Budd-Chiari syndrome. J Pathol 1971; 104:283.
51. Ozzello L, Stout AP, Murray MR: Cultural characteristics of malignant histiocytomas and fibrous xanthomas. Cancer 1963; 16:331.
52. Weiss SW: Malignant fibrous histiocytoma: a reaffirmation. Am J Surg Pathol 1982; 6:773.
53. Costa MJ, Weiss SW: Angiomatoid malignant fibrous histiocytoma: a follow-up study of 108 cases with evaluation of possible histologic predictors of outcome. Am J Surg Pathol 1990; 14:1126.
54. Bizer LS: Fibrosarcoma: report of 64 cases. Am J Surg 1971; 121:586.
55. Horn RC, Enterline HT: Rhabdomyosarcoma: a clinicopathological study of 39 cases. Cancer 1958; 11:181.
56. Cavazzana AO, Schmidt D, Ninfo V, et al: Spindle cell rhabdomyosarcoma: a prognostically favorable variant of rhabdomyosarcoma. Am J Surg Pathol 1992; 16:229.
57. Enzinger FM, Smith BH: Hemangiopericytoma: an analysis of 106 cases. Hum Pathol 1976; 7:61.
58. Zirkin RM: Retroperitoneal hemangiopericytoma. Int Surg 1977; 62:395.
59. Douglas JL, Mitchell R, Short DW: Retroperitoneal haemangiopericytoma. Br J Surg 1966; 53:31.
60. Ducatman BS, Scheithauer BW, Piepgras DG: Malignant peripheral nerve sheath tumors: a clinicopathologic study of 120 cases. Cancer 1986; 57:2006.
61. Smookler BM: Retroperitoneal synovial sarcoma: a report of four cases. Am J Clin Pathol 1982; 77:686.
62. Oda Y, Hashimoto H, Tsuneyoshi M, Takeshita S: Survival in synovial sarcoma: a multivariate study of prognostic factors with special emphasis on the comparison between early death and long-term survival. Am J Surg Pathol 1993; 17:35.
63. Miettienen M: Immunohistochemistry of soft-tissue tumors: possibilities and limitations in surgical pathology. A comprehensive survey of the usefulness and limitations of cellular markers in the differential diagnosis of these neoplasms. Pathol Annu 1990; 25(part 1):1–36.
64. Cohan RH, Baker ME, Cooper C, et al: Computed tomography of primary retroperitoneal malignancies. J Comput Assist Tomogr 1988; 12:804.
65. Fong Y, Coit DG, Woodruff JM, Brennan MF: Lymph node metastasis from soft tissue sarcoma in adults: analysis of data from a prospective database of 1772 sarcoma patients. Ann Surg 1993; 217:72.
66. Neifeld JP, Walsh JW, Lawrence W Jr: Computed tomography in the management of soft tissue tumors. Surg Gynecol Obstet 1982; 155:535.
67. DeSantos LA, Ginaldi S, Wallace S: Computed tomography in liposarcoma. Cancer 1981; 47:46.
68. Chang AE, Matory YL, Dwyer AJ, et al: Magnetic resonance imaging versus computed tomography in the evaluation of soft tissue tumors of the extremities. Ann Surg 1987; 205:340.
69. Bland KI, McCoy DM, Kinard RE, et al: Application of magnetic resonance imaging and computerized tomography as an adjunct to the surgical management of soft tissue sarcomas. Ann Surg 1987; 205:473.
70. Barth RJ, Merino MJ, Solomon D, et al: A prospective study of the value of core needle biopsy and fine needle aspiration in the diagnosis of soft tissue masses. Surgery 1992; 112:536.
71. Beahrs OH, Henson DE, Hutter RVP, Meyers MH: Soft tissues. *In* Beahrs OH, Henson DE, Hutter RVP, Myers MH (eds): Manual for Staging of Cancer, 3rd edition, p 127. Philadelphia, JB Lippincott Co, 1988.
72. Leyvraz S, Costa J: Histological diagnosis and grading of soft-tissue sarcomas. Semin Surg Oncol 1988; 4:3.
73. Kulander BG, Polissar L, Yang CY, et al: Grading of soft tissue sarcomas: necrosis as a determinant of survival. Mod Pathol 1989; 2:205.
74. Benjmark S, Hafstrom L, Jonsson PE, et al: Retroperitoneal sarcoma treated by surgery. J Surg Oncol 1980; 14: 307.
75. Catton CN, O'Sullivan B, Kotwall C, et al: Outcome and prognosis in retroperitoneal soft tissue sarcoma. Int J Radiat Oncol Biol Phys 1994; 29:1005.
76. Cody HS II, Turnbull AD, Fortner JG, et al: The continuing challenge of retroperitoneal sarcomas. Ann Surg 1984; 200:200.
77. Singer S, Corson JM, Demetri GD, et al: Prognostic factors predictive of survival of truncal and retroperitoneal soft-tissue sarcoma. Ann Surg 1995; 221:185.
78. Bevilacqua RG, Rogatoko A, Hajdu SI, Brennan MF: Prognostic factors in primary retroperitoneal soft-tissue sarcomas. Arch Surg 1991; 126:328.
79. Alvarenga JC, Ball AB, Fisher C, et al: Limitations of surgery in the treatment of retroperitoneal sarcoma. Br J Surg 1991; 78:912.
80. Fernandez-Trigo V, Surgarbaker PH: Sarcomas involving the abdominal and pelvic cavity. Tumori 1993; 79:77.
81. Skinner DG: Considerations for management of large retroperitoneal tumors: use of the modified thoracoabdominal approach. J Urol 1977; 117:605.
82. Wang YN, Zhu WQ, Shen ZZ, et al: Treatment of locally recurrent soft tissue sarcomas of the retroperitoneum: report of 30 cases. J Surg Oncol 1994; 56:213.
83. Shiloni E, Szold A, White DE, Freund HR: High-grade retroperitoneal sarcomas: role of an aggressive palliative approach. J Surg Oncol 1993; 53:197.
84. Suit HD, Mankin HJ, Wood WC, Proppe KH: Preoperative, intraoperative, and postoperative radiation in the treatment of primary soft tissue sarcomas. Cancer 1985; 55:2659.
85. Tepper JE, Suit HD, Wood WC, et al: Radiation therapy of retroperitoneal soft tissue sarcomas. Int J Radiat Oncol Biol Phys 1984; 10:825.
86. Fein DA, Corn BW, Lanciano RM, et al: Management of retroperitoneal sarcomas: does dose escalation impact on locoregional control? Int J Radiat Oncol Biol Phys 1995; 31:129.
87. Gunderson LL, Nagorney DM, McIlrath DC, et al: External beam and intraoperative electron irradiation for locally advanced soft tissue sarcomas. Int J Radiat Oncol Biol Phys 1993; 25:647.
88. Kiel KD, Won MH, Witt TR, et al: Preliminary results of protocol RTOG 85-07: phase II study of intraoperative radiation for retroperitoneal sarcomas. *In* Abe M, Takahasi M (eds): Intraoperative Radiation Therapy: Proceedings of the Third International Symposium of IORT, p 371. New York, Pergamon Press, 1991.
89. Sindelar WF, Kinsella TJ, Chen PW, et al: Intraoperative radiotherapy in retroperitoneal sarcomas: final results of a prospective, randomized, clinical trial. Arch Surg 1993; 128:402.
90. Willett CG, Suite HD, Tepper JE, et al: Intraoperative elec-

tron beam radiation therapy for retroperitoneal soft tissue sarcoma. Cancer 1991; 68:278.
91. Kinsella TJ, Sindelar WF, Lack E, et al: Preliminary results of a randomized study of adjuvant radiation therapy in resectable adult retroperitoneal soft tissue sarcomas. J Clin Ocol 1988; 6:18.
92. Greiner RH, Munkel G, Blattman H, et al: Conformal radiotherapy for unresectable retroperitoneal soft tissue sarcoma. Int J Radiat Oncol Biol Phys 1992; 22:333.
93. Goffman T, Tochner Z, Glatstein E: Large and massive adult sarcomas: primary treatment and iododeoxyuridine and aggressive hyperfractionated irradiation. Cancer 1991; 67:572.
94. Robertson JM, Sondak VK, Weiss SA, et al: Preoperative radiation therapy and iododeoxyuridine for large retroperitoneal sarcomas. Int J Radiat Oncol Biol Phys 1995; 31:87.
95. Sher HI: Chemotherapy for invasive bladder cancer: neoadjuvant versus adjuvant. Semin Oncol 1990; 17:555.
96. Elias AD, Antman KH: Adjuvant chemotherapy for soft-tissue sarcoma: a critical appraisal. Semin Surg Oncol 1988; 4:59.
97. Rosenberg SA, Tepper J, Glatstein E, et al: Prospective randomized evaluation of adjuvant chemotherapy in adults with soft tissue sarcomas of the extremities. Cancer 1983; 52:424.
98. Zalupski MM, Ryan JR, Hussein ME, et al: Systemic adjuvant chemotherapy for soft tissue sarcomas of the extremities. Surg Oncol Clin North Am 1993; 2:621.
99. Potter DA, Glenn J, Kinsella T, et al: Patterns of recurrence in patients with high grade soft-tissue sarcomas. J Clin Oncol 1985; 3:353.
100. Weingrad DW, Rosenberg SA: Early lymphatic spread of osteogenic and soft-tissue sarcomas. Surgery 1978; 84:231.
101. Putnam JB Jr, Roth JA: Resection of sarcomatous pulmonary metastases. Surg Oncol Clin North Am 1993; 2:673.
102. Gottlieb JA, Baker LJ, O'Bryan RM, et al: Adriamycin (NSC 123127) used alone and in combination for soft tissue and bone sarcoma. Cancer Chemother Rep 1975; 6: 271.
103. Borden EC, Amato DA, Rosenbaum C, et al: Randomized comparison of three Adriamycin regimens for metastatic soft tissue sarcomas. J Clin Oncol 1987; 5:840.
104. Luce JK, Thurman WG, Issacs BL, et al: Clinical trials with the antitumor agent 5-(3,3-dimethyl-1-triazeno)imidazole-4-carboxamide (NSC 45388). Cancer Chemother Rep 1970; 54:119.
105. Yap BS, Baker LH, Sinkovics JG, et al: Cyclophosphamide, vincristine, Adriamycin and DTIC (CyVADIC) combination chemotherapy for the treatment of advanced sarcomas. Cancer Treat Rep 1980; 64:93.
106. Edmonson JH, Ryan LM, Blum RH, et al: Randomized comparison of doxorubicin alone versus ifosfamide plus doxorubicin or mitomycin, doxorubicin, and cisplatin against advanced soft tissue sarcomas. J Clin Oncol 1993; 11:1269.
107. Antman KH, Crowley J, Balcerzak SP, et al: An intergroup phase III randomized study of doxorubicin and dacarbazine with or without ifosfamide and mesna in advanced soft tissue and bone sarcomas. J Clin Oncol 1993; 11:1276.
108. Santoro A, Tursz T, Mouridsen H, et al: Doxorubicin versus CYVADIC versus doxorubicin plus ifosfamide in first-line treatment of advanced soft tissue sarcomas: a randomized study of the European Organization for Research and Treatment of Cancer Soft Tissue and Bone Sarcoma group. J Clin Oncol 1995; 113:1537.
109. Edmonson JH: Chemotherapeutic approaches to soft tissue sarcomas. Semin Surg Oncol 1994; 10:357.
110. Golumbek PT, Axhari R, Jaffee EM, et al: Controlled release, biodegradable cytokine depots: a new approach in cancer vaccine design. Cancer Res 1993; 53:5841.
111. Edmonson JH: Needed: qualitative improvement in antisarcoma therapy. J Clin Oncol 1995; 13:1531.
112. Herr HW: Sarcoma of the urinary tract. *In* Dekernion JB, Paulson DF (eds): Genitourinary Cancer Management, p 259. Philadelphia, Lea & Febiger, 1987.
113. Tsukamoto T, Lieber MM: Sarcomas of the kidney, urinary bladder, prostate, spermatic cord, paratestis, and testis in adults. *In* Raaf JH (ed): Soft Tissue Sarcomas: Diagnosis and Treatment, p 201. St. Louis, Mosby, 1993.
114. Grignon DJ, Ayala AG, Ro JY, et al: Primary sarcoma of the kidney: a clinicopathologic and DNA flow cytometric study of 17 cases. Cancer 1990; 65:1611.
115. Mayes DC, Fechner RE, Gillenwater JY: Renal liposarcoma. Am J Surg Pathol 1990; 14:268.
116. Russo P, Brady MS, Conlon K, et al: Adult urological sarcoma. J Urol 1992; 147:1032.
117. Siniluotot TMJ, Paivansalo MJ, Hellstrom PA, et al: Hemangiopericytoma of the kidney: a case with preoperative ethanol embolization. J Urol 1988; 140:137.
118. Sen SE, Malek RS, Farrow GM, et al: Sarcoma and carcinosarcoma of the bladder in adults. J Urol 1985; 133:29.
119. Taylor RE, Busuttil A: Case report: adult rhabdomyosarcoma of bladder, complete response to radiation therapy. J Urol 1989; 142:1321.
120. Mills SE, Bova GS, Wick MR, Young RH: Leiomyosarcoma of the urinary bladder: a clinicopathologic and immunohistochemical study of 15 cases. Am J Surg Pathol 1989; 13:480.
121. Ahlering TE, Weintraub P, Skinner DG: Management of adult sarcomas of the bladder and prostate. J Urol 1988; 140:1397.
122. Harrison GSM: Malignant fibrous histiocytoma of the bladder. Br J Urol 1986; 58:457.
123. Oesterling JE, Epstein JI, Brendler CB: Malignant fibrous histiocytoma of the bladder. Cancer 1990; 66:1836.
124. Kerr KM, Grigor KM, Tolley DA: Rhabdomyosarcoma of the adult urinary bladder after radiotherapy for carcinoma. Clin Oncol 1989; 1:115.
125. Kawamura J, Sakurai M, Tsukamoto K, Tochigo H: Leiomyosarcoma of the bladder eighteen years after cyclophosphamide therapy for retinoblastoma. Urol Int 1993; 51:49.
126. Miettinen M: Rhabdomyosarcoma in patients older than 40 years of age. Cancer 1988; 62:2060.
127. Yum M, Miller JC, Agarwal BL: Leiomyosarcoma arising in atypical fibromuscular hyperplasia (phylloides tumor) of the prostate with distant metastasis. Cancer 1991; 68: 910.
128. Palmer MA, Viswanath S, Desmond D: Adult prostatic rhabdomyosarcoma. Br J Urol 1993; 71:489.
129. Skinner DG, Sherrod A: Total pelvic exenteration with simultaneous bowel and urinary reconstruction. J Urol 1990; 144:1433.
130. Sclama AD, Berger BM, Cherry JM, et al: Malignant fibrous histiocytoma of the spermatic cord: role of retroperitoneal lymphadenectomy in management. J Urol 1983; 130:577.
131. Heyn BR, Raney RB, Hays DM, et al: Late effects of therapy in patients with paratesticular rhabdomyosarcoma. J Clin Oncol 1992; 10:614.
132. Torosian MH, Wein AJ: Liposarcoma of the spermatic cord: case report and review of the literature. J Surg Oncol 1987; 34:179.
133. Grossman HB, Sonda LP, Lloyd RV, Gikas PW: Carcinosarcoma of bladder: evaluation by electron microscopy and immunohistochemistry. Urology 1984; 24:387.
134. Wick MR, Young RH, Malvesta R, et al: Prostatic carcinosarcomas. Am J Clin Pathol 1989; 92:131.

IX

URETHRA

38

URETHRAL CARCINOMA: DIAGNOSIS AND STAGING

MARIO C. BEDUSCHI, M.D., KENNETH I. WISHNOW, M.D., *and* JOSEPH E. OESTERLING, M.D.

Primary urethral carcinoma is a relatively rare tumor, accounting for less than 0.1% of all genitourinary neoplasms in both men and women. Although uncommon, urethral cancer displays an extremely diverse group of lesions, which differ substantially in mode of presentation, natural history, histopathology, and treatment. Due to its rarity, no single institution has a sufficient number of patients to prospectively evaluate different therapeutic options and establish treatment protocols. Until now, most previous reports on survival statistics were based on retrospective studies which, although helpful, have limitations.

Management of this pathology is done according to its size, stage, histopathology, and urethral location. Thus, in order to better understand, properly diagnose, and accurately stage this entity, it is desirable to have a thorough knowledge of the normal and abnormal features of the male and female urethra. In addition, because of the significant differences in presentation and anatomic features between both sexes, urethral carcinoma in men and women will be discussed separately.

MALE URETHRAL CARCINOMA

Anatomy

The male urethra acts as a conduit for both urinary and genital systems. It has an average length of 21 cm and extends from the bladder neck to the external urethral meatus. Classically, it is divided into three distinctive sections: penile, membranous, and prostatic urethra (Fig. 38–1). The prostatic segment, which is approximately 30 mm long, is also the widest and most distensible part of the urethra. It is closer to the anterior surface of the prostate as it courses its substance, and at the verumontanum level it displays an acute anterior angulation. Posteriorly, it shows a median longitudinal ridge of tissue formed by the epithelium of the mucosa and adjacent tissue called the crista urethralis, which represents an extension of the superficial bladder trigone. Alongside the crista urethralis lie the prostatic sinuses and the prostatic gland's excretory ducts. The verumontanum is located at the apex of the prostatic urethra and displays laterally a pair of ejaculatory ducts and medially the prostatic utricle (remnant of the müllerian duct). The membranous urethra is the thickest urethral segment and has an average length of 20 mm as it passes through the genitourinary diaphragm. It is a muscular organ, surrounded by smooth and striated muscle that composes the external urinary sphincter. Its anatomic integrity, after radical cystectomy and/or prostatectomy, seems to be closely related to urinary continence. The striated muscle involving this portion of the urethra has a posterior deficiency, so that it extends as an omega- or horseshoe-shaped structure from the prostate apex to the bulb of the penis. Its striated muscle fibers are mostly of the "slow twitch" type, allowing for sustained urethral compression. The pelvic fascia and ligaments sustain the membranous urethra and the prostatic apex. The deep dorsal vein of the penis courses the anterior aspect of the urethral sphincter between the transverse perineal ligament and the arcuate ligament of the pubis. The neurovascular bundles pass between the prostatic capsule and the lateral pelvic fascia at the 3- and 9-o'clock positions before they enter the penile crura.

The penile urethra, contained by the corpus spongiosum, is the longest urethral segment, with an average length of 15 cm in the adult male. It initiates at the membranous urethra and extends to the external urinary meatus. At the very proximal

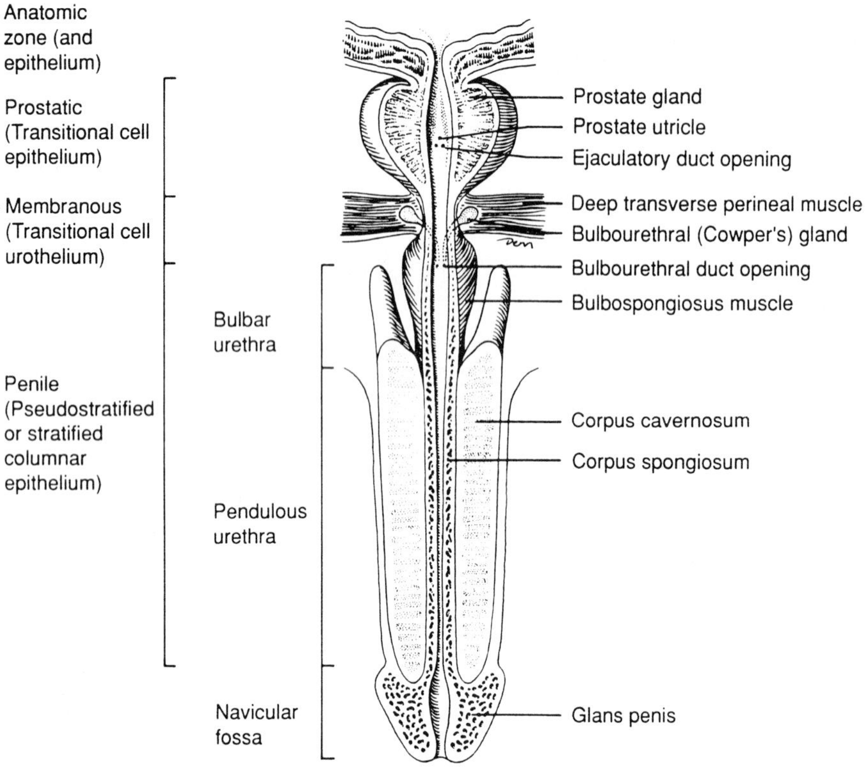
Anatomic zone (and epithelium)
Prostatic (Transitional cell epithelium)
Membranous (Transitional cell urothelium)
Penile (Pseudostratified or stratified columnar epithelium)
Bulbar urethra
Pendulous urethra
Navicular fossa
Prostate gland
Prostate utricle
Ejaculatory duct opening
Deep transverse perineal muscle
Bulbourethral (Cowper's) gland
Bulbourethral duct opening
Bulbospongiosus muscle
Corpus cavernosum
Corpus spongiosum
Glans penis

FIGURE 38–1. Anatomy of the male urethra. (From Carroll PR: Surgical management of urethral carcinoma. *In* Crawford ED, Das S [eds]: Current Genitourinary Cancer Surgery. Philadelphia, Lea & Febiger, 1990, with permission.)

portion, the pendulous urethra penetrates the corpus spongiosum and expands in a fusiform manner, forming the bulbar urethra. Both the corpus spongiosum and bulbar urethra are covered by the bulbospongiosus muscle. As the pendulous urethra enters the glans penis, it expands once more to form the fossa navicularis, and finally narrows down to open at the external meatus. The corpus spongiosum is a true vascular space consisting of sinusoidal tissue, lined by a continuous endothelial layer. This last structure is in close proximity to the urethral lumen, the result being that invasion of the tumor into this space provides direct access to vascular tissue and metastasis. The corpus spongiosum ends distally as the glans penis.

For diagnostic and therapeutic reasons, the urethra is divided into two portions: the posterior urethra, composed of the membranous and prostatic segments; and the anterior section, consisting of the pendulous and bulbar segments of the penile urethra.

Histology

Carefully described in 1972 by Bloom and Fawcett,[1] the histologic appearance of the male urethra varies along its extension. The prostatic segment is lined by the same type of transitional cells as the bladder neck. Stratified or pseudostratified columnar epithelium lines the pendulous, bulbous, and membranous urethra, whereas the mucosa of the meatus and fossa navicularis, as a rule, consist of squamous cells (Fig. 38–1). A great number of glands and ducts enter the urethra: the submucosal glands of Littre along the penile urethra, the ejaculatory and prostatic ducts in the prostatic urethra, and the bulbourethral glands (Cowper's glands) in the membranous urethra. The lamina propria of the mucosa is composed of loose connective tissue with a rich elastic network where numerous bundles of smooth muscle longitudinally oriented can be found. The outer layers show circular fibers as well. As described in the previous section, the membranous portion of the urethra is surrounded by a mass of striated muscle, a part of the urogenital diaphragm.

Lymphatic Drainage

Past reports have shown that 14 to 30% of male and female patients with urethral malignancy will present with lymph node spread at the moment of diagnosis.[2,3] It is well known that lymphatic channels of the anterior urethra preferentially drain into inguinal lymph nodes, and the posterior urethra into the pelvic chain. However, this feature may vary widely among patients depending on position, size, and extent of the tumor; and also, if the primary lymphatic route is obstructed by the disease.

Thus, a good knowledge of the specific locoregional lymphatic routes is important for accurate staging and adequate therapy. Lymphatics of the urethra and related structures drain into two major lymph node chains: those of the inguinal region (superficial and deep) and those of the pelvic region (obturator, external, and internal iliac) (Fig. 38–2).[4] Anterior urethral malignancy in male and female patients drains preferentially into the superficial inguinal lymph nodes. This chain of nodes is located in the subcutaneous tissue of the thigh, above the fascia lata. It is bounded superiorly by the inguinal ligament, the sartorius muscle laterally, and the abductor longus muscle medially.[4] The superficial inguinal nodes ultimately drain into the deep or external iliac lymph nodes. Deep inguinal nodes are found medially to the femoral vein and under the fascia lata, including Cloquet's node, which is located in the femoral canal medial to the lacunar ligament. Tumors of the posterior urethral segments drain into one or a combination of three pelvic chains: external, obturator, or presacral nodes (Fig. 38–2).[5,6]

Epidemiology and Etiology

Primary carcinoma of the urethra is the least frequent of the major urologic neoplasms, accounting for less than 1% of all male malignancies. Also, it is the only shared genitourinary cancer reported to have a higher incidence in females than in males, with a 4:1 predilection for women. Since its first description by Thiaudierre[7] in 1834, approximately 2,000 cases have been reported in the literature, 600 of them in men.[8] Even though there is a wide range of age presentation, from 13 to 90 years old, most of the patients are over 50 years of age when diagnosed with this pathology. No clear racial predisposition has been observed. Etiologic factors associated with this disease have not been definitively identified so far. Chronic urethral infections and/or irritation are frequent findings and are considered an important stimulus. Previous reports have shown that the majority of men with this pathology have a strong past history of strictures (35 to 88%), and recurrent urethral instrumentation and dilation.[9,10] It is noteworthy that the most frequent site of cancer, the bulbomembranous urethra, is also the prevalent region for stricture and metaplasia.[11] Urethritis, venereal disease, and trauma history are common findings and could be facilitating factors. The finding of viral particles in the urine of some patients with urologic malignancy suggest a pos-

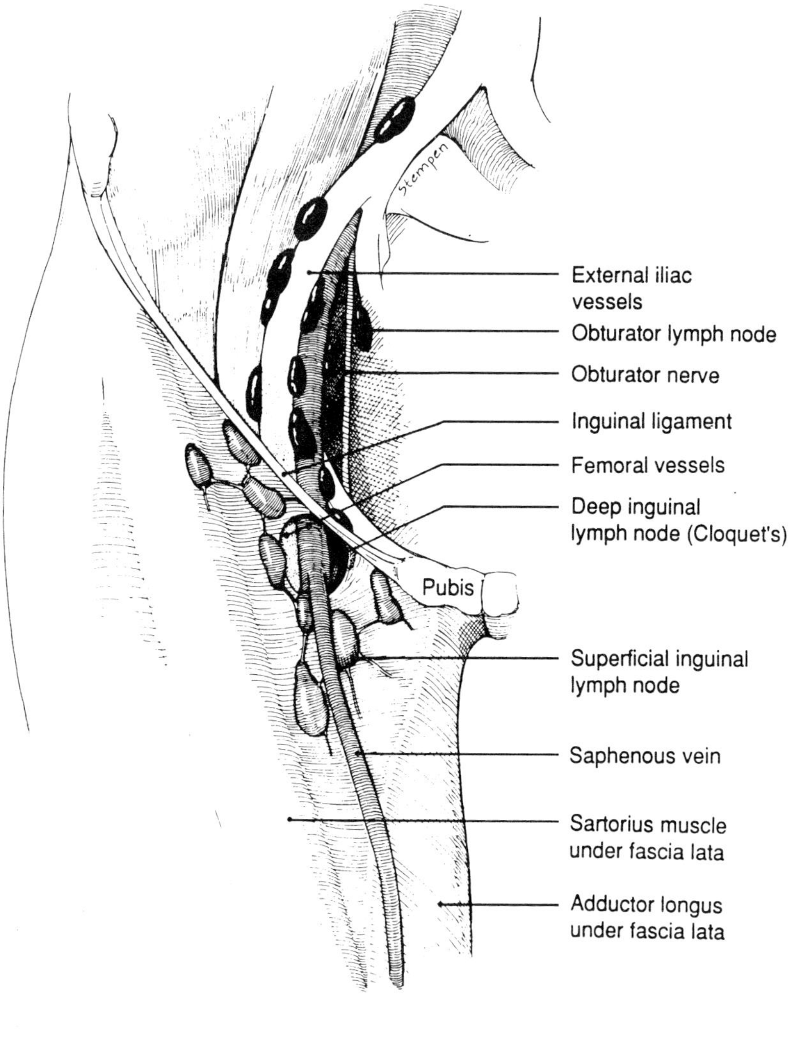
External iliac vessels
Obturator lymph node
Obturator nerve
Inguinal ligament
Femoral vessels
Deep inguinal lymph node (Cloquet's)
Pubis
Superficial inguinal lymph node
Saphenous vein
Sartorius muscle under fascia lata
Adductor longus under fascia lata

FIGURE 38–2. Lymphatic drainage of the urethra. (From Carroll PR, et al: Surgical anatomy of the male and female urethra. Urol Clin North Am 1992; 19(2):345, with permission.)

sible viral etiology, but no significant evidence has evolved so far.[12,13]

No etiologic role in the development of transitional cell carcinoma of the urethra has been identified, in contrast to the well-known association between aromatic amines, smoking, analgesic abuse, and bladder transitional cell carcinoma.[14] However, there is an unquestionable relationship with concominant or previous bladder cancer.[15,16]

Clinical Presentation

Clinical symptoms in the male differ widely, depending on the site and extension of the tumor, but they are usually vague and nondescript. When present, they frequently mimic those of more frequent and benign disorders such as stricture, fistula, and urethritis.[10] The most common symptoms in the penile segment are difficulty in urination and the presence of a nodule. With progression, the manifestations become the same as those of carcinoma of the prostatic urethra, which are symptoms associated with obstruction or incontinence secondary to overflow. Hematuria, urethral irritation, purulent discharge, decreased caliber and strength in the urinary stream, periurethral abscess, dysuria, straining to urinate, and fistula are other signs and symptoms found in combination with the previous picture.[17] Some patients may notice or present with penile erosion, priapism, impotence, and edema of the entire genital area. A ventral periurethral mass or fistula is frequently seen in anterior lesions, while a perineal mass is usually associated with large bulbar or bulbomembranous tumors. Anorexia, malaise, and weight loss are late and often terminal signs.

The interval between onset of symptoms and diagnosis is usually 5 to 6 months, but may be as long as 15 years.[10] Diagnosis is delayed, most of the time, due to the patients' failure to seek medical assistance, and also because of misdiagnosed conditions.

Diagnosis

The above-mentioned signs and symptoms of male urethral cancer are shared by other more common benign urethral lesions. This fact, combined with the rarity of this malignancy, imposes a high level of difficulty to the attending urologist, often resulting in diagnostic delays. In order to make the diagnosis, one must include urethral cancer among the list of differential diagnoses. A careful history and physical examination will identify high-risk individuals and/or misdiagnosed situations. Due to its high incidence, benign urethral stricture is often attributed as the cause of obstructive complaints, and traditional therapy is initiated. For such cases, it is good to keep in mind that every time a "stricture" requires frequent dilation or bleeds excessively after gentle manipulation, one must have a high index of suspicion and consider malignant process as a possibility.

In establishing diagnosis of urethral carcinoma, a tissue specimen is essential, and this is usually accomplished by urethroscopy and transurethral biopsy of any suspicious friable or necrotic-appearing tissue. Often, recurrent repeated deep biopsies are needed in areas of abscess or fistula for final confirmation; and occasionally, open or transperineal (Tru-cut) needle biopsy may be indicated.[18]

Other accessory diagnostic methods have been used, including retrograde urethrogram that was suggestive of urethral malignancy in 60% of patients in one series[19,20]; however, its use has not gained wide acceptance due to superior results obtained with the standard urethrocystoscopy. If available, long, irregular strictures with extravasation, obstruction, fistula formation, and intraluminal filling defects are among the abnormalities described. Urine cytology was used in two previous reports[10,19] and were positive for carcinoma in 88 and 100% of the cases, respectively, and may be considered as a screening procedure in high-risk subjects.

Transitional cell carcinoma of the prostate without concurrent or previous bladder cancer frequently presents with the irritative symptoms of frequency, urgency, and dysuria. If there is invasion of the stroma, the prostate may be nodular and indurated on palpation by rectal examination. Unlike the much more common adenocarcinoma of the prostate, the serum acid phosphatase level is normal and skeletal metastases are osteolytic rather than osteoblastic. Prostatic biopsies are necessary to adequately study the ducts and stroma for the presence of invasion or limitation to the epithelium.

Histopathology

Carcinoma of the urethra may arise from the surface epithelium of the urethra or from any of the local glands. The majority of male urethral carcinomas arising in the membranous or penile segment are of squamous cell origin (69 to 90%). On the other hand, the transitional cell type is most often seen in the posterior segment, accounting for 80% of the tumors originating in the prostatic urethra. Glandular, undifferentiated, and adenocarcinomatous are other tumor types that may be occasionally found. The incidence of male urethral carcinoma by tumor location within the urethra and the frequency of histopathologic types of each location is shown in Figure 38–3. Squamous cell carcinoma of the urethra resembles similar aspects seen in other organs. Usually, it is well or moderately differentiated with focal keratinization. The cells may display anaplastic and pleomorphic features with many mitoses (Fig. 38–4). Frequently, it

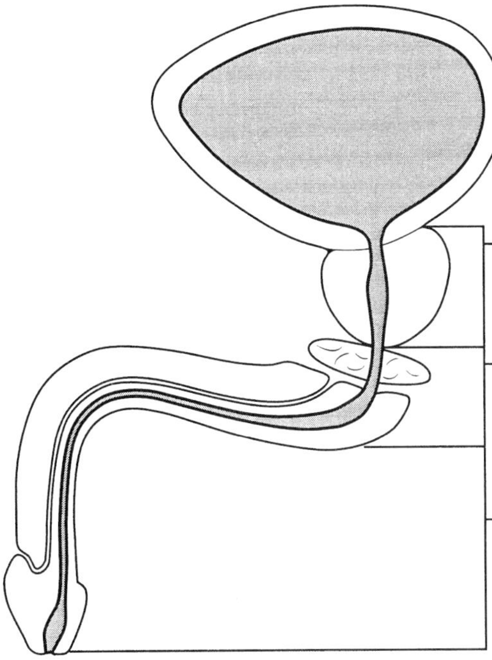
Prostatic (7%)
• Transitional 88%
• Squamous 14%
Bulbomembranous (59%)
• Squamous 82%
• Transitional 8%
• Adenocarcinoma 8%
• Undifferentiated 2%
Penile (34%)
• Squamous 90%
• Transitional 10%

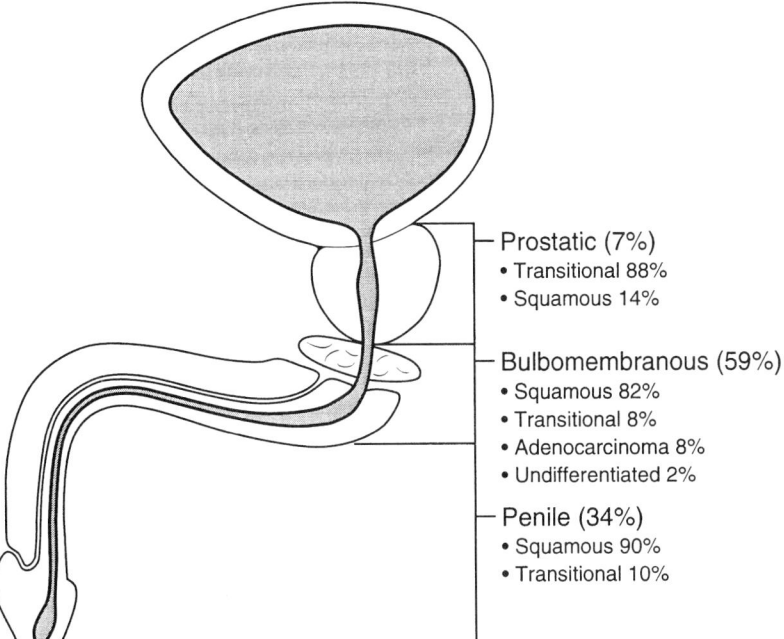

FIGURE 38–3. Incidence of male urethral carcinoma according to urethral location and frequency of histologic types. (From Johnson DE: Cancer of the male urethra. *In* Johnson DE, Bolieau M [eds]: Overview in Genitourinary Tumors: Fundamental Principles and Surgical Techniques. New York, Grune & Stratton, 1982, with permission.)

has an exophytic appearance, but it may become ulcerative and fungating with time.

Transitional cell carcinoma exhibits patterns identical to those seen in bladder cancer. Thus, the lesion may be a papilloma, carcinoma in situ (CIS), papillary, or infiltrating carcinoma (Fig. 38–5). Before the lesion has been ruled as a primary neoplasm of the urethra, it is absolutely essential to exclude transitional cell malignancy of the bladder, particularly CIS, since multicentric disease is an especially frequent feature in this pathology.[21,22] Adenocarcinomas of the urethra are rare, with numbers ranging from 6 to 10%. In the male, we find two different entities: first, in the prostatic urethra, a papillary adenocarcinoma has been described and posteriorly demonstrated to be a prostatic carcinoma due to the fact that their epithelial cells react to prostate-specific antigen (PSA) and prostatic acid phosphatase (PAP). It could originate from islands of prostatic secretory epithelium in the prostatic

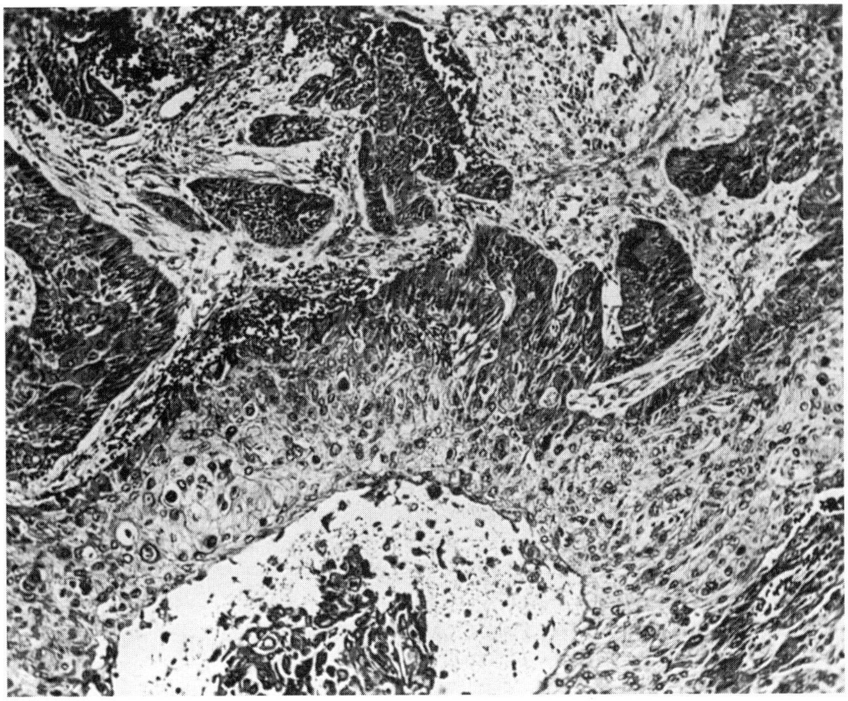

FIGURE 38–4. Squamous cell carcinoma of the urethra infiltrating the corpus spongiosum. (From Mostofi FK, et al: Carcinoma of the male and female urethra. Urol Clin North Am 1992; 19(2):347, with permission.)

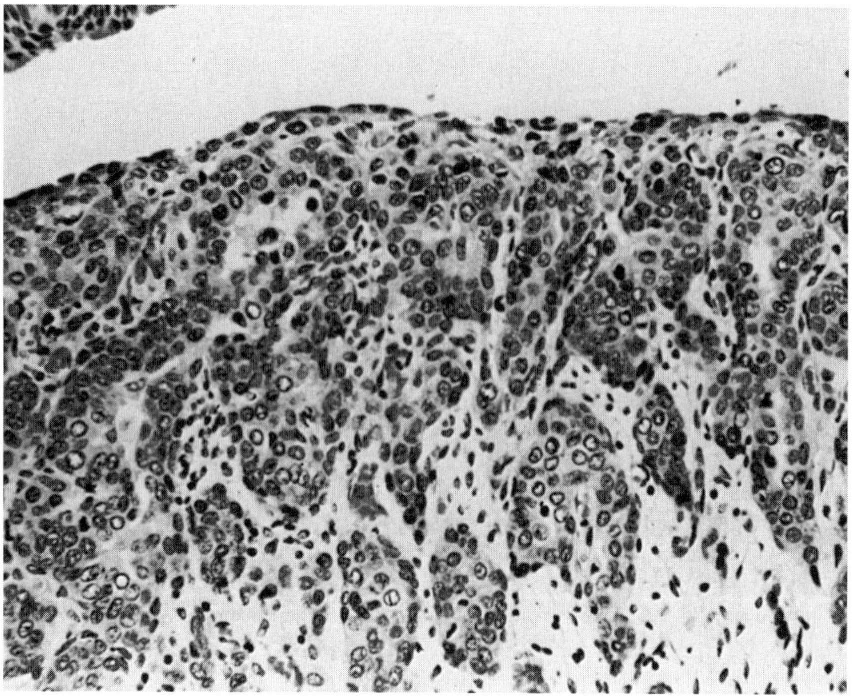

FIGURE 38–5. Infiltrating transitional cell carcinoma, grade II, of urethra. (From Mostofi FK, et al: Carcinoma of the male and female urethra. Urol Clin North Am 1992; 19(2):347, with permission.)

urethra, or from prostatic glands in the wall of the prostatic urethra. The second lesion is carcinoma of Cowper's glands. In contrast to the normal Cowper's gland, which consists of small regular acini lined by uniform high cuboidal cells with mucous cytoplasm and a small and delicate nucleus, in Cowper's adenocarcinoma, the glands are irregular and are lined by anaplastic epithelial cells.[22]

Stage

Accurate assessment of extent of disease and proper staging of the patient with urethral cancer is essential for a good therapeutic approach. This task should be accomplished through a complete clinical evaluation, and a careful physical examination is a fundamental step in this process. The assessment of the primary tumor should include the size, location, fixation, and involvement of nearby structures. The urethra should be carefully inspected and palpated, beginning at the meatus and extending to the urogenital diaphragm. Posterior urethral segments may be evaluated by invagination of the scrotum and by digital rectal examination (DRE). The corpora spongiosum and cavernosum should be meticulously inspected for masses and induration. Systematic palpation of the inguinal lymphatics should record the presence of lesions.

Urethrocystoscopy should be performed to obtain a good set of biopsy specimens for establishing diagnosis and evaluating the extent of disease. Palpation of the urethra over a cystoscope often assists in determining the degree of tumor invasion.

Since the above procedure is done under anesthesia, this is a good moment to perform a thorough physical examination, as described above, as well as a bimanual examination, which will assist in identifying associated prostatic abnormalities, trigonal invasion, or pelvic adherence.

The employment of computed tomography (CT) scanning or magnetic resonance imaging (MRI) should be considered in most cases of urethral cancer, in order to assess local progression of the disease. The exceptions would be the more distal and superficial lesions. MRI has shown promise in revealing an 83% accuracy in staging the disease in one recent study, but these results await definitive confirmation through larger study groups.[14] Due to its easy availability, CT and MRI have been tentatively used to assess pelvic and inguinal node involvement, but both lack specificity. In the event that enlarged nodes are present, and if clinically indicated, it is possible to perform CT-guided fineneedle aspiration for definition of node involvement. Lymphangiography offers several potential advantages over CT and MRI in assessing lymph node status, but its use continues to decline due to its invasiveness. Intravenous urography should be performed in all patients with tumors of transitional cell origin. Other screening studies such as bone scan, liver profile, chest x-ray, or chest CT should be dictated by the results. Despite all efforts, the index of understaging remains quite high.

There is no universally accepted staging system for male urethral cancer. The most commonly used system is the one developed by Ray and Guinan (Table 38–1).[23] A system proposed by the American Joint Committee on Cancer (AJCC) based on the

TABLE 38–1. STAGING SYSTEM FOR MALE URETHRAL CARCINOMA PROPOSED BY RAY AND ASSOCIATES*

Stage	Description
0	Tumor confined to mucosa
A	Tumor extension into but not beyond lamina propria
B	Tumor extension into but not beyond substance of corpus spongiosum or into but not beyond prostate
C	Direct extension into tissues beyond corpus spongiosum (corpora cavernosa, muscle, fat, fascia, skin, direct skeletal involvement) or beyond prostatic capsule
D1	Regional metastasis including inguinal and/or pelvic lymph nodes
D2	Distant metastases

*From Ray B, Canto SR, Whitmore WF: Experience with primary carcinoma of the male urethra. J Urol 1977; 117:591, with permission.

primary tumor and the presence or absence of regional lymph node involvement or dissemination (TNM) is presented in Table 38–2.

Natural History

Urethral carcinoma is a disease predominantly of middle age, and is often first diagnosed at an advanced stage due to local invasion and lymphatic metastases. Distant metastases by hematogenous routes are uncommon. The average age of the patient at presentation is 58 years. In the series by Ray et al.,[19] 26% of the patients had stage C disease at presentation, while 43% had stage D. This was especially true for patients with posterior lesions, which were either at stage C or D in 86% of cases at presentation. In contrast, stage A or B disease was identified in 55% of patients with anterior carcinoma. Carcinoma of the anterior urethra is thought to become symptomatic earlier in the disease process, which partially explains its earlier recognition and higher survival rate. Symptoms of carcinoma of the posterior urethra may be confused initially with stricture or some irritative process. The median elapsed time between development of symptoms and presentation for treatment was 5 months in one large series.

Urethral carcinoma spreads by direct extension to adjacent structures or to regional lymph nodes. Frequently, there is involvement of the corpora cavernosa or corpus spongiosum. Grabstald (1973) reported that skin ulceration is the primary finding on physical examination in many instances. The majority of patients have only local invasion or regional lymph node metastases when they die, with death occurring secondary to sepsis or bleeding.[24] Distant hematogenous spread is unusual, reported in 12% of patients in one study and 14% in another.[10,25] Of these patients, 62% had involvement of the corpora cavernosa when the diagnosis was made. The most common sites of distant metastases

TABLE 38–2. AMERICAN JOINT COMMITTEE ON CANCER STAGING SYSTEM FOR URETHRAL CANCER*

Primary Tumor (T) (Male)	
Tx	Primary tumor cannot be assessed
T0	No evidence of primary tumor
Tis	Carcinoma in situ
Ta	Noninvasive papillary, polypoid, or verrucous carcinoma
T1	Invades subepithelial connective tissue
T2	Invades corpus spongiosum or prostate or periurethral muscle
T3	Invades corpus cavernosum or beyond prostatic capsule or bladder neck
T4	Invades other adjacent organs
Regional Lymph Nodes (N)	
Nx	Regional lymph nodes cannot be assessed
N0	No regional lymph node metastasis
N1	Metastasis in a single lymph node, 2 cm or less in greatest dimension
N2	Metastasis in a single lymph node, >2 cm but no more than 5 cm in greatest dimension, or multiple lymph nodes, none >5 cm in greatest dimension
N3	Metastasis in a lymph node(s) >5 cm in greatest dimension
Distant Metastasis (M)	
Mx	Presence of distant metastasis cannot be assessed
M0	No distant metastasis
M1	Distant metastasis

*From Beahrs OH, et al (eds): Manual for Staging of Cancer, 4th edition. Philadelphia, JB Lippincott Co, 1992, with permission.

are the lungs, liver, and bones. Local ulceration with secondary infection and sepsis is a frequent cause of death.

Transitional cell carcinoma of the prostate behaves in a different fashion. It is usually regarded as being highly malignant, with a propensity for hematogenous dissemination. Carcinoma in situ begins in the prostatic ducts and is believed to be the precursor of invasive carcinoma.[26–28] Metastatic spread occurs by both hematogenous and lymphatic routes.

FEMALE URETHRAL CANCER

Anatomy

The female urethra is approximately 4 to 6 cm long and about 8 mm in diameter. It initiates at the internal meatus (vesical neck), and runs anteroinferiorly just below the symphysis, firmly adherent to the anterior wall of the vagina. It traverses the perineal membrane and ends at the external urethra, which is situated directly anterior to the vaginal introitus and 2 cm inferior to the glans clitoris (Fig. 38–6).

The female urethra represents the entire sphincteric mechanism for the bladder. It has a thick muscular wall, composed of two coats: an inner longi-

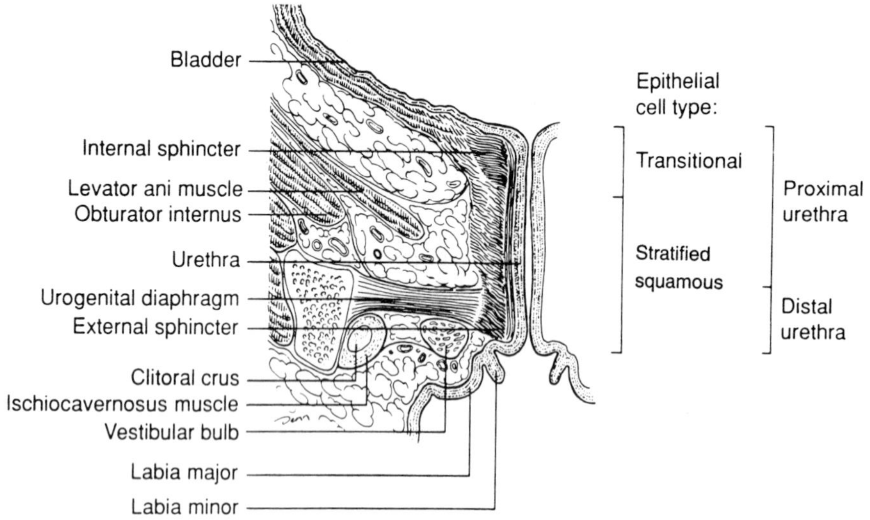
Bladder
Internal sphincter
Levator ani muscle
Obturator internus
Urethra
Urogenital diaphragm
External sphincter
Clitoral crus
Ischiocavernosus muscle
Vestibular bulb
Labia major
Labia minor
Epithelial cell type:
Transitional
Stratified squamous
Proximal urethra
Distal urethra

FIGURE 38–6. Anatomy of the female urethra. (From Carroll PR: Surgical management of urethral carcinoma. *In* Crawford ED, Das S [eds]: Current Genitourinary Cancer Surgery. Philadelphia, Lea & Febiger, 1990, with permission.)

tudinal layer continuous with the detrusor inner longitudinal musculature; and an outer semicircular layer continuous with the detrusor outer longitudinal musculature. At the middle urethral third, there is a dense condensation of striated muscle fibers, forming a ring. This last structure is related to voluntary continence. It is arbitrarily divided into an anterior segment (distal third) and a posterior segment (proximal two thirds). Practical importance of this arbitrary segmentation is that the distal one third of the urethra can be surgically excised and continence will be preserved.

Histology

The proximal third of the female urethra is lined by transitional cell epithelium, whereas the distal two thirds presents mainly stratified squamous epithelium. Submucosal glands lined by pseudostratified and stratified columnar epithelium are present throughout its length, including a vestigial prostate in the distal third of the urethra capable of reacting to PAP and PSA. The lamina propria is made of a loose connective tissue rich in elastic fibers, and a plexus of large vein. The muscularis layer consists of a double layer of smooth muscle distributed in a manner similar to that of the ureters, plus the reinforcement by a striated muscle at its orifice forming a sphincter.[22]

Epidemiology and Etiology

Primary carcinoma of the female urethra is a rare pathology, accounting for 0.02% of all malignancies in women. Wasserman, in 1895, reported the first 24 cases of female urethral tumor.[28] Since then, approximately 1200 such cases have been reported in the literature. It is the only genitourinary neoplasm shared by both sexes, with a 4:1 predilection for women. This has been an intriguing finding for the investigators, considering the greater length and higher complexity of the male urethra.

More than 35% of female urethral cancers occur in postmenopausal women between 50 and 70 years of age (average 60). However, occurrence has been reported at nearly any age (range, 4 to 90 years).[29,23] The neoplasm seems to have a higher incidence among white (84%) than among black women (12%) or Hispanics (4%).[30]

Precise etiologic factors for primary female urethral cancer have not been identified. Findings such as chronic irritation, fibrosis, caruncles, polyps, diverticula, coitus, parturition, and viral infection have been suggested as causative factors, but with no substantiating evidence.

Clinical Presentation

Symptoms of urethral carcinoma in women are nondescript. Urethral bleeding or spotting is the most commonly reported symptom, occurring in over 50% of the cases.[23,31–33] Other frequent symptoms include urgency, swelling, dysuria, frequency, pain, dyspareunia, incontinence, and palpable mass. Presence of urethrovaginal or vesicovaginal fistula or inguinal lymphadenopathy reveals advanced disease.[31] On physical examination, an anterior lesion may appear as a papillary, red, or meaty lump protruding through the meatus, or as a circumferentially indurated ring. Carcinoma is mistaken for benign caruncle in about 2% of clinically diagnosed caruncles. Larger and more extensive lesions may cause induration and fixation to the pubis or vagina.

Diagnosis

All the major symptoms of female urethral carcinoma are also common symptoms of other benign urethral lesions. These include caruncle, polyp, erosion, prolapse, hemangioma, diverticulum, fibroma, and urethrovaginal fistula. Thus, once faced by the signs and symptoms described above, one should include malignancy of the urethra in the differential diagnosis, in order to avoid delays in diagnosis and therapy. Survival depends on stage and size of the neoplasm at the time of diagnosis; for this reason, the liberal use of endoscopy and biopsy of any suspicious urethral lesion to evaluate lower tract symptoms is essential. The diagnostic approach in identifying this disease is similar to the one described for male diagnosis.

Histopathology

The three predominant cell types are squamous cell carcinoma, transitional cell carcinoma, and adenocarcinoma. Sullivan and Grabstald, in 1978, presented a revision of 584 patients where 70% were found to have squamous cell carcinoma, 10% had transitional cell carcinoma, and 18% had adenocarcinoma.[32] These were relatively equally distributed between the proximal and distal urethra, with 49% located in the anterior urethra and 51% classified as entire in location. In a more recent collective review of 568 cases, epidermoid or squamous cell carcinoma was seen in 55%, transitional cell carcinoma in 18%, adenocarcinoma in 16%, melanoma in 3%, anaplastic or undifferentiated in 1%, lymphoma in 0.5%, and others in 1%.[34]

The histologic characteristics of squamous cell carcinoma and transitional cell carcinoma are the same described elsewhere for male urethral cancer. Adenocarcinomas have two possible origins. The first, clear cell carcinoma, is frequently seen in female diverticula. The cells are usually cuboidal and form tubuloacinar structures similar to the ones observed in renal cell carcinoma. The tumor tends to metastasize and has a poor prognosis. The second and most interesting adenocarcinoma in the female urethra is prostatic carcinoma. It is located in the urethral external meatus, has a polypoid configuration, and is typically moderately differentiated. Its prostatic origin is confirmed by positive tissue reaction to PAP and PSA.[22]

Stage

Careful and accurate assessment of disease extension is important, as therapy and outcome depend more on stage and location of the tumor than on cell type or grade. Inspection of the meatus, labia, clitoris, vagina, and groin will identify possible areas of infiltration. Biopsies of the vulva, vagina, and bladder should be obtained according to findings on bimanual examination and cystourethroscopy.

Imaging assessment should be performed according to the parameters described elsewhere for male tumor staging.

TABLE 38–3. GRABSTALD STAGING SYSTEM FOR CARCINOMA OF THE FEMALE URETHRA*

Stage 0	In situ (limited to mucosa)
Stage A	Submucosal (not beyond submucosa)
Stage B	Muscular (infiltrating periurethral muscle)
Stage C	Periurethral
C1	Infiltrating muscular wall of the vagina
C2	Infiltrating muscular wall of the vagina with invasion of vaginal mucosa
C3	Infiltrating other adjacent structures (e.g., bladder, labia, clitoris)
Stage D	Metastasis
D1	Inguinal lymph nodes
D2	Pelvic lymph nodes below the bifurcation of the aorta
D3	Lymph nodes above the bifurcation of the aorta

*From Grabstald H, Hilaris B, Henschke U, et al: Cancer of the female urethra. JAMA 1966; 197:835, with permission. Copyright 1966, American Medical Association.

The clinical staging system proposed by Grabstald based on pathologic criteria at the Memorial Hospital[31] is widely used and is similar to that used for bladder cancer (Table 38–3). Grabstald has also described the location of the lesion as anterior, when limited to the meatus and distal third of the urethra, and as posterior (entire) when there is involvement of the proximal two thirds of the urethra, with or without extension to the anterior urethra. Anterior and posterior tumors occur with approximately equal frequency. Anterior tumors tend to be of lower grade and stage and have a better prognosis. Similarly, small lesions (<2 cm) and moderate size lesions (2 to 4 cm) have a better outcome than large (>5 cm) carcinomas.[31]

Table 38–4 presents the staging system proposed by the AJCC (TNM) in an attempt to establish a universal staging system.

Natural History

The natural history of urethral carcinoma in women is very similar to the natural history of the disease in men. Although urethral carcinoma has been reported in young individuals, more than 75% of patients are in the postmenopausal age group. Spread occurs by local extension to adjacent structures and to regional lymph nodes. Early invasion may involve the periurethral connective tissue, urethrovaginal septum, vagina, bladder neck, or vulva. Large, fungating meatal lesions may be difficult to differentiate from primary vulvar carcinoma. Involvement of the pubic bone is, surprisingly, unusual. Carcinoma of the entire urethra tends to be more locally advanced at initial presentation, possibly due to a delay in diagnosis. In one series, 13% of patients with an anterior lesion had metastases to lymph nodes in contrast to 30% of patients with carcinoma of the entire urethra.[35]

Lesions of the anterior urethra tend to metasta-

TABLE 38–4. FEMALE URETHRAL CANCER STAGING ACCORDING TO TNM

Primary Tumor (T) (Female)	
Tx	Cannot be assessed
T0	No evidence of primary tumor
Tis	Carcinoma in situ (CIS)
Ta	Noninvasive papillary, polypoid, or verrucous carcinoma
T1	Invades subepithelial connective tissue
T2	Invades periurethral musculature
T3	Invades anterior vagina or bladder neck
T4	Invades other adjacent organs
Regional Lymph Nodes (N)	
Nx	Regional lymph nodes cannot be assessed
N0	No regional lymph node metastasis
N1	Metastasis to a single lymph node, ≤2 cm in greatest dimension
N2	Metastasis to a single lymph, >2 cm but no more than 5 cm in greatest dimension, or multiple nodes involved with none >5 cm in greatest dimension
N3	Metastasis in a lymph node >5 cm in greatest dimension
Distant Metastases (M)	
Mx	Presence of distant metastasis cannot be assessed
M0	No distant metastasis
M1	Distant metastasis

*From Beahrs OH, et al (eds): Manual for Staging of Cancer, 4th edition. Philadelphia, JB Lippincott Co, 1992, with permission.

size to the inguinal nodes, while lesions of the posterior or entire urethra spread to the pelvic lymph nodes. Clinical evidence of inguinal adenopathy is seen in 35 to 56% of the patients, but pathologically proved metastasis occurs in only 12.5 to 35% of the total number of patients seen with this disease.[31,32,36] This has created controversy as to whether adenopathy usually represents metastatic disease rather than secondary infection. Grabstald found histologic evidence of cancer in 24 of 25 patients with enlarged nodes.[31]

Most authors consider inguinal adenopathy to represent metastatic disease. In those patients who underwent pelvic lymphadenectomy, 50% were found to have positive nodes.

As is the case with urethral carcinoma in men, distant metastatic spread is uncommon at the time of diagnosis.[31] Lung, liver, bone, and brain represent the most common areas of involvement. Of interest, several elderly patients have died as a result of the effects of a concomitant malignancy, rather than as a result of the primary urethral carcinoma.

SUMMARY

Carcinoma of the urethra is a disease characterized by extensive local invasion in both sexes. Although frequently advanced at presentation, distant metastatic spread beyond regional lymph nodes is unusual. Etiology is thought to be related to chronic irritation, stricture, infection, and diverticulum formation. Signs and symptoms are nondescript for carcinoma and are typical of the more common benign conditions, often resulting in a delay in diagnosis. Only with early recognition and prompt initiation of appropriate therapy can improvement in survival be achieved. The diagnosis of urethral carcinoma should be considered in any patient of either sex who presents with lower genitourinary tract or urethral symptoms.

REFERENCES

1. Bloom W, Fawcett DW: A Textbook of Histology, 10th edition. pp 799–804. Philadelphia, WB Saunders Co, 1975.
2. Anderson KA, McAninch JW: Primary squamous cell carcinoma of the anterior male urethra. Urology 1984; 23: 134–146.
3. Ray B, Canto AR, Whitmore WF: Experience with primary carcinoma of the male urethra. J Urol 1977; 117:591–594.
4. Johnson DE, Ames FC: Surgical anatomy and lymphatic drainage of the ilioinguinal region. *In* Johnson DE, Ames FC (eds): Groin Dissection. Chicago, Year Book Medical Publishers, 1985.
5. Sedgwick CE: Regional lymphatic dissection for malignancy of the extremity: radical goin dissection; radical axillary dissection. Surg Clin North Am 1956; 36:785–792.
6. Zacharin RA: The suspensory mechanism of the female urethra. J Anat Lond 1963; 97:423–427.
7. Thiaudierre PD, Cited by Hotchkiss RS, Amelar RD: Primary carcinoma of the male urethra. J Urol 1954; 72:1181.
8. Clark MO Jr, Kosanovich M: Primary carcinoma of the male urethra. South Med J 1972; 65:1339–1346.
9. Hotchkiss RS, Amelar RD: Primary carcinoma of the male urethra. J Urol 1954; 72:1181.
10. Kaplan GW, Buckley GJ, Grayhack JT: Carcinoma of the male urethra. J Urol 1967; 98:365.
11. Blandy JP: Urethroplasty in males. *In* Present Advances in Urology, p 208. New York, Churchill Livingstone, 1976.
12. Mellinger BC: Human papillomavirus in the male: an overview. AUA Update Series: Vol XIII, lesson 13, 1994.
13. Wiener JS, Walther PJ: A high association of oncogenic human papillomaviruses with carcinomas of the female urethra. J Urol 1994; 151:49–53.
14. Droller MJ: Bladder cancer. Curr Probl Surg 1981; 18:205.
15. Schellhammer PF, Whitmore WF Jr: Transitional cell carcinoma of the urethra in men having cystectomy for bladder cancer. J Urol 1976; 115:56.
16. Schellhammer PF, Whitmore WF Jr: Urethral meatal carcinoma following cystourethrectomy for bladder cancer. J Urol 1976; 115:61.
17. Fair WR, Perez CA, Anderson T: Cancer of the urethra and penis. *In* DeVita VT, Hellman S, Rosenberg S (eds): Cancer: Principles and Practice, 3rd edition. Philadelphia, JB Lippincott Co, 1989.
18. Zeidman EJ, Desmond P, Thompson IM: Surgical treatment of carcinoma of the male urethra. Urol Clin North Am 1992; 19:359–372.
19. Vapnek JM, Hricak H, Carroll PR: Recent advances in imaging studies for staging of penile and urethral carcinoma. Urol Clin North Am 1992; 19:257–266.
20. McCallum RW, Colapinto V: Urological Radiology of the Adult Male Lower Urinary Tract, p 111. Springfield, IL, Charles C Thomas, 1976.
21. Cordonier JJ, Spiut HJ: Urethral occurrence of bladder carcinoma following cystectomy. J Urol 1962; 87:398.
22. Mostofi FK, Davis CJ, Sesterhenn IA: Carcinoma of the male and female urethra. Urol Clin North Am 1992; 19: 347–358.
23. Levine RL: Urethral cancer. Cancer 1980; 45(Suppl):1965.
24. Grabstald H: Tumors of the urethra in men and women. Cancer 1973; 32:1236.

25. McLean LE, Furlong JH: Primary carcinoma of the male urethra. Urol Surv 1951; 1:1.
26. Ende N, Woods LP, Shelly HS: Carcinoma originating in ducts surrounding the prostatic urethra. Am J Clin Pathol 1963; 40:183.
27. Melicow MM, Hollowell JW: Intraurothelial cancer: carcinoma in situ: Bowen's disease of the urinary system: discussion of 30 cases. J Urol 1952; 68:763.
28. Ullman AS, Ross OR: Hyperplasia, atypism and carcinoma in situ in prostatic periurethral glands. Am J Clin Pathol 1967; 47:497.
29. Wasserman (quoted by McCrea and Furlong): Epithelioma primitif de l'urethre [these]. Paris, 1895.
30. Ray B, Guinan PD: Primary carcinoma of the urethra. *In* Javedpour N (ed): Principles and Management of Urologic Cancer, p 445–473. Baltimore, Williams & Wilkins, 1979.
31. Grabstald H, Hilaries B, Henschke U, et al: Cancer of the female urethra. JAMA 1966; 197:835.
32. Desai S, Libertino JA, Zurman L: Primary carcinoma of the female urethra. J Urol 1983; 129:873.
33. Sullivan J, Grabstald H: Management of carcinoma of the urethra. *In* Skinner DG, DeKernion JB (eds): Genitourinary Cancer, p 419. Philadelphia, WB Saunders Co, 1978.
34. Narayan D, Kanery B: Surgical treatment of female urethral carcinoma. Urol Clin North Am 1992; 19:373–382.
35. Antoniades J: Radiation therapy in carcinoma of the female urethra. Cancer 1969; 29:70.
36. Bracken RB, Johnson DE, Miller LS, et al: Primary carcinoma of the female urethra. J Urol 1976; 116:188.

39

URETHRAL CARCINOMA IN THE MALE AND FEMALE: MANAGEMENT AND PROGNOSIS

PATRICIA J. TERRY, M.D. *and* MICHAEL F. SAROSDY, M.D.

Primary urethral carcinoma is an extremely rare neoplasm. Since the mid-1850s, around 1200 cases of urethral carcinoma in females and 600 cases in males have been reported.[1] In general, the prognosis for such patients has been ominous, possibly because many patients have delayed initial presentation.

Because this condition is so rare, it has been difficult to develop a standardized treatment approach, and many reports are based on anecdotal successes. This discussion offers a summary of the important aspects of the management and prognosis of male and female patients with urethral carcinoma.

MANAGEMENT OF CARCINOMA OF THE FEMALE URETHRA

Urethral carcinoma is especially unusual in that it is the only urologic neoplasm that occurs more frequently in women than in men. Accounting for only 0.02% of all malignancies in women, most urethral cancer occurs in patients between the ages of 50 and 70 years.[2] The incidence is higher among Caucasians (88%) than African Americans (12%).[3]

The female urethra is approximately 4 to 6 cm in length. Although various terms have been used to classify female urethral tumors, the TNM classification is becoming widely accepted (Table 39–1). Anatomically, the female urethra is divided into the anterior segment (distal one third) and the posterior segment (proximal two thirds). The distal two thirds is lined by stratified squamous epithelium, and consequently carcinoma of this portion of the urethra is most often of the squamous cell type. The proximal one third is lined by transitional cell epithelium. Therefore, the most common tumor of the female proximal urethra is transitional cell carcinoma. Adenocarcinoma occurs infrequently in both the anterior and posterior urethra.[4]

Knowledge of the lymphatic drainage of the urethra is important when surgical therapy is being considered because lymphatic metastases are clinically present in 20 to 50% of patients at the time of presentation.[3] The distal or anterior female urethra and the labia drain primarily to the superficial inguinal lymph nodes, which then drain into either the deep inguinal nodes or the external iliac lymph nodes. The node of Cloquet or Rosenmüller, located in the femoral canal, is considered part of the deep inguinal lymph node chain. The proximal or posterior urethra drains into the external iliac, obturator, presacral, or para-aortic nodes.[5]

Diagnosis

Diagnosis is generally made by transurethral biopsy of the lesion. Because there is frequently significant inflammation surrounding distal lesions, the importance of a deep, adequate biopsy cannot be overemphasized.

After initial biopsy has been obtained, the disease is staged. In contrast to penile cancer patients, palpable inguinal lymph nodes will be malignant in 80% of patients with urethral carcinoma. Needle aspiration or node biopsy is usually indicated for evaluation of palpable nodes.[6]

Computed tomography (CT) of the pelvis may be useful to evaluate the deep inguinal nodes and to rule out pelvic metastatic disease. Common sites of metastasis include the lung, liver, and bone, so bone scan and/or CT of the chest and abdomen may also be indicated.[7]

TABLE 39–1. AMERICAN JOINT COMMITTEE ON CANCER STAGING FOR FEMALE AND MALE URETHRAL CARCINOMA

Primary Tumor (T)	
Tx:	Primary tumor cannot be assessed
T0:	No evidence of primary tumor
Tis:	Carcinoma in situ (CIS)
Ta:	Noninvasive papillary, polypoid, or verrucous carcinoma
T1:	Invades subepithelial connective tissue
T2:	Invades periurethral musculature (corpus spongiosum or prostate)
T3:	Invades anterior vagina or bladder neck (corpus cavernosum or beyond prostate or bladder neck)
T4:	Invades other adjacent organs
Regional Lymph Nodes (N)	
Nx:	Regional lymph nodes cannot be assessed
N0:	No regional lymph node metastasis
N1:	Metastasis to a single lymph node, 2 cm or less in greatest dimension
N2:	Metastasis to a single lymph node, >2 cm but <5 cm in greatest dimension, or multiple nodes involved with none >5 cm in greatest dimension
N3:	Metastasis to a lymph node >5 cm in greatest dimension
Distant Metastasis (M)	
Mx:	Presence of distant metastasis cannot be assessed
M0:	No distant metastasis
M1:	Distant metastasis

Treatment

Because of the rarity of urethral carcinoma, attempts to develop standardized treatment based on prospective studies have been unsuccessful. In addition, larger series span 25 years or longer, as well as a broad variety of surgical techniques and changes in radiation therapy.[8] As a result, only generalizations can be made and therapy continues to be best approached on a case-by-case basis.

Therapy for urethral carcinoma in the female is usually based upon the stage of the disease. The histologic grade of the tumor seems to have little influence on choice of treatment or patient survival. Anterior cancers are more likely to present at a lower stage and grade than posterior cancers, although both occur with almost equal frequency. The surgical options based on stage include local resection, partial or total urethrectomy, and anterior exenteration.[9]

Low-Stage Disease

In superficial, low-stage urethral carcinoma, interstitial radiation therapy alone has resulted in cure rates of 60 to 80%.[8,10] Complication rates as high as 42% have been reported, with incontinence seen in 30% of patients treated with radiation therapy. Other problems include stricture, fistulae, urethral stenosis, cellulitis, and osteomyelitis.[11–13]

Urethral tumors confined to the mucosa have also been treated effectively with laser resection or fulgaration. The CO_2 laser has been used extensively for external lesions with excellent results, and the neodymium:YAG laser has proven effective for complete eradication of intraurethral lesions. Both have the advantages of minimal bleeding and rapid healing. Laser resection, in contrast to electrocautery, relies on vaporization of tissues. Therefore, an adequate biopsy must be obtained prior to laser treatment for appropriate initial staging.[14,15]

For low-stage external meatus tumors, local excision alone may be adequate treatment. Intraurethral lesions restricted to the mucosa or submucosa (Tis, Ta, or T1) also may be managed by transurethral resection alone. For superficial lesions and those invading the periurethral musculature (T2), partial urethrectomy also may be performed.[9] Resection of two thirds of the distal urethra may be performed without causing incontinence. Preoperative or postoperative interstitial radiation has been recommended for lesions with periurethral muscular invasion.[13,16]

Partial Urethrectomy. The technique of partial urethrectomy involves making a circumferential urethral incision to allow a wide surgical margin. The urethra is dissected from the anterior tissues and the vaginal wall by grasping the urethra with an Allis clamp and extending it outward until the lesion is completely exposed. The anterior urethra is then transected 0.5 to 1.0 cm proximal to the tumor. Frozen sections of the proximal edge should be sent to ensure a cancer-free margin. The urethral stump is sutured to the vaginal wall to reconstruct the meatus. The most common complication of this procedure is urethral stenosis, which may be avoided by intermittent catheterization for several weeks following the surgery.[9]

High-Stage Disease

Tumors of the proximal or entire urethra are rarely superficial. Patients with more advanced stages of urethral carcinoma require radical therapy, sometimes combining radiation and surgery. Radiation alone for advanced urethral cancer is associated with 5-year survival rates between 0 and 57%.[9,11,17–20] For surgery alone, results are also very poor, with survival rates of 10 to 17%.[21] Preoperative radiation followed by anterior exenteration has resulted in 5-year survival rates of around 50%.[18,19,22]

Anterior exenteration in the female with advanced urethral carcinoma involves removal of the pelvic lymph nodes, uterus and adnexa, the entire urethra and bladder, and the anterior and lateral vaginal walls and en bloc resection of the inferior or entire pubic symphysis and inferior pubic rami. The technique of anterior exenteration involves several basic surgical goals, including preoperative bowel preparation, antibiotic prophylaxis, and prevention of deep vein thrombosis. A modified low lithotomy or hyperextended frogleg position provides adequate perineal exposure.[8]

Pelvic lymphadenectomy is performed first, followed by lateral and posterior mobilization and excision of the uterus, adnexa, and bladder. The vagina is opened distal to the cervix and the lateral vaginal walls are incised, leaving the anterior vaginal wall attached to the anterior pelvic organs.[8] The incision is then carried over the pubis, around the clitoris, and along the vulva on both sides of the vagina. The dissection is continued down to the periosteum of the inferior pubic rami. The origins of the adductor muscles are freed and the lateral vaginal incisions joined with those started in the abdomen. One end of a Gigli saw is then passed through the obturator foramen and brought out around the ischial rim of the pubic ramus. This is repeated on the opposite side with a second Gigli saw. A third saw is passed around the pubis to allow horizontal division of the pubis. After all three cuts in the pubis are made, the anterior pelvic organs can be removed en bloc with the inferior rim of the pubis. This procedure leaves the anterior pubic ramus intact, providing improved pelvic stability without compromising the principles of cancer surgery.[8]

Musculocutaneous flaps may be required to reconstruct the vagina and close the perineal defect. Urinary diversion in the form of an ileal conduit or a continent diversion is then completed. Recently, Hedden et al. reported that anterior exenteration with bladder sparing resulted in the achievement of local control in five of five patients, although follow-up was short.[23] It remains to be seen if this treatment option will provide acceptable results.

Inguinal lymphadenectomy is performed unilaterally or bilaterally only for palpable inguinal nodes. Prophylactic inguinal dissection has not been shown to have a survival benefit over therapeutic dissection, but does have significant morbidity.[8,9] Stage D urethral carcinoma with extensive local invasion and distant metastases can be managed by palliative surgery, radiation, or both.

Chemotherapy

Because of the rarity of urethral carcinoma, data on the use of chemotherapy are insufficient to draw definitive conclusions. Most information on chemotherapy for urethral carcinoma is presented in combination with that for penile carcinoma.

Drugs that have demonstrated activity against penile and urethral cancers include cisplatin, bleomycin, methotrexate, mitomycin, and 5-fluorouracil (5-FU). Combinations of these agents, along with newer therapies including biologic response modifiers and immunotherapy, are under investigation. Promising results have been demonstrated in anal and esophageal squamous cell carcinomas using a combination of radiation, 5-FU, and mitomycin C, suggesting the possibility of success with urethral or penile squamous cell carcinomas.[12,24,25] Multi-institutional cooperative group investigations of chemotherapeutic agents are needed to develop organ-sparing therapeutic approaches to urethral carcinoma.

Prognosis

Clinical stage appears to be the most important prognostic factor in female urethral carcinoma independent of cell grade or type, except for malignant melanoma, which has the lowest survival rate.[26] Tumor depth or penetration correlates well with survival regardless of the type of therapy administered.[8] Five-year survival rates have been reported to be 45% for Ta or T1 lesions (stage A), 11% for T2 (stage B), 26% for T3 or T4 (stage C), and 18% for any T with metastatic disease (stage D).[11] Over half of women patients will present with advanced disease, and somewhere between 35 and 50% will have inguinal adenopathy.

Sarosdy[28] compared the 5-year survival rates of five published series for females with urethral carcinoma by tumor location and noted an average of 49% 5-year survival for anterior tumors and 13% 5-year survival for posterior or entire urethral tumors.[1,3,16,27,28] Local recurrence rates have been reported at between 66 and 100%.[9,11]

Tumor size has also been correlated to survival. In a study by Bracken et al., patients having tumors less than 2 cm had 5-year survival rates of about 60%, whereas those with tumors greater than 5 cm had 5-year survival rates of 13%.[11] Grigsby and Corn published similar results relating tumor size of less than 2 cm to improved prognosis regardless of the type of therapy.[29] The prognostic significance of tumor grade is still in question, although it has been noted that lower stage lesions tend to be of lower tumor grade.[30]

Because the prognosis for women with urethral carcinoma parallels the stage of the disease, accurate staging is crucial prior to instituting therapy. The age and medical condition of the individual patient must also be considered in planning the therapeutic approach. Continued studies of this rare tumor are warranted to track and report the results of different treatment modalities in an effort to establish future standards of care.

MANAGEMENT OF CARCINOMA OF THE MALE URETHRA

Urethral carcinoma in men occurs even less frequently than the rare female urethral carcinoma, with somewhere around 600 cases reported in the literature. Most patients present in the fifth to seventh decade, and no racial predisposition in men has been reported.[31] Because this tumor is so unusual, prospective study of treatment options is nearly impossible and most information on male urethral carcinoma is based on retrospective reviews.

The male urethra is divided anatomically into anterior and posterior segments. The anterior or distal urethra consists of the penile urethra, while the posterior segment is made up of the prostatic, membranous, and bulbous urethra.

The lymphatic drainage of the male anterior urethra follows that of the glans and corpus spongiosum into the deep inguinal nodes. If the tumor involves the penile skin, drainage to the superficial inguinal and external iliac nodes must be considered. The posterior urethra drains to the external iliac chain, obturator lymph nodes, internal iliac, and presacral nodes.[32]

Most series have shown that men with tumors of the distal urethra have improved survival rates compared to those patients with posterior urethral lesions. The reason for the significantly worse prognosis of patients with posterior tumors may be that these patients tend to have a lengthy delay to presentation. Anterior lesions are almost always palpable, and this may account for the finding that anterior urethral tumors generally present at a lower stage than proximal tumors.[31]

Treatment

As in the female patient, choice of therapy for the male with urethral carcinoma is dependent on adequate staging, beginning with a biopsy of the lesion. Most biopsies can be performed transurethrally but, if necessary, transperineal specimens may be adequate. Physical exam should note the presence or absence of inguinal lymphadenopathy and urethral induration or fixation to the pelvis. Urethroscopy and cystoscopy should be performed on all patients. Unless the lesion is very distal and small, a CT scan of the pelvis should be obtained prior to definitive surgery to evaluate for lymphadenopathy.

Radiation

Radiation therapy for the treatment of male urethral carcinoma has been reserved mainly for patients who have failed local control or refused surgery. Results from reports of radiation therapy for male urethral carcinoma have been dismal, and most authors agree that surgical excision currently remains the preferred mode of therapy.[31] The most promising results are from studies using radiation or combinations of radiation and chemotherapy for downstaging locally advanced disease prior to radical resection.[24]

Local Excision for Distal Urethral Tumors

In a few well-selected patients, local excision of urethral carcinoma may be adequate therapy. The lesions that may be suitable for transurethral resection, laser fulgaration, or local excision include low-grade, low-stage tumors. Patients who have concomitant medical comorbidity that precludes more extensive surgery should also be considered candidates for local excision. Tumor location is of less importance in making this decision because complete resection of the lesion is the key to local control in both the anterior and posterior urethra. Several studies have shown excellent outcomes in patients managed by local excision of even bulbar lesions.[33–35]

Local excision might be performed transurethrally at the same time as the initial biopsy. A cold-cup forceps biopsy for cautery-free tissue should be submitted to the pathologist; then the tumor should be completely excised with the cutting current if possible. The entire urethra should be examined and any suspicious areas biopsied. Close follow-up is essential for patients undergoing local excision of urethral carcinoma because the recurrence rate may be higher than with more extensive resections.

Complications from local excision are uncommon. Urethral perforation is managed by Foley catheter drainage for several days or until retrograde urethrography demonstrates resolution of extravasation. Stricture after transurethral resection of a tumor should prompt a biopsy of the area to rule out recurrence.[36]

Partial Penectomy

Several series of partial penectomies for distal urethral carcinomas report excellent survival rates and low recurrence rates.[21,34,37] The principle of this surgery is to perform partial amputation of the penis, allowing resection of the lesion with a 2-cm proximal margin. Patient selection requires careful inspection of the entire urethra, including urethroscopy, to ensure that a 2-cm margin provides adequate penile length to direct the urinary stream in the standing position.[36]

Partial penectomy can usually be performed with the patient in the supine position. If there is any question of preserving adequate penile length, the lithotomy position may be considered to allow for a perineal urethrostomy. A tourniquet is applied at the base of the penis and the circumferential incision is made at least 2 cm proximal to the urethral lesion. The dorsal artery and veins are ligated and the corpora cavernosa are divided. The stump of the urethra should be dissected distally about 0.5 to 1.0 cm and then transected. The specimen should be inspected and frozen sections of the proximal margin should be obtained. More tissue can be excised or a total penectomy performed if adequate length is in question. The dorsal edge of the urethral stump is then spatulated and the corpora are closed. The tourniquet is released and any bleeding controlled. The skin of the shaft is then advanced over the corpora and closed to the urethral stump to create the neomeatus. A urethral catheter is left in place for 1 or 2 days.[36]

Complications of partial penectomy are rare. Meatal stenosis can be avoided by appropriate eversion of the urethral edges and adequate spatulation. Some authors have reported that partial penectomy can preserve not only adequate penile length for standing urination, but potency as well.

Others have noted that fewer than 50% of their patients were able to perform sexually after partial penectomy.[38] Frank discussion of these issues with patients is obviously an important part of the preoperative planning.

Total or Radical Penectomy

Total penectomy has been employed for distal urethral lesions where 2-cm margins were not possible or penile length was inadequate, and for proximal urethral tumors. Because more proximal tumors tend to present later and at more advanced stages, the reported survival rates for radical penectomy are discouraging.[35,39,40] One of the reasons for the dismal results may be inappropriate patient selection. The only ideal candidate for total penectomy for urethral carcinoma is the man with a Ta, T1, or T2 lesion that does not extend beyond the mid-bulbar urethra, or the patient with a distal lesion in whom a partial penectomy would result in an inadequate penile stump.[36] The choice of a total penectomy should be based on careful urethroscopy and biopsies and palpation of the lesion to assure that there is no extension beyond the corpus spongiosum.

For radical penectomy, the patient is placed in the lithotomy position with a sacral roll. A circumferential incision is made around the base of the penis at the penoscrotal junction. The incision may be carried laterally at the base of the penis or in the midline above and below the penis. The tunics of the testes and the ventral surface of the penis are dissected free from surrounding tissues. The suspensory ligaments are then divided and the dorsal vein is ligated and divided. An inverted U incision is made in the perineum and the urethra is dissected out and transected 2 cm proximal to the lesion, leaving adequate urethral length for the perineal urethrostomy. A urethral catheter may be inserted to provide traction. The paired arteries to the bulbar urethra may be encountered during this dissection, and should be ligated and divided. The crura of the penis are then dissected, divided, and oversewn. Any remaining attachments of the penis are divided at this time and the specimen is removed. The proximal urethral stump is mobilized to the urogenital diaphragm, and an opening made in the perineal flap of skin. The urethra is then brought out through this opening, spatulated, and sutured to the edges of the perineal skin. The catheter should be inserted into the bladder if not already in place. The superior skin incision is then closed, leaving a small Penrose drain.[36]

Complications of radical penectomy include scrotal hematoma and wound infection, which can be minimized with adequate hemostasis and drainage at the time of penectomy. Perineal urethrostomy stenosis can be avoided by having adequate urethral length without tension, spatulation of the urethra, and careful placement of the opening in the perineal skin. Some patients require periodic dilation of the urethrostomy or even surgical reconstruction of the meatus.

En Bloc Resection of the Penis, Scrotum, and Anterior Pubis with Cystoprostatectomy

Early experience with radiation or local excision of extensive posterior urethral carcinoma was dismal.[41] Klein et al. reported the largest single-institution series of 12 patients treated with en bloc excision and cystoprostatectomy in 1983, with much improved survival rates.[27] Thus it appears that, for patients with T3 (stage C) urethral carcinoma, en bloc resection of the penis, pubis, bladder, and prostate may be the only hope for survival. Preoperative staging should be completed with cystoscopy, biopsies, and pelvic CT scan to evaluate for lymphadenopathy. The extent of the resection may be varied depending on the relationship of the lesion to the scrotal contents or involvement of other organs. For example, some authors advocate preservation of the testes if the scrotal wall is not involved.[36] In more advanced cases, complete pelvic exenteration may be required.

The patient is positioned in the extended lithotomy position with the perineum horizontal to the table. A midline incision is made first, and pelvic lymphadenectomy is completed. If appropriate, the cystectomy is begun by ligating and dividing the lateral pedicles of the bladder and mobilizing it off the anterior surface of the rectum. The endopelvic fascia is opened and the lateral aspects of the prostate mobilized. The puboprostatics are not taken down.

An incision is then made around the shaft of the penis and scrotum to the perineum. The perineal dissection is then performed by incising the central tendon, mobilizing the urethra, and dissecting the penile crura to their origins. The anterior dissection is then extended to expose and divide the spermatic cords and divide the penile suspensory ligaments. The surgeon must then decide whether to resect the inferior pubis or the entire anterior pubis. Inferior pubic resection may provide pelvic stability and decrease postoperative weakness and pain, but complete resection may be necessary to resect bulky tumors adequately.

If inferior pubic resection is chosen, the origins of the thigh muscles are divided as close to the bone as possible. The dissection is carried superiorly along the medial border of the obturator foramen to the superior ramus. The Gigli saw is then used to divide the inferior ramus. The inferior pubis is then divided from the symphysis using the Gigli saw or an osteotome. To complete the anterior resection, the medial insertions of the pectineus muscles are detached from the superior ramus and the ramus divided with the saw. The entire specimen is then removed en bloc. A urinary diversion is then completed, and the midline and perineal incisions closed using a myocutaneous flap if the defect is large.[36]

The potential complications of this type of surgery are numerous, including problems with wound healing, pelvic abscess, and herniation. Most patients report adductor weakness postoperatively, but this usually resolves over time.[27,42]

Role of Lymphadenectomy in Male Urethral Carcinoma

Many studies have reported that in more than 50% of cases palpable inguinal nodes will be positive for carcinoma. As with penile carcinoma, inguinal lymphadenectomy has been shown to provide long-term, disease-free survival in the face of positive nodes.[21,35,36,41] There have been a few series reporting long-term survival in patients with positive pelvic nodes, but follow-up of these patients was short.[27,41]

In view of the above, any patient with palpable inguinal lymph nodes should have formal inguinal lymphadenectomy. Prophylactic inguinal lymphadenectomy is not warranted by most authors, but some suggest bilateral sentinel node biopsies may contribute to increased survival rates.[43] The modified dissection sparing the saphenous vein, as described by Catalona, has led to markedly decreased postoperative lower extremity edema.[44] Full pelvic lymphadenectomy is recommended for those patients undergoing en bloc resection of the lesion with cystoprostatectomy.[36]

The best management of patients with positive inguinal nodes is yet to be determined. Efforts are being made to develop new modalities of treatment, including combination radiotherapy, chemotherapy, and surgery. Initial success in treating squamous cell carcinoma of the esophagus and anus has been reported using combined radiation and chemotherapy.[45,46] Similar studies have demonstrated limited success in cases of urethral carcinoma in men and women, with best responses seen in patients with transitional cell carcinomas.[28,47] Efficacy against penile and urethral carcinoma has also been demonstrated using the combination of cisplatin and 5-FU followed by inguinal and pelvic lymphadenectomy, but the numbers are small and follow-up short.[25]

Prognosis

Survival data for men with urethral carcinoma have been studied in terms of tumor stage, grade, and location. Five-year survival for all stages of urethral carcinoma is around 50%, but falls to 5 to 15% for posterior tumors.[28,35,43,48] As with urethral carcinoma in the female patient, the poor prognosis of posterior lesions may be attributed to a delay in diagnosis and to a tendency for such patients to present at a more advanced stage. Winkler and Leiber reported that 73% of penile urethral lesions presented as stage 0 or A, compared to only 32% of bulbourethral tumors.[49] It has been suggested that posterior tumors not only present at a more advanced stage, but may actually be more invasive lesions. Cytometric and ploidy studies have demonstrated that more proximal tumors tend to be nondiploid, suggesting a more aggressive nature.[49]

A recent review of 23 male patients with anterior urethral carcinomas revealed that survival was influenced by grade, stage, and location of the tumor, although, as noted by other investigators, the higher grade neoplasms presented at a higher stage.[43] Tumor location strongly influenced survival in this group. Patients whose lesions originated in the fossa navicularis showed a 100% disease-free and disease-specific survival rate. The disease-free survival for penile urethral lesions was 55% and fell to only 25% for bulbomembranous carcinomas.[43]

The key to improving survival rates seems to be related directly to local control of the disease. Ahlering and Lieskovsky reviewed the series published since 1981, and found that of 15 patients treated with radical extirpation with and without radiation, 60% were alive at a median follow-up of 40 months.[7] This may reflect selection bias because, historically, 5-year survival for patients who present with stage C or D disease has been about 10 to 33%.[21,27,33,48]

Conclusion

The natural history of male urethral carcinoma suggests that management should be based on the principles of adequate local control through aggressive surgical excision, especially in proximal lesions. Radiation may be useful as an adjunct to surgery, and further investigations using chemotherapy and immunotherapy are necessary. As is the case with carcinoma of the female urethra, prospective studies of male urethral carcinoma are difficult because of the scarcity of this disease. Therefore, advances in treatment must rely on careful retrospective review and accurate reporting of case management.

REFERENCES

1. Hopkins SC, Grabstald H: Benign and malignant tumors of the male and female urethra. *In* Walsh PC, Gittes RF, Perlmutter AD, Stamey TA (eds): Campbell's Urology, 5th edition, pp 1441–1448. Philadelphia, WB Saunders Co, 1986.
2. Fagan GE, Hertig AT: Carcinoma of the female urethra: review of the literature. Obstet Gynecol 1955; 6:1.
3. Ray B, Guinan BD: Primary carcinoma of the urethra. *In* Javadpour N (ed): Principles and Management of Urologic Cancer, pp 445–473. Baltimore, Williams & Wilkins, 1979.
4. Robertson CN: Urethral carcinoma. *In* Glenn JF (ed): Urologic Surgery, 4th edition, p 680. Philadelphia, JB Lippincott Co, 1991.
5. Carroll PR, Dixon CM: Surgical anatomy of the male and female urethra. Urol Clin North Am 1992; 19:343–345.
6. Droller MJ: Urethral carcinoma in females. *In* Resnick MI, Kursh ED (eds): Current Therapy in Genitourinary Surgery, p 162. St. Louis, Mosby–Year Book, 1992.

7. Ahlering TE, Lieskovsky G: Surgical treatment of urethral cancer in the male patient. *In* Skinner DG, Lieskovsky G (eds): Diagnosis and Management of Genitourinary Cancer, pp 622–623. Philadelphia, WB Saunders Co, 1988.
8. Skinner EC, Skinner DG: Management of carcinoma of the female urethra. *In* Skinner DG, Lieskovsky G (eds): Diagnosis and Management of Genitourinary Cancer, pp 492–497. Philadelphia, WB Saunders Co, 1988.
9. Narayan P, Konety B: Surgical treatment of female urethral carcinoma. Urol Clin North Am 1992; 19:273–382.
10. Grabstald H: Tumors of the urethra in men and women. Cancer 1973; 32:1236–1255.
11. Bracken RB, Johnson DE, Miller LS, et al: Primary carcinoma of the female urethra. J Urol 1976; 116:188.
12. Eisenberger MA: Chemotherapy for carcinomas of the penis and urethra. Urol Clin North Am 1992; 19:333–338.
13. Forman JD, Lichter AS: The role of radiation therapy in the management of carcinoma of the male and female urethra. Urol Clin North Am 1992; 19:388.
14. Schaeffer AJ: Use of CO_2 laser in urology. Urol Clin North Am 1986; 13:393–404.
15. Staehler G, Chaussy C, Jocham D, et al: The use of neodymium-YAG lasers in urology: indication, technique, and critical assessment. J Urol 1985; 134:1155–1160.
16. Prempree T, Wizenberg MJ, Scott RM: Radiation treatment of primary carcinoma of the female urethra. Cancer 1978; 42:1177–1184.
17. Antoniades J: Radiotherapy in carcinoma of the female urethra. Cancer 1969; 24:70–76.
18. Hahn P, Krepant G, Malaker K: Carcinoma of the female urethra: Manitoba experience 1958–1987. Urology 1991; 37:106–109.
19. Johnson DE, O'Connell JR: Primary carcinoma of the female urethra. Urology 1983; 21:42–45.
20. Johnson DE: Cancer of the female urethra: overview. *In* Johnson DE, Boileau MA (eds): Genitourinary Tumors: Fundamental Principles and Surgical Techniques, pp 267–274. New York, Grune & Stratton, 1982.
21. Bracken RB: Exenterative surgery for posterior urethral cancer. Urology 1982; 19:248–251.
22. Ali MM, Klein FA, Hazra TA: Primary female urethral carcinoma: a retrospective comparison of different treatment techniques. Cancer 1988; 62:54–57.
23. Hedden RJ, Husseinzadeh N, Bracken RB: Bladder sparing surgery for locally advanced female urethral cancer. J Urol 1993; 150:1135–1137.
24. Baskin LS, Turzan C: Carcinoma of the male urethra: management of locally advanced disease with combined chemotherapy, radiotherapy and penile preserving surgery. Urology 1992; 39:21–25.
25. Hussein AM, Benedetto P, Sridhar KS: Chemotherapy with cisplatin and 5-fluorouracil for penile and urethral squamous cell carcinoma. Cancer 1990; 65:433–438.
26. Katz JI, Grabstald H: Primary malignant melanoma of the female urethra. J Urol 1976; 116:454–457.
27. Klein FA, Whitmore WF Jr, Herr HW, et al: Inferior pubic rami resection with en bloc radical excision of invasive proximal urethral carcinoma. Cancer 1983; 51:1238–1242.
28. Sarosdy MF: Urethral carcinoma. AUA Update Ser 1987; 7(13):2–7.
29. Grigsby PW, Corn BW: Localized urethral tumors in women: indications for conservative versus exenterative therapies. J Urol 1992; 147:1516–1520.
30. Grabstald H, Hilaus B, Henschke U, Whitmore WF: Cancer of the female urethra. JAMA 1966; 197:835–842.
31. Fair WR, Yang C: Urethral carcinoma in males. *In* Resnick MI, Kursh ED (eds): Current Therapy in Genitourinary Surgery, 2nd edition, pp 157–161. St. Louis, Mosby–Year Book, 1992.
32. Mostofi FK, Davis CJ, Sesterhem IA: Carcinoma of the male and female urethra. Urol Clin North Am 1992; 19: 347–358.
33. Ray B, Canto AR, Whitmore WF Jr: Experience with primary carcinoma of the male urethra. J Urol 1977; 117: 591–594.
34. Kennack JW: Conservative management of low grade neoplasms of the male urethra: a preliminary report. J Urol 1980; 123:175–177.
35. Hopkins SC, Nag SK, Soloway MS: Primary carcinoma of the male urethra. Urology 1984; 23:128–133.
36. Zeidman EJ, Desmond P, Thompson IM: Surgical treatment of carcinoma of the male urethra. Urol Clin North Am 1992; 19:359–372.
37. Anderson KA, McAninch JW: Primary squamous cell carcinoma of the anterior male urethra. Urology 1984; 23: 134–140.
38. Hoppman HJ, Fraley EE: Squamous cell carcinoma of the penis. J Urol 1978; 120:393–398.
39. King LR: Carcinoma of the urethra in male patients. J Urol 1964; 91:555–559.
40. Mandler JI, Pool TL: Primary carcinoma of the male urethra. J Urol 1966; 96:67–72.
41. Marshall VF: Radical excision of locally extensive carcinoma of the deep male urethra. J Urol 1957; 78:252–265.
42. Shuttleworth KED, Lloyd-Davies RW: Radical resection for tumors involving the posterior urethra. Br J Urol 1969; 41: 739–743.
43. Dinney PN, Johnson DE, Swanson DA, et al: Therapy and prognosis for male anterior urethral carcinoma: an update. Urology 1994; 43:506–514.
44. Catalona WJ: Modified inguinal lymphadenectomy for carcinoma of the penis with preservation of saphenous veins: technique and preliminary results. J Urol 1988; 140:306–310.
45. Flam MS, John M, Lavalvo LJ, et al: Definitive nonsurgical therapy of epithelial malignancies of the anal canal: a report of 12 cases. Cancer 1983; 51:1378.
46. Leichman L, Steiger Z, Seydel G, et al: Pre-operative chemotherapy and radiation therapy for patients with cancer of the esophagus: a potentially curative approach. J Clin Oncol 1984; 2:75–81.
47. Dexeus FH, Logothetis CJ, Sella A, et al: Combination chemotherapy with methotrexate, bleomycin and cisplatin for advanced squamous cell carcinoma of the male genital tract. J Urol 1991; 146:1284–1287.
48. Kaplan GW, Bulkley GJ, Grayhack JT: Carcinoma of the male urethra. J Urol 1967; 98:365–371.
49. Winkler HZ, Leiber MM: Primary squamous cell carcinoma of the male urethra: nuclear deoxyribonucleic acid ploidy studied by flow cytometry. J Urol 1988; 139:298–303.

40

URETHRECTOMY

ROBERT C. FLANIGAN, M.D.

Urethrectomy in urologic oncology is used for the definitive treatment of primary urethral cancers involving both men and women. In addition, the urethra may be removed in association with the definitive treatment of bladder cancer. This chapter defines the indications for urethrectomy, reviews the pertinent anatomic structures, describes the surgical techniques required for successful performance, outlines the pre- and postoperative management of patients, and reviews the complications associated with this procedure as well as the results that may be anticipated.

INDICATIONS

The indications for urethrectomy in men or women are for the treatment of urethral carcinoma and as an associated procedure in the treatment of bladder carcinoma. Primary carcinoma of the urethra is a rare occurrence. Approximately 1200 cases have been described in women and approximately 600 cases in men.[1] In contrast, urethral involvement with transitional cell carcinoma is much more common. However, the indications for urethrectomy in relationship to bladder cancer have been modified over recent years so that the primary indication in men is the involvement of the prostatic urethra and/or stroma by the underlying primary bladder cancer. Although previous indications for urethrectomy included multifocal tumors, diffuse carcinoma in situ, bladder neck tumors, and prostatic urethral involvement, prostatic urethral involvement appears to be the most compelling indication for urethrectomy. In a series of 124 patients who underwent cystoprostatectomy and were followed for a mean of 67 months, Levinson et al.[2] found that urethrectomy was required in no patient who presented with a solitary tumor at the bladder neck, in only 1.5% of patients with multifocal tumor, and in only 4.5% of patients with diffuse carcinoma-in-situ. In contrast, urethrectomy was required in 17% of men who presented with disease extending into the prostate, including 30% of men in whom stromal invasion occurred.[2] In addition, with a trend toward orthotopic reconstruction following cystectomy, strategies to preserve the urethra in both men and women have become much more important.[3] A more comprehensive description of therapeutic decisions involving urethral and bladder cancers are found in Chapters 38 and 18, respectively.

ANATOMY/EMBRYOLOGY

The urethra develops from the caudal end of the urogenital sinus after its complete septation from the cloaca. In the male, the urethral segment of the urogenital sinus forms the prostatic and membranous urethra, whereas in the woman it forms the entire urethra as well as the vaginal vestibule. The male urethra extends from the internal meatus in the bladder to the external meatus at the tip of the glans penis. It is divided into four regional segments, the prostatic, membranous, bulbous, and penile segments (Fig. 40–1). The prostatic urethra makes an acute angulation of approximately 30 degrees at the level of the verumontanum, is approximately 3 cm long, and lies much closer to the anterior surface of the prostate than to the posterior surface.

The anatomic relationship of the cavernous nerves to the prostate and bladder has been described by Lepor and associates and by Schlegal and Walsh.[4,5] The cavernous nerves travel posterior and lateral to the membranous urethra to the level of the urogenital diaphragm and diverge laterally into the crura of the corpora cavernosa distal to the membranous urethra. Careful dissection of the membranous urethra from the urogenital diaphragm, therefore, may prevent injury to the cavernous nerves and allow for preservation of potency (Fig. 40–2).[6]

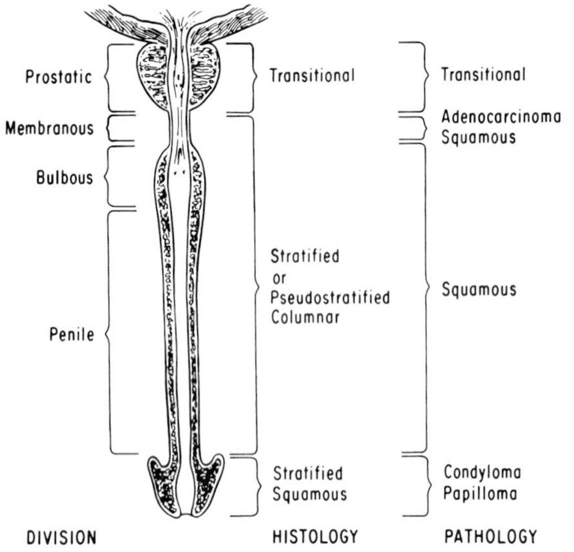
Prostatic
Membranous
Bulbous
Penile
Transitional
Stratified
or
Pseudostratified
Columnar
Stratified
Squamous
Transitional
Adenocarcinoma
Squamous
Squamous
Condyloma
Papilloma
DIVISION
HISTOLOGY
PATHOLOGY

FIGURE 40–1. Changes in the histology of the epithelial lining within the divisions of the male urethra tend to dictate the pathology of the tumor most likely to occur. (From Webster GD: The urethra. *In* Paulsen DF [ed]: Genitourinary Surgery, p 567. New York, Churchill Livingstone, 1983, with permission.)

The lymphatic drainage of the urethra in the male is similar to that of the penis. The meatus and anterior urethra drain to the inguinal nodes and thereafter to the pelvic nodes, whereas the proximal bulbomembranous and prostatic urethra drain primarily to the pelvic nodes (obturator, internal and external iliac nodes). Lymphatic drainage pathways must be taken into account when planning the extent of surgery necessary for the effective treatment of any urogenital cancer.[7]

In the male, the fossa navicularis and bulbar and penile urethra are lined by stratified or pseudostratified columnar epithelium that most often undergoes metaplastic change to squamous cell carcinoma, accounting for 75 to 80% of anterior urethral cancers (Fig. 40–1). Littre's glands and the paired Cowper's glands drain into the urethra and may undergo glandular metaplasia leading to adenocarcinomas of the urethra.

In women, transitional cell epithelium predominates in the proximal urethral portion, whereas squamous and stratified squamous epithelium predominate in the distal urethra (Fig. 40–3).[8] Therefore, in women, transitional cell carcinoma is more commonly found in the posterior urethra and squamous cell carcinoma in the area of the urethral meatus, while adenocarcinoma has been reported in either the posterior or anterior urethra (adenocarcinomas are derived from the periurethral glands or secondary to glandular metaplastic change of the urethral epithelium). The comparative anatomy of the female urethra and surrounding pelvic structures is shown in Figure 40–4.

The staging systems for female and male urethral carcinomas are depicted in Figures 40–5 and 40–6, respectively.

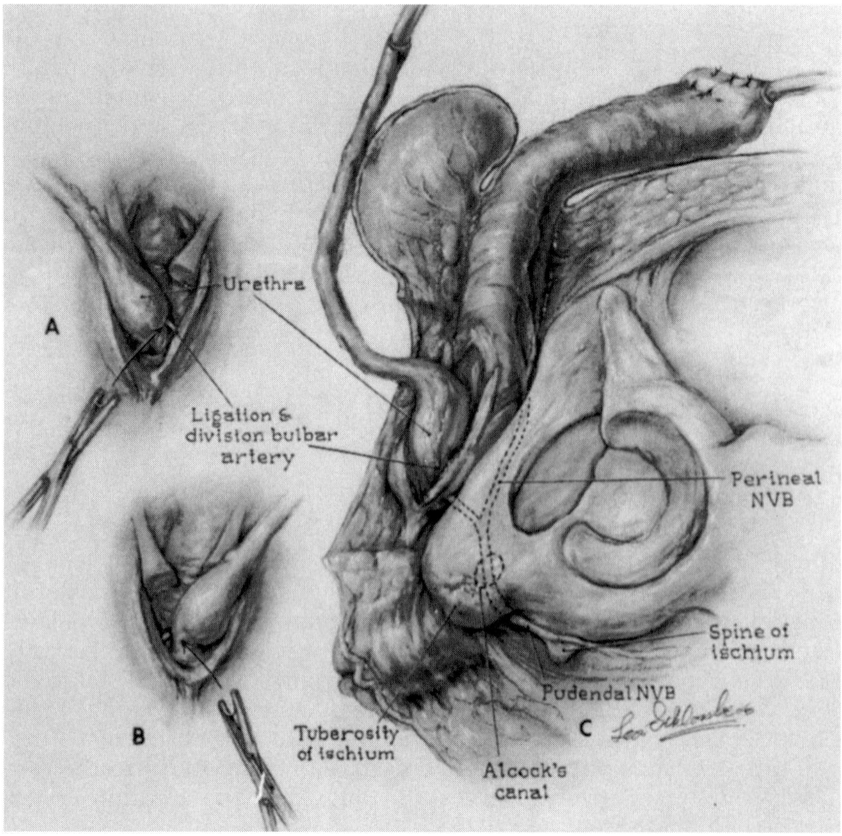
Urethra
A
Ligation &
division bulbar
artery
Perineal
NVB
Spine of
ischium
Pudendal NVB
B
Tuberosity
of ischium
C
Alcock's
canal

FIGURE 40–2. *A* and *B*, Ligation of bulbar urethral arteries with hemoclips. *C*, Lateral view shows relationship between internal pudendal and bulbar arteries, and ischium and inferior ramus of pubis. The bulbar arteries should not be fulgurated to prevent injury to internal pudendal arteries from which they arise and which provide arterial supply to corpora cavernosa. (From Brendler CB: Urethrectomy. *In* Walsh PC, Retik AB, Stamey TA, Vaughan ED Jr [eds]: Campbell's Urology, 6th edition, p 2779. Philadelphia, WB Saunders Co, 1992, with permission.)

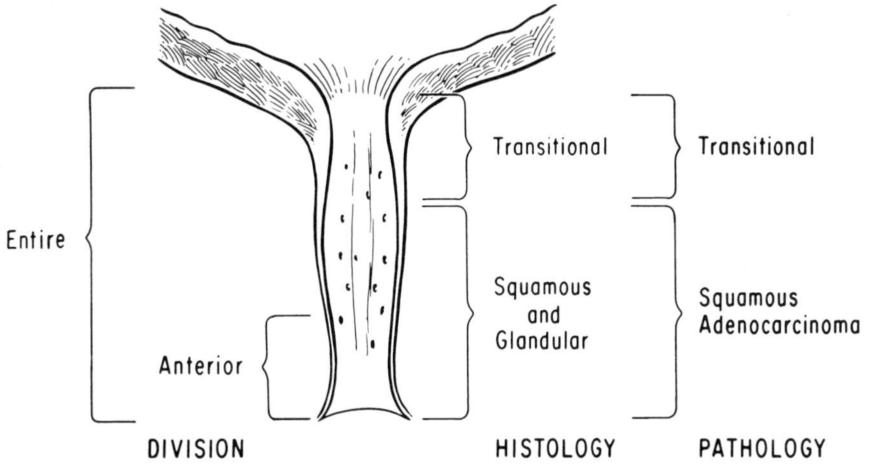
Entire
Anterior
Transitional
Squamous
and
Glandular
Transitional
Squamous
Adenocarcinoma
DIVISION
HISTOLOGY
PATHOLOGY

FIGURE 40–3. Urethral carcinomas in the female are classified according to whether they arise in the anterior portion or the entire urethra. The pathologic type of tumor occurring reflects the histology of the epithelium at the site of its occurrence. (From Webster GD: The urethra. *In* Paulsen DF [ed]: Genitourinary Surgery, p 567. New York, Churchill Livingstone, 1983, with permission.)

OPERATIVE TECHNIQUE

The operative techniques discussed in this chapter are divided into four sections: (1) partial and total urethrectomy in the female patient with primary urethral cancer, (2) partial and total urethrectomy in the male patient with primary urethral cancer, (3) total urethrectomy in the male patient in association with cystectomy, and (4) total urethrectomy in the female patient in association with cystectomy.

Partial and Total Urethrectomy in the Female Patient with Primary Urethral Cancer

The female patient with primary urethral cancer is prepared for anterior exenteration with mechanical and antibiotic bowel preparation, systemic antibiotics, and intravenous hydration. In those patients presenting with tumors of the distal third of the urethra that are confined to the mucosa, sub-

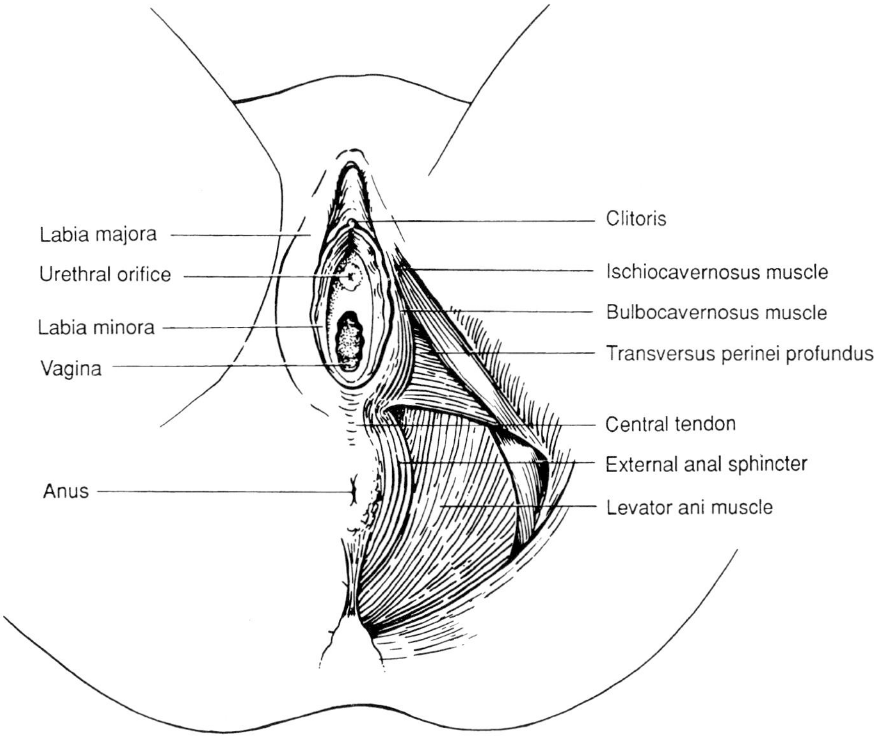
Labia majora
Urethral orifice
Labia minora
Vagina
Anus
Clitoris
Ischiocavernosus muscle
Bulbocavernosus muscle
Transversus perinei profundus
Central tendon
External anal sphincter
Levator ani muscle

FIGURE 40–4. Anatomy of the female perineum. (From Robertson C: Urethral carcinoma. *In* Glenn JF [ed]: Urologic Surgery, 4th edition, p 683. Philadelphia, JB Lippincott Co, 1991, with permission.)

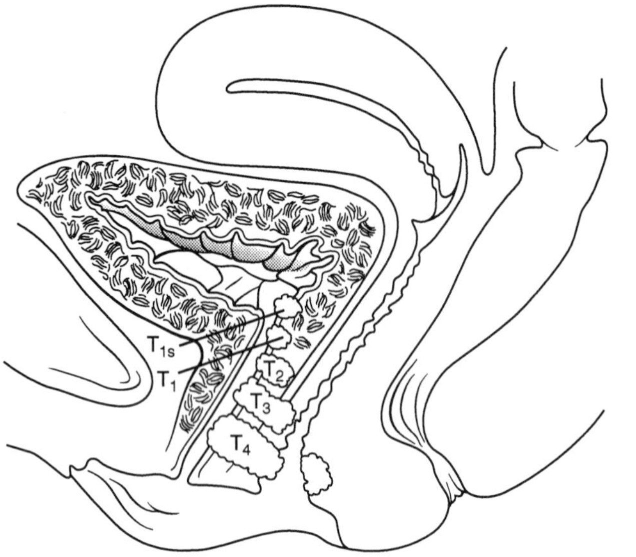
T1s
T1
T2
T3
T4

FIGURE 40–5. Staging of female urethral cancer.

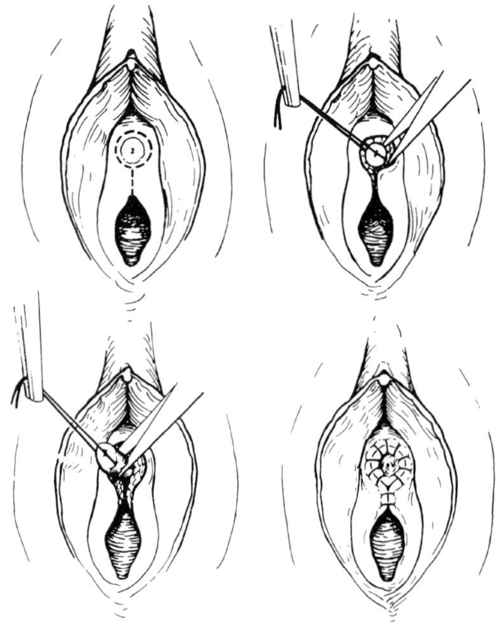

FIGURE 40–7. Technique for resection of the distal third of the female urethra. (From Robertson C: Urethral carcinoma. *In* Glenn JF [ed]: Urologic Surgery, 4th edition, p 685. Philadelphia, JB Lippincott Co, 1991, with permission.)

mucosa, or periurethral musculature, a distal urethrectomy may be appropriate. Distal urethrectomy is performed with the patient in the lithotomy position after full vaginal and abdominal preparation. A weighted speculum is used to improve visualization of the urethral orifice. A traction suture ligature of 0 or 2-0 silk is passed through the urethral meatus or the surrounding periurethral tissue. An encircling incision is then made around the meatus (Fig. 40–7). After sharp dissection of the urethral meatus, a longitudinal incision is made on the vaginal mucosa overlying the epithelium to approximately 2 cm beyond the point of palpable induration (Fig. 40–7). Sharp dissection then circumscribes the urethra, which is transected at the

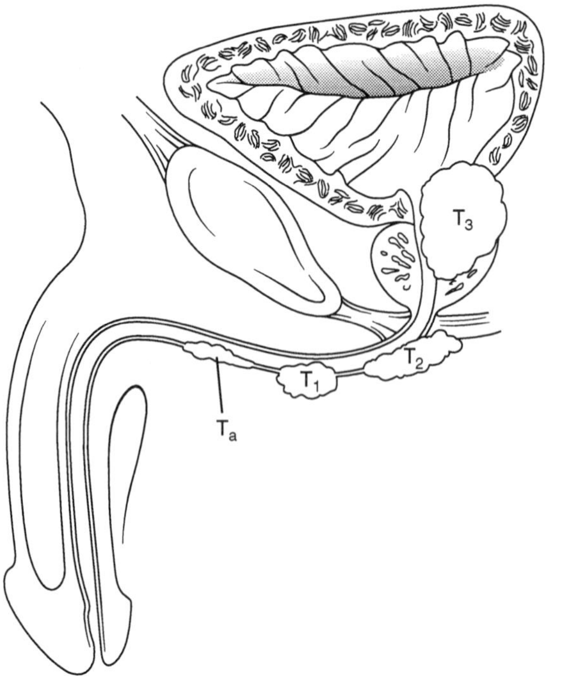
T3
T2
T1
Ta

FIGURE 40–6. Staging of male urethral cancer.

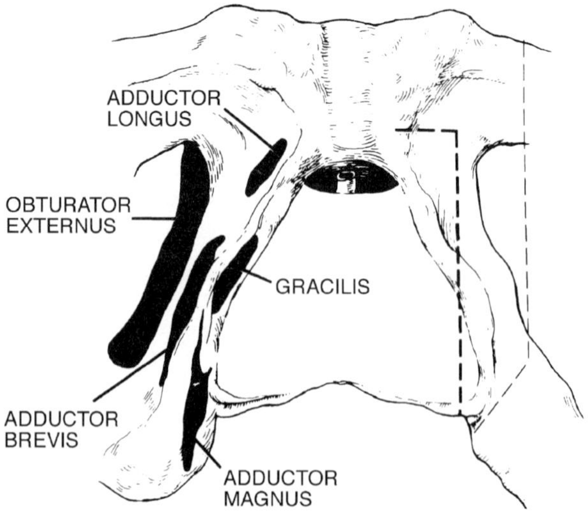
ADDUCTOR
LONGUS
OBTURATOR
EXTERNUS
GRACILIS
ADDUCTOR
BREVIS
ADDUCTOR
MAGNUS

FIGURE 40–8. In extensive pelvic/perineal exenteration, the urethra and external genitalia in continuity with the pelvic structures are removed. The pubic rami are identified and prepared for excision by freeing the overlying subcutaneous tissue, the suspensory ligament of the penis, and the various muscular attachments. The outlines of exenteration of the bone are indicated by the dotted lines. (From Schellhammer PF, Jordan GH: Surgery for urethral cancer. *In* Droller MJ [ed]: Surgical Management of Urologic Disease, p 841. St. Louis, Mosby Year Book, 1992, with permission.)

previously determined proximal extent of dissection. Frozen sections of the proximal urethral margin should be evaluated to document the absence of microscopic involvement of the urethra at that point. Mucosal edges of the remaining urethra may then be approximated to the vaginal mucosa using 3-0 chromic or polyglycolic acid (PGA) sutures. A 16- to 18-French Foley catheter is inserted into the bladder to provide urinary drainage. Vaginal repair is then completed using an interrupted or running 2-0 or 3-0 chromic or PGA suture. Povidone-iodine soaked vaginal packing is left within the vaginal vault and is removed on postoperative day 1.

In those patients in whom tumor extends microscopically beyond the point of palpable induration, and/or those patients with proximal urethral cancers in whom proximal urethral involvement of the tumor is established preoperatively, total urethrectomy, vulvectomy, clitorectomy, and anterior exenteration may be required to remove the tumor with an adequate margin.[9] In selected cases, resection of the pubic rami may also be necessary.[10] The female candidate for total urethrectomy is prepared in a fashion similar to that described for partial urethrectomy. The operation is generally begun abdominally, where radical cystectomy and pelvic lymph node dissections are performed in the standard fashion. In addition, salpingo-oophorectomy and hysterectomy are also performed in most cases. Resection of the anterior urethra en bloc with the abdominal structures proceeds along the lines described previously. Complete excision of the anterior compartment of the perineum may require a gracilis flap to provide for adequate pelvic floor support (Fig. 40–8).[11] Resection of the pubic rami is undertaken only in very extensive tumors because it may be associated with significant complications, including sacroiliac joint disruption and perineal hernia formation.[12] It is important to preserve vulvar skin whenever possible and to remove the specimen en bloc so as to avoid contamination of the operative field by tumor spillage. After completion of the extirpative aspects of the procedure, urinary diversion is completed.

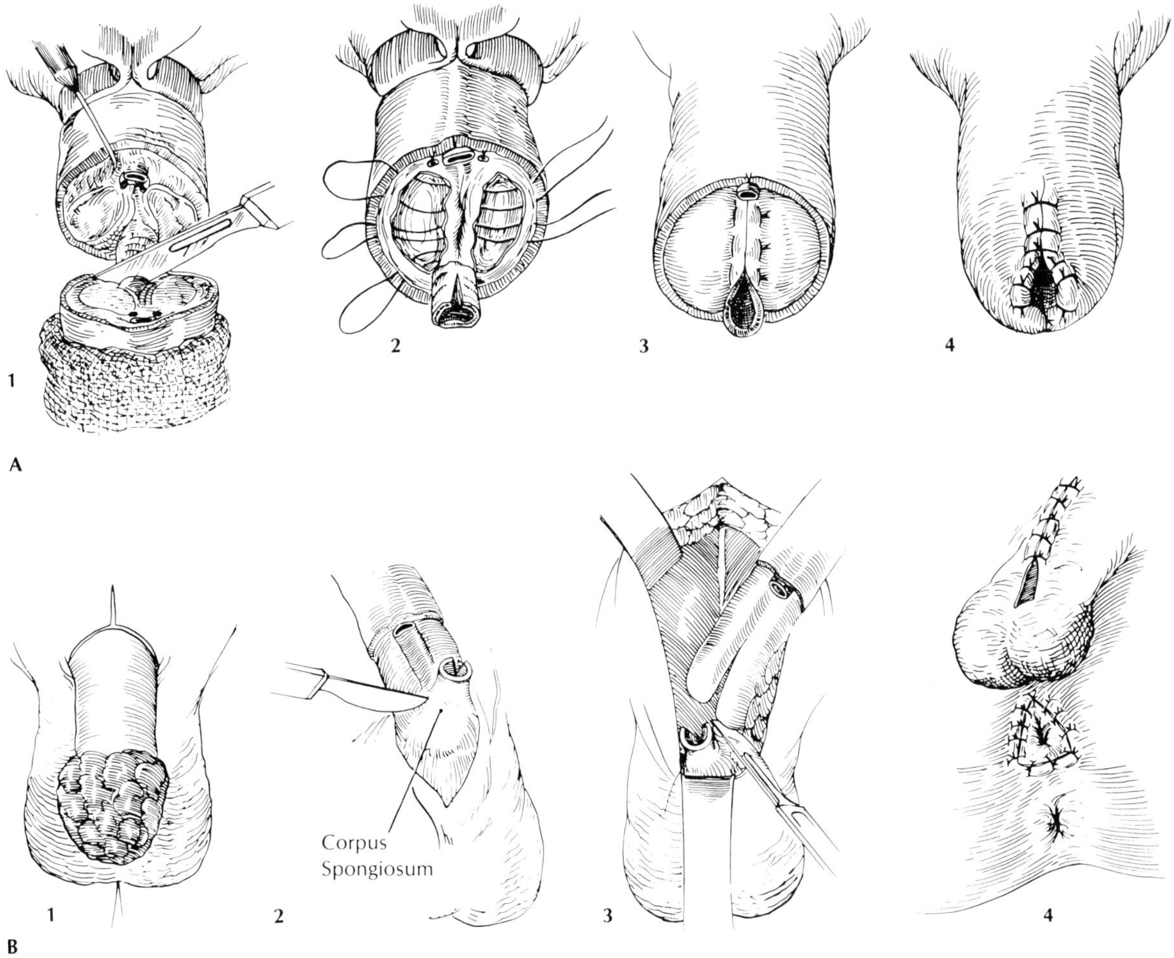
1
2
3
4
A
Corpus
Spongiosum
1
2
3
4
B

FIGURE 40–9. *A*, Techniques for distal amputation of the penis. *B*, Techniques for total amputation of the penis. (From Robertson C: Urethral carcinoma. *In* Glenn JF [ed]: Urologic Surgery, 4th edition, p 687. Philadelphia, JB Lippincott Co, 1991, with permission.)

Partial and Total Urethrectomy in the Male Patient with Primary Urethral Carcinoma

Distal urethral carcinoma in the male includes all tumors distal to the bulbous urethra.[13] These tumors may be managed by transurethral resection, partial penectomy, or partial penectomy with perineal urethrostomy. Standard techniques for penectomy are described in Chapter 4 and are pictured in Figure 40–9.

For patients with posterior urethral cancers, total urethrectomy with cystoprostatectomy is typically undertaken. The patient is placed in the lithotomy position with special attention to abduction of the legs (Fig. 40–10). After radical cystectomy and lymphadenectomy is completed, the membranous urethra is dissected from the urogenital diaphragm using finger dissection. Tension is then directed to the perineum. A midline or inverted Y incision is made in the anterior perineum overlying the central tendon (Fig. 40–11). The superficial and deep fascia are incised and the bulbocavernosus muscle divided in the midline and reflected laterally to expose the bulbous urethra (Fig. 40–13). A perineal ring retractor (Turner-Warwick) provides good exposure. After a segment of urethra is isolated by incising Buck's fascia overlying the inferior lateral grooves between the corpus spongiosum and the corpus cavernosum and dividing its superomedial attachments, a Penrose drain is advanced through the defect and used to create countertraction on the corpus spongiosum during the remaining distal dissection (Fig. 40–11). The plane between corpus spongiosum and corpus cavernosus is remarkably easy to develop in most cases, although inadvertent laceration of the tunica albuginea of the corpora cavernosa may produce considerable hemorrhage, which is most readily controlled with continuous 3-0 chromic or PGA sutures.

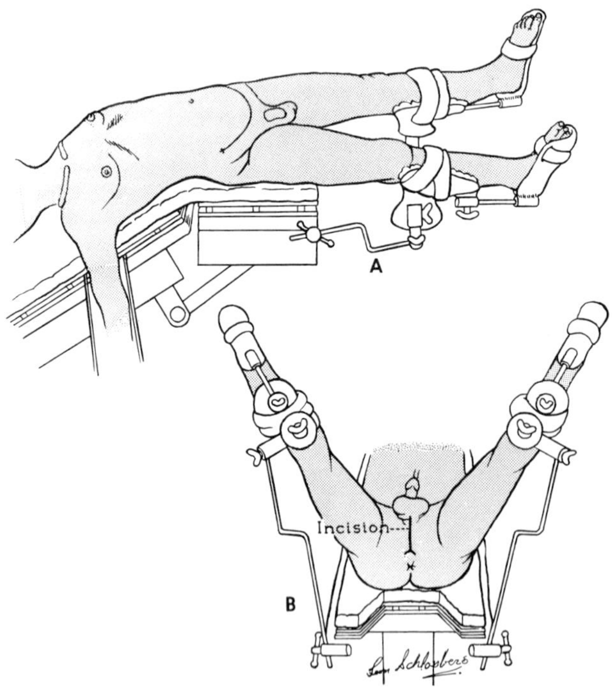
A
Incision
B

FIGURE 40–10. *A,* Patient position for radical cystoprostatectomy. Umbilicus is placed over break of table, and table is fully flexed and tilted into Trendelenburg's position, until legs are parallel to floor. *B,* Patient position for urethrectomy. Leg braces are elevated until hips are flexed 60 degrees and knees are fully extended. (From Brendler CB: Urethrectomy. *In* Walsh PC, Retik AB, Stamey TA, Vaughan ED Jr [eds]: Campbell's Urology, 6th edition, p 2775. Philadelphia, WB Saunders Co, 1992, with permission.)

During distal dissection, the penis becomes inverted and the plane between the corpus spongiosum and corpora cavernosa is lost. A decision must be made whether or not to preserve the fossa navicularis at this point. Preservation of the fossa navicularis may be helpful in allowing for more adequate placement and seating of the tips of a penile prosthesis at a later date. If the fossa navicularis is to be resected, the penile meatus is circumscribed using a tear-shaped incision and the fossa navicularis is mobilized from the glans penis and pulled into the perineal incision (Fig. 40–12). Defects in the glans penis are closed with interrupted 2-0 chromic or PGA sutures. Isolation of the proximal urethra at the bulbomembranous junction is the most difficult aspect of the procedure. Dissection is carried in a posterior and lateral direction with special care to identify and secure branches of the pudendal arteries entering at the 4- and 8-o'clock positions (Fig. 40–13). Small hemoclips or 3-0 chromic/PGA sutures are particularly useful for this maneuver. The urethrectomy is completed by mobilizing the most proximal bulbous urethral spongiosum and by dissecting the remaining membranous urethra from the urogenital diaphragm. At this point, the appropriate plane of dissection may be best appreciated by combined perineal and abdominal palpation and inspection.

The perineal wound is carefully irrigated and a suction or Penrose drain is positioned in the bed of the bulbous urethra and brought out through a separate stab wound (Fig. 40–14). Reapproximation of the bulbocavernosus muscle is undertaken in the midline using 2-0 chromic or PGA sutures. The subcutaneous tissue is closed with interrupted 3-0 chromic or PGA sutures and the skin is closed with interrupted 3-0 nylon sutures. The shaft of the penis is wrapped loosely with gauze or is covered with a self-adhering dressing of some variation. Exposure of the tip of the glans penis in order to permit prompt identification of postoperative ischemia is important.

Total Urethrectomy in the Male Patient in Association with Cystectomy

The procedure for concomitant urethrectomy at the time of cystoprostatectomy is very similar to that described previously for the treatment of pri-

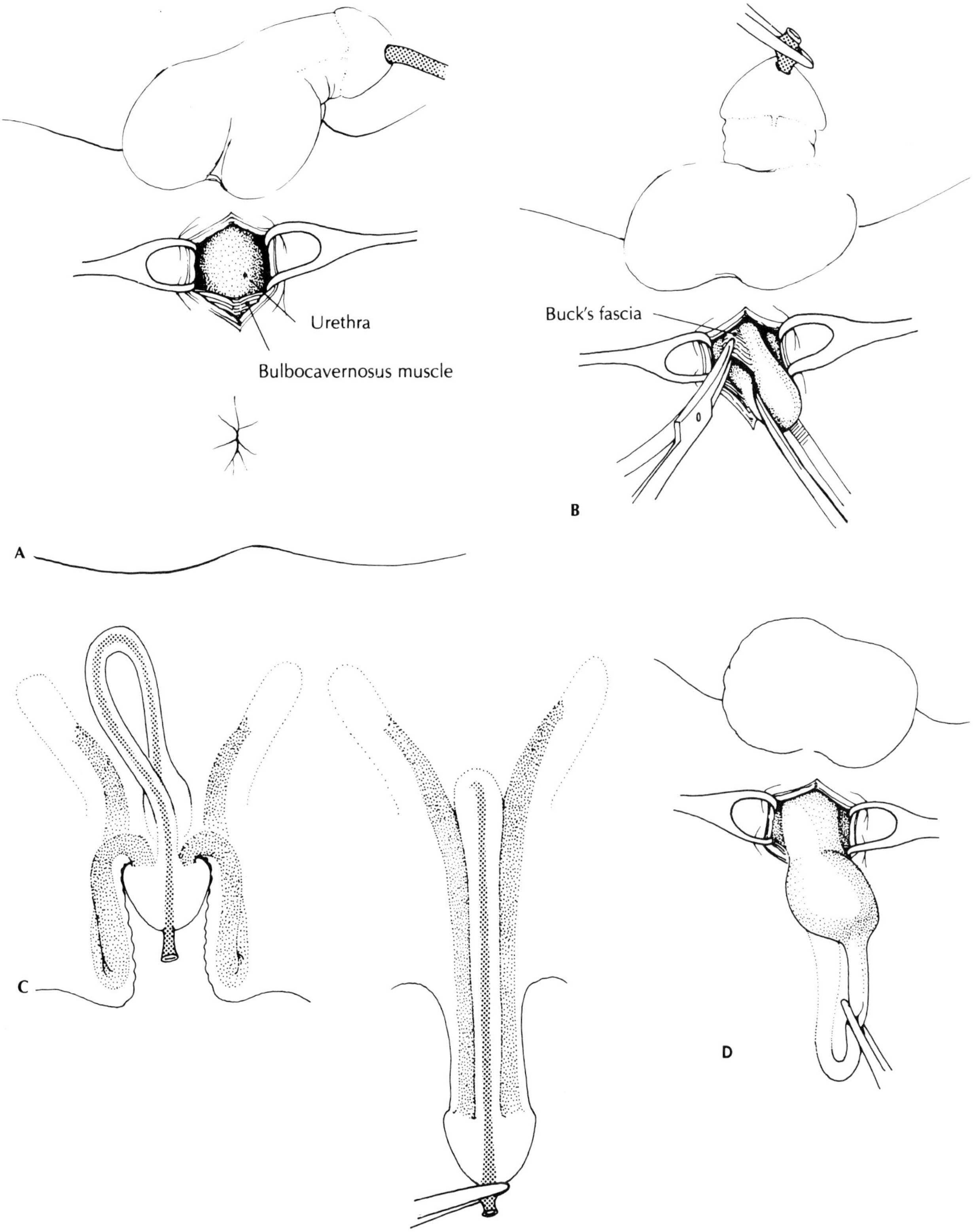
Urethra
Bulbocavernosus muscle
A
Buck's fascia
B
C
D

FIGURE 40–11. Total urethrectomy with cystoprostatectomy. (From Robertson C: Urethral carcinoma. *In* Glenn JF [ed]: Urologic Surgery, 4th edition, p 688. Philadelphia, JB Lippincott Co, 1991, with permission.)

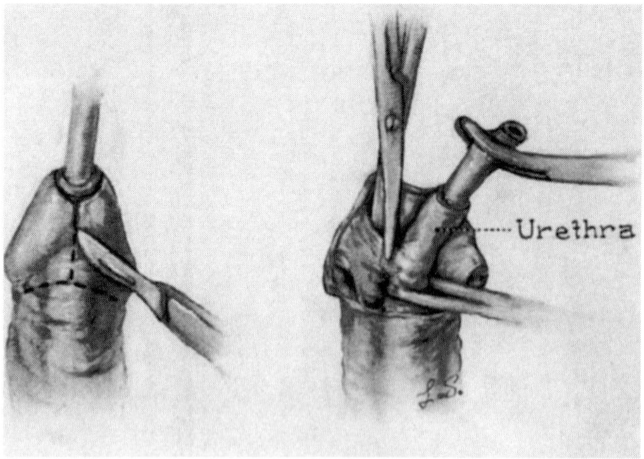
Urethra

FIGURE 40–12. Inverted T-incision on glans penis and dissection of glanular urethra. (From Brendler CB: Urethrectomy. *In* Walsh PC, Retik AB, Stamey TA, Vaughan ED Jr [eds]: Campbell's Urology, 6th edition, p 2778. Philadelphia, WB Saunders Co, 1992, with permission.)

mary urethral cancer. The bulbomembranous and prostatic urethral segments are those most often involved by extension of the primary bladder cancers; thus careful dissection of these areas is essential. This part of the dissection can be considerably more difficult when urethrectomy follows cystoprostatectomy by more than several weeks.[14] In such cases, a Foley catheter must be placed to the proximal end of the urethra and secured in place by suturing to the meatus, and dissection carried to the proximal extent of the catheter. Dissection of the proximal urethra should be done carefully and methodically because extensive traction on the urethra may avulse the proximal portion as a result of extensive fibrosis in this area. Drainage of the proximal urethral bed using a Jackson-Pratt or Penrose drain is suggested.

Total Urethrectomy in the Female Patient in Association with Cystectomy

Total urethrectomy in the woman with concomitant bladder cancer is very similar to that described for total urethrectomy for primary urethral cancer in the female patient. In this case, however, consideration should be given to removing a cuff of vagina underlying the urethral segment so as to ensure complete resection. When this is accomplished, reapproximation of the superior urethral margins should be initiated at the meatal extent of the excision, using 2-0 chromic G-U (5/8ths) needles to reconstrict the vagina superiorly. After transvaginal suturing to the level of the cephalad aspect of the pubis, the suture may be passed into the abdominal wound and the superior vaginal closure continued transabdominally, using a running suture.

POSTOPERATIVE CARE

In the male, penile and perineal drains can typically be removed after 24 to 48 hours and normal activity may be resumed within 1 to 2 days after

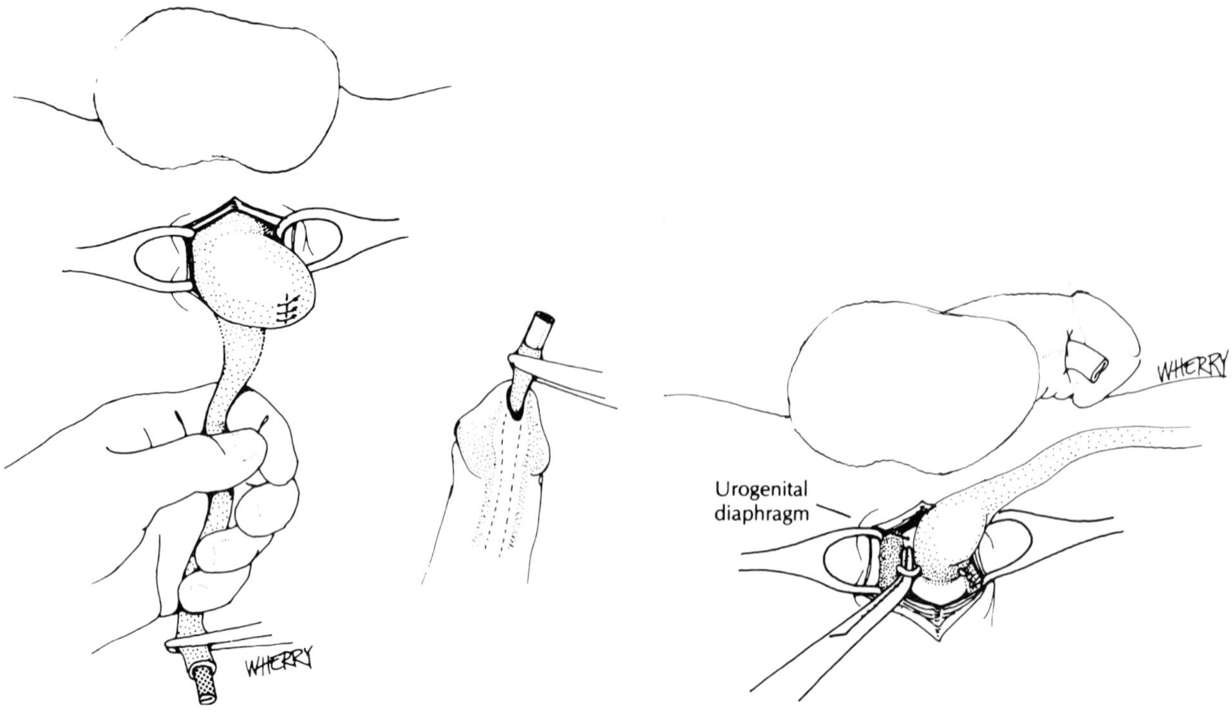
WHERRY
WHERRY
Urogenital
diaphragm

FIGURE 40–13. Control of the bulbar arteries during urethrectomy. (From Robertson C: Urethral carcinoma. *In* Glenn JF [ed]: Urologic Surgery, 4th edition, p 689. Philadelphia, JB Lippincott Co, 1991, with permission.)

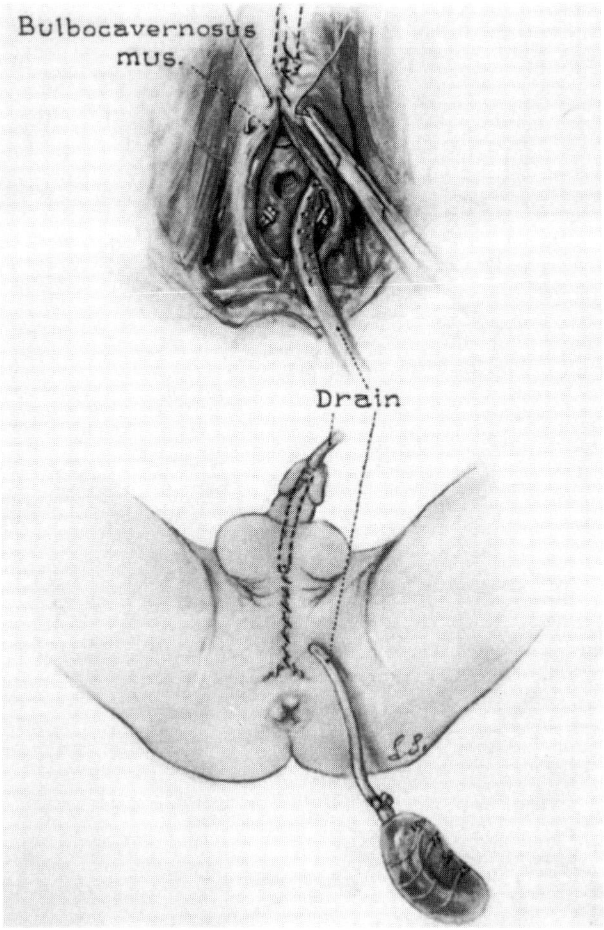
Bulbocavernosus mus.
Drain

FIGURE 40–14. Closure of the perineal incision and placement of the Jackson-Pratt drain. (From Brendler CB: Urethrectomy. *In* Walsh PC, Retik AB, Stamey TA, Vaughan ED Jr [eds]: Campbell's Urology, 6th edition, p 2780. Philadelphia, WB Saunders Co, 1992, with permission.)

surgery. The tip of the glans penis is periodically inspected during the early convalescence to rule out penile strangulation caused by the circumferential pressure dressing. Any absence of sensation or ischemic discoloration mandates redressing of the wound. When total urethrectomy is undertaken, a T-type perineal pressure dressing is helpful in decreasing postoperative bleeding in the perineal area.

Drainage of the urethrectomy incision in the female patient is typically not necessary. As mentioned previously, povidone-iodine vaginal packing is typically employed and removed the morning after surgery. One must be careful not to pack the dressing too tightly so as to prevent pressure necrosis of the reapproximated vaginal mucosa.

COMPLICATIONS

In both sexes, complications from total urethrectomy are typically those secondary to the abdominal/intestinal aspects of the dissection, including intestinal injury, fistula formation, pelvic abscess,

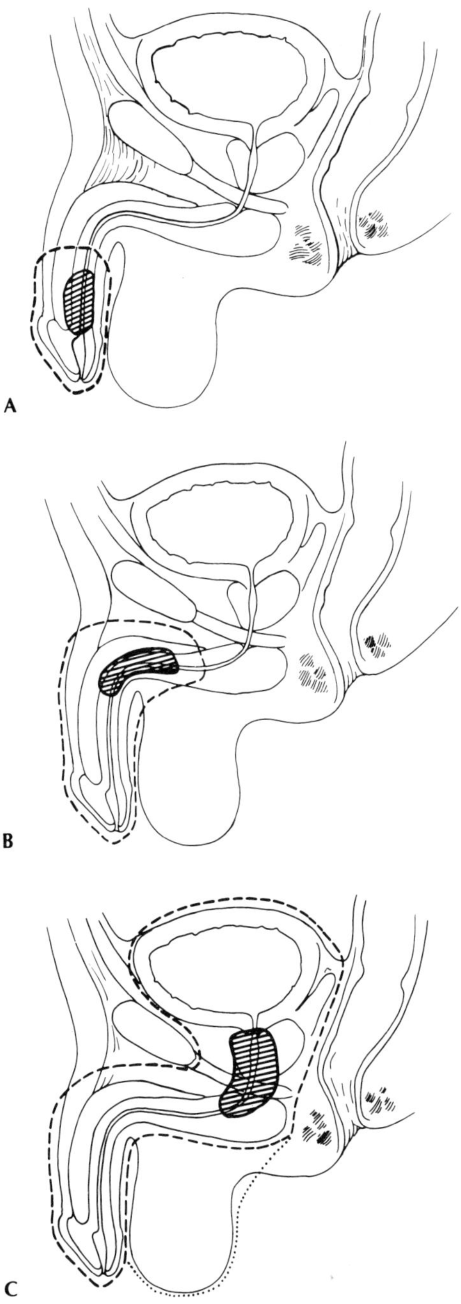
A
B
C

FIGURE 40–15. Boundaries of surgical management of distal penile (*A*), proximal penile (*B*), and prostatomembranous (*C*) male urethral carcinoma. (From Robertson C: Urethral carcinoma. *In* Glenn JF [ed]: Urologic Surgery, 4th edition, p 691. Philadelphia, JB Lippincott Co, 1991, with permission.)

and intestinal adhesions with small bowel obstruction. In the male, ecchymosis and edema of the penile skin are the rule after both primary and secondary urethrectomy. These changes typically resolve within 1 to 2 weeks after surgery. In the female, if complete excision of the anterior compartment of the perineum is required, muscle flap placement to reconstitute the pelvic floor may be necessary. If not undertaken, evisceration through the pelvic floor may be a secondary complication of this procedure.

TABLE 40-1. CARCINOMA OF THE FEMALE URETHRA: RELATION OF SURVIVAL AND SITE*,†

Authors	Anterior	Entire	Total
Staubirz et al.	8/22 (36%)	1/5 (20%)	9/27 (33%)
Grabstald et al.	9/28 (32%)	5/57‡ (9%)	14/85 (16%)
Desai et al.	4/10 (40%)	1/6 (17%)	5/16 (31%)
Peterson et al.	12/23 (57%)	5/24 (21%)	18/47 (38%)

*Modified from Ray B, Guinan CB: Primary carcinoma of the urethra. *In* Javadpour N (ed): Principles and Management of Urologic Cancer, pp 445–473. Baltimore, Williams & Wilkins, 1979, with permission.
†Five-year survival with no evidence of disease.
‡One alive, with cancer.

TABLE 40-2. CARCINOMA OF THE MALE URETHRA: RELATION OF TYPE, SITE, AND SURVIVAL*,†

	Location			
Type	Penile	Bulbomembranous	Prostate	Total
Squamous	12/27 (44%)	4/40 (10%)	0/1 (0%)	16/68 (24%)
Transitional	1/3 (33%)	0/4 (0%)	4/13 (31%)	5/20 (25%)
Adenocarcinoma	—	1/4 (25%)	—	1/4 (25%)
Undifferentiated	—	0/1 (0%)	—	0/1 (24%)
Total	13/30 (43%)	5/49 (10%)	4/14 (29%)	22/93 (24%)

*Modified from Ray B, Guinan CB: Primary carcinoma of the urethra. *In* Javadpour N (ed): Principles and Management of Urologic Cancer, pp 445–473. Baltimore, Williams & Wilkins, 1979, with permission.
†Five-year survival with no evidence of disease.

RESULTS

Boundaries for the surgical management of urethral cancer in the male are given in Figure 40–15. Male urethral cancers involving the anterior urethra can usually be treated by partial penectomy, whereas more proximal tumors typically require total penectomy with perineal urethrostomy, or cystoprostatectomy with urethrectomy (Fig. 40–15). A 2-cm tumor-free margin is typically undertaken and is desirable. When such guidelines are followed, local failure for anterior urethral carcinomas is unusual and the 5-year survival rate exceeds 50%.[15–17] In contrast, despite extensive surgery for posterior urethral cancers in men, local recurrence occurs frequently and is often associated with distant failure. The 5-year survival rate in these patients is only approximately 10 to 20% (Table 40–1).[15–17] Five-year survival rates for primary urethral cancer in women are also related to the site of the cancer and are also less common in patients with proximal urethral lesions (Table 40–2).[18]

The prognosis of various stages of bladder cancers extending to the urethra are discussed in Chapter 39.

REFERENCES

1. Ali MM, Klein FA, Hazva TA: Primary female urethral carcinoma. Cancer 1988; 62:54–57.
2. Levinson AK, Johnson DE, Wishnow KI: Indications for urethrectomy in an era of continent urinary diversion. J Urol 1990; 144:73.
3. Hickey DP, Soloway MS, Murphy WM: Selective urethrectomy following cystoprostatectomy for bladder cancer. J Urol 1986; 136:828.
4. Lepor H, Gregerman M, Crosby R, et al: Precise localization of the autonomic nerves from the pelvic plexus to the corpora cavernosa: a detailed anatomical study of the adult male pelvis. J Urol 1985; 133:207.
5. Schlegel PN, Walsh PC: Neuroanatomical approach to radical cystoprostatectomy with preservation of sexual function. J Urol 1987; 138:1402.
6. Brendler CB, Schlegel PN, Walsh PC: Urethrectomy with preservation of potency. J Urol 1990; 144:270.
7. Schellhammer PF, Jordan GH: Surgery for urethral cancer. *In* Droller MJ (ed): Surgical Management of Urologic Disease, pp 833–842. St. Louis, Mosby Year Book, 1992.
8. Schellhammer PF: Urethral carcinoma. Semin Urol 1989; 1: 835–840.
9. Grabstald H, Hilaris B, Henschke U, Whitmore WF: Cancer of the female urethra. JAMA 1966; 197:835–842.
10. Klein FA, Whitmore WF, Herr HW, et al: Inferior pubic rami resection with en bloc radical excision for invasive proximal urethral carcinoma. Cancer 1983; 51:1238–1242.
11. Johnson DE, Lo RR: Tumors of the penis, urethra and scrotum. *In* deKernion JB, Paulson DF (eds): Genitourinary Cancer Management, pp 219–270. Philadelphia, Lea & Febiger, 1987.
12. MacKenzie AR, Whitmore WF: Resection of the pubic rami for urologic cancer. J Urol 1968; 100:546–551.
13. Mandler JI, Pool TL: Primary carcinoma of the male urethra. J Urol 1966; 96:67–72.
14. Brendler CB: Urethrectomy. *In* Walsh PC, Retik AB, Stamey TA, Vaughan ED Jr (eds): Campbell's Urology, 6th edition, pp 2774–2781. Philadelphia, WB Saunders Co, 1992.
15. Ray B, Canto AR, Whitmore WF Jr: Experience with primary carcinoma of the male urethra. J Urol 1977; 117:591.
16. Ray B, Guinan PD: Primary carcinoma of the urethra. *In* Javadpour N (ed): Principles and Management of Urologic Cancer, pp 445–473. Baltimore, Williams & Wilkins, 1979.
17. Sullivan J, Grabstald H: Management of carcinoma of the urethra. *In* Skinner DG, deKernion JB (eds): Genitourinary Cancer, pp 419–429. Philadelphia, WB Saunders Co, 1978.
18. Ray B, Guinan CB: Primary carcinoma of the urethra. *In* Javadpour N (ed): Principles and Management of Urologic Cancer, pp 445–473. Baltimore, Williams & Wilkins, 1979.

X

PENIS

41

SQUAMOUS CELL CARCINOMA OF THE PENIS: DIAGNOSIS AND STAGING

KEVIN R. LOUGHLIN, M.D.

INCIDENCE

The incidence of squamous cell carcinoma of the penis varies widely according to geographic distribution. In the United States and most industrialized countries, squamous cell carcinoma of the penis is a rare malignancy, accounting for less than 1% of all male cancers.[1,2] The incidence in the United States has been estimated to be 1 to 2 cases per 100,000 males per year.[2,3] However, in societies that are more agrarian and where circumcision is less common, the incidence of squamous cell cancer of the penis is much higher. Reddy et al.[4] have reported that penile cancer comprises 16.7% of all cancer in parts of India, and Dodge and Linsell[5] have reported that penile cancer accounts for 12.2% of all cancers diagnosed in Uganda.

EPIDEMIOLOGY

Squamous cell carcinoma of the penis is virtually unknown in populations where neonatal circumcision is routinely practiced. Maden et al.[6] have reported that the risk for penile cancer was 3.2 times greater in men who were never circumcised and 3.0 times greater in men who underwent circumcision after the neonatal period. These authors also identified a 2.8 times increased risk for penile cancer among current smokers compared to men who never smoked.[6]

Penile squamous cell carcinoma most typically occurs in men in the sixth and seventh decades of life; however, it can occur in men below the age of 40.[3] Racial predilection has not been clearly proven, and any observed racial differences are more likely due to socioeconomic or environmental factors.[7]

There appears to be an infectious component to the etiology of squamous penile cancer. Maden et al.[6] have reported a strong correlation between a history of genital warts and subsequent development of penile cancer. These authors reported that the risk of penile cancer among men who reported a history of genital warts was 5.9 times that of men who reported no such history.[6]

Beyond the link between a history of condylomata and subsequent penile cancer, there is strong molecular biologic evidence demonstrating an association between human papillomavirus (HPV) infection and subsequent penile cancer. Iwasawa et al.[8] examined 111 untreated penile carcinomas retrospectively and found 70 to be positive for HPV DNA by polymerase chain reaction. Of these tumors, 68 were identified as type 16 and the other two as type 18. Of more interest, HPV type 16 was also detected in lymph node metastases of penile carcinoma and the DNA type matched that in the primary carcinoma.[8] In situ hybridization analysis found the HPV to be localized in the nuclei of the malignant cells.

Similar findings have been published by Scinicariello et al.[9] They demonstrated that HPV 16 DNA was incorporated into the host's genome in a primary squamous cell carcinoma and its lymph node metastases using Southern blot analysis and two-dimensional gel electrophoresis. These findings suggest a causal relationship between HPV and penile squamous cell carcinoma. Other reports have shown a similar relationship between HPV 16 and cervical cancer.[10] Such relationships raise the question of whether penile and cervical carcinomas may, in some instances, be considered venereal disease.[11]

DIFFERENTIAL DIAGNOSIS

The clinician must be aware of several pathologic conditions of the penis that may mimic squamous cell carcinoma. Buschke-Lowenstein tumor may grossly be indistinguishable from squamous cell carcinoma. Buschke-Lowenstein tumors also resemble condyloma acuminatum and have been referred to as "giant condyloma." However, they differ in that Buschke-Lowenstein tumors can invade and penetrate tissue, whereas condyloma acuminatum cannot. Despite the ability to invade locally, Buschke-Lowenstein tumors rarely metastasize. However, as with condylomata acuminatum and squamous cell carcinoma, the etiology of some Buschke-Lowenstein tumors appears to be viral. HPV types 6 and 11 have been identified in some of these lesions.[12]

Erythroplasia of Queyrat and Bowen's disease are both considered carcinoma in situ of the penis. Erythroplasia was first described by Queyrat as a red, velvety lesion found on the glans penis or prepuce.[13] The lesion may be ulcerative or painful. Histologically, the mucosa appears to be replaced by atypical, hyperplastic cells with hyperchromatic nuclei and mitotic figures.

Bowen's disease refers to an intraepithelial neoplasm of the skin associated with a high occurrence of subsequent internal malignancy.[14] However, the terms "Bowen's disease of the penis" and "erythroplasia of Queyrat" are used interchangeably. Visceral disease is not associated with carcinoma in situ of the penis. HPV has also been identified in carcinoma in situ of the penis.[15]

PRESENTATION

Squamous cell carcinoma of the penis occurs almost exclusively in uncircumcised men. The cancer typically begins as a small lesion on the glans. The primary lesion may be either exophytic or flat and ulcerative. The local lesion can grow to invade the entire glans, shaft, and corpora. The only reliable means of diagnosis is biopsy and histologic examination. No definite therapy, surgical or medical, should be instituted prior to histologic diagnosis. It is not unusual for many of these patients to delay seeking medical attention, and it has been reported that 15 to 50% of patients have the penile lesion for greater than 1 year prior to diagnosis.[16,17] Pain is usually not a presenting complaint, although weakness, weight loss, and fatigue can be present as a result of chronic suppuration.

The physical exam should note the size and extent of the local lesion. In addition, there should be careful palpation of the inguinal areas to determine if adenopathy is present.

LABORATORY STUDIES AND STAGING

There are no tumor markers for penile carcinoma. However, several investigators have reported an association between penile carcinoma and hypercalcemia.[18,19] Sklaroff and Yagoda[19] reported that 17 of 81 patients with penile carcinoma treated at Memorial Sloan-Kettering were hypercalcemic. Hypercalcemia seemed to be related to the bulk of the disease and may resolve with surgical excision of inguinal metastases.[20] Parahormone-like substances can be produced by the primary tumor or metastases.[21]

The most common sites of metastatic spread of penile cancer are the inguinal lymph nodes, the pelvic lymph nodes, lung, and bone. Cavernosography, lymphangiography, computed tomography (CT), ultrasonography, and magnetic resonance imaging (MRI) have all been utilized to stage the local lesion and metastatic extent of penile cancer. Despite reports of its accuracy, cavernosography is normally not performed because of the invasive nature of the technique.[22]

Horenblas et al.[23] examined the role of lymphangiography, CT, and fine-needle aspiration in penile cancer staging. In 98 patients with penile cancer, they found that CT scan provided accurate local staging in 74% of the patients. Lymphangiography was utilized in 19 patients to assess regional (inguinal and pelvic) lymph node status. All 6 patients with pathologically proven negative nodes had negative lymphangiograms; however, of the 13 patients with pathologically proven positive nodal involvement, 9 had negative lymphangiograms and 4 were positive, for a sensitivity of 31% and a specificity of 100%. These same investigators used CT scans to evaluate the nodal (inguinal and pelvic) status of 14 patients. CT scan was no better than lymphangiography, with a sensitivity of 36% and a specificity of 100%. Fine-needle aspiration was used to evaluate the inguinal nodes only in 18 patients. In this cohort, aspiration cytology had a sensitivity of 71% and a specificity of 100%.

The use of ultrasound in the staging of primary penile cancer was first reported in two patients in 1989.[24] A larger experience was reported by Horenblas et al.[25] In their group of 16 patients, accurate assessment of the depth and extent of the primary lesion was only achieved in 7 patients (44%). Ultrasound was most limited in differentiating invasion of subepithelial tissue from corpus spongiosum in the glans. However, determination of invasion into the corpus cavernosum was clearly demonstrated in all cases where it was present.

MRI has also been used to stage penile carcinoma. DeKervilier et al.[26] reported their preliminary experience with MRI and staging penile cancer. They found that MRI correctly staged local tumors in seven of nine cases. T2-weighted sequences were most useful, and they recommended that spin-echo T2-weighted sequences should be used in evaluating such patients.

TABLE 41–1. CLASSIFICATION FOR CARCINOMA OF THE PENIS*

Stage I (A)	Tumors confined to glans, prepuce, or both
Stage II (B)	Tumors extending onto shaft of penis
Stage III (C)	Tumors with inguinal metastasis that are operable
Stage IV (D)	Tumors involving adjacent structures; tumors associated with inoperable inguinal metastasis or distant metastasis

*From Jackson SM: The treatment of carcinoma of the penis. Br J Surg 1966; 53:33, with permission.

In addition to radiographic staging of penile cancer, Cabanas[27] introduced the concept of "sentinel node biopsy." This concept was based on the belief that penile cancer first spreads to a group of nodes located superomedial to the junction of the saphenous and femoral veins in the area of the superficial epigastric vein. However, subsequent reports[28–30] have failed to confirm the efficacy of the sentinel node biopsy and such a staging procedure is no longer recommended. Finally, in addition to staging the local lesion and regional lymph nodes, all patients with penile cancer should have a baseline chest x-ray and bone scan.

Staging Systems

Two major staging systems have been commonly employed to stage penile cancer. The Jackson system, introduced in 1966,[31] is the oldest system used (Table 41–1). A newer system, the TNM classification, is widely accepted and is now more commonly used than the Jackson system (Table 41–2).

TABLE 41–2. TNM CLASSIFICATION OF PENILE CARCINOMA*

Primary Tumor (T)	
Tx:	Primary tumor cannot be assessed
T0:	No evidence of primary tumor
Tis:	Carcinoma in situ
Ta:	Noninvasive verrucous carcinoma
T1:	Tumor invades subepithelial connective tissue
T2:	Tumor invades corpus spongiosum or cavernosum
T3:	Tumor invades other adjacent structures
Regional Lymph Nodes (N)	
Nx:	Regional lymph nodes cannot be assessed
N0:	No regional lymph node metastasis
N1:	Metastasis in single superficial inguinal lymph node
N2:	Metastasis in multiple or bilateral superficial inguinal lymph node
N3:	Metastasis in deep inguinal or pelvic lymph node(s), unilateral or bilateral
Distant Metastases (M)	
Mx:	Presence of distant metastasis cannot be assessed
M0:	No distant metastases
M1:	Distant metastases

*Adapted from Unio International Contre le Cancer: TNM Atlas: Illustrated Guide to the TNM/pTNM Classification of Malignant Tumors, 3rd edition, pp 237–244. New York, Springer-Verlag, 1989; *and* American Joint Committee on Cancer: from Manual Staging for Cancer, 3rd edition, p 189. Philadelphia, JB Lippincott, 1988.

SUMMARY

Penile cancer is a rare malignancy in regions where circumcision is routinely practiced. A careful physical exam and radiographic imaging are necessary to stage local and distant involvement of the tumor. A biopsy and pathologic confirmation of the diagnosis must be obtained prior to initiating treatment.

REFERENCES

1. Grabstald H: Cancer of the penis. J Cont Ed Urol 1979; 18: 15.
2. Sufrin G, Huben R: Benign and malignant lesions of the penis. *In*: Gillenwater JY, Grayback JT, Howard SS, Duckett JW (eds): Adult and Pediatric Urology, 2nd edition, pp 1643–1681. St. Louis, Mosby–Year Book, 1991.
3. Schellhammer PF, Jordon GH, Schlossberg SM: Tumors of the penis. *In* Walsh PC, Retik AB, Stamey TA, Vaughan ED Jr (eds): Campbell's Urology, 6th edition, pp 1264–1298. Philadelphia, WB Saunders Co, 1992.
4. Reddy CRRM, Raghavaigah NV, Mouli KC: Prevalence of carcinoma of the penis with special reference to India. Int Surg 1978; 60:470.
5. Dodge OG, Linsell CA: Carcinoma of the penis in Uganda and Kenya Africa. Cancer 1963; 16:1255.
6. Maden C, Sherman KJ, Beckmann AM, et al: History of circumcision, medical conditions, sexual activity and risk of penile cancer. J Natl Cancer Inst 1993; 85:19.
7. Hall NEL, Schottenfeld D: Penis. *In* Shottenfeld D, Fraumens JF Jr (eds): Cancer Epidemiology and Prevention, p. 964. Philadelphia, WB Saunders Co, 1982.
8. Iwasawa A, Kumamoto Y, Fujnaga K: Detection of human papilloma virus deoxyribonucleic acid in penile carcinoma by polymerase chain reaction and in situ hybridization. J Urol 1993; 149:59.
9. Scinicariello F, Rudy P, Saltzstein D, et al: Human papilloma virus 16 exhibits a similar integration pattern in primary squamous cell carcinoma of the penis and its metastasis. Cancer 1992; 70:2143.
10. Rohan T, Mann V, McLaughlin J, et al: PCR detected genital papilloma virus infection: prevalence and association with risk factors for cervical cancer. Int J Cancer 1991; 49: 856.
11. Loughlin KR: Penile cancer. Curr Opin Urol 1993; 3:415.
12. Boshart M, zor Hausen H: Human papilloma virus (HPV) in Buschke-Lowenstein tumors: physical state of the DNA and identification of a tandem duplication in the noncoding region of a HPV 6 subtype. J Virol 1986; 58:963.
13. Queyrat L: Erythroplasia du gland. Sec Franc Dermatol Syphilol 1911; 22:378.
14. Bowen J: Precancerous dermatoses: a review of two cases of chronic atypical epithelial proliferation. J Cutan Dis 1912; 30:241.
15. Pfister H, Haneke E: Dermonstration of human papilloma virus type 2 DNA in Bowen's disease. Arch Dermatol Res 1984; 276:123.
16. Hardner GJ, Bhanalaph T, Murphy GP, et al: Carcinoma of the penis: analysis of therapy in 100 consecutive cases. J Urol 1972; 108:428.
17. Gursel EO, Georgourtzos C, Uson AC, et al: Penile cancer. Urology 1973; 1:569.
18. Rudd FV, Rott RK, Skoglund RW, Ansell JS: Tumor induced hypercalcemia. J Urol 1972; 107:986.

19. Sklaroff RB, Yagoda A: Penile cancer: natural history and therapy. *In* Chemotherapy and Urological Malignancy, pp 98–105. New York, Springer-Verlag, 1982.
20. Block NL, Rosen P, Whitmore WF: Hemipelvectomy for advanced penile cancer. J Urol 1973; 110:703.
21. Malakoff AF, Schmidt JD: Metastatic carcinoma of penis complicated by hypercalcemia. Urology 1975; 5:519.
22. Raghavaiah NV: Corpus cavernosogram in the evaluation of carcinoma of the penis. J Urol 1978; 120:423.
23. Horenblas S, Van Tinteren H, Delemarre JF, et al: Squamous cell carcinoma of the penis: accuracy of tumor, nodes and metastasis classification system and role of lymphangiography, computerized tomography scan and fine needle aspiration cytology. J Urol 1991; 146:1279.
24. Yamashita T, Ogawa A: Ultrasound in penile cancer. Urol Radiol 1989; 11:174.
25. Horenblas S, Kroger R, Gallee MPW, et al: Ultrasound in squamous cell carcinoma of the penis: a useful addition to clinical staging. Urology 1994; 43:702.
26. deKervilier E, Ollier P, Desgrandchamps F, et al: Magnetic resonance imaging in patients with penile carcinoma. Br J Radiol 1995; 68:704.
27. Cabanas R: An approach to the treatment of penile carcinoma. Cancer 1977; 39:456.
28. Catalona WJ: Role of lymphadenectomy in carcinomas of the penis. Urol Clin North Am 1980; 7:785.
29. Perinetti EP, Crane DC, Catalona WJ: Unreliability of sentinel lymph node biopsy for staging penile carcinoma. J Urol 1980; 124:734.
30. Wespes E, Simon J, Schulman CC: Cabanas' approach: is sentinel node biopsy reliable for staging of penile carcinoma? Urology 1986; 28:278.
31. Jackson SM: The treatment of carcinoma of the penis. Br J Surg 1966; 53:33.

42

SUPERFICIAL CARCINOMA OF THE PENIS: MANAGEMENT AND PROGNOSIS

JOSEPH F. HARRYHILL, M.D., F.A.C.S. *and* VICTOR L. CARPINIELLO, M.D.

Penile squamous cell carcinoma accounts for only 2 to 5% of all genitourinary malignancies.[1] Because of its uncommon occurrence in the United States, it is difficult to assemble large, prospective trials that compare partial and total penectomy to organ-sparing alternatives in the management of the primary lesion. Even more controversy has appeared in the literature over the proper indications for, and timing of, inguinal lymphadenectomy for low-stage epidermoid tumors of the penis.

Because penectomy has a potentially significant impact on the psychosocial well-being and sexual function of the patient with penile cancer,[2] many alternative treatments that propose to accomplish tumor ablation with organ preservation have been described (Table 42–1). In carefully selected patients with clinically localized disease and small superficial lesions, it appears that complete tumor excision and local control can be accomplished successfully with conservative resection or organ-sparing ablative techniques.[3]

Although the patient's concern in penile cancer is focused on the surgical management of the primary lesion, it is the presence or absence of inguinal lymph node dissemination of tumor that largely determines prognosis.[1] When lymph nodes were clinically involved with tumor at the time of presentation (Jackson stage III), the 5-year survival rate in a compiled series of studies was 27%.[4] When relapse after treatment of the penile lesion occurs, the site of relapse (penile versus nodal) is an important prognostic feature. Hardner et al. noted an overall mean 7-year survival in patients with locally recurrent disease, but only a mean survival of 2 years when relapse occurred in the groin.[5]

This chapter reviews treatment alternatives and prognosis in superficial squamous cell cancer of the penis, as well as premalignant and in situ lesions. Although therapeutic methods may change, the objectives in penile cancer treatment remain constant: accurate diagnosis with biopsy and clinicopathologic assessment of lymph nodes status, disease eradication, and meticulous follow-up. Organ preservation, although important, should not compromise these objectives.

PREMALIGNANT LESIONS OF THE PENIS (TABLE 42–2)

Leukoplakia

Leukoplakia typically appears as a whitish plaque involving the glans and meatus, and may be indistinguishable from other inflammatory entities, including balanitis xerotica obliterans and candidiasis. On occasion, leukoplakia may be found adjacent to squamous cell carcinoma.[6] For these reasons, clinicians should perform biopsy and histopathologic examination routinely when presented with raised, inflammatory lesions of the penis. Treatment of leukoplakia is conservative; excision may be required for persistent lesions, and circumcision to remove a contributing source of inflammation is advisable.[4]

Balanitis Xerotica Obliterans

Also known as lichen sclerosis et atrophicus, this lesion appears white and atrophic and involves the glans and urethral meatus, sometimes with significant stenosis. In one series of 80 patients with cancer of the penis, 17 (21%) had a previous history of balanitis xerotica obliterans, thus highlighting the

TABLE 42–1. ALTERNATIVES TO PENECTOMY IN SUPERFICIAL PENILE CANCER

- Partial penectomy
- Circumcision
- Wide local excision
- Laser ablation
  - Neodymium:YAG
  - Carbon dioxide
- Cryoablation
- Radiation therapy
  - External beam (XRT)
  - Brachytherapy (surface mold; interstitial)
- Mohs micrographic surgery
- Chemotherapy
  - Topical (5-fluorouracil)
  - Systemic

putative premalignant nature of this entity.[7] Meatotomy and/or excision may be required; the use of topical or intralesional steroids has been suggested.[8] Laser therapy has also been used with satisfactory, although not perfect, cosmetic results.[9]

Bushke-Lowenstein Tumor

The Bushke-Lowenstein tumor develops as a locally destructive verrucous mass usually involving the glans and prepuce, and has a histologic appearance that is indistinguishable from benign condyloma acuminata.[4] However, in some cases, microscopic foci of invasive squamous cell carcinoma have been identified in these lesions.[10] Treatment generally involves local excision; partial or total amputation is sometimes required when significant destruction of the glans and penile shaft has occurred. Mohs micrographic surgery has also been recommended in treatment of this entity because its method of histopathologic examination of each resected layer can confirm negative margins.[6] Radiation therapy is reported to have only limited efficacy for this process,[11] and is therefore not advised.[8] In addition, there have been rare case reports of anaplastic transformation of verrucous carcinoma following treatment with radiation therapy.[12]

The term "verrucous carcinoma" is also used to describe such exophytic lesions, sometimes regarded as a true carcinoma but a variant that is less aggressive than typical squamous cell carcinoma. In a study by Seixas et al. of 32 cases of this unusual lesion, most patients were treated with surgical excision of the primary tumor, and none developed recurrent disease or died of cancer.[13] Of 17 patients who underwent inguinal lymphadenectomy, none had nodal involvement. Similarly, the remainder of patients managed without node dissection did not subsequently relapse with groin metastasis. This would support a conservative approach toward the patient with palpable adenopathy in verrucous carcinoma, and no need for sentinel node biopsy or prophylactic lymphadenectomy.[13,14]

TABLE 42–2. PREMALIGNANT AND IN SITU PENILE LESIONS

Premalignant Lesions
- Leukoplakia
- Balanitis xerotica obliterans
- Bushke-Lowenstein tumor (verrucous carcinoma)

Carcinoma in Situ Lesions
- Erythroplasia of Queyrat
- Bowen's disease
- Bowenoid papulosis

CARCINOMA IN SITU LESIONS OF THE PENIS (TABLE 42–2)

Erythroplasia of Queyrat

This form of in situ carcinoma typically presents as a painless, raised, erythematous, velvety plaque without ulceration found on the glans or prepuce. The median age of onset was 51 years in a large series of 100 cases.[15] The presence of ulceration in such lesions usually signifies the presence of invasive carcinoma, and thorough biopsies are thus indicated.[6] Erythroplasia of Queyrat has been treated in limited series with topical 5-fluorouracil with good results.[16] Twice-daily application of 2% fluorouracil solution or 5% ointment for 3 to 4 weeks is recommended. Erythroplasia of Queyrat is also amenable to laser therapy, and both the carbon dioxide (CO_2) (5- to 15-W setting) and neodymium:YAG laser (20- to 30-W setting) have been used successfully for ablation of such in situ lesions of the penis.[17–20]

Bowen's Disease

Unlike erythroplasia of Queyrat, which tends to involve the mucocutaneous surfaces of the glans and inner prepuce, Bowen's disease is histologically defined as carcinoma in situ involving the epithelial, follicle-bearing skin of the penis. It presents as a solitary raised, scaly plaque that may be found on the shaft or sometimes on the glans. Some literature has suggested an association between Bowen's disease and an increased risk of visceral malignancy,[15] while other sources find no such link.[21] Because of possible involvement of the deeper hair follicles, topical chemotherapy with 5-fluorouracil is discouraged.[22] Excision of the lesion with 5-mm margins is recommended instead.[3] Alternatively, Bowen's disease appears to be well suited for laser photoradiation. In one series using neodymium:YAG laser therapy, five patients with carcinoma in situ of the penis had no evidence of recurrence for more than 2 years.[23] The chemosurgery method of Mohs should also result in effective local control of such lesions.

Bowenoid Papulosis

In contrast to the above in situ entities, bowenoid papulosis, as described by Wade et al., presents with multiple small red violaceous lesions of the anogenital region in younger patients—a mean age of 28 years in a series of 11 subjects.[24] Bowenoid papulosis is noted in sexually active men and women, and the disease has been linked to the presence of human papillomavirus (HPV).[25,26] The association between HPV and dysplasia of the uterine cervix, and the presence of bowenoid papulosis in male sexual partners, has led to a growing body of evidence linking the virus causally to the development of squamous cell carcinoma of the male genital tract.[27] In a study by Sarkar et al., all samples of bowenoid penile carcinoma in situ as well as 9 of 11 cases of invasive squamous cell carcinoma tested positive for HPV type 16 DNA.[28] With the rising incidence of HPV genital infections, Malek and associates have predicted that an increase in the incidence of squamous cell carcinoma of the penis in the United States will occur.[29–31]

Although histologically similar to other carcinoma in situ lesions of the penis, bowenoid papulosis is a decidedly "benign" entity that is unlikely to progress to invasive carcinoma. Therefore, local therapy such as topical 5-fluorouracil, laser vaporization or photocoagulation, electrodissection, or cryoablation should be adequate for primary therapy, with rebiopsy and surgical excision indicated for persistent lesions. It is vital to stress the importance of careful clinical follow-up to patients treated for carcinoma in situ of the penis in its various forms[29] because untreated or recurrent lesions may progress to invasive, and ultimately metastatic, disease.[32]

SUPERFICIAL PENILE CARCINOMA

Treatment

Amputation and Partial Penectomy

The standard procedure in the ever-growing armamentarium of options for treatment of localized penile cancer remains amputation. In a series by deKernion et al., no local recurrences were reported in 48 cases managed with partial penectomy or wide local excision.[33] Partial penectomy is indicated if a distal penile tumor is present, and a 2-cm tumor-free margin can be achieved while maintaining adequate cosmetic and functional phallic length. Frozen section examination of the proximal margin is recommended at the time of partial penectomy.[8] Lesions of the glans penis have been managed with local excision, but the incidence of recurrence is high.[34]

Primary lesions of the proximal shaft and base of the penis are unusual; these cases have been handled with total penectomy and creation of a perineal urethrostomy if a satisfactory proximal margin is not possible.[33] Alternatively, selected patients with superficial disease on the penile shaft can be treated with wide excision of the skin and subcutaneous tissue.[3,35] Reconstruction with skin grafting or scrotal skin advancement may be necessary if a large defect remains following wide local excision of a superficial neoplasm on the penile shaft.[36] Experience shows that, when adequate excision of the cancer is performed, the prognosis then depends primarily on the characteristics of the neoplasm (depth of penetration; grade) rather than on the method used for its removal.[3,7]

Circumcision

Small, noninvasive tumors located on the distal prepuce can be managed with circumcision, provided a 2-cm margin can be achieved.[3,36] If a foreskin carcinoma cannot be excised with adequate clearance, the incidence of local tumor recurrence is quite high. Overall, McDougal et al. noted a local recurrence rate of 32% in patients treated with local excision or circumcision,[34] and Narayana et al. reported recurrence in 50% of cases, requiring subsequent partial amputation.[37] An earlier study by Hardner and associates is notable in that all patients managed with circumcision had local recurrence.[5] These statistics should be considered when circumcision is contemplated in the management of preputial cancers, and they highlight the need for continued assessment and close follow-up in patients with superficial carcinoma of the penis.

Circumcision is also an important adjunct in the treatment of premalignant penile lesions, such as leukoplakia, because the foreskin may be a source of chronic irritation.[8] Removal of the foreskin is also advised in patients prior to undergoing radiation therapy (either external beam treatments or brachytherapy) for penile neoplasms, to avoid development of foreskin sclerosis and secondary infection.[7,38,39]

Laser Therapy

Prior to technical advances that have made tissue ablation with laser energy possible, therapeutic options in treatment of penile tumors were limited to amputation and excision of lesions. The first use of laser photoradiation for cancer of the penis was reported in 1968. Parsons et al. published a single case of ablative treatment using a ruby laser in a patient who refused partial amputation for invasive epidermoid cancer.[40] A satisfactory cosmetic result was achieved, but subsequent partial penectomy revealed residual tumor. Since that time, much interest in laser phototherapy for cutaneous penile lesions has centered on the use of neodymium:YAG and CO_2 lasers; an understanding of the effects of these lasers on soft tissue is important in determining the appropriate use and limitations of this modality. As has been stated previously, eradication of tumor takes priority over achievement of a pleasing

TABLE 42–3. STAGING SYSTEMS FOR PENILE CANCER

Jackson Stage[43]	TNM UICC System[44]	Lesion
I	Tis, T1N0M0, T2N0M0*,†	Tumor limited to glans penis and/or prepuce
II	T3–4N0M0	Invasion into shaft or corpora
III	T1–4N1–3M0	Tumor confined to shaft, with proven regional node metastasis
IV	T1–4N1–3M1,2	Inoperative regional node involvement or distant metastasis

*T1, less than 2 cm; T2, 2 to 5 cm with minimal infiltration.
†TNM staging system allows for "subclassification" of patients with Jackson stage I lesions.

cosmetic result and phallic preservation.[19] It is the responsibility of the clinician to select patients whose lesions are most appropriately treated with organ-sparing laser therapy[41]; that is, tumors that are small (2 cm or less)[42] and noninvasive clinical stage Tis or T1 (Jackson stage I) lesions (see Table 42–3). Experience has shown that laser ablation of larger or invasive tumors is possible but is limited by a high local recurrence rate.[18,23,42,45] Malloy et al.[23] found the neodymium:YAG laser to be ineffective in the recurrence-free ablation of stage II (2- to 5-cm) lesions.

CO_2 LASER. This laser has an emission of 10,600 nm and is strongly absorbed by water with minimal scatter.[46] This allows for instantaneous vaporization of tissue at the site of laser impact, with boiling of intracellular water; the majority of incident energy is absorbed in less than 0.1 mm tissue depth.[47] Because of its intense absorption by water, CO_2 laser energy cannot be delivered through an irrigation medium, and thus cannot be used in cystoscopic procedures.[48] The CO_2 beam can be focused to a pinpoint spot size, which allows accurate scalpel-like incision of tissue and satisfactory hemostasis.[46] This may allow for debulking of a large lesion. The handpiece is then defocused to effect coagulation of the base of the resected lesion. Ablation of benign lesions, such as condyloma, can be carried out at low power (5 to 15 watts), whereas penile carcinoma will require a higher output (25 to 40 watts).[48,49]

NEODYMIUM:YAG LASER. Having a wavelength of 1060 nm, this laser is characterized by minimal absorption by water or biologic pigments such as hemoglobin.[41,49] Thus there is significant depth of penetration from forward scatter of the laser energy, resulting in coagulative necrosis of 4 to 6 mm of tissue. The treated area becomes characteristically white and firm, consistent with denaturization of protein, a process that occurs when the temperature exceeds 60°C.[41] Small blood vessels are coagulated by the process, making for adequate hemostasis. A power setting of 25 to 38 watts is suggested for treatment of superficial penile cancer, using the focusing handpiece.[23,49] The treated area is not closed; rather, healing occurs by secondary re-epithelization. Malloy et al. recommend circumcision in all patients undergoing laser ablation of superficial penile tumors on the glans and distal shaft.[50]

Tissue penetration of photocoagulation energy delivered by the neodymium:YAG laser can be enhanced by application of iced saline to the area during laser exposure. This cools the skin surface and prevents surface carbonization and vaporization, thus increasing depth of penetration.[50,51] Perhaps the most important limitation of laser therapy in the management of penile carcinoma is lack of tissue confirmation of negative margins.[41] This limits the usefulness of this modality to a select group of patients having small, superficial, well-delineated tumors. Nonetheless, use of neodymium:YAG may be preferable to CO_2 laser vaporization in squamous cell carcinoma of the penis because it achieves deeper penetration.[49] Malek has recommended reserving CO_2 treatment for premalignant lesions of the penis showing histologic evidence of dysplasia, while neodymium:YAG is used for in situ lesions and carcinoma.[18]

SUMMARY. Laser therapy appears to be well suited for treatment of penile carcinoma; in selected patients with superficial disease this modality can provide eradication of the primary lesion while avoiding the mutilating effects of penectomy or radiation[4] (Fig. 42–1). Close clinical follow-up is urged after laser ablation procedures because re-epithelialization of skin may take several months. Areas that heal poorly or incompletely should undergo repeat biopsy to rule out persistent disease.

Mohs Micrographic Technique

The concept of microscopically controlled frozen section excision of sequential thin layers of cutaneous lesions in Mohs surgery derives from the observation that cancer often extends beyond the clinically visible or palpable lesion.[52] Often, squamous carcinoma can infiltrate subjacent tissue by way of thin cords of cells. This phenomenon could explain the high local recurrence rate of cancers located on the prepuce, when an adequate (2-cm) tumor-free margin is not achieved. Das[36] has stressed the importance of a 2-cm margin in penile amputation because of this phenomenon of "noncontiguous" tumor growth.

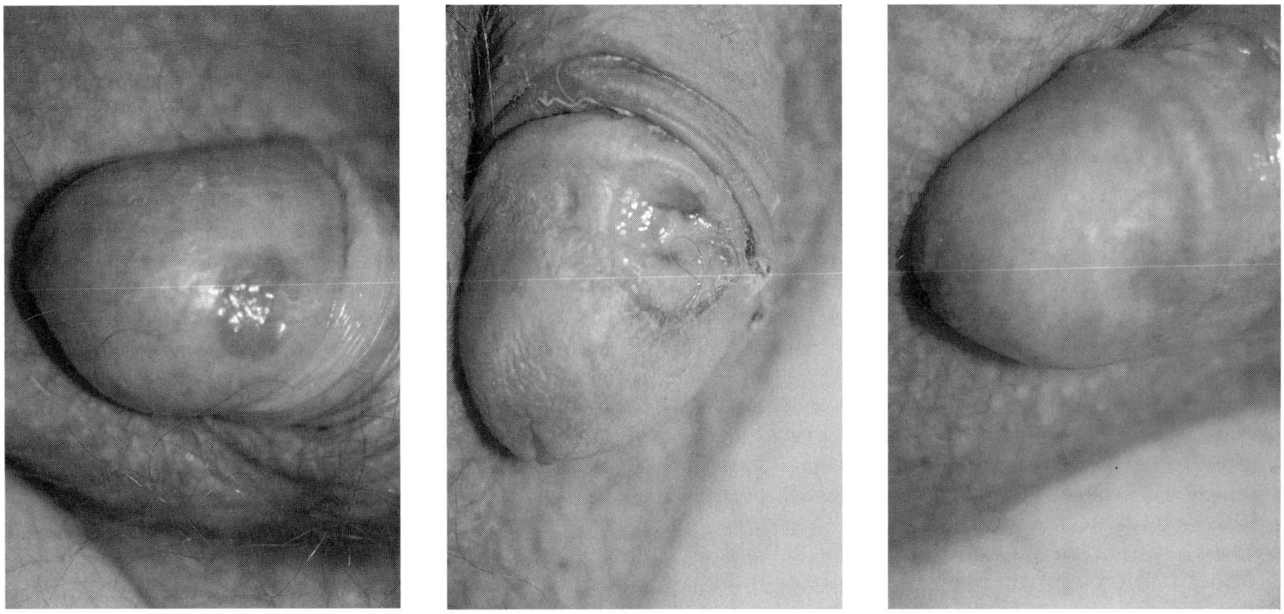
A
B
C

FIGURE 42–1. *A*, Squamous cell carcinoma of glans penis. *B*, Postoperative appearance 2 weeks following CO_2 laser ablation of lesion. *C*, Appearance 8 weeks postoperatively. (From Finkelstein LH: CO_2 laser surgery in urology. Surg Clin North Am 1984; 64:913–930, with permission. © by WB Saunders Co, Philadelphia.)

The fixed-tissue technique of Mohs surgery for lesions of the glans penis and prepuce usually involves initial debulking, if the lesion is large. Then, a keratinolytic (dichloroacetic acid) is applied to the base of the lesion and its surrounding rim under local anesthesia, followed by a fixative paste. After appropriate interval for a fixation, the treated layer is excised and examined microscopically for tumor. Depending on lesion size and depth of penetration, the total process may take several days and can be performed on an outpatient basis.[52] In a study of 29 patients with penile cancer treated by this technique, 18 patients who had Jackson stage I lesions enjoyed a 5-year cure rate of 81%.[53] It is notable that treatment failures presented with metastatic disease, not local recurrence. Prognosis was also found to be related to the size of the primary lesion; all patients with tumors less than 1 cm remained free of disease, whereas recurrence was 50% in lesions larger than 3 cm. As previously mentioned, Mohs surgery, either by fresh tissue or fixed technique, has proved to be successful in the eradication of penile carcinoma in situ and verrucous carcinoma.[22,52]

Radiation Therapy

Radiotherapy, either in the form of external beam radiation or brachytherapy (surface molds or interstitial), has been utilized as an organ-preserving alternative to surgery for management of the primary lesion in penile cancer.

EXTERNAL BEAM THERAPY. Several studies have demonstrated safety and efficacy in the use of external beam irradiation (XRT) for penile cancer. A series by Sagerman et al. was notable for a 3-year disease-free interval in seven of nine patients with Jackson stage I tumors.[54] The incidence of radiation necrosis after XRT requiring amputation is reported at 5 to 10%.[54,55] Patients should be informed that the rate of local disease control in penile preservation is approximately 60 to 80%,[54–58] and that surgical excision (i.e., partial penectomy) is advised in patients with local recurrence or radiation necrosis. Dosage delivered to the penis in various studies ranges from 35 to 65 Gy. Gerbaulet and Lambin recommend use of 2-Gy daily fractions in XRT to a total of 65 to 70 Gy,[39] noting that local complications will occur more frequently when larger fraction sizes are implemented. They also advise pretreatment circumcision.

A theoretical concern in the use of XRT for penile cancer focuses on the length of time required to achieve a therapeutic dose, often up to 7 weeks, and the possibility of disease spread in an aggressive lesion before tumoricidal dosage is achieved.[39,54] However, numerous studies have shown that radiation of the primary tumor does not adversely affect survival in penile cancer, even in patients with local recurrence following therapy.[39,43,56] It would appear that XRT, with surgical excision reserved for local recurrence, can be an acceptable alternative in the management of cancer of the penis, which can result in disease control and preservation of penile structure and function.[56] Several authors suggest comparable results with surgery and radiation (either XRT or brachytherapy) for small lesions but recommend amputation for larger, bulky tumors.[39,55,58]

Brachytherapy. Compared to XRT, brachytherapy appears to provide somewhat better local disease control in the treatment of penile cancer. Both surface molds and interstitial implantation have been used to deliver tumoricidal radiation energy to penile neoplasms. El-Demiry et al. utilized iridium mold therapy as the treatment of choice for squamous cell carcinoma in a series of 80 patients.[7] In subjects with Jackson stage I disease, local recurrence requiring surgical excision occurred in 21% and meatal strictures were noted in 17%. Patients did well, with a 5-year survival rate of 89%. The technique involves placement of the mold on the penis by the patient, to be worn intermittently for a length of time calculated to deliver a dose of approximately 60 Gy, usually over a 1-week period.[39]

Interstitial therapy using an iridium-192 wire afterloading technique has been used extensively in France because the anatomy of the penis makes it uniquely amenable to such treatment.[59] Under regional or general anesthesia, nonradioactive hypodermic or Henschke's needles are placed through a perforated Plexiglas template box through the penis in a line or matrix configuration. The number and geometry of needles required depends upon the size and depth of the tumor. Subsequently, active iridium wires are loaded into the hollow needles, to deliver a dose of 50 to 70 Gy over a 5- to 7-day period. An indwelling Foley catheter remains throughout the procedure, and prior circumcision should be well healed. Local control of T1 tumors exceeds 90%,[58,59] and survival rates according to stage are comparable to those with other treatment methods.

Complications of Radiotherapy. Complications that arise from the various radiation therapies in penile carcinoma include desquamation and acute edema, as well as occasional late effects such as foreskin sclerosis or phimosis in uncircumcised subjects, urethral and meatal stricture, and radionecrosis. Because surgery and radiation therapy of the primary tumor in penile cancer provide similar stage-for-stage survival results, advocates of radiotherapy emphasize its potential for organ preservation in recommending radiation as first-line therapy.

Other Modalities

Cryoablation of benign cutaneous lesions is widely practiced, but application of cryosurgical techniques in treatment of superficial penile carcinoma has received scant attention in the literature.[60]

Chemotherapy has been utilized in treatment of advanced disease in penile carcinoma. Bleomycin, cisplatin, and methotrexate are the most effective agents, but complete responses are rare.[61] A recent study examining the effectiveness of combination cisplatin and interferon-$\alpha 2_B$ in a neoadjuvant setting included seven patients with nonmetastatic stage T2 lesions.[62] This regimen showed significant antitumor activity in 75% of subjects, many of whom were able to then undergo a lesser surgical procedure than originally planned. The rationale for use of recombinant human interferon-α in penile carcinoma in this study is based on the theory of HPV in the pathogenesis of this neoplasm.[26–28,62]

Local Recurrence of Penile Cancer

It is well established that organ-sparing alternatives to penile amputation for cancer lead to higher local relapse rates. Such recurrences should be approached with aggressive resection of tumor, as well as a thorough reassessment of the patient's nodal status. The risk of local recurrence in truly superficial disease (TNM stages Tis, T1) is summarized in Table 42–4.

Recurrence of carcinoma in situ treated with topical chemotherapy may be amenable to Mohs surgery or laser ablation, if the patient still has noninvasive disease.[63] Local relapse following laser treatment, radiation therapy, or Mohs technique is probably best handled with partial or total penectomy. Wound healing in surgery of irradiated tissue may be somewhat compromised, and this fact serves to stress the need for proper patient selection of low-stage disease when offering primary radiotherapy in the treatment of penile cancer.[65]

When organ-sparing modalities are utilized in larger tumors, the rate of tumor persistence or local recurrence is predictably higher. In fact, Fraley et al. have advocated the use of local excision only in carcinoma in situ and for well-differentiated tumors confined to the foreskin. In a retrospective analysis of 66 patients with low-stage (Jackson stage I) disease, they note that treatment failure and death can occur if initial management of the primary tumor is overly conservative.[66]

Nodal Disease and Prognosis

As stated earlier, overall prognosis in all stages of penile cancer depends largely upon the presence or absence of inguinal lymph node metastasis. Many authors have noted that the incidence of histologically positive ilioinguinal lymph nodes in pa-

TABLE 42–4. LOCAL RECURRENCE RATES IN SUPERFICIAL (Tis, T1) PENILE CANCER TREATED BY VARIOUS MODALITIES

Treatment Modality	Recurrence Rate (%)
Partial penectomy	0–7[34]
Circumcision	32–50[34,37]
Laser ablation	15–30[23,63]
Mohs surgery	6[52]
Radiation therapy (XRT)	30[64]
Brachytherapy	
Surface mold	21[7]
Iridium interstitial*	9[38]

*Includes stage T1 and T2 lesions.

tients with palpably negative groins in penile cancer is approximately 20%.[4,5,8,34,67–69] In stage I disease, enlarged nodes are frequently due to inflammation, and reactive adenopathy should resolve within 3 to 6 weeks of treatment of the tumor and appropriate antibiotic therapy.[69] McDougal et al. noted no cancer deaths in 19 patients with Jackson stage I lesions who were managed with local treatment alone (i.e., no node dissection).[34] In an earlier study with 3-year follow-up by deKernion et al. only 1 patient in 13 (7%) with stage I tumor succumbed to metastatic disease.[33] Therefore, it would seem unnecessary to subject all patients with superficial disease to lymphadenectomy, given the well-known potential morbidity of such a procedure. However, it is vital that patients with superficial disease and palpable nodes at presentation return for clinical follow-up after treatment of the primary lesion. Inguinal lymph node dissection is advocated in such patients if nodal enlargement persists.[69] Obviously, lymph node dissection is also indicated in stage I disease if clinically negative nodes subsequently become palpable upon routine follow-up.

Alternatively, if patient compliance with regular follow-up is questionable, bilateral superficial "prophylactic" inguinal lymphadenectomy has been suggested by some.[69–71] In countries where close patient follow-up is not possible, bilateral clearance of inguinal and iliac nodes in all patients with penile cancer is practiced. Ayyappan et al. argue for such aggressive management of regional nodes, noting that many patients in India present with inguinal adenopathy that cannot be distinguished as reactive or metastatic, and that nodal spread is not reliably predicted by the characteristics of the primary tumor.[72]

In a summary of studies compiled by Thompson and Fair,[1] 12% of patients with Jackson stage I tumors progressed to adenopathy or cancer-related death, highlighting the need for close clinical follow-up of patients treated expectantly after removal of the primary tumor. Such a study also underscores the need for more accurate, noninvasive means of assessing nodal status in predicting progression in patients diagnosed with superficial penile cancer.

Cabanas has outlined the rationale and technique of sentinel lymph node biopsy in clinically negative groins.[73] However, another report found a 25% incidence of nodal metastasis following a negative "sentinel lymph node dissection" a median of 10 months following surgery.[74] The clinical failures included two of six patients with superficial (stage T1) disease. Alternatively, fine-needle aspiration of lymph nodes under fluoroscopic or CT guidance following lymphangiography has been described,[75] but a negative cytologic examination does not necessarily assure the absence of metastatic disease in these patients.

Histologic grade (moderate to poorly differentiated) as well as size of the primary lesion (greater than 2 cm) may predict local failure and higher risk of nodal spread in Jackson stage I disease.[66,67] Such "high-risk" patients might warrant consideration of more aggressive therapy, including the use of ilioinguinal lymphadenectomy as part of initial therapeutic management.

In summary, disease-free survival of 90 to 95% in patients with superficial, well-differentiated penile cancer who undergo adequate treatment of the primary tumor is expected. This would not seem to justify the routine use of ilioinguinal lymph node dissection for the management of Jackson stage I disease. In higher risk stage I patients with larger or high-grade tumors, or patients whose follow-up and compliance may be questionable, early lymphadenectomy may warrant consideration.

All patients with stage I tumors need close follow-up after excision of the primary lesion, with clinical examination of the penis and groin nodes every 2 to 3 months, especially within the first 3 years, when the risk of recurrence and nodal spread is highest.

REFERENCES

1. Thompson IM, Fair WR: Penile carcinoma. AUA Update Ser 1990; 9(1):1–8.
2. Opjordsmoen S, Fossa SD: Quality of life in patients treated for penile cancer: A follow-up study. Br J Urol 1994; 74:652–657.
3. Bissada NK: Conservative extirpative treatment of cancer of the penis. Urol Clin North Am 1992; 19:283–290.
4. Sufrin G, Huben RP: Benign and malignant lesions of the penis. *In* Gillenwater JY, Grayhack JT, Howards SS, Duckett JW (eds): Adult and Pediatric Urology, 2nd edition, pp 1643–1681. St. Louis, Mosby–Year Book, 1991.
5. Hardner GJ, Bhanalaph T, Murphy GT, et al: Carcinoma of the penis: analysis of therapy in 100 consecutive cases. J Urol 1972; 108:428–430.
6. Mikhail GR: Cancers, precancers, pseudocancers on the male genitalia. J Dermatol Surg Oncol 1980; 6:1027–1035.
7. El-Demiry MIM, Oliver RTD, Hope-Stone HF, et al: Reappraisal of the role of radiotherapy and surgery in the management of carcinoma of the penis. Br J Urol 1984; 56: 724–728.
8. Schellhammer PF, Grabstald H: Tumors of the penis. *In* Walsh PC, Gittes RF, Perlmutter AD, Stamey TA (eds): Campbell's Urology, 5th edition, pp 1583–1606. Philadelphia, WB Saunders Co, 1986.
9. Rosemberg SK, Jacobs H: Continuous wave carbon dioxide treatment of balanitis xerotica obliterans. Urology 1982; 19: 539–541.
10. Johnson DE, Lo RK, Srigley J, et al: Verrucous carcinoma of the penis. J Urol 1985; 133:216–218.
11. Fair WR, Fuks ZY, Scher HI: Cancer of the urethra and penis. *In* De Vita VT, Hellman S, Rosenberg SA (eds): Cancer: Principles and Practice of Oncology, 4th edition, pp 1114–1125. Philadelphia, JB Lippincott Co, 1993.
12. Fukunaga M, Yokoi K, Miyazawa Y, et al: Penile verrucous carcinoma with anaplastic transformation following radiotherapy: a case report with human papillomavirus typing and flow cytometric DNA studies. Am J Surg Pathol 1994; 18:501–505.
13. Seixas ALC, Ornellas AA, Marota A, et al: Verrucous carcinoma of the penis: retrospective analysis of 32 cases. J Urol 1994; 152:1476–1479.
14. McDougal WS: Verrucous carcinoma of the penis: retro-

spective analysis of 32 cases [editorial comment]. J Urol 1994; 152:1478–1479.
15. Graham JH, Helwig EB: Erythroplasia of Queyrat: a clinicopathologic and histochemical study. Cancer 1973; 32: 1396–1414.
16. Goette DK, Elgart M, DeVillez RL: Erythroplasia of Queyrat: treatment with topically applied fluorouracil. JAMA 1975; 232:934–937.
17. Rosemberg SK, Fuller TA: Carbon dioxide rapid superpulsed laser treatment of erythroplasia of Queyrat. Urology 1980; 16:181–182.
18. Malek RS: Laser treatment of premalignant and malignant squamous cell lesions of the penis. Lasers Surg Med 1992; 12:246–253.
19. Smith JA: Laser treatment of urologic cancers. Semin Surg Oncol 1989; 5:30–37.
20. Bandieramonte G, Santoro O, Boracchi P, et al: Total resection of glans penis surface by CO_2 laser microsurgery. Acta Oncol 1988; 27:575–578.
21. Andersen SL, Neilsen A, Reymann F: Relationship between Bowen disease and internal malignant tumors. Arch Dermatol 1973; 108:367–370.
22. Grossman HB: Premalignant and early carcinomas of the penis and scrotum. Urol Clin North Am 1992; 19:221–226.
23. Malloy TR, Wein AJ, Carpiniello VL: Carcinoma of penis treated with neodymium:YAG laser. Urology 1988; 31:26–29.
24. Wade TR, Kopf AW, Ackerman AB: Bowenoid papulosis of the penis. Cancer 1978; 42:1890–1903.
25. Gross G, Hagedorn M, Ikenberg H, et al: Bowenoid papulosis: presence of human papillomavirus (HPV) structural antigens and of HPV 16-related DNA sequences. Arch Dermatol 1985; 121:858.
26. Rosemberg SK, Herman G, Elfont E: Sexually transmitted papillomaviral infection in the male. VII. Is cancer of the penis sexually transmitted? Urology 1991; 37:437–440.
27. Obalek S, Jablonska S, Beaudenon S, et al: Bowenoid papulosis of the male and female genitalia: risk of cervical neoplasia. J Am Acad Dermatol 1986; 14:433–444.
28. Sarkar FH, Miles BJ, Plieth DH, et al: Detection of human papillomavirus in squamous neoplasm of the penis. J Urol 1992; 147:389–392.
29. Malek RS, Goellner JR, Smith TF, et al: Human papillomavirus infection and intraepithelial, in situ, and invasive carcinoma of the penis. Urology 1993; 42:159–170.
30. Aynaud O, Ionesco M, Barrasso R: Penile intraepithelial neoplasia: specific clinical features correlate with histologic and virologic findings. Cancer 1994; 74:1762–1767.
31. Barrasso R, DeBrux J, Croissant O, et al: High prevalence of papillomavirus-associated penile intraepithelial neoplasia in sexual partners of women with cervical intraepithelial neoplasia. N Engl J Med 1987; 317:916–923.
32. Eng TY, Petersen JP, Stack RS, et al: Lymph node metastasis from carcinoma in situ of the penis: a case report. J Urol 1995; 153:432–434.
33. deKernion JB, Tynberg P, Persky L, et al: Carcinoma of the penis. Cancer 1973; 32:1256–1262.
34. McDougal WS, Kirchner FK, Edwards RH, et al: Treatment of carcinoma of the penis: the case for primary lymphadenectomy. J Urol 1986; 136:38–41.
35. Rotolo JE, Lynch JH: Penile cancer: curable with early detection. Hosp Prac 1991; June 15:131–138.
36. Das S: Penile amputations for the management of primary carcinoma of the penis. Urol Clin North Am 1992; 19: 277–282.
37. Narayana AS, Olney LE, Loening SA, et al: Carcinoma of the penis: analysis of 219 cases. Cancer 1982; 49:2185–2191.
38. Delannes M, Malavaud B, Douchez J, et al: Iridium-192 interstitial therapy for squamous cell carcinoma of the penis. Int J Radiat Oncol Biol Phys 1992; 24:479–483.
39. Gerbaulet A, Lambin P: Radiation therapy of cancer of the penis: indications, advantages, and pitfalls. Urol Clin North Am 1992; 19:325–332.
40. Parsons RJ, Campbell JB, Thomley MW: Carcinoma of the penis treated by the ruby laser. J Urol 1968; 100:38–39.
41. von Eschenbach AC: The neodymium–yttrium aluminum garnet (Nd:YAG) laser in urology. Urol Clin North Am 1986; 13:381–391.
42. Blatstein LM, Finkelstein LH: Laser therapy for the treatment of squamous cell carcinoma of the penis. J Am Osteopath Assoc 1990; 90:338–344.
43. Jackson SM: The treatment of carcinoma of the penis. Br J Surg 1966; 53:33–35.
44. Spiessl B, Scheibe O, Wagner G (eds): TNM-Atlas: Illustrated Guide to the Classification of Malignant Tumours, pp 166–169. Berlin, Springer-Verlag, 1982.
45. Horenblas S, van Tinteren H, Delemarre JFM, et al: Squamous cell carcinoma of the penis. II. Treatment of the primary tumor. J Urol 1992; 147:1533–1538.
46. Olbricht SM, Arndt KA: Carbon dioxide laser treatment of cutaneous disorders. Mayo Clin Proc 1988; 63:297–300.
47. Schaffer AJ: Use of the CO_2 laser in surgery. Urol Clin North Am 1986; 13:393–404.
48. Finkelstein LH: CO_2 laser in urology. Surg Clin North Am 1984; 64:913–930.
49. Carpiniello VL, Schoenberg M: Laser treatment of condyloma and other external genital lesions. Semin Urol 1991; 9:175–179.
50. Malloy TR, Zderic S, Carpiniello VL: External genital lesions. *In* Smith JA, Stein BS, Benson RC (eds): Lasers in Urologic Surgery, 2nd edition, pp 23–34. Chicago, Year Book Medical Publishers, 1989.
51. Stein BS: Laser physics and tissue interaction. Urol Clin North Am 1986; 13:365–380.
52. Mohs FE, Snow SN, Larson PO: Mohs micrographic surgery for penile tumors. Urol Clin North Am 1992; 19: 291–304.
53. Mohs FE, Snow SN, Messing EM, et al: Microscopically controlled surgery in the treatment of carcinoma of the penis. J Urol 1985; 133:961–966.
54. Sagerman RH, Yu WS, Chung CT, et al: External-beam irradiation of carcinoma of the penis. Radiology 1984; 152: 183–185.
55. Ravi R, Chaturvedi HK, Sastry DVLN: Role of radiation therapy in the treatment of carcinoma of the penis. Br J Urol 1994; 74:646–651.
56. McLean M, Akl AM, Warde P, et al: The results of primary radiation therapy in the management of squamous cell carcinoma of the penis. Int J Radiat Oncol Biol Phys 1993; 25: 623–628.
57. Haile K, Delclos L: The place of radiation therapy in the treatment of carcinoma of the distal end of the penis. Cancer 1980; 45:1980–1984.
58. Mazeron JJ, Langlois D, Lobo PA, et al: Interstitial radiation therapy for carcinoma of the penis using iridium 192 wires: the Henri Mondor experience (1970–1979). Int J Radiat Oncol Biol Phys 1984; 10:1891–1895.
59. Daly NJ, Douchez J, Combs PF: Treatment of carcinoma of the penis by iridium 192 wire implant. Int J Radiat Oncol Biol Phys 1982; 8:1239–1243.
60. Madej G, Meyza J: Cryosurgery of penile carcinoma: short report on preliminary results. Oncology 1982; 39:350–352.
61. Kattan J, Culine S, Droz JP, et al: Penile cancer chemotherapy: twelve years' experience at Institut Gustave-Roussy. Urology 1993; 42:559–562.
62. Mitropoulos D, Dimopoulos MA, Kiroudy-Voulgari A, et al: Neoadjuvant cisplatin and interferon-alpha 2B in the treatment and organ preservation of penile carcinoma. J Urol 1994; 152:1124–1126.
63. Lerner SE, Jones JG, Fleischmann J: Management of recurrent penile cancer following partial or total penectomy. Urol Clin North Am 1994; 21:729–737.
64. Wan J, Grossman HB: Penile and urethral carcinoma: an overview. *In* Crawford ED, Das S (eds): Current Genitourinary Cancer Surgery, pp 358–366. Philadelphia, Lea & Febiger, 1990.
65. Koch MO, Smith JA: Local recurrence of squamous cell carcinoma of the penis. Urol Clin North Am 1994; 21: 739–743.

66. Fraley EE, Zhang G, Sazama R, et al: Cancer of the penis: prognosis and treatment plans. Cancer 1985; 55:1618–1624.
67. Fraley EE, Zhang G, Manivel C, et al: The role of ilioinguinal lymphadenectomy and significance of histologic differentiation in treatment of carcinoma of the penis. J Urol 1989; 142:1478–1482.
68. Catalona WJ: Surgical staging of genitourinary tumors. Cancer 1987; 60:459–463.
69. Mukamel E, deKernion JB: Early versus delayed lymph node dissection versus no lymph node dissection in carcinoma of the penis. Urol Clin North Am 1987; 14:707–711.
70. Abi-Aad AS, deKernion JB: Controversies in ilioinguinal lymphadenectomy for cancer of the penis. Urol Clin North Am 1992; 19:319–324.
71. Fowler JE: An approach to the management of penile cancer. Surg Ann 1992; 24:139–156.
72. Ayyappan K, Ananthakrishnan N, Sankaran V: Can regional lymph node involvement be predicted in patients with carcinoma of the penis? Br J Urol 1994; 73:549–553.
73. Cabanas RM: Anatomy and biopsy of sentinel lymph nodes. Urol Clin North Am 1992; 19:267–276.
74. Pettaway CA, Pisters LL, Dinney CPN, et al: Sentinel lymph node dissection for penile carcinoma: the MD Anderson Cancer Center experience. J Urol 1995; 154:1999–2003.
75. Scappini P, Piscioli F, Pusiol T, et al: Penile cancer: aspiration biopsy cytology for staging. Cancer 1986; 58:1526–1533.

43

INVASIVE CARCINOMA OF THE PENIS: MANAGEMENT AND PROGNOSIS

ANTONIO PURAS BAEZ, M.D., F.A.C.S. *and*
JORGE RIVERA HERRERA, M.D., F.A.C.S.

Carcinoma of the penis is usually an epidermoid tumor arising in the glans penis or mucosal lining of the prepuce. It is rarely seen in western industrialized countries and accounts for less than 1% of all male cancers.[1,2] However, in some regions of Africa, South America, and the tropics, it represents a significant health hazard. Survival appears to be directly related to tumor stage and grade. Patients diagnosed at an early stage can be adequately treated, and their survival compares favorably with that of an age-matched population. Prognosis will be grim for those patients with deeply infiltrating tumors and/or ilioinguinal node metastasis.

INCIDENCE AND EPIDEMIOLOGY

The incidence of squamous cell carcinoma of the penis follows a distinct geographic and racial distribution. It has been reported to constitute up to 16.7% of all cancers in Vishakhaptanam, India,[3] and 12.2% of cancers in Uganda.[4] In Brazil it represents 2.1% of all male malignancies, although in some regions of the country it constitutes up to 17% of all malignant tumors.[5] The Puerto Rico Cancer Registry reported an age-adjusted incidence of 5.5 per 100,000 males in 1980,[6] whereas in the United States the incidence is only around 0.9 per 100,000.[7]

The relatively high incidence in certain regions of India and Africa may relate to a large Hindu population who do not routinely practice circumcision, as contrasted to the lower occurrence in Moslems, who practice circumcision.[8–11] In a large Hispanic series, Marcial and colleagues found that 92% of patients with penile carcinoma presented with an unretractable prepuce.[12] Although penile carcinoma is uncommon in the United States, age-adjusted incidence suggests an increase in frequency of this lesion in blacks and Hispanics compared to white males.[13] Ornellas and colleagues[14] reported their experience with 414 patients with invasive squamous cell carcinoma of the penis at the Brazilian National Cancer Institute; the majority of the patients were white (68%), followed by mulatto (22%), while only 10% were blacks. These variations probably reflect cultural and socioeconomic conditions rather than specific racial differences.

This neoplasm is usually diagnosed between the fifth and seventh decades of life.[14–19] Figure 43–1 demonstrates the age distribution at diagnosis of 496 patients with carcinoma of the penis treated at the University of Puerto Rico.[20] The youngest patient was 20 years of age and the oldest 104 years, with a mean age of 57 years. This illness appears to be age related, showing an age-specific rate increase with each decade, having its peak at the sixth decade. Fifty-one per cent of our patients were younger than 60 years of age.

ETIOLOGY

Numerous factors have been associated with the risk of developing invasive squamous cell carcinoma of the penis. The most important appear to be the presence of an intact foreskin, phimosis, smegma, and viruses.

Presence of Foreskin, Phimosis, Circumcision

The precise etiology of penile carcinoma remains undetermined, although the most consistent de-

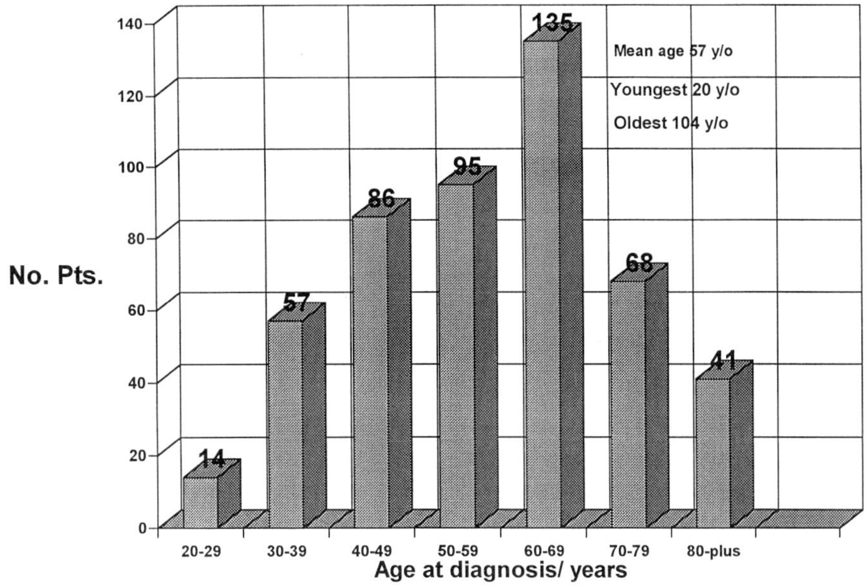
No. Pts.
140
120
100
80
60
40
20
0
14
57
86
95
135
68
41
Mean age 57 y/o
Youngest 20 y/o
Oldest 104 y/o
20-29
30-39
40-49
50-59
60-69
70-79
80-plus
Age at diagnosis/ years

FIGURE 43–1. Age distribution of 496 patients with penile cancer. (From Puras A, González-Flores B, Rodríguez R: Treatment of carcinoma of the penis. *In* Stevenson HG [ed]: Proceedings of the Kimbrough Urological Seminar, Vol 12, pp 143–152. Utical, NY, Bradock Press, 1979, with permission.)

nominator in this tumor is the presence of an intact foreskin. Of 169 patients with penile cancer seen at the Mayo Clinic, 69% had phimosis.[17] Marcial and colleagues reported unretracted prepuce or phimosis in 92% of the patients with invasive carcinoma of the penis.[12] Conversely, this tumor is rarely seen in populations performing ritual neonatal circumcision. It is extremely rare among Jews, who practice circumcision at birth; only solitary cases have been reported in the literature.[2,21,22] Penile cancer occurs infrequently in Moslems, who undergo circumcision between 4 and 9 years of age, although the incidence is somewhat higher than in Jews.[21–25] Although, this neoplasm can occur in men who were circumcised at birth, such reported cases involve patients who had incomplete circumcision or occurrence of scars in traumatic procedures.[24,26] Table 43–1 represents cumulative reported data of 1581 patients with penile carcinoma; 90% of these patients were not circumcised. Of the circumcised group, only five had the procedure early in life, whereas 95% were circumcised as adults. It appears that circumcision at birth will prevent carcinoma of the penis, but circumcision practiced later in life does not confer the same protection.

TABLE 43–1. CIRCUMCISION AND CARCINOMA OF THE PENIS

Not Circumcised		**1427**	**90%**
Circumcised		**154**	**10%**
Infancy	1		
Childhood	4		
Adolescence	2		
Adult	147		
TOTAL		1,581	100%

Data from references 14, 18, 20, 48, and 81.

Smegma

For years, retained smegma has been considered to play a role in the development of carcinoma of the penis.[27,28] Smegma appears to represent the debris of desquamated epithelial cells from the glans and inner surface of the foreskin[29] and secretions of sebaceous glands. Biochemical analysis of smegma revealed 26% fat and 13% proteins, consistent with necrotic epithelial debris.[30] Some authors believe that the effect of *Mycobacterium smegmatis* causes the degradation of smegma into potent carcinogens, such as hydrocarbons or sterols.[31,32] Experimental animal models have been used to document the carcinogenic actions of smegma, and have shown only a 3% incidence of carcinoma in the buried skin tunnel of mice and a 10% incidence of carcinoma of the uterine cervix following direct application of smegma.[32] There appears to be no convincing evidence demonstrating smegma as a carcinogenic factor in carcinoma of the penis, although its presence, in combination with chronic infection and irritation beneath a phimotic ring, may play a significant role.

Viruses

It has been reported that women whose spouses suffer from carcinoma of the penis have a higher incidence of carcinoma of the cervix compared to a controlled population[33–35]; however, these findings have been challenged by other authors.[36,37] The possible association of these two types of cancer has raised the strong suggestion of a sexually transmitted agent. Human papillomavirus (HPV), especially types 16 and 18, has been detected in around 50% of penile carcinomas. It has also been suggested that cervical carcinoma in women relates to penile or genital HPV infection in male sexual partners.[38] In the past 10 years, numerous reports have demonstrated a strong association between HPV and penile carcinoma.[39–41] In situ hybridization techniques have identified the E6 region of HPV DNA integrated into the DNA of cervical and penile squamous cell carcinoma cells.[42,43] A recent series reported by Cupp and colleagues[44] analyzed 42 cases of invasive squamous cell carcinoma of the penis; 13 patients presented with carcinoma in situ, 12 with intraepithelial neoplasia, 3 verrucous carcinoma, and 25 patients with balanitis xerotica obliterans, as well as 29 neonatal and 32 adult circumcision specimens. The overall detection rate for HPV in invasive squamous cell carcinoma was 55%: 92% for carcinoma in situ and for penile intraepithelial neoplasia, 4% for balanitis xerotica obliterans, and 9% for adult circumcision specimens. None of the patients with verrucous carcinoma and no neonatal circumcision specimens were positive for HPV. Cupp et al. concluded that the prevalence of HPV DNA is significantly greater in carcinoma of the penis than in control tissue; however, the prevalence is greater in noninvasive lesions than in invasive carcinoma. Strohmeyer[45] identified HPV 16 sequences integrated into the genome of primary and metastatic penile tumors, suggesting a theoretical significance of HPV 16 in the development of penile cancers. The cumulative evidence suggests that HPV may have a causative role, probably requiring other carcinogenic factors, in the development of this tumor.

HISTOPATHOLOGY AND NATURAL HISTORY

Over 97% of patients with invasive penile cancers had squamous cell carcinomas[14,20,46,47] (Fig. 43–2). Tumors usually begin as a small lesion on an uncircumcised male with evidence of chronic irritation and/or poor genital hygiene (Figs. 43–3 and 43–4). If left unattended, the lesion will gradually grow to involve the entire glans and/or prepuce (Fig. 43–5). Buck's fascia, which is rich in elastic fibers, acts as a temporary natural barrier, protecting the corporeal bodies and urethra from tumor invasion. As the malignant process progresses, there will be infiltration of Buck's fascia and the tunica albuginea, with possible invasion of cavernous erectile tissue and potential vascular dissemination. Untreated tumors usually continue to grow, producing progressive erosion and destruction of the penis (Fig. 43–6). Most lesions will develop secondary infection resulting in a foul-smelling discharge with or without cellulitis of the

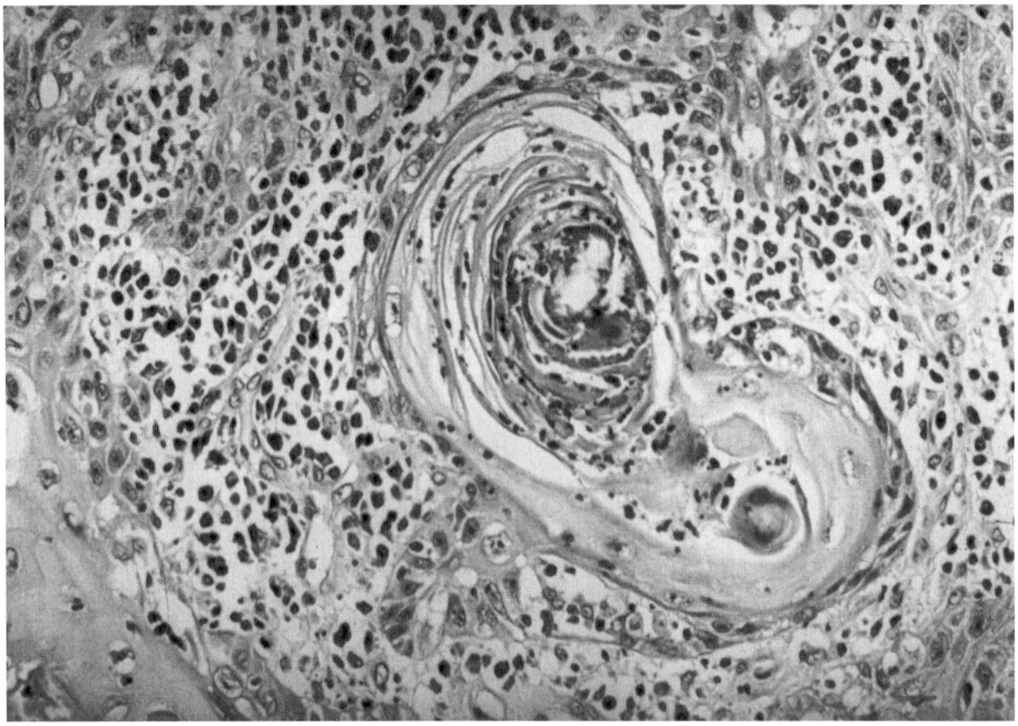

FIGURE 43–2. Squamous cell carcinoma of the penis, moderately differentiated tumor. Note keratinizing whorls with central degeneration (Pearl formation). Hematoxylin-eosin, ×80. (Courtesy of Antonio Puras Baez, M.D.)

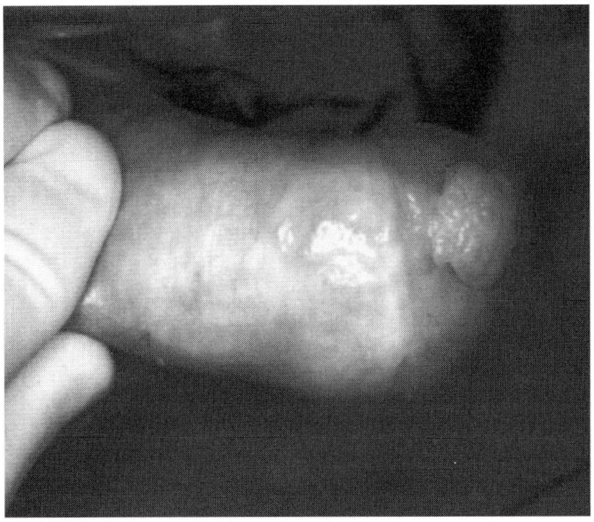

FIGURE 43–3. Exophytic lesion at the glans on an uncircumcised patient. (Courtesy of Antonio Puras Baez, M.D.)

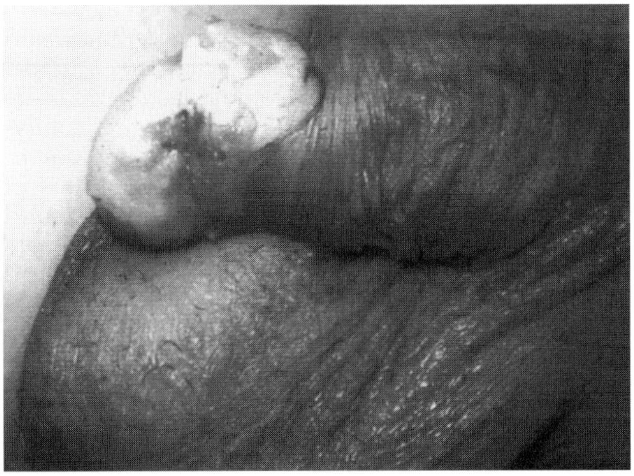

FIGURE 43–4. Small ulcerative epidermoid carcinoma at the coronal sulcus on an uncircumcised male. Note abundant smegma formation. (Courtesy of Antonio Puras Baez, M.D.)

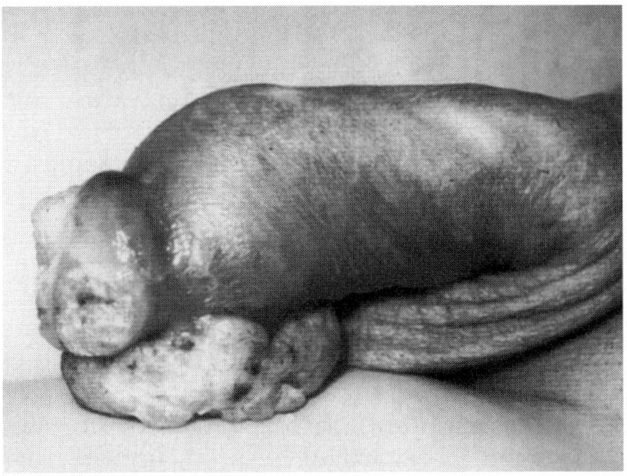

FIGURE 43–5. Large, fungating, exophytic tumor involving the glans and foreskin on an uncircumcised, phimotic penis. Note erosion through the prepuce and purulent discharge. (Courtesy of Antonio Puras Baez, M.D.)

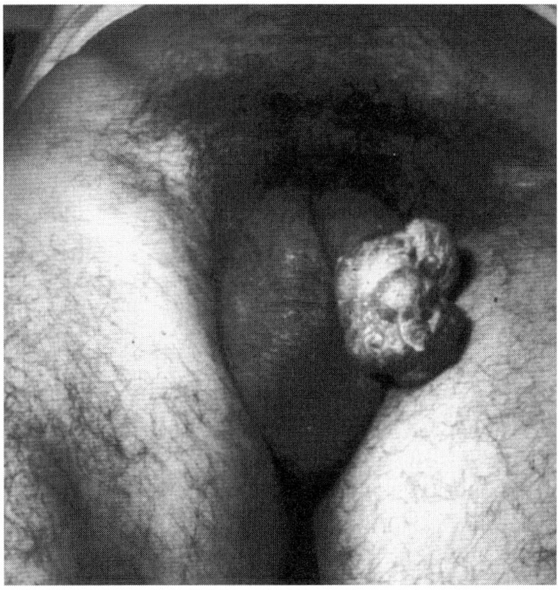

FIGURE 43–6. Extensive invasive carcinoma of the penis causing autoamputation of the glans. (Courtesy of Antonio Puras Baez, M.D.)

surrounding tissue. Table 43–2 demonstrates cumulative reported data on the location of the primary lesion of patients with penile cancer. Most tumors develop in the glans (52%).[20,48,49] The lesions may be fungating, exophytic, papillary, flat, and/or ulcerative. Ulcerative tumors are usually less differentiated, have a tendency for earlier nodal metastasis, and are associated with poor 5-year survival rates.[12,16,50,51]

The cumulative reported 5-year survival of patients with carcinoma of the penis is around 52%.[13] Table 43–3 demonstrates the 5-year survival rate for patients with penile cancer, which varies from 41 to 72%.[12,14,18,19,48,52–56] It should be noted that, although the overall survival is around 55%, the disease-specific survival is 72%.

In an attempt to correlate the histologic appearance of the lesion and survival, Marcial and colleagues[12] classified the lesion into five major histologic types. The 5-year survival for intraepithelial and leukoplakic lesions was over 67%, that for the verrucous type was 52%, that for the compact type was 36%, and that for the plexiform type was only

TABLE 43–2. LOCATION OF THE PRIMARY LESION IN PATIENTS WITH PENILE CARCINOMA

Site	No. Patients	%
Glans	326	52
Prepuce	93	15
Glans/Prepuce	207	33
Shaft	2	0.32
TOTAL	628	100

Data from references 20, 77, and 48.

TABLE 43–3. REPORTED FIVE-YEAR SURVIVAL IN CARCINOMA OF THE PENIS

Year	Reference	No. of Patients	% of Patients Surviving 5 Years Histologic Grade 1	2	3	Total
1955	Staubitz et al.[48]	204				41
1962	Marcial et al.[12]	210	64	40	25	53
1972	Hardner et al.[52]	100	51		39	49
1982*	Nelson et al.[53]	95				73
1987	Srinivas et al.[54]	119				43
1989	Fraley et al.[19]	54	95	47	10	56
1993	Kamat et al.[55]	150	90	59	17	59
1994*	Horenblas et al.[64]	118	79	68	47	72
1994	Ornellas et al.[14]	328	63	58	32	60
1995*,†	McDougal[56]	76	84	55	42	70

*Disease specific survival.
†Patients living 3 or more years without evidence of disease.

17%. The later lesion was almost always encountered in association with deeply infiltrating high-grade (grade III) cancers. Most of the high-grade tumors were of compact and plexiform types. There was also a strong correlation between histologic grade and inguinal node metastasis. Patients with low-grade tumors had only 5% incidence of positive inguinal nodes, whereas those with grade II and III tumors revealed 43 and 40% incidences, respectively. The 5-year survival for patients with grade I tumors was 64%, compared to 25% for high-grade lesions.

Cubilla and colleagues examined whole-organ penile sections of 66 patients with epidermoid carcinoma of the penis.[51] They classified the tumors into four major types; superficially spreading, vertical growth, verrucous, and multicentric. In 73% of the cases, the tumor exhibited histologic grades of moderate and poor differentiation, and histologic confirmation of lymph node metastasis was demonstrated in 49% of the 66 patients. Forty-eight per cent of patients with vertical growth pattern had involvement of two anatomic compartments (glans and foreskin). The metastatic rate was higher in vertical growth carcinoma (82%) than in superficial spreading tumors (42%). No evidence of metastasis was found in verrucous carcinoma. Six of eight patients (75%) with superficial spreading pattern and grade III tumors had lymph node metastasis; none of the patients with superficial spreading and grade I carcinoma showed metastasis. All six patients with vertical growth and poorly differentiated carcinomas had positive lymph nodes. Cubilla et al. concluded that tumor type and histologic grade have major significance in predicting lymph node metastasis.

Most recently, McDougal reviewed the records of 76 patients with carcinoma of the penis from four major teaching hospitals.[56] The disease-specific survival for these patients was 70%. He noticed a direct correlation between survival and tumor differentiation. The 5-year disease-specific survival for poorly differentiated tumors was 42%, compared to 84% for low-grade cancers. These data suggest that the likelihood of regional lymph node metastasis can be predicted based on differentiation of the primary tumor and depth of invasion. Of 24 patients with well- or moderately differentiated noninvasive primary tumors, only 1 (4%) had regional metastasis, compared to 43 of 52 patients (82%) with poorly differentiated or invasive tumors.

These data clearly establish the significance of patterns of tumor growth, tumor differentiation, and depth of invasion in predicting regional spread and survival.

CLINICAL PRESENTATION AND EVALUATION

Most patients with carcinoma of the penis will initially present with induration or erythema on the glans or foreskin, an exophytic lesion, a warty growth, or a purulent discharge with cellulitis and erythema of the foreskin on an uncircumcised penis. These lesions are usually nonpainful, and there is usually a delay in patient presentation to a physician because of personal neglect and self-denial.

In order to assess the clinical manifestations of squamous cell carcinoma of the penis, Sufrin and Huben[13] reviewed reports of more than 3500 patients with carcinoma of the the penis and found that the presenting symptoms consisted of a penile mass, lump, or nodule in 47% of patients, a penile ulcer or sore in 35%, and an inflammatory lesion or bleeding from the external surface of the penis in 17%. Only 0.7% of the patients were found incidentally during the course of an adult circumcision. The average age at diagnosis was 60.1 years (range 15 to 92 years). Similar findings were observed upon review of 496 patients with penile cancer at the University of Puerto Rico.[20]

The most frequent location of the primary lesion is on the glans, the coronal sulcus, and the prepuce. Only a few lesions have been identified on the shaft (see Table 43–2). A possible explanation for this finding may be that the shaft and meatus, unlike the glans, coronal sulcus, and inner surface of the prepuce, are not constantly exposed to smegma and other active carcinogenic irritants contained within the preputial sac.[57]

Other penile lesions, such as erythoplasia of Queyrat, tuberculosis, condyloma acuminatum, balanitis xerotica obliterans, and syphilitic chancre, may resemble penile carcinoma and must be considered in the differential diagnosis.

A penile lesion should be examined thoroughly and assessed in regard to location, tumor growth, size, and infiltration of the corporal bodies or the urethra. A rectal and bimanual pelvic examination as well as careful examination of the groins is of extreme importance. The lesion should be cultured and the patient started on appropriate antibiotic therapy. Any suspicious growth or ulceration should be biopsied and the depth of invasion assessed. Swelling or discharge of the distal penis, in the presence of phimosis, should be viewed with suspicion. A dorsal slit of the prepuce will permit adequate examination of the preputial sac and the glans as well as biopsy of any suspicious lesion.

LABORATORY STUDIES

Patients with suspicious nondetermined lesions should undergo routine skin tests, serology, cultures, and special tissue stains in order to identify any infectious process. In the early stages, patients with penile cancer will have normal routine laboratory chemistry. Patients with large infiltrative lesions and/or inguinal node metastasis may have anemia, leukocytosis, and hypoalbuminemia. Some may develop a paraneoplastic syndrome with hypercalcemia in the absence of detectable osseous metastasis.[58,59] In a report from the Memorial Sloan-Kettering Cancer Center, Sklaroff and Yagoda[60] reported that 17 of 81 patients (20.9%) with penile carcinoma had hypercalcemia; but, in the presence of inguinal metastasis, 16 of 17 patients (94%) had elevation of the serum calcium level. It appears that hypercalcemia is associated with tumor volume. It has been suggested that parahormone-like substances may be produced by the primary tumor and its metastasis.[61] In some patients hypercalcemia resolves following surgical removal of the groin nodes.[62]

IMAGING STUDIES

Radiologic studies in the evaluation of a patient with penile cancer should include a chest x-ray and upper tract imaging. The role of imaging studies in evaluating the extent of the primary lesion is not well established. The use of cavernosography,[63] ultrasound,[64] computed tomography (CT),[65] and magnetic resonance imaging (MRI)[66] have been used in order to assess the extent of the primary tumor. Raghavaiah performed preoperative cavernosography in 10 patients with carcinoma of the penis in order to determine the extent of the primary tumor.[63] He was able to upstage the disease in 3 of 10 (30%) patients. Subsequent pathologic analysis of the tissue specimen demonstrated complete correlation with the radiologic findings in all 10 patients. Using a 7.5-mHz linear array ultrasound, Horenblas and associates examined the extent of invasion to the corpora in patients with carcinoma of the penis.[64] They described the lesions as hypoechoic, and concluded that ultrasonography was not accurate enough for staging small lesions located at the glans, although it may be useful for larger tumors invading the tunica albuginea, corpora cavernosa, and urethra.

CT has been used extensively to evaluate nodal metastasis but appears to be of limited use for the primary lesion. In a report of 13 patients, Maiche found no improvement in the diagnostic capacity between CT scan and physical examination in the assessment of the primary lesion.[65] All penile tumors were detected by palpation, whereas some neoplasms were missed by CT. MRI appears to provide superior tissue contrast and is able to image the lesion in any plane. De-Kervileu and colleagues were able to correctly assess six of nine lesions (67%) compared to clinical evaluation.[66] In T2-weighted images, the contrast between the tunica and the corpora cavernosa appeared to be increased,[67] T2-weighted images are more useful than T1-weighted images in delineating the margins of the tumor.[66] In some patients with large inguinal metastases or ulcerated nodes, MRI will thoroughly detail the extent of the tumor, especially the presence or absence of tumor thrombus extending into the femoral vein.[68]

THERAPY

Survival in carcinoma of the penis depends primarily on the tumor grade,[12,14,18,19,52,55,56] depth of invasion,[12,51] and status of the regional nodes.[69–71] The primary therapeutic goal in the management of penile carcinoma should be complete tumor excision, regional lymphatic control, and a functional penis. In this chapter we mainly address the therapeutic alternatives in the treatment of the primary tumor.

Various therapeutic modalities, including surgery, radiotherapy, chemotherapy, and combinations of these, have been used in the treatment of the primary lesion. In order to evaluate survival of patients with carcinoma of the penis who underwent treatment of the primary lesion, Sufrin and Huben analyzed reports of over 4000 patients with penile cancer.[13] They found that, irrespective of tumor stage, grade, or type of therapy rendered, the average 3-, 5-, and 10-year survival rates of patients with penile cancer who received some form of treatment for this disease were 59, 52, and 32%, respectively; in contrast, the 5-year survival for patients with untreated penile cancer is around 6%.[13,20]

Surgery

Surgical excision plays a prominent role in the management of the primary lesion. If adequately performed, it will assess the histologic grade and depth of tumor invasion.

Circumcision and Excision

In some patients with small lesions involving the prepuce, complete tumor excision can be accomplished by a radical circumcision. It is important to obtain tumor-free margins because of the high incidence of recurrence.[12,54,69,72] Any suspicious lesion at the glans or coronal sulcus should be biopsied and proved to be free of tumor. Selected patients with superficial tumors of the penile shaft can be managed with a wide excision, excising around 2 cm of normal skin. The skin defect can be covered by a full-thickness skin graft or scrotal skin.

Micrographic Excision (Mohs Microsurgery)

Some invasive tumors of the glans can be excised layer by layer using microscopic examination of the entire undersurface of each layer and systematic use of frozen sections.[73,74] Microscopic guidance appears to provide histologic assurance of eradication of the primary tumor, and permits preservation of maximal amounts of normal tissue and normal function. Mohs and associates[73,74] described two techniques by which microscopic control of the tumor is achieved: the fixed tissue technique, in which the tissues are subjected to in situ chemical fixation prior to the excision of successive layers; and the fresh tissue technique, in which a local anesthetic is injected and the tissues are excised in the fresh, unfixed state. The fresh tissue technique is recommended for small penile tumors, whereas for larger infiltrative lesions, the fixed tissue technique will provide control of bleeding from the relatively noncontractile vessels of the erectile tissues of the glans, corpora cavernosa, and corpora spongiosa.[74]

In a series of 29 patients with carcinoma of the penis,[73] the 5-year cure rate among 25 determinant cases was 68%, while the primary carcinoma was eradicated in 23 of the 25 lesions (92%). It appears that microscopically controlled tumor excision provides an effective means to manage some types of penile cancers with excellent cosmetic and functional results.

Laser Surgery

Laser therapy using carbon dioxide and neodymium:yttrium-aluminum-garnet (Nd:YAG) lasers has been used to treat stage Tis, Ta, T1, and some T2 and T3 penile cancers. Major advantages of laser therapy for carcinoma of the penis are destruction of the tumor with penile preservation and function; it also gives the advantage of tissue destruction with sealing of small vessels and nerve endings, reducing the incidence of postoperative bleeding and pain.[75] The main disadvantage of laser surgery is the difficulty of obtaining histologic documentation and determining the depth of penetration by the tumor. It appears that the site and depth of penetration of the primary lesion correlate with its curability by Nd:YAG laser. Malloy and associates were able to cure five out of five patients with Tis of the penis but only six of nine patients with T1 lesions.[76] Bandieramonte and associates were able to resect T1 tumors at the glans penis by using a very short pulse and high peak power at the base of the lesion and at the meatus, providing precise excision of the specimen for pathologic examination.[77,78] However, a 15% recurrence rate was reported.[78] Boon reported an 81% success rate using laser excision with the aid of a sapphire tip followed by laser coagulation of the base of the tumor.[79] A large series[80] using the Nd:YAG laser for Tis, T1, T2, and T3 tumors reported a 5-year survival of 89% for node-negative and 25% for node-positive patients.[80] Only 2 of 28 patients (7%) with invasive tumor who were followed for 5 years developed local recurrence. Windahl and Hellsten reported their experience in the management of 32 patients with squamous cell carcinoma of the penis.[81] Thirteen patients received conventional surgery and 19 patients were treated with carbon dioxide and/or combined carbon dioxide and Nd: YAG laser. Although the two groups of patients are different with regard to age and tumor stage, the results in the laser group appear to be promising. All 19 patients who received laser treatment were tumor free with a mean follow-up of 31 months, and only 2 of 19 (11%) developed recurrent tumor later. The authors concluded that combined carbon dioxide and Nd:YAG laser therapy is an excellent organ-sparing treatment for stages Tis to T2N0M0, grade I and II squamous cell carcinoma of the penis, with low morbidity and excellent cosmetic and functional results.

We believe that larger controlled studies with longer follow-up are necessary before establishing laser therapy as a standard treatment for patients with invasive carcinoma of the penis.

Partial and Total Amputation

Invasive tumors involving the glans or distal shaft of the penis can be adequately managed by partial penile amputation, excising 1.5 to 2 cm of normal tissue proximal to the margin of tumor infiltration (Fig. 43–7). This should leave a functional penis that can allow standing micturition and often enough rigidity and length for vaginal penetration. Frozen sections of the proximal margins are necessary to confirm a tumor-free resection margin. The recurrence rate in these patients should be 10% or less[13,67,82] (Fig. 43–8).

Patients with large, extensive, and infiltrating tumors involving the glans and mid-shaft of the penis are managed with radical penile amputation and a perineal urethrostomy. Lesions involving the scrotum, perineum, and anterior abdominal wall may need adjuvant preoperative chemotherapy in an attempt to downsize the tumor. If no adequate response is observed, the patient will need complete removal of the neoplasm, with total emasculation. In some instances, cystoprostatectomy with urinary diversion will be necessary.

All penile lesions should be cultured and adequate antibiotic therapy established before surgical

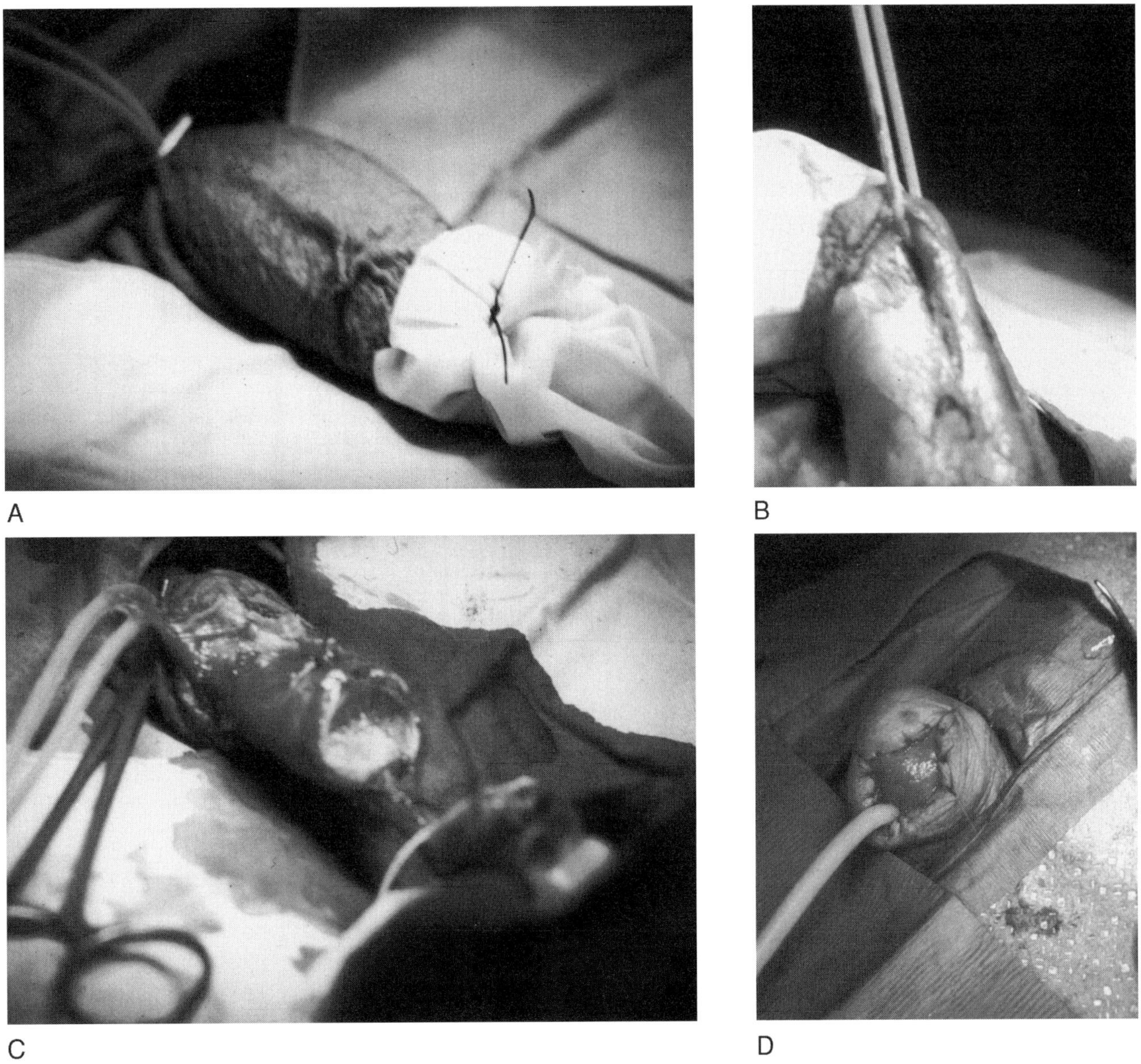
A
B
C
D

FIGURE 43–7. Partial amputation for penile cancer demonstrating total destruction of the glans penis. *A*, The tumor is covered with a rubber condom and a circumferential incision is made around 1.5 cm from the tumor margin. A soft rubber catheter serves as a tourniquet. *B*, The skin is retracted proximally. Corpora cavernosa and corpus spongiosum are identified. The urethra is separated from the corpora. *C*, The dorsal venous complex is ligated. The corpora cavernosa bodies are transected around 0.5 cm proximal to the original skin incision. The urethral stump is dissected and amputated around 1 cm beyond the corporal transection. The corpora cavernosa are closed with 2-0 polyglycolic sutures. The urethra is incised ventrally and spatulated toward the corporal bodies. *D*, The skin is approximated around the spatulated urethra using chromic 4-0 catgut. (Courtesy of Antonio Puras Baez, M.D.)

intervention. Following surgery of the primary lesion, we continue oral antibiotics for a period of 4 weeks.

Radiotherapy

Radiation therapy has been proposed as an alternative in the management of the primary lesion in order to preserve an intact penis with as much function as possible. The 5-year survival for patients receiving some form of radiotherapy to the primary lesion is around 60%.[13] Different types of delivery and radiation dosages have been utilized in the treatment of the primary tumor. This lack of uniformity in treatment makes it difficult to analyze the effectiveness of the radiation therapy. The choice of technique depends a great deal on the radiotherapist's preference and expertise and availability of radiation sources. The most common ra-

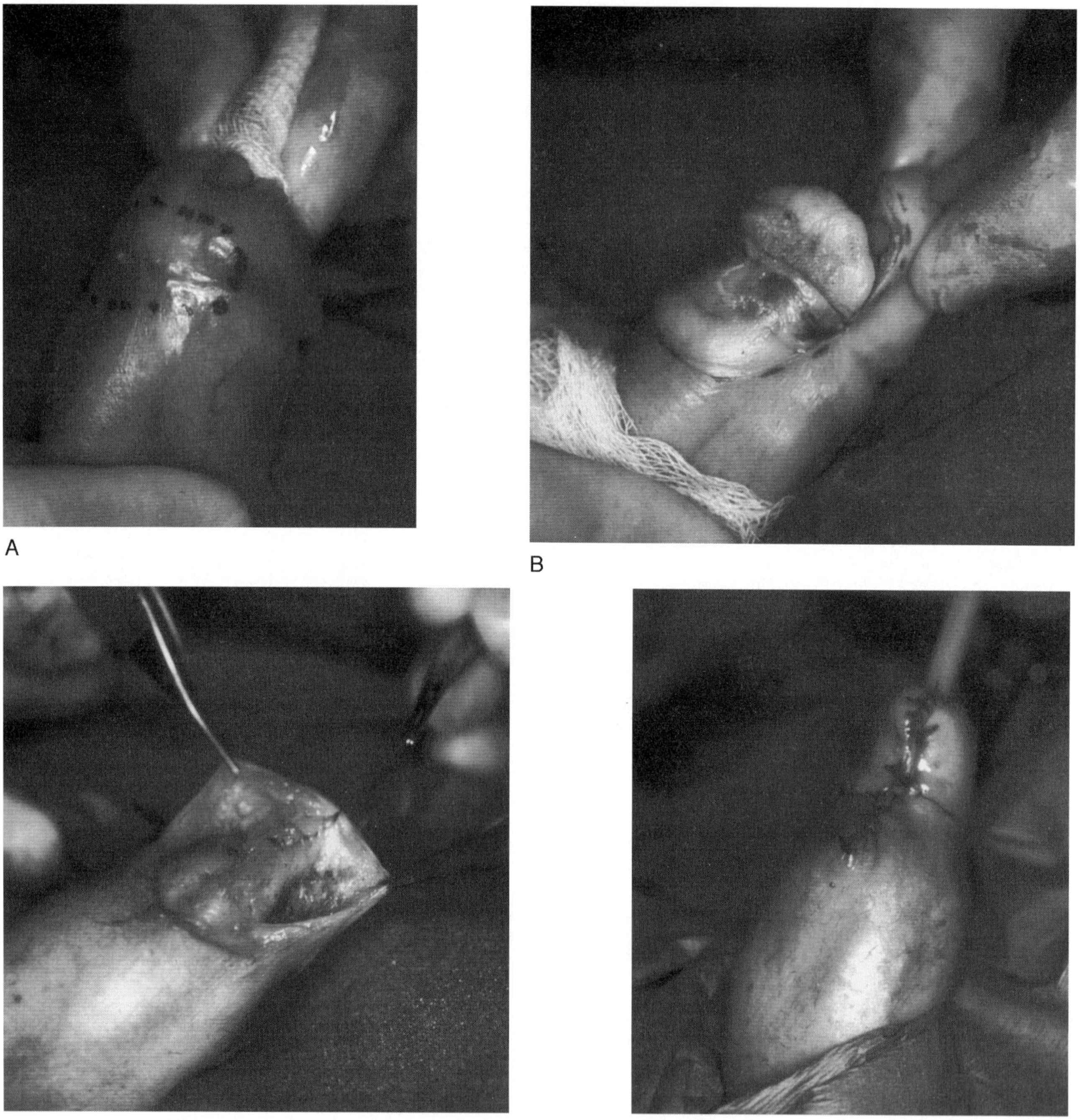

A B C D

FIGURE 43–8. *A,* Recurrent invasive squamous cell carcinoma at the coronal sulcus following circumcision for penile carcinoma. *B,* The lesion was removed entirely down to the corpora cavernosa and urethra. Frozen sections at the base of the corpora and urethra demonstrated negative margins. *C,* the urethra is repaired with 5-0 Vicryl. *D,* The glans is enclosed and the skin approximated. (Courtesy of Antonio Puras Baez, M.D.)

diation sources used have been external beam, with direct and/or parallel opposed fields, and brachytherapy, utilizing molds or interstitial implants. Direct field radiation treatment is recommended only for small superficial tumors and carcinoma in situ.[6,83] Parallel opposed fields have been used in order to radiate the entire thickness of the penis by encasing the lesion and the shaft of the penis in a block of wax or Perspex. Local control rates using this technique for T1 tumors vary between 60 and 84%.[84,85]

High-dose radiation can be administered to a tumor from a short distance by placing radioactive sources into (interstitial) or around (mold) the tumor. Danczak reported a series of 48 patients with penile carcinoma who underwent brachytherapy at the Institute of Oncology in Warsaw.[86] Thirty patients were treated with radium therapy and 18 with iridium-192. All patients were followed for a minimum of 3 years. The 3-year survival for patients treated with radium molds was 83%, and that for the group of patients treated with iridium seeds was 89%. The incidence of local recurrence for each group was 11 and 7%, respectively.

The main disadvantages of radiation therapy in the treatment of penile lesions are the side effects, including edema, mucositis, urethral stenosis, and ulceration with necrosis of the penis. It is imperative that all patients with carcinoma of the penis who will undergo radiation therapy be circumcised and started on appropriate antibiotics prior to treatment. In our series at the University of Puerto Rico,[20] 8 of 25 patients (32%) who received radiation therapy as treatment of the primary lesion recurred. The amputation rate for recurrent or persistent disease following radiation therapy for the primary lesion varies from 5 to 40%.[86–90]

In summary, radiation therapy can be considered in the management of small penile lesions (T1) in young sexually active patients. In the presence of persistent or recurrent disease (radiation failure), surgical amputation will be necessary in order to control the local lesion.

Chemotherapy

It has been demonstrated that squamous cell carcinoma of the penis is responsive to a variety of cytotoxic agents such as bleomycin, cisplatin, methotrexate, vincristine, and 5-fluorouracil (5-FU). These active cytotoxic agents have been used to treat the primary tumor and its metastases.

Single-Agent Therapy

The most widely used agent is bleomycin. In 1969, Ichikawa et al.[91] described their initial experience using bleomycin in the treatment of tumors of the penis and scrotum. Based on the observation that bleomycin is distributed and accumulates in squamous cell carcinoma, Ichikawa treated 8 patients with penile cancer using systemic bleomycin.[92] Complete resolution of the primary lesion was observed in two patients, partial response in four, and no response in two. Kyalwazi and colleagues reported their experience using single-agent bleomycin in 15 patients with squamous cell carcinoma of the penis.[93] Five patients were stage I, eight had tumor invading the shaft (stage II), and two were stage III/IV. They were treated with bleomycin at a dose of 30 to 60 mg twice a weak. Complete tumor regression was observed in 3 patients and partial regression in 11. It appears that the greatest response rate is observed in low-grade, low-stage tumors.

Sklaroff and Yagoda reported their experience with high-dose methotrexate (250 to 1500 mg) and citrovorum rescue in eight patients with epidermoid carcinoma of the penis.[94] Three of eight patients (38%) achieved complete or partial remission that persisted 11, 3, and 2 months. They concluded that methotrexate appears to be an active agent in the treatment of advanced penile cancer. Garnick and colleagues reported a complete remission using high-dose methotrexate followed by citrovorum factor rescue on a 46-year-old male with disseminated metastatic epidermoid carcinoma of the penis.[95]

Cisplatin has also been used as a single agent in the management of penile cancer. Gagliano and associates[96] reported their experience with 26 patients with advanced squamous cell carcinoma of the penis treated with cisplatin, 50 mg/m^2 intravenously, on days 1 and 8, repeated in 28-day cycles. Four of 26 (15%) achieved a partial response. The median survival was 4.7 months. The Memorial Sloan-Kettering Cancer Center experience using cisplatin in the management of penile cancer includes 14 patients.[97–99] Three of these patients had shown progression on bleomycin, nine had previously received methotrexate therapy, and six had previously received radiation therapy. Twelve of 14 patients were considered adequately treated. Of these, one achieved complete remission that lasted 7 months and two had a partial response.

Combination Therapy

Combinations of different active cytotoxic agents have been used in an attempt to increase the response rate. The most frequent combinations utilized have been bleomycin, vincristine, and methotrexate (VBM); methotrexate, bleomycin, and cisplatin; and cisplatin and 5-FU.

Pizzocaro and associates reported their experience with 17 patients with advanced squamous cell carcinoma of the penis using VBM.[100] Twelve patients underwent inguinal lymphadenectomy and were found to have lymph node metastasis, and underwent adjuvant chemotherapy. They received vincristine, 1 mg intravenously on day 1; bleomycin, 15 mg intramuscularly 6 and 24 hours after the vincristine administration; and methotrexate, 30 mg orally on day 3. The cycle was repeated weekly for 12 weeks. Of the 12 patients treated with adjuvant VBM, 11 had no evidence of disease for an average of 40 months and 1 patient relapsed and died of his disease.

In a case report from Japan, Inagaki and colleagues reported their experience in the management of a patient with stage IV penile cancer and ulcerated left inguinal metastasis.[101] He was given a combination of vincristine, peplomycin, methotrexate, and cisplatin. The cycle was repeated every 14 days; following four cycles the patient underwent partial penectomy and ilioinguinal lymphadenectomy. He was alive without evidence of disease 30 months following the surgical procedure.

A combination of cisplation and 5-FU was used in the treatment of six patients with penile cancer; of these, four had recurrent penile carcinoma, one had unresectable tumor at the time of diagnosis, and one had squamous cell carcinoma of the urethra that was unresectable at the time of presentation.[102] They received cisplatin at a dose of 100 mg/m^2 followed by continuous infusion of 5-FU at a dose of 960 mg/m^2 daily for 5 days. The cycle was repeated every 3 to 4 weeks. The patient with unresectable urethral carcinoma achieved complete clinical response after two cycles and underwent bilateral ileoinguinal lymphadenectomy after four cycles. The pathologic diagnosis showed evidence of microscopic disease in two of the inguinal nodes. He refused radiation therapy and experienced relapse 12 months after chemotherapy. He subsequently received two additional cycles of cisplatin and 5-FU with 4500 cGy of radiation therapy to the pelvis; he was free of disease 32 months after treatment. Partial response was observed in the five patients with squamous cell carcinoma of the penis. However, four of the five had unresectable tumors and were treated with radiation therapy. The median survival of this group was 15 months.

Shammas and associates reported their experience in the management of eight patients with advanced squamous cell carcinoma of the penis.[103] Two patients had stage IV disease at the time of presentation, four patients had recurrent disease and were stage IV at the time of entrance into the study, and two patients were classified as stage III. They were treated with cisplatin, 100 mg/m^2 intravenously on day 1, and 5-FU, 1000 mg/m^2 by continuous infusion daily for 5 days. The cycle was repeated every 3 to 4 weeks. Only three of the eight patients were able to tolerate the combination chemotherapy well enough to receive more than two cycles. None of the patients who relapsed following surgery of the primary lesion achieved an objective response. The patients with newly diagnosed stage IV disease achieved a partial response following chemotherapy. One patient with regional lymph nodes and multiple pulmonary metastases received two cycles of chemotherapy and had complete disappearance of his lung metastases. After three additional cycles of chemotherapy, he underwent partial penectomy and inguinal lymphadenectomy. Following neoadjuvant chemotherapy and surgery, he has been free of disease for 32 months. The other patient with stage IV disease achieved a partial response to the combination chemotherapy and was subsequently treated with radiation therapy followed by emasculation. He was alive and free of disease for 57 months.

Fisher and associates reported the use of cisplatin and 5-FU as neoadjuvant therapy in five patients with stage III squamous cell carcinoma of the penis.[104] They received cisplatin, 100 mg/m^2 on day 1, and 5-FU, 1000 mg/m^2 daily for 5 days, for two cycles prior to lymphadenectomy. Four of five (80%) were classified as responders and were able to undergo groin lymph node dissection. Two of these had no viable tumor in the pathologic specimen and two had microscopic disease. Follow-up ranged from 6 to 40 months; the four patients who achieved response to the neoadjuvant chemotherapy had no evidence of local or distant metastasis at the time of publication.

Mitropoulos and associates reported their experience using neoadjuvant cisplatin and interferon-α 2B in the treatment of 13 patients with nonmetastatic histologically confirmed invasive squamous cell carcinoma of the penis.[105] All patients were treated with a combination of 20 mg/m^2 cisplatin intravenously and 5×10^6 IU/m^2 of human interferon-α 2B subcutaneously daily for 5 consecutive days. An equivalent dose of interferon was then administered subcutaneously every 2 days for 3 weeks and the regimen was repeated at 28-day intervals. Of the 12 evaluable patients, 9 responded; 4 achieved a pathologically confirmed complete remission of 38, 21, 10, and 7 months' duration (two with relapse were treated with local therapy and remained with no evidence of disease). The five patients who achieved partial response underwent surgical removal of residual disease and remained disease free for 14 to 24 months. The most significant toxicities were anemia in five patients and reversible renal impairment in three. No patient had neutropenic fever or required platelet transfusion. The authors concluded that the combination of neoadjuvant cisplatin and interferon-α 2B induced responses in 75% of the 12 patients with penile carcinoma and allowed for a less radical operation than originally scheduled.

The known synergism between chemotherapy and radiation has led some researchers to utilize combinations of bleomycin and radiation therapy in order to attempt control of the primary tumor and regional lymphatics.[106–108] Edsmyr and colleagues were able to treat 47 patients with penile cancer using this combination.[106] Seven patients with stage I or II disease were treated with bleomycin, 50 mg intramuscularly per day for 5 days, during the first, third and fifth week. Bleomycin was followed after 1 to 2 hours by radiation therapy. Six of the seven patients (86%) achieved a complete clinical response. One patient developed a recurrence after 7 years and underwent surgery. One patient developed a recurrence 8 months following the treatment and required partial penile amputation. This patient has been free of disease for 10 years. Sexual function was preserved in all but one of the patients. A second group included 35 patients who were treated with the same combination using bleomycin and a total radiation dose of 5800 cGy; 33 of 35 patients (94%) achieved a complete response, and 11 of these developed recurrent disease and died.

It appears that combined surgery, chemotherapy, and/or radiotherapy may play a significant role in the management of large, invasive T2, T3, and T4 penile cancers. This multimodal treatment appears to improve organ preservation, penile integrity and function, and patient survival. Prospective randomized clinical trials are still needed in order to determine the optimal therapy in squamous cell carcinoma of the penis.

REFERENCES

1. Muir C, Waterhouse J, Mack T, et al: Cancer Incidence in Five Continents (Publication No. 88). Lyon, International Agency for Research on Cancer, 1987.
2. Persky L: Epidemiology of cancer of the penis. Recent Results Cancer Res 1977; 60:97–109.
3. Reddy CRRM, Raghavaiah NV, Mouli KC: Prevalence of carcinoma of the penis with special reference to India. Int Surg 1975; 60:470–476.
4. Dodge OG, Linsell CA: Carcinoma of the penis in Uganda and Kenya Africa. Cancer 1963; 16:1255–1263.
5. Brumini R: *In* Cancer in Brazil: Histopathological Data, 1976–1980. Rio de Janeiro, Ministry of Health, 1982.
6. Marcial V, Puras A, Marcial VA: Neoplasms of the penis. *In* Holland JF, Frei E, Bast R Jr, et al (eds): Cancer Medicine, 4th edition, pp 2165–2175. Baltimore, Williams & Wilkins, 1996.
7. National Cancer Institute, Division of Cancer Prevention and Control Surveillance Program: Cancer Statistics Review—1973–1981 (NIH Publication No. 90-2788). Bethesda, MD, National Institutes of Health, 1990.
8. Kyalwazi SK: Carcinoma of the penis. East Afr Med J 1966; 13:415–425.
9. Jussawalla DJ, Jain DK: Cancer Incidence in Greater Bombay, 1970–72. Bombay, The Indian Cancer Society, 1976.
10. Bleich AR: Prophylaxis of penile carcinoma. JAMA 1950; 143:1054–1057.
11. Wolbarst AL: Circumcision and penile carcinoma. Lancet 1932; 1:150–153.
12. Marcial VA, Figueroa J, Marcial RA, et al: Carcinoma of the penis. Radiology 1962; 79:209–220.
13. Sufrin G, Huben R: Benign and malignant lesions of the penis. *In* Gillenwater JY, Grayhack JT, Howards SS, et al (eds): Adult and Pediatric Urology, 2nd edition, pp 1643–1678. St Louis, Mosby–Year Book, 1991.
14. Ornellas AA, Correia AL, Marota A, et al: Surgical treatment of invasive squamous cell carcinoma of the penis: retrospective analysis of 350 cases. J Urol 1994; 151:1244.
15. National Cancer Institute: Surveillance, Epidemiology, End Results (NCI Monograph #57), pp 10–73. Bethesda, MD, National Cancer Institute, 1981.
16. Jensen MS: Cancer of the penis in Denmark 1942–1962. Dan Med Bull 1977; 24:66.
17. Hanash KA, Furlow WL, Utz DC, et al: Carcinoma of the penis: a clinicopathologic study. J Urol 1970; 104:291.
18. Horenblas S, Van Titeren H: Squamous cell carcinoma of the penis. IV. Prognostic factors of survival: analysis of tumor, nodes and metastasis classification system. J Urol 1994; 151:1239–1243.
19. Fraley EE, Zhang G, Manivel C, Niehaus GA: The role of ilioinguinal lymphadenectomy and significance of histological differentiation in treatment of carcinoma of the penis. J Urol 1989; 142:1478.
20. Puras A, González-Flores B, Rodríguez R: Treatment of carcinoma of the penis. *In* Stevenson HG (ed): Proceedings of the Kimbrough Urological Seminar, Vol 12, pp 143–152. Utical, NY, Bradock Press, 1979.
21. Leiter E, Lefkovitis AM: Circumcision and penile carcinoma. NY State J Med 1975; 75:1520.
22. Kochen M, McCurdy S: Circumcision and the risk of cancer of the penis: a life-table analysis. Am J Dis Child 1980; 134:484–486.
23. Shabad AL: Some aspects of the etiology and prevention of penile cancer. J Urol 1964; 92:696–702.
24. Bissada NK, Morcos RR, El-Senoussi M: Post-circumcision carcinoma of the penis I. Clinical aspects. J Urol 1986; 135:283–284.
25. Waterhouse J, Shanmugaratnam K, Muir C, et al (eds): Cancer incidence in Five Continents. IRAC Sci Publ 1982; 4:750–751.
26. Rogus BJ: Squamous cell carcinoma in a young circumcised man. J Urol 1987; 138:861–862.
27. Reddy D, Baruah I: Carcinogenic action of human smegma. Arch Pathol 1963; 75:414–420.
28. Plaut A, Kohn-speger A: The carcinogenic action of smegma. Science 1947; 195:391.
29. Shabad AL: The experimental production of penis tumors. Neoplasm 1965; 12:635.
30. Parkash S, Jeyakumar S, Subramanyan K, et al: Human subpreputial collection—its nature and formation. J Urol 1973; 110:211–212.
31. Melicow MM, Ganem EJ: Cancerous and precancerous lesions of the penis: a clinical and pathological study based on 23 cases. J Urol 1946; 55:486–514.
32. Pratt-Thomas HR, Heins HC, Latham E, et al: The carcinogenic effect of human smegma: an experimental study. Cancer 1956; 9:671–680.
33. Martínez I: Relationship of squamous cell carcinoma of the cervix uteri to squamous cell carcinoma of the penis among Puerto Rican women married to men with penile carcinoma. Cancer 1969; 24:777–780.
34. Graham S, Priore R, Graham M, et al: Genital cancer in wives of penile cancer patients. Cancer 1979; 44:1870–1874.
35. Smith PG, Kinlen LJ, White GC, et al: Mortality of wives of men dying with cancer of the penis. Br J Cancer 1980; 41:422.
36. Hellberg D, Nilsson S: Genital cancer among wives of men with penile cancer. Br J Obstet Gynecol 1989; 96: 221–225.
37. Maiche AG, Pyrhonen S: Risk of cervical cancer among wives of men with carcinoma of the penis. Acta Oncol 1990; 29:569–571.
38. Barrasso R, De Brux J, Croissant O, Orth G: High prevalence of papillomavirus-associated penile intraepithelial neoplasia in sexual partners of women with cervical intraepithelial neoplasia. N Engl J Med 1987; 317:916–923.
39. McCance DJ, Kalache A, Ashdown K, et al: Human papillomavirus types 16 and 18 in carcinomas of the penis from Brazil. Int J Cancer 1986; 37:55.
40. Villa LL, Lopes A: Human papillomavirus DNA sequences in penile carcinomas in Brazil. Int J Cancer 1986; 37:853.
41. Sarkar FH, Miles BJ, Plieth DH, Crissman JD: Detection of human papillomavirus in squamous neoplasm of the penis. J Urol 1992; 147:389.
42. Kristiansen E, Jenkins A, Holm R: Coexistence of episomal and integrated HPV16 DNA in squamous cell carcinoma of the cervix. J Clin Pathol 1994; 47:253.
43. Scinicariello F, Rady P, Saltzstein D, et al: Human papillomavirus 16 exhibits a similar integration pattern in primary squamous cell carcinoma of the penis and in its metastasis. Cancer 1992; 70:2143.
44. Cupp M, Malek R, Goellner J, et al: The detection of human papillomavirus deoxyribonucleic acid in intraepithelial, in situ, verrucous and invasive carcinoma of the penis. J Urol 1995; 154:1029.
45. Strohmeyer T: Penis cancer: the etiologic importance of papilloma virus. Hantarzt 1993; 44:133–134.
46. Lucia MS, Miller GJ: Histopathology of malignant lesions of the penis. Urol Clin North Am 1992; 19:227–246.
47. Burgers JK, Badalament RA, Drago JR: Penile cancer: clinical presentation, diagnosis, and staging. Urol Clin North Am 1992; 19:247–256.
48. Staubitz WJ, Lent MH, Oberkircher OJ: Carcinoma of the penis. Cancer 1955; 8:371.
49. Riveros M, García R, Cabanas R: Lymphadenography of the dorsal lymphatics of the penis. Cancer 1967; 20: 2026–2031.

50. Beggs JH, Spratt JS Jr: Epidermoid carcinoma of the penis. J Urol 1964; 91:166.
51. Cubilla AL, Barreto J, Caballero C, et al: Pathologic features of epidermoid carcinoma of the penis: a prospective study of 66 cases. Am J Surg Pathol 1993; 17:753–763.
52. Hardner GJ, Bhanalaph T, Murphy GP, et al: Carcinoma of the penis: analysis of therapy in 100 consecutive cases. J Urol 1972; 108:428.
53. Nelson R, Derrick F, Allen W: Epidermoid carcinoma of the penis. Br J Urol 1982; 54:172–175.
54. Srinivas V, Morse MJ, Herr HW, et al: Penile cancer: relation of extent of nodal metastasis to survival. J Urol 1987; 137:880.
55. Kamat MR, Kulkarni JN, Tongaonkar HB: Carcinoma of the penis: the Indian experience. J Surg Oncol 1993; 52:50.
56. McDougal W: Carcinoma of the penis: improved survival by early regional lymphadenectomy based on the histological grade and depth of invasion of the primary lesion. J Urol 1995; 154:1364–1366.
57. Schellhamer PF, Jordan GH, Schlossberg SM: Tumors of the penis. *In* Walsh PC, Retik AB, Stamey TA, Vaughan ED Jr (eds): Campbell's Urology, 6th edition, pp 1264–1291. Philadelphia, W B Saunders Co, 1992.
58. Anderson EE, Glenn JF: Penile malignancy and hypercalcemia. JAMA 1965; 192:128.
59. Rudd FV, Rotl RK, Skoglund RW, Ansell JS: Tumor induced hypercalcemia. J Urol 1972; 107:986.
60. Sklaroff RB, Yagoda A: Penile cancer: natural history and therapy. *In* Chemotherapy and Urological Malignancy, pp 98–105. New York, Springer-Verlag, 1982.
61. Malakoff AF, Schmidt JD: Metastatic carcinoma of penis complicated by hypercalcemia. Urology 1975; 5:519.
62. Block NL, Rosen P, Whitmore WF: Hemipelvectomy for advanced penile cancer. J Urol 1973; 110:703.
63. Raghavaiah NV: Corpus cavernosogram in the evaluation of carcinoma of the penis. J Urol 1978; 120:423.
64. Horenblas S, Kroger R, Galleo MP, et al: Ultrasound in squamous carcinoma of the penis: a useful addition to clinical staging? A comparison of ultrasound with histopathology. Urology 1994; 43:702–707.
65. Maiche AG: Computer tomography in the diagnosis and staging of cancer of the penis. Eur J Cancer 1993; 29A:779.
66. deKervilier E, Ollier P, Desgradchamp F, et al: Magnetic resonance imaging in patients with penile carcinoma. Br J Radiol 1995; 68:704–711.
67. Hricak H, Marotti M, Gilbert TJ, et al: Normal penile anatomy and abnormal penile conditions: evaluation with MR imaging. Radiology 1988; 169:683.
68. Puras A, Rivera J: Inguinal and pelvic lymphadenectomy for penile cancer. Urol Clin North Am 1995; 3:81–104.
69. McDougal WS, Kirchner FK Jr, Edwards RN, et al: Treatment of the penis: the case for primary lymphadenectomy. J Urol 1986; 136:38.
70. Cabanas RM: An approach for the treatment of penile carcinoma. Cancer 1977; 39:456.
71. Puras A, González-Flores B, Fortuño F, et al: Staging lymphadenectomy in the treatment of carcinoma of the penis. *In* Stevenson HG (ed): Proceedings of the Kimbrough Urological Seminar, Vol. 14, p 15. Utica, NY, Bradock Press, 1981.
72. Narayana AS, Olney LE, Loening SA, et al: Carcinoma of the penis: analysis of 219 cases. Cancer 1982; 49:2185.
73. Mohs FE, Snow SN, Messing EM, et al: Microscopically controlled surgery in the treatment of carcinoma of the penis. J Urol 1985; 133:961–966.
74. Mohs FE, Snow SN, Larson PO: Mohs micrographic surgery for penile tumors. Urol Clin North Am 1992; 19: 291–304.
75. Ascher PW, Ingolitsch E, Walter G, Oberbauer RW: Ultrastructural findings in CNS tissue with CO2 laser. *In* Kaplan I (ed): Laser Surgery, pp 81–90. Jerusalem, Jerusalem Academic Press, 1978.
76. Malloy TR, Wein AJ, Carpiniello VL: Carcinoma of the penis treated with neodymium:YAG laser. Urology 1988; 31:26.
77. Banderiamonte G, Cepera P, Marchesini R, et al: Laser microsurgery of superficial lesions of the penis. J Urol 1987; 138:315.
78. Bandieramonte G, Santoro O, Boracchi P, et al: Total resection of glans penis surface by CO2: laser microsurgery. Acta Oncol 1988; 27:575.
79. Boon TA, Sapphire probe laser surgery for localized carcinoma of the penis. Eur J Surg Oncol 1988; 14:193.
80. Kriegmar M, Rothenberger KW, Splizenpfell B, et al: Neodymium-YAG-laser treatment for carcinoma of the penis [Abstract 650]. J Urol 1990; 143:351A.
81. Windahl T, Hellsten S: Laser treatment of localized squamous cell carcinoma of the penis. J Urol 1985; 154:1020–1023.
82. deKernion JB, Tynbery P, Persky L, Fegen JP: Carcinoma of the penis. Cancer 1973; 32:1256.
83. Jones WG, Elwell CM: Radiation therapy for penile cancer. *In* Vogelzang NJ, Shipley WU, Scardino PT, Coffey DS (eds): Comprehensive Textbook of Genitouriary Oncology, pp 1109–1114. Baltimore, Williams & Wilkins, 1996.
84. McLean M, Akl AM, Warde P, et al: The results of primary radiation therapy in the management of squamous cell carcinoma of the penis. Int J Radiat Oncol Biol Phys 1993; 25:623–628.
85. Pointon RC: Carcinoma of the penis: external beam therapy. Proc R Soc Med 1975; 68:779–781.
86. Danczak E: Treatment of penis carcinoma with interstitially administered iridium: comparison with radium therapy. Recent Results Cancer Res 1977; 60:127–134.
87. Daly NJ, Douchez J, Combes PF: Treatment of carcinoma of the penis by iridium 192 wire implant. Int J Radiat Oncol Biol Phys 1982; 8:1239.
88. Sagerman RH, Yu WS, Chung CT, Puranki A: External beam irradiation of cancer of the penis. Radiology 1984; 152:183.
89. Mazeron JJ, Langlois D, Lobo PA, et al: Interstitial radiation therapy for carcinoma of the penis using iridium 192 wires: the Henri Mondor experience (1970–1979). Int J Radiat Biol Phys 1984; 10:1891.
90. Fossa SD, Hall KS, Johannessen MB, et al: Carcinoma of the penis: experience at the Norwegian Radium Hospital 1974–1985. Eur Urol 1987; 13:372.
91. Ichikawa T, Nakano I, Hirokawa I: Bleomycin treatment of the tumors of penis and scrotum. J Urol 1969; 102: 699–707.
92. Ichikawa T: Chemotherapy of penis carcinoma. Recent Results Cancer Res 1977; 60:140–156.
93. Kyalwazi S, Bhana D, Harrison N: Carcinoma of the penis and bleomycin chemotherapy in Uganda. Br J Urol 1974; 46:689.
94. Sklaroff R, Yagoda A: Methotrexate in the treatment of penile carcinoma. Cancer 1980; 45:214.
95. Garnick MB, Skarin AT, Stecle GD Jr: Metastatic carcinoma of the penis: complete remission after high dose methotrexate chemotherapy. J Urol 1979; 122:26.
96. Gagliano R, Blumenstein B, Crawford E, et al: Cis-diamminedichloroplatinum in the treatment of advanced epidermoid carcinoma of the penis: a South-west West Oncology Group study. J Urol 1989; 141:66.
97. Ahmed T, Sklaroff R, Yagoda A: Sequential trials of methotrexate, cisplatin and bleomycin for penile cancer. J Urol 1984; 132:464.
98. Sklaroff R, Yagoda A: Cis-diamminedichloride platinum II (DDP) in the treatment of penile carcinoma. Cancer 1979; 44:1563.
99. Yagoda A: Phase II trials with cis-dichlorodiammine platinum (II) in the treatment of urothelial cancer. Cancer Treat Rep 1979; 63:1565.
100. Pizzocaro G, Piva L: Adjuvant and neoadjuvant vincristine, bleomycin and methotrexate for inguinal metastases from squamous cell carcinoma of the penis. Acta Oncol 1988; 27:823.
101. Inagaki N, Hashimoto H, Nakata Y, et al: A case of ad-

vanced penile cancer treated with multimodal therapy. Acta Urol Jpn 1988; 34:1661.

102. Hussein A, Benedetto P, Sridhar K: Chemotherapy with cisplatin and 5-fluorouracil for penile and urethral squamous cell carcinoma. Cancer 1990; 65:433.

103. Shammas FV, Ous S, Fossa SD: Cisplatin and 5-fluorouracil and advanced cancer of the penis. J Urol 1992; 630:147.

104. Fisher HAG, Barada JH, Horton J, van Roemeling R: Neoadjuvant therapy with cisplatin and 5-fluorouracil for stage III squamous cell carcinoma of the penis [Abstract 633]. J Urol 1990; 143:332A.

105. Mitropoulos D, Dimopoulos MA, Koroydivoulgari A, et al: Neoadjuvant cisplatin and interferon-A2B in the treatment and organ preservation of penile carcinoma. J Urol 1994; 152:1124–1126.

106. Edsmyr F, Anderson L, Esposti P: Combined bleomycin and radiation in carcinoma of the penis. Cancer 1985; 56: 1257.

107. Maiche AG: Combined bleomycin and radiation treatment of penile carcinoma. Acta Oncol 1989; 28:548.

108. Stephens F: Bleomycin—a new approach in cancer chemotherapy. Med J Aust 1973; 1:1277.

44

PENECTOMY AND ILIOINGUINAL DISSECTION

DONALD F. LYNCH, JR., M.D. *and* PAUL F. SCHELLHAMMER, M.D.

The goal of surgery for carcinoma of the penis, as in other cancers, is complete excision of the tumor with adequate tissue margins. The size of the primary tumor, its location on the penis, the grade of the tumor, and the depth of invasion determine the extent of surgery that will be required. As has been discussed (see Chapter 42), some superficial lesions of the glans may be amenable to wide excision or to management with laser surgery or Mohs' micrographic surgery, and superficial tumors limited to the prepuce may sometimes be managed with circumcision.[1,2] For larger tumors (>2.0 cm), lesions located so as to preclude an adequate margin of resection, or cancers invading the tunica albuginea, corpora, or urethra, limited resection is not possible and partial or total penectomy will be required. Additionally, patients who develop recurrent tumor following unsuccessful attempts at wide excision or laser therapy require penectomy. Some patients with Buschke-Lowenstein tumor or Kaposi's sarcoma may also be candidates for penectomy, when problems with local management of the lesion necessitate intervention.

SURGICAL PROCEDURES FOR THE PRIMARY LESION

Biopsy

It is essential to confirm both the histology of the tumor and the stage or extent of the lesion with an adequate biopsy. Most penile cancers are squamous cell carcinomas, which spread by local invasion early in their course. These tumors metastasize to regional lymph nodes as they progress in size and depth and involve the highly vascular structures of the penis. Histologic confirmation of tumor depth is important in assessing the need for inguinal lymphadenectomy, as well as in determining whether adequate margins of resection can be obtained to allow organ-sparing surgery. Additionally, recent studies suggest that tumor grade also is a significant determinant in prognosis, and is an important consideration in assessing the risk of inguinal metastases.[3,4] Penile biopsy may be done as a separate procedure, or may be done in conjunction with frozen section confirmation as a prelude to definitive penile amputation. Full informed consent must be obtained prior to such a procedure.

Biopsy is performed by excising a 1- to 1.5-cm wedge of tissue that includes the margin of the tumor and provides normal tissue adjacent to the lesion to be examined for tumor infiltration (Fig. 44–1). The incision may be closed with interrupted 2-0 or 3-0 chromic gut, after which a sterile compressive dressing is applied. There have been no reports of tumor dissemination from biopsy of penile cancers.[5]

Partial Penectomy

Partial penectomy is appropriate in the treatment of tumors of the glans and distal penile shaft where a margin of at least 2 cm of normal tissue can be achieved. In the appropriately selected patient, this procedure should provide a penile stump of sufficient length to allow the patient to void while standing. If an adequate stump cannot be assured, total penectomy with a perineal urethrostomy is preferable.

The incidence of recurrent tumor following partial penectomy has been reported as ranging from 0 to 6%. Five-year survival rates of 70 to 80% following a properly performed partial penectomy have been noted when inguinal nodes are free of metastatic disease.[6,7]

If the patient has not been receiving antibiotic

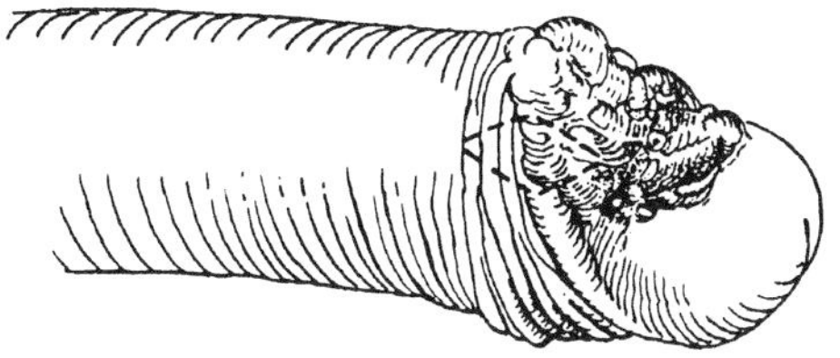

FIGURE 44–1. Wedge biopsy of the primary tumor. (From Das S, Crawford ED: Carcinoma of the penis: management of the primary. *In* Crawford ED, Das S [eds]: Current Genitourinary Cancer Surgery, p 367. Philadelphia, Lea & Febiger, 1990, with permission.)

therapy prior to surgery, intravenous antibiotics are administered preoperatively. A broad-spectrum cephalosporin that can be converted to oral therapy 48 to 72 hours following surgery is preferred. With the patient in the supine position, the entire penis and scrotum are scrubbed with povidone-iodine solution, and the lesion is then covered with a sterile glove or sponge secured with a sterile rubber band. A 1/4- to 1/2-inch Penrose drain is used as a tourniquet about the base of the penis.

A transverse incision is made over the dorsum of the penis 2.0 cm proximal to the most proximal tumor margin and carried circumferentially around the shaft (Fig. 44–2*A*). The superficial dorsal vessels are fulgurated, and the corpora are then sharply divided down to the urethra, taking care to ligate the deep dorsal vessel complex and each cavernosal artery (Fig. 44–2*B*). The distal urethra is dissected free approximately 1 cm proximally and distally, maintaining the 2-cm margin, to allow for spatulation and creation of a neomeatus. The amputation is then completed.

The corporal stumps are closed by approximating tunica albuginea with interrupted mattress sutures of 2-0 Vicryl (Fig. 44–2*C*). The tourniquet is then removed and further hemostasis obtained. The urethra is spatulated and sutured to the skin of the shaft with 3-0 or 4-0 Vicryl or Dexon. The remaining shaft skin is closed using 3-0 absorbable suture (Fig. 44–2*D*). An 18-French Foley catheter is placed to straight drainage for 24 to 48 hours, and the wound is dressed.

Alternatively, the penile shaft skin can be excised to create a flap dorsally. This can be folded ventrally to cover the stump of the penis, and the urethra spatulated and brought through a buttonhole in the flap. The flap edges are sutured with 3-0 Vicryl, and excess flap skin is then excised as needed (Fig. 44–3).

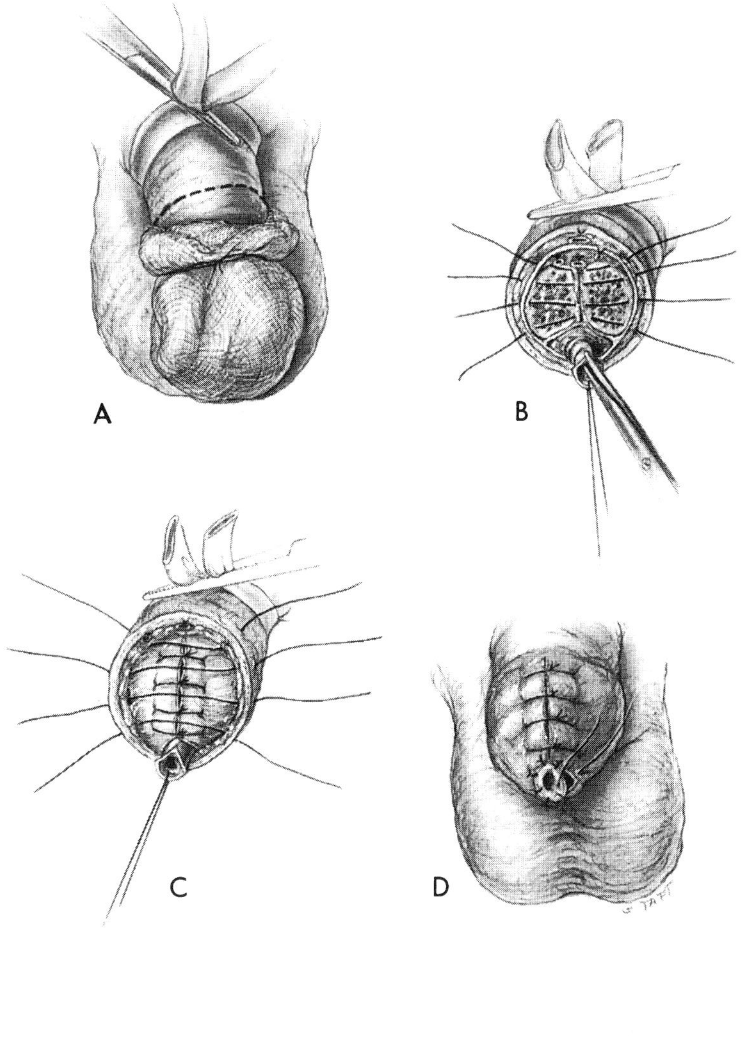
A
B
C
D

FIGURE 44–2. Classic technique for partial penectomy. *A*, Circumferential incision around the shaft with a margin of 2 cm from the lesion. *B*, Transection of the penis with closure of the corpora cavernosa. The urethral segment is made slightly longer to allow spatulation. *C*, Closure of the shaft skin. *D*, Securing the urethra. (From Herr HW: Surgery of the penile and urethral carcinoma. *In* Walsh PC, Retik AB, Stamey TA, Vaughan ED Jr [eds]: Campbell's Urology, 6th edition, p 3076. Philadelphia, WB Saunders Co, 1992, with permission.)

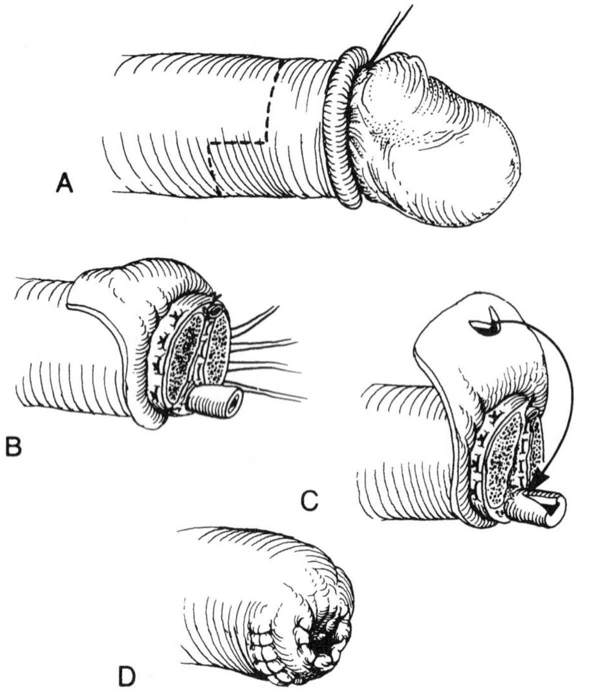
A
B
C
D

FIGURE 44–3. Variation of partial penectomy. *A*, Skin incision. *B*, Corporal bodies transected and closed with mattress sutures. Urethral stump dissected 1 cm beyond corpora. *C*, Buttonhole made in skin flap to allow for urethral anastamosis. Skin flap closed. *D*, Urethra spatulated and secured. This technique may decrease meatal stricture formation. (From Das S, Crawford ED: Carcinoma of the penis: management of the primary. *In* Crawford ED, Das S [eds]: Current Genitourinary Cancer Surgery, p 367. Philadelphia, Lea & Febiger, 1990, with permission.)

Additional stump length can sometimes be gained by dividing the suspensory ligament of the penis, dividing the ischiocavernosus muscle, and mobilizing the crura from the inferior pubis. The scrotum is incised along the raphe and reconstructed superior to the transported phallus.[8] These maneuvers may provide 1 to 2 cm of additional length and avoid the need for a total penectomy in carefully selected cases.

Total Penectomy

Total penectomy is the treatment of choice in patients in whom the lesion is located too proximally on the shaft to permit a partial amputation. The patient is placed in standard lithotomy position, and the penis, scrotum, lower abdomen, and perineum are prepared with povidone-iodine solution. The tumor is covered with a glove or dressing.

An elliptical incision is begun over the pubis and carried around the base of the penis to the midportion of the scrotal raphe (Fig. 44–4*A*). The corpus spongiosum is exposed ventrally and mobilized to the urogenital diaphragm. It is transected distal to the bulb, taking care to assure a 2-cm margin from the lesion (Fig. 44–4*B* and *C*). Dorsally, the incision is carried down through Buck's fascia, and the deep dorsal venous complex is identified and traced to the symphysis pubis (Fig. 44–4*D*). The dorsal vein complex is clamped, ligated with 2-0 silk suture, and divided at this point. The suspensory ligament of the penis is divided, and, with downward traction on the penile shaft, the corpora cavernosa are identified and dissected from their attachments to the inferior pubis. The corpora are individually ligated with 0 Vicryl suture and divided behind the pubis.

Following amputation of the penis, a 1-cm ellipse of skin is excised from the region of the perineal body midway between the rectum and scrotum. With blunt dissection, a tunnel is developed in the perineal subcutaneous tissue, and the urethra grasped and directed through this passage, taking care not to create excessive angulation. Excess urethra is excised and the urethral stump spatulated and secured to the perineal skin with 3-0 chromic or Vicryl sutures (Fig. 44–4*E*). After 3/4-inch Penrose drains are placed in the subcutaneous space, the primary incision is sutured with interrupted 3-0 Vicryl transversely, which closes the suprapubic wound and serves to elevate the scrotum off of the perineum (Fig. 44–4*E* and *F*). The wound is dressed and an 18-French Foley catheter is placed to straight drainage for 48 to 72 hours. The patient is maintained on broad-spectrum antibiotic therapy for 7 to 10 days.

MANAGEMENT OF REGIONAL DISEASE

If the initial battle against squamous cancer of the penis is waged on the penile integument, the war is lost or won in the regional nodes. A thorough understanding of the lymphatic drainage of the penis is essential to stage the patient, to monitor his progress following surgical intervention, and to deal with regional disease if it is present at diagnosis or develops subsequent to primary treatment. Although penile cancer, like testis cancer, remains one of the few malignancies for which regional lymphadenectomy can be curative, controversy exists regarding the timing and indications for inguinal and pelvic lymphadenectomy as well as the extent of the surgery required.

Anatomic Considerations

A thorough knowledge of the anatomy of the groin region is essential for the surgeon performing inguinal lymphadenectomy. The surgical anatomy has been described by Daseler and colleagues, who performed a series of 450 inguinal lymphadenectomies for a variety of tumors and whose technique has been viewed as the standard for penile cancer.[9]

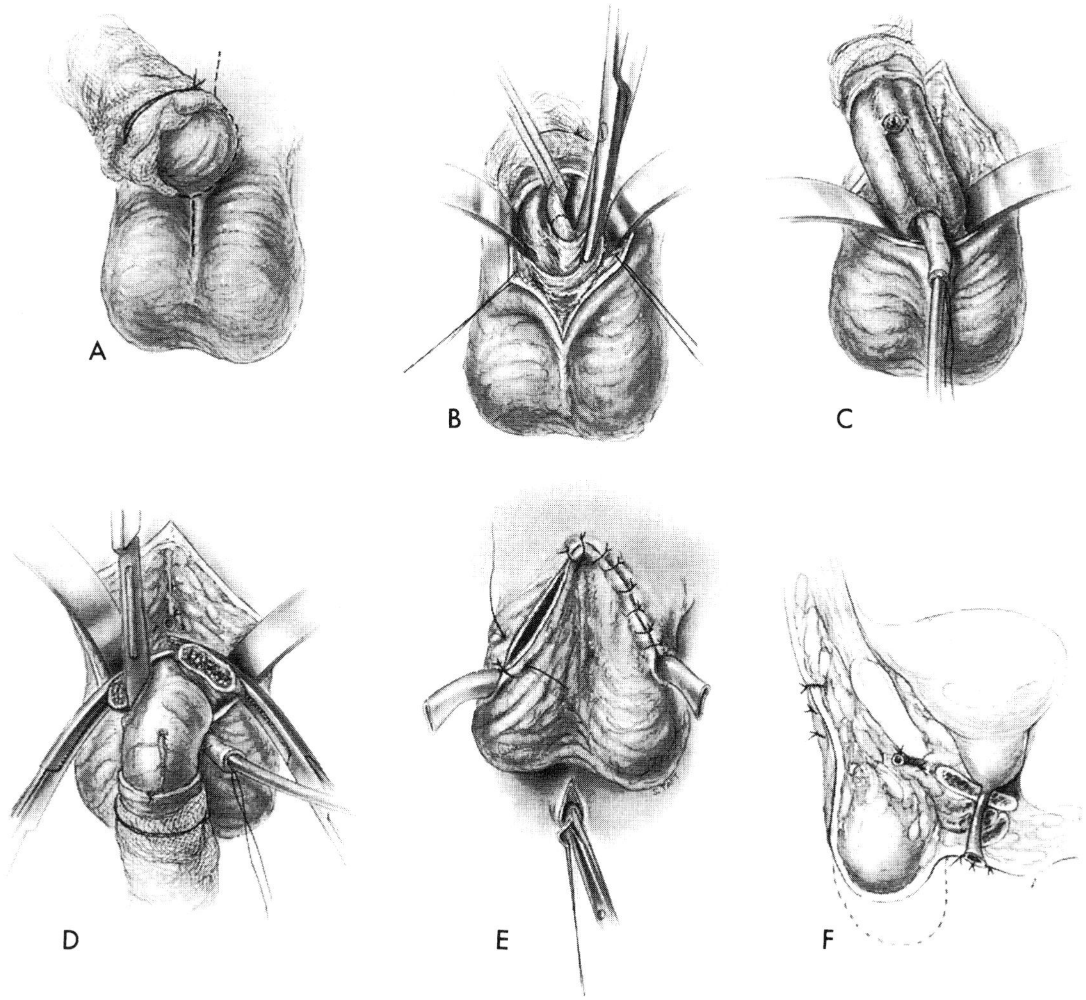
A
B
C
D
E
F

FIGURE 44–4. Technique of total penectomy. *A*, Elliptical incision around the base of the penis. *B*, Urethra isolated 2 cm proximal to tumor. *C*, Suspensory ligament divided. Urethra dissected from corpora and transected. *D*, Ligation of dorsal vessels. Transection of crura with ligation of the stumps. *E*, Perineal urethrostomy created. Urethra transposed, spatulated, and secured. *F*, Drains placed and incision closed horizontally to elevate scrotum away from urethrostomy. (From Herr HW: Surgery of penile and urethral carcinoma. *In* Walsh PC, Retik AB, Stamey TA, Vaughan ED Jr [eds]: Campbell's Urology, 6th edition, p 3077. Philadelphia, WB Saunders Co, 1992, with permission.)

The boundaries of the classic lymphadenectomy and their relationship to significant anatomic landmarks are illustrated in Figure 44–5.

Fascial Planes

The lower abdomen has two superficial fascial compartments, Scarpa's and Camper's fasciae. Camper's fascia is a fibrofatty layer that is continuous from the lower abdomen onto the thigh. At the scrotum, it fuses with the deeper Scarpa's fascia to form the tunica dartos. Scarpa's fascia is composed of a distinct fibrous sheath. From the abdomen, it crosses the inguinal ligament and fuses with the fascia lata of the thigh about 1 cm inferior to Poupart's ligament, forming Holden's line.

Within the pelvis, the iliac fascia invests the iliopsoas muscle and also covers the femoral nerve. The iliac fascia fuses with the transversalis fascia at the inguinal ligament. The inguinal ligament is formed by the aponeurosis of the external oblique muscle and runs from the anterior superior iliac spine to the pubic tubercle. The internal oblique muscle attaches to the lateral half of the inguinal ligament, and the transversus abdominis to its outer third.

Femoral Triangle (of Scarpa)

The femoral triangle is formed by the inguinal ligament, the medial margin of the sartorius muscle, and the medial border of the adductor longus muscle. It is covered by the fascia late except for the fossa ovalis, an opening through which the greater saphenous vein passes to empty into the femoral vein below. Passing through the femoral triangle are the femoral vessels and nerve. The vessels are invested within the femoral sheath, which is formed by extensions of the transversalis fascia, which passes below the inguinal ligament. This

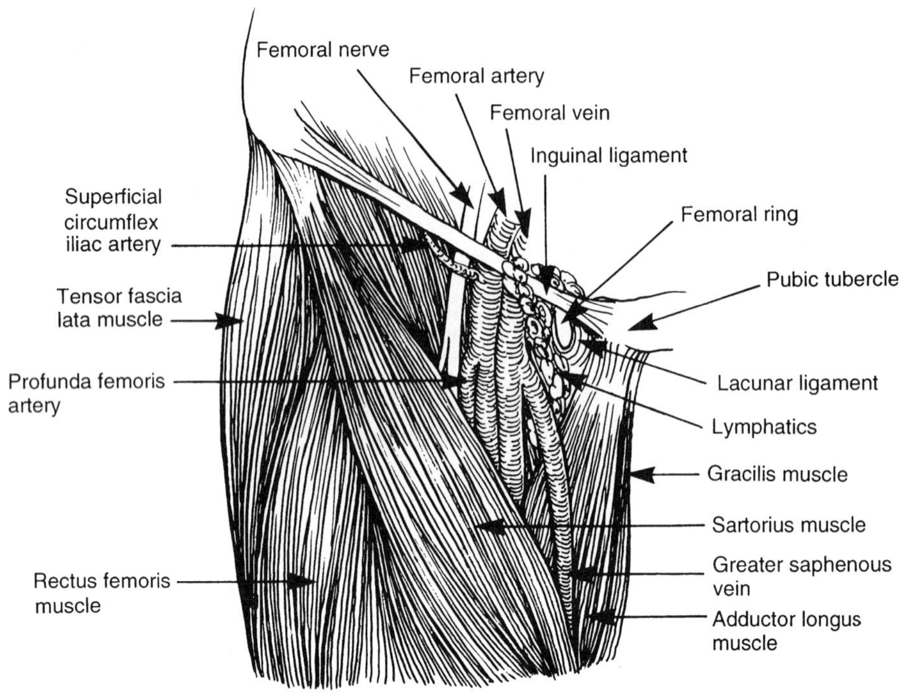
Femoral nerve
Femoral artery
Femoral vein
Inguinal ligament
Femoral ring
Pubic tubercle
Superficial circumflex iliac artery
Tensor fascia lata muscle
Profunda femoris artery
Lacunar ligament
Lymphatics
Gracilis muscle
Sartorius muscle
Greater saphenous vein
Rectus femoris muscle
Adductor longus muscle

FIGURE 44–5. Anatomic landmarks and groin dissection. (From Puras A, Rivera J: Inguinal and pelvic lymphadenectomy for penile cancer. Atlas Urol Clin North Am 1995; 3:81, with permission.)

sheath is composed of three compartments: the medial, containing the lymph nodes and lymphatic trunks; the middle, containing the femoral vein; and the lateral, containing the femoral artery. Lateral to the artery within the iliac fascia is the femoral nerve (Fig. 44–6).

Veins

The femoral vein enters the femoral triangle at its apex, medial to the femoral artery. About 4 cm below Poupart's ligament, it receives the greater saphenous vein anteriorly and the profunda femoris vein posteriorly. The greater saphenous vein originates at the dorsal venous arch of the foot and ascends medially, passing posterior to the medial epicondyle at the knee. It ascends in the superficial fascia of the thigh and empties into the femoral vein after passing through the fossa ovalis. Just before the fossa ovalis, it receives the superficial epigastric and external pudendal veins medially and the accessory saphenous and circumflex iliac veins laterally (Fig. 44–7). The femoral vein passes below the inguinal ligament to become the external iliac vein, which joins with the internal iliac (hypogastric) vein at the level of the sacroiliac joint to form the common iliac vein. The paired common iliac veins empty into the inferior vena cava at the level of the fifth lumbar vertebra.

Arteries

The common iliac arteries arise from the terminal aorta and divide at the level of the sacral promontory into the internal and external iliac arteries. The internal iliac passes posteromedially and divides to supply the pelvic musculature and pelvic organs. The external iliac artery passes below the inguinal ligament to become the femoral artery, which supplies the lower limb. Just prior to passing beneath the inguinal ligament, the external iliac artery gives off the medial inferior epigastric artery and the lateral circumflex iliac artery. Just after passing beneath the inguinal ligament, the femoral artery gives off the superficial epigastric artery, the superficial circumflex iliac artery, the superficial and deep external pudendal arteries, and the profunda femoris artery (Fig. 44–5). The femoral artery continues past the apex of the femoral triangle and terminates in the lower third of the adductor magnus, where it becomes the popliteal artery.

Nerves

The femoral nerve lies beneath the iliac fascia lateral to the femoral vessels and outside of the femoral sheath. It is usually not visualized in the inguinal dissection because the femoral nodal tissue lies medial to the vessels within the femoral sheath. Other nerves that may be encountered in the groin are the ilioinguinal and lateral cutaneous nerve of the thigh. The obturator nerve and genitofemoral nerves are encountered in the course of the pelvic lymphadenectomy.

Lymphatics

Lymphatic drainage of the penis is to the superficial and deep inguinal lymph nodes and to the

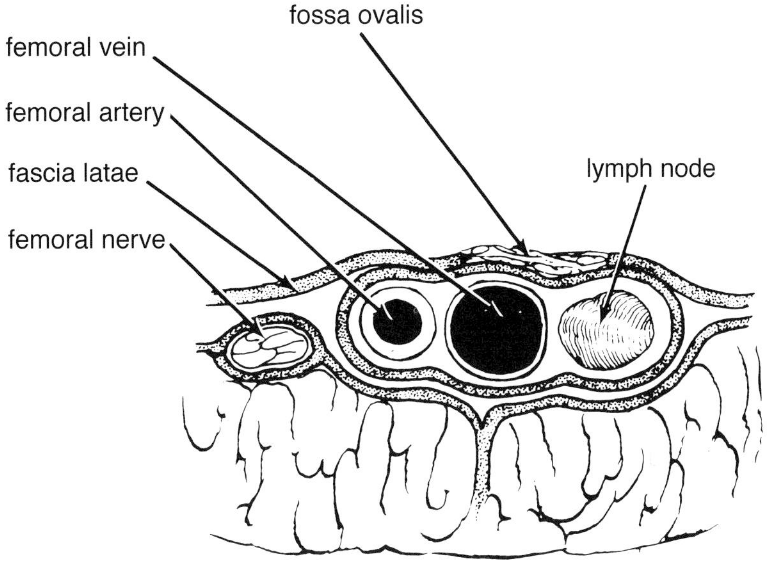
fossa ovalis
femoral vein
femoral artery
fascia latae
lymph node
femoral nerve

FIGURE 44–6. Anatomy of the femoral sheath. (From Das S, Crawford ED: Carcinoma of the penis: management of the primary. *In* Crawford ED, Das S [eds]: Current Genitourinary Cancer Surgery, p 375. Philadelphia, Lea & Febiger, 1990, with permission.)

pelvic nodes. The superficial inguinal nodes comprise from 4 to 25 nodes lying below Scarpa's fascia, superficial to the deep fascia of the thigh and closely associated with the saphenous vein (Fig. 44–7). Rouviere's classic study of inguinal anatomy divides the superficial inguinal nodes into five zones (Fig. 44–8) with the sentinel nodes lying within zone 2, just medial to the femoral vein around the superficial epigastric and superficial external pudendal veins.[9,10] The deep inguinal nodes —usually one to three on a side—lie below the fascia lata medial to the femoral vein (Fig. 44–9).

Lymphatic drainage of the prepuce and penile skin commences in the ventral penile skin, drains superficial to Buck's fascia in a dorsolateral direction, and then courses proximally along the dorsum of the penis to the superficial inguinal nodes. Drainage from the glans penis coalesces at the frenulum and passes laterally to the dorsal penis, deep to Buck's fascia paralleling the deep dorsal vein. One pathway is to the deep femoral node chain, which includes the femoral node of Cloquet or Rosenmüller. An additional lymphatic pathway may course along the inguinal canal to the lateral retrofemoral node, the most superficial of the external iliac chain.

The drainage of the corporal bodies also accompanies the deep dorsal vein of the penis, anastamosing freely with the presymphyseal lymphatic plexus at the base of the penis and draining into both superficial and deep inguinal nodes. Because of this network, metastatic involvement of both inguinal regions is possible. Further drainage from the base of the penis occurs via channels following the femoral canals proximally into the external iliac and pelvic nodes.[9–12]

The pelvic nodes include the external iliac group, the internal iliac or hypogastric nodes, and the common iliac chain (Fig. 44–10). The external iliac group (usually 8 to 10 nodes) lies anterior and medial to the external iliac vein. The hypogastric nodes (four to six in number) are located around the hypogastric vein, and the common iliac chain (4 to 10 nodes) is located anterolateral to or sometimes posterior to the common iliac vessels. Metastasis to the pelvic lymph nodes without involvement of the inguinal nodes is an extremely rare event, and appears to be based on a single report by Schreiner.[13] Such metastatic spread has not been observed in many recent studies.[3,14–17] Therefore, in the setting of negative superficial and deep inguinal node dissections and a negative pelvic computed tomography (CT) scan, resection of the pelvic nodes is not required.

Sentinel Node Biopsy

The concept of the sentinel node was proposed by Cabanas, who postulated that there is a node or group of nodes—lying between the superficial external pudendal vein and the superficial epigastric vein—where the earliest metastasis from a penile tumor will occur consistently (Fig. 44–11).[12,17] A negative sentinel node biopsy in the presence of clinically negative groins was thought to indicate that further inguinal dissection was unnecessary. Five-year survivals of 90% have been reported in

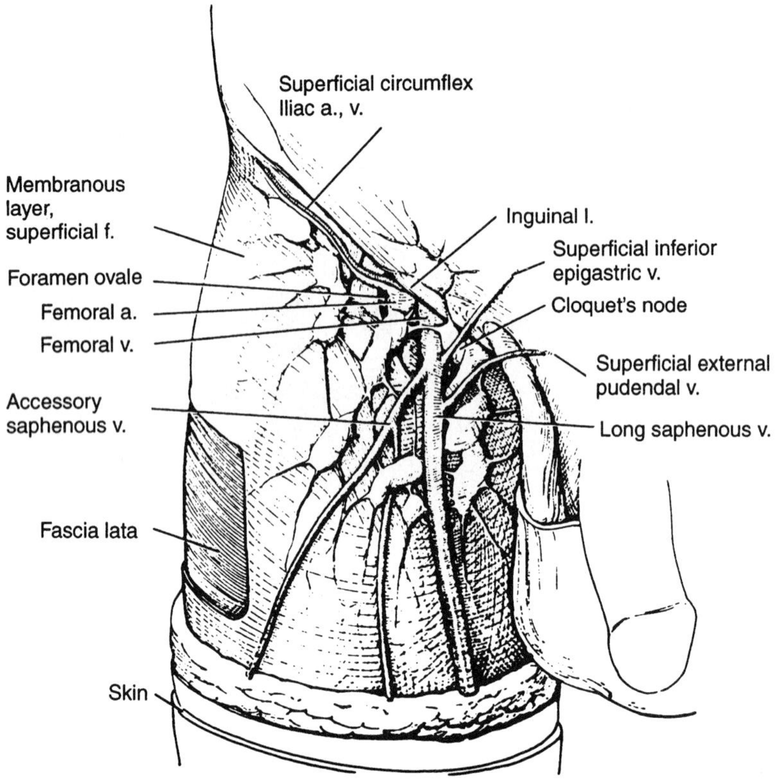
Superficial circumflex
Iliac a., v.
Membranous
layer,
superficial f.
Foramen ovale
Femoral a.
Femoral v.
Accessory
saphenous v.
Fascia lata
Skin
Inguinal l.
Superficial inferior
epigastric v.
Cloquet's node
Superficial external
pudendal v.
Long saphenous v.

FIGURE 44–7. Superficial inguinal nodes and arteriovenous system. (From Hinman F Jr, Stemphen PH: Atlas of UroSurgical Anatomy. Philadelphia, WB Saunders Co, 1993 *and* Seay TM, Peretsman SJ: Lymphatic anatomy for the urologist. *In* Seay TM, Peretsman SJ, Klein EA [eds]: Atlas Urol Clin North Am 1995; 3:8, with permission.)

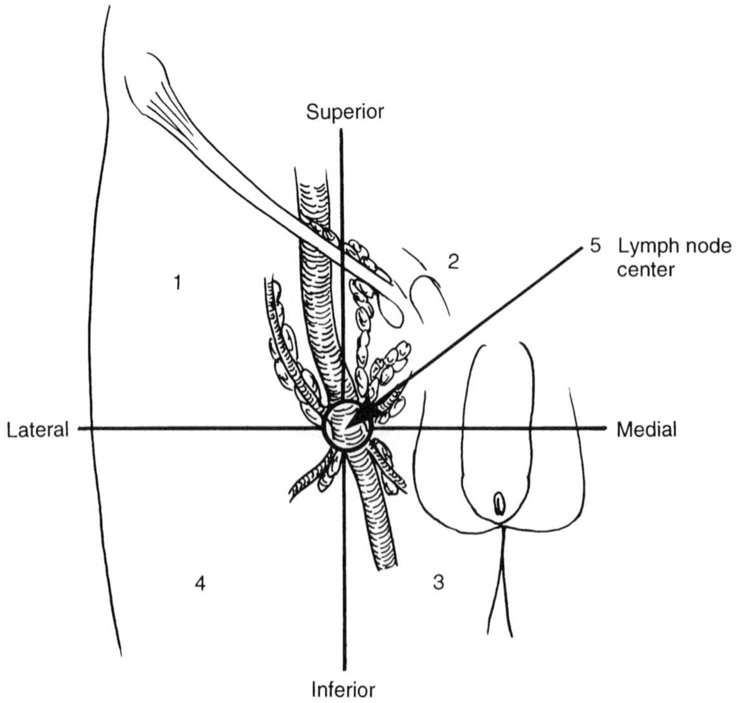
Superior
1
2
5 Lymph node
center
Lateral
Medial
4
3
Inferior

FIGURE 44–8. Divisions of the superficial inguinal nodes (after Rouviere). (From Puras A, Rivera J: Inguinal and pelvic lymphadenectomy for penile cancer. Atlas Urol Clin North Am 1995; 3:81, with permission.)

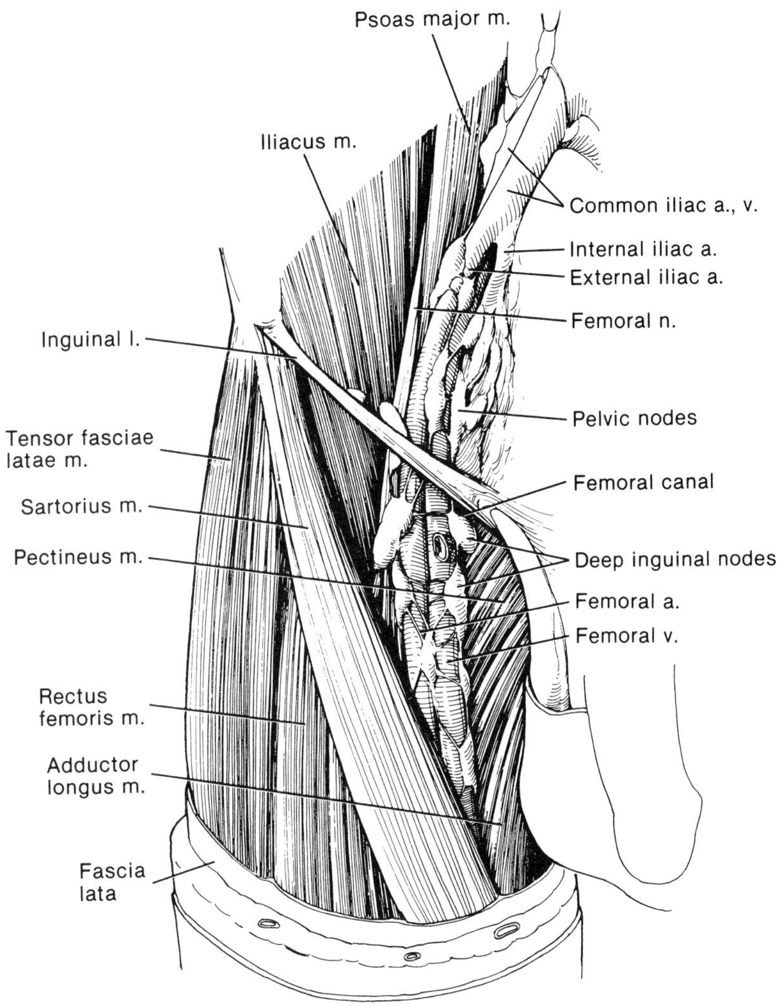
Psoas major m.
Iliacus m.
Common iliac a., v.
Internal iliac a.
External iliac a.
Femoral n.
Inguinal l.
Pelvic nodes
Tensor fasciae latae m.
Femoral canal
Sartorius m.
Pectineus m.
Deep inguinal nodes
Femoral a.
Femoral v.
Rectus femoris m.
Adductor longus m.
Fascia lata

FIGURE 44–9. Deep inguinal and iliac nodes. (From Hinman F Jr, Stemphen PH: Atlas of UroSurgical Anatomy. Philadelphia, WB Saunders Co, 1993 *and* Seay TM, Peretsman SJ: Lymphatic anatomy for the urologist. *In* Seay TM, Peretsman SJ, Klein EA [eds]: Atlas Urol Clin North Am 1995; 3:9, with permission.)

this setting. However, subsequent reports of the development of metastases following a negative sentinel node biopsy have suggested that sentinel node biopsy may not be consistently reliable.[18–20] Further evaluation of this technique continues. Sentinel node biopsy is not appropriate in the presence of clinically suspicious nodes; rather, full superficial and deep inguinal dissections should be performed. When the sentinel node biopsy is performed, the incision should be placed so that, if a full formal inguinal lymphadenectomy is later required, the original sentinel node biopsy incision can be excised with the lymphadenectomy specimen.

Considerations in Inguinal and Ilioinguinal Lymphadenectomy

Figure 44–12 summarizes our approach to the patient who has undergone surgery of the primary lesion and who is being considered for lymphadenectomy.

Because lymph node enlargement and lymphangiitis resulting from infection of the primary tumor is common at the time of diagnosis, all patients with penile cancer should receive 4 to 6 weeks of antibiotic therapy before undergoing inguinal lymphadenectomy. At the completion of this course of treatment, the groins are carefully examined for the presence of abnormal nodes. Thirty to 60% of patients who present with penile cancer have palpable inguinal nodes and, following antibiotic therapy, half of these nodes will harbor metastases.[21] When metastases are detected clinically in one groin, contralateral metastases will be present in 60% of cases because of the crossover of lymphatics at base of the penis.[5] Consequently, in this situation contralateral inguinal lymphadenectomy should be performed.

It is generally accepted that patients with low-grade, noninvasive tumors and clinically negative inguinal nodes may safely be managed expectantly if close follow-up with careful groin examinations

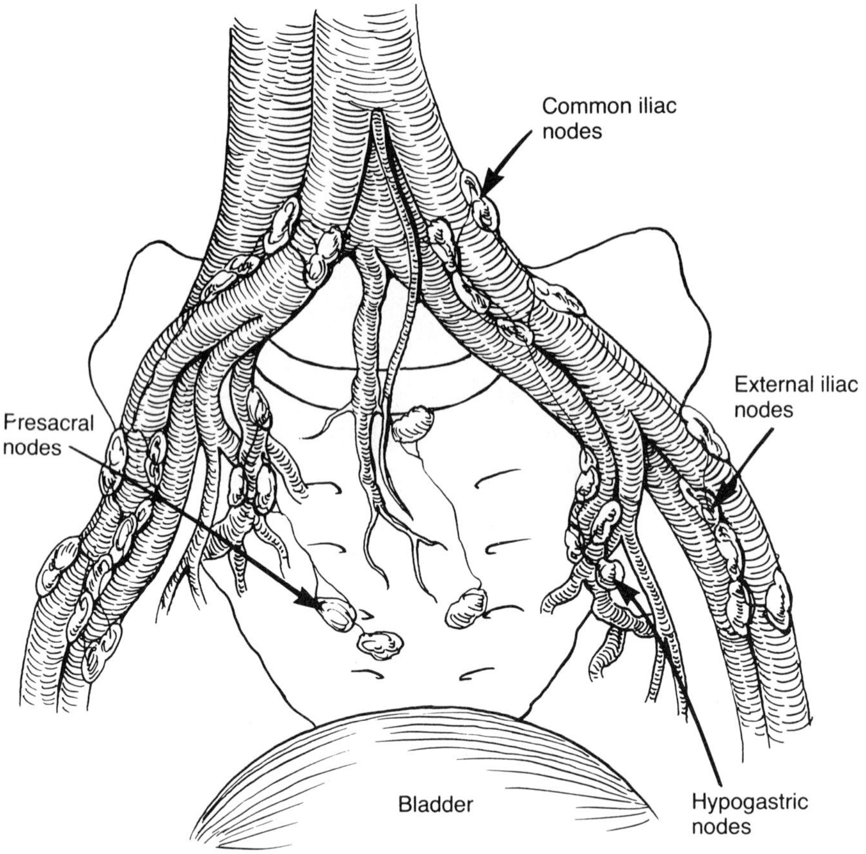
Common iliac
nodes
External iliac
nodes
Fresacral
nodes
Bladder
Hypogastric
nodes

FIGURE 44–10. Pelvic nodes (common iliac, external iliac, and hypogastric groups). (From Hinman F Jr, Stemphen PH: Atlas of UroSurgical Anatomy. WB Saunders Co, 1995 *and* Seay TM, Peretsman SJ: Lymphatic anatomy for the urologist. *In* Seay TM, Peretsman SJ, Klein EA [eds]: Atlas Urol Clin North Am 1995; 3:6, with permission.)

every 2 months for at least 2 years can be assured.[3,4,6,14] Unreliable patients or others who cannot be followed adequately are best served by prompt inguinal lymphadenectomy. Considerable debate has raged over the years regarding immediate or delayed lymphadenectomy in other patients with clinically negative groins. There has been support for expectant management of patients with invasive (T2 to T4) lesions and no palpable inguinal adenopathy, with surgical intervention undertaken only when lymphadenopathy develops. This avoids the substantial morbidity that can be associated with groin dissection. In those patients who later develop clinically positive nodes, delayed lymphadenectomy can provide care in 30 to 50%.[5,22–24] However, other series support immediate lymphadenectomy in these cases, citing higher mortality rates in patients who are followed until they develop clinically positive nodes before undergoing inguinal exploration.[3–6,14,22,25,26] It is clear that, in these patients, the window of opportunity to provide a cure has been lost.

Immediate groin irradiation in patients having clinically negative groins has been investigated, and the incidence of subsequent inguinal metastases was found not to be reduced significantly by this treatment.[5,27–29] Furthermore, irradiation makes subsequent physical examination of the groins difficult, and markedly increases problems with surgery and wound healing if a groin dissection later becomes necessary.

In the event that unilateral groin metastases develop some time after surgical treatment of the primary, inguinal lymphadenectomy of only the involved groin is required.[5] Although this would seem to contradict the recommendations outlined previously, bilateral occult metastases present from diagnosis that become clinically apparent later should manifest themselves at about the same time. Consequently, the lack of clinically detectable nodes on the side contralateral to a late-developing groin metastasis suggests that the contralateral nodes were not involved from the outset.

Preoperative staging of the pelvic, common iliac, and para-aortic nodes with CT scan and, where indicated, with needle biopsy is essential. Although survival has followed resection of tumor limited to the external iliac nodes, no patient with common iliac or para-aortic metastases has survived.[30] Fine-needle aspiration of suspicious nodes in these areas may confirm metastatic tumor and thus avoid unnecessary surgery. The most important predictor of

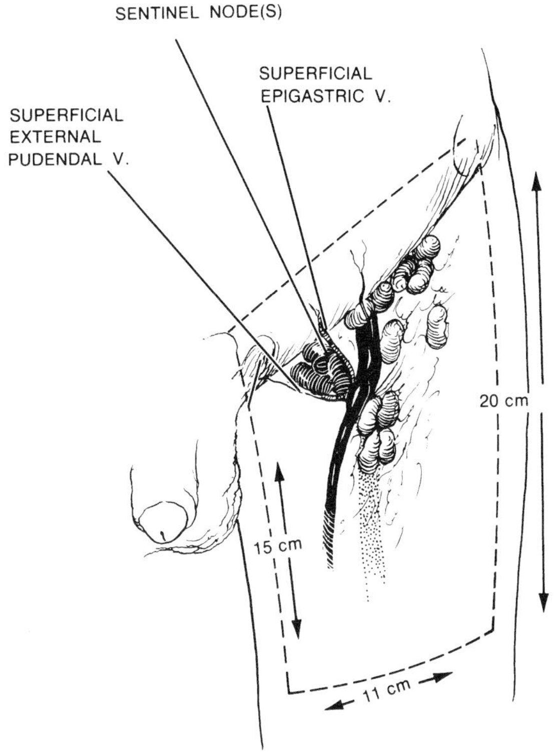
SENTINEL NODE(S)
SUPERFICIAL EPIGASTRIC V.
SUPERFICIAL EXTERNAL PUDENDAL V.
20 cm
15 cm
11 cm

FIGURE 44–11. Sentinel node anatomy. Biopsy is performed 2 cm lateral and 2 cm inferior to the pubic tubercle. (From Spaulding J: Tumors of the penis. *In* Javadpour N [ed]: Principles and Management of Urologic Cancer, p 488. Baltimore, Williams & Wilkins, 1979, with permission.)

ultimate survival continues to be the stage of the primary tumor and the presence or absence of nodal metastases.[4,31]

Occasionally, palliative groin dissection is performed even in the face of extensive regional or distant metastases. Lymphadenopathy that threatens to erode through the inguinal skin or invade into the femoral vessels may need to be removed to avoid pain, inguinal infection, or serious hemorrhage.

Avoiding Complications from Inguinal Lymphadenectomy

Despite the encouraging prognosis for many patients with inguinal metastases who undergo inguinal or ilioinguinal lymphadenectomy, there has been a longstanding reluctance on the part of surgeons to subject patients to this procedure because of the 30 to 50% incidence of major morbidity associated with it.[23,25,32,33] Complications include lymphocele, substantial lower limb lymphedema, skin loss, and infection. Skin flap necrosis can be minimized by selecting the appropriate incision, by careful tissue handling, by careful attention to skin flap thickness with excision of ischemic flap margins, and by transporting the head of the sartorius muscle to cover the defect left over the femoral vessels. Use of intravenous fluorescein dye and a Wood's lamp intraoperatively to assess viability of wound edges is a useful adjunct.[34] Lower limb lymphedema can be reduced by careful attention to intraoperative ligation of lymphatics, by immobilization of the limb or limbs in the postoperative period, and by suction drainage of the lymphadenectomy site. Elastic support hose should be used in the immediate postoperative period and may be required long term in many patients. Wound infection can be minimized by intensive preoperative antibiotic therapy to reduce infection and inflammation from the primary, and by the use of prophylactic antibiotics.[35] Thrombotic problems may be avoided through the use of subcutaneous heparin in the perioperative period, particularly when the classic inguinal and pelvic dissection is combined with prolonged bed rest postoperatively.

Technique of Inguinal Lymphadenectomy

Figure 44–13 shows the various incisions described for inguinal and ilioinguinal lymphadenectomy. We prefer the oblique incision below and parallel to the inguinal crease because it maintains the integrity of the inguinal ligament, and because it preserves the cutaneous blood supply that runs parallel to the inguinal ligament (Fig. 44–13*B* and *C*).

The indications for inguinal and ilioinguinal lymphadenectomy are outlined in Figure 44–12. When the lesion is stage Tis, T0, or T1, the tumor is of low grade (grade 1), the groins are negative, and the patient can be relied upon to participate in a program of close follow-up, we observe the patient with bimonthly exams for 2 years.[36] Similarly, if the lesion is of low grade at diagnosis and the inguinal nodes are enlarged but normalize following antibiotic therapy, we will follow the patient expectantly.

If the tumor demonstrates invasiveness (stage ≥T2) or is of high histologic grade (grade 2 or 3), and the groins are negative or normalize following antibiotic therapy, we recommend a modified bilateral superficial inguinal dissection with frozen section evaluation similar to that described by Catalona.[37] If these nodes are negative, we close and follow the patient expectantly as outlined previously. If these nodes are positive, we proceed with a classic inguinal lymphadenectomy, extending the limits of the groin dissection to those illustrated in Figure 44–14 and including a bilateral pelvic node dissection. If metastatic disease is found in the deep inguinal nodes, pelvic lymphadenectomy should be performed. Some surgeons prefer to operate on the more involved groin and do the pelvic lymphadenectomy as one procedure, performing the contralateral inguinal dissection several weeks later.[35]

If bilateral palpable inguinal nodes persist fol-

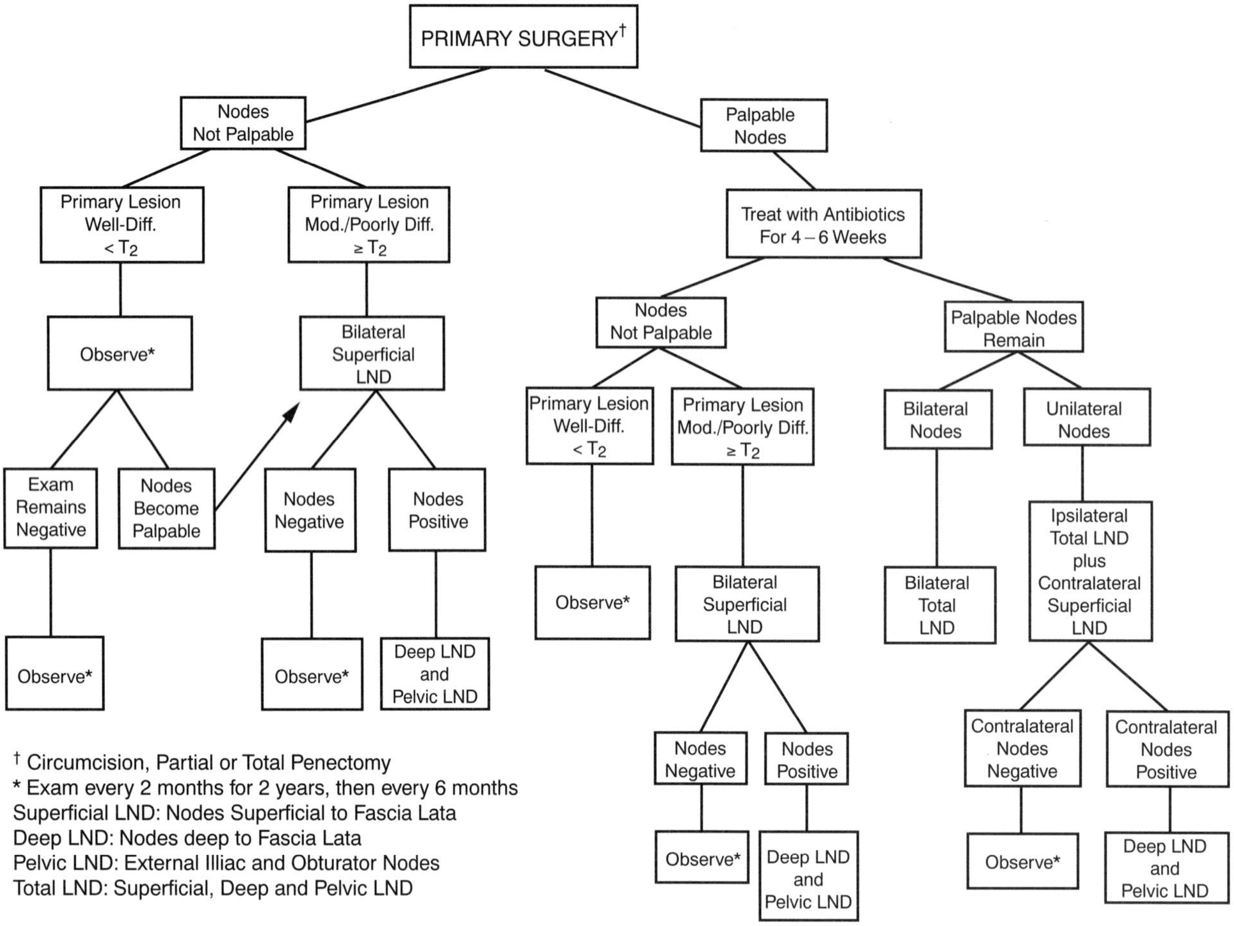
PRIMARY SURGERY†
Nodes Not Palpable
Palpable Nodes
Primary Lesion Well-Diff. < T2
Primary Lesion Mod./Poorly Diff. ≥ T2
Treat with Antibiotics For 4 – 6 Weeks
Observe*
Bilateral Superficial LND
Nodes Not Palpable
Palpable Nodes Remain
Primary Lesion Well-Diff. < T2
Primary Lesion Mod./Poorly Diff. ≥ T2
Bilateral Nodes
Unilateral Nodes
Exam Remains Negative
Nodes Become Palpable
Nodes Negative
Nodes Positive
Ipsilateral Total LND plus Contralateral Superficial LND
Observe*
Bilateral Superficial LND
Bilateral Total LND
Observe*
Observe*
Deep LND and Pelvic LND
Nodes Negative
Nodes Positive
Contralateral Nodes Negative
Contralateral Nodes Positive
† Circumcision, Partial or Total Penectomy
* Exam every 2 months for 2 years, then every 6 months
Superficial LND: Nodes Superficial to Fascia Lata
Deep LND: Nodes deep to Fascia Lata
Pelvic LND: External Illiac and Obturator Nodes
Total LND: Superficial, Deep and Pelvic LND
Observe*
Deep LND and Pelvic LND
Observe*
Deep LND and Pelvic LND

FIGURE 44–12. Algorithm for inguinal lymphadenectomy. (From Lynch DF, Schellhammer PF: Tumors of the penis. *In* Walsh PC, Retik AB, Stamey TA, Vaughan ED Jr [eds]: Campbell's Urology, 7th edition. Philadelphia, WB Saunders Co, in press, with permission.)

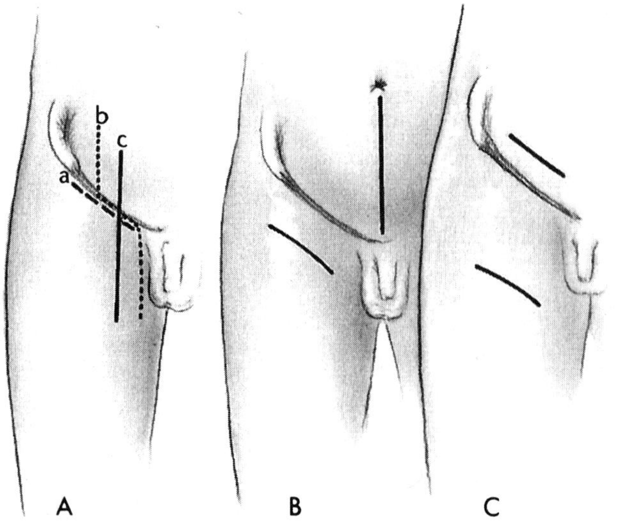
b
c
a
A
B
C

FIGURE 44–13. Incisions for radical inguinal lymphadenectomy. *A*, Single incision approaches: (a) oblique, (b) *S*-shaped, (c) vertical. *B*, Double incision, lower midline and inguinal. *C*, For unilateral pelvic lymphadenectomy, oblique abdominal incision combined with inguinal incision. (From Herr HW: Surgery of penile and urethral carcinoma. *In* Walsh PC, Retik AB, Stamey TA, Vaughan ED Jr [eds]: Campbell's Urology, 6th edition, p 3080. Philadelphia, WB Saunders Co, 1992, with permission.)

lowing antibiotic therapy, we proceed with bilateral ilioinguinal lymphadenectomy, using the classic limits of dissection. Some prefer to perform the pelvic node dissection first, aborting the inguinal dissection if grossly positive nodes are found.[14,38] Modern preoperative imaging procedures can often identify abnormal pelvic nodes preoperatively, however, allowing the surgeon to proceed from superficial to deep inguinal nodes, and then to the pelvic nodes if metastatic disease is encountered in the deep inguinal nodes.

In the event that one groin normalizes following antibiotic therapy but the other remains abnormal, we proceed with a superficial inguinal dissection on the normal side with frozen section evaluation. If this is negative, we proceed with a full ilioinguinal dissection on the contralateral abnormal side. Generally, pelvic node dissection is done through a low midline incision giving access to both right and left pelvic node groups (Fig. 44–13*B*). The dissection technique for this part of the operation is familiar to urologists because it is similar to that used in bladder cancer staging, except that the dissection of the external iliac nodes is carried more distally under the inguinal ligament to

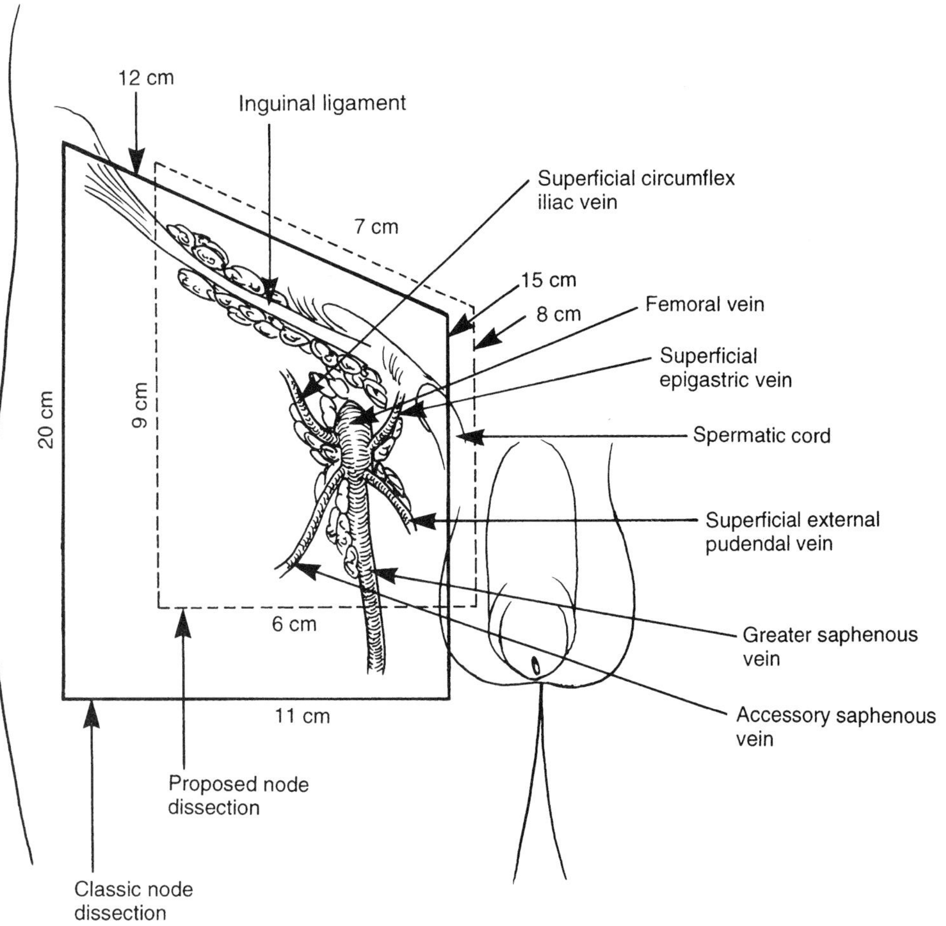
12 cm
Inguinal ligament
Superficial circumflex iliac vein
7 cm
15 cm
8 cm
Femoral vein
Superficial epigastric vein
20 cm
9 cm
Spermatic cord
Superficial external pudendal vein
6 cm
Greater saphenous vein
11 cm
Accessory saphenous vein
Proposed node dissection
Classic node dissection

FIGURE 44–14. Limits of the classic and modified inguinal lymphadenectomies. (From Puras A, Rivera J: Inguinal and pelvic lymphadenectomy for penile cancer. Atlas Urol Clin North Am 1995; 3:89, with permission.)

include all iliac and deep inguinal nodes there. If only one groin is involved, a unilateral pelvic node dissection may be done through an oblique low abdominal incision (Fig. 44–13C) and may provide some diminished patient morbidity.[39]

Modified Inguinal Lymphadenectomy

Although some patients with clinically negative groins will have impalpable metastatic disease, many will not. This coupled with the morbidity associated with the classic inguinal lymphadenectomies described by Daseler and Baranofsky has made surgeons reluctant to subject patients to these procedures, even when tumor characteristics indicate that lymphadenectomy would be advisable.[9,40] Both Catalona[37] and Puras and Rivera[41] have described modifications of the classic dissection that are aimed at reducing many of the unpleasant sequelae of the classic operation.

All patients are treated with 4 to 6 weeks of oral broad-spectrum antibiotics following excision of the primary tumor. A clear liquid diet the day prior to surgery is prescribed, and the patient is given cleansing enemas the night before surgery. Antiembolism compressive stockings are used.

The patient is placed in a supine position after spinal anesthesia is first administered. A Foley catheter is placed to straight drainage. The scrotum and penis are then retracted out of the field and draped off. The legs are then abducted and externally rotated to best expose the anteromedial thigh and groin. A pillow is placed beneath the knees for support. A 6- to 8-cm incision is then made 3 to 4 cm below the inguinal ligament and parallel to it (Fig. 44–15*A*). The incision is carried down to Scarpa's fascia and the plane immediately under Scarpa's fascia is developed. Gentle sponge traction is used to separate the skin edges (Fig. 44–15*B*). The subcutaneous tissue in Camper's layer is carefully preserved, and meticulous handling of these tissues and the skin edges must be observed throughout. Stay sutures of 2-0 or 3-0 silk and skin hooks are helpful to avoid injuring the wound edges.

The saphenous vein and its tributaries are iden-

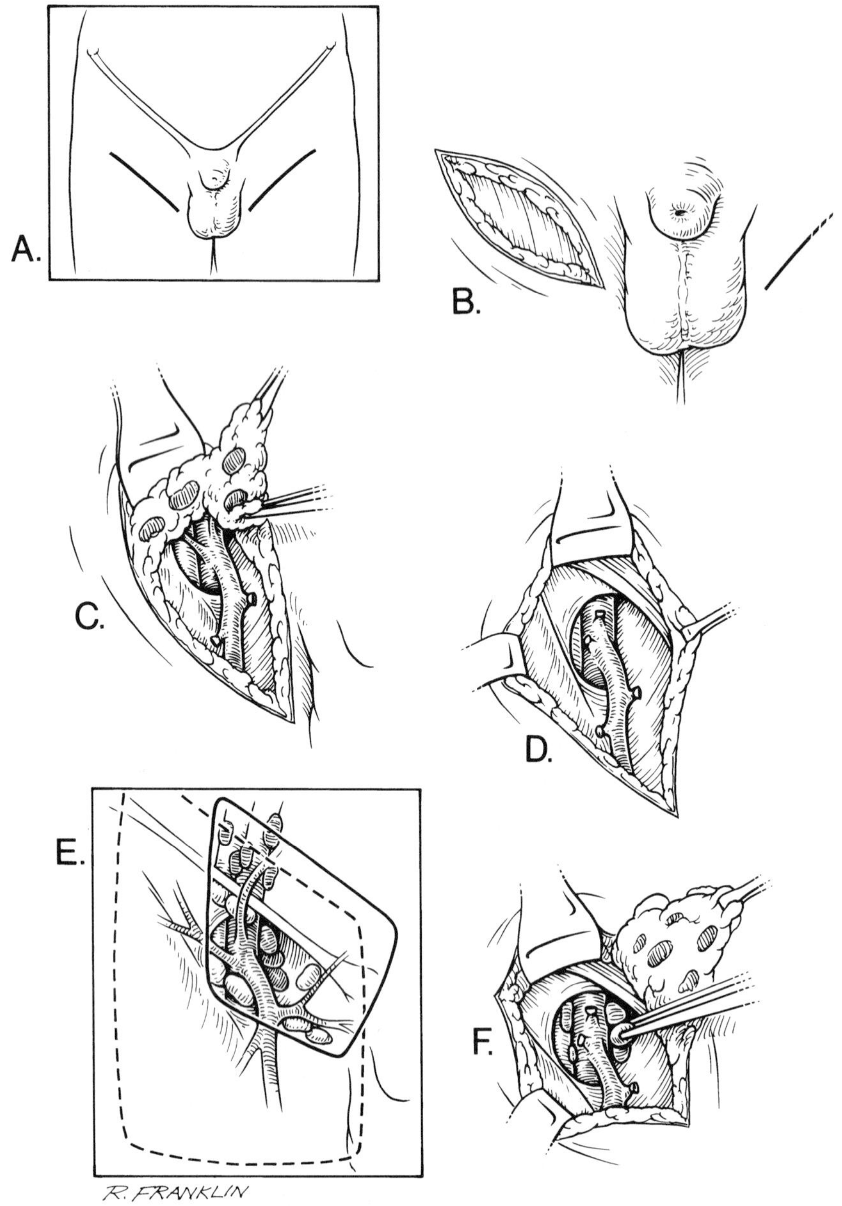
A.
B.
C.
D.
E.
F.
R. FRANKLIN

FIGURE 44–15. Technique of modified inguinal lymphadenectomy. *A*, Placement of inguinal incisions. *B*, Incising to Scarpa's fascia. *C*, Cephalad en bloc dissection of nodal package. Dissection of the saphenous vein with ligation of its tributaries. *D*, View following dissection of the superficial inguinal nodes. Fascia lata is intact. Dissection extends from 2 cm superior to the incision inferiorly to 4 cm below the lower edge of the incision. *E*, Catalona's modified inguinal lymphadenectomy. Lower dissection ends at the lower limit of the fossa ovalis. *F*, Detail of Catalona's dissection, when deep inguinal nodes are included. (Parts *A* through *D* from Puras A, Rivera J: Inguinal and pelvic lymphadenectomy for penile cancer. Atlas Urol Clin North Am 1995; 3:81, with permission; parts *E* and *F* from Catalona WJ: Modified inguinal lymphadenectomy for carcinoma of the penis with preservation of the saphenous veins: technique and preliminary results. J Urol 1988; 140:306, with permission. Copyright DF Lynch, Jr. and PF Schellhammer.)

tified, and the superficial areolar and node-bearing tissue is gently dissected off the vein downward to the fascia lata (Fig. 44–15*C*). The venous branches emptying into the saphenous vein are carefully ligated and divided. The saphenous vein is preserved (Fig. 44–15*D*). Particular attention is paid the tissue supermedial to the saphenous vein around the superficial epigastric vein because this is the area of the sentinel node tissue. Large lymphatics and small venous branches must be carefully and meticulously ligated or fulgurated. The dissection is carried superiorly to approximately 2 cm superior to the inguinal ligament, where it is carried down to the fascia of the external oblique muscle (Fig. 44–15*E*).

The dissection is carried inferiorly to about 4 cm below the incision. In the Catalona operation, the lower limit of dissection is the lower border of the fossa ovalis (Fig. 44–15*F*). We, as well as Puras and Rivera, carry our dissections slightly lower, although there is not much superficial nodal tissue in this area. The specimen of superficial nodal tissue is oriented, labeled by quadrant (Fig. 44–8), and sent for frozen section evaluation.

If the nodes are negative, the wound is thoroughly irrigated with sterile water and closed in layers, taking care to eliminate any potential spaces. A closed suction drainage system is placed (Fig. 44–16*D*) and remains for 5 to 7 days, during which time the patient is maintained at complete bed rest.

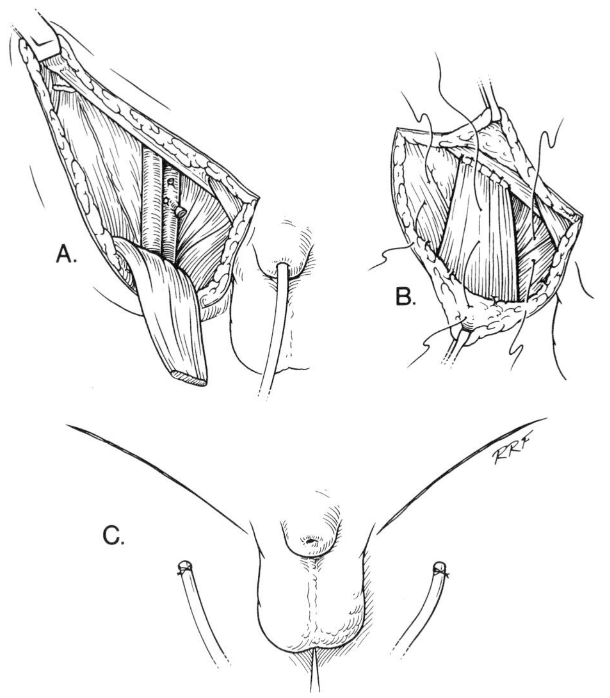
A.
B.
C.
RRF

FIGURE 44–16. Technique of classic inguinal lymphadenectomy. *A*, View following excision of the fascia lata, division of the saphenous vein, and dissection of the deep inguinal nodes. The sartorious muscle has been dissected free of its origin. *B*, Transposition of the sartorious muscle to cover the femoral vessels. Mattress sutures to muscle to close potential space to avoid lymphocele formation. *C*, Closed drainage system in place. This is maintained for 5 to 7 days. (Parts *A* and *C* from Puras A, Rivera J: Inguinal and pelvic lymphadenectomy for penile cancer. Urol Clin North Am 1995; 3:81, with permission; part *B* from Ferrigni RG, Novicki DE: Complications of lymphadenectomy in urologic surgery. Atlas Urol Clin North Am 1995; 3: 105. By permission of Mayo Foundation. Copyright DF Lynch, Jr. and PF Schellhammer.)

Classic Inguinal Lymphadenectomy (after Daseler)

When positive nodes are present or metastatic disease is confirmed by frozen section during a limited inguinal dissection, a classic radical inguinal lymphadenectomy is performed with the exception that the lateral limit is not carried to the anterior superior iliac spine because nodal tissue is not found there and the potential morbidity is increased.[9] An incision of 6 to 8 cm is made parallel to the inguinal ligament and about 3 to 4 cm inferior to it. The incision is carried down to Scarpa's fascia, and the saphenous vein is identified. This is ligated with 2-0 silk sutures and divided. The superficial nodal tissue is systematically mobilized, beginning in the superomedial quadrant, freeing the tissue toward the junction of the saphenous vein with the femoral vein at the fossa ovalis. The sentinel node tissue is identified and tagged with a suture. This dissection is extended above the inguinal ligament for 2 cm, and the limits of the standard dissection, as outlined in Figure 44–5, are utilized.

Next, the venous tributaries of the saphenous vein are meticulously ligated and divided, as well as any large lymphatics. The saphenous vein carefully dissected down to the fossa ovalis, and the junction with the femoral vein is identified, clamped, divided, and doubly ligated or suture ligated. The fascia lata is opened and excised with all the nodal tissue superficial to it. This exposes the femoral sheath and Scarpa's triangle. The lateral aspect of this dissection is the medial border of the sartorius, and the medial border of the adductor longus is the medial side.

The femoral sheath is opened from the inguinal ligament to the apex of the femoral triangle. Within the sheath are the femoral vein, the femoral artery lateral to it, and fatty areolar tissue containing the deep inguinal nodes medially (Fig. 44–6). The femoral nerve is lateral to the artery and is not encountered in the usual dissection (Fig. 44–16*A*). The vein is gently retracted laterally to allow dissection of tissue from the lateral and anterolateral aspect of the vein, and nodal and areolar tissue is dissected from the anterior artery and between the artery and vein. The nodes are dissected to below the inguinal ligament, to the node of Cloquet (or Rosenmüller), the most proximal of the deep inguinal chain. One to five nodes are usually encountered. About 5 to 8 cm below the inguinal ligament, the profunda femoris artery arises on the lateral aspect of the femoral artery. This must be carefully preserved, especially if myocutaneous flap coverage may later be required.

The wound is then irrigated carefully and careful attention is given to all bleeders and lymphatics. The sartorious muscle is separated sharply from its origin on the anterior superior iliac spine and mobilized medially to cover the now exposed femoral vessels[40,41] (Fig. 44–16*B*). Several sutures are used to secure Camper's fascia to the anterior aspect of the muscles to close potential space and discourage lymphocele formation[42] (Fig. 44–16*C*). The skin edges are carefully assessed, using intravenous fluorescein and the Wood's lamp if necessary, and any questionably viable skin is excised. Drainage using a closed suction catheter apparatus is placed, and the wound is then meticulously closed in layers (Fig. 44–16*D*).

The patient is maintained at complete bed rest with compressive stockings in place for 5 to 7 days. Subcutaneous heparin, begun prior to the procedure, is continued until the patient is ambulatory. The Foley catheter is discontinued after 24 to 48 hours. Closed suction is maintained for 5 days.

Management of Enlarged or Ulcerated Nodes and Femoral Vessel Involvement

Squamous cell carcinoma is characterized by aggressive local invasion into surrounding tissues. Large inguinal nodes, particularly when presented for treatment late or following an extended period of neglect, will have invaded the overlying skin of

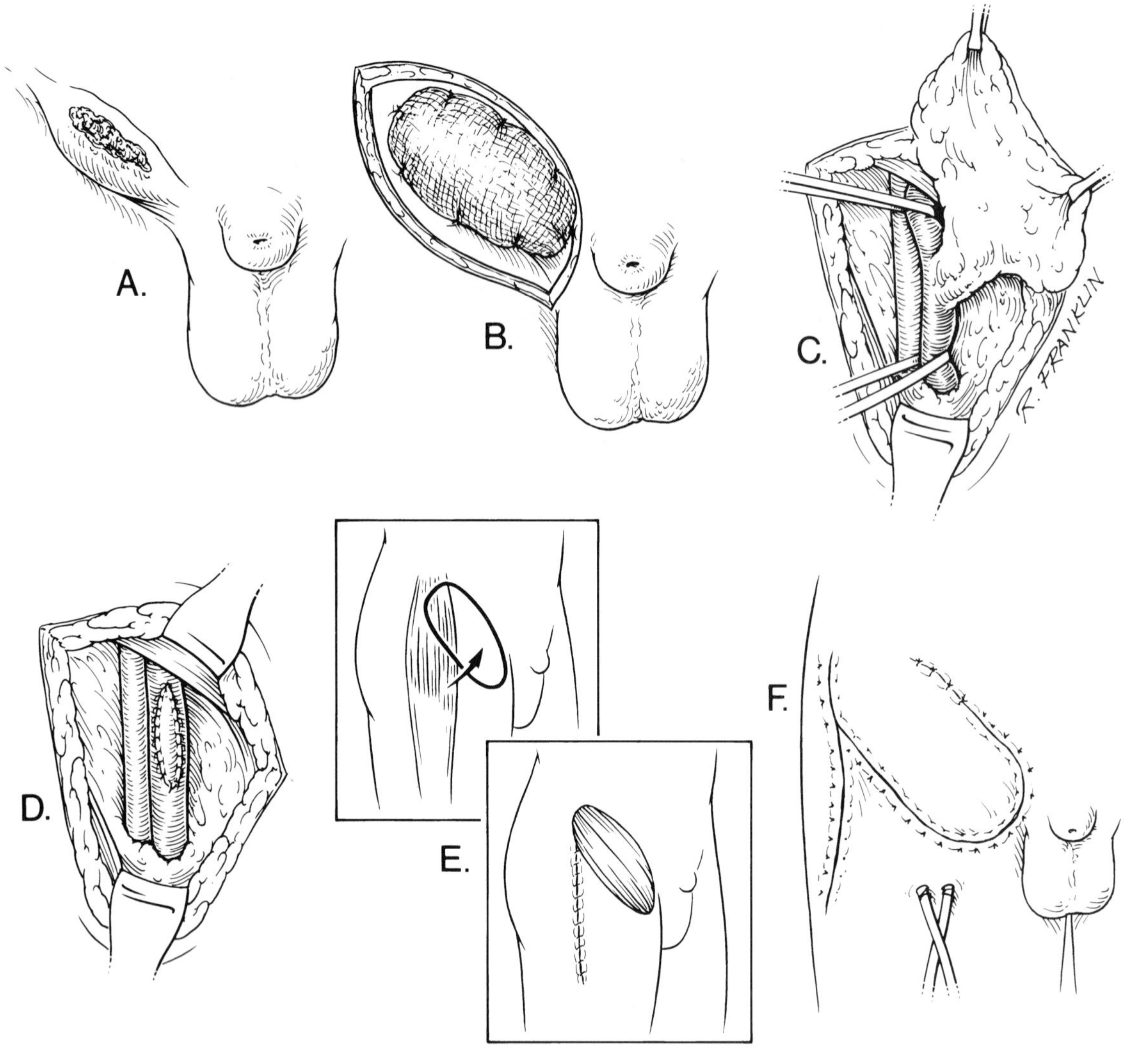
A.
B.
C.
R. FRANKLIN
D.
E.
F.

FIGURE 44–17. Excision of an enlarged, ulcerated node. *A*, Ulcerated node in groin. *B*, Tumor covered with gauze and dissected with a 2-cm margin of normal skin. *C*, Dissection of the femoral vessels with demonstration of tumor invasion of the femoral vein. *D*, View following excision of tumor with saphenous vein patch in place on the femoral vein. *E*, Rotation of tensor fascia lata as a myocutaneous flap to cover groin defect. *F*, Closure of groin with myocutaneous flap. (From Puras A, Rivera J: Inguinal and pelvic lymphadenectomy for penile cancer. Atlas Urol Clin North Am 1995; 3:81, with permission. Copyright DF Lynch, Jr. and PF Schellhammer.)

the groin and may ulcerate through it in extreme cases (Fig. 44–17*A*). Induration of the skin is suggestive of such local invasion. In this setting, the tumor is excised leaving a 2-cm margin of normal skin around the indurated or ulcerated area (Fig. 44–17*B*). A radical ilioinguinal lymphadenectomy is performed, and all tumor is completely resected.

In some instances, there may be involvement of the femoral vessels, particularly the vein. Resection of the anterior wall of the vein with reconstruction using a saphenous vein graft or Gore-Tex patch may be required[41] (Fig. 44–17*C* and *D*). In some instances of severe involvement, the vein may be ligated and excised.

Large skin defects may be closed with a tensor fascia lata or gracilis myocutaneous graft[43,44] (Fig. 44–17*E*). Such a graft may be based over the hip and swung medially and superiorly to cover a groin defect (Fig. 44–17*F*). Again, all postoperative precautions recommended for the classic radical lymphadenectomy should be employed for patients undergoing this procedure.

REFERENCES

1. Bissada NK: Conservative extirpative treatment of cancer of the penis. Urol Clin North Am 1992; 19:283.
2. Mohs FE, Snow SN, Messing EM, et al: Microscopically controlled surgery in the treatment of carcinoma of the penis. J Urol 1985; 133:961.
3. Fraley EE, Zhang G, Manivel C, et al: The role of ilioinguinal lymphadenectomy and the significance of histolog-

ical differentiation in the treatment of carcinoma of the penis. J Urol 1989; 142:1478.
4. McDougal WS: Carcinoma of the penis: improved survival by early regional lymphadenectomy based on the histological grade and depth of invasion of the primary lesion. J Urol 1995; 154:1364.
5. Ekstrom T, Edsmyr F: Cancer of the penis: a clinical study of 229 cases. Acta Chir Scand 1958; 115:25.
6. McDougal WS, Kirchner FK Jr, Edwards RH, et al: Treatment of carcinoma of the penis: the case for primary lymphadenectomy. J Urol 1986; 136:38.
7. Puras A, Gonzalez-Flores B, Rodriguez R: Treatment of carcinoma of the penis. *In* Stevenson HG (ed): Proceedings of the Kimbrough Urological Seminar, Vol 12, pp 143–152. Utica, NY, Bradock Press, 1979.
8. deSouza LJ: Subtotal amputation for carcinoma of the penis with reconstruction. Ann R Coll Surg 1976; 58:398.
9. Daseler E, Anson B, Riemann A: Radical excision of the inguinal and iliac lymph nodes. Surg Gynecol Obstet 1948; 87:679.
10. Rouviere HA: Anatomy of the Human Lymphatic System (Tobias MJ, trans). Ann Arbor, MI, Edward Bros, 1938.
11. Dewire D, Lepor H: Anatomic considerations of the penis and its lymphatic drainage. Urol Clin North Am 1992; 19: 211.
12. Riveros M, Garcia R, Cabanas RM: Lymphangiography of the dorsal lymphatics of the penis: technique and results. Cancer 1967; 20:2026.
13. Schreiner BF: Treatment of epithelioma of the penis based on a study of 60 cases. Radiology 1929; 13:353.
14. Srinivas V, Morse MJ, Herr HW, et al: Penile cancer: relation of extent of nodal metastases to survival. J Urol 1987; 137:880.
15. Horenblas S, Van Tinteren H, Dellemarre JFM, et al: Squamous cell carcinoma of the penis III. Treatment of regional lymph nodes. J Urol 1993; 149:492.
16. Kamat MR, Kulkani JN, Tongaonkar HB: Carcinoma of the penis: the Indian experience. J Surg Oncol 1993; 52:50.
17. Cabanas RM: An approach for the treatment of penile carcinoma. Cancer 1977; 39:456.
18. Perinetti EP, Crane DC, Catalona WJ: Unreliability of sentinel node biopsy for staging penile carcinoma. J Urol 1980; 124:734.
19. Wespes E, Simon J, Schulman CC: Cabanas approach: is sentinel lymph node biopsy reliable for staging penile carcinoma? Urology 1986; 28:278.
20. Fowler JE Jr: Sentinel lymph node biopsy for staging penile cancer. Urology 1984; 23:352.
21. Johnson DE, Lo RK: Management of regional lymph nodes in penile carcinoma: five-year results following therapeutic groin dissections. Urology 1984; 24:308.
22. Catalona WJ: Role of lymphadenectomy in carcinoma of the penis. Urol Clin North Am 1980; 7:85.
23. Narayana AS, Olney LE, Loening SA, et al: Carcinoma of the penis: analysis of 229 cases. Cancer 1982; 49:2185.
24. Lesser JH, Schwarz H II: External genital carcinoma: results of treatment at Ellis Fischel State Cancer Hospital. Cancer 1955; 8:1021.
25. Beggs JH, Spratt JS Jr: Epidermoid carcinoma of the penis. J Urol 1964; 91:166.
26. Fossa SD, Hall KS, Johanessen MB, et al: Carcinoma of the penis: experience at the Norwegian Radium Hospital: 1974–1985. Eur Urol 1987; 13:372.
27. Murrell DS, Williams JL: Radiotherapy in the treatment of carcinoma of the penis. Br J Urol 1965; 35:211.
28. Jensen MS: Cancer of the penis in Denmark: 1942 to 1962 (511 cases). Dan Med Bull 1977; 24:66.
29. Staubitz WJ, Melbourne HL, Oberkircher OJ: Carcinoma of the penis. Cancer 1955; 8:371.
30. Ornellas AA, Correia AL, Marota A, et al: Surgical treatment of invasive squamous cell carcinoma of the penis: retrospective analysis of 350 cases. J Urol 1994; 141:1244.
31. deKernion JB, Tynbery P, Persky L, et al: Carcinoma of the penis. Cancer 1973; 32:1256.
32. Skinner DG, Leadbetter WF, Kelley SB: The surgical management of squamous cell carcinoma of the penis. J Urol 1972; 107:273.
33. Hardner GJ, Bhanalaph T, Murphy GP, et al: Carcinoma of the penis: analysis of therapy in 100 consecutive cases. J Urol 1972; 108:428.
34. Smith JA, Middleton RG: The use of fluorescein in radical inguinal lymphadenectomy. J Urol 1979; 122:754.
35. Herr HW: Surgery of penile and urethral carcinoma. *In* Walsh PC, Retik AB, Stamey TA, Vaughan ED Jr (eds): Campbell's Urology, 6th edition, pp 3073–3089. Philadelphia, WB Saunders Co, 1992.
36. Lynch DF, Schellhammer PF: Tumors of the penis. *In* Walsh PC, Retik AB, Stamey TA, Vaughan ED Jr (eds): Campbell's Urology, 7th edition. Philadelphia, WB Saunders Co, in press.
37. Catalona WJ: Modified inguinal lymphadenectomy for carcinoma of the penis with preservation of the saphenous veins: technique and preliminary results. J Urol 1988; 140: 306.
38. Fowler JE: Mastery of Surgery: Urology. Boston, Little, Brown, 1991.
39. Spratt JS Jr, Shieber W, Dillard BM: Anatomy and Surgical Techniques of Groin Dissection. St. Louis, CV Mosby, 1965.
40. Baranofsky ID: Technique of inguinal node dissection. Surgery 1948; 24:555.
41. Puras A, Rivera J: Inguinal and pelvic lymphadenectomy for penile cancer. Urol Clin North Am 1995; 3:81.
42. Ferrigni RG, Novicki DE: Complications of lymphadenectomy in urologic surgery. Urol Clin North Am 1995; 3:105.
43. Hill HL, Nahai F, Vasconez LO: The tensor fascia lata myocutaneous free flap. Plast Reconstr Surg 1978; 61:517.
44. McCraw JB, Dibbell DG, Carraway JH: Clinical definition of independent myocutaneous vascular territories. Plast Reconstr Surg 1977; 60:341.

XI

PEDIATRIC MALIGNANCIES

45

NEUROBLASTOMA

MICHAEL C. CARR, M.D., PH.D. *and* MICHAEL E. MITCHELL, M.D.

Neuroblastoma is the second most common solid tumor in infants and children. Virchow, in 1864, was the first to speculate that its origin was neural, and he considered it a glioma.[1] Marchand, in 1891, noted the histologic similarities between neuroblastoma and developing sympathetic ganglia.[2] Following Wright's use of the term "neuroblastoma" in 1910, there has been little debate with regard to origin of the tumor. Herxheimer demonstrated in 1914 that fibrils in neuroblastoma stained with a specific neural silver stain, helping to establish the true origin of this tumor.[3] There was little published in the literature earlier this century, with Blacklock noting only 116 cases in the literature, to which he added 18 of his own.[4] At that time, neuroblastoma was fourth in order of frequency of malignant tumors in children. The number of cases described increased to 623 by 1953,[5] and today it remains the fourth most common malignancy in childhood, being less common than leukemia, brain tumors, and lymphoma.

Cushing and Wolbach, in 1927, reported for the first time a transformation of neuroblastoma into benign ganglioneuroma,[6] laying the foundation for a greater understanding of its biologic variability. Later descriptions noted that this event generally occurred in infants less than 6 months of age. Beckwith and Perrin noted microscopic foci of neuroblastoma cells in the adrenal glands in a number of infants under 3 months of age who died from other causes. These were termed "neuroblastoma in situ," and were estimated to occur approximately 40 times more frequently than the number of neuroblastoma cases clinically diagnosed. Recession of these foci appeared to be complete after 3 months of age.[7] Biochemical activity associated with neuroblastoma was initially noted as a result of elevated levels of urinary pressor amines.[8] It has subsequently been recognized that elevated levels of norepinephrine and its precursors and metabolites occur in patients with this tumor.

ETIOLOGY

Neuroblastoma develops from neural crest cells in the embryo. These cells give rise to sympathetic neuroblasts, which are found in the adrenal medulla, autonomic ganglia, and peripheral nerve sheaths. Other tumors that can arise from these cells include ganglioneuroma and ganglioneuroblastoma. The former may cause considerable morbidity secondary to spread to contiguous organs but does not metastasize. The latter is known to metastasize about 20% of the time and has greater malignant potential than ganglioneuroma.

Knudson and Strong, noting the apparent genetic influence, suggested that 20% of cases arise in children predisposed to the tumor by a dominant transmittable mutation.[9] Later work suggested that familial cases result from a prezygotic mutation and that nonfamilial cases result from a postzygotic somatic mutation.

Neuroblastomas are characterized cytogenetically by deletion of the short arm of chromosome 1, double-minute chromatin bodies (dmins) and homogeneously staining regions (HSRs).[10,11] The latter two abnormalities reflect gene amplification, whereas the former may represent deletion of a tumor suppressor gene. No other specific karyotypic abnormalities have been detected thus far.

Flow cytometry of DNA content provides a way of measuring total DNA content, which correlates with the modal chromosome number. Determination of the DNA index (DI) of neuroblastomas from infants provides important information that may be predictive of response to particular chemotherapeutic regimens as well as outcome.[12–14] Tumors with "hyperdiploid" DNA content (DI $\geq$ 1) are more likely to have lower stages of disease and to respond to cyclophosphamide and doxorubicin, whereas those with a "diploid" DNA content (DI = 1) are more likely to have advanced stages of disease and do not respond to this combination.[15] This analysis provides no information about specific chromosome rearrangements (deletions, translocation, or gene amplification), but does correlate with biologic behavior.

The discovery of extrachromosomal dmins and chromosomally integrated HSRs is a cytogenetic manifestation of gene amplification.[16,17] The region amplified is derived from the distal short arm of chromosome 2, containing the proto-oncogene N-*myc*. Brodeur and colleagues have demonstrated that N-*myc* amplification occurs in 25 to 30% of primary neuroblastomas from untreated patients, and amplification is associated primarily with advanced stages of disease.[18] Subsequent studies have shown that N-*myc* amplification was associated with rapid tumor progression and a poor prognosis. Amplification was found in only 5 to 10% of patients with low-stage disease or stage IV-S but in 30 to 40% of advanced disease patients.[19] It is almost always present at the time of diagnosis and, thus, appears to be an intrinsic biologic property in a distinct subset of patients with a poor prognosis.[20] There is a correlation between N-*myc* copy number and expression, and tumors with amplification express N-*myc* at much higher levels than are seen in tumors without amplification. Finally, there is heterogeneity in the level of expression among the tumors that have a single copy of N-*myc*, but higher expressing single-copy tumors do not appear to be a particularly aggressive subset.[21,22]

Deletions of the short arm of chromosome 1 are found in 70 to 80% of the near-diploid tumors that have been karyotyped. This cytogenetic finding is commonly associated with more advanced stages of disease, whereas tumors from patients with lower stages are more likely to be hyperdiploid or triploid, with very few structural rearrangements. The deletions of chromosome 1 are variable, but generally map to a region (1p36) that may contain a suppressor gene important in malignant transformation or progression. Recent molecular studies have shown a strong correlation between loss of heterozygosity for chromosome 1p and N-*myc* amplification, suggesting that these two events may be related.[23] An allelic loss on the long arm of chromosome 14 also has been noted, suggesting that there may be another suppressor gene involved in the pathogenesis of neuroblastomas.

INCIDENCE

Neuroblastoma accounts for 8 to 10% of all childhood tumors and is the most common malignant tumor of infancy. In the United States the incidence is 10.5 per million per year in white children and 8.8 per million per year in black children less than 15 years of age.[24,25] Male predominance is noted, but is slight (1.1:1). The incidence is underestimated because of the occurrence of spontaneous regression of neuroblastoma in situ. Approximately one third of cases are diagnosed in the first year of life and another quarter between 1 and 2 years of age. This is a younger age of presentation than that for Wilms' tumor. Unlike other childhood tumors, a low incidence of associated congenital anomalies exists. However, brain and skull defects have been noted in 2% of patients with neuroblastoma.[26] An association with neurofibromatosis and Hirschprung's disease has been noted.[27]

PATHOLOGY

Arising from primitive, pleuripotential sympathetic cells (sympathogonia) derived from the neural crest, neuroblastomas are found in a variety of locations. The adrenal medulla or cells in the adjacent retroperitoneal tissues on the posterior abdominal wall account for 50 to 80% of neoplasms in most reported series. The second most common location is within the posterior mediastinum, usually in paravertebral sites. The remaining neoplasms occur in derivatives of the neural crest within the pelvis, cervical region, and lower abdominal sympathetic chain, rarely within the posterior cranial fossa, or in other locations.

Macroscopically, the growths are lobular, and soft in consistency and weigh between 80 and 150 g. The cut surface is red-gray in color, and areas of hemorrhage and necrosis may be obvious as the tumor increases in size. Calcification is not infrequent, and this can help in the radiologic localization (Fig. 45–1).

Histologically, the cells are small and dark, like lymphocytes, and frequently are arranged in masses without any true pattern. It is one of the "small blue round cell" tumors of childhood. In characteristic lesions, rosettes are formed when the

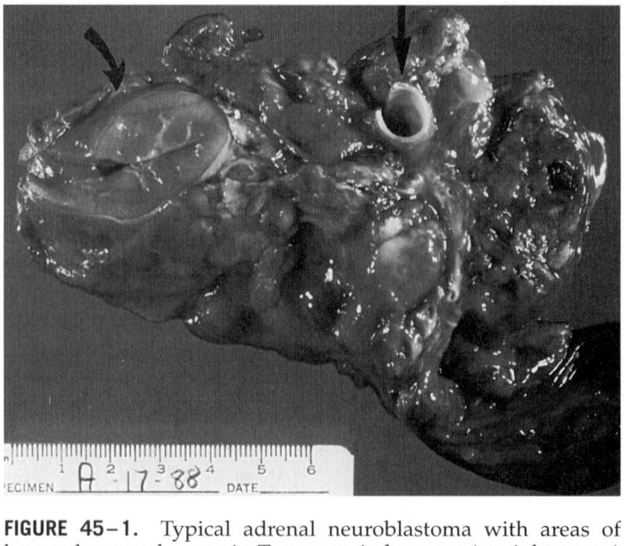

FIGURE 45–1. Typical adrenal neuroblastoma with areas of hemorrhage and necrosis. Tumor encircles aorta (straight arrow) with kidney seen at left (curved arrow). (Courtesy of Dr. Kathleen Patterson, Seattle, WA.)

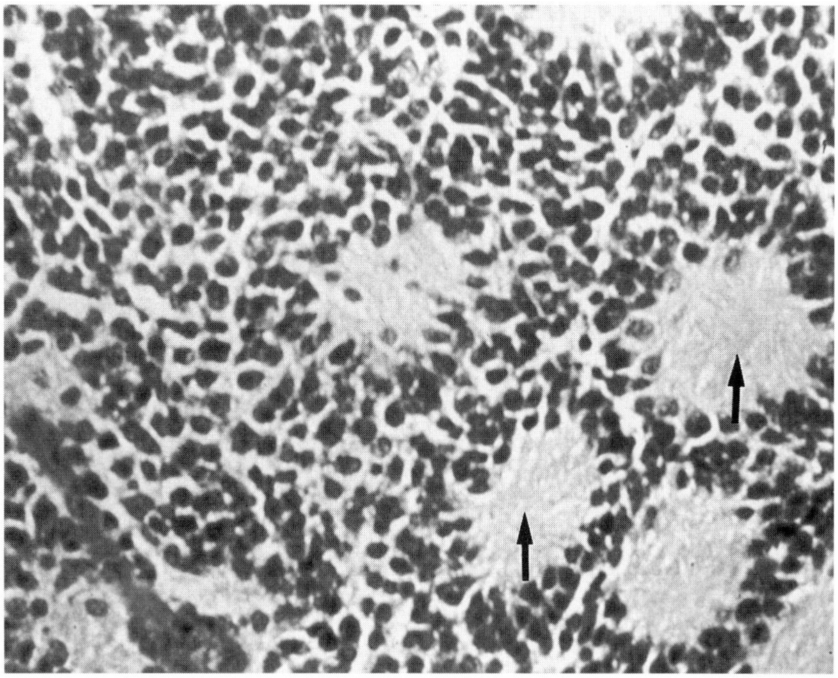

FIGURE 45–2. Histologically, the cells comprising neuroblastoma are small, with darkly staining nuclei and inconspicuous cytoplasm. Rosettes composed of tumor cells surround neuropil material (arrows). (Courtesy of Dr. Kathleen Patterson, Seattle, WA.)

tumor cells occupy the periphery and the young nerve fibrils grow into the center of each rosette (Fig. 45–2).

The fully differentiated, and benign, counterpart of neuroblastoma is the ganglioneuroma, composed principally of mature ganglia, neuropil, and schwannian cells. Ganglioneuroblastoma defines a heterogeneous group of tumors with histopathologic features reflecting the spectrum of maturation of neuroblastoma and ganglioneuroma. These may be either focal or diffuse, depending on the pattern seen, but diffuse ganglioneuroblastoma is associated with less aggressive behavior. Multiple sections should be examined to categorize these tumors accurately because viability and histopathologic features are variable.

Hematoxylin-eosin staining and light microscopy is often not enough to distinguish these tumors from other "small round blue cell" tumors of childhood. Immunohistochemical techniques and electron microscopy are helpful additions to light microscopy. Monoclonal antibodies recognizing neural filaments, synaptophysin, and neuron-specific enolase will stain neuroblastoma.[28] Electron microscopy visualizes the dense core and membrane-bound neural secretory granules in addition to microfilaments and parallel arrays of microtubules within the neuropil[29] (Fig. 45–3).

A histology-based prognostic classification that has gained widespread acceptance was developed by Shimada and colleagues.[30] The system is formulated around patient age and the following histologic features: the presence or absence of schwannian stroma, the degree of differentiation, and the mitosis-karyorrhexis index. A retrospective evaluation of the Shimada method in 295 patients treated by the Children's Cancer Study Group identified favorable and unfavorable patient subsets. The histologic patterns were independently predictive of outcome, whereas stage was prognostically less important than histologic grade.[31,32]

A simplified system has been devised, that predicts a favorable outlook based upon presence of calcification and a low mitotic rate ($\leq$10 mitoses/10 high power fields).[33] A grading system was developed for finding tumors with both features (grade 1), with the presence of only one of these features (grade 2), or the absence of both features (grade 3). When these grades were combined with age ($\leq$ 1 or > 1 year) and surgicopathologic staging, low- and high-risk groups emerged, that were clearly correlated with the Shimada favorable and unfavorable groups. Further prospective evaluation will be needed to assess either one of these classifications, taking into account histologic modifiers such as level of serum ferritin and neuron-specific enolase, N-*myc* copy number, and tumor DNA content.

PRESENTATION

Neuroblastoma most often presents as an abdominal mass (65% are discovered at the time of routine medical examination or by the parents). Infants tend to have more thoracic and cervical primary tumors. The tumor is usually asymmetric and located in the supraumbilical region, the hypochondrium, or the flank, often extending beyond the midline. Tumors that arise from the adrenal or suprarenal sympathetic chain are more lateral, whereas the medially located tumors may arise

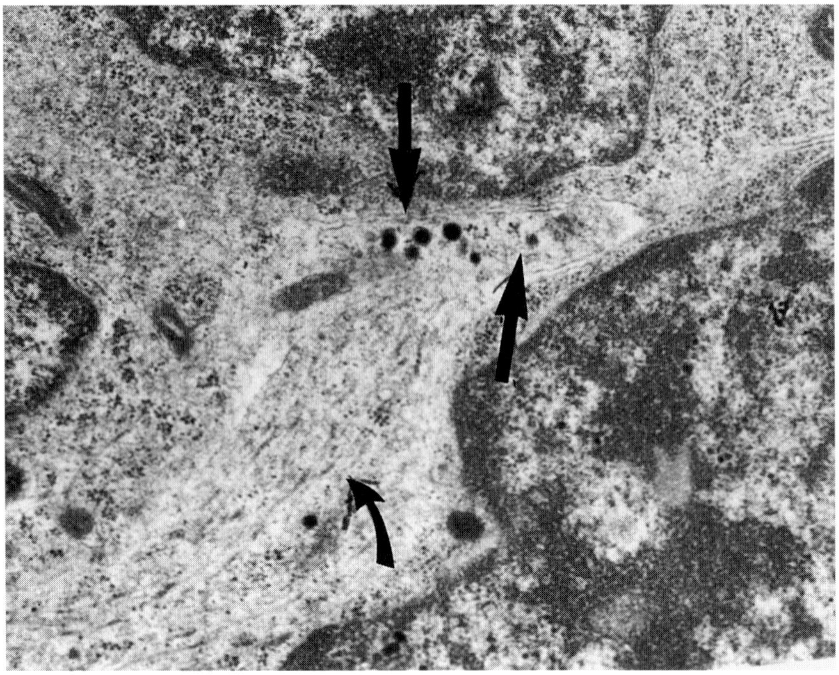

FIGURE 45–3. Electron microscopy showing dense core neural secretory granules (straight arrows) with microtubules (curved arrow) characteristic of neuroblastoma. (Courtesy of Dr. Kathleen Patterson, Seattle, WA.)

from the periaortic sympathetic chain. These tumors may then grow through the intervertebral foramina and produce spinal cord compression.

Neuroblastomas can arise from anywhere along the sympathetic chain; about 14% arise in the chest in infants over 1 year of age, but only 0.5% in the cervical region. Tumors arising from the cervical sympathetic ganglion may produce Horner's syndrome. In about 1% of patients, a primary tumor cannot be found. The majority of children with neuroblastoma are diagnosed by the age of 5 years, and it rarely occurs after age 10.

Metastatic extension of neuroblastoma occurs in two patterns, lymphatic and hematogenous. Regional lymph node metastasis will be noted in 35% of patients with apparently localized disease. Tumor spread to lymph nodes outside the cavity of origin is considered to be disseminated disease. These children may have a better prognosis if no other metastatic disease is found.[34] Hematogenous metastasis occurs most often to bone marrow, bone, liver, and skin. Rarely, disease may spread to lung and brain parenchyma, usually as a manifestation of relapsing or end-stage disease. The proportion of patients presenting with localized, regional, or metastatic disease is age dependent. The incidences for localized tumors, regional lymph node spread, and disseminated disease are 39, 18, and 25%, respectively, in infants (18% with stage 4S) compared to 19, 13, and 68%, respectively, in older patients.

The size and symptoms of neuroblastoma reflect the location of primary regional and metastatic disease. Complaints of fullness, discomfort, and, rarely, gastrointestinal tract dysfunction are due to abdominal disease. Bowel and bladder dysfunction can result from tumors arising from the organ of Zuckerkandl. Massive involvement of the liver in metastatic disease (Pepper syndrome) is particularly frequent in infants and may result in respiratory compromise.

Several classic signs and symptoms have been associated with metastatic neuroblastoma. Proptosis and periorbital ecchymosis are frequent and result from retrobulbar and orbital infiltration with tumor. Hutchinson syndrome describes widespread bone marrow and bone disease, causing bone pain, limping, and irritability in the younger child. Skin involvement is seen exclusively in infants with Evan's stage IV-S tumors[35] and is characterized by nontender, bluish subcutaneous nodules. Disseminated disease may manifest as failure to thrive and fever, the latter observed most often in the presence of bone metastasis. These are usually seen as lytic lesions on skeletal radiographs. Rarely, patients may present with the complications of catecholamine secretion by the neuroblastoma, which may include headache, hypertension, palpitations, and diaphoresis. The tumor may also lead to watery diarrhea secondary to vasoactive intestinal polypeptide.

DIAGNOSTIC EVALUATION

Minimum criteria for establishing the diagnosis of neuroblastoma include[36]

1. An unequivocal pathologic diagnosis made from tumor tissue by standard methods, including immunohistology or electron microscopy if necessary.
2. Bone marrow containing unequivocal tumor

cells (i.e., syncytia) and urine containing increased urinary catecholamine metabolites (>3 standard deviations above the mean, corrected for age).

Because neuroblastoma often secretes catecholamines, urinary levels of vanillylmandelic acid (VMA) or homovanillic acid (HVA) should be elevated.[37] A 24-hour urine collection was previously recommended, but normalizing VMA and HVA excretion to the milligram of creatinine in the sample makes a timed collection unnecessary and it avoids false-negative results caused by dilution.

Table 45–1 outlines the minimum testing to define the clinical stage of disease.[36] The evaluation often begins with an abnormal ultrasound, which demonstrates the mass and distinguishes a solid mass from a hydronephrotic kidney. It can also demonstrate lymph node enlargement, tumor extension, and liver metastasis, although computed tomography (CT) or magnetic resonance imaging (MRI) provide greater sensitivity (Figs. 45–4 through 45–6).

Most centers in the United States rely upon ^{99m}Tc-labeled diphosphonate scintigraphy for the evaluation of bone disease. Because of the biochemical activity of neuroblastoma, *meta*-iodobenzylguanidine scintigraphy becomes an attractive tool.[38] The compound is taken up by catecholaminergic cells, which include most neuroblastomas. Thus it becomes a very specific and sensitive method of assessing the primary tumor and focal metastatic disease.

There exists great variability in the number of bone marrow aspirates or biopsies done at different institutions. Data support the increased yield of bone marrow biopsies versus aspirates.[39] The international conferees on neuroblastoma staging recommended two bone marrow aspirates and two biopsies—that is, one of each from each of the posterior iliac crests.[36]

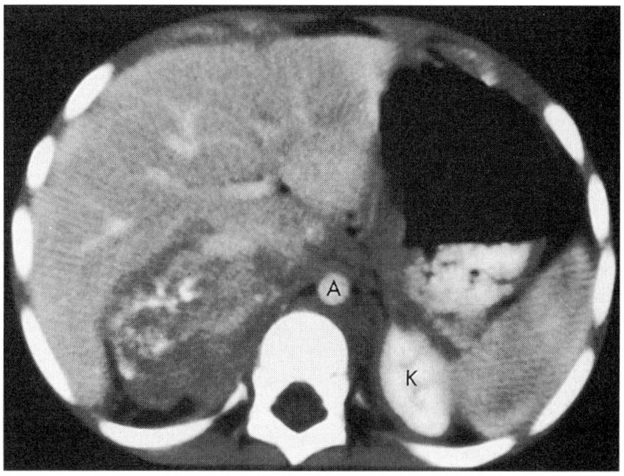
A
K

FIGURE 45–4. CT scan of 4-year-old with intravenous contrast showing right adrenal neuroblastoma with diffuse calcification, seen adjacent to liver. A, aorta; K, left kidney. (Courtesy of Dr. Edward Weinberger, Seattle, WA.)

STAGING

The current, favored staging system is based on clinical, radiographic, and surgical evaluation of children with neuroblastoma. The International Neuroblastoma Staging System (INSS) allows for uniformity in staging of patients, facilitating clinical trials and biologic studies around the world[36] (Table 45–2).

TABLE 45–1. MINIMUM RECOMMENDED TESTS FOR DETERMINING EXTENT OF DISEASE*,†

Tumor Site	Tests
Primary	Three-dimensional measurement of tumor by CT scan, MRI, or ultrasound
Metastases	Bilateral posterior iliac bone marrow aspirates and core biopsies (4 adequate specimens necessary to exclude tumor)
	Bone radiographs and either scintigraphy by ^{99m}Tc-labeled diphosphonate or ^{131}I- (or ^{123}I-) *meta*-iodobenzylguanidine (MIBG) or both
	Abdominal and liver imaging by CT scan, MRI, or ultrasound
	Chest radiograph (anteroposterior and lateral) and chest CT scan
Markers	Quantitative urinary catecholamine metabolites (VMA and HVA)

*From Brodeur GM, Castleberry RP: Neuroblastoma. *In* Pizzo PA, Poplack DG (eds): Principles and Practice of Pediatric Oncology, 2nd edition, p 750. Philadelphia, JB Lippincott, 1993, with permission.

†Note: For evaluation of bone metastases, ^{99m}Tc-labeled diphosphonate scintigraphy is recommended for all patients and is essential if MIBG scintigraphy is negative in bone.

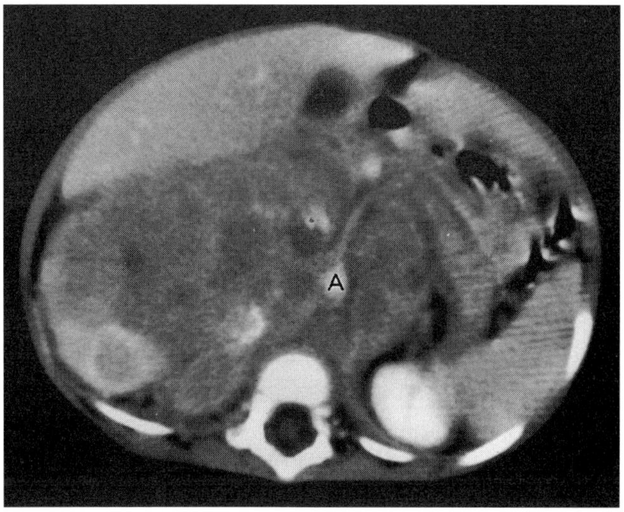
A

FIGURE 45–5. CT scan of 1-year-old with intravenous contrast showing extensive right adrenal neuroblastoma invading into right kidney, encircling aorta (A), and extending beyond the midline. (Courtesy of Dr. Edward Weinberger, Seattle, WA.)

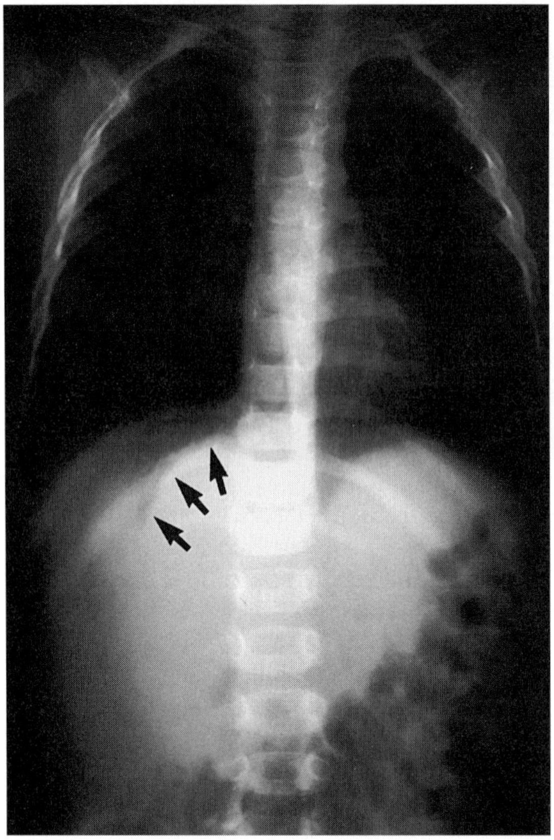

A

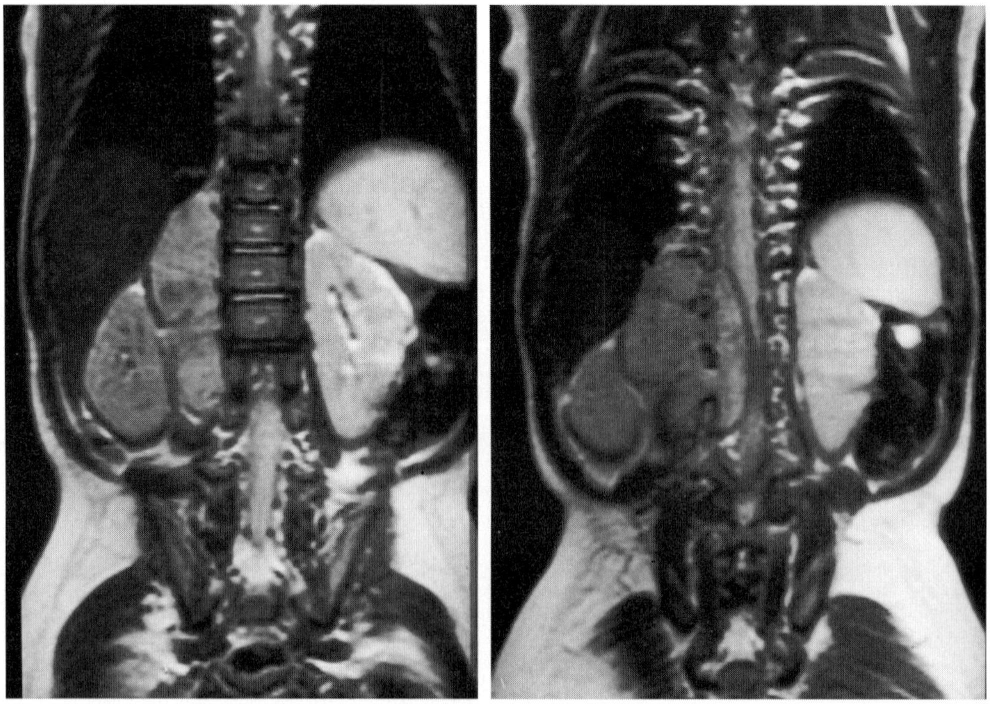

B C

FIGURE 45–6. Chest x-ray with subtle right paravertebral curvilinear stripe (arrowheads) raising possibility of right paravertebral mass. *B* and *C*, Coronal T1-weighted MRI images. *B* represents a more posterior view showing large mass between right kidney and vertebral bodies. *C* demonstrates multilobulated right paravertebral mass extending through three contiguous neural foramina into spinal canal with effacement of spinal cord. (Courtesy of Dr. Edward Weinberger, Seattle, WA.)

PROGNOSTIC CONSIDERATIONS

Stage of disease, the age of the patient at diagnosis, and site of the primary tumor are the most important clinical variables.[40–42] The overall prognosis of patients with stage 1, 2, and 4S is between 75 and 90%, whereas those with stage 3 and 4 have only a 10 to 30% 2-year disease-free survival. Age

TABLE 45-2. INTERNATIONAL NEUROBLASTOMA STAGING SYSTEM

Stage	Description
1	Localized tumor confined to the area of origin; complete gross excision, with or without microscopic residual disease; identifiable ipsilateral and contralateral lymph nodes negative microscopically
2A	Unilateral tumor with incomplete gross excision; identifiable ipsilateral and contralateral lymph nodes negative microscopically
2B	Unilateral tumor with complete or incomplete gross excision; with positive ipsilateral regional lymph nodes; identifiable contralateral lymph nodes negative microscopically
3	Tumor infiltrating across the midline with or without regional lymph node involvement; *or*, unilateral tumor with contralateral regional lumph node involvement; *or*, midline tumor with bilateral lymph node involvement
4	Dissemination of tumor to distant lymph nodes, bone, bone marrow, liver, and/or other organs (except as defined in stage 4S)
4S	Localized primary tumor as defined for stage 1 or 2 with dissemination limited to liver, skin, and/or bone marrow

is a sufficient prognostic variable, with the outcome of infants under 1 year of age being substantially better than the outcome of those greater than 1 year. Origin of the tumor is another important variable because patients with adrenal primaries have poorer outcomes than those with primaries from other origins.

A number of biologic variables have been assessed that may help predict the ultimate outcome for a patient. Histology, serum ferritin, neuron-specific enolase, gangliocyte G_{D2}, lactate dehydrogenase (LDH), DNA index, N-*myc* amplification, and deletion of chromosome 1p all have been described to provide clues of clinical behavior.[43,44]

TREATMENT

Surgery

As with most solid malignant neoplasms, complete surgical removal is the most effective form of therapy. Surgery is also used to make a diagnosis, provide tissue for biologic studies, surgically stage the tumor, and attempt excision of the tumor. Delayed primary or second-look surgery determines the response to therapy.

Based upon the INSS criteria, the operative protocol incorporates the following:

1. The resectibility of primary or metastatic tumor should be determined in light of tumor location, mobility, relationship to major vessels, ability to control blood supply, and overall prognosis of patient. Modern chemotherapy effectively consolidates and decreases the size of primary tumors and large lymph node metastases. Therefore, there is little place for the less predictable surgical assaults of previous years.

2. Nonadherent, intracavitary lymph nodes should be sampled. Gross examination during surgery may be inaccurate for detecting or ruling out lymph node metastasis in up to 25% of cases.[45] Lymph nodes adherent to and removed en bloc with the primary tumor do not alter the outcome of the patient.[46] Ideally, lymph nodes superior and inferior to the primary tumor should be sought and sampled, and their location documented. Lymph node sampling in patients with high thoracic, low cervical, or large abdominal primary tumors that are unresectable may be problematic. Other prognostic factors may be utilized in these situations, and, thus, the value of additional information regarding lymph node involvement is questionable.

3. Routine biopsy of the liver in situations involving an abdominal neuroblastoma without evidence of metastatic disease has been advocated. This practice has come into question, particularly because of the sensitivity of clinical staging by CT or MRI. Until the INSS criteria for staging are prospectively studied in all age groups, routine biopsy of liver during initial surgery in patients with primary abdominal tumors remains appropriate.

The surgical approach to neuroblastoma is best regarded as a vascular-type procedure. Neuroblastoma rarely invades the tunica media of large blood vessels but can involve the tunica adventitia. The appropriate plane of dissection usually exists beneath the tunica adventitia. Following partial exposure of the circumference of each vessel, the tumor is segmentally removed as complete vessel dissection occurs.[47]

The approach to an extensive *left-sided* abdominal tumor or preaortic tumor is through a long, supraumbilical, transverse incision. The left colon is reflected medially, followed by mobilizing of spleen, stomach, and pancreas. This is best accomplished by maintaining the plane between the mesocolon and Gerota's fascia. The viscera are reflected as far as the midline and placed in an intestinal bag, so that the tumor is exposed.

The first stage of the operation involves exposure of the arterial wall from below the distal limit of the tumor to just above the proximal limit of the tumor. The origin of the main visceral arteries are often noted at this time. Further dissection focuses on the distal extent of the tumor, along the external or common iliac artery. The surgeon and an assistant each pick up the adventitia, allowing longitudinal dissection along the middle of the vessel. The subadventitial plane has been entered, establishing the plane for the remainder of the operation. Proximal dissection proceeds to the tumor, incising along the middle of the vessel down to tunica media. Bipolar cautery is of considerable benefit.

Sympathetic nerves on the left will be transected, and an attempt should be made to preserve the nerves on the right. The aortic bifurcation is encountered and the dissection proceeds to the inferior mesenteric artery. If there is a large bulk of tumor, retrograde dissection may be helpful. Further dissection cephalad leads to the origin of the gonadal arteries and left renal vein crossing the aorta at the same level. Considerable tumor bulk can be encountered in this area. It is usually possible to identify the vein before entering the lumen. Dissection of 4 to 5 cm of vein will allow for retraction and adequate dissection beneath the aorta. Aortic dissection may be difficult at this level because of tumor adherence and the two gonadal arteries. Dividing the gonadal arteries and maintenance of the appropriate plane of dissection allow for safe dissection. Cephalad to the vein is the origin of the left renal artery, and just proximal to this is the superior mesenteric artery (SMA). Thus, at the level of the renal artery, the plane of dissection should become perpendicular to the anterolateral wall of the artery rather than directly anteriorly. This plane is then maintained as far as the diaphragm, where normal tissue is usually encountered.

With clearing of the anterior surface of the proximal aorta, the origins of the celiac artery and SMA are identified. These vessels are exposed and cleared, with the SMA usually being the easier vessel to dissect free. Once this artery is mobilized, the celiac and its branches are given attention. This area can be difficult, but by dissecting as before and maintaining the subadventitial plane, success is achieved. Frequently, two diaphragmatic branches arise from the trunk of the celiac artery or just proximally from the aorta, and these are divided. The left gastric artery may also be sacrificed without concern. Once the two main intestinal arteries are immobilized, the right side of the aorta may be exposed, with the right renal artery next being encountered. The tumor at this location may be attached posteriorly to the crus of the hemidiaphragm. Once its main attachments are divided, the tumor is removed. The tumor that has been attached between the celiac and SMA usually adheres to the posterior surface of the pancreas as well. In dissecting this from the pancreas, the termination of the splenic vein and its junction with the superior mesenteric vein are exposed. It is uncommon to see dense adherence in this region.[47] Following the removal of the preaortic tumor proximally, the left renal artery should be exposed and dissected free. This can be fairly tedious but is possible. When tumor is deep within the renal hilum, nephrectomy may be necessary. Once the renal artery is displayed, the primary tumor can be mobilized and excised. The remaining areas to be cleared lie below the level of the renal vessels and posterior to the length of the aorta. These areas do not present any unusual difficulty. As many as possible of the lumbar arteries should be preserved, but no untoward consequences have followed division of up to five arteries.[47] Finally, if there is considerable tumor bulk posterior to the inferior vena cava, reflection of the ascending colon may be necessary to achieve complete tumor clearance.

In general, thoracic procedures become more an exercise of rib clearance rather than a vascular-type operation. Pelvic tumors may provide some difficulty with regard to access. An extended Pfannenstiel-type incision, altered in that the recti are detached from the pubis, provides optimal exposure, but access may still be difficult. The anatomy is complicated by the presence of nerves of the sacral plexus, particularly with formal dissection of the internal iliac vessels. Once again, formal systematic and planned exposure of the important structures before tumor removal is of great value.[47]

Surgical complication rates in neuroblastoma range from 5 to 25%.[48, 49] The incidence increases in instances of aggressive abdominal resection of tumors at diagnosis. Reported complications include nephrectomy, hemorrhage, postoperative intussusception or adhesions, injury to renal vessels with subsequent renal failure, and neurologic defects, such as Horner's syndrome. Avoidance of surgical risk in infants who have better survival is recommended. Downstaging of the tumor with chemotherapy followed by surgical resection is the favored approach.

Chemotherapy

The mainstay of management in neuroblastoma is chemotherapy. A number of effective chemotherapeutic agents have been identified, including cyclophosphamide, cisplatin, doxorubicin, vincristine, etoposide, and teniposide, which alone yield complete response or partial response rates ranging from 34 to 45%. A combination of agents are used to take advantage of drug synergism, mechanisms of cytotoxicity, and differences in side effects. Cyclophosphamide and cisplatin are non–cell-cycle-specific agents often used in combination with cell cycle–dependent drugs (doxorubicin, teniposide). Using these combinations has resulted in improved response rates in children with advanced neuroblastoma. The chemotherapy is given in phases, which include induction, consolidation, and maintenance. The recently closed Children's Cancer Study Group 3881 protocol included the use of cisplatin, etoposide, doxorubicin, and cyclophosphamide. Typically, induction chemotherapy lasts 127 days, followed by 28 days of consolidation. It is during this period that the primary tumor is surgically resected. Unresectable primary and metastatic tumor is irradiated, and one course of chemotherapy is given to control micrometastasis during the debulking phase. Phase 3 is the maintenance phase (113 days), during which additional chemotherapy is given to all patients who do not have progressive disease following surgery and radiation. Those patients who had residual disease following their initial surgery will undergo surgical exploration in order to achieve a complete response and to determine whether active neuroblastoma is present. Metastatic lesions are biopsied to look for evidence of active disease.

Treatment Based on Risk Group

In recent years, the trend has been to group patients into prognostic categories based upon outcome data so that therapy is developed that accounts for risk of recurrent disease. Thus, patients with similar risk are then treated in a similar manner. The risk categories continue to evolve as a better understanding of tumor biology is obtained and more effective treatment strategies are developed. Based upon an extensive evaluation by the Pediatric Oncology Group (POG), three distinct risk groups (low, intermediate, and high) emerged.[50] The POG stages have been converted to INSS stages, with age stratification being infants less than or equal to 1 year versus children greater than 1 year.

Treatment of Low-Risk Disease

The following patients comprise this group: infants and children with localized and resected tumors (INSS stage 1) and partially resected tumors (INSS stage 2A), infants with regional disease (INSS stage 2B/3), and infants with INSS stage 4S disease (over 8 weeks of age). Complete surgical resection (stage 1) affords a disease-free survival of greater than 90% so that chemotherapy is needed only in the event of recurrence.[51] Surgery and minimal postoperative chemotherapy are required for all patients with INSS stage 2A and infants with INSS stage 2B/3 disease.[52] Radiation therapy is reserved for those patients who fail to respond to either primary or secondary chemotherapy. Management of infants with INSS 4S tumors is not standardized but may involve minimal chemotherapy and local radiation.

Treatment of Intermediate-Risk Disease

This group comprises children with metastatic disease to regional lymph nodes only (INSS stages 2B/3) and infants with INSS stage 4 tumors. Moderately aggressive chemotherapy and radiation have led to improvement in disease-free survival.[48] Intensive multiagent chemotherapy, along with irradiation of metatastic sites in selected patients, led to an event-free survival of 75% in infants with INSS stage 4 disease.[53] A further cooperative study of a similar group of patients combining chemotherapy and delayed removal of the primary tumor demonstrated 60% disease-free survival.[54]

TABLE 45–3. DISEASE-FREE SURVIVAL (2 YEARS) BASED UPON RISK CATEGORY AND AGE*

Risk Category	Patient Age (Yr)	INSS Stage	2-Year Disease-Free Survival (%)	Ref.
Low	All	1	>90	51
	All	2A	85	36
	<1	2B/3	87/89	†
	<1	4S	57–90	57,58
Intermediate	>1	2B/3	59	48
	<1	4	75	53
High	>1	4	40/15‡	56

*Modified from Brodeur GM, Castleberry RP: Neuroblastoma. *In* Pizzo PA, Poplack DG (eds): Principles and Practice of Oncology, 2nd edition, p 759. Philadelphia, JB Lippincott, 1993, with permission.

†R.P. Castleberry, personal observation.

‡Difference relates to complete versus partial surgical resection, respectively.

Treatment of High-Risk Disease

INSS stage 4 patients are those patients with disseminated disease. Intensification of treatment has included multiagent therapy of various combinations, but overall survival has remained disappointingly low (less than 15%). Therefore, the use of high-dose chemotherapy, surgery, intraoperative radiation, and bone marrow transplantation has resulted in 3-year survival rates showing definite improvement.[55] Benefit has been shown in complete surgical resection combined with aggressive chemotherapy, radiation, and bone marrow transplantation versus patients with only partial surgical resection (3-year survival of 40% versus 15%).[56] These single institutional studies await confirmation by other centers before definite conclusions can be drawn (see Table 45–3 for summary).

Radiation Therapy

Despite the radiosensitive nature of neuroblastoma in culture models, clinical response has been variable.[59] Historically, radiation has been used in the multimodality management of residual neuroblastoma, bulky unresectable tumors, and disseminated disease. More recent experience has demonstrated the efficacy of radiation in children with regional lymph node metastases (INSS stages 2B and 3),[48] in infants with isolated metastatic involvement of liver (INSS stage 4S) to initiate spontaneous tumor regression,[60] or in instances of total body irradiation in doses of 7.5 to 12 Gy as a precursor for autologous bone marrow transplantation.[61–63]

FUTURE CONSIDERATIONS

The identification of various prognostic markers of neuroblastoma allows for a more precise determination of biologic potential. A statistically significant association has been noted with tumors of low histologic grade along with a DI of more than 1 (hyperdiploid), a single copy of N-*myc* gene per haploid genome, and a serum LDH level of less than 1500 IU/L. High histologic grade was associated with a DI of 1, an amplified N-*myc* gene, and a serum LDH level of 1500 IU/L or more, factors that are associated with aggressive behavior.[64] The use of these prognostic factors allows for appropriate risk-specific therapy and the development of optimal treatment protocols for childhood neuroblastoma. Prospective studies are underway to confirm these findings with the addition of serum ferritin level (150 mg/ml or less)[65] as a further prognostic marker.

Identification of individuals who are predisposed to develop the tumor has become increasingly important. Cytogenetic studies have demonstrated alterations of chromosome 1p, reaching a frequency of more than 70%.[66] Alterations of 1p are also seen in significant frequency in other types of cancers, including colon cancer, alveolar rhabdomyosarcoma, hepatoblastoma, and ductal carcinoma of the breast.[67] Progress is being made that should reveal whether specific genetic information is commonly altered in neuroblastomas and, if so, what its significance is for tumorigenesis.

Urinary catecholamine metabolites are commonly elevated in neuroblastoma, but unfortunately are not as reliable tumor markers as α-fetoprotein or β-human chorionic gonadotropin for following germ cell tumors. Other markers, such as serum ferritin, neuron-specific enolase, and chromogranin A, have been identified, but none has proven superior. With greater understanding of the tumor biology, new markers may be identified that could prove useful for following response to therapy as well as early relapse.

Treatment strategies continue to evolve as clinical response improves. The goals now are to maximize the response and yet minimize the overall morbidity of treatment. This includes incorporating new principles of chemotherapy, such as continuous infusion of agents including doxorubicin, cisplatin, and etoposide. The current Children's Cancer Study Group study is comparing response using intensive high-dose consolidation therapy in order to eliminate residual tumor with chemoradiotherapy followed by bone marrow transplantation. Adjuvent postintensive therapy with a biologic response modifier, the differentiating agent 13-*cis*-retinoic acid, is being tested for effect on relapse after cytoreduction. The knowledge gained from the ongoing biologic studies will continually be applied to the clinical arena, as mechanisms of neuroblastoma transformation and progression are elucidated.

REFERENCES

1. Virchow R: Die Krankenhaften Geschwulste, 11:149. Berlin, Hirschwald, 1864.
2. Marchand F: Beitrage zur Kenntniss der normalen und pathologischen Anatomic der Glandula carotica und der Nebennieren Festschriff fur Rudolph. Virchows Arch 1891; 5:578.
3. Herxheimer G: Uebur Tumoren des Nebennierenmarkes, insbesondere das Neuroblastoma sympaticum. Beitr Pathol Anat 1914; 57:112.
4. Blacklock JWS: Neurogenic tumours of the sympathetic system in children. J Pathol Bacteriol 1934; 39:27–48.
5. Phillips R: Neuroblastoma. Ann R Coll Surg Engl 1953; 12: 29–47.
6. Cushing H, Wolbach SB: The transformation of a malignant paravertebral sympathicoblastoma into a benign ganglioneuroma. Am J Pathol 1927; 3:203.
7. Beckwith J, Perrin E: In situ neuroblastoma: a contribution to the natural history of neural crest tumors. Am J Pathol 1963; 43:1089.
8. Mason GH, Hart-Nercer J, Miller EJ, et al: Adrenaline-secreting neuroblastoma in an infant. Lancet 1957, 2:322.
9. Knudson AGJ, Strong LC: Mutation and cancer: statistical study of retinoblastoma. J Natl Cancer Inst 1976; 57:675.
10. Brodeur GM, Fong CT: Molecular biology and genetics of human neuroblastoma. Cancer Genet Cytogenet 1989; 41: 153.
11. Balaban-Malenbaum G, Gilbert F: Relationship between homogeneously staining regions and double minute chromosomes in human neuroblastoma cell lines. Prog Cancer Res Ther 1980; 12:97.
12. Look AT, Hayes FA, Nitschke R, et al: Cellular DNA content as a predictor of response to chemotherapy in infants with unresectable neuroblastoma. N Engl J Med 1984; 311: 231.
13. Gansler T, Chatten J, Varello M, et al: Flow cytometric DNA analysis of neuroblastoma: correlation with histology and clinical outcome. Cancer 1986; 58:2453.
14. Taylor SR, Locker J: A comparative analysis of nuclear DNA content and N-*myc* gene amplification in neuroblastoma. Cancer 1990; 65:1360.
15. Look AT, Hayes FA, Schuster JJ, et al: Clinical relevance of tumor cell ploidy and N-*myc* gene amplification in childhood neuroblastoma: a Pediatric Oncology Group Study. J Clin Oncol 1991; 9:581.
16. Biedler JL, Ross RA, Shanske S, Spengler BA: Human neuroblastoma cytogenetics: search for significance of homogeneously staining regions and double minute chromosomes. Prog Cancer Res Ther 1980; 12:81.
17. Brodeur GM: Neuroblastoma—clinical applications of molecular parameters. Brain Pathol 1990; 1:47.
18. Brodeur GM, Seeger RC, Schwab M, et al: Amplification of N-*myc* in untreated human neuroblastomas correlates with advanced disease stage. Science 1984; 224:1121.
19. Brodeur GM: Molecular Biology and Genetics of Human Neuroblastoma. Boca Raton, FL, CRC Press, 1990.
20. Brodeur GM, Hayes FA, Green AA, et al: Consistent N-*myc* copy number in simultaneous or consecutive neuroblastoma samples from sixty individual patients. Cancer Res 1987; 47:4248.
21. Nisen PD, Waber PG, Rich MA, et al: N-*myc* oncogene RNA expression in neuroblastoma. J Natl Cancer Inst 1988; 80:1633.
22. Slavc I, Ellenbogen R, Jung W-H, et al: N-*myc* gene amplification and expression in primary human neuroblastoma. Cancer Res 1990; 50:1459.
23. Fong C, White PS, Peterson K, et al: Loss of heterozygosity for chromosomes 1 to 14 defines subsets of advanced neuroblastomas. Cancer Res 1992; 52:1780.
24. Young JLJ, Ries LG, Silverberg E, et al: Cancer incidence, survival and mortality for children younger than 15 years. Cancer 1986; 58:598.
25. Voute PA: Neuroblastoma. *In* Sutow WW, Fernbach DJ, Vietti TJ (eds): Clinical Pediatric Oncology, p 559. St. Louis, CV Mosby, 1984.
26. Miller RW, Fraumeni JF, Hill JA: Neuroblastoma: epidemiologic approach to its origin. Am J Dis Child 1968; 115: 253.

27. Hope JW, Borns PF, Berg PK: Roentgenologic manifestations of Hirschprung's disease in infancy. Am J Roentgenol Radium Ther Nucl Med 1965; 95:217.
28. Dehner LP: Pathologic anatomy of classic neuroblastoma: including prognostic features and differential diagnosis. *In* Pochedly C (ed): Neuroblastoma: Tumor Biology and Therapy, p 111. Boca Raton, FL, CRC Press, 1990.
29. Triche TJ, Askin FB, Kissane JM: Neuroblastoma, Ewing's sarcoma and the differential diagnosis of small-, round-, blue-cell tumors. *In* Finegold M (ed): Pathology of Neoplasia in Children and Adolescents, p 145. Philadelphia, WB Saunders Co, 1986.
30. Shimada H, Chatten J, Newton WA Jr, et al: Histopathologic prognostic factors in neuroblastic tumors: definition of subtypes of ganglioneuroblastoma and an age-linked classification of neuroblastomas. J Natl Cancer Inst 1984; 73:405.
31. O'Neill JA, Littman P, Blitzer P, et al: The role of surgery in localized neuroblastoma. J Pediatr Surg 1985; 20:708.
32. Evans AE, D'Angio GJ, Propert K, et al: Prognostic factors in neuroblastoma. Cancer 1987; 59:1853.
33. Joshi V, Canto A, Altshuler G, et al: Prognostic significance of histopathologic features of neuroblastoma: a grading system based on the review of 211 cases from the Pediatric Oncology Group [Abstract]. Proc Am Soc Clin Oncol 1991; 10:311.
34. Rosen EM, Cassady JR, Frantz CN, et al: Neuroblastoma: the Joint Center for Radiation Therapy/Dana-Farber Cancer Institute/Children's Hospital experience. J Clin Oncol 1984; 2:714.
35. Evans AE, D'Angio GJ, Randolph JA: A proposed staging for children with neuroblastoma. Children's Cancer Study Group A. Cancer 1971; 27:374.
36. Brodeur GM, Seeger RC, Barrett A, et al: International criteria for diagnosis, staging and response to treatment in patients with neuroblastoma. J Clin Oncol 1988; 6:1874.
37. LaBrosse EH, Com-Nougue C, Zucker JM, et al: Urinary excretion of 3-methoxy-4-hydroxymandelic acid and 3-methoxy-4-hydroxyphenylacetic acid by 288 patients with neuroblastoma and related neural crest tumors. Cancer Res 1980; 40:1995.
38. Voute PA, Hoefnagel CA, Marcuse HR, de Kraker J: Detection of neuroblastoma with ^{131}I-meta-iodobenzylguanidine. Prog Clin Biol Res 1985; 175:389.
39. Bostrom B, Nesbit ME, Brunning RD: The value of bone marrow trephine biopsy in the diagnosis of metastatic neuroblastoma. Am J Pediatr Hematol Oncol 1985; 7:303.
40. Carlsen NLT, Christensen IJ, Schroeder H, et al: Prognostic factors in neuroblastomas treated in Denmark from 1943 to 1980: a statistical estimate of prognosis based on 253 cases. Cancer 1986; 58:2726.
41. Grosfeld JL, Schatzlein M, Ballantine TVN, et al: Metastatic neuroblastoma: factors influencing survival. J Pediatr Surg 1978; 13:59.
42. Jerev B, Bretsky SS, Vogel R, Helson L: Age and prognosis in neuroblastoma: review of 112 patients younger than 2 years. Am J Pediatr Hematol Oncol 1984; 6:233.
43. Schengrund CL, Repman MA, Shochat SJ: Ganglioside composition of human neuroblastomas—correlation with prognosis: a Pediatric Oncology Group Study. Cancer 1985; 56:2640.
44. Bourhis J, De Vathaire F, Wilson GD, et al: Combined analysis of DNA ploidy index and N-*myc* genomic content in neuroblastoma. Cancer Res 1991; 51:33.
45. Wilson ER, Altshuler GI, Smith EI, et al: Gross observation does not predict regional lymph node metastasis in the surgicopathologic staging of neuroblastoma [Abstract]. Proc Am Soc Clin Oncol 1989; 8:304.
46. Smith EI, Nitschke R, Shochat S, et al: Lack of significance of involved lymph nodes attached to localized neuroblastoma: a Pediatric Oncology Group study [Abstract]. Proc Am Soc Clin Oncol 1987; 6:219.
47. Kiely EM: The surgical challenge of neuroblastoma. J Pediatr Surg 1994; 29:128.
48. Castleberry RP, Kun L, Shuster JJ, et al: Radiotherapy improves the outlook for children older than one year with POG stage C neuroblastoma. J Clin Oncol 1991; 9:789.
49. Azizkjan RG, Shaw A, Chandler JG: Surgical complications of neuroblastoma resection. Surgery 1985; 97:514.
50. Nitschke R, Smith EI, Altshuler G, et al: Treatment of grossly unresectable localized neuroblastoma: a Pediatric Oncology Group study. J Clin Oncol 1991; 9:1181.
51. Matthay KK, Sather HN, Seeger RC, et al: Excellent outcome of stage II neuroblastoma is independent of residual disease and radiation therapy. J Clin Oncol 1989; 7:236.
52. Green AA, Hustu HO, Kumar M: Sequential cyclophosphamide and doxorubicin for induction of complete remission in children with disseminated neuroblastoma. Cancer 1981; 48:2310.
53. Paul SR, Tarbell NJ, Korf B, et al: Stage IV neuroblastoma in infants. Cancer 1991; 67:1493.
54. Castleberry RP, Shuster JJ, Smith EI: The Pediatric Oncology Group experience with the international staging system criteria for neuroblastoma. J Clin Oncol 1994; 12:2378.
55. Mugishima H, Iwata M, Okabe I, et al: Autologous bone marrow transplantation in children with advanced neuroblastoma. Cancer 1994; 74:972.
56. Chamberlain RS, Guinones R, Dinndorf P, et al: Complete surgical resection combined with aggressive adjuvant chemotherapy and bone marrow transplantation prolongs survival in children with advanced neuroblastoma. Ann Surg Oncol 1995; 2:93.
57. Nickersen HJ, Nesbit ME, Grosfeld JL, et al: Comparison of stage IV and IV-S neuroblastoma in the first year of life. Med Pediatr Oncol 1985; 13:261.
58. Altman AJ, Schwartz AD: Tumors of the sympathetic nervous system. *In* Shafer AJ, Markowitz M (eds): Malignant Diseases of Infancy, Childhood and Adolescence, p 368. Philadelphia, WB Saunders Co, 1983.
59. Weichselbaum RR, Epstein J, Little JB: *In vitro* cellular radiosensitivity of human malignant tumors. Eur J Cancer 1976; 36:47.
60. Stephenson SR, Cook BA, Mease AD, Ruymann FB: The prognostic significance of age and pattern of metastases in stage IV-S neuroblastoma. Cancer 1986; 58:372.
61. Philip T, Zucker JM, Bernard JL, et al: Bone marrow transplantation in an unselected group of 65 patients with stage IV neuroblastoma. *In* Dicke KA, Spitzer G, Jagannath S (eds): Autologous Bone Marrow Transplantation III, p 407. Houston, University of Texas, 1987.
62. Graham-Pole J, Casper J, Elfenbein G, et al: High-dose chemoradiotherapy supported by marrow infusions for advanced neuroblastoma: a Pediatric Oncology Group study. J Clin Oncol 1991; 9:152.
63. August CS, Serota FT, Koch PA, et al: Treatment of advanced neuroblastoma with supralethal chemotherapy, radiation and allogeneic or autologous marrow reconstruction. J Clin Oncol 1984; 2:609.
64. Joshi VV, Cantor AB, Brodeur GM, et al: Correlation between morphologic and other prognostic markers of neuroblastoma. Cancer 1993; 71:3173.
65. Hann HW, Evans AE, Siegel SE, et al: Prognostic importance of serum ferritin in patients with Stages III and IV neuroblastoma: the Children's Cancer Study Group experience. Cancer Res 1985; 45:2843.
66. Brodeur GM, Green AA, Hayes FA, et al: Cytogenetic features of human neuroblastomas and cell lines. Cancer Res 1981; 41:4678.
67. Schwab M: Amplification of N-*myc* as a prognostic marker for patients with neuroblastoma. Semin Cancer Biol 1993; 4:13.

46

WILMS' TUMOR

MICHAEL L. RITCHEY, M.D. *and* MAX J. COPPES, M.D., PH.D.

The management of Wilms' tumor has evolved considerably since its description nearly a century ago by Max Wilms. Wilms, a German surgeon,[1] was the first to propose that all the various elements of the tumor were derived from the same cell. His careful pathologic description of this tumor, also referred to as nephroblastoma, led to the association of his name with this tumor.

Initially, surgery held the only hope of cure. The surgical removal of one kidney became technically possible thanks to the pioneering work of Gustave Simon, a surgeon in Heidelberg, Germany. The first attempt at nephrectomy in a child was probably performed by Hueter in 1876.[2] Unfortunately the patient died during the surgical procedure. Ten years later, Kocher in Bern, Switzerland, performed the first successful nephrectomy in a child. Subsequently, several reports followed and surgery became the cornerstone of Wilms' tumor treatment. At first the ultimate outcome for patients with Wilms' tumor remained poor. Even by the late 1930s, survival was only 30%. The introduction of radiotherapy as an effective adjuvant treatment resulted in improved survival,[3] although it was not until the introduction of effective chemotherapy in the 1950s that a dramatic improvement in survival could be noted.[4] First, Farber from Boston reported the effectiveness of dactinomycin, and then workers at M.D. Anderson Cancer Center introduced vincristine for the treatment of this disease.[5] Because of the rarity of this tumor, it was recognized in the early 1970s that multicenter randomized trials would be necessary to conduct the needed clinical research to improve outcome. The cooperative group studies conducted by the National Wilms' Tumor Study Group (NWTSG) in North America, and the International Society of Paediatric Oncology (SIOP) in Europe have ultimately provided excellent survival rates for children with this malignant disorder.[6] This chapter reviews the major contributions of these clinical trials and some of the molecular genetics changes associated with this tumor and examines some of the new treatment strategies planned.

EPIDEMIOLOGY

Although childhood cancers comprise only 1% of all cancers, certain pediatric tumors have provided important information regarding cancer development. This is particularly true for the embryonal neoplasms of childhood, named because their morphologic appearance resembles that observed during embryogenesis. Of particular interest are the Wilms' tumors, which comprise up to one third of pediatric embryonal tumors.[7] Wilms' tumor is the most common malignant renal tumor of childhood. In North America the annual incidence in children under the age of 15 years is 7 per million.[7] Therefore, approximately 450 new cases should be expected each year. The overall median age at diagnosis is 3 1/2 years, although for boys it is 6 months lower than for girls. The disease occurs nearly equally in girls and boys worldwide.[8] There is some ethnic variation in its incidence, with slightly higher rates reported for the black populations and a lower incidence in Asian children. Paternal exposure to hydrocarbons and lead were initially implicated in the development of Wilms' tumor, but a more recent study suggests that environmental factors are not that important in the etiology of Wilms' tumor.[9]

Of greater interest is the genetic epidemiology of Wilms' tumor. For many years Wilms' tumor has been associated with a number of congenital abnormalities, including sporadic aniridia, hemihypertrophy, and genitourinary malformations.[10,11] The incidence of these conditions for children registered to the NWTSG is reported in Table 46–1.

The incidence of aniridia in patients with Wilms' tumor is 1.1%, much higher than the incidence in

TABLE 46-1. INCIDENCE OF CONGENITAL ANOMALIES ASSOCIATED WITH WILMS' TUMOR PATIENTS REPORTED TO THE NWTS

Anomaly	Rate (per 1000)
Aniridia	7.6
Beckwith-Wiedemann syndrome	8.4
Hemihypertrophy	33.8
Genitourinary anomalies	
Hypospadias	13.4
Cryptorchidism	37.3
Hypospadias and cryptorchidism	12.0

the general population, which is estimated at 1: 50,000 to 1:100,000. Wilms' tumor is seen in over 30% of children with *a*niridia, *g*enitourinary malformations, and mental *r*etardation (AGR syndrome). In the presence of Wilms' tumor, the term "WAGR syndrome" is used (*W*ilms' tumor and AGR). Most children with the WAGR syndrome suffer from a constitutional deletion on chromosome 11p13.[12]

Genitourinary abnormalities, such as hypospadias, cryptorchidism, and renal fusion anomalies, are also seen in association with Wilms' tumor independent of the WAGR syndrome. These anomalies are present in 4.5% of patients with Wilms' tumor.[13] However, because many of these genitourinary malformations are quite common in children, their presence seldom leads to searching for a syndrome diagnosis. Of particular interest is the recognition of the Denys-Drash syndrome[14,15] in children presenting with ambiguous genitalia. The Denys-Drash syndrome is characterized by ambiguous genitalia; renal mesangial sclerosis, usually resulting in end-stage renal failure; and Wilms' tumor.[16] Over 60 cases have now been reported in the literature, and genetic studies indicate that the Denys-Drash syndrome is associated with specific mutations of *WT1*, one of the Wilms' tumor genes on chromosome 11p.[17,18]

Hemihypertrophy occurs in 3% of patients with Wilms' tumor.[13] Isolated involvement of the leg is the most common manifestation in these patients and may be ipsilateral or contralateral to the tumor.[19] The risk of Wilms' tumor development in patients with hemihypertrophy is estimated to be on the order of 3 to 5%.[20] Patients with Beckwith-Wiedemann syndrome (BWS), a rare congenital overgrowth disorder characterized by visceromegaly (splenomegaly, hepatomegaly), macroglossia, and hyperinsulinemic hypoglycemia,[21,22] can also present with hemihypertrophy. Most cases of BWS are sporadic, but 15% exhibit heritable characteristics with apparent autosomal dominant inheritance. Patients with BWS are predisposed for certain cancers, in particular embryonal neoplasms. The incidence of Wilms' tumor in this patient population is less than 5%.[23]

GENETICS

The genetics of Wilms' tumor was once thought to be very similar to that of retinoblastoma (a childhood tumor of the retina), in particular because both tumors can occur bilaterally or in several members of the same family. Also, again as in retinoblastoma, when Wilms' tumor occurs bilaterally, the age at presentation is younger than in cases where the disease is limited to one kidney, suggesting a constitutional defect that predisposes that child to tumor formation. A younger age at diagnosis is also encountered in children with specific, Wilms'-tumor-predisposing congenital anomalies, such as aniridia.[13]

Analysis of the different median ages at presentation between groups of Wilms' tumor patients led Knudson and Strong in 1972 to propose a "two-hit" model for the development of Wilms' tumor similar to that proposed earlier for the development of retinoblastoma.[24] Their hypothesis predicts that two rate-limiting genetic events are necessary for tumor formation. Children with a genetic susceptibility would have a constitutional (prezygotic) lesion, either inherited from one of the parents or resulting from a spontaneous (de novo) mutation. In these children, only one additional somatic (postzygotic) event would be required for the development of Wilms' tumor, greatly increasing the likelihood of tumor formation as compared with *sporadic* cases in which two rare independent somatic mutations are required. However, it is now clear that the genetic alterations leading to the development of Wilms' tumor are more complex than those of retinoblastoma, and in fact involves multiple genes.[23]

The first evidence of a specific chromosomal region (locus) associated with Wilms' tumor development was the detection of cytogenetically visible deletions in patients with the WAGR syndrome. These patients were demonstrated to lack band 13 of the short arm of chromosome 11 (11p13) not only in their Wilms' tumor cells but in all body cells (i.e., constitutional deletions).[12] In these patients, the constitutional 11p13 deletion was thought to represent the first of two events proposed in Knudson and Strong's two-hit hypothesis; the second event could not be visualized cytogenetically and was assumed to consist of a smaller, cytogenetically invisible, alteration. By contrast, the loss of heterozygosity (LOH) for 11p13 DNA markers demonstrated in approximately one third of sporadic Wilms' tumors[25,26] was presumed to represent the second event, the first one being inactivation of the putative Wilms' tumor suppressor gene at this locus by a mutation or very small deletion. However, both observations implied the presence of a tumor suppressor gene at 11p13, involved in the development of Wilms' tumor. This was confirmed in 1990.[27-29] Subsequently, alterations of the Wilms' tumor suppressor gene *WT1* at 11p13 were shown in tumor DNA obtained from patients with sporadic Wilms' tumors, as well as in the constitutional DNA of patients with a genetic predisposition to Wilms' tumor.[30] *WT1*, which is expressed transiently in the developing kidney and also in specific cells of the gonads, is required for normal genitourinary development and is specifically of importance for the differentiation of the renal blastema.[31,32]

A second Wilms' tumor locus (already designated *WT2*) has been identified on chromosome 11p15.5.[33] This same chromosomal region has also been linked to the BWS.[34] For now, it is not known whether a single gene is responsible for both disorders or adjacent genes are independently responsible for each disease. Of particular interest with regard to this second Wilms' tumor locus is the observation that, in Wilms' tumors found to have LOH for DNA markers in this particular chromosomal region, it is invariably the maternal allele that is lost.[35] Also, some BWS patients have been shown to have two paternal copies of chromosome 11p in addition to the maternal copy (trisomy 11p15), whereas in certain patients with BWS who seem to have grossly normal karyotypes (i.e., no trisomy), both copies of chromosome 11 are in fact found to be inherited from the father, a condition termed uniparental isodisomy.[36] These observations suggest an inequality of the maternal and paternal 11p15 alleles. Apparently, in BWS expression is required from two paternal 11p15 alleles, whereas in Wilms' tumor the first of two events almost always occurs on the paternal 11p15 allele.

Other molecular abnormalities have been and still are being studied in Wilms' tumor patients. One of the more important observations has turned out to be the finding that approximately 20% of tumors apparently lose chromosomal material, as determined by LOH, on the long arm of chromosome 16,[35,37] and another 11% show LOH for DNA markers on the short arm of chromosome 1.[38] In a preliminary study, tumor-specific loss of either region (16q or 1p) was correlated with poor outcome, independent of stage or histology at initial presentation.[38] A larger group of patients must be studied to confirm this observation. The latest National Wilms' Tumor Study (NWTS-5) will therefore compare relapse-free survival percentages among patients whose tumors demonstrate tumor-specific LOH at 16q, 1p, or any other site, and those whose tumors are informative for these sites but do not show LOH.

CLINICAL PRESENTATION

The typical presentation of Wilms' tumor is that of an asymptomatic abdominal swelling or mass in a child, often found incidentally by a family member. The mass is generally quite large, frequently crossing the midline. Other presentations include abdominal pain mimicking appendicitis, or an acute abdomen resulting from rupture of the tumor with hemorrhage into the free peritoneal cavity. Hematuria is found in approximately one fourth of children at diagnosis, but only gross hematuria warrants further evaluation to exclude tumor extension into the renal pelvis and ureter. Hypertension is also present in about 25% of cases. The exact etiology for hypertension in this patient population remains unclear although several explanations have been proposed.[39]

Vascular tumor extension into the renal vein and inferior vena cava (IVC) can result in atypical presentations.[40] For example, a varicocele, particularly one that persists when the child is supine, may be secondary to obstruction of the spermatic vein as a result of tumor thrombus. However, varicocele, hepatomegaly resulting from hepatic vein obstruction, ascites, and congestive heart failure are only found in less than 10% of patients with intracaval or atrial tumor extension.[40] Very rarely the tumor can embolize to the pulmonary artery, with catastrophic consequences.[41]

PREOPERATIVE EVALUATION

Laboratory evaluation should include a complete blood count, liver function tests, and renal function tests. Serum calcium should also be checked. Hypercalcemia should alert the physician for the possible presence of either congenital mesoblastic nephroma or rhabdoid tumor of the kidney, rather than Wilms' tumor.[39] Finally, the 5 to 10% incidence of acquired von Willebrand's disease in newly diagnosed Wilms' tumor patients[42] mandates obtaining a coagulation screen, including a platelet count, and measurement of the bleeding time, prothrombin time, and activated partial thromboplastin time prior to surgery. The coagulation defect underlying the acquired von Willebrand's disease in patients with Wilms' tumor can be corrected preoperatively with the administration of DDAVP.[42]

There have been tremendous advances in body imaging techniques in recent years. As a consequence, children and adults alike are now usually subjected to more diagnostic studies before surgery than a decade ago. In recent years, there has been considerable debate regarding the role of certain imaging studies in the staging and management of children with Wilms' tumor.[43,44] Nevertheless, imaging studies can often establish the correct diagnosis before surgery (Fig. 46–1). This will help the surgeon to plan for a major surgical procedure. There is an increased incidence of surgical complications in Wilms' tumor patients with an incorrect preoperative diagnosis.[45] An equally important goal of preoperative imaging is to establish the presence of a functioning contralateral kidney prior to performing a nephrectomy. Historically, this information has been provided by an intravenous pyelogram. This imaging study will typically

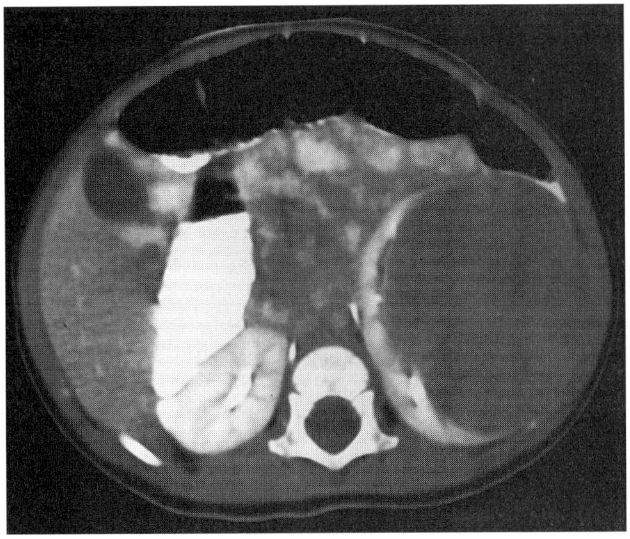

FIGURE 46-1. Computed tomographic scan of a large left Wilms' tumor with a small rim of functioning renal parenchyma.

demonstrate splaying of the collecting system by the intrarenal mass. However, nonopacification of the kidney is also common because of obstruction of the collecting system by tumor, intravascular tumor extension, or complete replacement of the renal parenchyma with neoplasm.[46] A nonfunctioning kidney was found in 28% of NWTSG patients with IVC or atrial extension.[40]

Usually, ultrasonography is the initial investigation performed in a child with a palpable abdominal mass. Ultrasound is readily available and can distinguish between solid and cystic lesions. Ultrasound can generally also determine if the mass is of intrarenal or extrarenal origin. One important role for ultrasound is to evaluate the patency of the IVC because extension of tumor thrombus into the IVC (Fig. 46-2) occurs in 4% of Wilms' tumor patients.[40] Color Doppler ultrasonography can assess flow and identify compression of the IVC. Ultrasound has replaced inferior venacavography, which is now used sparingly. Computed tomography (CT) visualization of the IVC is often hindered by unopacified blood resulting from an inadequate bolus injection of contrast. Magnetic resonance imaging (MRI) has been shown to be very helpful in detecting intravascular tumor in patients with both renal cell carcinoma and Wilms' tumor.[47,48] MRI is recommended for patients in whom ultrasound is inconclusive in establishing IVC patency.

One of the unanswered questions regarding imaging is the role of CT and MRI scans in determining the extent of disease (i.e., stage).[43,44] Because survival is correlated with stage (and histology), NWTSG investigators continually stress the need for accurate staging.[49] The current NWTSG staging system utilizes surgical and pathology findings only. It is unclear how imaging studies could contribute to more accurate staging. For example, there have been no studies to compare data obtained by imaging to those obtained by the surgeon during nephrectomy in assessing extrarenal extent. Occasionally, preoperative CT can suggest extracapsular tumor extension when there is irregularity of the tumor margin or evidence of regional adenopathy when lymph nodes are demonstrated physically separate from the tumor mass. However, enlarged retroperitoneal lymph nodes are common in children and often reactive. Moreover, even intraoperative (i.e., surgical) lymph node evaluation does not correlate well with histopathologic findings,[50] and one would therefore expect similar serious discrepancies when correlating histopathology with imaging studies.

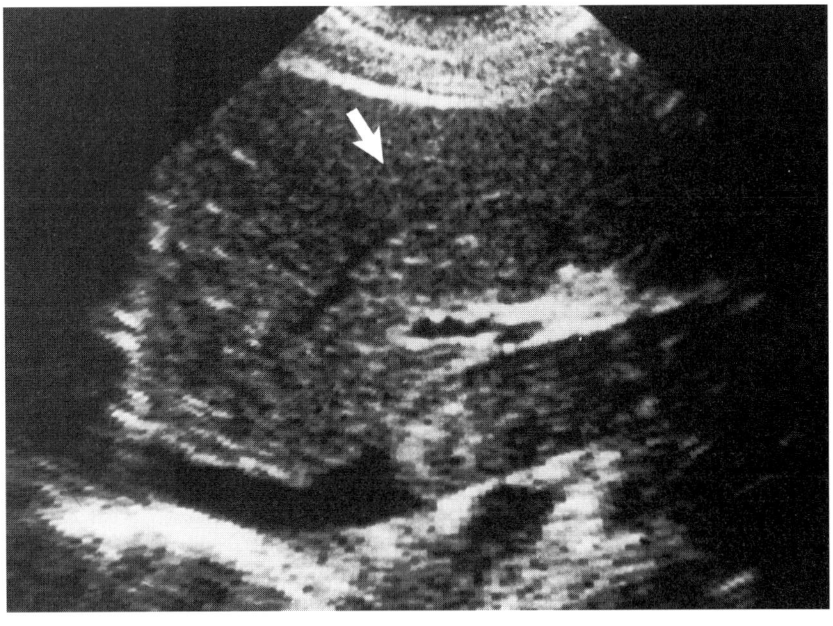

FIGURE 46-2. Ultrasound depicting intracaval thrombus (arrow).

In recent years, several groups of patients have been identified in whom primary surgical excision is not recommended. These include children who present with bilateral disease[51] or extensive intravascular tumor extension,[52] and tumors that require en bloc resection of other organs to achieve complete excision. Primary nephrectomy in the latter two groups of patients is associated with an increased incidence of surgical complications.[45] If the preoperative imaging evaluation could predict which tumors would be inoperable at surgical exploration, that information would greatly benefit the surgeon. Visceral involvement is uncommon in Wilms' tumor, but infiltration of the liver, colon, or spleen does occur.[45] Infiltration of the bowel or liver invasion by right-sided tumors is particularly difficult to assess by CT. The majority of children identified as having possible invasion of the liver on CT later prove to be negative at surgery.[53] CT is more predictive for absence of liver invasion, and, although deep-seated liver metastases are uncommon at presentation, early detection of liver metastases at diagnosis seems to improve prognosis.[54]

Detection of bilateral Wilms' tumor is important because the recommended treatment for these children is preoperative chemotherapy to shrink the tumors rather than upfront surgery. This approach facilitates preservation of renal parenchyma.[51,55] Only formal exploration of the contralateral kidney can provide an accurate assessment, although some reports have suggested that preoperative imaging can adequately evaluate the contralateral kidney.[56,57] A recent review of 122 patients with synchronous bilateral Wilms' tumor enrolled in NWTS-4 demonstrated that 7% of bilateral lesions were missed by the preoperative imaging studies.[58] Although CT was more sensitive than ultrasound in detecting bilaterality, neither technique was able to detect more than 50% of lesions less than 1 cm in diameter. Consequently, the NWTSG continues to recommend formal exploration of the contralateral kidney with both palpation and inspection of all surfaces.

The most common site of distant metastases is within the lungs, present at diagnosis in 8% of patients. The majority of these lesions can be identified on routine chest x-ray films. If the patient is documented to have metastases on chest radiographs, chest CT is unnecessary because even if additional smaller metastases are discovered, the CT findings will not alter the adjuvant treatment required. However, there is some controversy regarding the need for chest CT in children with negative chest x-ray films.[59,60] Clearly, some stage IV patients will only be identified by chest CT.[61,62] However, not all CT lesions result from metastatic disease. Some lesions identified on CT only represent benign lesions (e.g., histoplasmosis, granuloma, or round atelectasis). Therefore, lesions detected by CT scan only require histopathologic evaluation. A more important question is whether chest x-ray–negative, CT-positive patients require the same adjuvant treatment as those with a positive x-ray. Green et al. reviewed 32 children enrolled in NWTS-3, who had a negative chest roentgenogram but were identified with metastatic lesions on chest CT.[60] Surprisingly, survival in those patients treated according to the local extent of the abdominal disease alone was equivalent to that in those receiving treatment for stage IV disease (i.e., additional pulmonary irradiation). Green's results would suggest that chest x-ray–negative patients should be treated according to their local tumor stage, regardless of CT chest findings. Other investigators disagree. Wilimas et al. found that 40% of favorable histology patients with pulmonary densities detected on CT alone developed recurrent disease when pulmonary irradiation was omitted,[61] suggesting the need for additional therapy in such patients.

Uncommon sites of metastases can occur in renal tumors other than Wilms' tumor. A radionuclide bone scan and skeletal survey are both recommended if a histologic diagnosis of clear cell sarcoma of the kidney (CCSK) or renal cell carcinoma is confirmed. Both of these lesions have a propensity to metastasize to the skeleton.[41] Both rhabdoid tumor of the kidney (RTK) and CCSK are associated with brain metastases, and MRI of the brain should be obtained in the early postoperative period.

DIFFERENTIAL DIAGNOSIS

Even the most exhaustive imaging evaluation will not be able to confirm the histologic diagnosis of the renal mass prior to laparotomy. Neuroblastoma is the most common solid abdominal malignancy in childhood, but in most cases can be distinguished by its extrarenal location. Rarely, neuroblastoma will arise within the kidney, making the distinction difficult. RTK, CCSK, and renal cell carcinoma do not have any distinguishing radiographic features that will allow a preoperative diagnosis unless unusual sites of metastases (bone, brain) are evident.[63–65] Renal cell carcinoma generally presents after age 5 years, and it is the most common renal malignancy in the second decade of life.[63,66] RTK is more typically seen in infants and very young children with a mean age of 13 months.

Another tumor commonly seen in infancy is congenital mesoblastic nephroma. This is generally a benign lesion found in approximately 2% of childhood renal tumors. Most patients are under the age of 6 months at the time of diagnosis.[67] In fact, the typical presentation is that of a newborn with an abdominal mass. A number of cases have been diagnosed prenatally[68] (Fig. 46–3). However, favorable histology Wilms' tumor and RTK can also present in the first few months of life.[69] Nephrectomy is curative for most patients with congenital mesoblastic nephroma,[70] although there have been re-

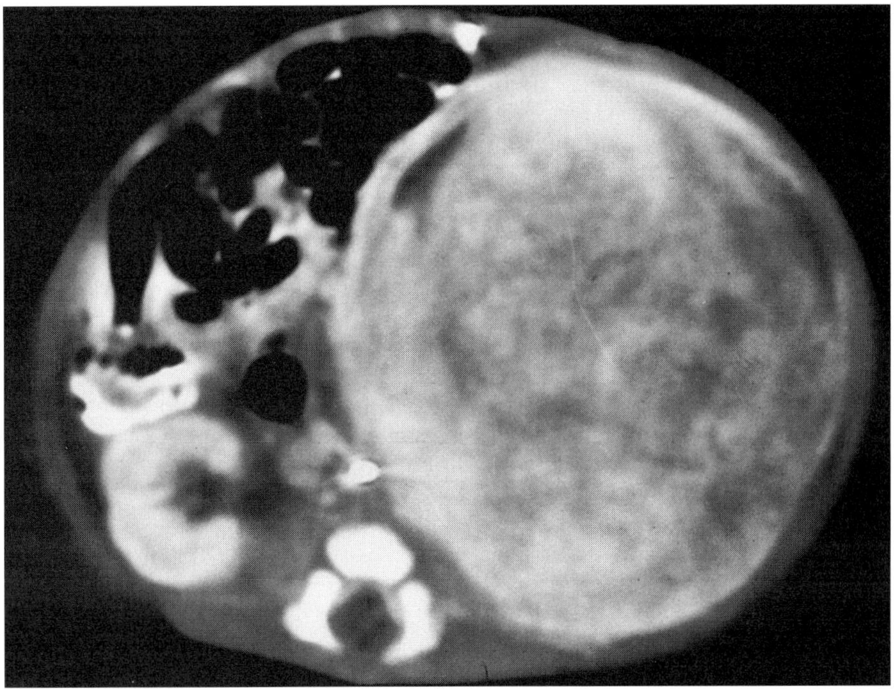

FIGURE 46–3. CT scan of a large congenital mesoblastic nephroma in a 2-day-old infant that was detected on antenatal ultrasound.

ports of local recurrence and occasionally metastases.[71–73] Adequacy of surgical resection and age at diagnosis in these patients appear to be more important predictors of relapse than histology.[74]

Renal angiomyolipoma is only rarely seen in childhood and is associated with tuberous sclerosis.[75] Demonstration of fat within a renal lesion by CT scan preoperatively should alert the surgeon to the presence of this tumor.

In addition to age at presentation, other clinical parameters can aid the clinician in narrowing the diagnostic possibilities. For example, a renal mass developing in a child with hemihypertrophy, BWS, or aniridia is most likely a Wilms' tumor. Bilateral or multicentric renal tumors are also highly suggestive of Wilms' tumor.

PATHOLOGY

On gross examination, Wilms' tumor is usually soft, lobulated, and tan or light gray in color. Hemorrhagic or necrotic areas are frequently noted. The microscopic features of Wilms' tumor classically consist of three components in varying proportions: blastema, stroma, and epithelium. Tumors that consist predominately of only one of these elements are encountered in 60% of cases and still are considered Wilms' tumor.[76] Blastema-predominant tumors are important in that they behave more aggressively, with early metastatic spread and more advanced disease at presentation. The stromal component can differentiate into striated muscle, cartilage, or fat. Wilms' tumors with predominant rhabdomyomatous elements were once thought to behave less aggressively, but recent evidence suggests that they are no different from the typical triphasic Wilms' tumor.[76]

The most important determinants of outcome are histopathology and tumor stage. Analysis of early NWTS patients identified a group of patients with unfavorable histopathologic features, associated with increased rates of relapse and death.[77] These "unfavorable histology" tumors are responsible for 50% of tumor deaths in the NWTSG studies but account for only 10% of patients.[78] Four distinct tumors are included in this unfavorable subgroup: (1) Wilms' tumor with extreme nuclear atypia (anaplasia), (2) those with monomorphic sarcomatous-appearing tumors, (3) RTK, and (4) CCSK. The latter two tumor groups have been reclassified and are now considered to be distinct entities from Wilms' tumors. CCSK accounts for 3% of renal tumors reported to the NWTSG. The age at diagnosis and location are the same as for Wilms' tumor. Its recognition is quite important in order that appropriate adjuvant therapy be instituted. In particular, doxorubicin should be used because its addition has resulted in a significant improved outcome for these children.[49] RTK is a highly malignant tumor that accounts for 2% of renal tumors registered to the NWTSG. RTK is now considered a sarcoma of the kidney and not of metanephric origin.[49] The prognosis of RTK remains dismal with conventional chemotherapeutic regimens, and new treatment strategies are being developed for the management of these children.

Anaplasia is a feature of Wilms' tumor that is associated with resistance to chemotherapy. It is therefore not surprising that the incidence of anaplasia reported by the NWTSG investigators (5%) is very similar to that reported in the SIOP studies

(5.3%),[76] where all tumors are pretreated with chemotherapy but the anaplasia persists after treatment.[79] Anaplastic features are rare in the first 2 years of life, but the incidence increases to 13% in children age 5 years or older.[80] Anaplastic Wilms' tumors are further stratified into focal and diffuse anaplasia. The definition of focal anaplasia was recently changed and is now based upon a topographic principle.[81] Focal anaplasia requires that the anaplastic nuclear changes be confined to the lesion. Diffuse anaplasia is diagnosed when anaplasia is present in more than one portion of the tumor or is found in any extrarenal or metastatic site. Confirming the notion that anaplasia is more a marker of chemoresistance than inherent aggressiveness of the tumor, outcome is generally excellent only if the tumor is completely removed (i.e., stage I tumor).[82]

Precursor Lesions

Lesions apparently representing Wilms' tumor precursors are found in 30 to 40% of kidneys removed for Wilms' tumor.[83] The current preferred term for these lesions is "nephrogenic rests," defined as foci of abnormally persistent nephrogenic cells that can develop into Wilms' tumor.[84] Two distinct categories of nephrogenic rests have been identified. The most common is the perilobar nephrogenic rest (PLNR), which is found in the periphery of the kidney. There is a higher prevalence of PLNR in children with Wilms' tumor and hemihypertrophy or BWS (Table 46–2). Intralobar nephrogenic rests (ILNRs), in contrast, can be found anywhere within the renal lobe (Fig. 46–4). Children with the WAGR syndrome or the Denys-Drash syndrome are more likely to have ILNRs. In the presence of multiple or diffuse nephrogenic rests, the term "nephroblastomatosis" is used.

TABLE 46–2. PREVALENCE OF NEPHROGENIC RESTS*

Patient Population	ILNR (%)	PLNR (%)
Infant autopsies	0.01	1
Renal dysplasia	Unknown	3.5
Unilateral Wilms' tumor	15	25
Synchronous bilateral Wilms' tumor	34–41	74–79
Metachronous bilateral Wilms' tumor	63–75	42
Beckwith-Wiedemann, hemihypertrophy	47–56	70–77
Aniridia	84–100	12–20
Drash syndrome	78	11

*Adapted from Beckwith JB: Precursor lesions of Wilms' tumor: clinical and biological implications. Med Pediatr Oncol 1993; 21: 158–168, with permission.

The natural history of nephrogenic rests, which occasionally are also found in kidneys without tumors,[85] is not entirely clear. Some undergo spontaneous regression and others hyperplastic changes, producing relatively large tumors. Although the histopathologic differential diagnosis between hyperplastic nephrogenic rests and Wilms' tumor can be very difficult (the exact criteria for distinguishing these two lesions remain to be defined),[76] the surgical management of both disorders is similar.

Multiple rests in one kidney are highly suggestive of the presence of nephrogenic rests in the other kidney because these lesions usually involve both kidneys. Consequently, the presence of ILNRs or PLNRs identifies patients at risk for the development of contralateral Wilms' tumor. Such children need careful follow-up imaging of the contralateral kidney (Table 46–3).

Biologic Parameters

As survival of children with favorable histology Wilms' tumor has continued to improve, it has be-

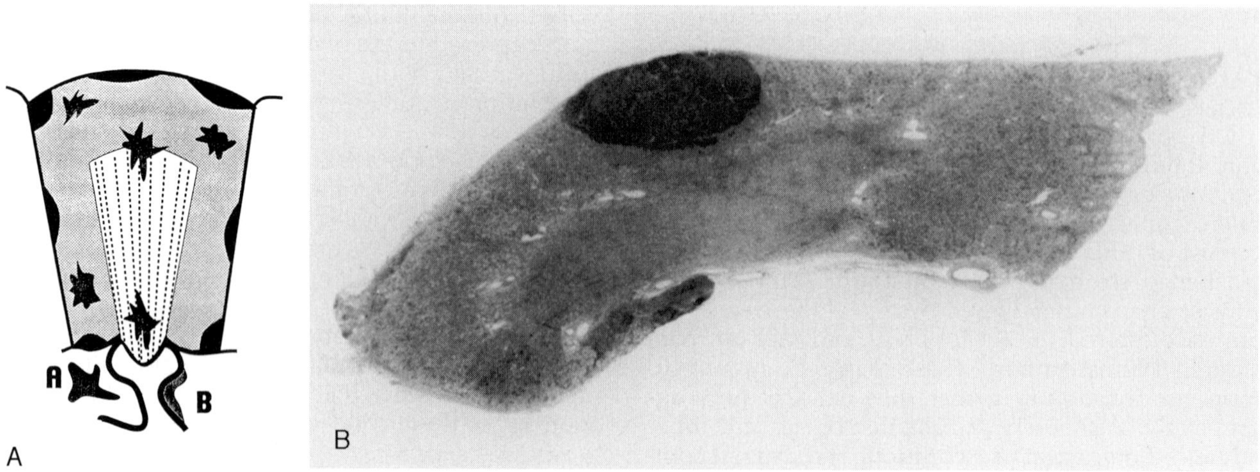
A
B
A
B

FIGURE 46–4. *A*, Illustration of renal lobe showing characteristic locations of intralobar nephrogenic rest (dark gray) and perilobar nephrogenic rest (black). (From Beckwith JB: Precursor lesions of Wilms' tumor: clinical and biological implications. Med Pediatr Oncol 1993; 21:158–168, with permission.) *B*, Perilobar nephrogenic rest composed of blastemal cells just beneath the renal capsule. Hematoxylin and eosin, × 40.

TABLE 46–3. RECOMMENDED FOLLOW-UP IMAGING STUDIES FOR CHILDREN WITH RENAL NEOPLASMS OF PROVEN HISTOLOGY AND FREE OF METASTASES AT DIAGNOSIS*

Tumor Type	Study	Schedule Following Therapy
Favorable histology Wilms' tumor; stage I anaplastic Wilms' tumor	Chest films	6 wk and 3 mo postop; then q 3 mo × 5, q 6 mo × 3, yearly × 2
Irradiated patients only	Irradiated bony structures†	Yearly to full growth, then q 5 yr indefinitely‡
Without nephrogenic rests (NRs) stages I and II	Abdominal ultrasound	Yearly × 3
Without NRs, stage III	Abdominal ultrasound	As for chest films
With NRs, any stage§	Abdominal ultrasound	q 3 mo × 10, q 6 mo × 5, yearly × 5
Stage II and III anaplastic	Chest films	As for favorable histology
	Abdominal ultrasound	q 3 mo × 4, q 6 mo × 4
Renal cell carcinoma	Chest films	As for favorable histology
	Skeletal survey and bone scan	As for CCSK
Clear cell sarcoma (CCSK)	Brain MRI and/or opacified CT	When CCSK is established; then q 6 mo × 10
	Skeletal survey and bone scan	
	Chest films	As for favorable histology
Rhabdoid tumor	Brain MRI and/or opacified CT	As for CCSK
	Chest films	As for favorable histology
Mesoblastic nephroma (MN)‖	Abdominal ultrasound	q 3 mo × 6

*Modified from D'Angio GJ, Rosenberg H, Sharples K, et al: Position paper: Imaging methods for primary renal tumors of childhood: cost versus benefits. Med Pediatr Oncol 1993; 21:205–212, with permission.

†To include any irradiated osseous structures.

‡To detect second neoplasms, benign (osteochondromas) or malignant.

§The panelists at the first International Conference on Molecular and Clinical Genetics of Childhood Renal Tumors, Albuquerque, New Mexico, May 1992, recommended a variation: q 3 mo for 5 yr or until age 7, whichever comes first.

‖Data from the files of Dr. J. B. Beckwith reveal that 20 of 293 MN patients (7%) relapsed or had metastases at diagnosis (4 of the 20 in the lungs, 1 of the 4 at diagnosis). All but one of the 19 relapses occurred within 1 year. Chest films for MN patients may be elected on a schedule such as q 3 mo × 4, q 6 mo × 2.

come increasingly difficult to find histologic features that will predict which patients are at risk for relapse. Stratification of favorable histology Wilms' tumor patients into low- and high-risk groups for relapse, independent of tumor stage, would allow intensification of treatment for those with an increased risk of relapse. Research has now focused on molecular or biologic factors.

As noted previously, LOH for a portion of the long arm of chromosome 16 has been found in 20% of Wilms' tumor patients.[23,37] A prospective study of 232 patients registered on the NWTS found that patients with 16q LOH had statistically significantly poorer 2-year relapse-free and overall survival than those without LOH for chromosome 16q.[38] In addition, LOH for chromosome 1p markers, occurring in approximately 11% of Wilms' tumors,[38] is also associated with an increased risk of relapse, although of borderline statistical significance. The hypothesis that molecular markers can be used to stratify patients for therapy will be tested in the recently opened NWTS-5.

Several studies have correlated cell DNA content, measured by flow cytometry, and prognosis in Wilms' tumor patients. Normal somatic cells have a diploid DNA content, cells in mitosis are tetraploid, and tumor cells with gross karyotypic abnormalities in number are labeled aneuploid. Aneuploid DNA histograms are found more commonly in anaplastic Wilms' tumors,[86] although this is not necessarily associated with poor prognosis.[87] Although tetraploid histograms in stage III and IV patients are indicative of poor outcome, it remains to be determined whether DNA ploidy is a more accurate predictor of survival than histology and stage.[88]

Nuclear morphometric techniques have been evaluated in Wilms' tumor and other urologic solid tumors to predict clinical outcome.[89] In a preliminary report of 27 favorable histology Wilms' tumor patients, multivariate analysis found that nuclear morphometry could indeed be used to separate patients with a poor prognosis. This finding was confirmed in a second study of 108 Wilms' tumor patients with favorable histology.[90] However, in the second study, which was performed by the same investigators who reported the first study, the shape descriptors of the nuclei predictive of outcome were different than in the first study.

In Wilms' tumor there are no biologic markers available yet that could mimic the function of α-fetoprotein in the management of germ cell tumors. Nevertheless, several biologic markers have been studied, including serum renin and prorenin, serum erythropoietin, neuron-specific enolase, and hyaluronic acid, hyaluronic acid stimulating activity, and hyaluronidase.[39] Of these, hyaluronic acid, HASA, and hyaluronidase are probably the most promising.[91]

PROGNOSTIC CONSIDERATIONS

Histopathology and tumor stage are the most important predictors of survival in Wilms' tumor patients. The staging system used by the NWTSG has undergone refinement over the years. The current staging system is summarized in Table 46–4. In NWTS-3, the distribution by stage of favorable histology tumors was stage I, 47%; stage II, 22%; stage III, 22%; and stage IV, 9%.[49] Both the surgeon and pathologist have responsibility for determining local tumor stage. Stage I tumors are limited to the kidney and can be completely resected. The first signs of spread outside the kidney are in the renal sinus or intrarenal blood or lymphatic vessels. Tumor extension into the soft tissues of the sinus or the presence of tumor cells in blood or lymphatic vessels of the renal sinus is considered stage II. Penetration through the renal capsule is the next most common site of extrarenal spread. Tumors that penetrate the renal capsule or the presence of tumor cells in the perirenal fat is also classified as stage II tumor.

In addition to the histopathologic features described above, the NWTSG pathologists have identified several pathologic variables predictive of tumor relapse in patients with stage I favorable histology tumors.[92] These "microsubstaging" variables are invasion of the tumor capsule, presence of an inflammatory pseudocapsule, renal sinus invasion, and tumor in the intrarenal vessels. Analysis of these microsubstaging variables found that one or more of these features was present in 24 stage I favorable histology patients from NWTS-3 who developed tumor relapse.[92] In a control group of 48 stage I patients, none had relapse if all four microsubstaging variables were negative. Approximately 40% of stage I patients would meet the latter criteria. A subsequent study of NWTS-4 favorable histology stage I patients found that the absence of adverse microsubstaging variables correlated not only with excellent survival but also with age at diagnosis (<2 years) and tumor weight (<550 g).[93] In NWTS-5, the more easily obtained variables of age and weight will be used to stratify stage I favorable histology patients for treatment.

Wilms' tumor usually metastasizes to regional lymph nodes, the lungs, and the liver. Patients with lymph node metastases are classified as stage III and require local radiotherapy following surgery. Because the presence of lymph node metastases mandates more intensive treatment and is associated with poorer outcome, it is important for the surgeon to obtain adequate lymph node sampling during nephrectomy in order to allow appropriate staging. Approximately 85% of hematogenous metastases at presentation are reported in the lungs, and about 15% of patients present with liver involvement.[94] Other sites of metastases, such as bone, mediastinum, and spinal cord, are uncommon. Fortunately, outcome even for patients with hematogenous metastases at diagnosis is far from poor, provided appropriate adjuvant therapy is supplied.

Tumor size and patient age have in the past been predictive of tumor recurrence. For NWTS-1 patients, the relapse rate was 14.8% for children less than 2 years of age, which was significantly better than for older children.[95] However, these variables have not proven to be of significance in subsequent NWTS trials, presumably because of overall improvement in treatment efficacy.[78] The only exception is the group of children less than 2 years of age at diagnosis and whose tumors weigh less than 550 g.[93]

TABLE 46–4. STAGING SYSTEM OF THE NWTS*

Stage	Description
I	Tumor limited to the kidney and completely excised. The renal capsule is intact and the tumor was not ruptured prior to removal. There is no residual tumor. The vessels of the renal sinus are not involved.
II	Tumor extends beyond the kidney but is completely excised. There is regional extension of tumor (i.e., penetration of the renal capsule, extensive invasion of the renal sinus). The tumor may have been biopsied or there may be local spillage of tumor confined to the flank. Extrarenal vessels may contain tumor thrombus or be infiltrated by tumor.
III	Residual nonhematogenous tumor confined to the abdomen: lymph node involvement, diffuse peritoneal spillage either before or during surgery, peritoneal implants, tumor beyond surgical margin either grossly or microscopically, or tumor not completely removed.
IV	Hematogenous metastases (lung, liver, bone, brain, etc.) or lymph node metastases outside the abdominopelvic region are present.
V	Bilateral renal involvement at diagnosis.

*Abstracted from Protocol.

SURGICAL MANAGEMENT

Although most of the improvement in survival of children with Wilms' tumor is attributable to introduction of effective chemotherapy and radiotherapy, surgery continues to play a very important role in successful treatment. The preoperative evaluation of a child with an abdominal mass can generally be completed in 48 hours in most medical centers. Emergent operation is not necessary unless there is evidence of active bleeding. The surgeon is responsible for safely removing the tumor and assessing the local tumor stage. This requires a thorough exploration of the abdominal cavity via a generous transperitoneal incision. The flank approach should not be used because regional staging and examination of the contralateral kidney are not possible. The liver is palpated and regional lymph nodes are examined for evidence of tumor spread. Exploration of the contralateral kidney should be performed prior to ipsilateral nephrectomy. As noted previously, one cannot rely entirely on the preoperative imaging studies to exclude bilateral disease.[58] Patients with bilateral tumors are managed with biopsy followed by chemotherapy without attempts at primary resection (see later).[55] The colon is reflected and Gerota's fascia opened so that the kidney can be palpated and inspected on all surfaces. Any abnormalities of the contralateral kidney should be biopsied to exclude occult Wilms' tumor or the presence of nephrogenic rests.

The colon and its mesentery are then reflected off the tumor and a radical nephrectomy is performed with sampling of regional lymph nodes. Formal lymph node dissection is not required.[50] Ligation of the renal vessels is performed prior to mobilization of the tumor, but only if exposure is adequate. More importantly, the surgeon should be certain that the contralateral renal vessels, aorta, and iliac or superior mesenteric arteries have not been mistakenly ligated.[96] Gentle handling of the tumor throughout the procedure is mandatory to avoid tumor spillage because spillage results in a sixfold increase in local abdominal relapse.[49] Additionally, patients with diffuse tumor spill are considered stage III and require more intensive therapy with whole abdominal irradiation and the use of doxorubicin.

Prior to ligation of the renal vein, palpation of the vein and IVC should be performed to exclude intravascular tumor extension. The majority of patients with IVC extension will fortunately be identified by imaging studies obtained prior to surgery.[40,97] Extension of tumor into the extrarenal vessels does not adversely affect prognosis if it is completely excised. For vena caval involvement below the level of the hepatic veins, the caval thrombus can be removed via cavotomy after proximal and distal vascular control is obtained. Generally the thrombus will be free floating, but, if there is adherence of the thrombus to the caval wall, the thrombus can often be delivered with the passage of a Fogarty or Foley balloon catheter. Patients with atrial extension may require cardiopulmonary bypass for thrombus removal.[98] Certain operative findings may suggest intravascular extension when it has not been correctly diagnosed preoperatively. For example, excessive bleeding from dilated superficial and retroperitoneal collaterals is a clue to obstruction of the vena cava. More ominous is the finding of sudden unexplained hypotension, which can result from embolization of the tumor thrombus.[99]

Primary surgical resection of IVC or atrial tumor extension is associated with increased surgical morbidity.[45] Several reports have demonstrated that these patients can best be managed by shrinkage of tumor and thrombus with preoperative chemotherapy.[52,100,101] This approach facilitates complete removal of the tumor with decreased morbidity. Although there has been one report of tumor embolus during chemotherapy,[102] this complication can also occur prior to or during surgical removal of the tumor.[41,99]

Occasionally, patients will present with massive tumors that are surgically unresectable. Heroic surgery with radical en bloc resection of the tumor and adjacent organs is not justified. Such operations are associated with increased surgical morbidity. In addition, the gross appearance of the tumor at the time of surgery can be misleading in interpreting tumor extent. These tumors often compress and adhere to adjacent structures without frank invasion, and in the majority of cases tumor invasion is not confirmed after the adjacent visceral organs are removed.[45] The appropriate management of tumors that are inoperable at presentation is tumor biopsy followed by chemotherapy. This approach almost always reduces the bulk of the tumor and renders it resectable.[103,104] Usually, there is adequate size reduction within 6 weeks. Serial imaging studies are helpful in assessing response. Patients who fail to respond to chemotherapy can subsequently be considered for preoperative irradiation, which may produce enough shrinkage to facilitate nephrectomy. One disadvantage of using preoperative therapy is that there is loss of important staging information (see later). Patients with unresectable tumors treated with preoperative chemotherapy with or without additional radiotherapy should be considered stage III and treated accordingly.[104] Therefore, it is very important that tumors not be determined to be unresectable on the basis of preoperative imaging alone.

The morbidity of the surgical procedure should not be overlooked in the management of children with Wilms' tumor. NWTSG investigators found a 20% incidence of surgical complications in a review of all NWTS-3 patients undergoing primary nephrectomy.[45] The most common complications were intestinal obstruction and hemorrhage.[105] Factors associated with an increased risk for surgical complications were higher local tumor stage, incorrect preoperative diagnosis, intravascular extension, and en bloc resection of other visceral organs. As noted previously, primary surgical resection is no longer recommended for patients in the latter two categories. It is hoped that selective use of preoperative chemotherapy will reduce surgical morbidity while maintaining excellent patient survival.

COOPERATIVE GROUP TRIALS

National Wilms' Tumor Study Group

Many early accomplishments in the treatment of children with Wilms' tumor were made by individuals or large single institutions but, as survival improved, larger numbers of patients were needed to conduct prospective randomized trials to answer therapeutic questions. Thus in North America, both pediatric cooperative groups, the Children's Cancer

Study Group and the Pediatric Oncology Group, initially initiated clinical trials within their own group but subsequently decided to collaborate within the NWTSG. Four intergroup studies have been completed and a fifth is underway.

NWTS-1 and NWTS-2

Many important findings resulted from the early clinical trials NWTS-1 (1969–1973) and NWTS-2 (1974–1978).[106,107] For example, postoperative local irradiation was shown to be unnecessary for group I patients. Also, combination chemotherapy of vincristine (VCR) and dactinomycin (AMD) was found to be more effective than the use of either drug alone. The addition of doxorubicin (DOX) was shown to improve survival of higher stage patients. However, even more important findings were the identification of unfavorable histologic features of Wilms' tumor and of prognostic factors that allowed refinement of the staging system, stratifying patients into high-risk and low-risk treatment groups.[108] After the completion of NWTS-1 and NWTS-2, it was recognized that the presence of lymph node metastases had an adverse outcome on survival. Children with lymph node metastases as well as those with diffuse tumor spill were found to be at increased risk of abdominal relapse. Therefore, such patients were considered stage III and given whole abdominal irradiation. These findings were incorporated into the design of NWTS-3 to try to decrease the intensity of therapy for the majority of low risk patients while maintaining overall survival.

NWTS-3

In NWTS-3, patients with stage I, favorable histology Wilms' tumor were treated successfully with a 10-week regimen of VCR and AMD, considerably decreasing the amount of chemotherapy administered and, as a consequence, the total duration of treatment.[49] The 4-year relapse-free survival was 89%, and the overall survival was 95.6%. Stage II favorable histology patients treated with AMD and VCR without postoperative radiation therapy had a survival rate (4-year overall survival of 91.1%) equivalent to patients who received the same treatment plus DOX, demonstrating that the cardiotoxic drug DOX is not necessary for the successful treatment of this group of patients. The dosage of abdominal irradiation for stage III favorable histology patients was reduced to 1080 cGy. This was shown to be as effective as 2000 cGy in preventing abdominal relapse if DOX was added to VCR and AMD. The 4-year relapse-free survival for stage III patients was 82% in NWTS-3, and the 4-year overall survival 90.9%. Patients with stage IV favorable histology tumors received abdominal (local) irradiation based on the local tumor stage. In addition, they all received 1200 cGy to both lungs. For radiotherapy in combination with VCR, AMD, and DOX, the 4-year relapse-free survival in this group was 79% and the overall survival 80.9%.[109] There was no statistically significant improvement in survival when cyclophosphamide was added to the three-drug regimen.

NWTS-4

The goals of the most recent intergroup study, NWTS-4 (1986–1994), were to further decrease treatment intensity for patients with favorable prognosis while trying to maintain their excellent survival. In addition, this was the first clinical pediatric cancer trial to evaluate the economic impact of two different treatment approaches (Table 46–5). Pulse-intensive regimens utilize simultaneous administration of agents at more frequent intervals to decrease the number of clinic visits and hence the cost of cancer treatment. NWTS-4 demonstrated

TABLE 46–5. PROTOCOL FOR NWTS-4*

	Radiotherapy	Chemotherapy Regimen Randomization
Stage I, FH and anaplasia	None	EE (AMD plus VCR; 24 wk) EE-4A (pulse-intensive AMD plus VCR; 18 wk)
Stage II, FH	None	K (AMD plus VCR; 22 or 65 wk)† K-4A (pulse-intensive AMD plus VCR; 18 or 60 wk)†
Stage III, FH	1080 cGy	DD (AMD, VCR, and DOX; 26 or 65 wk)† DD-4A (pulse-intensive AMD, VCR, and DOX; 24 or 54 wk)†
Stage IV, FH	Yes‡	DD or DD-4A as above†
CCSK, stage I–IV	Yes‡	DD or DD-4A as above†
Stage II–IV, UH	Yes‡	DD (65 wk) J (AMD, VCR, CPM, and DOX; 65 wk)

*Abreviations: FH, favorable histology; UH, unfavorable histology; AMD, dactinomycin; VCR, vincristine; DOX, doxorubicin; CPM, cyclophosphamide.

†A second randomization is carried out at 5 months postnephrectomy to determine if these patients will stop therapy or continue to 54 weeks or beyond.

‡Radiation therapy is given to all clear cell sarcoma patients. Stage IV FH patients are given radiation based on the local tumor stage.

that, although the administered drug dose intensity was greater on pulse-intensive regimens, these regimens, which indeed are cost effective, produce less hematologic toxicity than the standard regimens.[110] Patients treated with pulse-intensive regimens achieved equivalent survival compared to those treated with standard chemotherapy regimens.[111] Overall, the 4-year survival for patients with favorable histology Wilms' tumor now approaches 90%.[6]

NWTS-5

The recently opened intergroup study, NWTS-5, will be a single-arm therapeutic trial. Patients will not be randomized for therapy, but instead biologic features of the tumors will be assessed. This study will attempt to verify the preliminary findings that LOH for chromosomes 16q and 1p are useful in identifying patients who are at increased risk for relapse.[38] If these molecular genetic markers are indeed found to be predictive of clinical behavior, this information will then be used in subsequent NWTSG clinical trials to further stratify patients for therapy. Current recommendations for treatment to be utilized in NWTS-5 are outlined in Table 46–6. Treatment for patients with stage I or II favorable histology and stage I anaplastic Wilms' tumor is the same. They are to receive a pulse intensive regimen of VCR and AMD for 18 weeks.

Based on the results of the previous study (NWTS-4), which indicated that the 2-year relapse-free survival rate for patients under age 2 years and with tumor weights under 550 g was 95.5%,[93] a select group of patients (i.e., those 2 years of age with stage I favorable histology tumors weighing under 550 g) has been selected for management with surgery alone in NWTS-5.[112] However, because the excellent survival obtained in this specific patient group was only achieved by surgery followed by postoperative chemotherapy, NWTSG investigators recommend careful postoperative surveillance of this group of children so that, if they occur, relapses can be detected at an early stage and subsequently immediately treated.

Patients with stage III favorable histology and stage II or III focal anaplasia are to be treated with AMD, VCR, and DOX and 1080 cGy abdominal irradiation. Patients with stage IV favorable histology tumors receive abdominal irradiation based on the local tumor stage and 1200 cGy to both lungs.

Children with stage II through IV diffuse anaplasia and stage I through IV CCSK will be treated with a new chemotherapeutic regimen combining VCR, DOX, cyclophosphamide, and etoposide in an attempt to further improve the survival of this high-risk group. All these patients will receive irradiation to the tumor bed. Children with all stages of RTK will be treated with carboplatin, cyclophosphamide, and etoposide. These patients will also receive abdominal irradiation.

International Society of Paediatric Oncology

Investigators in Europe formed SIOP (the Société Internationale d'Oncologie Pédiatrique) in an attempt to improve the outcome of children with Wilms' tumor. The randomized trials conducted by SIOP differ from those of the NWTSG in that patients receive preoperative therapy prior to surgery. Also, no routine histopathologic diagnosis is ob-

TABLE 46–6. PROTOCOL FOR NWTS-5*

	Radiotherapy	Chemotherapy Regimen
Stage I, FH <24 mo and <550 g tumor weight	None	None (surgery only for this group)
Stage I, FH >24 mo and/or >550 g tumor weight Stage II, FH Stage I, anaplasia	None	EE-4A (AMD plus VCR; 18 wk)
Stage III–IV, FH Stage II–IV, focal anaplasia	Yes†	DD-4A (AMD, VCR, and DOX; 24 wk)
Stage II–IV, diffuse anaplasia	Yes†	I (VCR + DOX + CPM + E; 24 wk)
Stage I–IV CCSK	Yes†	I as above
Stage I–IV RTK	Yes†	RTK (Carbo + E + CPM; 24 wk)
Stage V, bilateral: biopsy or limited surgery, both kidneys		
Stage I or II, FH		EE-4A as above
Stage III or IV, FH		DD-4A as above
Stage I–IV, anaplasia		I as above

*Abbreviations: FH, favorable histology; AMD, dactinomycin; VCR, vincristine; DOX, doxorubicin; CPM, cyclophosphamide; E, etoposide; carbo, carboplatin.

†Consult protocol for details regarding radiation therapy.

tained prior to commencing treatment. The rationale for the SIOP approach is that preoperative chemotherapy will make the tumor less prone to intraoperative rupture or spill.[113,114] The European investigators also indicate that preoperative therapy leads to a more favorable stage distribution at the time of surgery,[115] as a result of which fewer patients will require postoperative radiation therapy. Preoperative treatment can indeed produce dramatic reduction in the size of the primary tumor, facilitating surgical excision (Fig. 46–5).

The SIOP investigators use tumor extent as found at the time of delayed (postchemotherapy) surgery to determine local tumor stage. However, this postchemotherapy stage may inadequately define the risk of intra-abdominal recurrence in unirradiated patients.[116] The SIOP staging system separates stage II into "node-negative" and "node-positive" groups. In SIOP-6, patients who were "postchemotherapy stage II" were randomized to receive or not receive abdominal irradiation. The investigators found that there was an unacceptable increase in the number of intra-abdominal recurrences in nonirradiated patients, although there was no significant difference in survival rates.[117] As a result, stage II node-negative patients are now

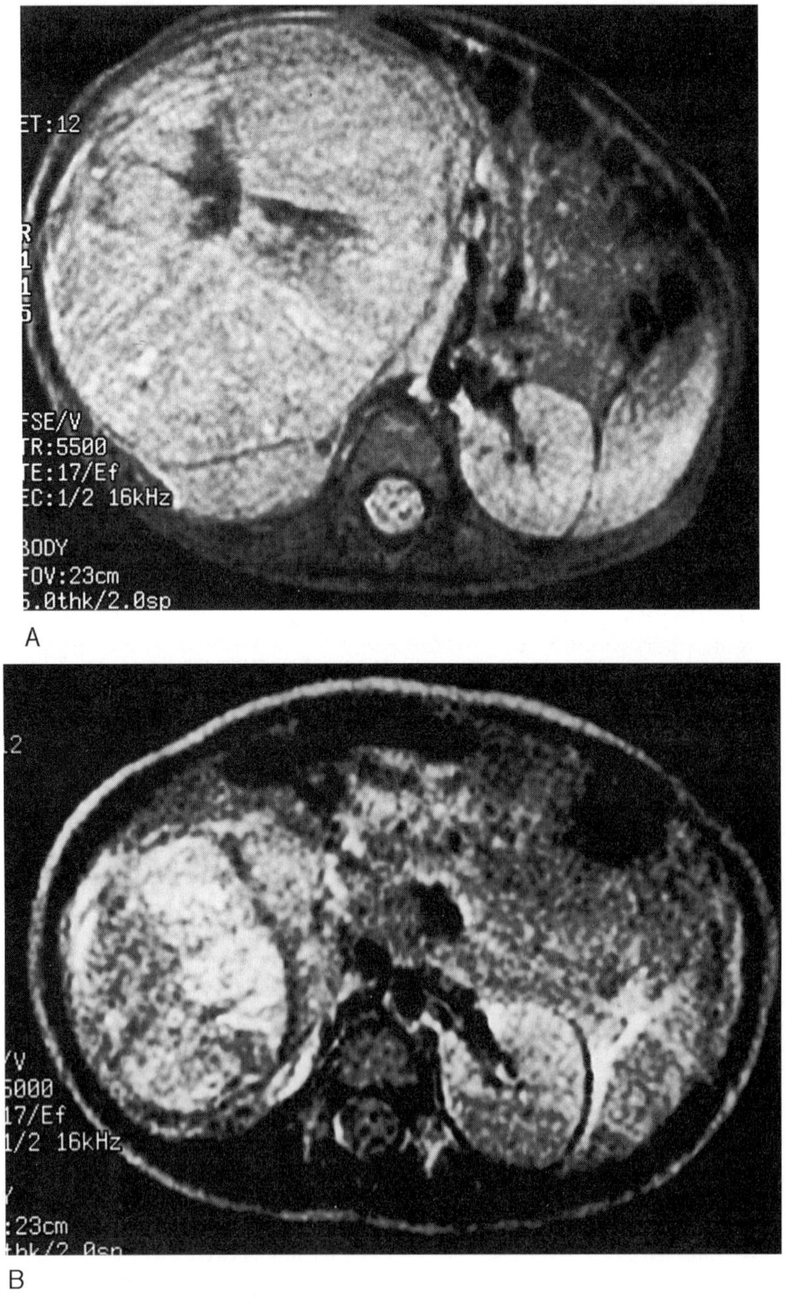
A
B

FIGURE 46–5. *A*, MRI scan of a large inoperable Wilms' tumor. *B*, After 6 weeks of chemotherapy the tumor has dramatically decreased in size.

given an anthracycline as part of the chemotherapy regimen. Consequently, a larger percentage of SIOP patients are now receiving a cardiotoxic drug than do patients registered to NWTSG studies. The significance of this is discussed later in the section on late effects. Of interest, when one compares the numbers of patients receiving abdominal irradiation, the incidence has decreased for both groups; 16% of SIOP-9 patients, 24% of NWTS-4 patients (not significantly different). The overall survival figures are comparable between the SIOP and NWTSG. One recent report suggests that the incidence of surgical morbidity is decreased when nephrectomy is performed after a course of preoperative chemotherapy.[118]

The NWTSG does recommend preoperative chemotherapy only for selected groups of Wilms' tumor patients. This includes those with bilateral involvement,[51] tumors inoperable at surgical exploration,[104] and tumor extension into the IVC above the hepatic veins.[52] For all other children, the NWTSG continues to recommend primary nephrectomy. The NWTSG investigators believe that this approach allows precise staging of patients with the ability to modulate treatment for each individual, thereby decreasing the intensity of treatment when possible while maintaining excellent overall survival.

BILATERAL WILMS' TUMORS

Synchronous bilateral Wilms' tumor occurs in about 5% of children with metachronous lesions developing in only 1%.[51,55,119] It is essential that the contralateral kidney is examined prior to ipsilateral nephrectomy to exclude bilateral disease, because the whole therapeutic approach to synchronous bilateral Wilms' tumor is radically different from that of unilateral disease. Instead of upfront surgery, patients with synchronous bilateral Wilms' tumor should undergo biopsies to establish the correct diagnosis, followed by preoperative therapy.[120] Radical excision of the tumors should not be performed at diagnostic surgery. The advantage of this approach is that more renal units will be spared if surgery is deferred until after the tumor burden is reduced.[50,121] This is important because renal failure has been reported in as many as 5% of bilateral patients.[122] However, initial partial nephrectomy or wedge excision should be considered if all tumor can be removed with preservation of two thirds or more of the renal parenchyma on both sides.

At initial surgical exploration, bilateral biopsies should be obtained for histopathologic confirmation of disease in both kidneys and definition of the histologic subtype. Suspicious lymph nodes should be biopsied, and a surgical stage assigned. Patients with favorable histology and stage I or II disease are given AMD and VCR, whereas those with stage III or IV favorable histology should also receive DOX. The response to chemotherapy is assessed by serial imaging studies. Surgical exploration with definitive resection is deferred until there has been a significant reduction in tumor burden. At the time of the second-look procedure, partial nephrectomy or wedge excision of the tumor is performed where possible. However, this approach should never compromise complete tumor resection. The surgeon must ensure that negative tumor margins can be obtained.

There are two primary concerns regarding partial nephrectomy for the treatment of Wilms' tumor: first, the possibility of local tumor recurrence and thus decreased survival, and second, an increased incidence of surgical complications. A recent review of NWTS-4 patients with synchronous bilateral tumors indicated that the 4-year survival rate for stage V patients was 81.7%. Surgical morbidity following partial nephrectomy was comparable to that following complete nephrectomy in unilateral Wilms' tumor patients.

If extensive tumor involvement precluding partial resection is still present after preoperative therapy, complete excision of tumor from the least involved kidney is performed. If this leaves a viable kidney, nephrectomy of the other kidney is carried out. Occasionally, bilateral nephrectomy is indicated. This will result in the need for dialysis. Indeed, the most common cause of renal failure in NWTS patients is bilateral nephrectomy for persistent tumor.[122] If transplantation is later considered, a waiting period of 2 years is recommended to ensure that the patient does not develop metastatic disease.[123]

TREATMENT OF RELAPSES

Children with relapsed Wilms' tumor have a variable prognosis, depending on the initial stage, site of relapse, time from initial diagnosis to relapse, and prior therapy. Adverse prognostic factors include relapse less than 12 months after diagnosis, prior treatment with DOX, and intra-abdominal relapse in patients previously having received abdominal irradiation.[124] The risk of tumor relapse in NWTS-3 at 3 years was 9.6, 11.8, 22, and 22%, respectively, for stages I through IV. Relapses occurred in 36% of stage I through III and 45% of stage IV patients with unfavorable histology.[49]

LATE EFFECTS OF CANCER TREATMENT

One consequence of the tremendous improvement in survival of children with malignancies is that there are many long-term survivors who have been exposed to both radiation and chemotherapeutic agents. These children require long-term surveillance because the sequelae of this therapy may not be evident for many years. One of the more serious concerns is the increased risk for second malignant neoplasms. Investigators from the NWTSG have noted a 1.6% cumulative incidence of second malignant neoplasms at 15 years post-treatment.[125] Prior treatment for relapse, the amount of abdominal irradiation, and use of DOX were all associated with an increased incidence of second malignant neoplasms.

Another risk associated with DOX is cardiac toxicity. Congestive heart failure is a well-known acute complication of treatment with anthracycline, and the incidence is dose related.[126] In addition, there are now reports of cardiac failure occurring up to 20 years after treatment.[127] For NWTS-1, -2, and -3 patients, the frequency of congestive heart failure to date is 1.7% among DOX-treated patients.[128] The risk was increased if the patient also had received whole-lung irradiation.

Numerous other organ systems are subject to the late sequelae of anticancer therapy. An early report on NWTSG patients found that musculoskeletal problems such as scoliosis were seven times more common in children who were treated with radiation.[129] It should be noted that these were patients from NWTS-1 and -2, wherein treatment intensity was much greater than is currently recommended. Damage to reproductive systems can lead to problems with hormonal dysfunction and or infertility. Female Wilms' tumor patients who received abdominal radiation have a 12% incidence of ovarian failure.[130] In addition, women with prior abdominal radiation have the potential for adverse pregnancy outcomes. Perinatal mortality rates are higher, and infants are more likely to have low birth weights.[131] Gonadal radiation in males can result in temporary azoospermia and hypogonadism.[132] The severity of damage to the testis is dependent on the dose of radiation.

There has been concern about the late occurrence of renal dysfunction in children who have undergone nephrectomy. Patients have been found to develop proteinuria, hypertension and renal insufficiency secondary to focal glomerulosclerosis, which has been attributed to hyperfiltration injury.[133,134] There is both clinical and experimental evidence of hyperfiltration damage of remnant nephrons after a loss of renal mass.[135] Most experimental studies involve a loss of greater than three fourths of the total renal mass, but there are only limited data assessing renal function long term in children following unilateral nephrectomy.[136,137] Although several studies have found no significant alterations in renal function following unilateral nephrectomy for Wilms' tumor,[138,139] other reports have noted an increased incidence of proteinuria and decreased glomerular filtration rate.[136,137,140] However, clinically important hypertension or renal insufficiency is rare.

One of the more important risk factors for a decrease in glomerular filtration rate is the amount of radiation to the remaining kidney. The correlation of functional impairment with the renal radiation dose was reported by Mitus and others in a review of 100 children treated for Wilms' tumor.[141] The incidence of impaired creatinine clearance was significantly greater for children receiving greater than 1200 cGy to the remaining kidney, and all cases of overt renal failure occurred in patients who had received more than 2300 cGy.

The concern of renal dysfunction has led some centers to consider parenchyma-sparing procedures for unilateral tumors.[142] Because the majority of tumors are too large for partial nephrectomy at presentation, the patient must be given preoperative chemotherapy, after which less than 10% of patients may then be amenable to partial nephrectomy. However, in order to scientifically justify this approach, many children would have to be treated accordingly to demonstrate its benefits because the incidence of renal failure is quite low for unilateral Wilms' tumor. A review of the NWTSG data base found that less than 0.2% of unilateral Wilms' tumor patients developed renal failure. Moreover, the majority of these patients suffered from the Denys-Drash syndrome, a disorder wherein all patients invariably develop end-stage renal disease irrespective of the cancer therapy.[122]

REFERENCES

1. Zantinga AR, Coppes MJ: Max Wilms (1867–1918): the man behind the eponym. Med Pediatr Oncol 1992; 20: 515–518.
2. Zantinga AR, Coppes MJ: Historical aspects of the identification of the entity Wilms tumor, and of its management. Hematol Oncol Clin North Am 1995; 9:1145–1155.
3. Priestly JT, Schulte TL: The treatment of Wilms' tumor. Urology 1942; 47:7–10.
4. Farber S: Chemotherapy in the treatment of leukemia and Wilms' tumor. JAMA 1966; 198:826–836.
5. Sutow WW: Chemotherapy in childhood cancer (except leukemia): an appraisal. Cancer 1965; 18:1585.
6. Coppes MJ, Ritchey ML, D'Angio GJ: The path to progress in medical science: a Wilms tumor conspectus. Hematol Oncol Clin North Am 1995; 9:xiii–xviii.
7. Birch JM, Breslow N: Epidemiologic features of Wilms tumor. Hematol Oncol Clin North Am 1995; 9:1157–1178.
8. Breslow N, Olshan A, Beckwith JB, et al: Ethnic variation in the incidence, diagnosis, prognosis and follow-up of children with Wilms' tumor. J Natl Cancer Inst 1994; 86: 49–51.
9. Olshan AF, Breslow NE, Daling JR, et al: Wilms tumor and paternal occupation. Cancer Res 1990; 50:3212–3217.
10. Miller RW, Fraumeni JF, Manning MD: Association of Wilms tumor with aniridia, hemihypertrophy and other congenital malformations. N Engl J Med 1964; 270:922–927.
11. Clericuzio CL: Clinical phenotypes and Wilms tumor. Med Pediatr Oncol 1993; 21:182–187.
12. Riccardi VM, Sujansky E, Smith AC, Francke U: Chromosomal imbalance in the aniridia-Wilms' tumor association: 11p interstitial deletion. Pediatrics 1978; 61:604–610.
13. Breslow NE, Beckwith JB: Epidemiological features of Wilms' tumor: results of the National Wilms' Tumor Study. J Natl Cancer Inst 1982; 68:429–436.
14. Denys P, Malvaux P, Van Den Berghe H, et al: Association d'un syndrome anatomo-pathologique de pseudohermaphroditism masculin, d'une tumeur de Wilms, d'une ne-

phropathie parenchymateuse et d'un mosaicism XX/XY. Arch Fr Pediatr 1967; 24:729–739.
15. Drash A, Sherman F, Hartmann WH, Blizzard RM: A syndrome of pseudohermaphroditism, Wilms tumor, hypertension and degenerative renal disease. J Pediatr 1970; 76: 585–593.
16. Jadresic L, Leake J, Gordon I, et al: Clinicopathologic review of twelve children with nephropathy, Wilms tumor, and genital abnormalities (Drash syndrome). J Pediatr 1990; 117:717–725.
17. Pelletier J, Bruening W, Kashtan CE, et al: Germline mutations in the Wilms' tumor suppressor gene are associated with abnormal urogenital development in Denys-Drash syndrome. Cell 1991; 67:437–447.
18. Coppes MJ, Huff V, Pelletier J: Denys-Drash syndrome: relating a clinical disorder to genetic alterations in the tumor suppressor gene WT1. J Pediatr 1993; 123:673–678.
19. Green DM, Breslow NE, Beckwith JB, Norkool P: Screening of children with hemihypertrophy, aniridia, and Beckwith-Wiedemann syndrome in patients with Wilms' tumor: a report from the National Wilms Tumor Study. Med Pediatr Oncol 1993; 21:188–192.
20. Tank ES, Melvin T: The association of Wilms' tumor with nephrologic disease. J Pediatr Surg 1990; 25:724–725.
21. Sotelo-Avila C, Gonzalez-Crussi F, Fowler JW: Complete and incomplete forms of Beckwith-Wiedemann syndrome: their oncogenic potential. J Pediatr 1980; 96:47–50.
22. Beckwith JB: Macroglossia, omphalocele, adrenal cytomegaly, gigantism and hyperplastic visceromegaly. Birth Defects 1969; 5:188–196.
23. Coppes MJ, Haber DA, Grundy P: Genetic events in the development of Wilms tumor. N Engl J Med 1994; 331: 586–590.
24. Knudson AG, Strong LC: Mutation and cancer: a model for Wilms' tumor of the kidney. J Natl Cancer Inst 1972; 48:313–324.
25. Koufos A, Hansen MF, Lampkin BC, et al: Loss of alleles at loci on human chromosome 11 during genesis of Wilms' tumor. Nature 1984; 309:170–172.
26. Huff V: Inheritance and functionality of Wilms tumor genes. Cancer Bull 1994; 46:255–259.
27. Bonetta L, Kuehn SE, Huang A, et al: Wilms tumor locus on 11p13 defined by multiple CpG island-associated transcripts. Science 1990; 250:994–997.
28. Call KM, Glaser T, Ito CY, et al: Isolation and characterization of a zinc finger polypeptide gene at the human chromosome 11 Wilms' tumor locus. Cell 1990; 60:509–520.
29. Gessler M, Poustka A, Cavenee W, et al: Homozygous deletion in Wilms tumours of a zinc-finger gene identified by chromosome jumping. Nature 1990; 343:774–778.
30. Coppes MJ, Campbell CE, Williams BRG: The role of *WT1* in Wilms tumorigenesis. FASEB J 1993; 7:886–895.
31. Kreidberg JA, Sariola H, Loring JM, et al: WT-1 is required for early kidney development. Cell 1993; 74:679.
32. Van Heyningen V, Bickmore WA, Searwright A, et al: Role for the Wilms tumor gene in genital development. Proc Natl Acad Sci U S A 1990; 87:5383.
33. Reeve AE, Sih SA, Raizis AM, Feinberg AP: Loss of allelic heterozygosity at a second locus on chromosome 11 in sporadic Wilms' tumor cells. Mol Cell Biol 1989; 44:711–719.
34. Koufos A, Grundy P, Morgan K, et al: Familial Wiedemann-Beckwith syndrome and a second Wilms tumor locus both map to 11p15.5. Am J Hum Genet 1989; 44:711–719.
35. Coppes MJ, Bonetta L, Huang A, et al: Loss of heterozygosity mapping in Wilms tumor indicates the involvement of three distinct regions and a limited role for nondisjunction or mitotic recombination. Genes Chromosom Cancer 1992; 5:326–334.
36. Grundy P, Telzerow P, Haber D, et al: Chromosome 11 uniparental isodisomy predisposing to embryonal neoplasms. Lancet 1991; 338:1079.
37. Maw MA, Grundy PE, Millow LJ, et al: A third Wilms' tumor locus on chromosome 16q. Cancer Res 1992; 52: 3094–3098.
38. Grundy PE, Telzerow PE, Breslow N, et al: Loss of heterozygosity for chromosomes 16q and 1p in Wilms tumor predicts an adverse outcome. Cancer Res 1994; 54:2331–2333.
39. Coppes MJ: Serum biological markers and paraneoplastic syndromes in Wilms tumor. Med Pediatr Oncol 1993; 21: 213–221.
40. Ritchey ML, Kelalis PP, Breslow N, et al: Intracaval and atrial involvement with nephroblastoma: review of National Wilms' Tumor Study-3. J Urol 1988; 140:1113–1118.
41. Zakowski MF, Edwards RH, McDonough ET: Wilms' tumor presenting as sudden death due to tumor embolism. Arch Pathol Lab Med 1990; 114:605–608.
42. Coppes MJ, Zandvoort SWH, Sparling CR, et al: Acquired von Willebrand disease in Wilms tumor patients. J Clin Oncol 1993; 10:1–7.
43. Cohen MD: Staging of Wilms' tumor. Clin Radiol 1993; 47:77–81.
44. D'Angio GJ, Rosenberg H, Sharples K, et al: Position paper: imaging methods for primary renal tumors of childhood: cost versus benefits. Med Pediatr Oncol 1993; 21: 205–212.
45. Ritchey ML, Kelalis PP, Breslow N, et al: Surgical complications following nephrectomy for Wilms' tumor: a report of National Wilms' Tumor Study-3. Surg Gynecol Obstet 1992; 175:507–514.
46. Nakayama DK, Ortega W, D'Angio GJ, O'Neill JA: The nonopacified kidney with Wilms' tumor. J Pediatr Surg 1988; 23:152–155.
47. Weese DL, Applebaum H, Taber P: Mapping intravascular extension of Wilms' tumor with magnetic resonance imaging. J Pediatr Surg 1991; 26:64–67.
48. Roubidoux MA, Dunnick NR, Sostman HD, Leder RA: Renal carcinoma: detection of venous extension with gradient-echo MR imaging. Radiology 1992; 182:269–272.
49. D'Angio GJ, Breslow N, Beckwith JB, et al: Treatment of Wilms' tumor: results of the Third National Wilms' Tumor Study. Cancer 1989; 64:349–360.
50. Othersen HB Jr, DeLorimer A, Hrabovsky E, et al: Surgical evaluation of lymph node metastases in Wilms' tumor. J Pediatr Surg 1990; 25:1–2.
51. Blute ML, Kelalis PP, Offord KB, et al: Bilateral Wilms' tumor. J Urol 1987; 138:968–973.
52. Ritchey ML, Kelalis PP, Haase GM, et al: Preoperative therapy for intracaval and atrial extension of Wilms' tumor. Cancer 1993; 71:4104–4110.
53. Ng YY, Hall-Craggs MA, Dicks-Mireaux C, Pritchard J: Wilms' tumour: pre- and post-chemotherapy CT appearances. Clin Radiol 1991; 43:255–259.
54. Thomas PRM, Shochat SJ, Marical P, et al: Prognostic implications of hepatic adhesions, invasion, and metastases at diagnosis of Wilms' tumor. Cancer 1991; 68:2486–2488.
55. Montgomery BT, Kelalis PP, Blute ML, et al: Extended follow-up of bilateral Wilms' tumor: results of the National Wilms Tumor Study. J Urol 1991; 146:514–518.
56. Koo AS, Koyle MA, Hurwitz RS, et al: The necessity of contralateral surgical exploration in Wilms' tumor with modern noninvasive imaging technique: a reassessment. J Urol 1990; 144:416–417.
57. Goleta-Dy A, Shaw PJ, Stevens MM: Re: The necessity of contralateral surgical exploration in Wilms' tumor with modern noninvasive imaging technique: a reassessment. [Letter]. J Urol 1992; 147:171.
58. Ritchey ML, Green DM, Breslow NE, Norkool P: Accuracy of current imaging modalities in the diagnosis of synchronous bilateral Wilms tumor. Cancer 1995; 75: 600–604.
59. Cohen MD: Current controversey: is CT scan of the chest needed in patients with Wilms tumor? J Pediatr Hematol Oncol 1994; 16:191.
60. Green DM, Fernbach DJ, Norkool P, et al: The treatment of Wilms' tumor patients with pulmonary metastases de-

tected only with computed tomography: a report from the National Wilms' Tumor Study. J Clin Oncol 1991; 9: 1776–1781.
61. Wilimas J, Douglass EC, Magill HL, et al: Significance of pulmonary computed tomography at diagnosis in Wilms' tumor. J Clin Oncol 1988; 6:1144–1146.
62. Wooton SL, Rumack CM, Albano EA, et al: Pulmonary metastases in Wilms' tumor. Pediatr Radiol 1994; 24:463.
63. Broecker B: Renal cell carcinoma in children. Urology 1991; 38:54–56.
64. Glass RBJ, Davidson AJ, Fernbach SK: Clear cell sarcoma of the kidney: CT, sonographic and pathologic correlation. Radiology 1991; 180:715–717.
65. White KS, Grossman H: Wilms' and associated renal tumors of childhood. Pediatr Radiol 1991; 21:81–88.
66. Hartman D, Davis C, Madewell J, Friedman A: Primary malignant tumors in the second decade of life: Wilms tumor versus renal cell carcinoma. J Urol 1982; 127:888–891.
67. Coppes MJ, Tournade MF, Lemerle J, et al: Preoperative care of infants with nephroblastoma: the International Society of Pediatric Oncology 6 experience. Cancer 1992; 69: 2721–2725.
68. Ohmichi M, Tasaka K, Sugita N, et al: Hydramnios associated with congenital mesoblastic nephroma: a case report. Obstet Gynecol 1989; 74:469–471.
69. Ritchey ML, Azizkhan RG, Beckwith JB: Neonatal Wilms tumors. J Pediatr Surg 1995; 30:856–859.
70. Howell CJ, Othersen HB, Kiviat NE, et al: Therapy and outcome in 51 children with mesoblastic nephroma: a report of the National Wilms' Tumor Study. J Pediatr Surg 1982; 17:826–830.
71. Joshi VV, Kasznica J, Walters TR: Atypical mesoblastic nephroma: pathologic characterization of a potentially aggressive variant of conventional congenital mesoblastic nephroma. Arch Pathol Lab Med 1986; 110:100–106.
72. Gormley TS, Skoog SJ, Jones RV, Maybee D: Cellular congenital mesoblastic nephroma: what are the options? J Urol 1989; 142:479–483.
73. Heidelberger KP, Ritchey ML, Dauser RC, et al: Congenital mesoblastic nephroma metastatic to the brain. Cancer 1993; 72:2499–2502.
74. Beckwith JB: Congenital mesoblastic nephroma: when should we worry? Arch Pathol Lab Med 1986; 110:98–99.
75. Blute ML, Malek RS, Segura JW: Angiomyolipoma: a clinical metamorphosis and concepts for management. J Urol 1988; 139:20–24.
76. Schmidt D, Beckwith JB: Histopathology of childhood renal tumors. Hematol Oncol Clin North Am 1995; 9:1179–1200.
77. Beckwith JB, Palmer NF: Histopathology and prognosis of Wilms tumor: results from the National Wilms Tumor Study. Cancer 1978; 41:1937–1948.
78. Breslow NB, Churchill G, Beckwith JB, et al: Prognosis for Wilms' tumor patients with nonmetatastic disease at diagnosis—results of the Second National Wilms' Tumor Study. J Clin Oncol 1985; 3:521–531.
79. Weirich A, Schmidt D, Harms D, et al: Distribution of subtypes in standard Wilms tumor after pre-operative chemotherapy and its possible influence of the patients cure rate. Med Pediatr Oncol 1994; 23:217.
80. Bonadio JF, Storer B, Norkool P, et al: Anaplastic Wilms' tumor: clinical and pathological studies. J Clin Oncol 1985; 3:513–520.
81. Faria P, Beckwith JB: A new definition of focal anaplasia (FA) in Wilms tumor identifies cases with good outcome: a report from the National Wilms Tumor Study [Abstract]. Mod Pathol 1993; 6:3p.
82. Zuppan CW, Beckwith JB, Weeks DA, et al: The effect of preoperative therapy on the histologic features of Wilms' tumor: an analysis of cases from the Third National Wilms' Tumor Study. Cancer 1991; 68:385–394.
83. Bove KE, McAdams AJ: The nephroblastomatosis complex and its relationship to Wilms' tumor: a clinicopathologic treatise. Perspect Pediatr Pathol 1976; 3:185–223.
84. Beckwith JB, Kiviat NB, Bonadio JF: Nephrogenic rests, nephroblastomatosis, and the pathogenesis of Wilms' tumor. Pediatr Pathol 1990; 10:1–36.
85. Bennington JL, Beckwith JB: Tumors of the kidney, renal pelvis, and ureter. *In* Atlas of Tumor Pathology, Second Series, Fasicle 12, p 33. Bethesda, MD, Armed Forces Institute of Pathology, 1975.
86. Douglass EC, Look AT, Webber B, et al: Hyperdiploidy and chromosomal rearrangements define the anaplastic variant of Wilms tumor. J Clin Oncol 1986; 4:975.
87. Rainwater LM, Hosaka Y, Farrow GM, et al: Wilms tumors: relationship of nuclear deoxyribonucleic acid ploidy to patient survival. J Urol 1987; 138:974–977.
88. Layfield LJ, Ritchie AWS, Ehrlich R: The relationship of deoxyribonucleic acid content to conventional prognostic factors in Wilms' tumor. J Urol 1989; 142:1040–1043.
89. Partin AW, Walsh AC, Epstein JI, et al: Nuclear morphometry as a predictor of response to therapy in Wilms' tumor: a preliminary report. J Urol 1990; 144:1222–1226.
90. Partin AW, Gearhart JP, Leonard MP, et al: The use of nuclear morphometry to predict prognosis in pediatric urologic malignancies: a review. Med Pediatr Oncol 1993; 21:222–229.
91. Lin RY, Argent PA, Sullivan KM, et al: Urinary hyaluronic acid is a Wilms tumor marker. J Pediatr Surg 1995; 30: 304–308.
92. Weeks DA, Beckwith JB, Luckey DW: Relapse-associated variables in stage I, favorable histology Wilms' tumor. Cancer 1987; 60:1204–1212.
93. Green DM, Beckwith JB, Weeks DA, et al: The relationship between microsubstaging variables, tumor weight and age at diagnosis of children with stage I/favorable histology Wilms tumor: a report from the National Wilms Tumor Study. Cancer 1994; 74:1817–1820.
94. Breslow N, Churchill G, Nesmith B, et al: Clinicopathologic features and prognosis for Wilms' tumor patients with metastases at diagnosis. Cancer 1986; 58:574.
95. Breslow NB, Palmer NF, Hill LR, et al: Prognostic factors for patients without metatastes at diagnosis. Cancer 1978; 41:1577.
96. Ritchey ML, Lally KP, Haase GM, et al: Superior mesenteric artery injury during nephrectomy for Wilms' Tumor. J Pediatr Surg 1992; 27:612–615.
97. Ritchey ML, Othersen HB Jr, deLorimier AA, et al: Renal vein involvement with nephroblastoma: a report of National Wilms' Tumor Study—3. Eur Urol 1990; 17:139–144.
98. Nakayama DK, deLorimier AA, O'Neill JA Jr, et al: Intracardiac extension of Wilms' tumor: a report of the National Wilms' Tumor Study. Ann Surg 1986; 204:693–697.
99. Shurin SB, Gauderer MWL, Dahms BB, Conrad WG: Fatal intraoperative pulmonary embolization of Wilms tumor. J Pediatr 1982; 101:559–562.
100. Dykes EH, Marwaha RK, Dicks-Mireaux C, et al: Risks and benefits of percutaneous biopsy and primary chemotherapy in advanced Wilms' tumour. J Pediatr Surg 1991; 26:610–612.
101. Oberholzer HF, Falkson G, DeJager LC: Successful management of inferior vena cava and right atrial nephroblastoma tumor thrombus with preoperative chemotherapy. Med Pediatr Oncol 1992; 20:61–63.
102. Borden TA: Wilms tumor and pulmonary embolism. Soc Pediatr Urol Newsletter 1992, pp 27–29.
103. Bracken RB, Sutow WW, Jaffe N, et al: Preoperative chemotherapy for Wilms' tumor. Urology 1982; 19:55–60.
104. Ritchey ML, Pringle K, Breslow N, et al: Management and outcome of inoperable Wilms tumor: a report of National Wilms' Tumor Study. Ann Surg 1994; 220:683–690.
105. Ritchey ML, Kelalis P, Breslow N, et al: Small bowel obstruction following nephrectomy for Wilms' tumor. Ann Surg 1993; 218:654–659.
106. D'Angio GJ, Evans AE, Breslow N, et al: The treatment of Wilms' tumor: results of the National Wilms' Tumor Study. Cancer 1976; 38:633–646.
107. D'Angio GJ, Evans A, Breslow N, et al: The treatment of

Wilms' tumor: results of the Second National Wilms' Tumor Study. Cancer 1981; 47:2302–2311.

108. Farewell VT, D'Angio GJ, Breslow N, Norkool P: Retrospective validation of a new staging system for Wilms' tumor. Cancer Clin Trials 1981; 4:167–171.

109. Green DM, Breslow N, Evans I, et al: The treatment of children with stage IV Wilms tumor: a report from the National Wilms Tumor Study Group. Med Pediatr Oncol 1996; 26:147–152.

110. Green DM, Breslow NE, Evan I, et al: Effect of dose intensity of chemotherapy on the hematological toxicity of the treatment of Wilms tumor: a report from the National Wilms Tumor Study. Am J Pediatr Hematol Oncol 1994; 16:207–212.

111. Green DM, Breslow N, Beckwith JB, et al: A comparison between single dose and divided dose administration of dactinomycin and doxorubicin: a report from the National Wilms Tumor Study Group [Abstract]. Med Pediatr Oncol 1996; 27:218.

112. Larsen E, Perez-Atayde A, Green DM, et al: Surgery only for the treatment of patients with stage I (Cassady) Wilms' tumor. Cancer 1990; 66:264–266.

113. Lemerle J, Voûte PA, Tournade MF, et al: Preoperative versus postoperative radiotherapy, single versus multiple courses of actinomycin D, in the treatment of Wilms' tumor: preliminary results of a controlled clinical trial conducted by the International Society of Paediatric Oncology (SIOP). Cancer 1976; 38:647–654.

114. Lemerle J, Voûte PA, Tournade MF, et al: Effectiveness of preoperative chemotherapy in Wilms' tumor: results of an International Society of Paediatric Oncology (SIOP) clinical trial. J Clin Oncol 1983; 1:604–609.

115. de Kraker J, Weitzman S, Voûte PA: Preoperative strategies in the management of Wilms tumor. Hematol Oncol Clin North Am 1995; 9:1275–1286.

116. Green DM, Breslow NE, D'Angio GJ: The treatment of children with unilateral Wilms tumor. J Clin Oncol 1993; 11:1009–1010.

117. Tournade MF, Com-Nougue C, Voûte PA, et al: Results of the sixth International Society of Pediatric Oncology Wilms' Tumor Trial and Study: a risk-adapted therapeutic approach in Wilms' tumor. J Clin Oncol 1993; 11:1014–1023.

118. Godzinski J, Tournade M-F, DeKraker J, et al: Surgical complications after postchemotherapy nephrectomy in SIOP-9 Wilms tumor patients. Med Pediatr Oncol 1994; 23:172.

119. Coppes MJ, DeKraker J, Van Dijken PJ, et al: Bilateral Wilms' tumor: long-term survival and some epidemiological features. J Clin Oncol 1989; 7:310–315.

120. Ritchey ML, Coppes M: The management of synchronous bilateral Wilms tumor. Hematol Oncol Clin North Am 1995; 9:1303–1316.

121. Shaul DB, Srikanth MM, Ortega JA, Mahour GH: Treatment of bilateral Wilms' tumor: comparison of initial biopsy and chemotherapy to initial surgical resection in the preservation of renal mass and function. J Pediatr Surg 1992; 27:1009–1015.

122. Ritchey ML, Green DM, Thomas P, et al: Renal failure in Wilms tumor. Med Pediatr Oncol 1996; 26:75–80.

123. Penn I: Renal transplantation for Wilms' tumor: report of 20 cases. J Urol 1979; 122:793–794.

124. Grundy P, Breslow N, Green DM, et al: Prognostic factors for children with recurrent Wilms' tumor: results from the Second and Third National Wilms Tumor Study. J Clin Oncol 1989; 7:638–647.

125. Breslow NE, Takashima JR, Whitton JA, et al: Second malignant neoplasms following treatment for Wilms tumor: a report from the National Wilms Tumor Study Group. J Clin Oncol 1995; 13:1851–1859.

126. Gilladoga AC, Manuel C, Tan CT, et al: The cardiotoxicity of Adriamycin and daunomycin in children. Cancer 1976; 37:1070–1078.

127. Steinherz LJ, Steinherz PG, Tan CTC, et al: Cardiac toxicity 4 to 20 years after anthracycline therapy. JAMA 1991; 266:1672–1677.

128. Green DM, Breslow NE, Moksness J, D'Angio GJ: Congestive failure following initial therapy for Wilms tumor: a report from the National Wilms Tumor Study [Abstract]. Pediatr Res 1994; 35:161A.

129. Evans AE, Norkool P, Evans I, et al: Late effects of treatment for Wilms' tumor: a report from the National Wilms' Tumor Study Group. Cancer 1991; 67:331–336.

130. Stillman RJ, Schinfeld JS, Schiff I, et al: Ovarian failure in long term survivors of childhood malignancy. Am J Obstet Gynecol 1987; 139:62–66.

131. Li FP, Gimbrere K, Gelber RD, et al: Outcome of pregnancy in survivors of Wilms tumor. JAMA 1987; 257: 216–219.

132. Kinsella TJ, Trivette G, Rowland J, et al: Long-term follow-up of testicular function following radiation for early-stage Hodgkin's disease. J Clin Oncol 1989; 7:718–724.

133. Case records of the Massachusetts General Hospital, Weekly Clinicopathological Exercises. Case 17-1985. Scully RE, Mark EJ, McNeely BU (eds). N Engl J Med 1985; 312:1111–1119.

134. Welch TR, McAdams AJ: Focal glomerulosclerosis as a late sequela of Wilms tumor. J Pediatr 1986; 108:105–109.

135. Anderson S, Meyer TW, Brenner BM: The role of hemodynamic factors in the initiation and progression of renal disease. J Urol 1985; 133:363–368.

136. Argueso LR, Ritchey ML, Boyle ET Jr, et al: Prognosis of the solitary kidney after unilateral nephrectomy in childhood. J Urol 1992; 148:747–751.

137. Robitaille P, Mongeau JG, Lortie L, Sinnassamy P: Long-term follow-up of patients who underwent nephrectomy in childhood. Lancet 1985; 1:1297–1299.

138. Barrera M, Roy LP, Stevens M: Long-term follow-up after unilateral nephrectomy and radiotherapy for Wilms tumor. Pediatr Nephrol 1989; 3:430–432.

139. Bhisitkul DM, Morgan ER, Vozar MA, Langman CB: Renal functional reserve in long-term survivors of unilateral Wilms tumor. J Pediatr 1990; 118:698–702.

140. Levitt GA, Yeomans E, Dicks-Mireaux C, et al: Renal size and function after cure of Wilms tumor. Br J Cancer 1992; 66:877–882.

141. Mitus A, Tefft M, Feller FX: Long-term follow-up of renal function of 108 children who underwent nephrectomy for malignant disease. Pediatrics 1969; 44:912–921.

142. McLorie GA, McKenna PH, Greenberg M, et al: Reduction in tumor burden allowing partial nephrectomy following preoperative chemotherapy in biopsy proved Wilms' tumor. J Urol 1991; 146:509–513.

47

RHABDOMYOSARCOMA OF THE PELVIS AND PARATESTICULAR STRUCTURES

MARTIN KAEFER, M.D. *and* ALAN B. RETIK, M.D.

Rhabdomyosarcoma is an aggressive neoplasm with a propensity toward local infiltration early and eventual metastatic dissemination.[1] It is the most common sarcoma of childhood, comprising 5 to 15% of all childhood solid tumors and 4 to 8% of all childhood malignancies.[2] The incidence of genitourinary rhabdomyosarcoma is 0.5 to 0.7 cases per million children less than 15 years of age.[3] This entity is seen more often in males than in females (1.4:1) and more often in whites than in blacks (2.3:1).[4] Most cases present within the first decade of life, with two specific age peaks occurring between ages 2 and 6 and 15 and 19 years of age.[5]

Rhabdomyosarcoma arises from primitive totipotential embryonal mesenchyme. Many locations for the primary lesion are possible. Following the head and neck, the most common location is the genitourinary tract. Twenty per cent of all childhood rhabdomyosarcoma involves either the bladder, prostate, vagina, cervix, or paratesticular tissues. Tumors that primarily involve nongenitourinary pelvic sites have a worse prognosis overall, in part because of delays in presentation.[6]

A hereditary basis for rhabdomyosarcoma appears to exist. An association between rhabdomyosarcoma and several congenital disorders has been identified in as many as 32% of cases.[7] Included among the possible congenital disorders are von Recklinghausen's disease (neurofibromatosis type II), Gorlin's basal cell nevus syndrome, and the fetal alcohol syndrome.[8,9] Individuals with rhabdomyosarcoma also have an increased incidence of genitourinary anomalies similar to that in Wilms' tumor.[7] The increased incidence in siblings of children with central nervous system tumors and adrenocortical carcinoma, as well as familial aggregations of rhabdomyosarcoma with other sarcomas, breast tumors, and brain neoplasms, is also suggestive of a possible genetic factor.[8,10]

Untreated, this malignant condition will progress rapidly. In addition to its ability to rapidly invade local tissues, both lymphatic and hematogenous dissemination are possible. Lymphatic spread occurs in 20% of genitourinary rhabdomyosarcoma and may be as high as 40% with prostatic primaries.[11] Hematogenous metastases involve the lung, liver, bone, and bone marrow and are present in 20% of patients at the time of diagnosis.[11] Nearly 80% of patients who develop metastatic disease will do so within 1 year after diagnosis.[12] Prior to the advent of effective chemotherapy, surgery both with and without radiation proved to be only 20 to 30% effective in curing these children.[5,11] However, survival has improved from a dismal 10 to 15% in the late 1960s to over 70% at 3 years (Intergroup Rhabdomyosarcoma Study [IRS]-III). Two reasons for this remarkable improvement have been the formation of cooperative study groups and the development of combined modality approaches.

Intra-abdominal genitourinary sites share similar clinical manifestations, diagnosis, and management. Paratesticular rhabdomyosarcoma, because of its better prognosis and differences in management, is discussed separately.

PATHOLOGY

Rhabdomyosarcoma can arise from any site that has developed from embryonic mesenchyme. It is composed of rhabdomyoblasts, which are thought to be a neoplastic analog of premature striated muscle. Histologically the subtypes are considered to differ based on their extent of differentiation from the mesenchymal progenitor. The most widely recognized classification system is that proposed by Horn and Enterline.[13] Four main histologic subsets were included in their original system: embryonal, botyroid subtype of embryonal, alveolar, and pleomorphic.

Embryonal rhabdomyosarcoma is the most common variant overall, and constitutes 60% of childhood cases and roughly two thirds of rhabdomyosarcomas involving the genitourinary tract.[4] Grossly, it may resemble a bunch of grapes (sarcoma botyroides). Tumors with this appearance tend to arise from hollow organs such as the bladder or vagina. Microscopically, its architecture of spindle-shaped cells with abundant eosinophilic cytoplasm is considered to resemble skeletal muscle cells seen in the 7- to 10-week fetus.[14] One third of embryonal rhabdomyosarcoma will demonstrate a striated appearance. Cavazzana and colleagues described a new histologic appearance that they termed "spindle cell rhabdomyosarcoma."[15] This relatively rare variant of the embryonal form has been identified most often in men with low-stage paratesticular primaries. The IRS has confirmed the existence of this subtype, which appears to have a significantly better prognosis when compared with classic embryonal rhadomyosarcoma (95.5% versus 80% survival at 5 years).[16]

Alveolar rhabdomyosarcoma is the second most common histologic type seen in children (20% of all childhood cases). Its name is derived from its histologic architecture, reminiscent of pulmonary alveoli.[13] Microscopically it is composed of multiple small round cells with scanty amounts of eosinophilic cytoplasm resembling skeletal muscle at 10 to 21 weeks' gestation. It has the worst prognosis, with the highest rate of regional lymph node and bone marrow involvement. Alveolar histology also has the highest rate of tumor recurrence. Pleomorphic rhabdomyosarcoma, the type usually found in the adult population, is identified in only 1% of childhood cases. Both the alveolar and pleomorphic variants involve the trunk and extremities more frequently than the genitourinary system. Tumors composed of more than one histologic subtype are termed mixed. In addition, 10 to 20% of all cases lack histologic characteristics of muscle cells and are designated undifferentiated (anaplastic) rhabdomyosarcoma. The primitive round cells that make up this later variant resemble Ewing's sarcoma of the bone.

Recently a new international classification system has been proposed by the IRS[17] (Table 47–1). This system, termed the International Classification of Rhabdomyosarcoma (ICR), incorporates criteria from several known classification systems and is highly predictive of clinical outcome. Pleomorphic rhabdomyosarcoma is left out of the proposed system because it does not occur with any regularity in children. Histologic features of the most common variants are shown in Figure 47–1.

TABLE 47–1. IRC HISTOLOGIC CLASSIFICATION OF RHABDOMYOSARCOMA (RMS)

I.	**Superior prognosis**
	a. Botyroid RMS
	b. Spindle Cell RMS
II.	**Intermediate prognosis**
	a. Embryonal RMS
III.	**Poor prognosis**
	a. Alveolar RMS
	b. Undifferentiated sarcoma
IV.	**Subtypes whose prognosis is not presently evaluable**
	a. RMS with rhabdoid features

PRESENTATION

Specific signs and symptoms of rhabdomyosarcoma rely heavily on the organ of involvement and size of the primary at initial assessment.[18] Patients with early bladder or prostate involvement may experience symptoms of irritative voiding. As these tumors expand into the bladder or urethral lumen, obstructive symptoms may ensue, potentially leading to urinary retention, incontinence, or infection[19] (Fig. 47–2). Involvement of the trigone (the most common location in the bladder) may result in hydronephrosis and renal deterioration from obstruction. Hematuria arises as these neoplasms invade through the epithelial layer. Bladder primaries are more commonly seen in males (2:1) less than 5 years of age.[20] Prostatic primaries may present with symptoms of constipation. A mass is often appreciated on rectal exam. The average age of presentation for prostatic primaries is 3.5 years.[19]

Patients with vaginal primaries may present with a visible mass at the introitis, hemorrhage, vaginal discharge, or extrusion of tumor fragments from the introitus.[21] Urethral obstruction leading to urinary retention may result. Vaginal tumors generally arise from the anterior vaginal wall and have a mean age of presentation of less than 2 years. Patients with uterine tumors typically present in adolescence after the onset of menses.[21]

EVALUATION

Once the diagnosis of rhabdomyosarcoma is entertained, thorough radiographic assessment of both the primary and potential metastatic sites is mandatory. This diagnostic effort is important because of the significant prognostic differences between tumors arising from different sites.

Satisfactory evaluation of the genitourinary organs and potential intra-abdominal metastatic sites can be accomplished with ultrasound and computed tomography (CT) scanning of the abdomen and pelvis. The classic appearance on ultrasound is one of a lobulated soft tissue mass with homogeneous echogenicity and an echotexture suggestive of muscle[22] (Fig. 47–3). Focal areas of decreased

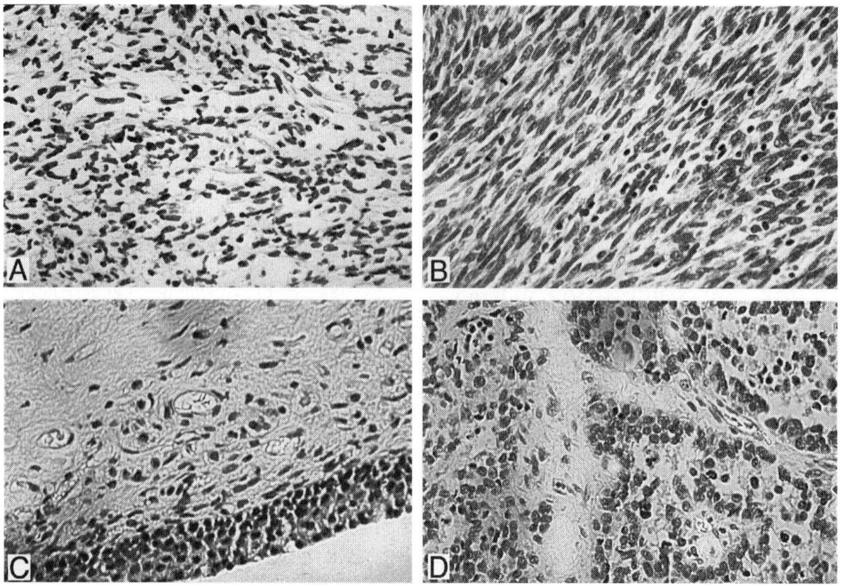
A
B
C
D

FIGURE 47–1. Histologic subtypes of rhabdomyosarcoma. *A*, embryonal; *B*, spindle cell; *C*, botyroid; *D*, alveolar. H & E stain, ×33 magnification. (Courtesy of Dr. Philip Faught.)

echogenicity within the mass are suggestive of hemorrhage or necrosis. The use of transrectal ultrasound in the evaluation of rhabdomyosarcoma has been proposed.[23] Unlike adenocarcinoma of the prostate, which exhibits a predominantly hypoechoic appearance, rhabdomyosarcoma is consistently isoechoic relative to normal prostate tissue. In older patients this modality can provide a safe and painless method for obtaining both diagnostic and follow-up (post-therapy) ultrasound-guided biopsies.

CT scanning has been the most widely used radiographic modality for evaluating genitourinary rhabdomyosarcomas (Fig. 47–4). Newer spiral CT technology allows faster and more accurate data acquisition. Scanning is performed with oral, rectal, and intravenous contrast. Bladder distention is important for detection of bladder wall invasion.

Recently, magnetic resonance imaging (MRI), with its improved contrast resolution, has offered new potential for staging tumors (Figs. 47–5 and 47–6). The use of longitudinal T1-weighted images reduces false impressions of tumor spread by reducing the partial-volume averaging effect encountered in CT scanning, while the enlarged field of view of the MRI images offers an additional advantage over ultrasound studies.[24] Adequate visualization of intravesical masses and invasion into neighboring pelvic structures requires the addition of contrast enhancement with gadolinium-DTPA and the use of more heavily weighted T2 images.

Recent advances in positron emission tomography scanning as well as immunoscans with ^{111}In-labeled monoclonal antibodies may also prove to be useful adjuncts to currently available imaging modalities.[25] However, even with the optimal use of available imaging modalities, the origin of tumors that have achieved a large size may not be appreciated preoperatively.

Because there are no known serologic tumor markers for rhabdomyosarcoma, an accurate diagnosis is dependent on tissue biopsy. Tumors in-

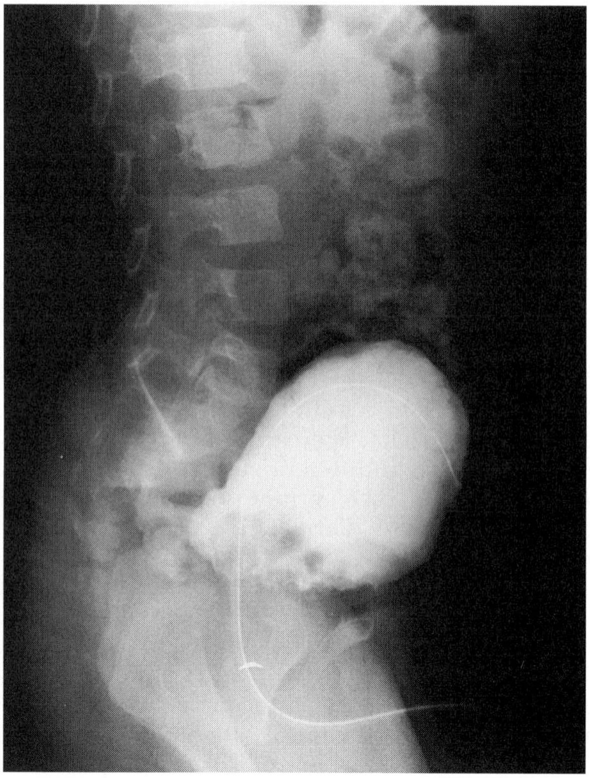

FIGURE 47–2. Oblique view of a cystogram showing a space-occupying mass at the base of the bladder that proved to be an embryonal (botyroid) rhabdomyosarcoma.

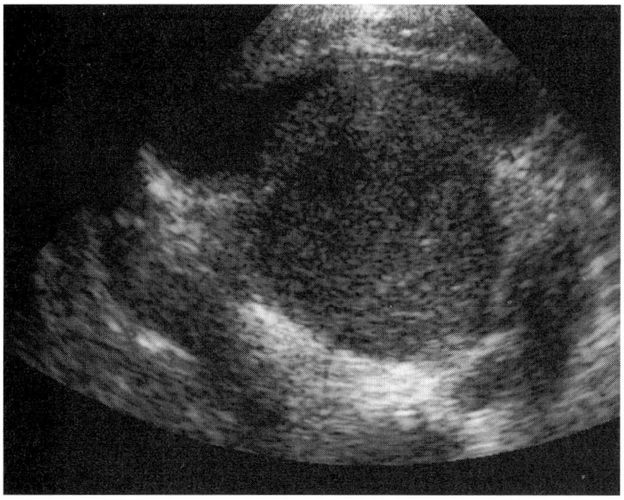

FIGURE 47–3. Bladder ultrasound of a rhabdomyosarcoma of the prostate demonstrating homogeneous echogenicity and an echotexture suggestive of muscle.

volving the bladder, prostate, and vagina may be amenable to endoscopic biopsy. Minimizing the use of the coagulating current will reduce the degree of tissue artifact. The use of cold-cup forceps through the 13-French cystoscope is therefore the preferred method for acquiring tissue. It is also important to maintain a high suspicion of urethral involvement. Submucosal extension of bladder or prostate rhabdomyosarcoma is not always evident on cystoscopy. This has led Loughlin and associates to recommend routine urethral biopsies at the time of endoscopic assessment.[26] Pelvic and retroperitoneal tumors not directly involving the inner surface of these hollow viscera may alternatively be biopsied either percutaneously (i.e., Tru-Cut needle), by transrectal or transvaginal ultrasound-guided biopsy, or by open laparotomy. Regardless of the method of obtaining the biopsy, the surgeon must be sure to perform a thorough sampling to avoid an error in diagnosis. The importance of optimal

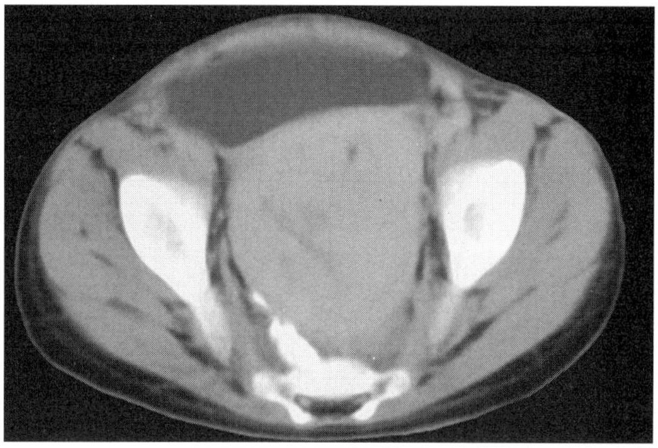

FIGURE 47–4. CT scan of the pelvis showing a solid mass posterior to the bladder that later proved to be a rhabdomyosarcoma of prostatic origin.

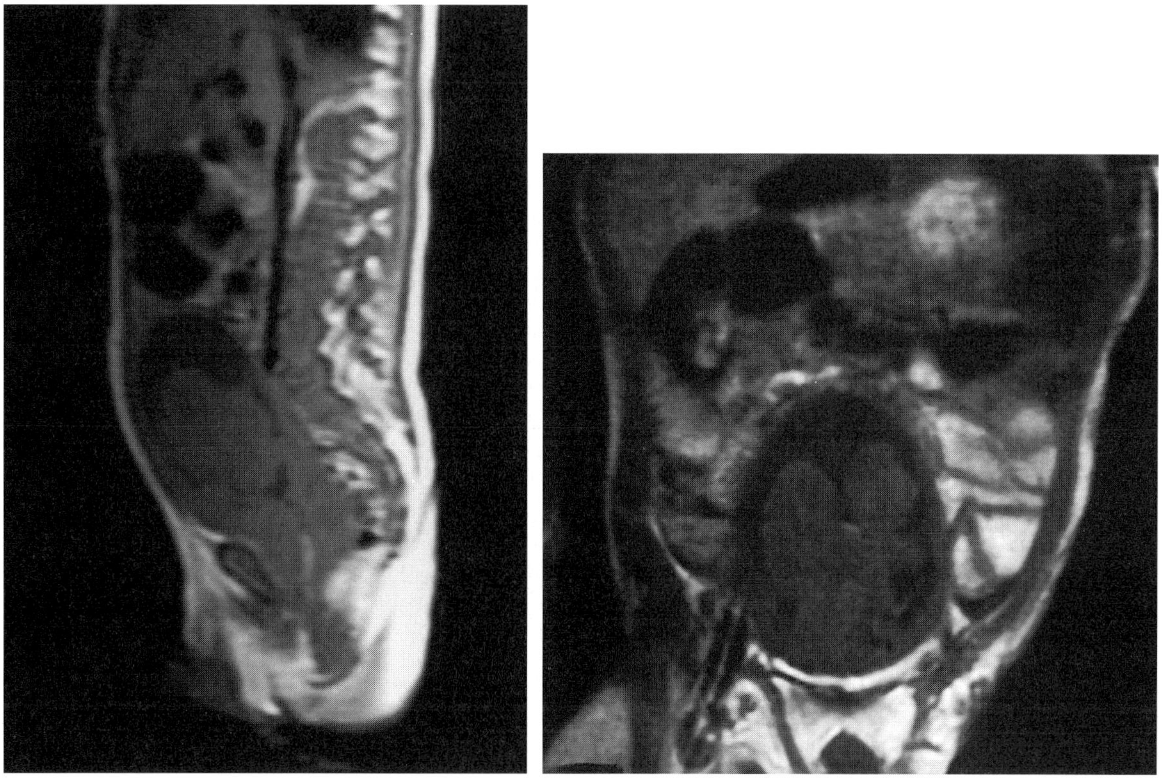

FIGURE 47–5. Sagittal (left) and coronal (right) MRI views showing a botyroid rhabdomyosarcoma of the bladder.

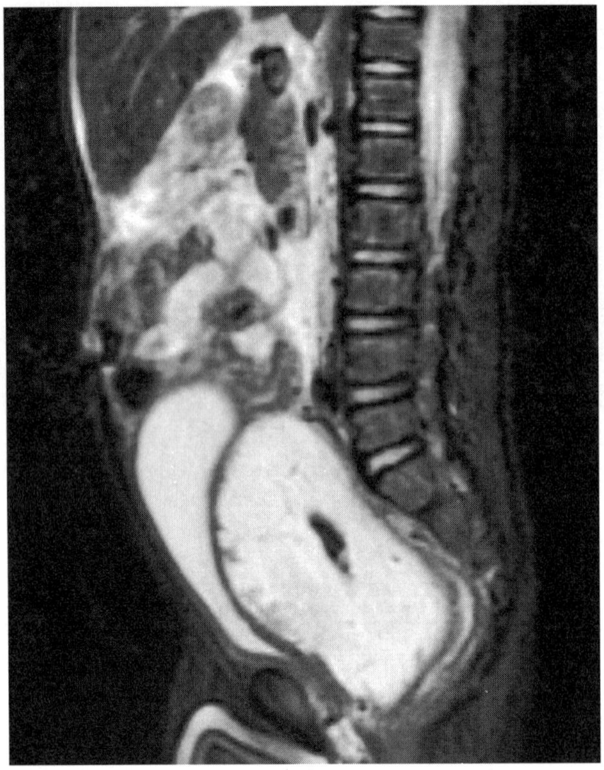

FIGURE 47–6. Sagittal MRI view demonstrating a large prostatic rhabdomyosarcoma.

staging is emphasized by the prognostic importance of stage and varying intensity of treatment.

The liver, lung, bone, and bone marrow are the most common sites for metastatic spread. Therefore, serologic evaluation (i.e., complete blood count, liver function tests), radiographic evaluation of the chest, technetium bone scanning, and bone marrow biopsy should be performed in every patient. Other potential sites of metastatic involvement exist (i.e., central nervous system) and should undergo further organ-specific evaluation as dictated by the history and physical findings.

STAGING

The staging of rhabdomyosarcoma has evolved with our understanding of tumor behavior. The system most commonly used today is derived from the ongoing experience of the major collaborative study of rhabdomyosarcoma in the United States, the IRS. Division into specific groups is dependent on two main factors: the resectability of the primary tumor and the status of the draining lymph nodes. Further stratification has been introduced in the IRS-IV protocol based on histology and site of primary involvement.

Group 1 is defined as local disease (without lymph node involvement) that has been completely removed both grossly and microscopically. The specific designation of a tumor confined to its muscle or organ of involvement (1A) or infiltrating into neighboring structures (1B) is made after microscopic evaluation.

Group 2 is comprised of those patients whose tumors are grossly removed yet have either microscopic residual (2A), regional nodal involvement with no microscopic residual disease (2B), or both nodal involvement and residual disease (2C).

Disseminated disease may take the form of either incomplete removal of gross disease (group 3) or distant metastatic involvement (group 4). Greater than 50% of patients have advanced disease at the time of diagnosis.

One clear shortcoming of this system is that it is dependent on the extent of surgical resection. As a result, two tumors of the same pathologic stage may be assigned to differing clinical groups.

The staging system used in IRS-IV has been designed to overcome some of these shortcomings. An important change is the inclusion of pretreatment stage (tumor, node, metastasis [TNM] classification). The format of this revised staging system is shown in Table 47–2.[27]

TREATMENT

Treatment of rhabdomyosarcoma has undergone significant change over the past three decades. Initial efforts to control this disease were primarily surgical. Typically, in the case of pelvic genitourinary rhabdomyosarcoma, this meant anterior or total pelvic exenteration with diversion of the urinary and fecal stream.[1] Extending the dissection to include the bulbomembranous urethra in males is often necessary because of its frequent involvement in prostatic primaries.[1,26] The observation that rhabdomyosarcoma cells were radiosensitive led to the introduction of radiotherapy into patient care in the early 1950s.[28] D'Angio and colleagues subsequently identified a synergistic action between actinomycin D and radiation.[29] This finding, along with subsequent identification of other effective chemotherapeutic agents, led Pinkel and Pickren to suggest the potential advantage of multimodality therapy.[30]

The benefit of combining surgical therapy with adjuvant radiation and chemotherapy was first demonstrated in 1972.[1,12] All patients who received combined modality therapy of radical surgery followed by chemotherapy and external beam radiotherapy (XRT) survived. In contrast, of seven patients with pelvic rhabdomyosarcoma who did not receive multimodality therapy, six died. Later series confirmed the value of combining radical local therapy, radiation therapy, and chemotherapy.[12] Heyn et al.'s experience with 43 patients treated with initial resection of all gross disease followed by local XRT with or without actinomycin D and vincristine for 1 year were revealing. Nearly a twofold increase in relapse-free 2-year survival was demonstrated with the addition of chemotherapy (85% versus 47%).[12]

TABLE 47–2. IRS IV STAGING

Stage	Tumor Location	TNM Classification T	Size	N	M
1	Favorable sites	T1 or T2	a or b	N0 or N1	M0
2	Unfavorable site	T1 or T2	a	N0	M0
3	Unfavorable site	T1 or T2	a	N1	M0
		T1 or T2	b	N0 or N1	M0
4	Metastatic disease	T1 or T2	a or b	N0 or N1	M1

*T1, confined to anatomic site of origin; T2, extension and/or fixation to surrounding tissue; Ta, tumor less than 5 cm in greatest diameter; Tb, tumor is 5 cm or larger; N0, regional lymph nodes are not clinically involved; N1, regional nodes are clinically involved by tumor; M0, no distant metastases; and M1, metastases are present. GU tumors considered to be favorable sites include the vulva and vagina. GU tumors considered to be unfavorable sites include the bladder, prostate, and uterus.

Intergroup Rhabdomyosarcoma Studies

As in the treatment of Wilms' tumor, it became clear that the limited experience of individual institutions would not allow for proper evaluation of a growing number of available treatment options. In an effort to combine the efforts of these institutions, the IRS was conceived. The primary objectives of IRS-I were to determine whether (1) postoperative irradiation of the tumor bed was necessary for disease control in group 1 patients; (2) chemotherapy with vincristine, actinomycin D, and cyclophosphamide (VAC) was superior to vincristine and actinomycin D alone (VA) in group 2 patients; (3) pulse VAC after initial irradiation in groups 3 and 4 was beneficial; and (4) Adriamycin provided some added benefit in those with advanced disease (groups 3 and 4).

The protocol of the IRS-I study group entailed initial surgical excision with subsequent radiation and chemotherapy. External beam radiation in doses ranging from 2000 to 5500 cGy were used. Patients in clinical group 1 were randomized to receive either VAC or VAC + radiation. Clinical group 2 patients were randomized to receive either VA + radiation or VAC + radiation. Patients with advanced disease (clinical groups 3 and 4) were randomized to receive either VAC + radiation or VAC + Adriamycin + radiation. The chemotherapeutic regimen was continued for 2 years in most cases. Neither postoperative radiation in group 1, cyclophosphamide in group 2, nor Adriamycin in groups 3 and 4 provided any statistically significant advantage.[31] It also was evident that groups 2 through 4 benefited from the added modality of radiation. However, moderately high doses of radiation were required to decrease the incidence of local recurrence.[32]

Of the 686 patients entered into IRS-I, 62 presented with either bladder, prostate, or vaginal primaries. The overall survival rate for those with primary genitourinary sites was 81% (50 of 62). Of these, 44% (22 of 50) originally retained the bladder. Relapse, either locally or with distant metastasis, usually occurred within the first 2 years. Relapse was a particularly ominous sign, with only 2 of 13 patients surviving long term.[19]

Following the favorable results of the IRS-I study and the enthusiasm over the initial follow-up of the patients with bladder salvage, IRS-II (1978–1984) set out to evaluate the feasibility of primary chemotherapy. Following confirmation of the diagnosis by biopsy, these patients were started on initial VAC chemotherapy followed by repetitive monthly courses with the same agents. If a response was evident, chemotherapy was continued out to 16 weeks. The mass was then resected and chemotherapy continued for 2 years on a monthly basis. If there was gross or microscopic disease following resection, then radiotherapy was added to the regimen. XRT as well as insertion of interstitial beads or rods into the vagina or bladder have been used with excellent results. A total of 109 patients in IRS-II presented with tumors of either bladder, prostate, vagina, or uterus. Disappointingly, chemotherapy alone provided relapse-free survival in only 10% of patients.

Although neoadjuvant chemotherapy led to a higher bladder salvage rate initially (97%), extended follow-up (3 years) revealed no significant difference between patients retaining their bladder between the two IRS studies (22% versus 23%).[33] However, the 3-year survival following partial cystectomy was almost identical to that for all patients with bladder rhabdomyosarcoma (79% and 78%, respectively).[34]

Although patients retain their native bladder, the ultimate impact on quality of life must be measured in terms of bladder function. Of patients who retained their bladders during IRS-I and IRS-II, 73% had satisfactory bladder function. Renal function was preserved in nearly every patient.[35] Others have reported between 50 and 80% success rates for preserving a normally functioning bladder.[36,37] However, of the patients who developed problems with bladder function, many received higher doses of local irradiation than is recommended in current protocols. Total dose prescriptions currently recommended are 4000 to 5000 cGy, because increased morbidity without increase in local control occurs at doses of 5500 cGy.[38] It was hoped that lower total radiation dose, along with smaller daily dose fractions, avoidance of radiosensitizing chemotherapeutic agents, and prevention of urinary tract infections, would all help to reduce late bladder morbidity.[39]

From these data, it may be concluded that partial cystectomy is a viable option when gross tumor removal can be assured (i.e., isolated dome lesions). Survival is not adversely affected if a radical operation is delayed until residual tumor is defined or progression is noted, but further delay is not recommended.[37,40] Careful monitoring of these children is essential to identify late bladder deterioration resulting from radiation and/or chemotherapy.[36,41] Primary augmentation at the time of partial cystectomy may also improve the chances of the patient retaining an adequate functional capacity. For the young patient in whom bladder preservation is not feasible, the initial construction of a nonrefluxing colon conduit serves as an appropriate temporizing measure. In most patients, a later continent urinary diversion, fashioned from the original conduit, may then be planned as the patient achieves a long-term disease-free status and demonstrates the proper motivation to perform self-catheterization.[42,43]

Despite a change in basic approach in IRS-II (from initial radical surgery to initial chemotherapy), the success of organ sparing was similar to that of IRS-I. However, the mortality rate rose from approximately 10% to 25%, a difference that could be attributed to the elimination of the group of patients that had primary radical surgery.[33] This study emphasized the need for improved induction chemotherapy if improved long-term results were to be achieved. The objectives of IRS-III (1984–1988) were to address five specific issues regarding chemotherapeutic protocols and response to therapy. Prior to randomization, patients were divided into favorable or unfavorable histology.[31] The alveolar, anaplastic, and monomorphous types were included in the unfavorable category. All other histologic types were considered to be in the favorable category. The study objectives included whether (1) the duration of chemotherapy with VA could be reduced to only 1 year in group 1 and 2 patients with "favorable" histology, (2) the addition of cisplatinum and doxorubicin had an advantage over standard VAC chemotherapy, (3) the addition of cisplatinum ± etoposide had an advantage over standard VAC chemotherapy in groups 3 and 4, (4) patients who demonstrated only a partial response by week 20 would benefit from the addition of additional cell cycle–specific agents, and (5) second- and third-look surgery to assess response in groups 3 and 4 would improve local control. It was hoped that the addition of these additional chemotherapeutic agents to pulse VAC for pelvic tumors would help avoid radical surgery in more patients. Because of the poorer prognosis of prostate over bladder primaries, earlier institution of radiotherapy in cases of prostate and bladder neck primaries tumors was also instituted.

The results of IRS-III have been strikingly superior to those of IRS-I and -II.[33] Rate of retention of functional bladder at 4 years from diagnosis was approximately 60%, a greater than 100% improvement over results in IRS-I and -II (22% and 25%, respectively). Mortality in patients with nondisseminated disease (groups 1 through 3) has declined to less than 10%.

Female Genital Tract Rhabdomyosarcoma

In 1988, Hays et al. reported on the results of 47 primary tumors of the vagina, uterus, or vulva that had been treated under IRS-I and IRS-II protocols.[21] Treatment of vaginal primaries consisted of initial chemotherapy followed by delayed hysterectomy and/or partial vaginectomy in the majority of cases. The primary treatment objective of achieving equivalent or better outcomes with less extensive ablative surgery (i.e., anterior exenteration) were realized. The uniquely favorable response to therapy that was realized in the treatment of vaginal primaries (90% survival) distinguishes them from uterine primaries. Primary tumors of the uterus, although managed with similar chemotherapeutic regimens, proved to have a worse prognosis. Superficial polypoid involvement of the uterus faired substantially better than those lesions that presented with more extensive local disease. (All patients with extensive local disease had succumbed to their disease within 1 year of diagnosis.) Tumors of the vulva were managed with local en bloc resection and chemotherapy with or without adjunctive chemotherapy. Eight of the nine patients were disease free at a mean follow-up of 6.4 years, with the remaining patient demonstrating recurrence 2.5 years after initial treatment.

Treatment: Future Directions

The objectives of IRS-IV (1989 to the present) include a plan to evaluate the validity of treatment based on the pretreatment stage. Staging has been modified to include favorable versus unfavorable primary sites as well as size of the primary. New chemotherapeutic agents to be evaluated include etoposide and ifosfamide. The benefit of hyperfractionated radiation on local control will be evaluated in group 3. This method of radiation delivery has the theoretical advantage of increased tumor kill with reduced injury to normal tissue.[38]

PARATESTICULAR RHABDOMYOSARCOMA

Paratesticular primaries are associated with a good prognosis and are considered separately from pelvic primaries because of differences in treatment.[44] The primary histology is favorable (embryonal) in the majority (97%).[6] Lymphatic spread is noted in 28%.[6] The majority of patients present with a palpable mass in the scrotum, and most patients present with clinical group 1 and 2 disease (81%). Initial evaluation should include serum tumor markers (α-fetoprotein and the β subunit of human chorionic gonadotropin) to help differentiate paratesticular rhabdomyosarcoma from a testicular primary. Scrotal ultrasonography is ideal for characterizing the scrotal mass. Although paratesticular tumors rarely involve the testis itself, initial therapy usually consists of radical orchiectomy. An inguinal approach with early control of the vasculature prevents cross-contamination of the inguinal lymphatics in cases of tumor spillage (Fig. 47–7). If the primary has been removed through a scrotal incision, then scrotectomy should also be done at the time of definitive resection.

Controversy still surrounds the need for staging retroperitoneal lymphadenectomy in patients with a negative radiographic evaluation of the retroperitoneum and chest. Evaluation of 121 paratesticular tumors entered into IRS-III have provided some valuable information to help rationally assess this issue.[45] Preoperative radiographic evaluation had only a 57% sensitivity (43% of patients who demonstrated node positivity were negative on radiographic evaluation). This finding is profoundly important when considering that node positivity is associated with decreased patient survival.[45]

As an analogy to the use of chemotherapy in clinical stage A nonseminomatous germ cell tumors, the staging retroperitoneal lymph node dissection will prevent undertreatment of false-negative clinical group 2 patients. The patient with localized group 1 pathology may avoid radiotherapy if found to have negative retroperitoneal lymph nodes.[26] In addition, the proper identification of clinical group 1/pathologic group 2 patients (false-negative radiographic staging of the retroperitoneum) will allow these patients to receive postoperative radiation therapy—an adjunct that has increased 2-year relapse-free survival to 90%.

The first three IRS studies advocated staging RPLND in all cases of paratesticular rhabdomyosarcoma. However, excellent survival statistics without RPLND in patients with negative computerized tomography have brought into question the need for routine RPLND in this patient subset.[46] Lymph node dissection is not recommended in current IRS-IV trials in children with localized, completely resected tumors whose imaging study results are negative. These patients are being closely monitored for node relapse.

Overall survival for patients treated with IRS-I and -II protocols is 89% at 3 years. This apparent survival advantage over rhabdomyosarcoma involving other primary sites may be due in part to earlier detection. With such favorable outcomes, especially within groups 1 and 2 (93% and 90% cure rates, respectively), attention has been focused on reducing side effects. Staging and proposed treatment as outlined by IRS-IV are seen in Table 47–3.[47] Newer studies identifying biologic characteristics associated with low metastatic potential may in the future help to reduce or eliminate the use of systemic therapy in specific subsets of patients (i.e., surgically staged group 1 patients).[48]

OUTCOME

Prognostic Factors

Identification of prognostic variables is of great importance for stratifying patients in order to permit valid comparison of alternative therapies and for tailoring therapy according to risk of relapse. Univariate and multivariate analysis of the 1688 patients enrolled in IRS-I and IRS-II has led to the identification of specific prognostic criteria as well as improved staging. Clinical group (disease extent)

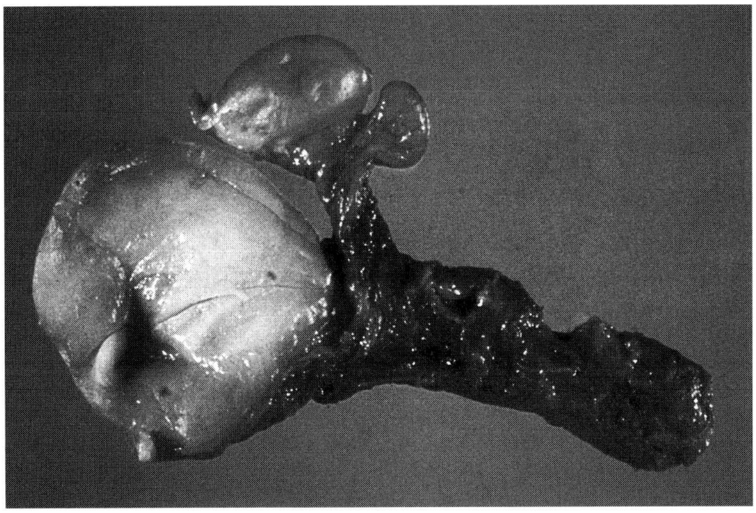

FIGURE 47–7. A large paratesticular rhabdomyosarcoma removed through an inguinal incision, with early control of the cord and vessels. (Courtesy of Dr. Philip Faught.)

TABLE 47–3. IRS-IV STAGING AND TREATMENT OF PARATESTICULAR RHABDOMYOSARCOMA

Clinical Group	Tumor Status	Therapy
1	Tumor completely excised* (not alveolar subtype)	Vincristine and actinomycin D for 1 yr†
2	Tumor excised with microscopic residual disease at margin and/or positive lymph nodes involving ipsilateral hilar–para-aortic chain	Vincristine plus actinomycin D plus cyclophosphamide versus vincristine plus actinomycin D plus ifosfamide for 1–2 yr plus radiation therapy to involved region‡
3	Gross residual local and/or regional disease (retroperitoneal nodes), which is not surgically removable	Three- to 7-drug regimen plus radiation therapy to involved region§
4	Distant metastasis	Same as group 3

*If there has been scrotal contamination, hemiscrotectomy and relocation of the contralateral testis into the thigh are advised to avoid the effects of local radiation on the remaining gonad.

†No radiation for group 1 patients.

‡Conventional radiation.

§Conventional or hyperfractionated radiation.

proved to be the most important patient characteristic related to survival in both IRS-I and IRS-II.[49] Survival decreased in a progressive fashion from clinical group 1 to clinical group 4 (82% versus 24%). Specific characteristics that make up these groups have been shown to be important prognostic factors in and of themselves. Rodary and associates demonstrated that outcome is improved if the tumor is less than 5 cm in size and noninvasive and the lymph nodes are not involved.[50]

The site of the primary tumor is important—so much so that it has been incorporated into the current staging system of IRS-IV. Genitourinary sites have a survival advantage over nongenitourinary sites, with the difference noted to be most significant in clinical group 4 cases.[49] Paratesticular and female external genitalia are highly favorable sites. Bladder, prostate, and uterus share an intermediate prognosis, and nongenitourinary pelvic sites have a relatively poor prognosis.[50] Although bladder primaries have been reported to have a more favorable outcome than prostate primaries, it is in fact often difficult to determine the exact site of origin in many cases.[51]

The IRS has recently demonstrated that histology is predictive of outcome. After studying the survival rates of all histologic subtypes in 800 patients from IRS-II, a new system based on prognosis (the ICR) was formulated. The ICR has been tested in both a univariate and multivariate model and found to be highly reproducible and predictive of outcome. The best survival is noted in botyroid rhabdomyosarcoma (95% survival at 5 years). Nonbotyroid embryonal rhabdomyosarcoma has a survival rate in the intermediate range (67% at 5 years), with alveolar and undifferentiated sarcoma having the poorest prognoses (54% and 47%, respectively).[17] The difference in prognosis is most significant in patients with localized disease.[49]

Survival

Overall, the survival rate for genitourinary primary tumors has been second only to that of orbital lesions, with nearly 75% of the patients in IRS-I having long-term survival.[31] Paratesticular tumors have the best prognosis, with 89% of patients surviving long-term.[52] Most have favorable histology and present with clinical group 1 and 2 pathology. The current survival for bladder and prostate tumors is 80% when treated with conservative surgery.[33] These results, although improvements over IRS-II statistics, still fall short of the 90% survival noted in these tumors when managed by anterior pelvic exenteration and support the belief that present chemotherapy and radiotherapy has not yet substituted for radical surgical procedures in many of these children.[11] Patients with vaginal tumors have a greater than 90% survival, but only 40% of patients with uterine tumors survive.[21] Most patients who relapse with distant metastasis die of disease.[53]

Side Effects

Dramatic improvements in the survival rates of rhabdomyosarcoma patients have led to a greater emphasis on improving the quality of life for these children. The efforts directed at reducing surgical morbidity by introducing organ-sparing surgery in properly selected patients have been previously discussed. Additional side effects are grouped based on the primary treatment modality from which they result.

Problems related to surgical procedures used in the treatment of paratesticular rhabdomyosarcoma include loss of normal ejaculatory function, hydrocele, small bowel obstruction, and lymphedema of the leg.[54] In all cases of ejaculatory incompetence, the patient had undergone a full bilateral retroperitoneal lymph node dissection. The improved understanding of the relationship between sympathetic innervation and retroperitoneal anatomy has subsequently resulted in modified procedures designed to spare these sympathetic nerves.[55] Results of prechemotherapy nerve-sparing procedures have yielded intact ejaculatory rates of as high as 99%. Problems related to surgical procedures used in the treatment of pelvic rhabdomyosarcoma to a large extent reflect the type of reconstructive effort undertaken. Patients who received urinary conduits after total cystectomy for pelvic primaries developed upper tract deterioration twice as often as the patients who were managed with partial cystectomy.[35] This finding is in agreement with the past experience of the urologic community with ileal and colon conduits in the pediatric population.[56,57] Radical surgical procedures used in treating bladder and prostate primaries in males have a high likelihood of resulting in impotence. When surgical intervention entails resection of the prostate or bladder, familiarization with the anatomy of the neurovascular bundle can prove invaluable in preserving erectile function.[58]

Specific radiotherapy injury is difficult to separate from the influence of other treatment modalities. Along with potentially influencing the previously listed surgical complications and potentiating the damaging effects of doxorubicin and cyclophosphamide, side effects of bone/soft tissue hypoplasia, short stature, chronic diarrhea, and urethral strictures have been documented.[59] Despite radiation doses as high as 5280 cGy, the kidneys were believed to generally have retained normal function after having therapy directed to the para-aortic or iliac lymph nodes during treatment for paratesticular primaries.[54] Secondary malignancies can arise as late as 20 years following retroperitoneal radiation.[60] One patient with a concomitant diagnosis of neurofibromatosis developed a fibrosarcoma of the retroperitoneum 14 years after treatment. With an increasing number of patients now experiencing durable remissions, close monitoring will be required to identify these possible late complications.

Late effects of chemotherapy from the IRS-I and IRS-II study groups primarily related to hemorrhagic cystitis and gonadal dysfunction resulting from cyclosphosphamide. Significant hematuria was identified in between 29 and 33% of patients who received this drug.[35,54] Mesna (sodium 2-mercaptoethane sulfonate), which binds acrolein (the toxic metabolite of cyclophosphamide), may be used to prevent this complication. Early institution of continuous bladder irrigation has recently been shown to reduce the incidence of significant hemorrhagic cystitis. If significant hematuria does occur (>50 red blood cells per high-power field), these alkylating agents should be withheld until the hematuria resolves. Once the hematuria has resolved, these agents may be resumed. A review of the combined IRS-I and IRS-II patients with pelvic genitourinary primaries who underwent bladder preservation revealed one fourth to be suffering from irritative bladder symptomatology.[35] However, because the majority of patients received both radiation and chemotherapy, it is difficult to define specific individual contributions to either modality.

Although effects of cyclophosphamide on testicular function have not been systematically evaluated in the majority of genitourinary rhabdomyosarcoma patients, the elevation of follicle-stimulating hormone levels or known azoospermia in 50% of patients tested is in agreement with known side effects in the treatment of nonseminomatous germ cell tumors with this agent.[61] Newer chemotherapeutic agents will likely lead to further issues in patient management (i.e., myelosuppression).

MOLECULAR BIOLOGY OF RHABDOMYOSARCOMA

Recent advances in the molecular understanding of rhabdomyosarcoma hold promise of developing improved diagnostic and prognostic criteria so as to better apply future therapeutic alternatives.

As stated previously, the diagnosis of rhabdomyosarcoma is based on the application of light and electron microscopy. Rhabdomyosarcoma has classically been included under the histologic grouping of small round cell neoplasms of childhood—a category that includes such diverse malignancies as Ewing's sarcoma, medulloblastoma, and hepatoblastoma.[62] The differential diagnosis of rhabdomyosarcoma relies on the identification of rhabdomyoblasts and characteristic cross-striations of skeletal muscle. Morphometric techniques that utilize several shape descriptors of the cell nucleus have also been used to characterize these tumors.[63] However, a significant proportion of these malignancies are poorly differentiated and lack clearly discernible characteristics to support the diagnosis of rhabdomyosarcoma.[64]

Efforts to identify immunohistochemical differences between other small round cell tumors have centered around muscle-specific proteins. Monoclonal antibodies to muscle cell–specific proteins (i.e., the muscle-specific intermediate filament desmin and muscle-specific actin) have been beneficial in diagnosing poorly differentiated cases of rhabdomyosarcoma. Other monoclonal probes appear to recognize only one specific histologic subtype, a characteristic that may help further differentiate between favorable (i.e., embryonal) and unfavorable (i.e., alveolar) subtypes.[65]

Cytogenetic abnormalities, most notably translocations, have been identified in many pediatric malignancies and have been shown to have both diagnostic and prognostic relevance.[66] Molecular heterogeneity has likewise been shown in rhabdomyosarcoma.[67] A loss of heterozygosity at chromosome 11 has been noted in the embryonal subtype, whereas tumors in the alveolar group have frequently been found to exhibit a t(2;13)(q37;q14) translocation.[68,69] Evaluation of nuclear DNA content by flow cytometric techniques has demonstrated that diploidy is a poor prognostic finding, whereas tumors that demonstrate aneuploid patterns are associated with a more favorable outcome.[48,70]

The molecular significance of these and other chromosomal alterations are presently under investigation. A chimeric protein involving the *PAX3* and *FKHR* gene products has been identified in alveolar rhabdomyosarcomas with t(2;13) translocations. The fusion of genes coding for both a transcription factor and a DNA binding domain may have important implications in the events surrounding transcriptional control and development of rhabdomyosarcoma.[71] Perhaps the most exciting advance has been the identification of a master gene regulatory protein (Myo D1) that is normally only expressed in myoblasts and skeletal muscle cells.[72] This protein has been shown to bind to the regulatory regions of several muscle-specific genes and control their transcription. Transfection of this gene into a fibroblast converts it to a muscle cell.[72] This gene is found in all rhabdomyosarcomas and is a valuable differential marker for diagnosis. Moreover the Myo D1 locus maps to chromosome 11, the site of chromosomal alteration noted in patients with the embryonal subtype of rhabdomyosarcoma.[73]

Amplification of specific growth regulatory molecules such as the proto-oncogene N-*myc* have been extensively studied in other pediatric tumors and shown to correlate with prognosis.[74] Identification of N-*myc* gene amplification in the alveolar variant of rhabdomyosarcoma may prove to be an important prognostic indicator in patients with this disease as well.[75,76] The presence of P glycoprotein (a molecule associated with multidrug resistance), and mutations of the tumor suppresser gene *p53* have likewise been demonstrated in these tumors.[77–79]

In vitro experiments with human rhabdomyosarcoma cell lines have demonstrated the presence of multiple peptide growth factors thought to play a role in tumor formation and maintenance.[65] Secretion of specific heparin-binding growth factors has recently been identified. Specific inhibitors of these growth factors may have therapeutic potential in patients with rhabdomyosarcoma. An in vivo animal xenograft model (nude mice with the human A-204 rhabdomyosarcoma cell line) has been developed and has so far shown promise in determining sensitivity as well as resistance mechanisms toward various agents designed to inhibit these growth-related protein molecules.[80] The heparin analog pentosan polysulfate has been shown to inhibit tumor growth both in vitro and in vivo. Phase I trials using this agent in other tumors have provided encouraging results.[81]

SUMMARY

The treatment and prognosis of the child with rhabdomyosarcoma has experienced dramatic improvements over the past two decades. As our understanding of tumor behavior has evolved, it has become possible to not only improve survival but also focus on important quality-of-life issues. Future therapeutic advances will depend largely on an improved molecular understanding of altered cell behavior and the continued efforts of multi-institutional studies.

REFERENCES

1. Grosfeld JL, Clatworthy JP: Pelvic rhabdomyosarcoma in infants and children. J Urol 1972; 107:673.
2. Young JL, Miller RW: Incidence of malignant tumors in U.S. children. J Pediatr 1975; 86:254.
3. Lacey SR, Jewett TC Jr, Karp MP, et al: Advances in the treatment of rhabdomyosarcoma. Semin Surg Oncol 1986; 2:139.
4. Maurer JM, Moon T, Donaldson M: The Intergroup Rhabdomyosarcoma Study: a preliminary report. Cancer 1977; 40:2015.
5. Sutow WW: Prognosis in childhood rhabdomyosarcoma. Cancer 1970; 25:1384.
6. Raney B Jr, Carey A, Snyder HM, et al: Primary site as a prognostic variable for children with pelvic soft tissue sarcomas. J Urol 1986; 136:874.
7. Ruymann FB, Maddux HR, Ragab A, et al: Congenital anomalies associated with rhabdomyosarcoma: an autopsy study of 115 cases. A report from the Intergroup Rhabdomyosarcoma Study Committee. Med Pediatr Oncol 1988; 16:33.
8. Pizzo PA, Horowitz ME, Poplack DG, et al: Solid tumors of childhood. De Vita VT Jr, Hellman S, Rosenberg SA (eds): Cancer: Principles and Practice of Oncology, 3rd edition, p 1647. Philadelphia, JB Lippincott Co, 1989.
9. McKeen EA, Bodurtha J, Meadows AT: Rhabdomyosarcoma complicating multiple neurofibromatosis. J Pediatr 1978; 93:992.
10. Li FP, Fraumeni JF: Soft tissue sarcomas, breast cancer and other neoplasms: a familial syndrome. Ann Intern Med 1969; 71:747.
11. Grosfeld JL, Weber TR, Weetman RM, et al: Rhabdomyosarcoma in childhood: analysis of survival in 98 cases. J Pediatr Surg 1983; 18:141.
12. Heyn RM, Holland R, Newton WA Jr: The role of combined chemotherapy in the treatment of rhabdomyosarcoma in children. Cancer 1974; 34:2128.
13. Horn RC Jr, Enterline HT: Rhabdomyosarcoma: a clinicopathological study and classification of 39 cases. Cancer 1958; 11:181.
14. Patton RB, Horn RC Jr: Rhabdomyosarcoma: clinical and pathological features and comparison with human fetal and embryonal skeletal muscle. Surgery 1962; 52:572.
15. Cavazzana AO, Schmidt D, Ninfo V, et al: Spindle cell rhabdomyosarcoma: a prognostically favorable variant of rhabdomyosarcoma. Am J Surg Pathol 1992; 16:229.
16. Leuschner I, Newton WJ, Schmidt D, et al: Spindle cell variants of embryonal rhabdomyosarcoma in the parates-

ticular region: a report of the Intergroup Rhabdomyosarcoma Study. Am J Surg Pathol 1993; 17:221.
17. Newton WA Jr, Gehan EA, Webber BL, et al: Classification of rhabdomyosarcomas and related sarcomas. Cancer 1995; 76:1073.
18. Hays DM: Pelvic rhabdomyosarcoma in childhood: diagnosis and concepts of management reviewed. Cancer 1980; 45:1811.
19. Hays DM, Raney RJ, Lawrence WJ, et al: Bladder and prostatic tumors in the Intergroup Rhabdomyosarcoma Study (IRS-I): results of therapy. Cancer 1982; 50:1472.
20. Kramer SA, Kelalis PP: Pediatric urologic oncology. *In* Gillenwater JY, Grayhack JT, Howards SS, et al (eds): Adult and Pediatric Urology, p 2001. Chicago, Year Book Medical Publishers, 1987.
21. Hays DM, Shimada H, Raney RJ, et al: Clinical staging and treatment results in rhabdomyosarcoma of the female genital tract among children and adolescents. Cancer 1988; 61:1893.
22. Bahnson RR, Zaontz MR, Maizels M, et al: Ultrasonography and diagnosis of pediatric genitourinary rhabdomyosarcoma. Urology 1989; 33:64.
23. Terris MK, Eigner EB, Briggs EM, et al: Transrectal ultrasound in the evaluation of rhabdomyosarcoma involving the prostate. Br J Urol 1994; 74:341.
24. Fletcher BD, Kaste SC: Magnetic resonance imaging for diagnosis and follow-up of genitourinary, pelvic, and perineal rhabdomyosarcoma. Urol Radiol 1992; 14:263.
25. Reuland P, Koscelniak E, Ruck P, et al: Application of an anti-myosin antibody for scintigraphic differential-diagnosis of infantile tumors. Int J Rad Appl Instrum 1991; 18:89.
26. Loughlin KR, Retik AB, Weinstein HJ, et al: Genitourinary rhabdomyosarcoma in children. Cancer 1989; 63:1600.
27. Snyder HM, D'Angio GJ, Evans AE, et al: Pediatric oncology. *In* Walsh PC, Retik AB, Stamey TA, Vaughan ED Jr (eds): Campbell's Urology, 6th edition, p 2001. Philadelphia, WB Saunders Co, 1992.
28. Stobbe GC, Dargeon HW: Embryonal rhabdomyosarcoma of the head and neck in children and adolescents. Cancer 1950; 3:826.
29. D'Angio GJ, Farber S, Maddock CL: Potentiation of x-ray effects by actinomycin D. Radiology 1959; 73:175.
30. Pinkel D, Pickren J: Rhabdomyosarcoma in children. JAMA 1961; 175:293.
31. Maurer HM, Beltangady M, Gehan EA, et al: The Intergroup Rhabdomyosarcoma Study-I: a final report. Cancer 1988; 61:209.
32. Tefft M: Radiation of rhabdomyosarcoma in children: local control in patients enrolled into the Intergroup Rhabdomyosarcoma Study. NCI Monogr 1981; 56:75.
33. Hays DM: Bladder/prostate rhabdomyosarcoma: results of the multi-institutional trials of the Intergroup Rhabdomyosarcoma Study. Semin Surg Oncol 1993; 9:520.
34. Hays DM, Lawrence WJ, Crist WM, et al: Partial cystectomy in the management of rhabdomyosarcoma of the bladder: a report from the Intergroup Rhabdomyosarcoma Study. J Pediatr Surg 1990; 25:719.
35. Raney BJ, Heyn R, Hays DM, et al: Sequelae of treatment in 109 patients followed for 5 to 15 years after diagnosis of sarcoma of the bladder and prostate: a report from the Intergroup Rhabdomyosarcoma Study Committee. Cancer 1993; 71:2387.
36. Hicks BA, Hensle TW, Burbige KA, et al: Bladder management in children with genitourinary sarcoma. J Pediatr Surg 1993; 28:1019.
37. Hays DM: New approaches to the surgical management of rhabdomyosarcoma in childhood. Chir Pediatr 1990; 31:197.
38. Thames HD Jr, Withers RH, Peters LJ, et al: Changes in early and late radiation reponses with altered dose fractionation: implications for dose-survival relationships. Int J Radiat Oncol Biol Phys 1982; 8:219.
39. Broecker BH, Plowman N, Pritchard J, et al: Pelvic rhabdomyosarcoma in children. Br J Urol 1988; 61:427.
40. Shapiro E, Strother D: Genitourinary rhabdomyosarcoma in childhood: current treatment alternatives and controversies in management. Cancer Treat Res 1992; 59:1.
41. Yeung CK, Ward HC, Ransley PG, et al: Bladder and kidney function after cure of pelvic rhabdomyosarcoma in childhood. Br J Cancer 1994; 70:1000.
42. Lander EB, Shanberg AM, Tansey LA, et al: The use of continent diversion in the management of rhabdomyosarcoma of the prostate in childhood. J Urol 1992; 147:1602.
43. Duel BP, Hendren WH, Bauer SB, et al: Reconstructive options in genitourinary rhabdomyosarcoma. J Urol 1996; 156:1798.
44. Blyth B, Mandell J, Bauer S, et al: Paratesticular rhabdomyosarcoma: results of therapy in 18 cases. J Urol 1990; 144:1450.
45. Wiener ES, Lawrence W, Hays D, et al: Retroperitoneal node biopsy in paratesticular rhabdomyosarcoma. J Pediatr Surg 1994; 29:171.
46. Goldfarb B, Khoury AE, Greenberg ML, Churchill BM, et al: The role of retroperitoneal lymphadenectomy in localized paratesticular rhabdomyosarcoma. J Urol 1994; 152:785.
47. Shapiro E, Strother D: Pediatric genitourinary rhabdomyosarcoma. J Urol 1992; 148:1761.
48. Shapiro DM, Parham DM, Douglass EC, et al: Relationship of tumor-cell ploidy to histologic subtype and treatment outcome in children and adolescents with unresectable rhabdomyosarcoma. J Clin Oncol 1991; 9:159.
49. Crist WM, Garnsey L, Beltangady MS, et al: Prognosis in children with rhabdomyosarcoma: a report of the Intergroup Rhabdomyosarcoma Studies I and II Intergroup Rhabdomyosarcoma Committee. J Clin Oncol 1990; 8:443.
50. Rodary C, Gehan EA, Flamant F, et al: Prognostic factors in 951 nonmetastatic rhabdomyosarcoma in children: a report from the International Rhabdomyosarcoma Workshop. Med Pediatr Oncol 1991; 19:89.
51. Raney RJ, Gehan EA, Hays DM, et al: Primary chemotherapy with or without radiation therapy and/or surgery for children with localized sarcoma of the bladder, prostate, vagina, uterus, and cervix: a comparison of the results in Intergroup Rhabdomyosarcoma Studies I and II. Cancer 1990; 66:2072.
52. Raney RB Jr, Tefft M, Lawrence W Jr, et al: Paratesticular sarcoma in childhood and adolescence: a report from the Intergroup Rhabdomyosarcoma Studies I and II, 1973–1983. Cancer 1987; 60:2337.
53. Raney RB Jr, Crist WM, Maurer HM, et al: Prognosis of children with soft tissue sarcoma who relapse after achieving a complete response. Cancer 1983; 52:44.
54. Heyn R, Raney RJ, Hays DM, et al: Late effects of therapy in patients with paratesticular rhabdomyosarcoma. Intergroup Rhabdomyosarcoma Study Committee. J Clin Oncol 1992; 10:614.
55. Donohue J, Foster R, Rowland R: Nerve-sparing retroperitoneal lymphadenectomy with preservation of ejaculation. J Urol 1990; 144:287.
56. Elder DD, Moisey CU, Rees RWM: A long-term follow-up of the colonic conduit operation in children. Br J Urol 1979; 51:462.
57. Shapiro SR, Lebowitz R, Colodny AH: Fate of 90 children with ileal conduit urinary diversion a decade later: analysis of complications, pyelography, renal function and bacteriology. J Urol 1975; 114:289.
58. Walsh PC, Lepor J, Eggleston JC: Radical prostatectomy with preservation of sexual function: anatomical and pathological considerations. Prostate 1983; 4:473.
59. Hughes LL, Baruzzi MJ, Ribeiro RC, et al: Paratesticular rhabdomyosarcoma: delayed effects of multimodality therapy and implications for current management. Cancer 1994; 73:476.
60. Dieckmann KP, Wegner HE, Krain J: Multiple primary neoplasms in patients with testicular germ cell tumor. Oncology 1994; 51:450.
61. Johnson D, Hainsworth J, Linde R: Testicular function fol-

lowing combination chemotherapy with cisplatin, vinblastine, and bleomycin. Med Pediatr Oncol 1984; 12:233.
62. Winters JL, Geil JD, O'Connor WN: Immunohistology, cytogenetics, and molecular studies of small round cell tumors of childhood. Ann Clin Lab Sci 1995; 25:66.
63. Partin AW, Gearhart JP, Leonard MP, et al: The use of nuclear morphometry to predict prognosis in pediatric urologic malignancies: a review. Med Pediatr Oncol 1993; 21: 222.
64. Enzinger F, Weiss S: Soft Tissue Tumors, 3rd edition, p 1120. St. Louis, CV Mosby, 1995.
65. Houghton JA, Meyer WH, Houghton PJ: Scheduling of vincristine: drug accumulation and response of xenografts of childhood rhabdomyosarcoma determined by frequency of administration. Cancer Treat Rep 1987; 71:717.
66. Fletcher JA, Kozakewich JP, Hoffer FA, et al: Diagnostic relevance of clonal cytogenetic aberrations in malignant soft-tissue tumors. N Engl J Med 1991; 324:436.
67. Wang-Wuu S, Soukup S, Ballard E, et al: Chromosomal analysis of sixteen rhabdomyosarcomas. Cancer Res 1988; 48:983.
68. Ture-Carel C, Lizard-Nacol S, Justrabo E, et al: Consistent chromosomal translocation in alveolar rhabdomyosarcoma. Cancer Genet Cytogenet 1986; 19:361.
69. Scrable JJ, Witte DP, Lampkin BC, et al: Chromosomal localization of the human rhabdomyosarcoma locus by mitotic recombination mapping. Nature 1987; 329:645.
70. Wijnaendts LCC, van der Linden JC, van Diest PJ, et al: Prognostic importance of DNA flow cytometric variables in rhabdomyosarcomas. J Clin Pathol 1993; 46:948.
71. Barr FG, Galili N, Holick J, et al: Rearrangement of the PAX3 paired box gene in the paediatric solid tumor alveolar rhabdomyosarcoma. Nat Genet 1993; 3:113.
72. Davis RL, Weintraub J, Lassar AB: Expression of a single tranfected cDNA converts fibroblasts to myoblasts. Cell 1987; 51:987.
73. Scrable J, Witte D, Shimada J, et al: Molecular differential pathology of rhabdomyosarcoma. Genes Chromosom Cancer 1989; 1:23.
74. Schwab M, Ellison J, Busch M, et al: Enhanced expression of the human gene N-myc consequent to amplification of DNA may contribute to malignant progression of neuroblastoma. Proc Natl Acad Sci U S A 1984; 81:4940.
75. Driman D, Thorner PS, Greenberg ML, et al: MYCN gene amplification in rhabdomyosarcoma. Cancer 1994; 73:2231.
76. Garson JA, Clayton J, McIntyre P, et al: N-myc oncogene amplification in rhabdomyosarcoma at relapse. Lancet 1986; 1:1496.
77. Felix CA, Kappel CC, Mitsudomi T, et al: Frequency and diversity of p53 mutations in childhood rhabdomyosarcoma. Cancer Res 1992; 52:2243.
78. Diller L, Sexsmith E, Gottliev A, et al: Germline p53 mutations are frequently detected in young children with rhabdomyosarcoma. J Clin Invest 1995; 95:1606.
79. Chan JSL, Thorner PS, Haddad G, et al: Immunohistochemical detection of P-glycoprotein: prognostic correlation of soft tissue sarcoma of childhood. J Clin Oncol 1990; 8:689.
80. Zugmaier G, Lippman ME, Wellstein A: Inhibition by pentosan polysulfate (PPS) of heparin-binding growth factors released from tumor cells and blockage by PPS of tumor growth in animals. J Natl Cancer Inst 1992; 84:1716.
81. Nguyen NM, Lehr JE, Peinta KJ: Pentosan inhibits angiogenesis in vitro and suppresses prostate tumor growth in vivo. Anticancer Res 1993; 13:2143.

48

PEDIATRIC TESTICULAR TUMORS

FRANCIS X. SCHNECK, M.D. *and* CRAIG A. PETERS, M.D.

Any solid scrotal mass in a child must be considered a tumor until proven otherwise, because the majority of testicular tumors will be malignant. Testis tumors in infants and children are rare; however, the incidence of testicular cancer has steadily increased since 1940.[1,2] Because testicular cancer develops in only about 1 per 100,000 children, the relative incidence of tumor subtypes and their natural history and demographics are difficult to analyze based on the experience of any one children's center. Useful information has been generated, however, from the Prepubertal Testicular Tumor Registry, which has now collected over 330 patients since 1980. The registry has helped to demonstrate the important basic differences between testicular cancer in children and adults.

The natural history of testis cancer in children is in vivid contrast with that of adult testis tumors. Most prepubertal testis tumors are cured by local radical extirpation alone, in sharp contrast to the behavior, treatment, and outcome in postpubertal children or adults with testis tumors. About two thirds of pediatric testicular tumors are malignant. This chapter discusses the classification, diagnosis, pathology, natural history, and treatment of intratesticular tumors of childhood. (Paratesticular tumors are addressed in Chapter 47.) Changing trends in the management of testicular tumors in children are also discussed.

PATHOGENESIS AND CLASSIFICATION

Classification systems have organized testis tumors into two subtypes, those of either germ cell or non–germ cell origin. Germ cell tumors of the testis arise from premeiotic germ cells, and are divided into two major histologic subtypes, seminomas and nonseminomas. Primordial germ cells arise from the yolk sac near the allantois and migrate to the gonadal ridges during the sixth week of embryogenesis. Arrest during migration possibly explains the extragonadal sites of germ cell tumor development, including the mediastinum, retroperitoneum, and pineal gland. Non–germ cell testis tumors arise from specialized stromal cells (Sertoli and Leydig cells) and nonspecialized supporting connective tissue and blood vessels.

The pathogenesis of testis tumors has helped define the classification systems, which are based mostly on the adult cancer experience. This did not fully satisfy the different spectrum or behavior of tumors seen in children, and therefore modification was made to these classification schemes to better serve pediatric testis tumors. Ninety to 95% of all adult testis tumors are of germ cell origin, whereas in children only 77% of tumors are of germ cell origin and 23% are of non–germ cell origin. Yolk sac tumor, a malignant germ cell tumor rarely seen in adults, is the most common testicular neoplasm in children, accounting for 63% of all reported cases, while teratomas make up 14% and all others account for 5% or less. The most common germ cell testicular neoplasm in adults, seminoma, is rarely seen in children. Choriocarcinoma, a highly metastatic postpubertal testis germ cell tumor, has never been reported in children. Testicular germ cell tumors of childhood and those in postpubertal children and adults may therefore arise from different precursor cells.

Classification of prepubertal testis tumors is based on a synthesis of the experience of the Prepubertal Testicular Tumor Registry and the World Health Organization classification of adult testis tumors, and is adopted by the Section of Urology of the American Academy of Pediatrics,[3] as shown in Table 48–1.

GERM CELL TESTICULAR TUMORS

Yolk Sac Tumors

These tumors derive their name from the histologic similarity to the endodermal sinus of the rat

TABLE 48–1. HISTOLOGIC CLASSIFICATION OF PEDIATRIC TESTIS TUMORS

Germ Cell Tumors
Yolk sac
Teratoma
Mixed germ cell
Seminoma
Gonadal Stromal Tumors
Leydig cell
Sertoli cell
Juvenile granulosa cell
Mixed
Gonadoblastoma
Tumors of Supporting Tissues
Fibroma
Leiomyoma
Hemangioma
Tumor-like Lesions
Epidermoid cysts
Hyperplastic nodule secondary to adrenogenital syndrome
Lymphomas and Leukemias
Secondary Tumors
Tumors of the Adnexa

yolk sac[4] (Fig. 48–1). Yolk sac tumors are the most common testicular neoplasm in childhood, and have a multitude of synonyms (embryonal cell carcinoma, endodermal sinus tumor [of Teilum], orchioblastoma, adenocarcinoma of the testis). The incidence of yolk sac tumor in selected children's testicular cancer series ranges from 39 to 62%.[5–9] These germ cell malignancies present in children as a pure tumor that may have variable histologic patterns, whereas, in postpubertal and adult patients, yolk sac tumors are rarely found in their pure form but instead appear as a component of approximately 30% of mixed nonseminomatous germ cell tumors.[10] Yolk sac tumors in prepubertal children follow a different clinical path than germ cell tumors in adults. The relatively benign course of prepubertal yolk sac tumors, compared to the invasive nature of adult germ cell tumors, has led to the belief that these tumors arise from a different process of tumorigenesis. This has recently been challenged by the discovery of intratubular germ cell neoplasia associated with infantile yolk sac tumors, a form of carcinoma in situ considered a precursor lesion to frankly invasive germ cell neoplasia. Intratubular germ cell neoplasia was believed not to have coexisted with infantile yolk sac tumors, although it is found in almost all patients with adult nonseminomatous germ cell testicular tumors and in over 85% of patients with seminoma.[11] Intratubular germ cell neoplasia is also strongly associated with cryptorchidism and gonadal dysgenesis, conditions that have a malignant potential. The finding of intratubular germ cell neoplasia associated with prepubertal yolk sac tumor underscores the notion that these tumors may not actually have a different tumorigenic pathway than adult germ cell tumors; rather, the respective hosts account for the differences in biologic potential.

Immunohistopathology

Grossly, yolk sac tumors usually appear as a yellow-white, bulging multinodular tumor. The mucinous cut surface may appear multicystic and spongy. Necrosis and hemorrhage are uncommon. These tumors microscopically can have multiple architectural patterns that are commonly mixed. Alveolar, papillary, and solid patterns may be observed; however, the reticular pattern is most commonly seen and is characterized by a lace-like pattern of elongated cells. No particular pattern of yolk sac tumor can be related to prognosis. The most distinctive histologic element of yolk sac tumor is the Schiller-Duval body, a glomeruloid structure with a parietal layer of plump cells surrounding a central vascular core. This is present in about 50% of tumors. Immunohistochemically, yolk sac tumors exhibit keratin and placental alkaline phosphatase. The expression of α_1-fetoprotein (AFP), however, is diagnostic. AFP is seen in the cytoplasm of the cell, particularly in the hyaline droplets, intracytoplasmic eosinophilic bodies that may also be seen extracellularly and that are present in over four fifths of yolk sac tumors.[10]

AFP, a 70-kDa single peptide chain glycoprotein, is produced by the fetal yolk sac, liver, and gastrointestinal tract. It is an albumin precursor and the dominant serum binding protein in the fetus. AFP is elevated in 90% of children with yolk sac tumors, and therefore is a clinically useful postoperative tumor marker. AFP levels may be as high as 61,000 ng/dl at presentation[5]; however, elevated levels do not correlate with tumor volume, stage, or recurrence. Persistent elevation postorchiectomy represents possible residual tumor, and metastatic disease must therefore be suspected. AFP serum levels are normally elevated in newborns, and may remain mildly elevated above the normal adult baseline (<10 ng/dl) up to 8 months of age.[12] AFP levels may therefore not be helpful preoperatively in neonates and infants with a suspected testicular tumor because elevated levels do not necessarily confirm the presence of malignancy, and may possibly mask a hormonally active tumor until the predicted serum levels fall to their appropriate range.[13] Measurements of AFP levels at birth have a mean value of 48,406±34,718 ng/ml and decrease to 2654±3080 ng/ml by 4 weeks of age, 323±278 ng/ml by 2 months of age, and 8.5±5.5 ng/ml by 8 months of age.[14] AFP has a serum half-life of about 5 days. It is reasonable, therefore, to initiate a metastatic work-up if AFP levels do not approach normal levels after five half-lives, or about 4 to 6 weeks after surgery. A normal AFP level, however, does not definitively rule out the possibility of residual disease because false-negative levels have been seen in the face of metastasis.

Presentation

Yolk sac tumors usually present as a painless testicular mass incidentally found on physical exam.

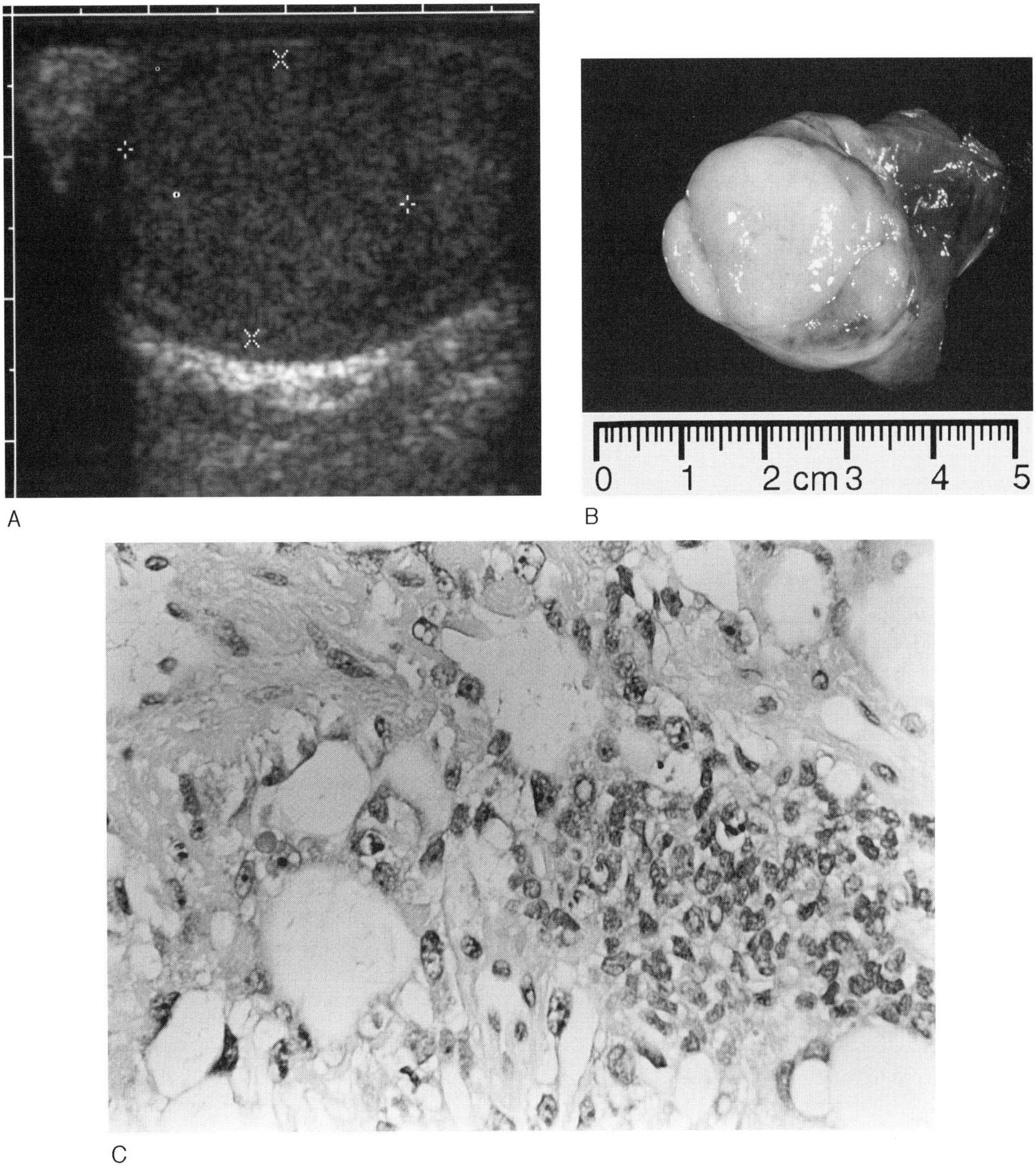
A
0 1 2 cm 3 4 5
B
C

FIGURE 48–1. A yolk sac tumor was found in a 1-year-old boy presenting with an enlarged hemiscrotum and a firm testicle. *A*, Ultrasonographic examination revealed a homogeneous mass within the testis. *B*, Gross appearance of the cut testis following radical orchiectomy. A smooth yellowish surface without cysts or hemorrhage was seen, although these features may be present. *C*, Histologic appearance of a yolk sac tumor (endodermal sinus tumor) from a 1-year-old boy, showing a loose reticular pattern with irregular cystic spaces. AFP staining is positive in these tumors, and hyaline globules may be seen both intracellularly and extracellularly. Hematoxylin and eosin, ×400. *Illustration continued on following page*

Diagnosis has been reported as early as birth and as late as up to 15 years; however, the average age is 3 years. It had been suggested that children diagnosed under the age of 2 have a better prognosis; however, age was not found to be of prognostic significance in the Prepubertal Testicular Cancer Registry of 207 enrolled children with yolk sac tumor.[5] In that same study, 16% developed metastatic disease; of those children, the metastasis rate was 25% for boys greater than 2 years and 14% for those under 2, although the difference did not reach statistical significance. This suggests that there may be a higher incidence of metastasis in children diagnosed under the age of 2. There is often as much

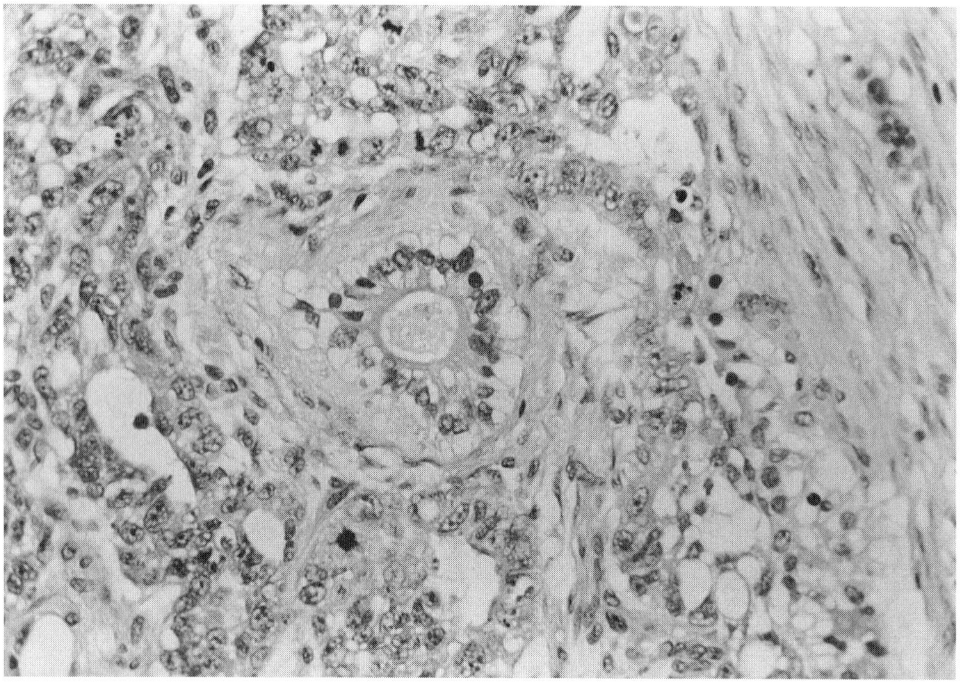

D

FIGURE 48–1. *Continued* *D*, Schiller-Duval body (endodermal sinus) from a yolk sac tumor showing a characteristic flattened layer of cells surrounding a tuft of cuboidal cells having a central capillary. Hematoxylin and eosin, ×250.

as a 4-month delay in diagnosis. The most common misdiagnosis is hydrocele, and it is therefore important to carefully evaluate the testicle in any child with a new hydrocele, either at the time of presentation or at surgery, so as not to miss a possible malignancy.

Diagnostic Investigations

When a child presents with a testicular mass, the diagnostic investigation of choice is surgical exploration. Ultrasonography may be useful in the evaluation of testicular masses when the clinical presentation is uncertain and the differential diagnosis of testicular torsion or trauma is possible; however, ultrasonography should not replace surgical intervention when there is any possibility of tumor. A radical orchiectomy is performed through an inguinal incision. The spermatic cord is clamped atraumatically prior to manipulation and delivery of the testicle from the scrotum. After delivery of the testicle with its surrounding tunics, the cord is divided and transected high at the internal ring. The surgical field should be re-draped around the cord prior to transection, and sterile water used to irrigate the inguinal wound. Permanent suture is used to ligate the stump of the cord for possible later identification if retroperitoneal lymph node dissection (RPLND) is performed. Scrotal orchiectomy is contraindicated because of the possibility of scrotal contamination, which has been well described.[3]

Staging

After the pathologic diagnosis of yolk sac tumor is certain, staging of disease extent must be undertaken. The staging system for yolk sac tumor is based on Kaplan et al.'s modification[3] of the system proposed by Boden and Gibb.[15] Stage I tumors are those limited to the testis. Stage IIA tumors include radiographically unrecognized metastasis to the retroperitoneal lymph nodes discovered at the time of RPLND, or persistent elevation of AFP without evidence of metastasis. Stage IIB tumors have bulky retroperitoneal disease. Stage III disease involves distant metastatic disease outside of the retroperitoneum. Yolk sac tumors spread via lymphatic and hematogenic routes, or both, and hematogenous dissemination appears to be more common.[16] Common sites of tumor spread are the lungs, retroperitoneal lymph nodes, liver, and bone. The Prepubertal Testicular Tumor Registry recently reported on 212 patients with yolk sac tumor of whom 33 (15.6%) presented with metastatic disease.[16] Involved metastatic sites included the retroperitoneum (lymphatic spread) in 27% and hematogenous spread in 40%, and 19% had a combination of both lymphatic and hematogenous metastatic disease. The most common site of hematogenous spread is to the lungs.

The initial staging investigations should include a preoperative AFP level, followed by a chest x-ray and computed tomography (CT) of the abdomen, pelvis, and chest. Serial determinations of AFP are performed monthly after orchiectomy. The argument has been made that monitoring serial AFP levels is adequate to assess for residual or recurrent disease after orchiectomy. Serial AFP levels are useful not only in assessing patients with stage I disease under surveillance for relapse, but useful as well in patients with stage II or III disease to assess the affects of adjuvant therapy. Ehrlichman and associates reported that CT scanning in the assessment of intra-abdominal metastatic disease has limited usefulness, and found a false-negative rate of 40%, a false-positive rate of 50%, and overall accuracy of 69% in patients with stage I or II nonseminomatous testicular tumors.[17] Kaplan et al.,[3] in contrast, reported from the Prepubertal Testicular Tumor Registry that, in 85 children with yolk sac tumor who had CT scan performed as part of their metastatic work-up, accuracy was better. Five (6%) had studies suspicious for disseminated disease in the retroperitoneum, and two of those five children (40%) were found to have false-positive scans. In 80 children with originally normal scans, only 2 (2.5%) had false-negative results.

Treatment

The treatment of children with yolk sac tumor begins with expeditious radical orchiectomy. Serial AFP levels and CT of the abdomen and chest are then important for staging and subsequent monitoring of disease. Thereafter, treatment is based on the stage of disease.

Between 80 and 100% of children with testicular yolk sac tumor will present with organ-confined stage I disease, and debate exists as to the management of these patients.[7–9,16,18,19] The controversy centers around whether RPLND is routinely indicated if the metastatic work-up (CT scan and AFP levels) is negative. The management of adult nonseminomatous testis cancers often include RPLND because of the aggressive nature of these tumors and the high incidence of regional spread; however, in contrast, only a small percentage (approximately 4 to 12%) of children with yolk sac tumor will have metastatic retroperitoneal disease.[6,16,19,20] More commonly, children will have hematogenous spread, and therefore RPLND would not be of therapeutic or diagnostic value in the majority of patients. RPLND also is associated with significant morbidity, including late bowel obstruction, anejaculation, and vascular and lymphatic complications. Complication rates from the few series that report complications are between 19 and 27%.[3,16]

Overall, relapse in patients with clinical stage I disease who are treated with radical orchiectomy and surveillance is about 10 to 20%.[21] AFP is an exceptionally useful monitoring test for relapse or for the presence of residual disease after orchiectomy. However, it does not always correlate with tumor volume, and false-negative results have been reported in the presence of metastatic disease. In light of the fact that a sensitive and specific biologic tumor marker exists, as well as an effective salvage chemotherapy for those patients who do relapse, surveillance is a more reasonable option for follow-up of children with stage I disease. Based on the recent literature, it is becoming more evident that close surveillance after radical orchiectomy is the treatment of choice for stage I disease. Monitoring of these patients should include serial AFP determinations obtained monthly for the first year, then bimonthly for the second year. CT scan of the chest and abdomen is also obtained every 3 months for the first year, and every 6 months in the second year.

Approximately 15% of children with testicular yolk sac tumor will present with metastatic disease.[16,21] The true percentage of those with retroperitoneal micrometastatic disease is probably underestimated because many children with clinical stage I disease are under surveillance after radical orchiectomy, and CT scan cannot completely be relied upon to diagnose metastatic disease. The treatment of children with metastatic disease depends on the site(s) and extent of spread. For those patients with either stage IIA or IIB disease, both RPLND and chemotherapy have been used alone and in combination.

RPLND has a well-defined diagnostic and therapeutic role in the management of adult patients with germ cell testicular tumors. At present, the role of RPLND in children believed to have stage IIA or IIB disease is controversial and has not been examined in a systematic fashion. As already discussed, there is no clear indication to perform RPLND in children with stage I disease because surveillance is playing a more significant and logical role with excellent results. The exceptions are in those children who in follow-up are thought to have relapsed based on suspicious abdominal CT scan or the progressive elevation of AFP levels without evidence of hematologic metastasis. There is no role for RPLND in children with stage III disease because chemotherapy is the mainstay of treatment. The likelihood of RPLND being positive for metastatic disease with elevated AFP levels and a negative CT scan is decreased, however, because hematogenous spread has been shown to be more common. This is borne out by the reviews of children with yolk sac tumor who underwent RPLND for clinical stage I disease; only a small percentage (<10%) were upgraded to a higher pathologic stage. Added to this relapse rate of about 10%, greater than 80% of children are cured of stage I disease by radical orchiectomy alone without having to suffer the morbidity and possible long-term complications of RPLND.

Because few children with yolk sac tumor present with metastatic disease, reports of patients in whom RPLND has been applied as treatment for stage IIA and IIB disease are few and results difficult to extrapolate within this subgroup. The Prepubertal Testis Tumor Registry recently reported a review of all children with yolk sac tumors (212 patients), and only 2% had biopsy-proven metastatic spread to the retroperitoneum and would therefore have benefited from RPLND.[16] This review also reported that in the 11 of 212 patients who underwent RPLND, 5 were positive for metastatic disease, and 6 had negative RPLNDs, 1 of whom later had a relapse in the lung. Of those patients with negative node dissections, all had negative CT scans. In contrast, in the five children with pathologically proven metastatic retroperitoneal spread, only one child was reported to have a positive CT scan, although three of these children had no CT scan reported to the registry. The complication rate of RPLND from this review was 27%, which was equal to the positive yield of the procedure itself. RPLND has also been advocated in children with an elevated AFP level after chemotherapy without any radiographic evidence of persistent disease.

Salvage chemotherapy plays a vital role in the management of patients with metastatic yolk sac tumor; however, no standard chemotherapeutic protocol exists. Most regimens are based on adult protocols for nonseminomatous germ cell tumors, which include a combination of two or more agents. The advent of effective multiagent chemotherapy has improved the overall survival of children with testicular tumors. Before 1979, reports of survival in children with metastatic yolk sac tumor were uncommon, especially if treatment did not include combination therapy.[22,23] Fernandes and colleagues showed a survival rate of 50% in patients treated before, and 100% in patients treated after, the introduction of new chemotherapeutic protocols and diagnostic imaging techniques.[7] The most effective combinations are vincristine, actinomycin D, and cyclophosphamide or cisplatin, bleomycin, and vinblastine. Children with hematogenous metastatic disease have been treated successfully with combination chemotherapy, with salvage rates approaching 100%.[7,9,18,24–27] Relative indications for chemotherapy include evidence for gross metastatic disease, especially hematogenous spread, as well as indications similar to those for RPLND, which include suspicious retroperitoneal lymph node spread or persistently elevated AFP levels after orchiectomy without an obvious source of disease. A residual retroperitoneal mass has been described in a child after chemotherapy for metastatic disease.[28] Although AFP levels normalized, the mass was excised and found to contain fibrous tissue, necrosis, and calcification. Some reports recommend adjuvant chemotherapy in all patients; however, chemotherapy should be reserved for patients with documented disease because there are significant complications from chemotherapy, including hemorrhagic cystitis and testicular damage.

In conclusion, children who have been treated for yolk sac tumor of the testis should be regularly monitored by a physician who is familiar with the natural history of this tumor and the complications of therapy. The overwhelming consensus is that children with stage I yolk sac tumors should be managed with surveillance and close follow-up. The spectre of relapse affects the minority of patients; however, the application of recently improved multiagent chemotherapeutic salvage regimens have improved survival rates to near 100%. Compared to adult testicular tumors, RPLND has fewer indications and less impact in the management of metastatic disease, and should be reserved for patients with nonbulky tumor mass confined to the retroperitoneum, or for persistently elevated AFP levels anytime in follow-up after orchiectomy without any evidence of disease elsewhere. With long-term relapse rates reported as between 0 and 13%, the overall prognosis for children with metastatic disease is excellent, largely because of modern chemotherapeutic regimens, protocols for which have only recently have begun to be tested in a standardized fashion.[3,9,24]

Teratoma

Testicular teratoma represents the second most common germ cell tumor in prepubertal boys and accounts for 14% of all prepubertal testicular tumors; however, it represents only 5% of all testicular tumors diagnosed in newborn infants[5] (Fig. 48–2). The mean age at presentation is 18 months. By definition, these tumors are derived from the three germ layers—endoderm, mesoderm, and ectoderm—and may develop into almost any tissue or organ seen in the fetus or adult. Grossly, teratomas are heterogeneous masses, most often composed of firm, solid areas with intervening variably sized cysts. The cystic characteristics of this tumor help to differentiate it by ultrasound from other testicular lesions. Teratomas are well encapsulated; hemorrhage and necrosis are not uncommon, and there may be small areas of calcification. Although reported, it is rare to see the hair, teeth, and sebaceous material that are more often seen in ovarian dermoid cysts.

Microscopically, teratomas are categorized as either mature or immature, depending on whether the histologic pattern is that of an adult or embryologic tissue type or a mixture of both, as is usually the case. Prepubertal testicular teratomas are most often mature and well-differentiated tumors characterized by cystic areas lined by respiratory, intestinal, or squamous epithelium. Cartilage, bone, muscle, neural tissue, epidermoid tissue, salivary glands, and ciliated and intestinal epithelium can be found, admixed with fibroblastic or smooth muscle stroma. Immature teratomas are uncommon tumors that are histologically more primitive, less organoid, and usually composed of neural tissue, intestinal glands, cartilage, squamous epithelium, or ocular anlage. The stroma is composed of a fetal

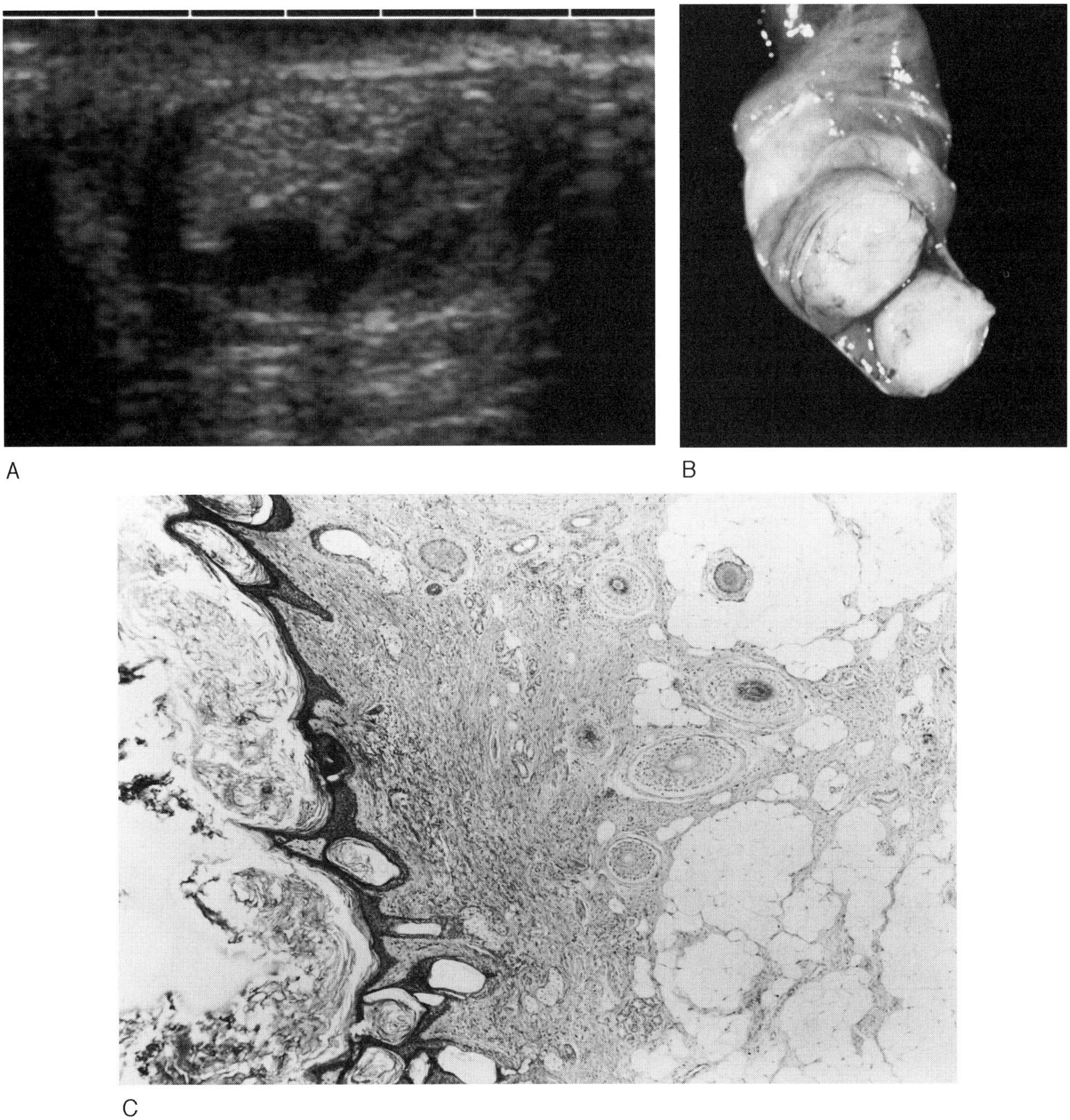
A
B
C

FIGURE 48–2. A 1-year-old boy with an enlarged left hemiscrotum was found to have a mature teratoma. *A*, Ultrasonographic examination showed a heterogeneous testicular mass with solid and cystic areas. *B*, Gross examination of the encapsulated tumor revealed an irregular surface with multiple small cystic areas. *C*, Histologic examination showed multiple mature elements as seen here, including epidermis, hair follicles, adipose tissue, muscular elements, and cartilage. No immature elements were identified. Hematoxylin and eosin, ×40.

mesenchyme of loose spindle cells in a mucopolysaccharide matrix. Immunohistochemically, teratomas do not express AFP, and patients with these tumors have never been reported to have elevated AFP serum levels.

Prepubertal teratomas are benign lesions that have never been reported to metastasize. This sharply contrasts the biologic potential and malignant behavior of teratomas found in postpubertal adolescents and adults. Curative treatment for prepubertal teratoma is radical orchiectomy alone. For children with testicular tumors that are strongly suspected to be teratomas based on characteristic preoperative ultrasonographic findings and a negative hormonal work-up, testis-sparing enucleation is a reasonable alternative to orchiectomy. This technique is carried out through an inguinal incision, and the testis and spermatic cord are mobilized, delivered, and isolated from the surgical field in a fashion similar to radical orchiectomy. Only after the spermatic cord is occluded is the tunica vaginalis opened and enucleation performed. The tunica albuginea of the testis is opened and the encapsulated lesion gently shelled out with blunt dissection. The tunica albuginea is then closed while waiting for the frozen-section results, and spermatic cord occlusion is released only after the confirmation of a benign lesion. If the diagnosis of a benign lesion cannot be made with confidence, then a radical orchiectomy should be performed. There have been no reports of local recurrence or distant spread using this technique.[29,30] Enucleation is only recommended in prepubertal children; it must be emphasized that teratomas in postpubertal males are biologically malignant and have the potential to metastasize.

GONADAL STROMAL TUMORS

Testicular tumors of the interstitium are derived from a common mesenchymal stem cell and are not of germ cell origin. These neoplasms are more common in children than adults and include Leydig cell, Sertoli cell, and juvenile granulosa cell tumors. Gonadal stromal tumors account for 8% of all prepubertal testicular tumors; however, they make up 27% of all tumors that present in the neonatal period.[13] An important clinical aspect of these tumors is the possibility of hormonal activity, in which case the child might present with precocious puberty. Children with gonadal stromal tumors usually present with a painless testicular mass. In general, these tumors are considered benign and are cured with orchiectomy alone. Leydig cell tumors are the most common gonadal stromal tumor in children and adults. The following discussion covers gonadal stromal tumors in children only. In general, preoperative evaluation should include transcrotal ultrasound, chest x-ray, and serum AFP level.

Leydig Cell Tumor

Leydig cells normally produce testosterone under stimulation of the gonadotropin luteinizing hormone (LH) and regulation of the hypothalamic-pituitary axis. When these cells undergo malignant change, abnormal testosterone synthesis may occur autonomously without regulatory control from the hypothalamic-pituitary axis. These hormonally active tumors most commonly synthesize testosterone, and are rarely associated with elevated estrogen, cortisol, or 17-hydroxyprogesterone (17-OHPG). Leydig cell tumors often cause precocious puberty, or the appearance of secondary sex characteristics prior to the ninth or tenth year of age in boys. The peak incidence of Leydig cell tumors occurs between 4 and 10 years of age. The diagnosis is delayed for up to 1 year in 70% and up to 5 years in 15% of children.[31,32] The most likely explanation for this is that Leydig cell tumors are slow growing and relatively small, and children may not present with a palpable testicular mass; there may be only a slight asymmetry in the affected testis (Fig. 48–3). Typically, children with Leydig cell tumors present with endocrine dysfunction (i.e., precocious puberty) as their first sign before any testicular abnormality is diagnosed.

Precocious puberty often manifests as accelerated somatic growth and progressive virilization, including phallic growth and the development of pubic hair. Less commonly, patients present with facial hair, acne, and deepening of the voice.[33] Gynecomastia is present in about 30% of postpubertal adolescents and adults but is uncommon in children. When present, gynecomastia is associated with increased estrogen or progesterone levels.[31,34] Leydig cell tumors are only responsible for 10% of precocious puberty in boys.[33,35] Precocious puberty is due to an intracranial tumor in over 50% of patients, and is characterized by elevation of gonadotropin levels (follicle-stimulating hormone [FSH] and LH). If gonadotropin levels are normal in the work-up of precocious puberty, the next most likely cause is either a primary adrenal or testicular abnormality.[32]

In children with precocious puberty, it is important to differentiate between Leydig cell tumors and congenital adrenal hyperplasia (CAH) because treatment is strictly surgical in the former and medical in the latter. Patients with CAH often develop hyperplastic testicular tumors if medical compliance is poor.[36] These children can present with bilateral testicular nodules, whereas Leydig cell tumors are unilateral in 97% of cases.[34,37] Both testicular tumors function independently of hypothalamic-pituitary axis regulation and produce steroids without tropic hormonal stimulation, plasma levels of which are normal or low. In patients with CAH, serum 17-OHPG and urinary pregnanetriol, the excretory product of 17-OHPG, are elevated in 21-hydroxylase deficiency, which is not present in patients with Leydig cell tumors.[35] Urinary 17-ketosteroid excretion is also elevated in CAH; in contrast, urinary 17-ketosteroid excretion is variable in patients with Leydig cell tumors and ranges from normal to markedly increased. Elevated levels of urinary 17-ketosteroid occur in patients with Leydig cell tumors that secrete large quantities of testosterone.

The biologic differences of these tumors can be exploited to make the differential diagnosis. Testicular tumors secondary to CAH respond to both corticotropin (ACTH) stimulation and dexamethasone suppression. The dexamethasone suppression test should cause clinical regression of the tumor in patients with CAH as well as decrease 17-OHPG levels, and administration of ACTH should either not change or accentuate the already elevated plasma and urinary levels of 17-ketosteroid, quite possibly exacerbating testicular symptoms. Therefore, it has

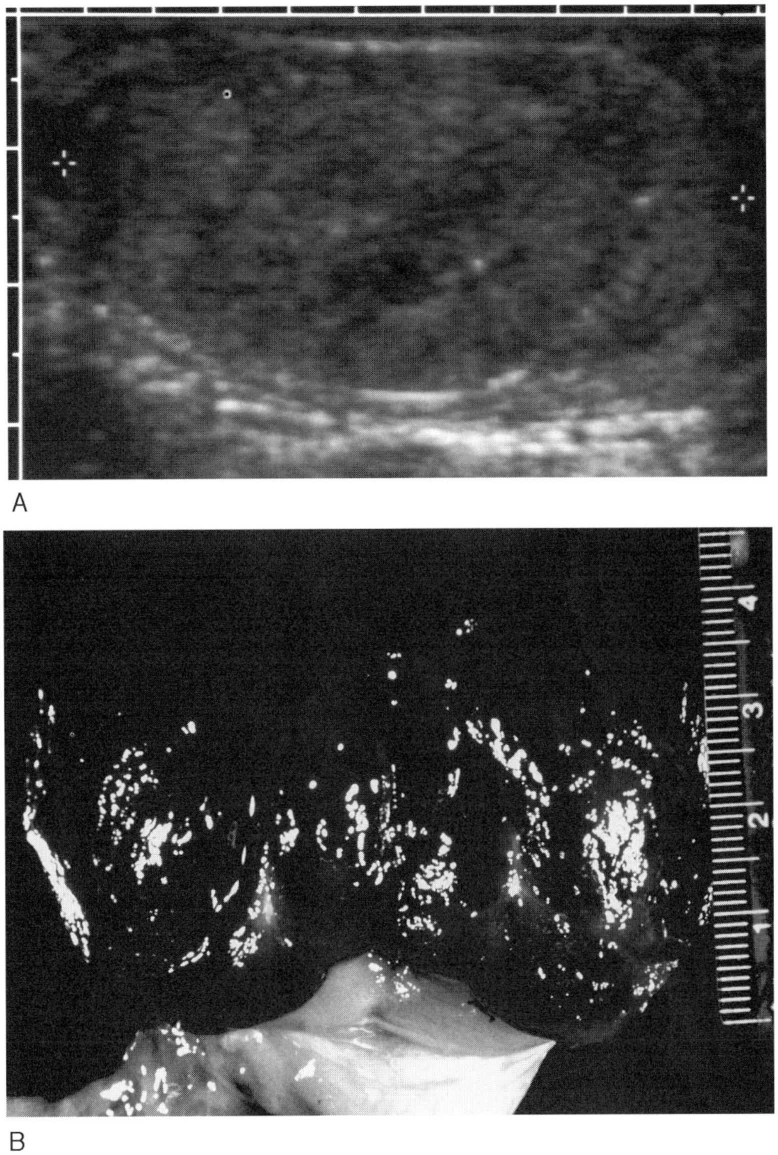
A
B

FIGURE 48–3. Leydig cell tumor from a 13-year-old boy with testicular enlargement and an atrophic contralateral testis. His serum testosterone was 1608 mg/dl, FSH was 0.1 IU/L, and LH was 0.12 IU/L. *A*, Ultrasonographic examination revealing inhomogeneous testicular parenchyma and marked disparity in testicular size, with the affected right testis measuring 5.0 × 3.4 cm while the left testis was 2.0 cm in length. *B*, Gross view of bivalved Leydig cell tumor revealing a gelatinous and hemorrhagic surface. A fibrous capsule was present.

Illustration continued on following page

been recommended that a reasonable method of differentiating Leydig cell tumors from CAH includes a dexamethasone suppression test and determination of plasma 17-OHPG as well as urinary pregnanetriol levels.[35] Leydig cell tumors are unresponsive to ACTH and dexamethasone as well as gonadotropin stimulation.

Grossly, Leydig cell tumors in children are small, well-encapsulated lesions that are generally solid and yellow-brown in appearance on cut section. Areas of hemorrhage and necrosis are not uncommon. Three basic cell types have been described in a review by Kim. Most commonly this includes a medium to large polygonal cell with an indistinct cell border and an eosinophilic, finely granular, or occasionally vacuolated cytoplasm that closely resembles a Leydig cell.[34] Nuclear characteristics include a round to oval nucleus, delicate chromatin, and a single prominent nucleolus. The second cell type resembles the zona fasciculata of the adrenal cortex—large in size with a vacuolated cytoplasm. The third type of cell is small, contains little cytoplasm, and has round, hyperchromatic nuclei. Some of these cells resemble plasma cells. Reinke's crystalloids, cytoplasmic acidophilic rectangular crystals that are present in about 35% of adult Leydig cell tumors, are absent in children.[34]

Work-up of children with Leydig cell tumors in-

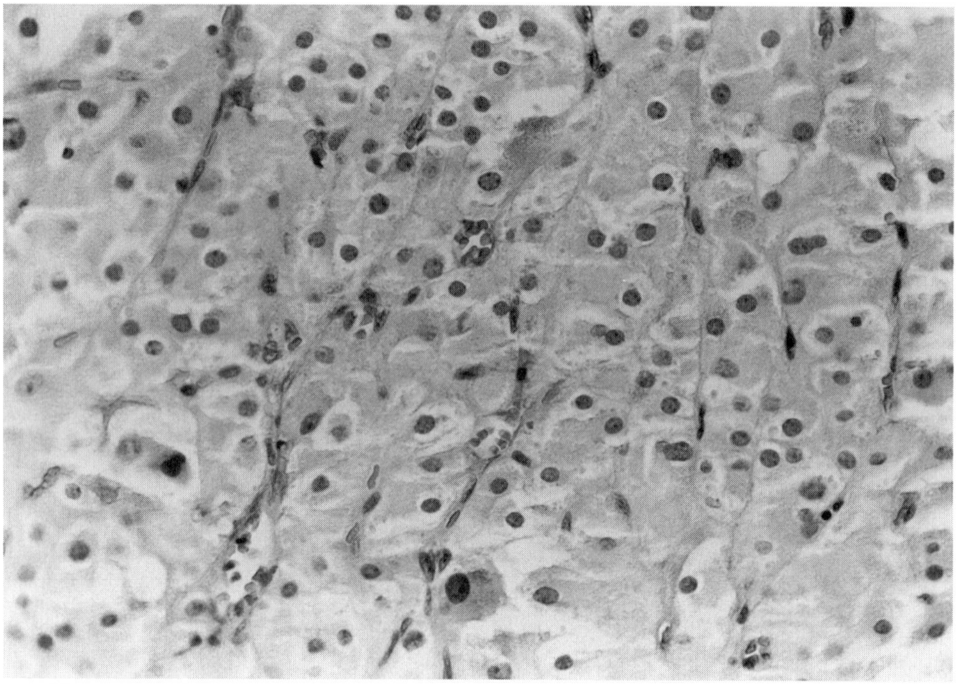

C

FIGURE 48–3. *Continued* C, Histologic appearance of the Leydig cell tumor showing sheets of uniform eosinophilic cells having a slightly granular cytoplasm. Occasional crystalloids of Reinke may be seen in these tumors. Hematoxylin and eosin, ×400.

cludes measurement of testosterone, FSH, and LH serum levels. Ultrasound may be particularly helpful in locating a suspected testicular lesion if none can be palpated. These have the ultrasonographic appearance of an intraparenchymal homogeneous, hypoechoic lesion.[38] Orchiectomy is adequate treatment alone because there has never been a reported case of relapse or metastasis in a child. In contrast, about 10% of Leydig cell tumors in adults are malignant, with documented metastasis most commonly to regional lymph nodes and less often to lung, liver, bone, and kidney.[39] A reasonable alternative to orchiectomy is enucleation of the tumor.[38] A testis-sparing approach is appealing, if the diagnosis is certain preoperatively, because of the benign nature of these tumors, and is technically possible because they are often small and encapsulated. Adrenogenital syndrome or a contralateral Leydig cell tumor should be suspected if hormonal abnormalities persist after orchiectomy. The hormonal manifestations of virilization, however, may not completely regress after tumor ablation, especially if the diagnosis was long unrecognized and untreated.[32]

Sertoli Cell Tumor

Although fatal malignant degeneration has been reported, Sertoli cell tumors are considered uniformly benign in prepubescent children.[40–42] The biologic characteristics of this tumor, like teratoma and Leydig cell tumor, transform to have a greater malignant potential in adulthood, when the incidence of metastasis is 30%.[43] Sertoli cell tumors account for about 1% of all prepubertal testis tumors and 17% of all non–germ cell tumors.[5,6] These tumors usually present as a unilateral painless testicular mass at any age—most commonly, however, in infants under 6 months of age.[6] Sertoli cell tumors have the potential to be hormonally active, and patients—more commonly adults—present with gynecomastia. In contrast to children with Leydig cell tumors, precocious puberty (virilization) is not superimposed with gynecomastia. It has been proposed that Sertoli cell tumors have steroidogenic potential to synthesize estrogen.[44] Sertoli cell tumors are usually small, firm, well-circumscribed intratesticular lesions that are gray, yellow, or white in color on cut section. Histologically, these tumors appear as uniform eosinophilic cells with rare mitotic figures that resemble the fetal testis.[6] The histopathologic criteria for this malignancy has yet to be determined except by definition of metastasis. Treatment of choice is orchiectomy with close follow-up to exclude retroperitoneal metastasis.

Juvenile Granulosa Cell Tumor

Juvenile granulosa cell tumor accounted for 1% of tumors reported to the Prepubertal Testicular Tumor Registry and is the most common testicular tumor discovered within the first few days of life[5,45]

(Fig. 48–4). Its frequency in the newborn period, up to 6 months of age, is further reflected by the fact that it accounts for 27% of all neonatal testicular tumors, thus making it the most common sex cord/gonadal stromal testicular tumor in infancy.[13] Because of their early presentation, it has been postulated that these tumors arise in utero.[45] Granulosa cell tumors derive from the stroma of the testis and are benign and hormonally inactive. Most tumors present within the first month of life and are cured by orchiectomy alone. Grossly, granulosa cell tumors appear as firm, solid, well-circumscribed intratesticular lesions that on cut section are gray-white or tan to yellow in color and contain multiple cysts of varying sizes. This architectural characteristic, however, does not specifically identify these tumors preoperatively by ultrasound, especially in the neonate, where ultrasound fails to demonstrate an abnormality in 40% of patients.[13] Other germ cell tumors, namely teratomas and yolk sac tumors, may have cystic elements as well, making ultrasonographic differentiation unreliable.[32] A significant portion of tumors, however, may have a predominantly solid nodular structure.[45] Histologically, granulosa cells are vacuolated and lipid rich, and both follicular and solid elements are seen. The cysts are lined by granulosa-like cells and often surrounded by theca-like cells. These tumors may be

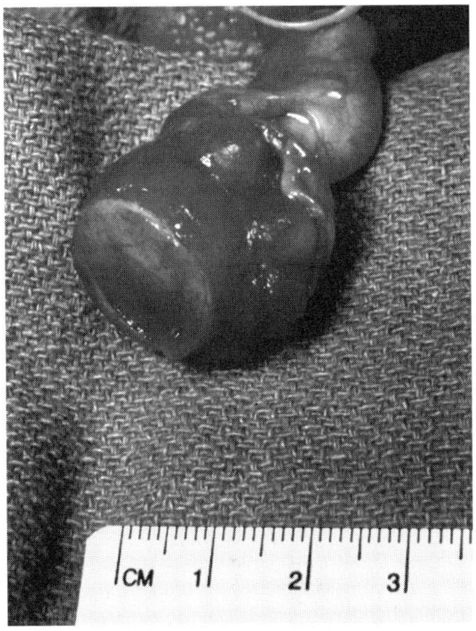
CM 1 2 3

A

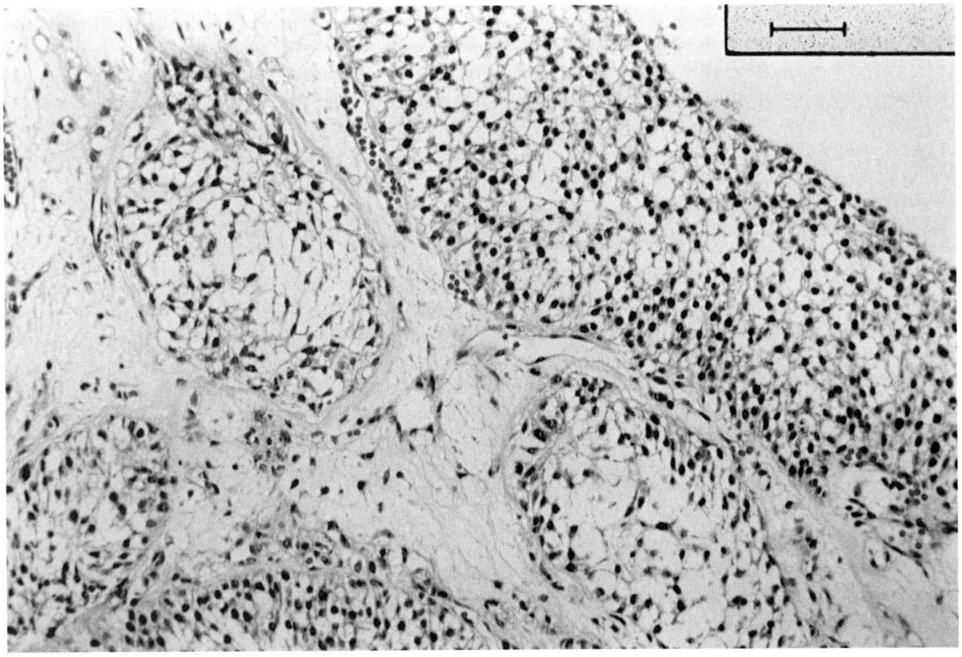

B

FIGURE 48–4. A newborn boy with a firm smooth left testicle was seen with dark coloration of his hemiscrotum. *A*, A firm tumor had replaced most of the testis and is shown on cut section. *B*, Histology showed this to be a juvenile granulosa cell tumor with vacuolar cells in cords. Hematoxylin and eosin, ×100.

termed granulosa-theca cell tumors if theca cell elements are identified.

Because of the histologic evidence of prominent mitotic activity in some tumors,[45] the potential for malignancy and metastasis may exist; however, this has not been reported in the prepubertal age group. Because of the small numbers of reported cases, uncertainty exists as to whether or not to classify these tumors as malignant.[13,45] AFP levels have limited value as tumor markers because granulosa cell tumors have not been shown to produce elevated serum levels. Therefore, follow-up with periodic chest x-ray and retroperitoneal imaging is reasonable. These tumors have been associated with cryptorchidism, testicular torsion, ambiguous genitalia, and chromosomal and endocrine abnormalities, as well as being identified in the fetal testis.[45–50]

GONADOBLASTOMA

Gonadoblastomas are rare tumors found in dysgenetic gonads of children with intersex. These tumors account for about 1% of all tumors reported to the Prepubertal Testicular Tumor Registry and 10% of all tumors discovered in the neonatal period.[5,13] Histologically, gonadoblastomas are made up of aggregates of germ cells and stromal cells. The stromal component is composed of immature cells similar to Sertoli or granulosa cells. Of tumors that are diagnosed in the pubertal period or later, two thirds of patients may have Leydig cell or theca-lutein cell elements present, and therefore the possibility of hormonal activity may exist. This usually causes virilization, although feminization has been reported. Gonadoblastomas are bilateral approximately one third of the time.

Children with a dysgenetic or streak gonad and a karyotype with a Y chromosome have the potential to develop a tumor, most commonly a gonadoblastoma. This most commonly occurs in phenotypic females with a 46,XY karyotype and intra-abdominal testes (testicular feminization syndrome) and accounts for 80% of cases of gonadoblastomas. Overall, the incidence of germ cell tumors in patients with testicular feminization is 5 to 10%.[51,52] These tumors are most often benign; however, the possibility of malignant transformation exists—usually a dysgerminoma, which resembles a seminoma of an adult that is not hormonally active. Concomitant germ cell malignancies that have been reported include choriocarcinoma, teratoma and teratocarcinoma, embryonal carcinoma, and seminoma. The risk of a gonadal tumor is much greater when patients are diagnosed during or after puberty, with a reported incidence of neoplasia as high as 44%.[49]

Other conditions in which tumors may arise are in children with pure gonadal dysgenesis and, more commonly, mixed gonadal dysgenesis with a karyotype of 45,X/46,XY mosaicism and tumor arising from the testis or streak gonad. In Scully's review of 74 children with gonadoblastoma, he found that 20% of children who developed tumors were phenotypic males, usually male pseudohermaphrodites with mixed gonadal dysgenesis.[53] A report was published that found gonadal dysgenesis, both mixed and pure, to carry a greater risk of tumor formation, with a prevalence of 64%.[49] Although the overall malignant potential is greatest in postpubertal patients, the potential also exists for prepubescent children to develop neoplasia associated with gonadal dysgenesis. Of those patients with gonadal dysgenesis diagnosed before the age of 5 (4 of 14), 3 of the 4 developed associated tumors, including a dysgerminoma in situ, a mucinous cystadenofibroma, and a juvenile granulosa cell tumor.[49] Overall, 33% of children from that series were under school age when their tumors were diagnosed. Testicular intratubular germ cell neoplasia, a premalignant condition, has been reported in 6% of patients with dysgenetic gonads at a median age of 13 years.[54]

Treatment is radical orchiectomy soon after the diagnosis is confirmed. Biopsy is not necessary and carries with it a high false-negative rate as a result of sampling error.[49] Laparoscopy has not only a diagnostic but a therapeutic role in the management of children with intersex. Gonadectomy can easily be performed laparoscopically. The general management recommendation would be removal of the streak or dysgenetic gonad in the prepubertal period before possible malignant progression.

TUMOR-LIKE LESIONS OF THE TESTIS

Epidermoid Cysts

These intratesticular tumors account for approximately 2% of all tumors reported to the Prepubertal Registry[5] (Fig. 48–5). Most patients with this tumor, however, present in their second to fourth decades of life. Epidermoid cysts are benign in both the prepubertal and postpubertal patient, and malignancies associated with these tumors have not been reported.[29,55] Histologically, epidermoid cysts are considered monophasic teratomas and are lined by squamous epithelium that contains keratinized material within. Intratubular germ cell neoplasia, a premalignant lesion, has not been observed in these patients.[56] A suggestive preoperative diagnosis can be made by the findings of a circumscribed, firm, smooth testicular mass on physical exam and a complex heterogeneous mass with a well-demarcated echogenic rim, smooth wall, and echogenic center on ultrasound, although it is possible for teratoma to have a similar appearance.[29,30] AFP and β-human chorionic gonadotropin serum levels are normal. Enucleative surgery with organ preservation has been applied to the management of

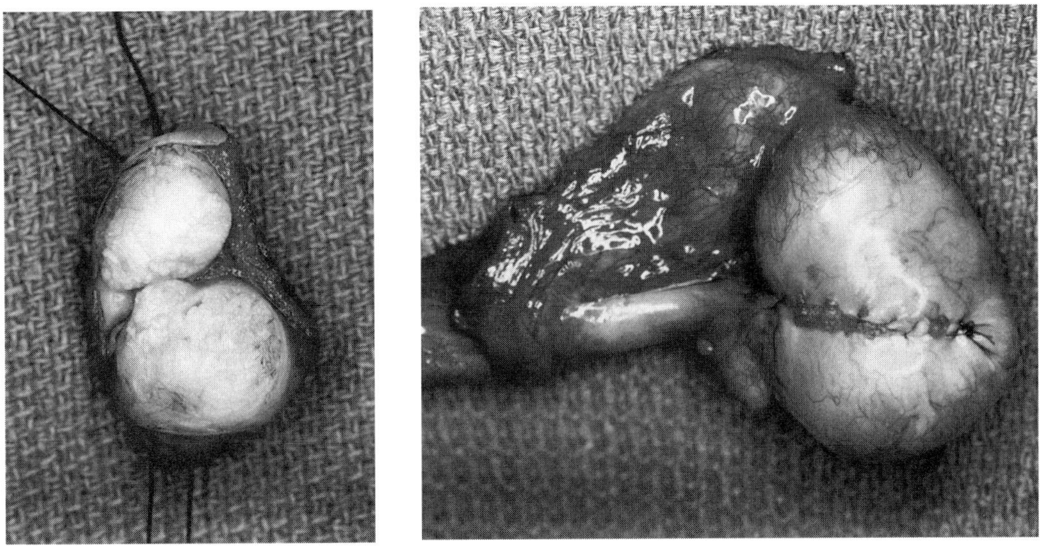

A B

FIGURE 48–5. Gross appearance of epidermoid tumor in a child, showing the enucleated mass (*A*) and the reconstructed testis (*B*).

these tumors with good results, and is presently the treatment of choice.[29,30] Heidenreich et al. found that 39% of all patients had been treated with an organ-preserving approach and had no reported long-term local recurrence or metastasis.[29] However, if the preoperative diagnosis is uncertain or at the time of surgery a suspicious lesion is encountered, then the most prudent course is a radical orchiectomy. After the tumor is enucleated and before the spermatic cord occlusion is released, a frozen section should be performed. This has been shown to be a reliable method of confirming the diagnosis of an epidermoid cyst and ruling out malignancy.[29]

Hyperplastic Nodule Secondary to Adrenogenital Syndrome

Children with this syndrome present with precocious puberty, markedly elevated serum 17-OHPG and urine 17-ketosteroid levels, and bilateral testicular tumors. Bilateral testicular masses are usually synchronous and present 83% of the time. A discrete testicular mass may be palpable; however, often only a difference in testicular volume may be appreciable. In contrast to most other testicular tumors, treatment of this syndrome is medical as opposed to surgical, and it is therefore critical to differentiate this disease from Leydig cell tumor. There have been no reports of relapse or distant metastasis. The biochemical defect is most often due to 21-hydroxylase deficiency, 65% of the time salt wasting and 35% of the time non–salt wasting.[37] The actual cell of origin of this nodule has been debated in the literature, and it is ascribed to poorly controlled adrenogenital syndrome (AGS) with ACTH-induced hyperplasia of either interstitial cells, ectopic intratesticular adrenal cortical rests, or putative pluripotential cells.[37,57,58] Ectopic adrenal rests are typically found in proximity to the epididymis or in the spermatic cord and have not been described in the testicular parenchyma. Rutgers et al. base their argument for ACTH-induced proliferation of pluripotential cells of the testicular hilus as the most probable cells of origin on embryologic and logistic considerations; however, confirmational evidence is lacking.

Hyperplastic nodules secondary to AGS most commonly present in early adulthood; however, about a third of cases present in children with most manifesting clinical features of AGS between birth and 9 years of age. In 18% of patients the diagnosis of AGS was not suspected until the discovery of testicular masses.[37] These tumors often develop in patients who are poorly compliant with medical therapy.[36] Small asymptomatic tumors tend to present in children, whereas large tumors are more common in young adults. Most tumors (86%) arise from the hilum of the testicle. These tumors are well demarcated although not encapsulated, lobulated, rubbery to firm, and brown-green in appearance.[37] Microscopically, the normal testicular architecture is usually obliterated and replaced by sheets or nests of cells separated by dense, fibrous bands of tissue.[37] The cells are large with abundant, finely granular, eosinophilic cytoplasm. Cytoplasmic lipochrome pigment is usually present, but crystals of Reinke are invariably absent. As mentioned in the discussion of Leydig cell tumors, AGS testicular tumors respond to both ACTH stimulation and dexamethasone suppression, whereas Leydig cell tumors are not responsive to exogenous hormonal factors. This biologic variance has been exploited to differentiate these two entities; administration of

TABLE 48–2. COMPARISON OF LEYDIG CELL TUMORS (LCT) AND HYPERPLASTIC TESTICULAR NODULES ASSOCIATED WITH ADRENOGENITAL SYNDROME (TTAGS)

	LCT	TTAGS
Precocious puberty	Yes	Yes
Bilateral tumors	No	Usually
Gynecomastia	Possible	No
17-Ketosteroids	Normal	Increased
Age at presentation	Older	2–3 yr
Hormonal autonomy	Yes	No
Malignant potential	Adult only	No
Treatment	Surgical	Medical
Cell of origin	Leydig	Pluripotential(?)

ACTH should result in exacerbation of symptoms (i.e., increase in tumor size and elevation of hormonal markers [17-OHPG]), and dexamethasone suppression should have an opposite effect. Failure of symptomatic resolution with adequate medical treatment warrants a tissue diagnosis. The distinguishing features of Leydig cell tumors and hyperplastic testicular nodules associated with AGS are shown in Table 48–2.

SECONDARY TUMORS

Lymphomas and Leukemias

Acute lymphoblastic leukemia (ALL) is the most common secondary tumor of the testis. The testicle is the second most common site of relapse after bone marrow, and between 10 and 30% of patients with ALL will have testicular leukemic relapse. One review showed that 25% of patients had testicular relapse, with 60% of these having no other evidence of disease.[59] Testicular leukemia presents as either a discrete testicular mass or enlargement, or more commonly as occult disease diagnosed by biopsy. Overt testicular relapse is rare and has been reported to be 2%.[60] The testes are a harbor for leukemic cells and are considered a privileged site where cancerous cells are postulated to be immune to the effects of chemotherapy. Therefore, testicular relapse indicates persistent or residual disease. This theory has been used to explain the improved survival rate in girls of 10 to 20%.[32] Overt testicular leukemia or occult relapse is typically treated by intensified chemotherapy and radiotherapy to the testes.

Because of the risk of relapse, testicular biopsy has been widely advocated in all boys with ALL after finishing treatment, with resumption of chemotherapy and addition of testicular radiotherapy if occult disease is detected. Testicular leukemia is very radiosensitive[61]; however, some authors advocate chemotherapy alone, which may help to limit the combined gonadotoxic effect of chemotherapy and irradiation.[62] Ultrasound and magnetic resonance imaging have not been shown to be clinically useful screening devices, with false-negative rates reported to be 50%, and should not replace testicular biopsy,[63] although biopsy has a false-negative rate of about 10%.[64,65] Based on the experience of the Children's Cancer Study Group, about 13% of boys will have occult disease diagnosed by testicular biopsy after 3 years of disease-free survival, and of those 38% will relapse despite conventional salvage therapy.[60] Disease-free survival was shown to be significantly better in the group of boys without occult testicular relapse, which represents the aggressive nature and adverse outcome associated with occult testicular leukemia. Routine testicular biopsy was therefore considered to be clinically prudent not only because it offered prognostic information, but in the hope that it would identify a group of children who would possibly benefit from an intensified salvage strategy. Many do not advocate biopsy, however, and base this on no apparent benefit on improved survival.[64,66,67]

Furthermore, intensified up-front chemotherapy has improved the overall survival of children with ALL, as well as decreased the incidence of testicular leukemic relapse and improved its salvage rate, resulting in controversy as to whether postchemotherapy screening for residual disease has a role in the management of boys with ALL.[64] Controversy surrounds the routine use of testicular biopsy, and it has yet to be decided whether these children will be better served by early identification and treatment of occult testicular leukemia versus retrieval therapy for those who develop overt testicular relapse.

REFERENCES

1. Adami HO, Bergstrom R, Mohner M, et al: Testicular cancer in nine northern European countries. Int J Cancer 1994; 59:33–38.
2. Brown LM, Pottern LM, Hoover RN, et al: Testicular cancer in the United States: trends in incidence and mortality. Int J Epidemiol 1986; 15:164–170.
3. Kaplan GW, Cromie WC, Kelalis PP, et al: Prepubertal yolk sac testicular tumors—report of the Testicular Tumor Registry. J Urol 1988; 140:1109–1112.
4. Telium G: Endodermal sinus tumors of the ovary and testis: comparative morphogenesis of the so-called mesonephroma overii (Schiller) and extraembryonic (yolk sac allantoic) structures of the rat's placenta. Cancer 1959; 12: 1092–1105.
5. Kay R: Prepubertal Testicular Tumor Registry. Urol Clin North Am 1993; 20:1–5.
6. Brosman SA: Testicular tumors in prepubertal children. Urology 1979; 13:581–588.
7. Fernandes ET, Etcubanas E, Rao BN, et al: Two decades of experience with testicular tumors in children at St. Jude Children's Research Hospital. J Pediatr Surg 1989; 24:677–681.
8. Bruce J, Gough DC: Long-term follow-up of children with testicular tumours: surgical issues. Br J Urol 1991; 67:429–433.
9. Haas RJ, Schmidt P, Gobel U, Harms D: Treatment of malignant testicular tumors in childhood: results of the German National Study 1982–1992. Med Pediatr Oncol 1994; 23:400–405.

10. Brodsky GL: Pathology of testicular germ cell tumors [Review]. Hematol Oncol Clin North Am 1991; 5:1095–1126.
11. Hu LM, Phillipson J, Barsky SH: Intratubular germ cell neoplasia in infantile yolk sac tumor: verification by tandem repeat sequence in situ hybridization. Diagn Mol Pathol 1992; 1:118–128.
12. Brewer JA, Tank ES: Yolk sac tumors and alpha-fetoprotein in first year of life [Review]. Urology 1993; 42:79–80.
13. Levy DA, Kay R, Elder JS: Neonatal testis tumors: a review of the Prepubertal Testis Tumor Registry. J Urol 1994; 151: 715–717.
14. Wu JT, Book L, Sudar K: Serum alpha-fetoprotein (AFP) levels in normal infants. Pediatr Res 1981; 82:50–52.
15. Boden G, Gibb R: Radiotherapy and testicular neoplasms. Lancet 1951; 2:1195–1197.
16. Grady RW, Ross JH, Kay R: Patterns of metastatic spread in prepubertal yolk sac tumor of the testis. J Urol 1995; 153:1259–1261.
17. Ehrlichman RJ, Kaufman SL, Siegelman SS, et al: Computerized tomography and lymphangiography in staging testis tumors. J Urol 1981; 126:179–181.
18. Huddart SN, Mann JR, Gornall P, et al: The UK Children's Cancer Study Group: testicular malignant germ cell tumours 1979–1988. J Pediatr Surg 1990; 25:406–410.
19. Griffin GC, Raney RJ, Snyder HM, et al: Yolk sac carcinoma of the testis in children. J Urol 1987; 137:954–957.
20. Carroll WL, Kempson RL, Govan DE, et al: Conservative management of testicular endodermal sinus tumor in childhood. J Urol 1985; 133:1011–1014.
21. Flamant F, Nihoul FC, Patte C, Lemerle J: Optimal treatment of clinical stage I yolk sac tumor of the testis in children. J Pediatr Surg 1986; 21:108–111.
22. Colodny AH, Hopkins TB: Testicular tumors in infants and children. Urol Clin North Am 1977; 4:347–358.
23. Exelby PR: Testis cancer in children. Semin Oncol 1979; 6: 116–120.
24. Pinkerton CR, Pritchard J, Spitz L: High complete response rate in children with advanced germ cell tumors using cisplatin-containing combination chemotherapy. J Clin Oncol 1986; 4:194–199.
25. Leonard MP, Jeffs RD, Leventhal B, Gearhart JP: Pediatric testicular tumors: the Johns Hopkins experience. Urology 1991; 37:253–256.
26. Mann JR, Pearson D, Barrett A, et al: Results of the United Kingdom Children's Cancer Study Group's malignant germ cell tumor studies. Cancer 1989; 63:1657–1667.
27. Marina N, Fontanesi J, Kun L, et al: Treatment of childhood germ cell tumors: review of the St. Jude experience from 1979 to 1988. Cancer 1992; 70:2568–2575.
28. Uehling DT, Phillips E: Residual retroperitoneal mass following chemotherapy for infantile yolk sac tumor. J Urol 1994; 152:185–186.
29. Heidenreich A, Engelmann UH, Vietsch HV, Derschum W: Organ preserving surgery in testicular epidermoid cysts [Review]. J Urol 1995; 153:1147–1150.
30. Rushton HG, Belman AB: Testis-sparing surgery for benign lesions of the prepubertal testis. Urol Clin North Am 1993; 20:27–37.
31. Kramer SA, Kelalis PP: Pediatric urologic oncology. *In* Gillenwater JY, Grayhack JT, Howards SS, Duckett JW (eds): Adult and Pediatric Urology, 2nd edition, pp 2245–2287. St. Louis, Mosby–Year Book, 1991.
32. Cortez JC, Kaplan GW: Gonadal stromal tumors, gonadoblastomas, epidermoid cysts, and secondary tumors of the testis in children [Review]. Urol Clin North Am 1993; 20:15–26.
33. Ducharme J, Collu R: Pubertal development: normal, precocious and delayed. Clin Endocrinol Metab 1982; 11:57–87.
34. Kim I, Young RH, Scully RE: Leydig cell tumors of the testis: a clinicopathological analysis of 40 cases and review of the literature. Am J Surg Pathol 1985; 9:177–192.
35. Urban MD, Lee PA, Plotnick LP, Migeon CJ: The diagnosis of Leydig cell tumors in childhood. Am J Dis Child 1978; 132:494–497.
36. Srikanth MS, West BR, Ishitani M, et al: Benign testicular tumors in children with congenital adrenal hyperplasia. J Pediatr Surg 1992; 27:639–641.
37. Rutgers JL, Young RH, Scully RE: The testicular "tumor" of the adrenogenital syndrome: a report of six cases and review of the literature on testicular masses in patients with adrenocortical disorders [Review]. Am J Surg Pathol 1988; 12:503–513.
38. Ilondo MM, van den Mooter F, Marchal G, et al: A boy with Leydig cell tumor and precocious puberty: ultrasonography as a diagnostic aid. Eur J Pediatr 1981; 137: 221–227.
39. Dilworth JP, Farrow GM, Oesterling JE: Testicular tumors of non-germ cell origin. AUA Update Ser 1992; 11:18–23.
40. Madsen E, Hultberg B: Metastasizing Sertoli cell tumours of the human testis: a report of two cases and a review of the literature. Acta Oncol 1990; 29:946–949.
41. Rosvoll R, Woodard J: Malignant Sertoli cell tumor of the testis. Cancer 1968; 22:8–13.
42. Sharma S, Seam RK, Kapoor HL: Malignant Sertoli cell tumor of the testis in a child. J Surg Oncol 1990; 44:129–131.
43. Brosman SA: Tumors: male genital tract. *In* Kelalis PP, King LR, Belman AB (eds): Clinical Pediatric Urology, 2nd edition, pp 1202–1219. Philadelphia, WB Saunders Co, 1985.
44. Gabrilove JL, Freiberg EK, Leiter E, Nicolis GL: Feminizing and nonfeminizing Sertoli cell tumors [Review]. J Urol 1980; 124:757–767.
45. Lawrence WD, Young RH, Scully RE: Juvenile granulosa cell tumor of the infantile testis: a report of 14 cases. Am J Surg Pathol 1985; 9:87–94.
46. Crump WD: Juvenile granulosa cell (sex cord-stromal) tumors of fetal testis. J Urol 1983; 129:1057–1058.
47. Marshall FF, Kerr WJ, Kliman B, Scully RE: Sex cord-stromal (gonadal stromal) tumors of the testis: a report of 5 cases. J Urol 1977; 117:180–184.
48. Raju U, Fine G, Warrier R, et al: Congenital testicular juvenile granulosa cell tumor in a neonate with X/XY mosaicism. Am J Surg Pathol 1986; 10:577–583. (Published erratum appears in Am J Surg Pathol 1986; 10:740)
49. Gourlay WA, Johnson HW, Pantzar JT, et al: Gonadal tumors in disorders of sexual differentiation. Urology 1994; 43:537–540.
50. Young RH, Lawrence WD, Scully RE: Juvenile granulosa cell tumor—another neoplasm associated with abnormal chromosomes and ambiguous genitalia: a report of three cases. Am J Surg Pathol 1985; 9:737–743.
51. Rutgers JL, Scully RE: Pathology of the testis in intersex syndromes [Review]. Semin Diagn Pathol 1987; 4:275–291.
52. Scully RE: Neoplasia associated with anomalous sexual development and abnormal sex chromosomes. Pediatr Adolesc Endocrinol 1981; 8:203–217.
53. Scully RE: Gonadoblastoma: a review of 74 cases [Review]. Cancer 1970; 25:1340–1356.
54. Ramani P, Yeung CK, Habeebu SS: Testicular intratubular germ cell neoplasia in children and adolescents with intersex [Review]. Am J Surg Pathol 1993; 17:1124–1133.
55. Shah KH, Maxted WC, Chun B: Epidermoid cysts of the testis: a report of three cases and an analysis of 141 cases from the world literature. Cancer 1981; 47:577–582.
56. Manivel JC, Reinberg Y, Niehans GA, Fraley EE: Intratubular germ cell neoplasia in testicular teratomas and epidermoid cysts: correlation with prognosis and possible biologic significance. Cancer 1989; 64:715–720.
57. Clark R, Albertson B, Munabi A: Steroidogenic enzyme activities, morphology, and receptor studies of a testicular adrenal rest in a patient with congenital adrenal hyperplasia. J Clin Endocrinol Metab 1990; 70:1408–1413.
58. Radfar N, Bartter FC, Easley T: Evidence for endogenous LH suppression in a man with bilateral testicular tumors and congenital adrenal hyperplasia. J Clin Endocrinol Metab 1977; 45:1194–1204.
59. Oakhill A, Mainwaring D, Hill FG, et al: Management of

leukaemic infiltration of the testis. Arch Dis Child 1980; 55: 564–566.
60. Miller DR, Leikin SL, Albo VC, et al: The prognostic value of testicular biopsy in childhood acute lymphoblastic leukemia: a report from the Childrens Cancer Study Group. J Clin Oncol 1990; 8:57–66.
61. Amendola BE, Hutchinson R, Grossman HB, Amendola MA: Isolated testicular leukemic relapse: response to radiation therapy. Urology 1987; 30:240–243.
62. Kim TH, Hargreaves HK, Brynes RK, et al: Pretreatment testicular history in childhood acute lymphocytic leukemia. Lancet 1981; 2:657–658.
63. Klein EA, Kay R, Norris DG, et al: Noninvasive testicular screening in childhood leukemia. J Urol 1986; 136:864–866.
64. Hudson MM, Frankel LS, Mullins J, Swanson DA: Diagnostic value of surgical testicular biopsy after therapy for acute lymphocytic leukemia. J Pediatr 1985; 107:50–53.
65. Chessells J, Leiper A, Rogers D: Outcome following late marrow relapse in childhood acute lymphoblastic leukemia. J Clin Oncol 1984; 2:1088–1091.
66. Pui CH, Dahl GV, Bowman WP, et al: Elective testicular biopsy during chemotherapy for childhood leukaemia is of no clinical value. Lancet 1985; 2:410–412.
67. Sutherland R, Dreyer ZE, Gonzales ET, Roth DR: Testicular biopsy in children with acute lymphoblastic leukemia: does it improve survival? [Abstract 53]. Presented to the American Academy of Pediatrics, Section of Urology, San Francisco, 1995.

XII

ADDITIONAL TOPICS

49

LAPAROSCOPIC ONCOLOGY

INDERBIR S. GILL, M.D., ELSPETH M. MCDOUGALL, M.D., F.R.C.S.(C), *and* RALPH V. CLAYMAN, M.D.

Despite the initial report of laparoscopic surgery in 1910 by Jacobeus,[1] it was not until 70 years later that laparoscopic urology was initiated. In 1976, Cortesi and associates reported using the laparoscope to search the abdomen in a patient with an undescended testicle.[2] Laparoscopic urology remained largely in the pediatric realm for the next 15 years. In 1990, Schuessler and Vancaillie, in collaboration with Griffith, brought laparoscopy into adult urology with their initial report of using the technique to perform a pelvic lymph node dissection in order to preoperatively stage prostate cancer.[3] The technique rapidly was adopted by the urologic community, and between 1992 and 1994 laparoscopic pelvic lymph node dissection became the leading laparoscopic procedure throughout the United States.

Other urologic surgeons became interested in extending the laparoscopic approach to myriad surgical problems. Thereafter, laparoscopic "firsts" were recorded for nearly every type of "open" urologic procedure for both benign and malignant disease.[4] Within a 3-year period, laparoscopy had been successfully applied to retroperitoneal lymph node dissection, radical nephrectomy, partial nephrectomy, nephroureterectomy, cystectomy, diverticulectomy, partial cystectomy, radical prostatectomy, adrenalectomy, and gonadectomy.

The focus of this chapter is on laparoscopic procedures as they relate to the field of urologic oncology. Each of the aforementioned procedures, both diagnostic and ablative, is reviewed with regard to its history, indication, technique, results, and overall efficacy/efficiency. The key question with any new surgical procedure remains: "It's new, but is it better?" The answer to this question rests in the hands of each of us, as we attempt to compare the "latest in technology" with the "tried and true." For laparoscopy, these phase III trials are as yet in their earliest stages.

LAPAROSCOPIC DIAGNOSTIC PROCEDURES IN UROLOGIC ONCOLOGY: STAGING LYMPHADENECTOMY

Staging lymphadenectomy as a "stand alone" procedure is most commonly performed for prostate and testis cancer. In the former, a pelvic lymphadenectomy is performed to determine suitability of the lesion for subsequent definitive therapy, whereas in the latter circumstance, a retroperitoneal lymph node dissection is viewed as both therapeutic and diagnostic. In addition, staging pelvic lymphadenectomy has also been used sparingly in patients with bladder and penile cancer.

Pelvic Lymph Node Dissection for Prostate Cancer

History

In 1990, laparoscopic surgery was propelled into the realm of adult urology as a result of the work of Griffith, Schuessler, and Vancaillie.[3] By performing a limited lymph node dissection in a patient with prostate cancer, this group identified a laparoscopic procedure with tremendous potential application. Indeed, within a short span of time, laparoscopic lymph node dissection became a widely accepted procedure, and thousands of urologists learned how to perform laparoscopy largely for this purpose.

In 1996, staging pelvic lymph node dissection (PLND) continues to be the "gold standard" method for evaluating pelvic nodal involvement in patients with prostate cancer. This is because radiologic techniques (ultrasonography, computed tomography [CT] scan, magnetic resonance imaging) have an unacceptably high (40 to 50%) false-negative rate in diagnosing metastatic nodal disease.[5] The recently described technique of radioimmunoscintigraphy of pelvic nodes with ^{111}In-labeled monoclonal antibody CYT-356 had an overall accuracy of 76% in 19 patients with prostate cancer.[6]

An evolving body of evidence suggests that the vast majority of contemporary patients with prostate cancer are presenting with node-negative disease. In two recent series of 200 and 521 consecutive patients undergoing radical prostatectomy for clinically localized prostate cancer, nodal involvement was present in only 3.4% and 6.7% of patients, respectively.[7,8] Accordingly, efforts are being increasingly focused toward refining patient selection criteria for PLND. Only patients with a reasonable chance of having nodal involvement should undergo a staging PLND; those with a low probability of metastatic disease in the first place should be spared an "unnecessary" lymphadenectomy.

In this regard, the recent discovery of prostate-specific antigen (PSA) as an excellent tumor marker has played an important role. Metastatic nodal disease has been shown to occur more frequently in patients with high PSA levels, advancing Gleason score, and increasing tumor volume.[9] Using logistic regression analyses, nomograms have been developed based on three criteria: serum PSA, primary Gleason grade, and local clinical stage.[10] Such nomograms allow the urologist to preoperatively predict the probability of pelvic nodal involvement on an individual basis with reasonable, but not absolute, accuracy.

Indications

In candidates for a radical **retropubic** prostatectomy, laparoscopic PLND is indicated only in those at high risk for lymphatic metastases, provided that confirmation of metastatic nodal disease would preclude a prostatectomy in those patients. Accordingly, current indications for laparoscopic PLND in patients opting for a retropubic prostatectomy are PSA level greater than 30 ng/ml *or* Gleason grade of 4 or higher *or* clinical stage B2, C, or D0 *or* CT-diagnosed, needle biopsy–negative pelvic lymphadenopathy.[5] Currently, only 5% of patients undergoing a radical retropubic prostatectomy satisfy the above criteria.

In contrast, radical **perineal** prostatectomy or definitive **radiotherapy** or **cryotherapy** should be preceded by a laparoscopic PLND in many, but not all, patients. In a current analysis of 191 consecutive patients with clinically localized prostate cancer, it was determined that a patient with a PSA level of 30 ng/ml or less *and* Gleason grade of 3 or lower was at minimal risk for nodal involvement.[11] Another study indicated that the combination of PSA level of 10 ng/ml or less, a Gleason grade of 3 or lower, *and* a low clinical stage (A, B1) will rarely (i.e., <4% for stage A and 2% for stage B1) be associated with malignant lymphadenopathy.[10] Finally, nonpalpable, ultrasound-diagnosed prostate cancer was not associated with metastatic pelvic nodes in any of 28 patients.[12] Only in patients not meeting these strict criteria is a PLND indicated currently. Under these circumstances, it is estimated that less than half of all prostate cancer patients prior to perineal prostatectomy or planned radiation therapy or cryotherapy would need a node dissection.

The hemipelvis more likely to have lymphatic involvement is dissected first: ipsilateral to the location of the prostate nodule, the side of positive biopsy, the side with enlarged lymph nodes on pelvic CT scan, or, in cases of bilateral prostatic lobe involvement, the side with the greater tumor burden or higher Gleason score. By obtaining a frozen section of the nodes from this side, a needless bilateral dissection can be avoided in 83% of patients with malignant lymphadenopathy.[13] Rarely, when lateralizing factors are absent, laparoscopic PLND is first performed on the right side because of technical ease, since there are usually colonic adhesions or sigmoid diverticulae present on the left side in most older men.[5,14]

Limited Node Dissection: Transperitoneal Approach

TECHNIQUE. The laparoscopic surgeon stands on the contralateral side and the assistant stands on the same side as the obturator fossa to be dissected.[15] The pelvis may be hyperextended with a roll under the sacrum. The patient is positioned in 30 degrees Trendelenburg, with the side to be dissected elevated by 30 degrees.

A four- or five-port approach is employed, as dictated by the patient's body habitus: the four-port "diamond" configuration affords better exposure in thin patients; the five-port "fan" array is reserved for obese patients or for an extended PLND. The anatomic extent of a laparoscopic dissection mirrors its open surgical counterpart (Table 49–1). The posterior parietal peritoneum is incised parallel and lateral to the medial umbilical ligament.[14] This in-

TABLE 49–1. ANATOMIC BOUNDARIES OF LIMITED AND EXTENDED PLND

Boundaries	Limited Node Dissection	Extended Node Dissection
Inferior	Pubis	Pubis
Medial	Bladder Medial umbilical ligament Pubic tubercle Ureter	Bladder Medial umbilical ligament Pubic tubercle Ureter
Lateral	Obturator internus muscle External iliac vein	Genitofemoral nerve External iliac artery
Superior	Bifurcation of common iliac vessels Medial umbilical ligament	Common iliac vessels Ureter
Posterior	Obturator nerve	Obturator nerve Presciatic tissue

cision is extended cephalad along the external iliac vein up to the bifurcation of the common iliac vein. Alternatively, an inverted-V peritoneotomy can be employed to obtain wider access into the pelvic retroperitoneum.[16] The horizontally oriented vas deferens is divided at the point just before it crosses the medial umbilical ligament. The medial and posterior aspects of the external iliac vein are skeletonized (lateral limit of the dissection). This dissection is extended toward the glistening white symphysis pubis, freeing the lymph node packet distally (caudal limit of dissection); an occasionally present aberrant obturator vein should be preserved. Cephalad traction on the nodal packet allows dissection along its posterior aspect, thus bringing the obturator nerve into view (posterior limit of the dissection). The nodal packet is then detached from its sole remaining attachment at the "V" area between the external iliac vein and the medial umbilical ligament.

RESULTS. The surgical adequacy of a laparoscopic PLND is similar to that of an open PLND (Table 49–2). The extent of anatomic dissection, number of lymph nodes retrieved (10 in laparoscopic PLND vs. 11 in open PLND),[17] and the node-positive rate (41% in the laparoscopic group vs. 47% in the open surgical group)[18] are comparable. However, the laparoscopic approach is associated with decreased patient morbidity as compared to the open approach. The laparoscopic approach results in decreased blood loss (100 vs. 212.5 ml; $p = 0.004$), faster resumption of oral intake (0.63 vs. 2.17 days; $p = 0.0001$), decreased analgesic requirement (1.55 vs. 47 mg MSO_4; $p = 0.0001$), and shortened hospital stay (1.7 vs. 5.37 days; $p = 0.0001$).[18]

Laparoscopic PLND is associated with a significant learning curve. In an analysis of 100 consecutive patients undergoing laparoscopic PLND, the complication rate decreased from 14% in the initial 50 cases to 4% in the latter 50.[19] In another study of 103 consecutive patients undergoing laparoscopic PLND, 10 dissections were aborted; 8 of these unsuccessful cases occurred in the first 40 patients undergoing laparoscopic PLND.[20] The multi-institutional report by Kavoussi and coworkers on 372 patients undergoing laparoscopic PLND also showed that the majority of the failed procedures were in the first 8 cases at each institution.[21]

At this writing, no perioperative mortality has been reported in over 500 patients undergoing a laparoscopic PLND.[12,17–24] The overall complication rate was 15%; vascular injury (2%) was the most common major intraoperative complication (10 patients). Urinary retention (1.6%) was the most common postoperative complication (Table 49–3).

Laparoscopic PLND has rekindled interest in the perineal approach for radical prostatectomy. Many studies have confirmed the feasibility and safety of combining laparoscopic PLND and radical perineal prostatectomy in a single anesthetic session[25–29] (Table 49–4). In a series of 86 patients undergoing one-stage laparoscopic PLND and radical perineal prostatectomy, mean total operative time was 246 minutes (laparoscopic PLND = 86 min, repositioning = 23 min, radical perineal prostatectomy = 129 min).[27] Four patients (5%) had a false-negative result on frozen section of the lymph nodes. Average hospital stay was 3.1 days; however, 19 patients (25%) were discharged within 48 hours and an additional 39 (51%) within 72 hours.[27] In another series of 37 patients, mean operative time for the combined procedure was 244 minutes (range, 150 to 350 minutes) and only 12 patients (32%) required a blood transfusion (mean, 1.7 units/patient). No patient had a false-negative result on frozen section evaluation of the lymph nodes. Liquid diet was resumed on the evening of surgery and average hospital stay was 5.3 days (range, 3 to 9 days).[29]

The value of a staging laparoscopic PLND prior to either a radical perineal or retropubic prostatectomy has been compared to open PLND and radical retropubic prostatectomy. In a nonrandomized study, 26 patients underwent laparoscopic PLND and radical perineal prostatectomy (group I), 24 underwent laparoscopic PLND and radical retropubic prostatectomy (group II), and a control group of 26 patients underwent standard open PLND and radical retropubic prostatectomy (group III).[26] Patients in group I had a shorter operative time (214 vs. 278 vs. 215 minutes; $p < 0.01$), decreased blood loss (576 vs. 1275 vs. 1100 ml; $p < 0.001$), lower rate of blood transfusions (23 vs. 79 vs. 77%; $p < 0.001$), and shorter hospital stay (4.6 vs. 9.6 vs. 7.3 days; $p < 0.001$) as compared to groups II and III, respectively. Of these 76 patients, 23 (30%) had positive surgical margins; no statistically significant difference in the incidence of positive surgical margins was found among the three groups. Complications occurred in two patients (8%) in group I, seven patients (29%) in group II, and one patient (4%) in group III. Complete urinary continence at 6 months (69 vs. 64 vs. 73%) and postoperative potency rates (25 vs. 29 vs. 29%) were similar among the three groups.[26] In a smaller study, combined laparoscopic PLND and total perineal prostatectomy (group I; $N = 12$) was compared with standard radical retropubic prostatectomy (group II; $N = 10$).[28] Of interest, in group I, after completing the laparoscopic PLND, the authors laparoscopically mobilized the seminal vesicles to facilitate the subsequent perineal prostatectomy. Patients in group I had similar operative time (237.5 vs. 237.5 minutes), decreased blood loss (450 vs. 1250 ml; $p = 0.001$), more rapid ambulation (1 vs. 2 days; $p = 0.002$), more rapid resumption of oral intake (1 vs. 3.5 days; $p < 0.001$), and shorter hospital stay (3 vs. 6 days; $p < 0.001$) as compared to the open group.[28] Overall, it appears that combined laparoscopic PLND and radical perineal prostatectomy can accurately assess pelvic nodes and afford satisfactory cancer control of organ-confined disease while avoiding an abdominal incision and minimizing patient morbid-

TABLE 49–2. LAPAROSCOPIC PLND—CURRENT EXPERIENCE*

Reference	No. of Pts.	Mean Age (yr)	Timing of Prostatectomy	Type of Radical Prostatectomy	No. of Ports	No. of Nodes Retrieved	Positive Nodes (%)	False-Negative Rate (%)	OR Time (min)	Estimated Blood Loss (ml)	Analgesia (mg of MSO_4)	Resume Diet (days)	Hospital Stay (days)	Convalescence (wk)	Conversion to Open Surgery: No. (%)	Complication Rate (%)
Transperitoneal																
Schuessler et al.[12]	147	71	—	—	4–5	45.3	23%	—	150	100	—	—	2	2	4 (8%)	31
Winfield et al.[17]	68	68	Simultaneous = 15 Delayed = 51	Perineal = 8 Retropubic = 15 XRT = 20	4	9.8	23%	4%†	150	<100	—	<1	1.5	1	11 (17%)	27
Kerbl et al.[18]	80	70	Simultaneous = 10 Delayed = 4	Retropubic = 14	4	—	41%	—	200	100	1.6	<1	1.7	1.5	0 (0%)	13
Rukstalis et al.[20]	103	—	Simultaneous = 20 Delayed = 78	Retropubic	4	9	19%	10%‡	158	94–134	6.0	—	1.8	—	10 (10%)	13.5
Guazzoni et al.[24]	80	65	Delayed	Retropubic	4–5	9	0%	10%	136	80–120	—	—	2	1	0 (0%)	18
TOTAL	378	86	—	—	4–5	18	21%	8%	158	168	3.8	<1	1.8	1.4	25 (7%)	13.5
Retroperitoneal																
Das and Tashima[35]	9	71	Simultaneous	Retropubic = 8 XRT = 2	4	12.8	11%	0%	50–110	—	—	—	1	—	0 (0%)	11
Villiers et al.[36]	10	62	Delayed	Retropubic = 1 Perineal = 7	5	—	20%	0%	84	—	—	—	2	<1	0 (0%)	20
Etwaru et al.[37]	12	65	Delayed	Perineal XRT	5	7	25%	—	180	—	—	—	—	—	0 (0%)	17
TOTAL	31		—	—	4–5	10	19%	8%	96	—	—	—	1.5	<1	0 (0%)	18

*Modified from Gill IS, Clayman RV, McDougall EM: State of the art: advances in urologic laparoscopy. J Urol 1995; 154:1275, with permission.
†Based on 28 patients subjected to open lymphadenectomy subsequently.
‡Based on 20 patients subjected to open lymphadenectomy subsequently.

TABLE 49–3. COMPLICATIONS OF TRANSPERITONEAL LAPAROSCOPIC PLND*,†

Total no. of patients	500
Total no. of complications	62 (12%)
Intraoperative Complications (*N* = 20)	
Anesthetic complications	1
Unable to access peritoneum	1
Organ injuries (18)	
Bowel	1
Ureter	2
Bladder	3
Vascular	10
Obturator nerve	2
Postoperative Complications (*N* = 42)	
Urinary retention	8
Lymphocele/lymphedema	5
Prolonged ileus	6
Deep venous thrombosis	5
Prolonged scrotal edema	3
Significant ecchymosis	2
Wound infection	2
Bleeding requiring transfusion	3
Delayed diagnosis of bowel injury	2
Small bowel obstruction	2
Anesthetic complication	1
Fascial dehiscence	1
Pelvic hematoma	1
Retroperitoneal abscess	1
Secondary open surgical intervention	13
Complete lymphadenectomy could not be done	17
(Causes: patient body habitus, adhesions, problems achieving pneumoperitoneum, prolonged anesthetic)	

*From Gill IS, Clayman RV, McDougall EM: State of the art: advances in urologic laparoscopy. J Urol 1995; 154:1275, with permission.

†This table includes patients from large series currently available in literature.

ity. These data have led to a resurgence of radical perineal prostatectomy at some centers.[25–29]

In addition to its use prior to surgical prostatectomy, laparoscopic PLND is technically feasible and safe in patients who have previously received external beam radiotherapy for prostate cancer. In two separate reports, a total of 16 men with elevated PSA levels or clinical failure following definitive radiotherapy were selected for laparoscopic PLND prior to salvage prostatectomy.[30,31] Average operative time ranged from 154 to 182 minutes and blood loss was 55 ml. Cancerous lymph nodes were identified in 3 of 16 patients (19%). Bowel perforation occurred in one patient. It was concluded that, although radiation therapy resulted in obliteration of tissue planes with some resultant increase in difficulty of the laparoscopic dissection, laparoscopic PLND could nevertheless be accomplished safely in this situation.[30,31]

Laparoscopic PLND has been combined with transperineal radioactive seed implantation of the prostate under real-time interactive transrectal ultrasound guidance.[32] Fifty-eight patients underwent the single-stage procedure: no patient had positive pelvic lymph nodes. Total operative time was 226 minutes and hospital stay was 2.2 days. At a 2-year follow-up, 16% of patients had biopsy-proven local failure. In patients electing radioactive seed implantation for definitive treatment of prostate cancer, same-session laparoscopic PLND can provide definitive assessment of pelvic nodal status.[32]

Laparoscopic PLND is more expensive than open PLND: \$9406 versus \$8399 if the nodes are positive, and \$9747 versus \$7812 if the nodes are negative.[33] Although preoperative costs were comparable (\$532 vs. \$693), intraoperative costs were 52% higher (\$8075 vs. \$5332) and postoperative costs were 280% lower (\$842 vs. \$2161) for the laparoscopic versus the open surgery group. Of note, the costs associated with laparoscopic PLND have not decreased from 1990–1991 to 1993–1994.[34] However, assessing the true financial impact of laparoscopy remains an inherently difficult task. Whereas pre-, intra-, and postoperative hospital dollar costs are easily calculated, subjective parameters, including decreased patient morbidity, more rapid return to work, and superior cosmetic result, are more difficult to assess monetarily.[34]

Limited Node Dissection: Extraperitoneal Approach

Technique. Pelvic lymphadenectomy can be performed by an entirely extraperitoneal laparoscopic approach[35–37] (Table 49–2). Through a 1.5-cm midline, subumbilical skin incision, the preperitoneal space is entered and blunt finger dissection performed. An open (Hasson) cannula is secured. A catheter-mounted balloon is introduced and inflated with 1 to 1.2 L of saline. Balloon expansion atraumatically displaces the peritoneal envelope cephalad and rapidly develops the pelvic extraperitoneal space. Additional ports are placed bilaterally, just below the midpoint of a line joining the anterior superior iliac spine and the umbilicus. The boundaries of the extraperitoneal PLND mirror those of the transperitoneal limited PLND.

Results. Extraperitoneal and transperitoneal laparoscopic PLND were compared in 75 patients.[38] Nodal yield (1 to 22 in the extraperitoneal group vs. 2 to 23 in the transperitoneal group), operative time (2.3 hours in both groups), and hospital stay (2.7 vs. 3.2 days) were similar between the two groups; however, postoperative ileus was reduced in the extraperitoneal group. The extraperitoneal approach was converted to an open or transperitoneal laparoscopic approach in 3% of the patients because of prior surgical adhesions. Complications in the extraperitoneal group included one lymphocele and one bowel injury; complications in the transperitoneal group included one lymphocele and one umbilical hernia. In another series of nine patients undergoing extraperitoneal laparoscopic PLND, operative time ranged from 50 to 110 minutes, mean number of lymph nodes retrieved was 12, and hospital stay was 1 day. Intraoperative end-tidal CO_2 levels did not exceed 48.5 mm Hg in any patient.[35]

TABLE 49–4. ONE-STAGE LAPAROSCOPIC PLND AND RADICAL PERINEAL PROSTATECTOMY

Reference	No. Pts	OR Time (hr)	EBL (ml)	Blood Transfusions: No. (%)		No. Lymph Nodes Retrieved	Node Pos. Rate (%)	Pos. Surg. Margins (%)	Hosp. Stay (days)	Complications		Follow-up (mos)	Continence Rate (%)	Potency Rate (%)
				Pts Without	Pts With					Major	Minor			
Lerner et al.[25]	31	4.5	593	23 (74)	8 (26)	—	11	18	6	4[†] (13%)	3[†] (10%)	23	—	23
Parra et al.[26]	26	3.6	576	20 (77)	6 (23)	—	5	—	4.6	2[‡] (8%)	—	6	69	25
Thomas et al.[27]	76	4.1	—	52 (69)	24 (31)	8.2	16	—	3	1[§] (1%)	6[§] (8%)	4.2	93	—
Teichman et al.[28]	10	4.0	450	9 (90)	1 (10)	—	17	25	3	0 (0%)	1[‖] (10%)	—	80	0
Levy and Resnick[29]	37	4.1	300–500	25 (68)	12 (32)	—	17	—	5.3	4[¶] (11%)	—	13.6	81	—
TOTAL	180	4.1	540	76	24	8.2	13	22	4.4	7%	9%	11.7	75	24

*EBL, estimated blood loss.
[†]Complications: major—myocardial infarction (1), trocar site hernia (1), lymphocele (1); minor—colitis (2), urine leak (1).
[‡]Complications: major—rectal injury (2).
[§]Complications: major—rectal injury (1); minor—ileus (2), wound complications (3), prolonged intubation (1).
[‖]Complications: minor—hematoma (1).
[¶]Complications: major—rectal injury (2), deep venous thrombosis (1), pelvic abscess (1).

In conclusion, for a standard PLND, the extraperitoneal approach allows a technically adequate dissection; however, as regards an extended dissection, exposure of the iliac bifurcation and common iliac lymph nodes may be more difficult by this technique. Although surgeon preference dictates whether the transperitoneal or the extraperitoneal technique is employed for PLND, the latter approach may be preferable in patients with suspected abdominal adhesions from prior surgery.

Extended Pelvic Lymph Node Dissection: Transperitoneal Approach

An extended PLND has also been performed by laparoscopic techniques.[12] The rationale of an extended lymphadenectomy is that lymphatic metastases may "skip" the primary landing site (i.e., obturator nodes) and selectively target the iliopsoas, presciatic, and/or presacral lymph nodes in up to 14% of patients with prostate cancer[39]; the latter lymph node groups are not excised during a limited PLND.

TECHNIQUE. The boundaries of an extended laparoscopic PLND are as follows: the terminal 2 cm of the common iliac artery (proximal), the genitofemoral nerve (lateral) (iliopsoas nodes), and the ureter as it crosses the common iliac vessels (medial) (Table 49–1). The posterior limit (obturator nerve) and the caudal limit (pubic bone) are identical to those of a limited PLND. The medial umbilical ligament is divided and the hypogastric artery is dissected in an attempt to retrieve the presacral lymph nodes. The ureter, as it crosses the common iliac vessels, is also identified. Finally, dissection between the obturator and sciatic nerves is performed to retrieve the presciatic nodes.

RESULTS. Laparoscopic extended PLND significantly increased the nodal yield (mean, 45 nodes/patient), with a node-positive rate of 23%.[12] Mean operative time and hospital stay were 2.5 hours and 2 days, respectively. Complications occurred in 31% of patients. Interestingly, in 30% of patients, the iliopsoas lymph nodes were the sole site of metastatic disease; thus a limited PLND would have missed the diagnosis of D_1 disease in these patients. Another study showed that a limited (standard) open surgical PLND misses solitary positive deep pelvic nodes in 14% of cases.[40] However, in a series of 96 patients undergoing laparoscopic PLND, 15 underwent an extended dissection; all 4 patients with positive nodes had positive nodes in the obturator group as well.[41] Of concern, of the nine major complications following laparoscopic PLND, four occurred in the extended PLND group. The authors believe that the extended technique directly contributed to the increased complication rate.[41] Accordingly, although the advantages of an extended PLND have been questioned, it seems reasonable to state that it will upstage 6 to 15% of patients, thereby saving these patients needless additional therapy.

Minilaparotomy for Limited Pelvic Lymph Node Dissection

In any current treatise on minimally invasive techniques for staging PLND, it is appropriate to discuss the technique of minilaparotomy PLND. In an effort to minimize patient morbidity without resorting to laparoscopic technology, extraperitoneal PLND has been performed through either bilateral 3- to 4-cm long McBurney point incisions[42,43] or a single 6-cm midline infraumbilical incision.[44,45] In the largest reported experience to date, 139 patients have undergone PLND by the bilateral incision technique in France since 1987.[42] Although detailed data were not reported in this abstract, operating time was approximately 1 hour and hospital stay ranged from 3 to 5 days. Complications occurred in eight patients (6%): deep vein thrombosis (four), lymphocele (three), and colonic injury (one). In a series of 11 patients, outpatient PLND was performed through two 3-cm incisions overlying the obturator fossae.[43] Operative time averaged 84 minutes and blood loss was 29 ml. Average number of lymph nodes retrieved was seven; metastatic disease was confirmed in four patients. Nine patients were treated on an outpatient basis. The lone complication was an external iliac venotomy, which was repaired by extending the skin incision to 6 cm. Hospital costs associated with outpatient PLND averaged $6813.[43] Similarly, PLND through a single 6-cm lower midline incision has been reported in 13 and 16 patients from two institutions.[44,45] In the first study, minilap PLND (N = 13) was compared with laparoscopic PLND (N = 20), and standard open PLND (N = 7). The minilap group had a shorter hospital stay (1.3 vs. 1.3 vs. 7 days) and decreased costs as compared to the laparoscopic and open PLND groups, respectively.[44]

Convalescence, analgesic use, and delayed complication data have not yet been reported in any series on minilap PLND. Nevertheless, in the current health care era of cost containment, minilap PLND is a reasonable alternative to laparoscopic limited PLND. Of note, to date, there have been no reports of a minilaparotomy extended PLND.

Limited Transperitoneal Pelvic Lymph Node Dissection for Penile Cancer

In patients with invasive penile cancer, evidence of pelvic nodal metastases is a poor prognostic feature, because it heralds likely incurable disease and limited patient survival. In one series of 30 patients with penile cancer, all 9 patients with pelvic nodal metastases died of disease progression within 7 months.[46] Persistent inguinal lymphadenopathy following postpenectomy antibiotic therapy is indicative of inguinal nodal metastases in up to 86% of patients. Furthermore, 30% of patients with malignant inguinal lymphadenopathy (particularly those with high tumor volume in the inguinal nodes) will have concomitant pelvic nodal metastases.[46]

Classically, patients with clinically persistent inguinal lymphadenopathy following standard postpenectomy antibiotic therapy undergo an extended (superficial and deep) inguinal lymph node dissection, a procedure associated with significant local morbidity. Following histologic confirmation of inguinal metastases, a staging pelvic lymphadenectomy is performed to rule out pelvic nodal involvement. However, Assimos and Jarrow have noted that an inguinal lymphadenectomy is of no therapeutic benefit if pelvic nodal metastases exist concurrently.[47] Accordingly, they proposed that, in patients with persistent inguinal lymphadenopathy following a course of antibiotic therapy, the pelvic nodes should be initially assessed by a laparoscopic PLND (Fig. 49–1). Their rationale is that a staging laparoscopic PLND causes considerably less morbidity than an inguinal lymphadenectomy. If pelvic nodal metastases are confirmed, the prognosis is grim, and further surgical intervention is not warranted except to palliate local symptoms. Conversely, if the pelvic nodes are free of disease, an open surgical inguinal lymphadenectomy should be performed, either in the same operating session or secondarily. The authors cautioned that, at the time of the subsequent inguinal lymphadenectomy, the vital lymphatic tissue in the vicinity of the circumflex iliac vessels must be excised; this tissue is technically difficult to retrieve during the laparoscopic pelvic lymphadenectomy.

In the series of Assimos and Jarrow, three patients with stage T3 (UICC staging system) squamous cell carcinoma of the penis and persistent inguinal lymphadenopathy underwent a staging laparoscopic PLND.[47] Average operating time was 3.3 hours and hospital stay was less than 24 hours. There were no perioperative complications. The average number of pelvic lymph nodes retrieved was eight; no tumor was found in any of the pelvic nodes. All three patients underwent secondary inguinal lymphadenectomy; metastases were found in the superficial inguinal nodes unilaterally in two patients. One patient developed recurrent groin disease at a follow-up of 5 months, requiring further therapy; the other two patients had no evidence of disease at follow-up of 10 and 18 months. There are two additional reports of laparoscopic node dissection in four patients with penile cancer.[19,48] Overall, it is clear that data on the application of laparoscopic PLND in the management of patients with suspected metastatic penile cancer are scant at the present time.

Retroperitoneal Lymph Node Dissection for Testis Cancer

Laparoscopic retroperitoneal lymph node dissection (RPLND) has been explored at a handful of centers as a minimally invasive alternative for definitive diagnosis and treatment of selected patients with clinical stage I nonseminomatous germ cell tumors of the testis.[49–55] The laparoscopic technique aims to avoid the discomfort and the 6 to 19% complication rate associated with an open RPLND[56,57] while eliminating the 30% recurrence rate associated with surveillance protocols.[58]

Technique

Via a four- to six-port transperitoneal approach, the ipsilateral colon is mobilized medially; the renal

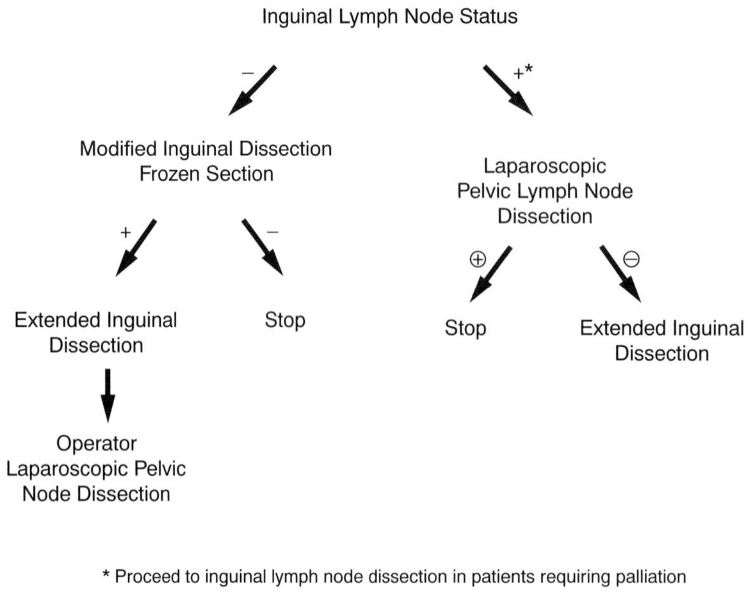
Inguinal Lymph Node Status
−
+*
Modified Inguinal Dissection
Frozen Section
Laparoscopic
Pelvic Lymph Node
Dissection
+
−
⊕
⊖
Extended Inguinal
Dissection
Stop
Stop
Extended Inguinal
Dissection
Operator
Laparoscopic Pelvic
Node Dissection
* Proceed to inguinal lymph node dissection in patients requiring palliation

FIGURE 49–1. Proposed role of laparoscopic pelvic lymphadenectomy in invasive penile cancer. (From Assimos DG, Jarow JP: Role of laparoscopic pelvic lymph node dissection in the management of patients with penile cancer and inguinal adenopathy. J Endourol 1994; 8:365, with permission.)

hilum, ureter, and great vessels are dissected. Lymphadenectomy is usually performed according to a modified template.[59] However, in an attempt to mirror the "split and roll" open technique of retroperitoneal lymphadenectomy, Janetschek et al. have developed a two-step ventral-lateral laparoscopic approach.[50] The ventral approach is employed to mobilize the colon, excise the spermatic cord remnant, and dissect the anatomic limits of the template. The lateral approach allows transection of the lumbar vessels and retrieval of the retroaortic and retrocaval nodes.

Results

Janetschek and coworkers performed a unilateral laparoscopic retroperitoneal lymphadenectomy in 15 patients with clinical stage I testicular tumors (Table 49–5). Mean operative time was 5.8 hours and hospital stay was 5.5 days. Complications occurred in four patients (27%). The node-positive rate was 20%. Antegrade ejaculation was preserved in 93% of patients.[50] In a U.S. multi-institutional analysis of 20 patients, mean operative time was 6 hours and the complication rate was 30%. The node-positive rate was 15%. Antegrade ejaculation was preserved in all patients.[51]

Currently, laparoscopic RPLND is an advanced laparoscopic procedure with a steep learning curve. Although it may be considered as an extension of clinical staging in stage I patients with certain risk factors (i.e., high T stage [TNM system], lymphovascular invasion of the primary tumor, absence of yolk sac elements, presence of embryonal elements),[60] there are many concerns about its use. First, the potential complication rate of a laparoscopic retroperitoneal lymphadenectomy (Table 49–6) exceeds that of its open counterpart. Second, there is definite uncertainty regarding its anatomic thoroughness and the overall accuracy of dissection. Because of these factors, we believe that laparoscopic RPLND remains an investigational technique best performed at recognized centers of laparoscopic urology; also, all patients with positive nodes diagnosed by a laparoscopic retroperitoneal lymphadenectomy should likely undergo subsequent chemotherapy because the therapeutic benefit of laparoscopic RPLND has yet to be demonstrated.

Concerns Regarding Tumor Implantation

As mentioned previously, laparoscopic PLND has been employed for staging prostate, bladder, penile, and testis cancer. Given the possibility of seeding of cancer cells, the issue of cutaneous metastases at the laparoscopic trocar site is an important one. Trocar site seeding has been reported following laparoscopy for gallbladder adenocarcinoma,[61] gastric tumors,[62] colonic tumors,[63] hepatocellular carcinoma,[64,65] and ovarian tumors.[66,67] In the urologic literature, one report each of subcutaneous implantation following laparoscopy for prostate[68] and bladder cancer[69] are available. Six months after laparoscopic PLND for a stage T3pN1M0, grade 2 adenocarcinoma of the prostate, a cutaneous nodule was noted at the trocar site that had been used for removal of the nodal packet; aspiration cytology confirmed metastatic adenocarcinoma.[68] In the second case, a patient with stage T1, grade 2 transitional cell carcinoma of the bladder underwent laparoscopic biopsy of a large bladder dome tumor that was possibly invading the abdominal wall. Subcutaneous metastasis was noted at the laparoscopic trocar site subsequently. Because this patient had previously undergone two endoscopic resections of the bladder tumor by the suprapubic route, it is unclear whether the subcutaneous metastasis represented tumor implantation secondary to the endoscopic resection, the laparoscopic biopsy, or hematogenous dissemination.[69] Nevertheless, the authors recommended that, given their propensity for seeding,[70] urothelial transitional cell cancers should not be biopsied laparoscopically. However, as regards renal cell carcinoma, in McDougall and colleagues' series of 17 patients undergoing laparoscopic radical nephrectomy, subcutaneous metastases have not occurred in any patient, throughout a follow-up of 4 years.[71]

Although the previously mentioned two papers are the only reports of port site metastatic implantation in the urologic literature, nevertheless, the use of laparoscopy in oncologic procedures has raised concern regarding its potential for facilitating malignant seeding of intraperitoneal and trocar sites. As a prerequisite, tumor cells must adhere to a tissue surface before they can survive and grow. In an attempt to inhibit tumor cell adherence, a novel polycationic copolymer, PLL-g-MPEG, was tested.[72] Mock laparoscopy (using a 16-gauge angiocatheter) was used in 10 mice to intraperitoneally inject murine bladder tumor cells with or without copolymer PLL-g-MPEG. At autopsy 16 days later, significantly smaller tumor volumes were noted in the group that had received PLL-g-MPEG. The reduced tumor volumes were noted both intraperitoneally and at trocar sites. The authors concluded that addition of PLL-g-MPEG to an intraperitoneal suspension of tumor cells resulted in decreased implantation compared to controls.[72] Clinical application of this technology awaits.

LAPAROSCOPIC ABLATIVE PROCEDURES IN UROLOGIC ONCOLOGY

The laparoscopic approach to renal and ureteral cancer remains investigational as well as controversial. However, at several centers throughout the country, the laparoscopic removal of these tumors is being performed on a routine basis. Phase III

TABLE 49–5. LAPAROSCOPIC RPLND FOR CLINICAL STAGE I TESTICULAR TUMORS

Reference	No. Pts	No. Ports	OR Time (min)	Blood Loss (ml)	No. Nodes	Node Pos. R. (%)	Hosp. Stay (days)	Convalescence (weeks)	Complications	Conversion to Open surgery	Antegrade Ejaculation (%)
Castillo et al.[49]	16	3	130	190	16	—	≤2	—	0	0	100
Janetschek et al.[50]	15	6	348	—	—	20	5.5	2.3	4 (27%)	2 (13%)	93
Gerber et al.[51]	20	4–6	360	250	14.5	15	3	2	3 (15%)	6 (30%)	100
Klotz[52]	6	—	265	600	15	—	1.2	1.5	0	2 (33%)	—
Henkel et al.[53]	6	5	287	—	0	6	—	—	1 (17%)	0	100
TOTAL	63	3–6	287	347	15.2	18	3.5	1.9	8 (13%)	10 (16%)	98

TABLE 49–6. COMPLICATIONS OF LAPAROSCOPIC RPLND (*N* = 63)*

Total no. of patients = 63	
Complications	**8 (13%)**
Lymphocele	2
Pressure sore	2
Edema	1
Subcapsular myonecrosis	1
Bleeding from trocar site	1
Ureteral stenosis	1
Conversion to Open Surgery	**10 (16%)**
Vascular injury	5
Gonadal vein (2)	
Lumbar vein (1)	
Aorta (1)	
SMA (1)	
Duodenal injury	1
Large metastasis	1
Reason not stated	3
Disease Recurrence	**4 (6%)**
Chest (3)	
Abdomen (1)	

*Data from references 49 through 55.

type studies comparing laparoscopic with open surgical therapy are just beginning to be published.

Renal Cell Cancer

Radical and Total Nephrectomy

HISTORY. The classic description of the radical nephrectomy for treating renal cell cancer was described by Robson and colleagues in 1969.[73] Laparoscopic surgery has recently been recognized as an option for removal of the kidney and adrenal gland necessitated by benign disease.[73–78] The use of this technique for performing a radical or total nephrectomy has only recently been reported. The first laparoscopic nephrectomy for renal tumor was performed at Washington University in June of 1990. Since then, the laparoscopic approach for performing a radical nephrectomy has been limited and remains somewhat controversial. Nonetheless, several institutions have now reported successful completion of both total and radical laparoscopic nephrectomies for renal cell cancer.

INDICATIONS. Presently, laparoscopic radical nephrectomy is best reserved for patients with stage T1N0M0 or T2N0M0 disease. The main controversy of this procedure centers on the risk of tumor spillage and seeding. Urban and colleagues have shown that the LapSac (Cook Urological, Inc., Spencer, IN), which is constructed of a durable double layer of impermeable plastic and nondistensible nylon, remains impermeable even after complete morcellation of an entrapped kidney.[79] The largest sack size presently available is the 8 × 10-inch sack. Accordingly, the procedure is limited to those patients with a specimen size less than approximately 16 cm in diameter, in most individuals this would translate into a tumor size of under 8 cm. Patients with a tumor thrombus involving the renal vein are in general not considered candidates for the laparoscopic radical nephrectomy, although there has been a solitary case report of successful laparoscopic radical nephrectomy under such circumstances. Patients with a tumor thrombus extending into the inferior vena cava are presently not candidates for a laparoscopic approach.

TECHNIQUE. Clinical experience indicates that a transperitoneal rather than retroperitoneal approach to laparoscopic radical or total nephrectomy is the more appropriate technique. After lateral insufflation with a Veress needle, five laparoscopic ports are placed: one 12-mm port at the level of the umbilicus on the midclavicular line, one 12-mm port on the anterior axillary line just below the costal margin, one 12-mm port on the anterior axillary line 2 to 3 cm below the level of the umbilicus, and two 5-mm ports on the posterior axillary line just below the costal margin and just above the iliac crest. The procedure most commonly includes dissection of the kidney and adrenal gland, within an intact Gerota's fascia, and individual dissection of the renal vessels. For lower pole tumors, adrenalectomy can be omitted. The renal artery is secured with five 9-mm vascular clips and transected between the third and fourth clip. Then the renal vein is secured and simultaneously transected with the vascular EndoGIA device (U.S. Surgical Corporation, Norwalk, CT), which lays down six 3-cm rows of 2.5-mm staples and cuts the tissue between the third and fourth staple lines. The hilar dissection is carried to the level of the inferior vena cava on the right side or the aorta on the left side, thereby including all of the hilar lymph nodes with the specimen. The ureter is then secured with four 9-mm clips and divided.

Following complete mobilization of the kidney, an appropriately sized (5 × 8-inch or 8 × 10-inch) entrapment sack is introduced into the abdomen. A locking grasping forceps is affixed to the ureteral stump of the specimen, and the specimen is then directed into the open entrapment sack.

Removal of the specimen may be performed using intracorporeal morcellation within the entrapment sack or alternatively, the entrapped kidney can be removed intact through a small incision. The **morcellation** technique includes placement of the surgical specimen within the entrapment sack and delivery of the sack opening through one of the 12-mm port sites. It is often helpful to replace the 12-mm port with a 15- or 18-mm port to facilitate the morcellation process. The port site and neck of the sack are then securely draped and isolated from the rest of the surgical sites and morcellation is performed using the 10-mm electrical tissue morcellator (Cook Urological, Inc., Spencer, IN) to reduce the risk of tumor cell spillage. Accurate pathologic diagnosis can be performed from the morcellated tissue; however, accurate staging is not possible. A separate paracaval and para-aortic node dissection can be performed to aid in the staging of the tumor if this is the practice of the operating surgeon.

The **intact** technique of specimen removal involves placement of the surgical specimen within the organ entrapment sack. An extension of a midline or subcostal port site incision is then created to approximately 5 to 7 cm, allowing extraction of the surgical specimen within the organ entrapment sack through this site.

Controversy continues as to the most appropriate technique for specimen removal. To date no case of tumor seeding of the port site has been reported using the technique of morcellation or intact removal. However, clinical follow-up of these patients is limited; further long-term follow-up will be necessary before this concern can be adequately answered.

Results. Twenty-four laparoscopic radical nephrectomies for renal tumors have been performed at Washington University School of Medicine. The average age of the patients was 63 years (range, 29 to 90 years). The average surgical specimen weight was 417 g (range, 190 to 1100 g). The average operative time and estimated blood loss were 6.2 hours (range, 4.5 to 9 hours) and 184 ml (range, 50 to 600 ml), respectively. The average hospital stay in this patient group was 4.2 days (range, 3 to 11 days). The patients resumed oral intake within 12 hours of their operative procedure and on average required 39 mg of morphine sulfate equivalents (range, 2 to 220 mg) for postoperative analgesia. The average time for the patients to return to their normal preoperative activities was 2.6 weeks (range 1 to 6 weeks).

On review of the literature, 75 laparoscopic radical nephrectomies for renal tumor have been performed[71,80–93] (Table 49–7). Overall, the mean operative time for the laparoscopic radical nephrectomy was 5.5 hours. The patients usually resumed oral intake within 24 hours of the surgical procedure and required on average 27 mg of morphine sulfate equivalents for postoperative pain management. The mean hospital stay was 6.7 days.

A cohort group of patients undergoing an open surgical radical nephrectomy for pT1 or pT2 renal tumor were retrospectively reviewed and compared to a group of laparoscopic radical nephrectomy patients at Washington University.[71] Twelve consecutive patients with stage pT1 and pT2 disease undergoing open radical nephrectomy, operated on between January 1993 and September 1994 and with a specimen weight of less than 850 g, were compared to 12 patients undergoing laparoscopy radical nephrectomy for stage pT1 or pT2 renal cell carcinoma during a similar time period and with a similar specimen weight. The two groups were similar with regard to age and American Society of Anesthesiologists (ASA) score. The patients undergoing laparoscopic radical nephrectomy had a significantly larger average specimen weight compared to the open radical nephrectomy group (514 vs. 311 g, respectively). The laparoscopic radical nephrectomy took significantly longer to perform compared to the open radical nephrectomy (6.9 vs. 2.2 hours, respectively). There was no significant difference in the average estimated blood loss for the two groups. However, 2 of the 12 open patients required an intraoperative blood transfusion of 2 units of packed red blood cells. One of these patients received an additional 2 units of packed red blood cells during the immediate postoperative period. A third patient also received a 2-unit transfusion during the immediate postoperative period. In the laparoscopic group, there were no intraoperative transfusions: two elderly patients received a postoperative transfusion. Postoperatively, the laparoscopic radical nephrectomy patients, in compar-

TABLE 49–7. LAPAROSCOPIC RADICAL NEPHRECTOMY FOR TUMOR

Reference	No. Pts	Pathologic Stage	Mean Operative Time (hrs)	Mean Blood Loss (ml)	Time to Oral Intake (days)	Postoperative Parenteral Analgesia (mg MSO_4)	Mean Hospital Stay (days)
Coptcoat et al.[75]	5	T2	4.5	—	—	—	4.8
Kavoussi et al.[80]	8	—	7.5	295	<1	15	5.2
Ono et al.[81]	5	T1 (3) T2 (2)	6.4	430	—	—	11
Tse and Knaus[82]	4	—	5	—	1	—	4.3
Tschada et al.[83]	11 7	— —	4–6* 2.5–5†	 —	— —	— —	— —
McDougall et al.[71]	24	T1 (11) T2 (12) T3b (1)	6.2	184	<1	39	4.2
Gill et al.[83]	11	—	5.5	471	—	—	10
TOTAL	75	T1–T3b	5.5	345	<1	27	6.7

*Specimen retrieval by morcellation within the organ entrapment sack.
†Specimen retrieval by manual assistance through pararectus incision.

ison to the open radical nephrectomy patients, required less postoperative parenteral analgesia (24 vs. 40 mg morphine sulfate equivalent, respectively), a shorter time to resume oral intake (1 vs. 3 days), and a briefer hospital stay (4.5 vs. 8.4 days). None of the laparoscopic radical nephrectomy patients received Toradol postoperatively. However, 8 of the 12 patients who had an open radical nephrectomy received Toradol (range, 60 to 390 mg) for postoperative discomfort.

In the 24 *laparoscopic* radical nephrectomy patients at Washington University there were several major complications (13%). A 71-year-old man with a 1100-g surgical specimen was converted to an open procedure as a result of intraoperative bleeding. He received a 2-unit transfusion. The bleeding site turned out to be back-bleeding from the already dissected specimen. A 91-year-old woman developed cardiac arrhythmias and an ileus during her postoperative recovery; she responded to medical management and nasogastric tube suction, respectively. She was also given 1 unit of blood postoperatively for dilutional anemia. One 85-year-old patient developed mild congestive heart failure; this occurred before the oliguria associated with a prolonged pneumoperitoneum was appreciated. This woman had received 4800 ml of intraoperative intravenous fluids in an attempt to stimulate urine output. Postoperatively, the hematocrit was diminished to 22.8% and she received 1 unit of blood while undergoing a diuresis.

Minor complications occurred in 3 of 24 laparoscopic patients (13%): ileus (1) and transient nerve paresthesias (2) related to the prolonged lateral decubitus position. All complications resolved with supportive care. Both nerve paresthesias occurred prior to our obtaining a specially padded operating table (Orthopedic Systems Inc., Hayward, CA).

There were two delayed laparoscopic complications (8%) both consisting of abdominal wall hernias at the flank incision site used for intact specimen removal in the entrapment sack. These two patients had body mass indices (weight in kilograms divided by height in meters, squared) of 36 and 32, respectively, categorizing them as morbidly obese and obese, respectively. In both cases the incision for specimen removal was along the lower flank region between the two lower trocar sites. We have since changed our site for intact retrieval to a subcostal or midline incision; to date, no other patients have developed this complication.

In the *open* radical nephrectomy patient group there was one major complication (8%) among the 12 patients. A 61-year-old woman with preoperatively recognized renal insufficiency developed postoperative renal failure, necessitating chronic hemodialysis following radical nephrectomy for a stage T1 renal cell carcinoma. Two minor complications (17%) occurred in the open radical nephrectomy patients, including a severe wound infection necessitating intensive care management for 6 days postoperatively and a 43-year-old man who developed postoperative bibasilar atelectasis and fever, which resolved with conservative management. In addition, two patients (17%) required chest tubes as a result of a postoperative pneumothorax and an intraoperative pleurotomy, respectively. Delayed complications occurred in several patients: one patient (8%) developed a wound hernia and two patients (12%) continued to complain of wound paresthesias or wound discomfort.

Gill and colleagues performed a multicenter review of 185 patients undergoing laparoscopic nephrectomy between June 1990 and July 1993.[84] Thirty-two patients underwent a radical or modified radical nephrectomy without adrenalectomy. Overall, there were 15 complications in this group, representing a complication rate of 47%. The complications included 1 access-related complication (hernia at a trocar site), 3 intraoperative complications, and 11 postoperative complications. The intraoperative complications included bleeding from the renal vein secondary to misfiring of the Endo-GIA stapler, laceration of an aberrant branch of the inferior vena cava during dissection of the renal hilum, and ligation of the superior mesenteric artery mistaken for the renal artery. All of these complications were managed by laparotomy (two emergently and one electively). The superior mesenteric artery ligation was managed by polytetrafluoroethylene (Gore-Tex) graft repair. The postoperative complications included ileus (one patient), bleeding duodenal ulcer (one), enterocutaneous fistula (one), congestive heart failure (two), atrial fibrillation (one), myocardial infarction (one), urinary retention (one), pneumonitis (two), and nonoliguric acute tubular necrosis (one). Of the 32 laparoscopic radical nephrectomies 5 (16%) were converted to an open operation. In addition to the three vascular injuries requiring laparotomy repair, two patients underwent elective open surgical intervention for technical inability to laparoscopically dissect the renal pedicle or the kidney.

The complication rate of laparoscopic radical nephrectomy is higher than the 19% complication rate noted for open transperitoneal radical nephrectomy.[85] A large part of this is attributable to the learning curve for laparoscopic radical nephrectomy; indeed, the largest number of complications occur during a given surgeon's initial 10 cases. Indeed, in our series, among the last 12 laparoscopic radical nephrectomy patients, there have been no major complications and the minor plus delayed complication rate has fallen to 16%.

A major drawback to laparoscopic surgery has been the problem of increased costs incurred. At Washington University the charges associated with 12 open and 12 laparoscopic contemporary radical nephrectomies for pT1 and pT2 tumors were evaluated with respect to the operating room charges and the overall charges to the patient (Table 49–8). The mean operating room charge for the open rad-

TABLE 49–8. COMPARISON OF CHARGES FOR OPEN AND LAPAROSCOPIC RADICAL NEPHRECTOMY FOR T1 AND T2 RENAL CANCER AT WASHINGTON UNIVERSITY MEDICAL SCHOOL

	Open	Laparoscopic
Time period	1993–1994	1990–1995
Number of patients	12	12
Operating time (hr)	2.3	6.6
Hospital stay (days)	8.1	4.2
Operating room charges	$3309	$10,090
OR charges/hour	$1390	$1597
TOTAL CHARGES	$16,620	$18,470

ical nephrectomy patients was $3309, with a mean hourly operating room charge of $1390. In comparison, the mean operating room charge for the laparoscopic radical nephrectomy patients was significantly higher at $10,090, although the mean hourly operating room charge was only slightly higher at $1597. The longer operative time for the laparoscopic radical nephrectomy resulted in significantly higher operating room charges. The mean *overall* charge for the open radical nephrectomy patients was $16,620 compared to a mean overall charge of $18,470 for the laparoscopic radical nephrectomy patients.

The significantly higher operating room charges for the laparoscopic radical nephrectomy compared to the open radical nephrectomy reflect the longer operative time required for the laparoscopic procedure. The operating room charges represent the most expensive component of the patient's hospitalization. Therefore, the reduction in hospital stay does not begin to compensate for the longer operative time of the laparoscopic procedure compared to the open radical nephrectomy.

Patients with an uncomplicated open radical nephrectomy incur far less expense than patients undergoing an uncomplicated laparoscopic radical nephrectomy. Although the overall difference between the two groups is only about $2000, if the uncomplicated patients in each group are compared, then the cost differential rises to nearly $4000.

CONCLUSIONS. Laparoscopic radical nephrectomy can duplicate the immediate effectiveness of open surgical management of low-stage renal cell carcinoma while providing the patient with less postoperative discomfort, a shorter hospital stay, and a more rapid return to regular activities. The controversy regarding the issue of long-term effectiveness with regard to tumor seeding or the development of local or distant recurrence remains to be resolved by further long-term follow-up in clinical studies. However, to date, with this technique there have been no reports of malignant seeding of any port site or of local recurrence.[71,80,81] To minimize the risk of tumor spillage and seeding and to allow for accurate grading and staging of the tumor, intact organ retrieval may be performed. The risk of a wound hernia may be reduced by performing the intact specimen removal through an extension of a midline umbilical port or by using a subcostal extension of a port site. The major limitations of the laparoscopic radical nephrectomy presently are the long operative time and the highly skilled surgical team necessary to complete the procedure. It would appear that, as surgeons become more facile in laparoscopy and as laparoscopic instrumentation becomes more automated and ergonomic, the complication rates will decrease and the operative time will be reduced. These changes must occur in order for laparoscopic radical nephrectomy to become a widespread accepted technique.

Partial Nephrectomy

HISTORY. Partial nephrectomy or nephron-sparing surgery has become a successful form of treatment for patients with localized renal cell carcinoma when there is a need to preserve functioning renal parenchyma.[86] The technical success rate with nephron-sparing surgery in several large studies has been reported and represents a 5-year cancer-specific survival rate of 87 to 90% in patients with sporadic renal cell carcinoma. The major disadvantage of nephron-sparing surgery for renal cell carcinoma is the risk of postoperative local tumor recurrence in the operated kidney, which has been observed in 4 to 6% of patients.[86]

Recent advances in radiologic procedures to image the kidney have resulted in a marked increase in the discovery of asymptomatic low-stage, small renal cell carcinomas. The low stage and size of these tumors combined with advances in surgical techniques have renewed interest in the possibility of diverging from radical nephrectomy in favor of nephron-sparing surgery. However, Whang and colleagues recently reported a prospective study performed to determine the *histologic* incidence of multifocal renal cell carcinoma in patients who would be considered candidates for partial nephrectomy.[87] In their patients, who had a primary tumor size of 2 cm or less, multifocal disease was found in 2 of 44 patients (5%), and in those patients with a primary tumor size between 2 and 5 cm, 8 of 44 patients (18%) were found to have multifocality. It would therefore appear that partial nephrectomy in patients with unilateral renal cell carcinoma should be approached with caution.

However, the clinical impact of Whang's study remains undetermined. In this regard, it is of interest that Licht and colleagues, using radiologic imaging studies, found the local recurrence rate to be 4% at a mean of 50.3 months among 216 patients undergoing nephron-sparing surgery for renal cell carcinoma; overall, 40% of these tumors were 4 cm or larger. Of interest, among patients with smaller (i.e., mean 3.6 cm) "incidental" carcinomas, only one had a local recurrence (1.1%).[88] The latter finding is identical to the incidence of renal cell cancer developing in the contralateral kidney.[89]

Laparoscopic partial nephrectomy was first done in 1992 by Winfield and associates.[90] Since that time, all reports of laparoscopic partial nephrectomy have been limited to only a few patients among whom the disease process has always been benign. To date, there have been no published reports of laparoscopic partial nephrectomy for renal tumor.

INDICATIONS. Indications for this approach include patients in whom radical nephrectomy would render the patient anephric with subsequent immediate need for dialysis (e.g., bilateral renal cell carcinoma or renal cell carcinoma involving a solitary functioning kidney). In addition, patients with unilateral renal cell carcinoma who have conditions that might threaten the future function of the opposite kidney, such as calculus disease, chronic pyelonephritis, renal artery stenosis, ureteral reflux, or systemic diseases such as diabetes and nephrosclerosis, may be candidates for nephron-sparing surgery.

TECHNIQUE. The main limiting factor for performing a laparoscopic partial nephrectomy for a renal tumor is the ability to maintain hemostasis and adequately resect the lesion. Investigative studies are presently being performed to evaluate various techniques and energy modalities for establishing adequate hemostasis while incising the kidney.

Port placement and the approach to the kidney are similar to that for the radical nephrectomy. Exposure of the surface of the kidney is important in order to identify the landmarks for the transection of the kidney. It is this requirement that may jeopardize the ability to perform the "radical" partial nephrectomy. Gerota's fascia is incised and peeled back over the anterior and posterior surfaces to expose the polar region of the kidney planned for partial nephrectomy.

Intraoperative laparoscopic ultrasound examination of the kidney is useful to identify the intraparenchymal lesion and determine the planned line of incision of the kidney in order to completely excise the tumor plus an adequate margin of normal tissue. The line of incision is scored circumferentially on the renal capsule using electrocautery.

Various cutting modalities have been utilized for performing partial nephrectomy. These include a combination of the cutting current of an electrosurgical blade followed closely by a 10-mm laparoscopic argon beam coagulation probe. Alternatively, the harmonic scalpel, which uses high-frequency ultrasound vibration of the blade to create tissue cutting and simultaneous coagulation, may be used. The cutting procedure is performed with the harmonic blade until the specimen has been completely excised. The raw parenchymal surface is then extensively fulgurated with the argon beam coagulator. The use of an argon beam coagulator is, in the authors' opinion, essential to the successful completion of laparoscopic partial nephrectomy in a nonduplicated system.

A preplaced ureteral catheter can be used to inject methylene blue to identify the opening(s) into the collecting system. These are then closed, using an intracorporeal suturing technique, with 2-0 or 3-0 chromic or Vicryl suture. An indwelling ureteral stent is usually left in place.

The specimen is placed within an organ entrapment sack and removed intact. Frozen section histologic analysis of the tumor margin is performed in order to determine if the tumor has been completely excised along with a "surrounding" cuff of normal tissue. The remainder of the operative procedure and postoperative care are similar to that for a radical nephrectomy, except that, prior to removal of the Foley catheter, a cystogram is performed to rule out reflux or extravasation.

RESULTS. Recent data indicate that radical nephrectomy and nephron-sparing surgery provide equal efficacy in terms of curative treatment in patients with a single, small (<4 cm), and clearly localized renal cell carcinoma. The long-term renal functional advantage of nephron-sparing surgery with a normal opposite kidney requires further study. The results of nephron-sparing surgery are less satisfactory in patients with larger (>4 cm) or multifocal renal cell carcinoma, and radical nephrectomy remains the treatment of choice in these clinical instances.[88]

There has been no report in the literature of a successful laparoscopic partial nephrectomy for a renal tumor. Winfield and colleagues reported successful laparoscopic partial nephrectomy for benign disease in four of six patients. In these four individuals, the average operative time was 6.1 hours, with an average hospital stay of 8.3 days. Convalescence occurred over 2.3 weeks. Of note, in one of the two failed patients, the indication was a renal mass; however, the mass was not wholly contained in the laparoscopic specimen and an open procedure ensued.[90]

CONCLUSIONS. As technological improvements are developed to allow excision of tissue and simultaneous hemostasis, the application of laparoscopy to partial nephrectomy may be extended to those patients who may be candidates for nephron-sparing surgery. However, the same concerns regarding tumor spillage and tumor seeding that have been addressed with the laparoscopic radical nephrectomy for renal cell carcinoma are even greater with laparoscopic partial nephrectomy because of the higher risk of tumor exposure or transgression. For benign disease, laparoscopic partial nephrectomy remains a difficult and tedious procedure that has only been performed at a handful of centers. For malignant disease, laparoscopic partial nephrectomy remains only a dim, as yet untested concept.

Enucleation/Wedge Resection

HISTORY. Studies comparing enucleation with partial nephrectomy for renal cell carcinoma have shown no statistically significant difference in the disease-free survival rates or local recurrence rates.[91] However, pseudocapsular invasion of renal cell carcinoma may not allow complete tumor excision by enucleation, especially if the tumor is larger than 3 cm. Accordingly, a wedge excision of the tumor that includes a rim of uninvolved renal parenchyma is, in general, preferred over simple tumor enucleation.[92]

Small (<2 cm) peripherally located lesions of the kidney suspicious for renal cell carcinoma have been managed in a handful of cases by laparoscopic wedge resection. This is particularly true in the patient with renal compromise or a solitary functioning kidney.

Indications. The extensive use of ultrasound and CT scanning has increased the occurrence of incidentally detected renal cell carcinoma. Ritchie and deKernion reviewed over 3000 malignant renal tumors found over a 13-year period and estimated that 15% of these masses were discovered incidentally.[93] These asymptomatic tumors tend to be smaller and of lower stage than symptomatic tumors. Surgical exploration is often necessary just to complete an accurate diagnosis because fine-needle aspiration of these small lesions can result in a significant number of false-negative results. Several studies have shown significantly improved survival rates for patients undergoing surgical excision of incidentally detected renal cell carcinoma.[94,95] The majority of the lesions are histologically malignant; albeit small, they still have the potential to metastasize. Surgical excision usually is curative.

Technique. In performing a laparoscopic wedge excision of a small renal lesion, two instruments are essential: a laparoscopic ultrasound unit and an argon beam coagulator with laparoscopic probes. The former is necessary to clearly identify the lesion, and the latter provides excellent hemostasis of the renal parenchyma.

Depending on the location of the lesion, the technique for laparoscopic wedge resection is performed using a retroperitoneal (posterior lesion) or transperitoneal (anterior tumor) approach.[96] For retroperitoneoscopy, balloon dilation of the retroperitoneal space is performed via a 12-mm port in the inferior lumbar triangle. Next, three additional trocars are placed: a 12-mm port at the lateral edge of the sacrospinalis muscle midway between the costal margin and iliac crest, a 12-mm port along the anterior axillary line just above the iliac crest, and a 5-mm port along the anterior axillary line just below the costal margin. For a transperitoneal approach, the port placement is similar to that used for a transperitoneal laparoscopic nephrectomy.

In either approach, Gerota's fascia is incised overlying the area of the kidney to be addressed and the perinephric fat is carefully removed to completely expose the surface of the kidney. The lesion may be well visualized if it is exophytic or on the surface of the kidney. However, intraoperative ultrasound examination of the kidney is very helpful in planning the approach. The argon beam coagulator or electrosurgical scissors is used to fulgurate and mark the renal capsule along the proposed line of excision, thereby broadly circumscribing the lesion and leaving a broad cuff of surrounding normal parenchyma. The electrosurgical scissors or, alternatively, a harmonic scalpel is used to cut the renal parenchyma, and the argon beam coagulator is used to further fulgurate the cut parenchymal surface.

The excised specimen may be retrieved using 10-mm grasping forceps or a small organ entrapment sack through a 12-mm port. The specimen must be removed intact; intraoperative frozen section analysis of the specimen margins is performed in order to assure complete excision of the lesion along with an appropriate margin of normal tissue. Provided there is no evidence of tumor in the resected margin, the base of the excision site is fulgurated with the argon beam coagulator. Additional hemostasis can be obtained by placing a plug of Avitene on the surgical site. Finally, the cavity is filled with a small piece of perirenal fat; this can be secured to the renal capsule with one or two intracorporeal sutures.

Results. There has been only one case report in the literature of laparoscopic wedge resection of a renal tumor.[96] A 69-year-old man was incidentally found to have a 1-cm mass along the posterior midportion of the right kidney that enhanced on gadolinium magnetic resonance imaging. His metastatic evaluation was negative, and he underwent a laparoscopic exploration of the right kidney and wedge resection of the lesion using a retroperitoneal approach. The operative time was 2 hours and the patient had an estimated blood loss of 75 ml. The patient was discharged from the hospital on the third postoperative morning. During his hospitalization he required no postoperative analgesics, and he returned to all of his regular activities within 1 week postoperatively. The final pathologic study revealed a low-grade granular renal cell carcinoma (i.e., oncocytoma) composed of tubules and small cystic spaces. The section of the base of the tumor, which had been sent as a separate specimen and was negative on frozen section, revealed a minute area of tumor involvement on the permanent slides. In 12 months of follow-up, there has been no recurrence.

Conclusion. Clearly, the controversy continues about the appropriateness of nephron-sparing surgery versus radical nephrectomy in the management of incidentally detected solid renal masses. With regard to wedge excision in particular, it is clear that this is only indicated for small renal tumors in which the entire tumor and a cuff of normal surrounding renal parenchyma can be excised. If this is not the case, then a formal partial nephrectomy or radical nephrectomy is indicated. Tumor "enucleation" is currently not a recommended procedure.

With regard to laparoscopic surgery, its use for wedge excision remains scant. Experience with this approach is minimal and its future remains uncertain.

Upper Tract Transitional Cell Cancer

The laparoscopic approach to upper tract transitional cell carcinoma has only recently been described. To date, all of the reports on this technique have consisted of patient series under 20 subjects. Only one open surgery comparative study has been published. Clearly, the use of laparoscopy in these patients is still in a state of evolution and, at present, almost all laparoscopic experience resides on the steep part of the learning curve.

Nephroureterectomy/Ureterectomy

HISTORY. Transitional cell carcinoma of the renal pelvis represents only 7% of all renal tumors and 5% of all urothelial tumors.[97] Approximately 30% of these patients presenting with upper tract urothelial tumors will have, at the time of presentation, extension beyond the renal pelvis or parenchyma and invasion of the peripelvic and perirenal fat, lymph nodes, hilar vessels, and adjacent or distant tissues. These patients have a poor cancer-free 5-year survival rate of less than 5 to 10%.[98] However, in the 70% of patients who present with the urothelial tumor localized to the kidney or urothelium, the 5-year survival rate following total nephroureterectomy exceeds 75%. A complete ureterectomy is an essential part of the procedure because of the 30 to 60% of recurrent tumor in any remaining portion of the ipsilateral ureter.[99] The gold standard of treatment for patients with upper ureteral or renal pelvis transitional cell carcinoma is total nephroureterectomy, with excision of the ipsilateral periureteral cuff of bladder mucosa.

The development of the technique for laparoscopic nephrectomy and the availability of the EndoGIA tissue stapler (U.S. Surgical Corporation, Norwalk, CT) allowed the first clinical laparoscopic nephroureterectomy to be performed at Washington University School of Medicine on May 30, 1991.[100] Since that time, laparoscopic nephroureterectomy has been successfully completed at many institutions throughout the world.

INDICATIONS. Notwithstanding recent developments in the endosurgical therapy of upper tract transitional cell cancer, the standard radical nephroureterectomy remains the treatment of choice in the majority of patients with transitional cell carcinoma of the pelvis and upper ureter.[101,102] The same extirpative nephroureterectomy procedure performed at open surgery can be duplicated laparoscopically. Likewise, in the rare patient who undergoes a simple nephrectomy for unsuspected upper tract transitional cell cancer, a subsequent complete ureterectomy must be accomplished in order to eliminate the high risk of tumor recurrence in the retained ureteral stump.

TECHNIQUE. The technique of laparoscopic nephroureterectomy and ureterectomy involves a preprocedural, transurethral unroofing of the affected distal ureter and placement of an external ureteral catheter (7-French occlusion balloon). Alternatively, the ureteral orifice and tunnel can be resected transurethrally. The advantage of ureteral resection is that the ureter can be rapidly "plucked" instead of tediously dissected distally; however, the chance of retroperitoneal or peritoneal seeding from the tumor cell–laden urine is a realistic concern.

In preparation for the laparoscopic portion of the procedure, the patient is placed in a lateral decubitus position. Lateral insufflation is performed and six trocars are placed: 12-mm trocar in the midclavicular line just off of the iliac crest, a 12-mm port just below the costal margin on the anterior axillary line, a 5-mm port 2 to 3 cm below the level of the umbilicus on the anterior axillary line, a 5-mm port just above the iliac crest on the posterior axillary line, a 12-mm port subcostal along the posterior axillary line, and a 12-mm port 2 cm above the symphysis pubis in the midline.

The renal part of the procedure is identical to that for a laparoscopic radical or total nephrectomy; an adrenalectomy is only considered in the case of tumor involvement of the upper calyces of the collecting system. The entire kidney is completely freed from the renal hilum and all of its retroperitoneal attachments except the ureter.

The ureter is identified as it crosses the iliac vessels and is dissected down into the pelvis. The vas deferens (male) or round ligament (female), superior vesical artery, and medial umbilical ligament often require transection and securing with 9-mm vascular clips to adequately expose the distal ureter and complete the caudal dissection down to the ureterovesical junction. The ureter is completely freed until the initial transurethrally made incision through the detrusor muscle fibers at the ureterovesical junction is identified. Grasping forceps through the lower anterior axillary line port are used to retract the ureter superiorly and laterally to expose the bladder at the ureterovesical junction. Once there has been satisfactory circumferential dissection of the ureterovesical junction, the 12-mm laparoscopic EndoGIA tissue stapler is inserted through the midline 12-mm port. The 7-French occlusion balloon catheter is deflated and removed along with the guidewire. The EndoGIA stapler is fired across the cuff of bladder; six 3-cm rows of titanium staples are laid down and the bladder is simultaneously incised by the EndoGIA device between the third and fourth rows of staples. This should completely free the specimen. Alternatively, in the case when the ureteral tunnel is initially "resected," at this point in the procedure upward traction on the middle ureter is usually sufficient to deliver the distal ureter and ureteral stump, without the aforedescribed dissection of the vas, etc.

Accurate staging and grading of patients with upper tract transitional cell carcinoma is thought to be crucial to both their prognosis and planned adjuvant therapy postoperatively. Patients with evidence of extension of tumor into the renal parenchyma or through the renal pelvis would be considered for adjuvant chemotherapy or radiation therapy. Accordingly, in the patient with a renal pelvis or ureteropelvic junction tumor, preparation is made for *intact* removal of the specimen. In addition, intact removal should, in theory, further decrease the chances of port site seeding from the tumor. However, in the patient with a middle or proximal ureteral tumor, the ureter can be removed intact and the kidney can then be morcellated in the sack, thereby precluding enlargement of any of the port sites.

A 5 × 8-inch or 8 × 10-inch organ entrapment sack is inserted through the 12-mm subcostal anterior axillary port and opened in the abdomen. The surgical specimen is secured at the ureteropelvic junction and manipulated into the entrapment sack. The distal end of the ureter is clipped to the edge of the entrapment sack. The table is turned to place the patient supine; the neck of the sack is delivered onto the abdominal wall at the 12-mm suprapubic site. If the patient has a middle or proximal ureteral tumor, then the clip is released from the bladder cuff and edge of the sack and the entire length of ureter is pulled upward out of the sack. Two clips are applied at the most proximal extent of the ureter and the ureteral specimen is cut. On a separate table, the ureter is cut longitudinally to see if the entire area of the tumor is contained in the specimen. If this is the case, then the area around the neck of the sack is draped off and the remaining entrapped kidney is morcellated with a high-speed tissue morcellator.

If the tumor is in the renal pelvis, then the suprapubic midline port through which the neck of the sack was delivered is extended inferiorly for 2 to 3 inches. The sack with its entrapped specimen is then slowly pulled out of the incision; Army/Navy retractors are helpful during this maneuver. After delivery of the specimen, the incision site and all port sites larger than 10 mm are closed with fascial sutures, subcuticular sutures, and adhesive skin strips. The 5-mm ports are closed just with adhesive strips.

Results. Since May 1991, 12 patients (8 male and 4 female) have undergone laparoscopic nephroureterectomy for transitional cell carcinoma of the upper tract at Washington University Medical School.[103] The average patient age has been 69 years (range, 58 to 83 years). The average ASA rating at the time of the surgical procedure was 3, with 55% of the patients having an ASA rating of 3 or 4. The average operative time was 8.2 hours (range, 6.7 to 10.6 hours). This *total* operative time included the time for cystoscopy and transurethral unroofing of the ureter, which averaged approximately 1 hour. The average specimen weight was 417 g (range, 229 to 730 g). The final pathologic diagnosis in 10 patients was transitional cell carcinoma: pTa in 7 patients, pT2 in 2 patients, and pT3b in 1 patient. In the remaining two patients only proximal ureteral atypia was found because these patients had undergone an endourologic resection of their tumor prior to the laparoscopic nephroureterectomy. The average time for patients undergoing laparoscopic nephroureterectomy to resume oral intake was 16 hours after their surgery (range, 6 to 72 hours). On average, patients required 18 mg of morphine sulfate equivalents for postoperative analgesia (range, 0 to 48 mg). Cystograms performed 2 to 10 days following the procedure have revealed no evidence of extravasation. The average hospital stay was 4.8 days (range, 4 to 8 days). In these patients, return to regular activities averaged 3 weeks (range, 1 to 4 weeks).

There were no intraoperative complications. The estimated blood loss was between 100 and 400 ml in the laparoscopic nephroureterectomy patients. There was one major postoperative complication: an ASA 4 patient underwent open surgical exploration 7 hours following his laparoscopic procedure for postoperative bleeding. The site of bleeding was from the inferior edge of the adrenal gland. Postoperatively, he developed adult respiratory distress syndrome (ARDS). Despite recovering from his ARDS, his cardiac status deteriorated and he developed a fatal dysrhythmia. He expired on postoperative day 66. One patient has developed a delayed complication; at 2.5 months after her procedure she noted the development of an incisional hernia. The intact organ specimen removal was performed through a horizontal extension of the port site incisions between the lower ports along the anterior axillary line and the posterior axillary line. Because of this case, we have changed our protocol: intact removal of the specimen is now done through a lower midline incision.

There was one technical complication in our first patient: a 1-cm ureteral stump remained postoperatively. In all the subsequent patients no ureteral stump was radiographically or cystoscopically detectable.

All patients have undergone surveillance cystoscopy, intravenous pyelography, and urine cytology on a regular basis. Eight patients have undergone an average follow-up of 25 months (range, 14 to 41 months). During this time no intravesical staples or stones have been noted within the bladder. Of note, in our initial patient, a small staple can be seen at the end of the 1-cm ureteral stump; to date, despite more than 4 years of follow-up, no stone has formed on this staple.

One patient was found on the final pathologic specimen to have microscopic spread of the transitional cell carcinoma into the perirenal fat. This patient underwent adjuvant postoperative chemotherapy; CT 9 months postoperatively revealed a recurrent tumor mass in the retroperitoneum, and the patient died 12 months postoperatively of metastatic disease. Three patients had recurrent transitional cell carcinoma in the bladder and were treated with transurethral resection. The pathology confirmed grade I–II, noninvasive transitional cell carcinoma in all of these patients. One other patient had bladder biopsies on two occasions that showed atypia. This patient and one of the patients who had recurrent bladder transitional cell carcinoma have undergone a 6-week course of intravesical bacille Calmette-Guérin therapy. Both of these patients are presently without evidence of disease. All patients have had normal intravenous pyelograms or CT scans during their surveillance.

Stephenson and colleagues have recently reported their experience with 13 patients undergoing laparoscopic nephroureterectomy for transitional cell carcinoma.[104] The mean age of the patients was 62.2 years. The mean operative time was only 2.8 hours, although this did not include the time to "resect" the ipsilateral ureteral tunnel. The mean hospital stay was 5.6 days and the patients received a mean of 0.3 units of blood transfused. There were two major complications (15%): one 77-year-old man died on postoperative day 2 of a myocardial infarction and multiorgan failure, and one patient required conversion to an open procedure following vascular trauma. There was one minor complication, a paralytic ileus for 5 days postoperatively that resolved with conservative management. The only significant difference in comparing the Washington University experience with the report by Stephenson and colleagues is the operative times (Table 49–9). It has been our experience that this is a long operative procedure requiring a highly skilled surgical team. However, both reports indicate that laparoscopic nephroureterectomy, compared to the open surgical approach, is a safe and effective procedure and provides the patient with minimal postoperative discomfort and a rapid resumption of normal activities.[103,104]

In comparing laparoscopic nephroureterectomy patients with patients undergoing an open surgical nephroureterectomy, the laparoscopic procedure was on average 2.5 times longer than the open nephroureterectomy at Washington University.[103] Surgeon experience does not appear to improve the operative time, although our 12 cases may yet represent our initial learning curve, and other investigators have reported shorter operative times.[103] However, the laparoscopic patients resume their oral intake more quickly and require less postoperative parenteral analgesia. In addition, hospital stay for the laparoscopic nephroureterectomy patients was significantly shorter. Also the laparoscopic nephroureterectomy patients convalesce more quickly; they return to work or regular activity in less than half the time (2.8 vs. 6 weeks) and are completely recovered five times more quickly (6 weeks vs. 7.4 months) than the open surgical group.[105]

Laparoscopic ureterectomy has been performed on two patients at Washington University Medical School for incidentally identified upper tract transitional cell carcinoma. In one patient a radical nephrectomy had been performed for a calcified renal mass suspicious for renal cell carcinoma. However, the final histologic diagnosis was transitional cell carcinoma. In the second patient a laparoscopic nephrectomy was performed for a nonfunctioning kidney with ureteropelvic junction obstruction and hematuria; a transitional cell cancer was found in the specimen. Preoperative evaluations had revealed no abnormality on urine cytologies or retrograde pyelography. Both patients subsequently underwent laparoscopic ureterectomy with a cuff of bladder for definitive therapy of their previously unsuspected upper tract transitional cell carcinoma.

In both patients the estimated blood loss during the procedure was less than 100 ml. The operative times were 7.3 and 3.5 hours, respectively. This time included the transurethral incision of the intramural ureter. The patients required 68 and 8 mg of morphine equivalent, respectively. They resumed their normal oral intake within 24 hours of the surgical procedure and had hospital stays of 7 days and 1 day, respectively. The final pathologic evaluation revealed a grade 2 out of 4 transitional cell carcinoma in the first patient's ureteral specimen, and in the other patient no pathologic abnormality was noted. One patient had bladder tumors at the

TABLE 49–9. LAPAROSCOPIC NEPHROURETERECTOMY FOR TRANSITIONAL CELL CARCINOMA

	No. Pts	Mean Operative Time (hr)	Time to Oral Intake	Postoperative Parenteral Analgesia (mg MSO_4)	Mean Hospital Stay (days)	Time to Regular Activity (weeks)
McDougall et al.[103]	12	8.2*	0.7	18	4.8	3
Stephenson et al.[104]	13	2.7	—	—	5.6	—
TOTAL	25	5.5	—	—	5.2	—

*Includes cystoscopic ureteral tunnel resection.

6-month surveillance cystoscopy. This patient underwent transurethral resection of these low-grade, superficial lesions and continues surveillance cystoscopy. The other patient has been free of recurrent disease.

Concerns have arisen regarding the security of the stapled bladder closure and the possibility that the staples may serve as a site for future stone formation. In this regard, Figenshau and colleagues established that the laparoscopic EndoGIA tissue stapler (U.S. Surgical Corp., Norwalk, CT) reliably secures the bladder and expeditiously incises the distal end of the surgical specimen.[105] This minimizes the risk of any possibility of tumor spillage because the bladder is never formally opened since the bladder cuff is immediately secured with staples as it is cut. Postoperative follow-up cystograms have confirmed that a watertight closure of the bladder is achieved using this technique. In neither animal studies nor our clinical experience have any staple-related problems occurred. Titanium is well tolerated in the urinary tract because of its corrosive-resistant nature, low toxicity, and excellent tissue and fluid biocompatibility.[106]

Because of the risk of tumor recurrence in the bladder, patients with a history of upper tract transitional cell carcinoma require endoscopic surveillance following their nephroureterectomy. We have had three patients (25%) with recurrent bladder tumor, which was satisfactorily managed with transurethral resection. The reported incidence of bladder tumors following nephroureterectomy ranges from 28 to 75% depending on the location of the primary lesion. Finally, to date, there has been no instance of port site or intraperitoneal seeding or local recurrence with laparoscopic nephroureterectomy.

Conclusions. Laparoscopic nephroureterectomy or ureterectomy is a feasible treatment option for patients with upper tract transitional cell carcinoma or a retained ureteral stump, respectively. The immediate efficacy of this procedure appears to be equal to that of an open nephroureterectomy. Two major drawbacks to the approach persist: the lengthy operative time and the need for significant laparoscopic experience on the part of the surgeon. However, even in this early phase of laparoscopic nephroureterectomy, the benefits to the patient are readily apparent: less postoperative discomfort, a rapid return to normal activities, and a brief convalescence. Further follow-up is needed to determine if the long-term efficacy of the laparoscopic approach is equivalent to that of open nephroureterectomy. Also, it is imperative that the currently excessive operating room time for these cases be reduced to a point that the laparoscopic procedure becomes competitive with the open approach. The use of the ureteral "pluck," as evidenced by Stephenson et al.'s data,[104] and a manual assist, as espoused by Coptcoat and coworkers,[75] are steps that have already had a significant impact in this regard.

Bladder Cancer

Lower Tract Transitional Cell Cancer

The application of laparoscopy to bladder cancer has been scant. Use of laparoscopy for cystectomy and diversion, partial cystectomy, bladder diverticulectomy, and delivery of laser energy to the bladder has been reported. However, none of these applications has been subjected to comparison with its open counterpart, nor have any of these techniques received widespread acceptance.

Cystectomy and Diversion

History. The first laparoscopic cystectomy was performed for benign disease by Parra and coworkers. This case was done in a female patient who already had a urinary diversion and was suffering from pyocystis[107]; a 22-g bladder was removed during a 130-minute procedure. The hospital stay was 5 days. These authors later performed a cystectomy in a male patient; this individual also had a urinary diversion and pyocystis. The operative time was 160 minutes and the hospital stay was only 3 days.[108]

Likewise, there have been very few reports of performing an ileal conduit laparoscopically. The initial publication on this technique was by Kozminiski and Partamian; they were successful in doing this procedure in two patients.[109]

Only three groups have put the two procedures together in order to perform a radical cystectomy and diversion for bladder cancer: Sanchez de Badajoz and colleagues ($N = 1$), Townell and associates ($N = 1$), and Puppo and colleagues ($N = 5$).[110–112] In Townell's and Puppo's reports, the procedure was actually laparoscopically assisted as both groups sought to facilitate the procedure via a transvaginal or transperineal incision, and the ileal diversion or cutaneous ureterostomies were performed via a minilaparotomy.[111,112] In Puppo's series, four of the patients also had bilateral ovariectomies and hysterectomy via the laparoscopic route.[112]

Indications. The indications for the few laparoscopic cystectomies that have been done for bladder cancer have been the same as for an open procedure. Specifically, each of the patients done to date have had muscle-invasive tumor ($N = 5$), carcinoma in situ with intolerance to BCG ($N = 1$), or high-grade, superficial disease ($N = 1$).[110–112]

Technique. The technique for laparoscopic cystectomy and ileal conduit diversion is highly variable. The dissection of the bladder is done after a transperitoneal approach usually via five or six trocar sites. The bladder pedicles are taken with an EndoGIA vascular stapler, as is the urethra. None of the specimens has been entrapped in an impermeable sack. Instead, each specimen was delivered intact by pulling it through a transabdominal (4 to 5-cm), transperineal (male patient), or transvaginal incision. In the latter two situations the use of a transvaginal or transperineal incision has facilitated not only delivery of the specimen but also dissection of the bladder. To occlude this opening and preserve the pneumoperitoneum, a fluid-filled glove is helpful.

The diversion, either cutaneous ureterostomies or, more commonly, ileal conduit, can be performed in several ways; however, it would appear that the easiest method is to deliver the ureters and bowel via the stoma site or via the 4 to 5-cm transabdominal minilaparotomy incision used to deliver the bladder. This allows for cutting the loop and performing the ureteral-enteral anastomoses on top of the abdomen using standard open surgical techniques. Alternatively, a transverse ileal conduit can be created, in which case the left ureter does not have to be tunneled beneath the sigmoid mesocolon. Only Kozminski and Partamian have reported doing the bowel anastomosis intra-abdominally using the EndoGIA stapler.[109]

Results. These few procedures were all quite lengthy: 6 to 8 hours. In only one report is the hospital stay given: an average of 12.1 days.[112] In none of the reports is the convalescence period given. Similarly, in only one report is there any follow-up; at 1 year the upper tracts apparently were normal.[110] To date there have been no reports of seeding of a trocar site in these few cases, but again the number of cases is small and the follow-up remains brief (6 to 18 months, average of 10.8 months). In this regard, the initial report of seeding of a trocar site from bladder cancer at the time of PLND or laparoscopic biopsy is quite worrisome.[69,113]

Conclusions. Laparoscopic cystectomy and diversion is an example of the potential of laparoscopic surgery. However, the actual incorporation of this technique into the routine approach to surgically treatable bladder cancer has not yet occurred in any center to the best of the authors' knowledge. Also, despite the passage of sufficient time since reports of this procedure, none of the three centers that initiated this procedure has as yet come forth with a follow-up report of laparoscopic cystectomy and diversion in a series of patients. The extended operative times and high skill requirements for this procedure, combined with the seeming necessity of a minilaparotomy and inability to perform a continent diversion have limited its spread to other institutions.

Laparoscopic Partial Cystectomy and Diverticulectomy

To date, there have been no reports of laparoscopic partial cystectomy or laparoscopic diverticulectomy for bladder cancer. However, both procedures have been done in a limited number of patients with benign disease. As with cystectomy and diversion, these are all anecdotal case reports comprising a variety of techniques. To date, there are no series or comparative studies.[114–117]

Laparoscopic Monitoring/Enhancement of Transurethral Nd:YAG Therapy

Gerber and colleagues have reported use of laparoscopy to facilitate transurethral Nd:YAG therapy in five patients with T2–T3b bladder cancer.[118] The small bowel was mobilized off of the serosal surface of the bladder, thereby precluding possible bowel injury during the Nd:YAG therapy. In addition, in two patients, the laser was used via the laparoscope to sandwich the tumor between the transurethral and transabdominal administration of laser energy, allowing for the delivery of high levels of energy (38,000 to 103,000 J). Of note, there were no perioperative bowel or bladder perforations.

However, the results of this therapy were disappointing. Within 4 months, locally recurrent disease was present in all but one patient; metastatic disease occurred within 9 months in three of the five patients and in both of the patients treated with "sandwich" therapy.

Prostate Cancer

The application of laparoscopic techniques to the direct treatment of prostate cancer has been rare. In this respect, laparoscopy has been used primarily to assist in the delivery of other forms of therapy: seminal vesicle dissection prior to perineal prostatectomy, enterolysis prior to radiation therapy, or prostate monitoring during cryotherapy. However, even in this regard, experience has been limited to reports from only a handful of centers.[28,119–121]

Laparoscopically Assisted Seminal Vesicle Dissection

History. The use of laparoscopy to facilitate definitive therapy for prostate cancer has been scant. There are two reports of using laparoscopy to dissect out the seminal vesicles immediately prior to radical perineal prostatectomy.[28,119]

Indications. Laparoscopic dissection of the seminal vesicles is only indicated as an extension of a preceding laparoscopic PLND in which the frozen section of the nodal tissue is negative and the urologist is planning to then proceed at the same session with a perineal prostatectomy.[28,119] In those cases in which a PLND is not indicated, there is no indication to proceed with laparoscopy solely to dissect the seminal vesicles.

Technique. After completing the PLND and while awaiting the results of the frozen section, the initial dissection of the seminal vesicles is begun. A transperitoneal incision is made extending from the peritoneal reflection over one vas deferens to the peritoneal reflection over the opposite vas deferens. Dissection is continued caudal along the vasa until the ampulla of each vas is identified. By dissecting just lateral and posterior to the proximal vasa, the seminal vesicles are identified. Dissection is continued along each seminal vesicle; it is essential to keep the dissection directly on the surface of the seminal vesicle in order to preclude injury to the rectum, ureter, or neurovascular bundle associated with the prostate. The artery at the base of each seminal vesicle is secured with a 9-mm clip.

Next, the dissection proceeds along the undersurface of the prostate. During this maneuver, it is helpful to have the assistant place a finger in the rectum to displace the rectum posteriorly. The dissection is carried caudal to the level of the rectourethralis muscle. At the end of the procedure, the peritoneum is reapproximated using a hernia stapler.

Results. There have been two series in which laparoscopic seminal vesicle dissection has been performed. Teichman et al. reported on 10 patients, among whom the procedure was successful in 6; inability to dissect the seminal vesicles laparoscopically was due to seminal vesicle involvement in two cases. The average time allowed for the dissection was 40 minutes. No complications were reported.[28] In contrast, Kavoussi and colleagues were successful in completing a seminal vesicle dissection in 15 of 16 patients; the lone failure was due to seminal vesicle tumor invasion. Their higher success rate was associated with longer operating room times: 1 to 2.5 hours. Again, no complications were noted.[119]

In Teichman's series, the results of laparoscopic lymph node dissection plus seminal vesicle dissection and perineal radical prostatectomy in 10 patients were compared to open radical retropubic prostatectomy in 12 contemporary patients. Of interest is that the actual operating time for the two procedures was identical at 237 minutes; however, because of the need for repositioning in the laparoscopy group, the average operating room time was 330 minutes versus 288 minutes in the radical retropubic prostatectomy group. Of interest, the laparoscopic patients experienced a statistically significant reduction in blood loss (450 vs. 1250 ml), blood tansfusions, ileus (1 vs. 2 days), pain medications (44 vs. 119 mg morphine sulfate equivalents), and hospital stay (3 vs. 6 days).[28]

Conclusions. Laparoscopically assisted perineal prostatectomy is a viable procedure in the patient who requires both a PLND and in whom the surgeon desires to proceed with definitive surgery at the same session. The method is well described and the operating time is not unreasonably lengthy. Difficulty in completing the dissection is most commonly due to spread of the prostate cancer into the seminal vesicles.

Laparoscopically Assisted Radiation Therapy and Cryotherapy

Laparoscopy has been used in two other situations to facilitate therapy for prostate cancer. In a report by Jarrett and colleagues, an enterolysis was performed laparoscopically prior to administering radiotherapy to an elderly male with a prior history of right colon resection.[120] On the treatment planning radiographs, a loop of small bowel was identified that appeared to be fixed directly over the treatment area. Using a three-port approach, the bowel was freed, and a 10 × 20-cm piece of synthetic mesh was stapled to the pelvic and abdominal sidewalls as well as to the posterior peritoneum, thereby creating a sling to prevent the small bowel from falling into the area of treatment.

A second novel use of the laparoscope was reported by Sklar and colleagues.[121] In their work, immediately following a laparoscopic PLND, they proceeded with planned cryotherapy. They used the laparoscopic access to place needle thermistors so they could both measure temperatures and visually assess the progress of the cryosurgical ablation in two patients. They recorded temperatures on the anterior surface of the prostate of −28° and −36° C, well below the −20° C needed to achieve cell death in the canine prostate. Of note, despite dissecting through the endopelvic fascia and dividing the puboprostatic ligaments, direct visualization of the anterior surface of the prostate never revealed any frost formation in either patient.[121]

Laparoscopic Radical Retropubic Prostatectomy

Among the most potent demonstrations of the potential of laparoscopic surgery was that presented to the urologic community in 1992 by Schuessler and colleagues when they reported the initial successful completion of a totally laparoscopic radical retropubic prostatectomy in a 65-year-old man.[122] Using a five-port approach, a standard prostatectomy was performed complete with intracorporeal suturing of the dorsal venous complex and a four suture urethral vesical anastomosis including urothelial eversion and a racquet-handle closure of the bladder. The procedure required 8 hours of operative time and the blood loss was 750 ml. No additional reports of laparoscopic radical retropubic prostatectomy have been forthcoming.

The major problem with this approach remains the difficulty of completing the vesicourethral anastomosis.[123] Traditional intracorporeal suturing and knot-tying make this approach very tedious. Perhaps with more experience, and as intracorporeal suturing equipment improves (e.g., Endo-Stitch, U. S. Surgical Inc., Norwalk, CT), this approach may be revisited. However, for the time being, given the average operating time of 2 to 3 hours for most open radical retropubic prostatectomies and the rising popularity of the minimally invasive radical perineal prostatectomy, the future of laparoscopic prostatectomy appears dim.

Adrenal Tumors

The vast majority of adrenalectomies are for a benign lesion: pheochromocytoma, aldosteronoma, functioning adenoma, adrenal hyperplasia, and the like. Primary adrenal cancer is quite rare and is usually limited to those lesions larger than 4 to 6 cm. Secondary adrenal cancer caused by metastatic disease is not uncommon; however, it is the exceptional patient who comes to adrenalectomy as a result of a solitary adrenal metastasis. In all of these surgical situations, the standard has been open adrenalectomy via an anterior abdominal or dorsal approach. Presently, each of the aforedescribed conditions has been successfully addressed laparoscopically.

Laparoscopic Adrenalectomy

HISTORY. Laparoscopic adrenalectomy was first described in the English literature in 1992. Gagner and colleagues successfully completed a laparoscopic adrenalectomy in two patients: one with Cushing's disease (bilateral adrenalectomy performed) and the other with a 3.5-cm pheochromocytoma. Both operations required only 2 to 3.5 hours, and both patients were discharged from the hospital in 3 to 4 days.[124] Quite soon thereafter, the technique was adopted at many centers in Japan. Independent reports by Go and coworkers,[125] Higashihara and associates,[126] Matsuda and coworkers,[127] and Suzuki and colleagues[128] all corroborated the safety and feasibility of laparoscopic adrenalectomy for a wide range of adrenal lesions: cysts, angiomyolipoma, adrenal hyperplasia, aldosteronoma, adenoma, and pheochromocytoma. To date there have been two cases of primary adrenal cancer removed laparoscopically and two cases of adrenalectomy in patients with a solitary metachronous metastasis from renal cell cancer.[124,125]

INDICATIONS. The indications for laparoscopic adrenalectomy have expanded rapidly. At first, it was thought that pheochromocytoma and adrenal cancer would be contraindications; likewise, it was written that the right adrenal was more amenable to this approach.[125] However, over the last 4 years, it has become apparent that all adrenal lesions requiring removal, regardless of etiology, size, (up to 10 cm), or side, can be successfully removed laparoscopically[126–129] (R. V. Clayman, unpublished data). Presently, the only contraindication to a laparoscopic approach would be an adrenal cancer with adrenal vein and/or vena caval involvement.

TECHNIQUE. For a **transperitoneal** adrenalectomy, anywhere from four to six trocars are placed in the abdomen.[130] The patient is placed supine or in a full lateral decubitus position.[131]

On the *right* side, the right triangular and posterior coronary ligaments of the liver are incised vertically and horizontally, respectively, thereby allowing cephalad retraction of the liver and immediate access to the supra-adrenal vena cava. From the medial limb of the posterior coronary ligament incision, a vertical incision can be made caudally, thereby incising Gerota's fascia over the adrenal gland and the upper pole of the kidney. The adrenal vein is then isolated and secured with three clips (two clips remain on the caval side), following which the inferior, lateral, and finally posterior surfaces of the adrenal gland are freed from the retroperitoneum and the superior pole of the right kidney.[130]

On the *left* side, the lateral attachments between the spleen and the diaphragm are incised, following which the splenorenal and splenocolic ligaments are divided, thereby affording safe retraction cephalad of the spleen. Gerota's fascia is then incised along the upper medial border of the kidney in order to expose the upper pole of the kidney and the adrenal gland. Dissection along the upper medial border of the kidney will usually reveal the left adrenal vein running cephalad from the main renal vein. The adrenal vein is circumferentially dissected and subsequently divided between two pairs of 9-mm clips. Finally, the left adrenal gland is mobilized from the kidney laterally and then from the retroperitoneum medially and posteriorly.[130]

The free adrenal gland is removed either by extending one of the port sites to 2 to 3 cm or by placing the adrenal gland into a laparoscopic entrapment sack. Once in the sack, the adrenal gland, if small, can be removed intact by tugging on the sack, or it can be morcellated with a Kelly clamp and extracted piecemeal via the port site.

Brunt and colleagues described a totally **retroperitoneal** approach to the adrenal via a pneumoretroperitoneum.[132] This study in the pig laid the groundwork for subsequent clinical trials. In the clinical realm, the use of this approach has been most extensively reported by Morita and colleagues.[133] Usually a four-port approach is used, with the patient in a lateral decubitus position. Mandressi and coworkers have reported a similar approach, albeit with the patient lying prone in a jackknife position.[134] The major difficulty with this approach is the small working space available in the retroperitoneum and the difficulty in the obese patient of delivering instruments high enough in the retroperitoneum to safely dissect the adrenal gland. In addition, in patients with Cushing's disease this approach is particularly difficult because of the amount of periadrenal adipose tissue.[133]

RESULTS. To date, over 200 **transperitoneal** laparoscopic adrenalectomies have been reported by 13 groups worldwide. The average operating room time has been 4.2 hours, with minimal blood loss (average <200 ml). The hospital stay in the United States and Canada has averaged 3 to 4 days, with convalescence occurring within 1 to 2 weeks. The conversion rate to open surgery has been low (0.6%) and complications have been few (6%)[124–144] R. V. Clayman, unpublished data). In contrast, experience with a **retroperitoneal** approach has been scant, less than 25 reported cases. However, among these patients the hospital stay has only been 2 to 3 days with only 83 ml blood loss. Convalescence averages 1.4 weeks. Although this approach is suitable for most adrenal problems in the *thin* patient, it is ill advised in the obese individual or in the patient with Cushing's disease, adrenal cancer, or a large adrenal tumor (>100 g).[133,137,144]

Comparison studies of laparoscopic adrenalectomy with contemporary open adrenalectomy have been published independently by two groups. In each instance the operating room time for the laparoscopic procedure has been longer by 20 to 80 minutes than for an open procedure; however, the blood loss, time to oral intake, use of parenteral analgesics, hospital stay, and convalescence has been decreased over 50% in each series.[128,138] In addition, it would appear that, with increased experience and improved instrumentation (e.g., argon beam coagulator, ultrasonic aspirator), the time for laparoscopic adrenalectomy will soon approach that for an open adrenalectomy, thereby making the procedure not only effective but also efficient.[139]

Conclusion. Laparoscopic adrenalectomy for benign tumors of the adrenal gland appears to be a reasonable first-line choice of therapy in the hands of skilled laparoscopists. The operating room time is only slightly longer than for an open procedure, while the decrease in postoperative analgesic use, ileus, hospital stay, and convalescence are highly significant. The experience with adrenal cortical carcinoma and with solitary metastases to the adrenal gland is still largely anecdotal; however, even in these two areas it would appear that laparoscopic adrenalectomy has a role.

Dysgenetic Gonad: Laparoscopic Gonadectomy

Another use of laparoscopy, albeit an unusual one, is to remove the intra-abdominal gonads in patients with male pseudohermaphroditism either resulting from a lack of müllerian inhibiting factor (i.e., Swyer's syndrome) or caused by testicular feminization resulting from androgen insensitivity. Overall, 20 to 30% of these patients develop gonadal neoplasias, usually a gonadoblastoma or more rarely a dysgerminoma. In patients with the more severe condition of Swyer's syndrome (i.e., lack of normal testis development and absence of müllerian inhibiting factor), the streak gonads should be removed as early as possible because tumors may develop as early as 6 months of life. A similar approach can be used in the patient with mixed gonadal dysgenesis, in whom a unilateral streak gonad is invariably present. In contrast, in patients with testicular feminization, the gonads are not removed until after puberty to allow for the normal growth spurt and because gonadal tumors in this group are rare during the prepubertal years.

The laparoscopic procedure is usually accomplished via four trocars with the patient in the supine position. The dysgenetic gonad is easily identified near the small fallopian tube (Swyer's syndrome) or by tracing the gonadal vessels to the gonad (testicular feminization). The specimens in general are quite small and it is rather straightforward to dissect and clip the gonadal vessels. The dissected gonads can be placed in a small 2×5-inch entrapment sack and delivered via one of the 10 to 12-mm ports.

Experience with this approach has been quite good, albeit limited to only eight cases in four reports.[145–148] Among three young patients (ages 18 to 25 years), in only one case had the gonad undergone malignant change to gonadoblastoma. Patients were usually discharged the same day as the procedure. Patient size appeared to be no contraindication because in one report bilateral gonadectomy was successfully performed in a 399-pound individual.

In conclusion, although male pseudohermaphroditism and mixed gonadal dysgenesis are rare conditions, the laparoscopic approach is an effective and efficient means of removing the potentially troublesome gonad(s). The patients treated in this manner have enjoyed a brief hospital stay and rapid convalescence.

FUTURE APPLICATIONS OF LAPAROSCOPY IN UROLOGIC ONCOLOGY

General Advances

The future of laparoscopy is dependent upon two factors: surgeon experience and advances in technology. To become proficient in laparoscopy, the urologist must be doing these procedures on a routine basis. The minimum requirement would be two cases a month, and even this caseload would likely be sufficient to only maintain, rather than truly advance, one's skills. To achieve a satisfactory laparoscopic caseload, it will likely become necessary for only one urologist in a group of six to eight to do all of the laparoscopy for the group. Only in this manner will a caseload sufficient for both maintenance and progress of abilities be assured.

From a technological standpoint, the actual performance of laparoscopy has tremendous room for improvement. Presently a surgical assistant rather than the surgeon controls the camera; therefore, a change in the line of sight of the surgeon occurs every 5.5 seconds.[149] Likewise, the absence of multiuse instruments forces frequent instrument changes; this alone accounts for 10% of the operative time and also contributes to the ongoing disturbance in the surgeon's line of sight.[149]

These problems are currently being addressed on several fronts. First, the development and eventual perfection of robotics in the operating room will allow the surgeon to operate with both hands while controlling the camera by voice or head movement. In the earliest studies, Kavoussi and associates have shown that use of the robot by the surgeon results in less need for cleansing the endoscope and less chance of inadvertent tissue contact by the laparoscope.[150] Along a similar line, developments are afoot to provide the surgeon with better instrumentation for performing rapid blunt dissection; the development of high-pressure pneumodissection is one step in this direction.[151] Also, newer instruments for incising tissue are allowing for rapid dissection in a bloodless field; the argon beam coagulator and the harmonic scalpel are both quite effective in achieving and maintaining hemostasis.[139,152] In addition, the further refinement of the ultrasonic aspirator may make it much easier for the surgeon to remove obscuring fatty tissue in order to more efficiently expose underlying vascular structures.[139] Also, the development of micromachines will eventually allow the surgeon to control a multiuse instrument capable of grasping, incising, and dissecting.[153] This alone would greatly reduce the "down" time currently associated with the more complicated laparoscopic approaches.

Finally, there has been a tremendous amount of work expended in trying to develop alternative energy sources for surgical and laparoscopic application. To this end, laser energy, high-intensity focused ultrasound, cryotherapy, and radiofrequency are all being currently investigated.

Lasers have been applied for tissue ablation in urologic oncology both during open surgery and endoscopically. A laparoscopic interstitial contact laser was used experimentally to ablate renal parenchyma in an acute porcine model.[154] Utilizing a synthetic sapphire interstitial Nd:YAG contact probe, various energy levels were tested under laparoscopic guidance. Whereas tissue effects were minimal at energy levels less than 240 J, grossly apparent renal parenchymal coagulation necrosis occurred at 480 J of energy. At 720 J, pronounced tissue vaporization surrounded by a 1.5-cm wide zone of coagulation necrosis was noted. No intraoperative hemorrhage from the renal parenchymal site was noted. The authors concluded that laparoscopic laser ablation may find application in selected patients with small renal lesions.[154]

Analogous to extracorporeal shock wave lithotripsy for stone disease, **high-intensity focused ultrasound** (HIFU) has been employed for controlled transcutaneous ablation of intra-abdominal organ tissues. HIFU accomplishes thermal destruction of tissue by concentrating ultrasonic waves in a narrow focal zone. Recently, Adams and colleagues employed HIFU to ablate renal tumors in the rabbit.[155] Kidney tumors were induced by angiographically implanting rabbit VX-2 papilloma-induced carcinoma cells in six animals. Two weeks later, tumor ablation was performed by HIFU. On histologic examination, tissue destruction was evident at all treatment sites; sharp demarcation was noted between the treatment and nontreatment areas. The authors concluded that extracorporeal HIFU can successfully and precisely ablate renal neoplasms in the rabbit model.[157]

Cryosurgery utilizes rapid, extreme cooling to achieve cell death. Until now limited to the treatment of superficial skin lesions, cryosurgery, under real-time ultrasound monitoring, has also been employed for treating visceral tumors. Reports of open and laparoscopic hepatic cryosurgery[156] have been published.

In urology, cryotherapy has been largely used for treating selected patients with prostate cancer.[157] However, four recent reports have explored the use of cryosurgery for ablating renal tumors.[158–161] Delworth and colleagues cryoablated renal tumors in two patients with the open surgical technique[160]; Uchida and colleagues employed percutaneous cryoablation to treat renal tumors in two patients.[161] However, histologic confirmation of complete tumor cell death and negative "surgical margins" was not mentioned in these reports.

Gill and coworkers recently demonstrated the technical feasibility of laparoscopic renal cryoablation under real-time, endoscopic, color flow Doppler ultrasound monitoring in 12 acute porcine kidneys.[162] The advancing edge of the ice ball could be clearly monitored by laparoscopic ultrasonography. Tissue cryodestruction was documented by light and electron microscopy. The authors concluded that laparoscopic renal cryosurgery is technically feasible; however, further studies are needed to assess its impact on long-term morbidity and renal function.[162] Clinical application of laparoscopic renal cryosurgery awaits.

Radiofrequency ablation of tissues with fine needle electrodes has been performed in neurosurgery for three decades. Hepatic radiofrequency ablation has been successfully performed, initially by open surgery and more recently by laparoscopic techniques.[163]

Gill and colleagues have recently evaluated laparoscopic radiofrequency ablation of the kidney.[164] Using a laparoscopically guided percutaneous, electrosurgical probe, radiofrequency ablation of the kidney was performed under real-time ultrasound monitoring. A spreading array electrode was used to deliver the electrosurgical waveform at various power settings. Continuous tissue temperature monitoring by thermistors documented transient temperatures of 100° C in the targeted renal parenchyma. Renal lesions of 2.5 to 3.5 cm were consistently obtained; the evolving lesion could be clearly monitored ultrasonographically. Histologic evaluation documented uniform cell necrosis. The authors concluded that radiofrequency energy can be delivered laparoscopically in order to ablate renal parenchyma under ultrasonographic monitoring.[164]

Overview

In the operating room of the 1990s efficiency is key; to this end, laparoscopic procedures must be streamlined to a point that the operating room time needed to perform a procedure laparoscopically is no longer than the time needed to perform the same procedure under open conditions. Until this goal is reached, the laparoscopic benefits to the patient of decreased convalescence, less pain, improved cosmesis, and shorter hospital stay will mean little to those who have to pay for these currently more expensive, equally effective, yet "kinder" procedures. The harsh realities of today's medical climate mandate that, for a "new" procedure to become the standard of care, the benefit that accrues must be to patient and payer alike.

REFERENCES

1. Jacobaeus HC: Uber die Moglichkeit, die Zystoskopie bei Untersuchung seroser Hohlungen anzuwenden. Munch Med Wochenschr 1910; 57:2090.
2. Cortesi N, Ferrari P, Zambarda E, et al: Diagnosis of bilateral abdominal cryptorchidism by laparoscopy. Endoscopy 1976; 8:33.
3. Griffith DP, Schuessler WW, Vancaillie TH: Laparoscopic lymphadenectomy—a low morbidity alternative for staging pelvic malignancies. J Endourol 1990; 4(Suppl 1):S-84.
4. Gill IS, Clayman RV, McDougall EM: Advances in urological laparoscopy. J Urol 1995; 154:1275.
5. Gill IS, Clayman RV: Laparoscopic pelvic lymphadenectomy. Surg Oncol Clin North Am 1994; 3:323.
6. Babaian, RJ, Sayer, J, Podoloff DA, et al: Radioimmunoscintigraphy of pelvic lymph nodes with ^{111}indium-labeled monoclonal antibody CYT-356. J Urol 1994; 152:1952.
7. Danella JF, deKernion JB, Smith RB, et al: The contemporary incidence of lymph node metastases in prostate cancer: implications for laparoscopic lymph node dissection. J Urol 1993; 149:1488.
8. Petros JA, Catalona WJ: Lower incidence of unsuspected lymph node metastases in 521 consecutive patients with clinically localized prostate cancer. J Urol 1992; 147:1574.
9. Bluestein DL, Bostwick DG, Bergstralh EJ, et al: Eliminating the need for bilateral pelvic lymphadenectomy in select patients with prostate cancer. J Urol 1994; 151: 1315–1320.
10. Partin AW, Yoo J, Carter HB, et al: Use of prostate specific antigen, clinical stage and Gleason score to predict pathologic stage in men with localized prostate cancer. J Urol 1993; 150:110.
11. Thomas R, Steele R, Ahuja S: Evolving role of laparoscopy in the management of prostate cancer: a one institution-one surgeon experience. J Urol 1995; 153:481A.
12. Schuessler WW, Pharand D, Vancaillie TG: Laparoscopic standard pelvic node dissection for carcinoma of prostate: is it accurate? J Urol 1993; 150:898.
13. Harrison SH, Seale-Hawkins C, Schun CW, et al: Correlation between side of palpable tumor and side of pelvic node metastasis in clinically localized prostate cancer. Cancer 1992; 69:750.
14. Winfield HN, Schuessler WW: Pelvic lymphadenectomy: limited and extended. *In* Clayman RV, McDougall EM (eds): Urologic Laparoscopy, pp 225–260. St. Louis, Quality Publishing, 1992.
15. Schuessler WW, Vancaillie TG, Reich H, et al: Transperitoneal endosurgical lymphadenectomy in patients with localized prostate cancer. J Urol 1991; 145:988.
16. See WA, Cohen M, Winfield HN: Inverted V peritoneotomy significantly improves nodal yield in laparoscopic pelvic lymphadenectomy. J Urol 1993; 149:772.
17. Winfield HN, Donovan JF, See WA, et al: Laparoscopic pelvic lymph node dissection for genitourinary malignancies: indications, techniques and results. J Endourol, 1992; 6:103.
18. Kerbl K, Clayman RV, Petros JA, et al: Staging pelvic lymphadenectomy for prostate cancer: a comparison of laparoscopic and open techniques. J Urol 1993; 150:396.
19. Lang GS, Ruckle HC, Hadley R, et al: One hundred consecutive laparoscopic pelvic lymph node dissections: comparing complications of the first 50 cases to the second 50 cases. Urology 1994; 44:221.
20. Rukstalis DB, Gerber GS, Vogelzang NJ, et al: Laparoscopic pelvic lymph node dissection: a review of 103 consecutive cases. J Urol 1994; 151:670.
21. Kavoussi LR, Sosa E, Chandhoke P, et al: Complications of laparoscopic pelvic lymph node dissection. J Urol 1993; 149:322–325.
22. Griffith DP, Schuessler WW, Nickell KG, et al: Laparoscopic pelvic lymphadenectomy for prostatic adenocarcinoma. Urol Clin North Am 1992; 19:407.
23. Parra RO, Andrus C, Boullier J: Staging laparoscopic pelvic lymph node dissection: comparison of results with open pelvic lymphadenectomy. J Urol 1992; 147:875.
24. Guazzoni G, Montorsi F, Bergamaschi F, et al: Open surgical revision of laparoscopic pelvic lymphadenectomy for staging of prostate cancer: the impact of laparoscopic learning curve. J Urol 1994; 151:930.
25. Lerner SE, Fleischmann J, Taub HC, et al: Combined laparoscopic pelvic lymph node dissection and modified Belt radical perineal prostatectomy for localized prostatic adenocarcinoma. Urology 1994; 43:493.
26. Parra RO, Boullier JA, Rauscher JA, et al: The value of laparoscopic lymphadenectomy in conjunction with radical perineal or retropubic prostatectomy. J Urol 1994; 151: 1599.
27. Thomas R, Steele R, Smith R, et al: One-stage laparoscopic pelvic lymphadenectomy and radical perineal prostatectomy. J Urol 1994; 152:1174.
28. Teichman JMH, Reddy PK, Hulbert JC: Laparoscopic pelvic lymph node dissection, laparoscopically assisted seminal vesicle mobilization, and total perineal prostatectomy versus radical retropubic prostatectomy for prostate cancer. Urology 1995; 45:823.
29. Levy DA, Resnick MI: Laparoscopic pelvic lymphadenectomy and radical perineal prostatectomy: a viable alternative to radical retropubic prostatectomy. J Urol 1994; 151:905.
30. Jarrard DF, Chodak GW: Prostate cancer staging after radiation utilizing laparoscopic pelvic lymphadenectomy. Urology 1995; 46:538.
31. Lund GO, Winfield HN, Donovan JF, et al: Laparoscopic pelvic lymph node dissection following definitive radiotherapy for prostate cancer. J Urol 1994; 151:344A.
32. Stone NN, Ramin SA, Wesson MF, et al: Laparoscopic pelvic lymph node dissection combined with real-time transrectal radioactive seed implantation of the prostate. J Urol 1995; 153:1555.
33. Troxel SA, Winfield HN: Comparative cost analysis of laparoscopic versus open pelvic lymph node dissection for men with cancer of the prostate. J Urol 1994; 151:675.
34. Troxel SA, Winfield HN: Comparative financial analysis of laparoscopic pelvic lymph node dissection (LPLND) performed in 1990–91 versus 1993–94. J Urol 1995; 153: 357A.
35. Das S, Tashima M: Extraperitoneal laparoscopic staging pelvic lymph node dissection. J Urol 1994; 151:1321.
36. Villiers A, Vannier JL, Abecassis R, et al: Extraperitoneal endosurgical lymphadenectomy with insufflation in the staging of bladder and prostate cancer. J Endourol 1993; 7:229.
37. Etwaru D, Raboy A, Ferzli G, et al: Extraperitoneal endoscopic gasless pelvic lymph node dissection. J Laparoendoscop Surg 1994; 4:113.
38. Hakim LS, Raboy A, Antario JM, et al: Extraperitoneal endoscopic pelvic lymph node dissection versus laparoscopy: advantages and selection criteria for the staging of localized prostate cancer. J Urol 1993; 149:415A.
39. McDowell GC, Johnson JW, Tenney DM, et al: Pelvic lymphadenectomy for staging clinically localized prostate

cancer; indications, complications and results in 217 cases. Urology 1990; 35:476.
40. Golimbu M, Morales P, Al-Askari S, et al: Extended pelvic lymphadenectomy for prostate cancer. J Urol 1994; 127: 452.
41. Parra RO, Hagood PA, Boullier JA, et al: Complications of urological laparoscopic surgery: experience at St Louis University. J Urol 1994; 151:681.
42. Fatton B, Guy L, Raynaud F, et al: Minimally invasive surgery for iliac node dissection. J Urol 1995; 153:516A.
43. Mohler JL: Outpatient pelvic lymph node dissection. J Urol 1995; 154:1439.
44. Perotti M, Gentle D, Kaufman RP Jr.: Mini lap pelvic lymph node dissection (MLPLND) minimizes morbidity, costs and hospitalization of pelvic lymph node dissection (PLND). J Urol 1994; 151:498A.
45. Steiner MS, Marshall FF: Mini-laparotomy staging pelvic lymphadenectomy (minilap): alternative to standard and laparoscopic pelvic lymphadenectomy. Urology 1993; 41: 201.
46. Srinivas V, Morse MJ, Herr HW, et al: Penile cancer: relation of extent of nodal metastasis to survival. J Urol 1987; 137:880.
47. Assimos DG, Jarow JP: Role of laparoscopic pelvic lymph node dissection in the management of patients with penile cancer and inguinal adenopathy. J Endourol 1994; 8: 365.
48. Holevas R, Lui P, Hadley R, et al: Laparoscopic management of metastatic penile carcinoma. J Urol 1993; 149: 502A.
49. Castillo O, Azocar G, Cauwelaert RV, et al: Laparoscopic retroperitoneal lymph node dissection in testicular cancer. J Urol 1995; 153:516A.
50. Janetschek G, Reissigl A, Peschel R, et al: Laparoscopic retroperitoneal lymphadenectomy for clinical stage I testicular tumor. J Endourol 1993; 7:S175.
51. Gerber GS, Bisada NK, Hulbert JC, et al: Laparoscopic retroperitoneal lymphadenectomy: multi-institutional analysis. J Urol 1994; 152:1188.
52. Klotz L: Laparoscopic retroperitoneal lymphadenectomy vs open lymphadenectomy for stage I NSGCT: a comparison. J Urol 1995; 153:356A.
53. Henkel TO, Potempa DM, Rassweiler JJ, et al: The Mannheim experience with laparoscopic retroperitoneal lymphadenectomy for testicular cancer. J Endourol 1993; 7:S140.
54. Hulbert JC, Fraley EE: Laparoscopic retroperitoneal lymphadenectomy: new approach to pathologic staging of clinical stage I germ cell tumors of the testis. J Endourol 1992; 6:123.
55. Stone NN, Schlussel RN, Waterhouse RL, et al: Laparoscopic retroperitoneal lymph node dissection in stage A nonseminomatous testis cancer. Urology 1993; 42:610.
56. Donohue JP, Rowland RG: Complications of retroperitoneal lymph node dissection. J Urol 1981; 125:338.
57. Babaian RJ, Bracken RB, Johnson DE: Complications of transabdominal retroperitoneal lymphadenectomy. Urology 1981; 17:126.
58. Peckham MJ, Barret A, Husband JE, et al: Orchidectomy alone in testicular stage I non-seminomatous germ cell tumors. Lancet 1982; 2:786.
59. Richie JP: Clinical stage I testicular cancer: the role of modified retroperitoneal lymphadenectomy. J Urol 1990; 144:1160.
60. Freedman LS, Jones WG, Peckham MJ, et al: Histopathology in the prediction of relapse of patients with stage I testicular teratoma alone. Lancet 1987; 2:294.
61. Drouard F, Delamarre J, Capron JP: Cutaneous seeding of gallbladder cancer after laparoscopic cholecystectomy [Letter]. N Engl J Med 1991; 325:1316.
62. Cava A, Roman J, Gonzalez Quintela A, et al: Subcutaneous metastasis following laparoscopy in gastric adenocarcinoma. Eur J Surg Oncol 1990; 16:63.
63. Alexander RJ, Jaques BC, Mitchell KC: Laparoscopically assisted colectomy and wound recurrence [Letter]. Lancet 1993; 341:249.
64. Keate RF, Shaffer R: Seeding of hepatocellular carcinoma to peritoneoscopy insertion site [Letter]. Gastrointest Endosc 1992; 38:203.
65. Russi EG, Pergolizzi S, Mesiti M, et al: Unusual relapse of hepatocellular carcinoma. Cancer 1992; 70:1483.
66. Hsiu JG, Given FT Jr, Kemp GM: Tumor implantation after diagnostic laparoscopic biopsy of serous ovarian tumors of low malignant potential. Obstet Gynecol 1986; 68(suppl):90S.
67. Stockdale AD, Pocock TJ: Abdominal wall metastasis following laparoscopy: a case report. Eur J Surg Oncol 1985; 11:373.
68. Bangma CH, Kirkels WJ, Chadha S: Cutaneous metastasis following laparoscopic pelvic lymphadenopathy for prostatic carcinoma. J Urol 1995; 153:1635.
69. Stolla V, Rossi D, Bladou F, et al: Subcutaneous metastases after coeliscopic lymphadenectomy for vesical urothelial carcinoma. Eur Urol 1994; 26:342.
70. Breul J, Block T, Breidenbach H, Hartung R: Implantation metastasis after a suprapubic catheter in a case of bladder cancer. Eur Urol 1992; 22:86.
71. McDougall EM, Clayman RV, Elashry OM: Laparoscopic radical nephrectomy for renal tumor: the Washington University experience. J Urol 1996; 155:1180.
72. Capelouto CC, Elbert D, Hubbell JA, et al: Inhibition of peritoneal tumor implantation during laparoscopy using a copolymer PLL-g-MPEG. J Endourol 1993; 7:S198.
73. Robson CJ, Churchill BM, Anderson W: The results of radical nephrectomy for renal cell carcinoma. J Urol 1969; 101:297.
74. Clayman RV, Kavoussi LR, Soper NJ, et al: Laparoscopic nephrectomy: initial case report. J Urol 1991; 146:278–282.
75. Coptcoat M, Joyce A, Rassweiler J, Popert R: Laparoscopic nephrectomy: the King's clinical experience [Abstract 881]. J Urol 1992; 147(part 2):433A.
76. Kerbl K, Clayman RV, McDougall EM, Kavoussi LR: Laparoscopic nephrectomy: the Washington University experience. Br J Urol 1994; 73:231.
77. Higashirha E, Tanaka T, Natahara K, et al: Laparoscopic adrenalectomy: technical review. Jpn J Endourol 1992; 5: 150.
78. Matsuda T, Terachi T, Yoshida O: Laparoscopic adrenalectomy: the surgical technique and initial results of 13 cases. Minim Invasive Ther 1993; 2:123.
79. Urban DA, Kerbl K, McDougall EM, et al: Organ entrapment and renal morcellation: permeability studies. J Urol 1993; 150:1792.
80. Kavoussi LR, Kerbl K, Capelouto C, et al: Laparoscopic nephrectomy for renal neoplasms. Urology, 1993; 42: 603.
81. Ono Y, Katoh N, Kinukawa T, et al: Laparoscopic nephrectomy, radical nephrectomy and adrenalectomy: Nagoya experience. J Urol 1994; 152:1962.
82. Tse ETW, Knaus RP: Laparoscopic nephrectomy: the learning curve experience. Can J Surg 1994; 37:153–157.
83. Tschada RK, Rassweiler JJ, Mannheim K, et al: Laparoscopic tumor nephrectomy—the German experiences. J Urol 1995; 154:479.
84. Gill IS, Kavoussi LR, Clayman RV, et al: Complications of laparoscopic nephrectomy in 185 patients: a multi-institutional review. J Urol 1995; 154:479.
85. Scott RF Jr, Selzman HM: Complications of nephrectomy: review of 450 patients and a description of a modification of the transperitoneal approach. J Urol 1966; 95:307.
86. Novick AC: Partial nephrectomy for renal cell carcinoma. Urology 1995; 46:149.
87. Whang M, O'Toole K, Bixon R, et al: The incidence of multifocal renal cell carcinoma in patients who are candidates for partial nephrectomy. J Urol 1995; 154:968.
88. Licht MR, Novick AC, Goormastic M: Nephron sparing surgery in incidental versus suspected renal cell carcinoma. J Urol 1994; 152:39.
89. Hawkins CA, Wollan PC, Grabner A, et al: Disease out-

come in patients with low grade, low stage renal cell cancer is similar when treated by nephron-preserving or radical surgery [Abstract 133]. J Urol 1994; 151:261A.
90. Winfield HN, Donovan JF, Lund GO, et al: Laparoscopic partial nephrectomy: initial experience and comparison to the open surgical approach. J Urol 1995; 153: 1409.
91. Stephens R, Graham SD Jr: Enucleation of tumor versus partial nephrectomy as conservative treatment of renal cell carcinoma. Cancer 1990; 65:2663.
92. Blackley SK, Ladaga L, Woolfitt RA, et al: Ex-situ study of the effectiveness of enucleation in patients with renal cell carcinoma. J Urol 1988; 140:6.
93. Ritchie AWS, deKernion JB: Incidental renal neoplasms: incidence in Los Angeles County, treatment and prognosis. Prog Clin Biol Res 1990; 269:347.
94. Tosaka A, Ohya K, Yamada K, et al: Incidence and properties of renal masses and asymptomatic renal cell carcinoma detected by abdominal ultrasonography. J Urol 1990; 144:1097.
95. Thompson IM, Peek M: Improvement in survival of patients with renal cell carcinoma—the role of the serendipitously detected tumor. J Urol 1988; 140:487.
96. McDougall EM, Clayman RV, Anderson K: Laparoscopic wedge resection of a renal tumor: initial experience. J. Laparoendosc Surg 1993; 3:577.
97. Nocks BN, Henry NM, Daly JJ, et al: Transitional cell carcinoma of the renal pelvis. Urology 1982; 19:472.
98. Wagle DG, More RH, Murphy GP: Primary carcinoma of the renal pelvis. Cancer 1974; 33:1642.
99. Cummings KB: Nephroureterectomy: rationale in the management of transitional cell carcinoma of the upper urinary tract. Urol Clin North Am 1980; 7:569.
100. Kerbl K, Clayman RV, McDougall EM, et al: Laparoscopic nephroureterectomy: evaluation of first clinical series. Eur Urol 1993; 23:431.
101. Jarrett TW, Sweetser PM, Weiss GH, et al: Percutaneous management of transitional cell carcinoma of renal collecting system: 9-year experience. J Urol 1995; 154:1629.
102. Blute ML, Segura IW, Patterson DE, et al: Impact of endourology on diagnosis and management of upper tract urothelial cancer. J Urol 1989; 141:1298.
103. McDougall EM, Clayman RV, Elashry OM: Laparoscopic nephroureterectomy for upper tract transitional cell cancer: the Washington University experience. J Urol 1995; 154:975.
104. Stephenson RN, Sharma NK, Tolley DA: Laparoscopic nephroureterectomy: a comparison with open surgery. J Endourol 1995; 9:S99.
105. Figenshau RS, Albala DM, Clayman RV, et al: Laparoscopic nephroureterectomy: initial laboratory experience. Minim Invasive Ther 1991; 1:93.
106. Williams DF: Titanium as a metal for implantation. Part II: biological and clinical applications. J Med Eng Technol 1977; 1:266.
107. Parra RO, Andrus CH, Jones JP, et al: Laparoscopic cystectomy: initial report on a new treatment for the retained bladder. J Urol 1992; 148: 1140.
108. Parra RO, Worischeck JH, Hagood PG: Laparoscopic simple cystectomy in a man. Surg Laparosc Endosc 1995; 5: 161.
109. Kozminiski M, Partamian, KO: Case report of laparoscopic ileal conduit. J Endourol 1992; 6:147.
110. Sanchez de Badajoz E, Gallego Perales JL, Reche Rosade A, et al: Laparoscopic cystectomy and ileal conduit: case report. J Endourol 1995; 9:59.
111. Townell NH, Rahman S, Matthews LK: Laparoscopic cystectomy and prostatourethrectomy: initial case report. Minim Invasive Ther 1994; 3:369.
112. Puppo P, Perachino M, Ricciotti G, et al: Laparoscopically assisted transvaginal radical cystectomy. Eur Urol 1995; 27:80.
113. Andersen JR, Steven K: Implantation metastasis after laparoscopioc biopsy of bladder cancer. J Urol 1995; 153: 1047.
114. Nadler RB, Pearle MS, McDougall EM, et al: Laparoscopic extraperitoneal bladder diverticulectomy: initial experience. Urology 1995; 45:524.
115. Parra RO, Jones JP, Andrus CH, et al: Laparoscopic diverticulectomy: preliminary report of a new approach for the treatment of bladder diverticulum. J Urol 1992; 148: 869.
116. Nezhat CR, Nezhat FR: Laparoscopic segmental bladder resection for endometriosis: a report of two cases. Obstet Gynecol 1993; 81:882.
117. Ferzli G, Wenof M, Giannakakos A, et al: Laparoscopic partial cystectomy for vesical endometrioma. J Laparoendosc Surg 1993; 3:161.
118. Gerber GS, Chodak GW, Rukstalis DB: Combined laparoscopic and transurethral neodymium:yttrium-aluminum-garnet laser treatment of invasive bladder cancer. Urology 1995; 45:230.
119. Kavoussi LR, Schuessler WW, Vancaillie TG, et al: Laparoscopic approach to the seminal vesicles. J Urol 1993; 150:417.
120. Jarrett TW, Pardalidis NP, Silverstein M, et al: Laparoscopic enterolysis and placement of an intestinal sling before radiation therapy for the treatment of prostate cancer. Urology 1995; 45:326.
121. Sklar GN, Koschorke G, Filderman PS, et al: Laparoscopic monitoring of cryosurgical ablation of the prostate. Surg Laparosc Endosc 1995; 5:376.
122. Schuessler WW, Kavoussi LR, Clayman RV, et al: Laparoscopic radical prostatectomy: initial case report. J Urol 1992; 147:246A.
123. Moran ME, Bowyer DW, Szabo Z: Laparoscopic suturing in urology: a model for vesicourethral anastomosis. Minim Invasive Ther 1993; 2:165.
124. Gagner M, Lacroix A, Bolte E: Laparoscopic adrenalectomy in Cushing's syndrome and pheochromocytoma [Letter]. N Engl J Med 1992; 327:1033.
125. Go H, Takeda M, Takahashi H, et al: Laparoscopic adrenalectomy for primary aldosteronism: a new operative method. J Laparoendosc Surg 1993; 5:455.
126. Higashihara E, Tanaka Y, Horie S, et al: Laparoscopic adrenalectomy: initial 3 cases. J Urol 1993; 149:973.
127. Matsuda T, Terachi T, Yoshida O: Laparoscopic adrenalectomy: the surgical technique and initial results of 13 cases. Minim Invasive Ther 1993; 2:123.
128. Suzuki K, Kageyama S, Daisuke U, et al: Laparoscopic adrenalectomy: clinical experience with 12 cases. J. Urol 1993; 150:1099.
129. Terachi T, Kawakita M, Yoshiyuki K, et al: Laparoscopic adrenalectomy: results of 47 cases. J Urol 1995; 153:513A.
130. Fernandez-Cruz L, Benarroch G, Torres E, et al: Laparoscopic approach to the adrenal tumors. J Laparoendosc Surg 1994; 3:541.
131. Gagner M, Lacroix A, Bolte E, et al: Laparoscopic adrenalectomy: the importance of a flank approach in the lateral decubitus position. Surg Endosc 1994; 8:135.
132. Brunt LM, Molmenti EP, Kerbl K, et al: Retroperitoneal endoscopic adrenalectomy: an experimental study. Surg Laparosc Endosc 1993; 3:300.
133. Morita K, Sakakibara N, Seki T, et al: Clinical study of 25 cases with adrenal tumor—comparison between transabdominal, translumbar, laparoscopic approach. Nippon Hinyokika Gakkai Zasshi 1994; 85:778.
134. Mandressi A, Buizz C, Zaroli A, et al: Laparoscopic nephrectomies and adrenalectomies by posterior retroextraperitoneal approach. J Endourol 1993; 7:S174.
135. Albala DA, Prinz RA: Laparoscopic adrenalectomy: results of eight patients. J Urol 1994; 151:393A.
136. Suzuki K, Ihara H, Kageyama S, et al: Laparoscopic adrenalectomy—clinical analysis of 25 cases. J Urol 1994; 151:498A.
137. Suzuki K, Ihara H, Kageyama S, et al: Laparoscopic adrenalectomy—comparative analysis of retroperitoneal vs. transperitoneal approach. J Urol 1995; 153:481A.
138. Guazzoni G, Montorsi F, Lanzi R, et al: Transperitoneal laparoscopic versus open adrenalectomy for benign hy-

perfunctioning adrenal tumors: a comparative study. J Urol 1995; 153:1597.
139. Takeda M, Go H, Imai T, et al: Experience with 17 cases of laparoscopic adrenalectomy: use of ultrasonic aspirator and argon beam coagulator. J Urol 1994; 152:902.
140. Yoshioka T, Yamaguchi S, Kokado Y, et al: Experience of laparoscopic adrenalectomy. J Endourol 1994; 8:S83.
141. Schichman S, McGillvay D, Malchoff C, et al: Laparoscopic adrenalectomy: a multi-institutional review. J Urol 1995; 153:516A.
142. Castilho LN, Ferreira U, Netto RN Jr, et al: Laparoscopic adrenalectomy. J Endourol 1995; 9:S84.
143. Nakagawa K, Murai M, Deguchi N, et al: Laparoscopic adrenalectomy: clinical results of 25 patients. J Endourol 1994; 8:S82.
144. Ono Y, Katoh N, Kinukawa T, et al: Laparoscopic nephrectomy, radical nephrectomy and adrenalectomy: Nagoya experience. J Urol 1994; 152:1962.
145. Kristiansen SB, Doody KJ: Laparoscopic removal of 46 XY gonads located within the inguinal canals. Fertil Steril 1992; 58:1076.
146. Wilson EE, Vuitch F, Carr BR: Laparoscopic removal of dysgenetic gonads containing a gonadoblastoma in a patient with Swyer syndrome. Obstet Gynecol 1992; 79: 842.
147. McDougall EM, Clayman RV, Anderson K, et al: Laparoscopic gonadectomy in a case of testicular feminization. Urology 1993; 42:201.
148. Yu TJ, Shu K, King FT, et al: Use of laparoscopy in intersex patients. J Urol 1995; 154:1193.
149. Wilson PD, Ribeiro B, Williams NS, et al: Safe handling of laparoscopic instruments. Minim Invasive Ther 1994; 3(Suppl 1):78.
150. Kavoussi LR, Moore RG, Adams JB, et al: Comparison of robotic versus human laparoscopic camera control. J Urol 1995; 154:2134.
151. Pearle MS, Nakada SY, McDougall EM, et al: Laparoscopic pneumodissection: initial clinical experience. Urology 1995; 45:882.
152. Amaral JF: Laparoscopic cholecystectomy in 200 consecutive patients using an ultrasonically activated scalpel. Surg Laparosc Endosc 1995; 5:255.
153. Fujimasa I: Micromachining technology and biomedical engineering. Appl Biochem Biotechnol 1993; 38:233.
154. Lofti MA, McCue P, Gomella LG: Laparoscopic interstitial contact laser ablation of renal lesions: an experimental model. J Endourol 1994; 8:153.
155. Adams JB II, Moore RG, Anderson JH, et al: High-intensity focused ultrasound ablation of rabbit kidney tumors. J Endourol 1996; 10:71.
156. McCall JL, Jorgensen JO, Morris P: Laparoscopic hepatic cryotherapy: a study of safety in rabbits. Surg Laparosc Endosc 1996; 6:29.
157. Miller RJ Jr, Cohen JK, Merlotti LA: Percutaneous transperitoneal cryoablation of the prostate for the primary treatment of clinical stage C adenocarcinoma of the prostate. Urology 1994; 44:170.
158. Onik GM, Reyes G, Cohen JK, Porterfield B: Ultrasound characteristics of renal cryosurgery. Urology 1993; 42:212.
159. Stephenson RA, King D, Rohr RL: Renal cryoablation in a canine model [Abstract 700]. J Urol 1995; 153:403A.
160. Delworth MG, Pisters LL, Fornage BD, von Eschenbach AC: Cryotherapy for renal cell carcinoma and angiomyolipoma. J Urol 1996; 155:252.
161. Uchida M, Imaide Y, Sugimoto K, et al: Percutaneous cryosurgery for renal tumours. J Urol 1995; 75:132.
162. Gill IS, Matamoros A, Heffron T, et al: Laparoscopic renal cryosurgery: feasibility studies. Urology (submitted).
163. Watanabe Y, Sato M, Abe Y, et al: Laparoscopic microwave coagulo-necrotic therapy for hepatocellular carcinoma: a feasible study of an alternative option for poor-risk patients. J Laparoendosc Surg 1995; 5:169.
164. Gill IS, Fox R, Matamoros A, et al: Laparoscopic radiofrequency ablation of the kidney: feasibility studies. (in preparation)

50

CREATIVE MODALITIES

MARK A. WAINSTEIN, M.D., BRUCE CARLIN, M.D.,
GREGORY W. BARAN, M.D., *and* MARTIN I. RESNICK, M.D.

Over the past two decades there has been a revolution of varied radiologic imaging modalities. Refinements in computed tomography (CT) that have allowed improved resolution with subsecond scans, the introduction and maturation of magnetic resonance imaging (MRI), and the arrival of clinical positron emission tomography (PET) have all expanded potential imaging applications. With the development of faster, more efficient computer technology, these imaging modalities have become less expensive and more available. In this chapter, applications of new imaging modalities in the evaluation and treatment of urologic oncology patients are discussed.

HELICAL (SPIRAL) COMPUTED TOMOGRAPHY

With the advent of new imaging modalities, the detection and diagnosis of neoplastic processes has markedly increased. Nowhere in the body has this been noted more than in the kidney.[1] Because of the widespread use of CT and ultrasound, it is well documented in the literature that renal lesions are being detected earlier, at reduced size and stage, and with increased frequency.[1–3] With this increased detection of what has been termed "incidental" renal lesions, the differentiation of neoplastic from nonneoplastic processes has become increasingly important in the interpretation of these studies.

Since its clinical introduction in the mid-1970s, CT has become the generally accepted modality for evaluating many renal masses that have usually been detected by intravenous urography or ultrasonography. Specific CT characteristics are utilized in assessing these masses, including the appearance of unenhanced scans, the amount and pattern of contrast enhancement, the presence and location of calcifications, the location and thickness of the cyst wall, and the presence of septation.[4–7] Respiratory misregistration and partial volume averaging are specific technical limitations of CT that have led to incomplete evaluation of small renal masses.[8,9] Respiratory misregistration is due to variations in tidal volumes between respiratory cycles, which result in "skip" areas of the imaged organ or lesion. Partial volume averaging represents an attenuation value composed of closely adjacent structures that are contained within the same image voxel and are therefore averaged.

Spiral CT, with the capability of performing multiple contiguous 1-second tube rotations coupled with continuous patient transport, has allowed volumetric images to be obtained during a single breath-holding period.[10,11] Three major technical refinements allow for spiral CT imaging: the development of the slip-ring gantry, improved detector efficiency, and greater tube cooling capability. The slip-ring gantries contain a set of rings and electrical components that allow imaging data to be obtained in a helical spatial distribution. Refinements in detector technology make it possible to reduce the dose of radiation while providing higher quality image acquisition.

Advantages of this technology are its ability to acquire contiguous imaging data with multiplanar reformations and almost eliminate respiratory misregistrations. In addition, this method has been combined with a dynamic intravenous contrast bolus, thus allowing imaging of the abdominal vasculature, specifically the aorta, renal arteries, and splanchnic circulation. Through innovative image reprocessing, it is possible to obtain excellent anatomic details of the abdominal vasculature. With further refinements, CT angiography may serve as a relatively inexpensive alternative to traditional angiography in the evaluation of the abdominal vasculature.

In studying the kidney, preliminary unenhanced scans are usually obtained to evaluate the density of a renal lesion. With enhanced scans, contrast material is injected at a rate of 1.5 to 2.0 ml/sec for a total of 120 ml, and scans are obtained with 5 to 7-mm collimations during a 30-second helical exposure. As with all imaging modalities, selection of the phase of enhancement—vascular, nephrogenic, or pyelographic—will determine which anatomic region will be depicted with greatest contrast. Vascular enhancement of the renal vein will peak well before the nephrogram. Unfortunately, because there is a lack of relative medullary enhancement on these very early scans, small renal lesions will often be overlooked. Because of this concern, the kidneys will be rescanned as conventional axial slices after completion of the 30-second helix. Regardless of the timing of the contrast bolus, helical CT can delineate lesions as small as 1 cm because of the lack of registration artifacts and the ability to reconstruct slices at overlapping intervals.[12]

Contrast-enhanced spiral CT with new surface rendering software creates three-dimensional surface images of the kidney that are virtually free of motion artifact and image reformats that closely resemble original structures (Fig. 50–1). This technology is the result of the growth and sophistication of computer software. Three-dimensional imaging promises to be both a valuable diagnostic

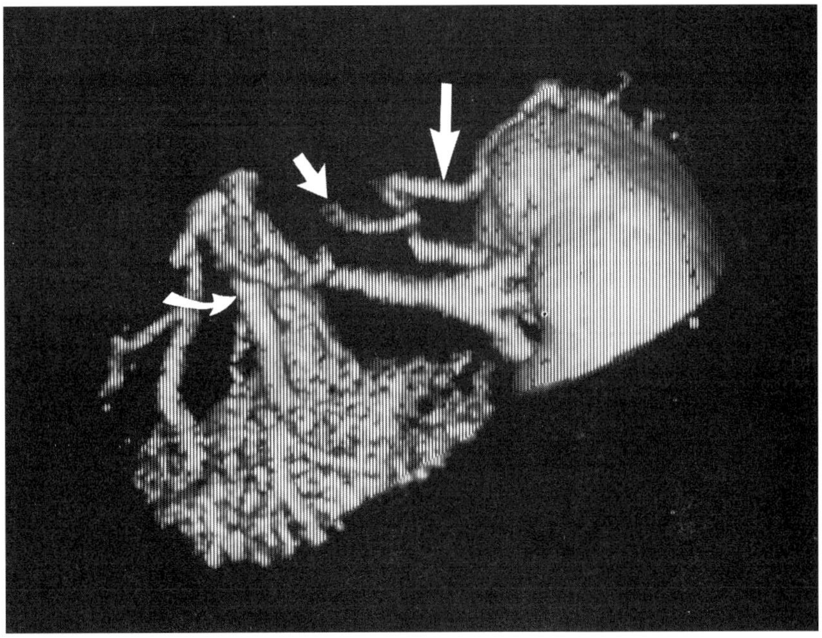

A

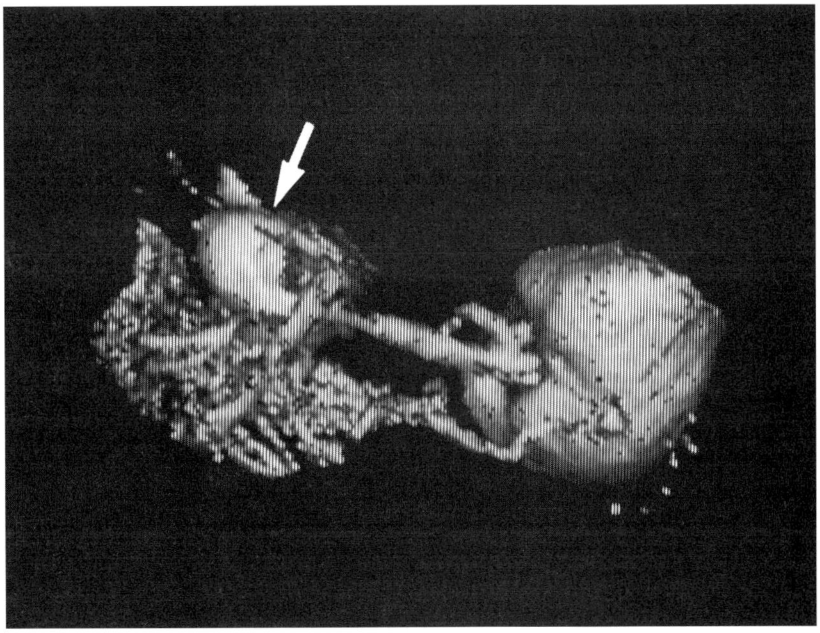

B

FIGURE 50–1. Three-dimensional reconstruction (*A*, anterior view; *B*, superior view) of the left kidney illustrating the left renal vein, renal artery (arrowhead), and adrenal artery (straight arrow). Note the superior mesenteric artery and vein (curved arrow). In *B*, there is an incidental aortic aneurysm (arrow).

and therapeutic modality, and already has found specific applications in radiation therapy, oncology, orthopedics, and general surgery.[13–19]

Spiral CT has already found value in urologic applications. By eliminating respiratory misregistrations and avoiding "skip lesions," small renal lesions can be accurately evaluated by this modality.[12,17,18] The typical spiral CT appearance of small renal cell carcinomas is that of a noncalcified mass with an attenuation value of 20 Hounsfield units (H) or more that enhances with intravenous contrast agents. Investigators have utilized the high-quality three-dimensional reconstructions in visualizing relationships between tumor, renal hilar vasculature, and collecting system prior to nephron-sparing surgery.[19] Although intraoperative ultrasound has been reported to aid in surgical strategies of partial nephrectomy, it does not provide the overall perspective provided by the three-dimensional spiral CT.[20,21] This technology has been applied in other surgical subspecialties in preoperative evaluation and surgical planning. Complete evaluation of the utility of three-dimensional imaging as a surgical planning tool will require further study.

TRANSRECTAL COLOR DOPPLER ULTRASOUND

Prostate cancer is the most common cancer in men and the second most common cause of cancer death.[22] The advent of endorectal ultrasound scanning brought early hope for an accurate means of diagnosing prostate cancer.[23–26] Unfortunately, transrectal ultrasound (TRUS) did not prove valuable as a screening study because of its poor sensitivity and specificity. Reported positive predictive values of malignant lesions are in the range of 18 to 60%.[27–29] Although investigations have shown that combining findings on digital rectal examination, serum prostate-specific antigen (PSA) level, and TRUS have improved detection of prostatic neoplasms, this method cannot identify all cancers.[26,30,31] TRUS is recognized as the method of choice for biopsy guidance.[32] Improving the predictive value of TRUS would enable more selective biopsies to be performed.

High-frequency color Doppler ultrasound has made it possible to noninvasively image the vascular architecture of superficial organs such as the testis and the thyroid.[33–35] The advent of transrectal probes with pulsed Doppler and color flow imaging at high frequencies has provided a new potential for improved diagnosis of prostate cancer. Color Doppler ultrasound analysis has added to the diagnostic capability of gray-scale ultrasound scanning for both the detection and distinction of different disease processes. Color Doppler imaging (CDI) is a convenient and integral adjunct to gray-scale ultrasound; however, the role of CDI in diagnosis and management of prostate cancer is currently under investigation.[36] Theoretically, color Doppler scanning should depict cancer by identifying tumor hypervascularity. Early and very preliminary data on Doppler ultrasound scanning of the prostate suggest limited improvement over gray-scale ultrasound in differentiating malignancies from benign disease processes.[37–42] Recent investigators have reported that color flow signal intensity is generally low or absent in normal prostatic tissue and that a focal hypervascularity in the peripheral zone should alert the examiner to the possible presence of a malignant lesion[38–42] (Fig. 50–2). Initial anecdotal experience suggests that increased color flow signal is consistent with prostate cancer,[39–42] with some investigators reporting a positive predictive value as high as 81%.[38,39]

Drawbacks to this imaging technique include examination subjectivity along with significant overlap in appearance between neoplastic and inflammatory processes.[42,43] Although these initial data demonstrate improved positive predictive values using color Doppler ultrasound, they are not sufficient to make decisions regarding the need for or against biopsy. Further studies are needed to evaluate this imaging modality as an adjunct to transrectal gray-scale ultrasound.

MAGNETIC RESONANCE IMAGING

Incidental adrenal masses often create a diagnostic dilemma. Since the use of CT has become widespread, adrenal masses of at least 1 cm in diameter have been discovered in 0.6 to 1.5% of the population.[44,45] In patients without known malignancies, these lesions may be managed conservatively with follow-up CT examination when there is no clinical or endocrine dysfunction.[46–49] In the previously diagnosed oncologic patient, clinical management often depends on whether an adrenal lesion represents a metastasis from a distant primary, which is not uncommon, or a benign process.[50,51] Establishing the nature of an adrenal mass less than 3 cm in diameter can be difficult, and CT scans lack adequate sensitivity or specificity to make an accurate diagnosis.[52,53] Several imaging features with CT or MRI are more common with benign cortical masses than with metastases, including small size, smooth margins, homogeneous enhancement, low attenuation on CT scan, and lack of high signal intensity on T2-weighted MRI images.[54–57] These signs are not specific enough in most instances to preclude biopsy or frequent radiologic reexamination. Percutaneous biopsy of the adrenal gland is not without complications,[58–60] and serial examination with CT or MRI to document instability is expensive and inconvenient.

In an attempt to differentiate benign from malignant lesions, many MRI techniques have been studied.[54,55,61–66] Early reports describe differences of adrenal masses on T1- or T2-weighted images.[55,61–64]

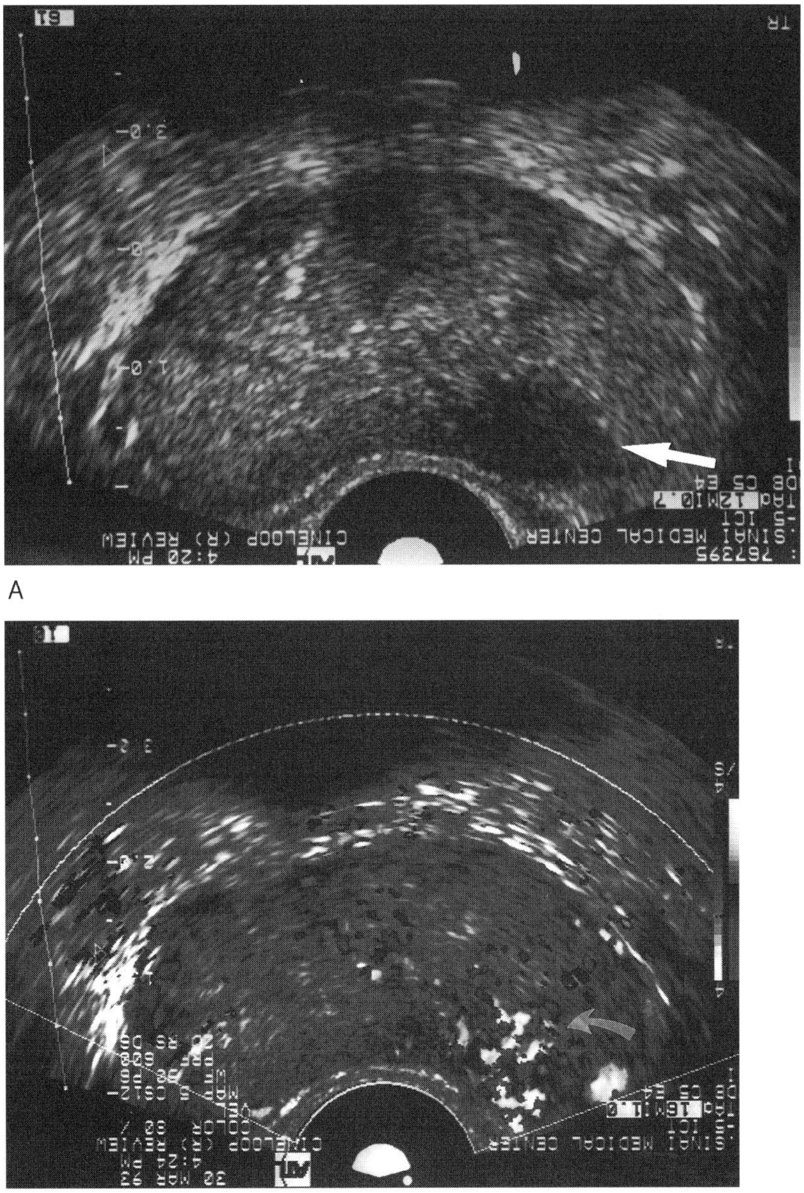

A

B

FIGURE 50–2. *A,* Transverse gray-scale image of the prostate demonstrating a focal hypoechoic lesion in the left peripheral zone (arrow). *B,* Corresponding slow-flow color Doppler sonograph illustrating an intense flow pattern filling the entire hypoechoid lesion, suggestive of adenocarcinoma of the prostate (curved arrow). Histologic specimen revealed a Gleason's 3+4 adenocarcinoma of the prostate.

Some investigators found that malignant adrenal lesions tend to have higher signal intensity on standard T2-weighted MR images than adenomas, but there was substantial overlap in signals between these groups.[55,67,68] Other investigators have used dynamic contrast-enhanced images, which attempt to utilize adrenal avidity for contrast material, and their rate of washout. Unfortunately this technique was also ineffective.[64,66,69]

Chemical Shift Magnetic Resonance Imaging

Findings with chemical shift MRI have shown improved ability to help characterize adrenal masses. High degrees of lipid accumulation occur in benign cortical masses such as adrenocortical nodules and adrenal adenomas, whereas metastatic deposits, pheochromocytomas, and adrenocorticocarcinomas generally show no lipid accumulation.[62,63,70,71] Protons in triglycerides and water possess different resonance frequencies when they are exposed to a given magnetic field, allowing chemical shift MRI techniques to reliably demonstrate small quantities of fat.[72–77] It has been shown that T1-weighted opposed-phase imaging techniques are sensitive for detecting small proportions of lipids within tissues.[77,78] Numerous studies have documented that the role of chemical shift MRI appears to be effective for characterization of many adrenal masses[60,62,63,79,80] (Fig. 50–3). Some investigators report close to 100% accuracy in differentiating adenomas from other lesions based on quantitative signal intensity measurements.[61,62,70,71]

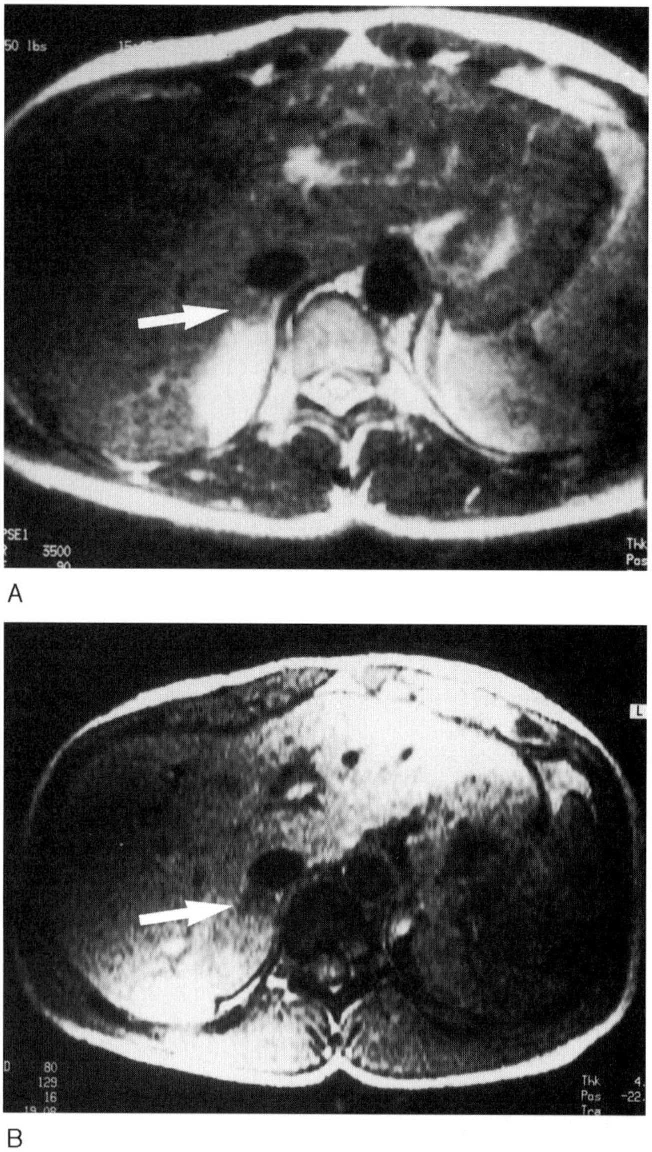
A
B

FIGURE 50–3. *A*, Axial MR image of the right adrenal gland demonstrating a round adrenal mass that is almost isointense with the liver (straight arrow). *B*, Corresponding opposed-phase gradient-echo image showing that the mass has decreased signal intensity indicative of a higher lipid content (curved arrow). Histology of the specimen revealed an aldosteronoma.

In conclusion, chemical shift MRI is a simple and noninvasive method that can help identify fat within adrenal lesions and therefore support a benign diagnosis and reduce the need for percutaneous biopsy and serial imaging. Appropriate use of this modality may decrease morbidity and cost of medical care to the patient.

Gadolinium-Enhanced Magnetic Resonance Imaging

Radiologic assessment of renal masses relies largely on CT and ultrasound, and the diagnostic accuracy of these two imaging modalities approaches 100%.[81–84] The demonstration of enhancement within renal masses, indicative of the tumor vascularity, is a key element in the diagnostic workup.[83,84] MRI in the evaluation of renal masses has been reserved for selected cases in which either a tumor thrombus within the renal vein and/or inferior vena cava or invasion of adjacent organs (e.g., liver) is suspected.[85–89]

Another group of patients in whom MRI has been useful are those with impaired renal function. A subset of patients with baseline renal insufficiency or contrast medium allergy are at increased risk for nephrotoxic reactions to iodinated contrast material.[90–99] Some degree of contrast material–induced renal failure has been reported to occur in 15 to 42% of patients with azotemia following administration of an iodinated contrast agent.[81,90] This risk appears to be related to the preinjunction creatinine levels.[96–99] Although most controlled studies have not shown a statistically significant difference in the incidence of adverse effects between ionic and nonionic compounds, lower osmolar agents do seem to cause less nephrotoxicity in patients with renal insufficiency.[98,99]

Gadolinium-enhanced MRI is an alternative

method for evaluating renal masses in this patient group. Gadolinium-DTPA for assessment of renal cell carcinomas has been demonstrated experimentally in both rabbits and humans,[81,82,96] and there are no reports of gadolinum-induced nephrotoxicity.[97–99] In addition, it has also been shown that this agent in its usual dosage is completely eliminated with hemodialysis.[100,101] Gadopentetate dimeglumine-DTPA, like technetium-99m-DTPA, is freely filtered and not reabsorbed by the kidney,[102,103] and the distribution and excretion of this agent is quite similar to that of iodinated contrast material. Although severe anaphylactoid reactions have been reported with gadopentetate dimeglumine, the frequency appears to be on the order of 1:750,000 doses.[104] Preliminary data suggest gadolinium-enhanced MRI is capable of demonstrating tumor enhancement in patients with renal failure, thus providing a noninvasive method of differentiating cysts from tumors in this select patient population.

POSITRON EMISSION TOMOGRAPHY

While the ability to detect oncologic processes using noninvasive cross-sectional imaging techniques has increased dramatically during the last two decades, significant insights have also occurred with methods that quantify tissue metabolism. PET is one noninvasive diagnostic technique that has the capacity to measure the metabolism of specific compounds in tissue. The basis of this technology is a radiotracer, a positron-emitting analogue of glucose, that provides a means of measuring physiologic functions. PET scanning with the glucose analogue 2-deoxy-2-[^{18}F]fluoro-D-glucose (FDG) was initially used to noninvasively assess cardiac and cerebral function.[105–108]

Malignant neoplasms demonstrate increased aerobic glycolysis and avidly take up FDG.[105,109,110] Within malignant cells, FDG is phosphorylated at the 6 position by hexokinase and is then metabolically trapped within the cell.[109,111–113] This increased uptake and retention of FDG has been documented in animal studies and in patients with a variety of tumors, including hepatomas, brain tumors, and thyroid and colon carcinoma.[114–117] Potential applications of this technology in treatment of oncology patients are limitless. PET will play a major role in the diagnosis and treatment of a variety of malignant processes by providing information on primary tumor stage as well as serving as a tool to monitor efficacy of therapy.

By utilizing different radiopharmaceuticals, varied information can be obtained, including quantification of tumor perfusion, evaluation of tumor metabolism, and the monitoring of radiolabeled cytostatic agents.[118] For example, quantification of tumor perfusion necessitates short-lived isotopes provided by copper compounds and oxygen-15–labeled pharmaceuticals.[118,119] PET studies of tumor metabolism are performed with either glucose derivatives or amino acids, including methionine, thyimidine, and tyrosine.[120–125] Cytostatic agents such as 5-fluorouracil have been radiolabeled and evaluated in treatment of different malignancies.[126–129] Because tumors are composed of a heterogeneous population of cells, multiple radiotracers will eventually be needed to evaluate different malignancies and monitor therapeutic responses.

Early experience with PET has provided encour-

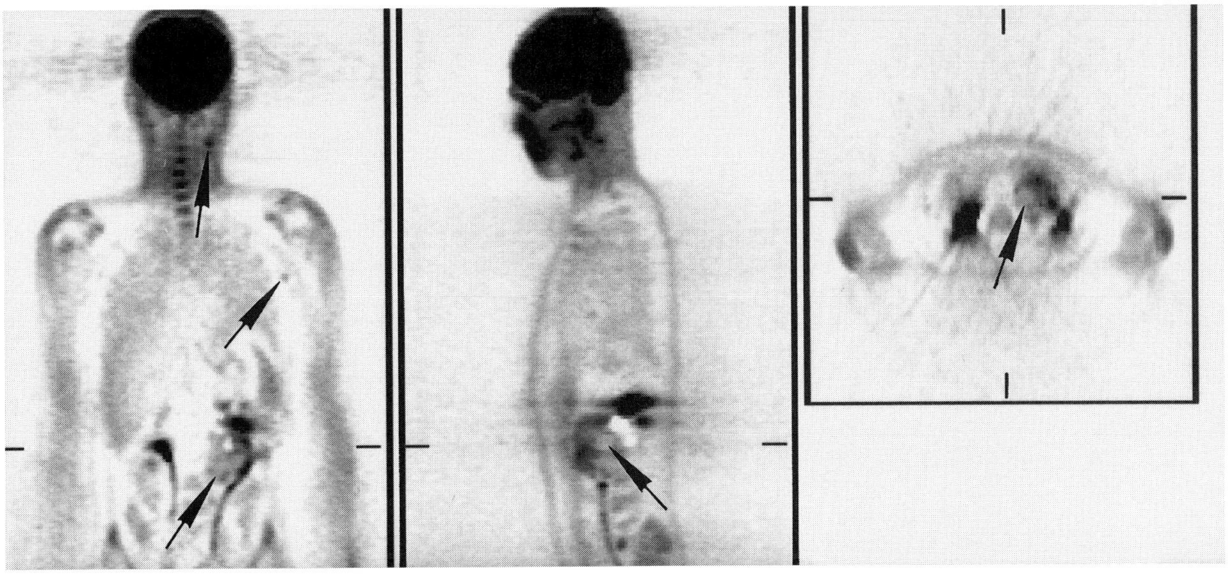

FIGURE 50–4. PET scan using fluorodeoxyglucose of a patient with a history of transitional cell carcinoma. The total body scan demonstrates several abnormal deposits consistent with metastatic disease. There is a large mass adjacent to the left kidney, as well as a left axillary and neck lymph node (demonstrated by the arrows). The sagittal and tomographic images also confirm the presence of metastatic disease in this patient.

aging accuracy in the identification of metastatic lesions associated with renal, bladder, and prostate cancer[105,110,130,131] (see Fig. 50–4). Interestingly, PET scans have demonstrated alterations in tumor metabolism that precede changes appearing on CT and MRI. In addition, PET scans have demonstrated the ability to identify metastases in the presence of normal-appearing radiologic studies, thus providing important staging information.[105,110,130] A decrease in FDG uptake following therapy has been shown to be an early predictor of chemosensitivity and radiosensitivity.[132–134] This ability to evaluate treatment efficacy will facilitate patient selections for continued observation or administration of additional treatment. The future of PET in urologic oncology promises to lead to improvements in diagnosis and therapy in a variety of malignancies.

Although PET has been available for over a decade, the high cost of a scanner and the need for a cyclotron to generate position-emitting radionucleotides, along with the poor resolution relative to other imaging modalities, have limited its application. Although its role may be only complementary to morphologic imaging modalities, including CT and MRI, PET scanning offers a multitude of research possibilities. The future of this technology and its role in the treatment of oncology patients remains to be defined.

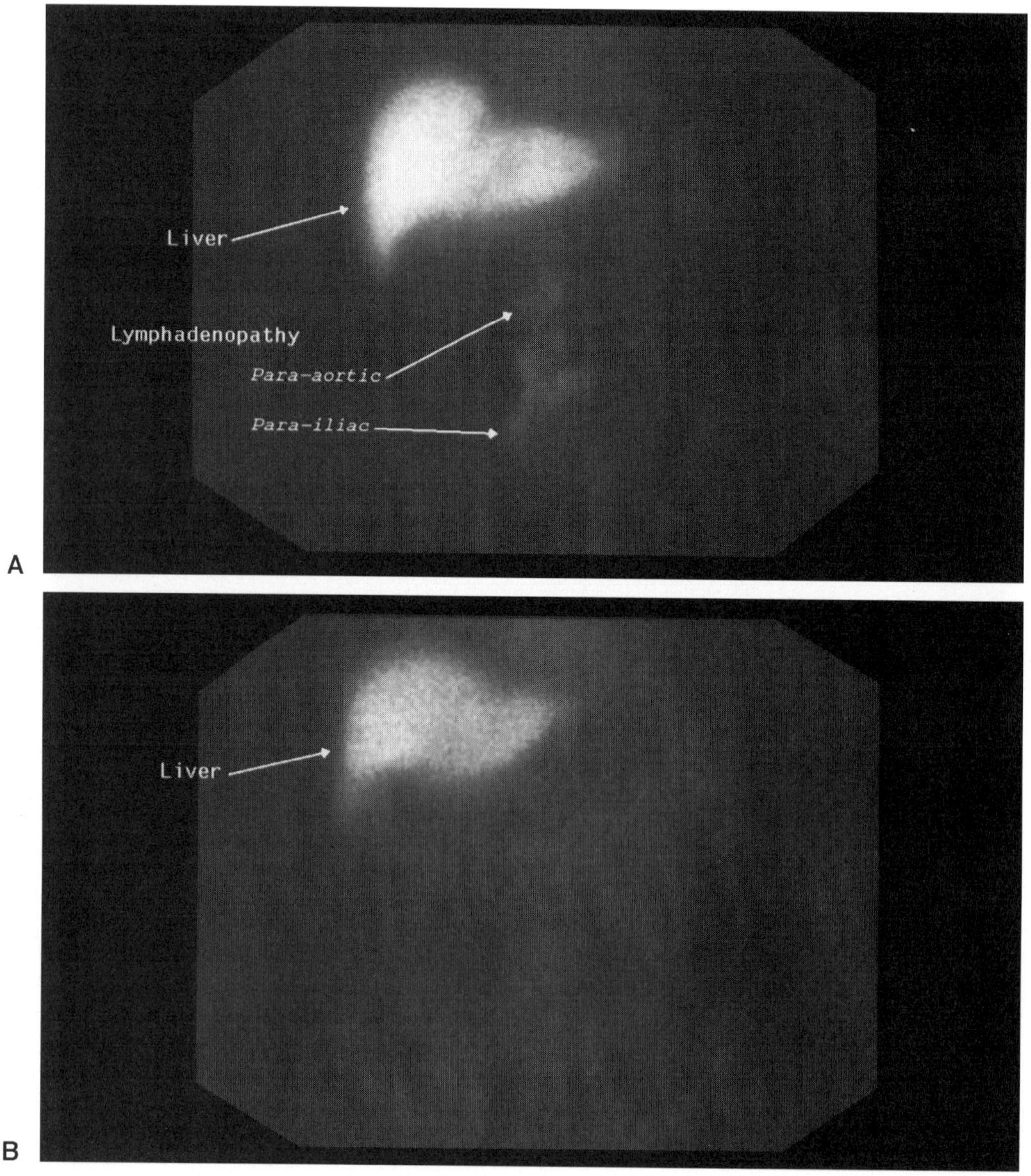
A
Liver
Lymphadenopathy
Para-aortic
Para-iliac
B
Liver

FIGURE 50–5. ^{111}In–CYT-356 immunoscintigraph revealing recurrent prostate cancer in the para-aortic and parailiac lymph nodes in a 57-year-old male with a rising PSA level after a radical prostatectomy and pelvic lymphadenectomy. *A*, Increased signal intensity in the abdominal lymph nodes. *B*, Normal scan from another patient for comparison.

RADIOIMMUNOSCINTIGRAPHY WITH INDIUM-111–LABELED CYT-356

The presence of occult lymphatic metastases in patients with clinically localized prostate cancer portends a worse prognosis and probable recurrence after radical prostatectomy or radiation therapy. Currently, the gold standard for the diagnosis of lymph node metastasis is pelvic lymph node dissection performed either as an open or a laparoscopic procedure. Noninvasive methods using cross-sectional imaging have been ineffective in identifying early lymph node metastasis. CT and MRI have been shown to lack sensitivity because, unless the involved lymph nodes are enlarged greater than 1.5 cm in diameter, they will be interpreted as normal.[135–138]

The presence of recurrent prostate cancer following attempted curative therapy is suggested by a rising serum PSA level and can be equally difficult to localize. The recurrence may be local (e.g., prostatic bed) or distant (e.g., regional lymph nodes) and cannot usually be determined by TRUS, nuclear bone scan, CT, or MRI.[139] A noninvasive method that provides accurate identification of recurrent disease would potentially allow the use of definitive treatment and, it is hoped, increase survival.

7E11-C5.3 is a murine immunoglobulin G1 monoclonal antibody that was produced at the Cytogen Corporation (Princeton, NJ) by establishing a hybridoma cell line from the fusion of murine myeloma cells and spleen cells from mice exposed to the prostate cancer xenograft LNCaP.[140] This antibody recognizes a prostate-specific membrane glycoprotein that is expressed by benign and malignant prostate tissue. Radiolabeling this antibody with ^{111}In has yielded a ^{111}In-CYT-356 conjugate that can be detected with whole-body immunoscintigraphy.

Radioimmunoscintigraphy using this conjugate is currently being used in clinical trials to identify patients with occult lymph node metastasis before definitive treatment and to localize recurrent disease in patients with rising PSA levels after definitive treatment (Figs. 50–5 and 50–6). In two pub-

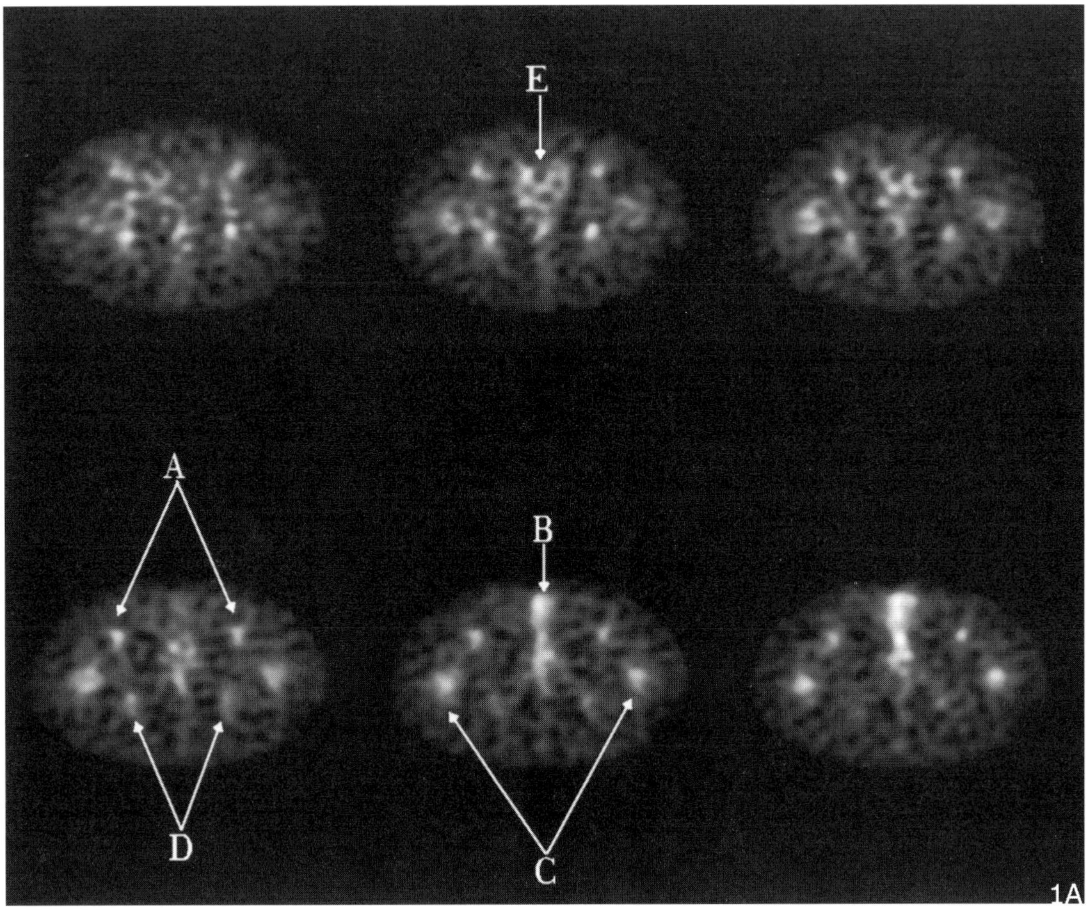
E
A
B
D
C
1A

FIGURE 50–6. ^{111}In–CYT-356 immunoscintigraph showing recurrent prostate cancer within the prostatic fossa in a 61-year-old male with a rising PSA level after radical prostatectomy and pelvic lymphadenectomy. *A*, femoral vasculature; *B*, base of the penis; *C*, head of the femur; *D*, ischial bone marrow; *E*, recurrent tumor in the prostatic fossa. Note that the prostatic fossa is usually found 2 to 3 cm cranial to the increased signal intensity at the base of the penis.

lished studies,[140,141] this technique was reported to be safe with no significant complications; two cases of mild hypotension and one allergic reaction were noted. In both studies, no patient developed human anti-murine antibodies (HAMA). In our current series, we found that no patient experienced a significant complication. However, to date four patients have developed HAMA.

The initial experience in the detection of occult lymphatic spread was reported by Babaian et al.[140] In that study, 19 patients with clinically localized prostate cancer underwent preoperative radioimmunoscintigraphy and the results of the scan were compared to the histologic analysis of the lymph nodes. Eight patients had lymph node metastases pathologically. Immunoscintigraphy detected four of eight of the cases (50%). Of the 11 patients without lymphatic spread, 9 (82%) had negative scans. Therefore, the accuracy of this test was reported as 76%, with a considerably higher specificity than sensitivity. This study established that the technique may be useful in detecting lymphatic spread but more expertise needs to be developed to increase its sensitivity.

The initial experience with the localization of recurrent disease was reported by Kahn et al.[141] In that study, 27 men were identified as having a rising PSA level greater than 0.8 ng/ml after pelvic lymphadenectomy and radical prostatectomy. These patients underwent immunoscintigraphy and the authors compared the results of the scan with previous CT and MRI studies as well as biopsy of the prostatic fossa. Twenty-two patients had abnormal scans. In 11 of 22 (50%), positive correlations were made with the aforementioned modalities. The other 11 patients had either negative radiologic studies or negative prostatic fossa biopsy. As noted previously, cross-sectional imaging is not accurate in evaluating microscopic spread; therefore, the actual sensitivity of this technique may be higher. Certainly, histologic evidence of recurrence either by open or percutaneous biopsy would be necessary to confirm the efficacy of immunoscintigraphy.

Our experience is similar to that of both Babaian and Kahn. We have found that immunoscintigraphy with ^{111}In-CYT-356 has a high specificity in detecting occult lymphatic spread, but that its sensitivity needs to be improved. Likewise, we have identified many cases of recurrent disease by immunoscintigraphy that are not confirmed by the available modalities and need histologic confirmation (Figs. 50–5 and 50–6). It is hoped that, with future efforts, this scan will prove to be useful in the diagnosis and treatment of patients with prostate cancer.

REFERENCES

1. Bosniak MA: The small (<3.0 cm) renal parenchymal tumor: detection, diagnosis, and controversies. Radiology 1991; 179:307–308.
2. Smith SJ, Bosniak MA, Megibow AJ, et al: Renal cell carcinoma: earlier discovery and increased detection. Radiology 1989; 170:699–703.
3. Amendola MA, Bree BL, Pollack HM, et al: Small renal cell carcinoma: resolving a diagnostic dilemma. Radiology 1988; 166:637–640.
4. Parenty RA, Pradel J, Parienty I: Cystic renal cancer: CT characteristics. Radiology 1985; 157:741–744.
5. Balfe DM, McClennan BL, Stanley RJ, et al: Evaluation of renal masses considered indeterminant on computed tomography. Radiology 1982; 142:421–428.
6. Curry NS, Schabel SI, Betstill WL Jr: Small renal neoplasms: diagnostic imaging, pathologic features, and clinical course. Radiology 1986; 158:113–117.
7. Hartman DS, Aronson SA, Frazer H: Current status of imaging renal masses. Radiol Clin North Am 1991; 29: 475–496.
8. Levine E, Huntrakoon M, Wetzell H: Small renal neoplasms: clinical, pathologic, and imaging features. AJR 1989; 153:69–73.
9. Birnbaum BA, Bosniak MA, Megibow AJ, et al: Observations on the growth of renal neoplasms. Radiology 1990; 176:695–701.
10. Kalender WA, Seissler W, Klotz E, et al: Spiral volumetric CT with single-breath-hold technique, continuous transport, and continuous scanner rotation. Radiology 1990; 176:181–190.
11. Villafana T: Technologic advances in computed tomography. Curr Opin Radiol 1991; 3:275–283.
12. Silverman SG, Seltzer SE, Adams DF, et al: Spiral CT of the small indeterminate renal mass: results in 48 patients [Abstract]. Radiology 1991; 181(P):125.
13. Fishman EK, Magid D, Ney DR, et al: Three dimensional CT imaging in orthopedics state of the art 1988. Orthopedics 1988; 2:1021–1026.
14. Pate D, Resnick D, Andre M, et al: Perspective: three dimensional imaging of the musculoskeletal system. AJR 1986; 147:545–551.
15. Burk DL Jr, Mears DC, Kennedy WH, et al: Three dimensional computed tomography of acetabular fractures. Radiology 1985; 155:183–186.
16. Fishman EK, Drebin RA, Magid D, et al: Volumetric rendering techniques: applications for three-dimensional imaging of the hip. Radiology 1987; 163:737–738.
17. Silverman SG, Lee BY, Seltzer SE, et al: Small (<3.0 cm) renal masses: correlation of spiral CT features and pathologic findings. AJR 1994; 163:597–605.
18. Zeman RK, Fox SH, Silverman, PM, et al: Helical (spiral) CT of the abdomen. AJR 1993; 160:719–725.
19. Chernoff DM, Silverman SG, Kikinis R, et al: Three-dimensional imaging and display of renal tumors using spiral CT: a potential aid to partial nephrectomy. Urology 1994; 43:125–129.
20. Assimos DG, Boyce H, Woodruff RD, et al: Intraoperative renal ultrasonography: a useful adjunct to partial nephrectomy. J Urol 1991; 146:1218–1220.
21. Gilbert BR, Russo P, Zirinsky K, et al: Intraoperative sonography: application of renal cell carcinoma. J Urol 1988; 139:582–584.
22. Boring CC, Squires TS, Tong T: Cancer statistics, 1993. CA 1993; 43:7–26.
23. Resnick MI, Willard JW, Boyce, WH: Ultrasonic evaluation of the prostatic nodule. J Urol 1981; 120:86–89.
24. Rifkin MD, Friedland GW, Shortliffe L: Prostatic evaluation by transrectal endosonography: detection of carcinoma. Radiology 1986; 158:85–90.
25. Dahnert WF, Hamper UM, Eggleston JC, et al: Prostatic evaluation by transrectal sonography with histopathologic correlation: the echopenic appearance of early carcinoma. Radiology 1986; 158:97–102.
26. Lee F, Littrup PJ, Kumasaka GH, et al: Use of transrectal ultrasound in the diagnosis, guided biopsy, staging, and screening of prostate cancer. Radiographics 1987; 7:627–644.
27. Rifkin MD, Choi H: Endorectal prostate ultrasound: im-

plications of the small peripherally placed hypoechoic lesion. Radiology 1988; 166:619–622.
28. Lee F, Torp-Pederson S, Littrup PJ, et al: Hypoechoic lesions of the prostate: clinical relevance of the tumor size, digital rectal examination, and prostate-specific antigen. Radiology 1989; 170:29–32.
29. Ragde H, Bagley CM Jr, Aldape HC, et al: Prostate cancer screening with high resolution transrectal ultrasound. J Endourol 1989; 3:115–123.
30. Catalona WJ, Smith DS, Ratliff TL, et al: Measurement of prostate specific antigen in serum as a screening test for prostate cancer. N Engl J Med 1991; 324:1156–1161.
31. Cooner WH, Mosley BR, Rutherford CL, et al: Prostate cancer detection in a clinical urological practice by ultrasonography, digital rectal examination and prostate specific antigen. J Urol 1990; 143:1146–1154.
32. Rifkin MD, Archibald AA, Pisarchik J, et al: Palpable masses in the prostate: superior accuracy of US-guided biopsy compared with the accuracy of digitally guided biopsy. Radiology 1991; 179:41–42.
33. Middleton WD, Thorne DA, Melson GL: Color Doppler ultrasound of the normal testis. AJR 1989; 152:293–297.
34. Middleton WD, Bell MW: Analysis of intratesticular arterial anatomy with emphasis on transmediastinal arteries. Radiology 1993; 189:157–160.
35. Solbiata L, Cioffi V, Ballarti E: Ultrasonography of the neck. Radiol Clin North Am 1992; 30:941–954.
36. Rifkin MD, Sudakoff GS, Archibald AA: Prostate: techniques, results, and potential application of color Doppler US scanning. Radiology 1993; 186:509–513.
37. Fornage BD: Transrectal duplex sonography of prostate carcinoma: preliminary experience [Abstract]. Radiology 1989; 173(P):81.
38. Baran GW, Parulekar SG, Alfidi MM, et al: Color Doppler imaging of the prostate: global pattern analysis of the external gland. (manuscript in preparation)
39. Parulekar SG, Baran GW, Cohen SM, et al: Doppler sonography of hypoechoic areas of the prostate. (manuscript in preparation)
40. Rifkin MD, Alexander AA, Helinek TG, et al: Color Doppler as an adjunct to prostate ultrasound. Scand J Urol Nephrol 1991; 137(Suppl):85–89.
41. Kelly IMG, Lees WR, Rickards D: Prostate cancer and the role of color Doppler US. Radiology 1993; 189:153–156.
42. Rifkin MD, Choi H: Implications of small, peripheral hypoechoic lesions of endorectal US of the prostate. Radiology 1988; 166:619–622.
43. Newman JS, Bree RL, Rubin JM: Prostate cancer: diagnosis with color Doppler sonography with histologic correlation of each biopsy site. Radiology 1995; 195:86–90.
44. Russi S, Blumenthal HT, Gray SH: Small adenomas of the adrenal cortex in hypertension and diabetes. Arch Intern Med 1945; 76:284–291.
45. Glazer HS, Weymn PJ, Sagel SS, et al: Nonfunctioning adrenal masses: incidental discovery on computed tomography. AJR 1982; 139:81–85.
46. Mitnick JS, Bosniak MA, Megibow AJ, et al: Nonfunctional adrenal adenomas discovered incidentally on computed tomography. Radiology 1983; 148:495–499.
47. Copeland PM: The incidentally discovered adrenal mass. Ann Intern Med 1983; 98:940–945.
48. Bernadino M: Management of the asymptomatic patient with a unilateral adrenal mass. Radiology 1988; 166:121–123.
49. Berland LL, Koslin DB, Kenney PJ, et al: Differentiation between small benign and malignant adrenal masses with dynamic incremental CT. AJR 1988; 151:95–101.
50. Pagani JJ: Normal adrenal glands in small cell lung carcinoma: CT-guided biopsy. AJR 1983; 140:949–951.
51. Sandler MA, Pearlberg JL, Madrazo BL, et al: Computed tomographic evaluation of the adrenal gland in the preoperative assessment of bronchogenic carcinoma. Radiology 1982; 145:733–736.
52. Hussian S, Belldegrun A, Seltzer SE, et al: Differentiation of malignant from benign adrenal masses: predictive indices on computed tomography. AJR 1985; 144:61–65.
53. Lee M, Hahn PF, Papanicolaou N, et al: Benign and malignant adrenal masses: CT distinction with attenuation coefficients, size, and observer analysis. Radiology 1991; 179:415–418.
54. Reinig JW, Doppman JL, Dwyer AJ, et al: MRI of indeterminate adrenal masses. AJR 1986; 147:493–496.
55. Baker ME, Blinder R, Spritzer C, et al: MR evaluation of adrenal masses at 1.5 T. AJR 1989; 153:307–312.
56. Miyake H, Maeda H, Tashiro M, et al: CT of adrenal tumor: frequency and clinical significance of low-attenuation lesions. AJR 1989; 152:1005–1007.
57. Kier R, McCarthy S: MR characterization of adrenal masses: field strength and pulse sequence considerations. Radiology 1989; 171:671–674.
58. Bernandino ME, Walther MM, Phillips VM, et al: CT-guided adrenal biopsy: accuracy, safety, and indications. AJR 1985; 144:67–69.
59. Casola G, Nicolet V, Van Sonnenberg E, et al: Unsuspected pheochromocytoma: risk of blood-pressure alterations during percutaneous adrenal biopsy. Radiology 1986; 159:733–735.
60. Reinig JW, Stutley JE, Leonhardt CM, et al: Differentiation of adrenal masses with MR imaging: comparison of techniques. Radiology 1994; 192:41–46.
61. Glazer GM, Woolsey EJ, Borello J: Adrenal tissue characterizations in MR imaging. Radiology 1986; 158:73–79.
62. Tsushima Y, Ishizaka H, Matsumoto M: Adrenal masses: differentiation with chemical shift, fast low-angle shot MR imaging. Radiology 1993; 186:705–709.
63. Mitchell DG, Crovello M, Matteucci T, et al: Benign adrenocortical masses: diagnosis with chemical shift MR imaging. Radiology 1992; 185:345–351.
64. Krestin GP, Friedmann G, Fischback R, et al: Evaluation of adrenal masses in oncologic patients: dynamic contrast-enhanced MR vs CT. J Comput Assist Tomogr 1991; 15:104–110.
65. Chezmar JL, Robbins SM, Nelson RC, et al: Adrenal masses: characterization with T1-weighted imaging. Radiology 1988; 166:357–359.
66. Krestin GP, Steinbrich W, Friedmann G, et al: Adrenal masses: evaluation with fast gradiant-echo MR imaging and GD-DTPA-enhanced dynamic studies. Radiology 1989; 171:675–680.
67. Remer EM, Weinfeld RM, Glazer GM, et al: Hyperfunctioning and nonhyperfunctioning benign adrenal cortical lesions: characterization and comparison with MR imaging. Radiology 1989; 171:681–685.
68. Chan TW, Listerud J, Kressel HY: Combined chemical-shift and phase-selective imaging for fat suppression: theory and initial clinical experience. Radiology 1991; 181: 41–47.
69. Semelka RC, Shoenut JP, Lawrence PH, et al: Evaluation of adrenal masses with gadolinium enhancement and fat-suppression MR imaging. J Magn Reson Imaging 1993; 3: 337–343.
70. Tsushima Y, Ishizaka H, Kato T, et al: Differential diagnosis of adrenal masses using out-of-phase flash imaging. Acta Radiol 1992; 33:262–265.
71. Bilbey JH, McLoughlin RF, Kurkjian PS, et al: MR imaging of adrenal masses: value of chemical-shift imaging for distinguishing adrenomas from other tumors. AJR 1995; 164:637–642.
72. Buxton RB, Wismer GL, Brady TJ, et al: Quantitative proton chemical shift imaging. Magn Reson Med 1986; 3: 881–890.
73. Dixon WT: Simple proton spectroscopic imaging. Radiology 1984; 153:189–194.
74. Levenson H, Greensite F, Hoefs J, et al: Fatty infiltration of the liver: quantification with phase-contrast MR imaging at 1.5 T vs biopsy. AJR 1991; 156:307–312.
75. Poon CS, Szumowski J, Plewes DB, et al: Fat/water quantitation and differential relaxation time measurement us-

ing chemical shift imaging technique. Magn Reson Med 1989; 7:369–382.
76. Rosen LR, Carter MA, Pykett LL: Proton chemical shift imaging: an evaluation of its clinical potential using an in vivo fatty liver mode. Radiology 1985; 154:469–472.
77. Mitchell DM, Kim I, Chang TS, et al: Chemical shift phase-difference and suppression magnetic resonance imaging techniques in animals, phantoms, and humans: fatty liver. Invest Radiol 1991; 26:1041–1052.
78. Leroy-Willig A, Bittoun J, Luton JP: A step forward in the characterization of adrenal cortical lesions [Letter]. Radiology 1993; 188:880–881.
79. Leroy-Willig A, Bittoun J, Luton JP, et al: In vivo MR spectroscopic imaging of the adrenal glands: distinction between adenomas and carcinomas larger than 15 mm based on lipid content. AJR 1989; 153:771–773.
80. Ichikawa T, Fujimoto H, Murakami K, et al: Adrenal tissue characterization with 0.-T MR imaging: value of T2*-weighted images. J Magn Reson Imaging 1993; 3:742–745.
81. Rofksy NM, Weinreb JC, Bosniak MA, et al: Renal lesion characterization with gadolinium-enhanced MR imaging: efficacy and safety in patients with renal insuffiency. Radiology 1991; 180:85–89.
82. Eileenberg SS, Lee JK, Brown JJ, et al: Renal masses: evaluation with gradiant-echo Gd-DTPA-enhanced dynamic MR imaging. Radiology 1990; 176:333–338.
83. Balfe DM, McClennan BL, Stanley RJ, et al: Evaluation of renal masses considered indeterminant on computed tomography. Radiology 1982; 142:421–428.
84. Sagel SS, Stanley RJ, Levitt RG, et al: Computed tomography of the kidney. Radiology 1977; 124:359–370.
85. Bosniak MA: The current radiological approach to renal cysts. Radiology 1986; 158:1–10.
86. Hricak H, Thoeni RF, Carroll PR: Detection and staging of renal neoplasms: a reassessment of MR imaging. Radiology 1988; 166:643–634.
87. Karstaed TN, McCullough DL, Wolfman NT: Magnetic resonance imaging of the renal mass. J Urol 1986; 136: 566–570.
88. Pritchett TR, Raval JK, Benson RC, et al: Preoperative magnetic resonance imaging of vena cava tumor thrombi: experience with five cases. J Urol 1987; 138:1220–1222.
89. Fein AB, Lee JKT, Balfe DM, et al: Diagnosis and staging of renal cell carcinoma: a comparison of MR imaging and CT. AJR 1987; 148:748–753.
90. McClennan BL: Ionic and nonionic iodinated contrast media: evolution and strategies for use. AJR 1990; 155:225–233.
91. Brezis M, Epstein FH: A closer look at radiocontrast-induced nephropathy [Editorial]. N Engl J Med 1989; 323: 179–182.
92. Schwab SJ, Hlatky MA, Pieper CJ, et al: Contrast nephrotoxicity: a randomized controlled trial of a nonionic and ionic radiographic contrast agent. N Engl J Med 1989; 323: 149–153.
93. Berns AS: Nephrotoxicity of contrast media. Kidney Int 1989; 35:730–740.
94. Cigarrao RG, Lange RA, Williams RH, et al: Dosing of contrast material to prevent contrast nephropathy in patients with renal disease. Am J Med 1989; 86:649–652.
95. Parfrey PS, Griffith SM, Barrett BJ, et al: Contrast material-induced renal failure in patients with diabetes mellitus, renal insufficiency; or both: a prospective, controlled study. N Engl J Med 1989; 320:143–149.
96. Yancey M, Ackerman MY, Kaude JV, et al: Gadolinium-DTPA enhancement of VX-2 carcinoma of the rabbit kidney on T1 weighted magnetic resonance images. Acta Radiol 1987; 28:479–482.
97. Carr DH, Brown J, Bydder GM, et al: Gadolinium-DTPA as contrast agent in MRI: initial clinical experience in 23 patients. AJR 1984; 143:215–224.
98. Lautin EM, Freeman NJ, Schoenfeld AH, et al: Radiocontrast-associated renal dysfunction: incidence and risk factors. AJR 1991; 157:49–58.
99. Bush WH Jr, Mclennan DL, Swanson DP: Contrast media reactions: prediction, prevention, and treatment. Postgrad Radiol 1993; 13:136–148.
100. Krahe T, Landwehr P, Gotz R, et al: The dialysability of gadolinium-DTPA [Abstract]. Radiology 1990; 177(P): 167.
101. Lackner K, Krahe T, Haustein J: The dialysability of Gd-DTPA. *In* Bydder G, Felix R, Buchelor E, et al (eds): Contrast Media in MRI, pp 321–327. Brinklaan, The Netherlands, Medicom, 1990.
102. Wesolowski CA, Conrad GR, Kirchner PT, et al: A direct modeling approach to the early renal vascular transit of Tc 99m chelates. Med Phys 1987; 14:1032–1041.
103. Chervu LR, Blaufox MD: Renal radiopharmaceuticals: an update. Semin Nucl Med 1982; 12:224–245.
104. Lufkin RB: Severe anaphylactoid reaction to Gd-DTPA [Letter]. Radiology 1990; 176:879.
105. Wahl RL, Harney J, Hutchins G, et al: Imaging of renal cancer using positron emission tomography with 2-deoxy-2-(18F)-fluoro-d-glucose: pilot animal and human studies. J Urol 1991; 146:1470–1473.
106. Phelps ME, Huang SC, Hoffman EJ, et al: Tomographic measurement of local cerebral glucose metabolic rate in humans with (F-18) 2-fluoro-2-deoxy-D-glucose: validation of method. Ann Neurol 1979; 6:371.
107. Gallagher BM, Ansari A, Atkins H, et al: Radiopharmaceuticals XXVII. F8-labelled 2-deoxy-2-fluoro-D-glucose as a radiopharmaceutical for measuring regional myocardial glucose metabolism in vivo: tissue distribution and imaging studies in animals. J Nucl Med 1977; 18:977.
108. Schelbert HR, Henze E, Phelps ME, et al: Assessment of regional myocardial ischemia by positron-emission computed tomography. Am Heart J 1982; 103:588.
109. Walburg O: The Metabolism of Tumors, pp 129–169. London, Constable and Co., Ltd, 1931.
110. Harney JV, Wahl RL, Liebert M, et al: Uptake of 2-deoxy,2-(18F) fluoro-D-glucose in bladder cancer: animal localization and initial patient positron emission tomography. J Urol 1991; 145:279–283.
111. Som P, Atkins HL, Bandopadhyay D, et al: A fluorinated glucose analog, 2-fluoro-2-deoxy-D-glucose (F-18): nontoxic tracer for rapid tumor detection. J Nucl Med 1980; 21:670.
112. Gallagher BM, Fowler JS, Gutterson NI, et al: Metabolic trapping as a principle of radiopharmaceuticals design: some factors responsible for biodistribution of [18F]-deoxy-2-fluoro-D-glucose. J Nucl Med 1978; 19:1154.
113. Monakhov NK, Neistadt EL, Shavlovski MM, et al: Physicochemical properties and isoenzyme composition of hexokinase from normal and malignant human tissues. J Natl Cancer Inst 1978; 61:27.
114. Francavilla TL, Miletich RS, DiChiro G, et al: Positron emission tomography in the detection of malignant generation of low-grade gliomas. Neurosurgery 1989; 24:1.
115. Larson SM, Weiden PL, Grunbaum Z, et al: Positron imaging feasibility studies. II: Characteristics of 2-deoxyglucose uptake in rodent and canine neoplasms. J Nucl Med 1981; 22:875.
116. Joensuu H, Ahonen A, Klemi P: 18 F-fluorodeoxyglucose imaging in the preoperative diagnosis of thyroid malignancy. Eur J Nucl Med 1988; 13:50.
117. Yonekura G, Benua RS, Brill AP, et al: Increased accumulation of 2-deoxy-2-[18]fluoro-D-glucose in liver metastases from colon carcinoma. J Nucl Med 1988; 23: 1133.
118. Strauss LG, Conti PS: The applications of PET in clinical oncology. J Nucl Med 1991; 32:623–648.
119. Mathias CJ, Welch MJ, Raichle ME, et al: Evaluation of a potential generator-produced PET tracer for cerebral perfusion imaging: single-pass cerebral extraction measurements and imaging with radiolabeled Cu-PTSM. J Nucl Med 1990; 31:351–359.
120. Bolster JM, Vaalburg W, Paans AM, et al: Carbon-11-labeled tyrosine to study tumor metabolism by positron emission tomography (PET). Eur J Nucl Med 1986; 29: 321–324.

121. Martiat P, Farrant A, Labar D, et al: In vivo measurement of carbon-11-thymidine uptake in non-Hodgkin's lymphoma using positron emission tomography. J Nucl Med 1988; 29:1633–1637.
122. Kubota K, Yamada K, Fukuda H, et al: Tumor detection with carbon-11-labeled amino acids. Eur J Nucl Med 1984; 9:136–140.
123. Kubota K, Matsuzawa T, Fujiwara T, et al: Differential diagnosis of solitary pulmonary nodules with positron emission tomography using [11C]-L-methionine. J Comput Assist Tomogr 1988; 12:794–796.
124. Strauss LG, Clorius JH, Schlag P, et al: Recurrence of colorectal tumors: PET evaluation. Radiology 1989; 170: 329–332.
125. Nagata Y, Yamamoto K, Hiroka M, et al: Monitoring liver tumor therapy with [18F]FDG positron emission tomography. J Comput Assist Tomogr 1990; 14:370–374.
126. Ischiwata K, Ido T, Abe Y, et al: Studies on F-labeled pyrimidine III. Biochemical investigation of F-labeled pyrimidines and comparison with H-deoxythymidine in tumor-bearing rats and mice. Eur J Nucl Med 1985; 10: 39–44.
127. Haberkorn U, Strauss LG, Dimitrakopoulou A, et al: PET studies of fluorodeoxyglycose metabolism in patients with recurrent colorectal tumors receiving radiotherapy. J Nucl Med 1991; 32:1485–1490.
128. Ginos JZ, Cooper AJL, Dhawan V, et al: [13N] cisplatin PET to assess pharmacokinetics of intra-arterial versus intravenous chemotherapy for malignant brain tumors. J Nucl Med 1987; 28:1844–1852.
129. Diksic MA, Mitsuka S, Conway T, et al: Use a PET to evaluate in vivo pharmacokinetics of chemotherapeutic agents BCNU and SarCNU in humans. Tumor Diagnostik Therapie 1988; 9:171.
130. Letocha H, Ahlstrom H, Malmstroms PU, et al: Positron emission tomography with L-methionine in the monitoring of therapy response in muscle-invasive transitional cell carcinoma of the urinary bladder. Br J Urol 1994; 74: 767–774.
131. Bachor R, Kleinschmidt K, Kocher F, et al: Positron emission tomography for the diagnosis of urological tumors [Abstract]. J Urol 1995; 153:954S.
132. Iosilevsky G, Front D, Bettman L, et al: Uptake of gallium-67 citrate and [2-H] deoxyglucose in tumor model, following chemotherapy and radiotherapy. J Nucl Med 1985; 26:278.
133. Minn H, Payl R, Ahonen A: Evaluation of treatment response to radiotherapy in head and neck cancer with fluorodeoxyglucose. J Nucl Med 1988; 29:1521.
134. Minn H, Soini I: [18-F] Fluorodeoxyglucose scintigraphy in diagnosis and follow up of treatment in advanced breast cancer. Eur J Nucl Med 1989; 15:61.
135. Hricak H, Dooms GC, Jeffrey RB, et al: Prostatic carcinoma: staging, clinical assessment, CT and MR imaging. Radiology 1987; 162:331–336.
136. Rifkin MD, Zerhouni EA, Gatsonis CA, et al: Comparison of magnetic resonance imaging and ultrasonography in staging early prostate cancer. N Engl J Med 1990; 323: 621–626.
137. Weinerman PM, Arger PH, Coleman BG, et al: Pelvic adenopathy from bladder and prostate carcinoma: detection by rapid sequence computed tomography. AJR 1983; 140: 95–99.
138. Wolf JS, Cher M, Dall'era M, et al: The use and accuracy of cross-sectional imaging and fine needle aspiration cytology for detection of pelvic lymph node metastases before radical prostatectomy. J Urol 1995; 153:993–999.
139. Spencer JA, Golding SJ: Patterns of lymphatic metastases at recurrence of prostate cancer: CT findings. Clin Radiol 1994; 49:404–407.
140. Babaian RJ, Sayer J, Podoloff DA, et al: Radioimmunoscintigraphy of pelvic lymph nodes with ^{111}indium-labeled monoclonal antibody CYT-356. J Urol 1994; 152: 1952–1955.
141. Kahn D, Williams RD, Seldin DW, et al: Radioimmunoscintigraphy with ^{111}indium labeled CYT-356 for the detection of occult prostate cancer recurrence. J Urol 1994; 152:1490–1495.

51

NUTRITIONAL ISSUES FOR THE CANCER PATIENT

TERRY W. HENSLE, M.D. *and* JAMES C. KU, M.D.

The close relationship between nutritional status and surgical outcome has been acknowledged for a number of years. It is now generally accepted that malnutrition significantly affects the hospital course of patients undergoing major surgery.[1-3] Malnutrition also has direct bearing on the morbidity and mortality of seriously traumatized and septic patients. Severe protein loss has been shown to impede tissue repair, reduce resistance to infections, and interfere with enzyme and plasma protein synthesis.

Malnutrition is a major risk factor for the development of infection in the general surgical population. Immune defects seen in malnutrition include low levels of complement, impaired opsonic and neutrophil function, impaired delayed hypersensitivity, decreased lymphoid mass and function, and a reprioritization of acute-phase proteins.[4] Nutritional repletion reverses this immune dysfunction, resulting in a decrease in infectious morbidity and mortality.

Recent studies have demonstrated that up to 50% of hospitalized general surgical or general medical patients are malnourished to some degree.[5,6] This demonstration of the wide prevalence of in-hospital malnutrition has brought the problem into focus. If urologists are to accept the responsibility for the delivery of optimal medical and surgical care, they must accurately establish the nature of the patients' nutritional status and the extent of their nutritional needs.

NUTRITIONAL ASSESSMENT: MEASUREMENT OF BODY COMPONENTS

Nutritional assessment should be an integral part of the evaluation of all patients who are scheduled for an extensive surgical procedure or for some form of antineoplastic therapy. It has been clearly demonstrated that such surveillance can minimize the risk of elective or semielective cardiac surgery or solid tumor surgery.[7] Therefore, it becomes essential for the surgeon to accurately establish the nature and extent of the individual patient's nutritional needs in order to formulate a reasonable plan of nutritional support. Nutritional assessment is an inexact science and is generally based on measurement of body mass, anthropomorphic measurements, biochemical parameters, and functional studies. Clearly a history of weight loss or gain, anorexia, vomiting, diarrhea, or any chronic illness provides valuable insight into the nutritional status of a patient. Additionally, careful physical exam may provide further clues to the nutritional status of a patient. Muscle wasting, weakness, loss of thenar muscles, loss of body fat, or edema of hypoproteinemia suggests malnutrition.

A nutritional assessment includes characterization of several components for comparison with standards of the key body constituents. Measurement of the weight-height ratio provides a rough estimate of nutritional status; however, changes in fluid balance can affect this estimate significantly. A history of weight loss also provides useful information regarding nutritional status; in general, a weight loss of 5% in 1 month or 10% in 6 months indicates severe weight loss.[8] This information alone, however, does not provide information regarding the nature of the weight loss; the loss may be secondary to fluid loss, protein depletion, or fat catabolism. Thus further investigative studies are necessary. In its simplest form, a nutritional assessment also includes the measurement of the body protein stores, fat stores, and energy expenditure.

Skeletal Muscle Protein

A simple and accurate method of assessing the skeletal muscle compartment is to measure the mid-arm muscle circumference and compare it to known standards for age and sex.[9] Estimation of creatinine-height index (CHI) also indicates the quantity of muscle stores and is a sensitive measure of protein depletion in cachectic and marasmic states.[10] In obese or edematous patients, the height-weight index may not provide an accurate estimate of the nutritional status and therefore, has limited application in nutritional assessment.

Visceral Protein

In stress conditions, loss of secretory or visceral protein occurs rapidly. Biochemical markers in nutritional assessment most commonly include albumin, transferrin, and prealbumin.[11] Other markers that have been studied include retinol-binding protein, C-reactive protein, complement, and fibronectin. Of the visceral proteins, albumin has been shown in multiple studies to be the best single predictor of outcome.[12] Serum albumin levels below 3.0 mg/dl generally represent a significant depletion. Levels can be depressed secondary to transcapillary leakage following periods of stress induced by sepsis, surgery, or other injury. Because of the long half-life of albumin (18 to 20 days), the utility of serum albumin in monitoring the effectiveness of nutritional support may be limited[13]; monitoring of acute changes may be facilitated by monitoring serum transferrin (half-life 7 days) and urinary nitrogen excretion. Serum transferrin also has limitations in that it is also affected by iron levels, stress, and blood transfusions in addition to nutritional status.[13] The cellular immune system also reflects important visceral function. Measurements of the total lymphocyte count, together with delayed cutaneous hypersensitivity reaction to recall skin test antigens (SKSD, mumps, *Candida*), are particularly useful indicators of the visceral protein compartment.[10]

Fat Stores

The major energy store in the body is fat, and fat mass can adequately be measured by tricep skinfold. This is not as accurate as weighing patients underwater; however, it is usually more readily tolerated by the patients and much easier to carry out. Given the fact that each pound of fat contains 3500 kcal, only a severe loss (<60% of standard) represents significant depletion of stored energy.

Extent of Hypermetabolism

It is interesting to note that the degree of hypermetabolism, as measured by urinary nitrogen loss, in the patient undergoing radical cystectomy places that patient in the same category of metabolic injury as patients with multiple long bone fractures and just below patients with severe sepsis and major body burns. Unless nutritional support is provided, this hypermetabolism can lead to extensive cumulative protein loss. The relationship between urea nitrogen excretion and metabolic rate is due to the obligatory oxidation of body cell mass that occurs with stress or starvation. Thus energy expenditure and extent of hypermetabolism (percentage above normal) can be predicted from a simple clinical determination of urea nitrogen in a 24-hour urine collection.[14] Generally, serum albumin, arm muscle circumference, and the CHI are not sensitive enough parameters to evaluate the efficacy of nutritional therapy over the short term. Nitrogen balance is one of the more sensitive methods to assess the effects of nutritional therapy on a daily basis.

Thus a wide variety of tests are available to determine nutritional status; these include anthropomorphic measurements, biochemical data, immunologic analyses, and muscle function tests. However, there is no clear consensus on the best method to interpret the available data.[15] One commonly used method is the prognostic nutritional index (PNI); this equation combines data from serum albumin, transferrin, triceps skinfold thickness, and delayed hypersensitivity results to assess nutritional status[16]:

$$\text{PNI} = 158 - 16.6(\text{ALB}) - 0.78(\text{TSF})$$
$$- 0.20(\text{TFN}) - 5.8(\text{DH})$$

In this formula, albumin (ALB) is measured in grams per liter, triceps skinfold (TSF) in millimeters, and serum transferrin (TFN) in milligrams per liter; delayed hypersensitivity (DH) is scored as 0 for nonreactive, 1 for less than 5 mm of induration, and 2 for over 5 mm of induration. Scores over 50 are defined as high risk, scores from 40 to 49 are intermediate risk, and scores less than 40 are low risk. Some investigators have suggested that careful history and physical examination are equally effective predictors of nutritional status.[17–19] Another commonly used measurement is the subjective global assessment (SGA).[20] The SGA assesses nutritional status based upon historical information (weight change, dietary change, gastrointestinal symptoms, functional capacity) and also objective data (subcutaneous fat loss, muscle wasting, ankle edema, and ascites).

Detsky and colleagues have evaluated the accuracy of various nutritional assessment methods in 59 surgical patients and concluded that the SGA has the highest sensitivity and specificity.[18] The SGA was superior to any single objective measurement tested (albumin, transferrin, delayed cutaneous hypersensitivity, anthropometry, and CHI) and also the PNI. Combining any of the objective measurements with the SGA did not improve sensitivity or specificity. The second best combination was either the PNI or the CHI.

TYPES OF IN-HOSPITAL MALNUTRITION

Nutritional assessment makes it possible to identify and categorize patients with in-hospital malnutrition. Kwashiorkor, a type of protein malnutrition, is a disease state associated with severe depletion of the visceral protein compartment, lowering of serum albumin and transferrin values, and a depression of cell-mediated immunity. There may be little or no associated change in anthropometric measurements or height-weight index in these patients.

Marasmus (protein-calorie malnutrition) is the more common form of in-hospital malnutrition. There may be some depression of the visceral protein compartment; however, there is marked loss of skeletal muscle compartment and body fat stores, demonstrated by reduction of all the anthropometric measurements. A combination of kwashiorkor and marasmus is a frequent accompaniment of chronic illness. This process leads to a depression of anthropometric measurements as well as measurements of the visceral protein compartment.

Once a nutritional defect has been identified, a period of at least 2 weeks is necessary for objective response to nutritional therapy. Only when there has been some measure of response (i.e., return of cellular immunity, increase in serum albumin levels, or weight gain) can a patient be considered an appropriate candidate for surgery. When one assesses the consequences of failing to treat malnutrition in terms of hospital cost and patient morbidity, it becomes essential to recognize malnutrition early, repair the deficit, and minimize complications.

CANCER CACHEXIA

Cancer cachexia refers to a constellation of symptoms characterized by inanition, anorexia, weakness, and weight loss. Anemia, impaired immunity, and organ dysfunction are often associated with this syndrome. Enhanced toxicity of chemotherapeutic drugs may also be present as a result of decreased drug clearance, decreased hepatic metabolism, and decreased biliary and serum clearance.[21] The true etiology of cancer cachexia is unclear, but evidence suggests that the cause is multifactorial. Up to 50% of cancer patients may have symptoms and signs of cachexia at the time of initial diagnosis.[22]

Inadequate caloric intake is the major contributor in most patients with weight loss. Nausea, vomiting, diarrhea, mucositis, and the presence of gastrointestinal malignancy may all promote malnutrition. Patients may also suffer from depression, altered taste sensation, and even food aversion. Clearly the presence of bowel obstruction, malabsorption, or odynophagia/dysphagia will adversely affect nutritional status. Although inadequate caloric intake is a major cause of malnutrition in cancer patients, other factors clearly are important in the development of the cancer cachexia syndrome. Some patients continue to experience weight loss despite an apparently adequate caloric intake.[23]

An increase in metabolic demands or an increase in the resting energy expenditure (REE) has been suggested as a factor in cancer cachexia. Tumor burden itself probably only plays a small role in REE because profound cachexia can be seen with tumors representing less than 0.1% of body mass. Studies of REE in cancer patients have suggested an increased REE, but results have been variable. No consistent elevation in REE has been seen in cancer patients.[22,24] In a study of 200 malnourished cancer patients by Knox et al.,[25] increased REE was seen in only 26% of patients; a normal or decreased REE was seen in the remaining 74% of patients.

Abnormalities in glucose metabolism and insulin resistance have also been demonstrated in cancer patients. Glucose intolerance, often seen in cancer patients, is related to reduced tissue sensitivity to insulin.[26] Increased glucose recycling from lactate has also been demonstrated.[27] This futile metabolic pathway, known as the Cori cycle, converts glucose to lactate and then reconverts the lactate to glucose by gluconeogenesis. This inefficient energy usage has been estimated to consume up to 250 to 300 kcal/day.[28] Increased protein catabolism has been seen with cancer by several investigators.[29–31] Protein turnover and hypermetabolism are generally elevated in patients with cancer cachexia. Increased lipolysis, hyperlipidemia, and decreased fat mass are also frequently seen in cancer cachexia.[32]

In addition, circulating factors either of host or tumor origin are believed to play a major role in the pathogenesis of cancer cachexia. Tumor necrosis factor (TNF), interleukin-1 (IL-1), and interleukin-6 (IL-6) have been all implicated as inducers of anorexia. IL-1, TNF, and IL-6 are potent inducers of anorexia, and IL-1 and TNF are known to promote proteolysis and skeletal muscle wasting.[21,33] In addition, TNF has been shown in cell culture studies to inhibit the transcription of several enzymes involved in lipogenesis.[34] Current evidence suggests that TNF may be the major cytokine involved in the pathogenesis of cancer cachexia.[21,33]

THE UROLOGIC ONCOLOGY PATIENT

There are several misconceptions regarding nutrition and cancer. Although many diseases, such as arteriosclerosis, hypertension, diabetes, degenerative diseases, and certain tumors, clearly have nutritional concomitants, there are no current data to support or refute any role for nutrition in the development or resolution of urologic cancers.

What is certain, however, is that protein-calorie malnutrition is the most common secondary diagnosis in all patients with malignant disease. This malnutrition is less a consequence of the tumor pathophysiology than of the patient's altered food intake. On initial presentation, many cancer patients have already lost weight as a result of tumor activity, anxiety, and pain. Treatment with chemotherapy, radiotherapy, immunotherapy, and surgery causes injury to tissue and a need for repair of tissue. Thus nutrition of the cancer patient is a serious challenge for the physician.

Cachexia in the cancer patient has been recognized for centuries. It has many causes. Both tumor dysfunction and hypermetabolism may well play at least some role; however, dysphagia, anorexia, nausea, and vomiting are the most important causes.

Diet and Prostate Cancer

The relationship between diet and prostate cancer is poorly understood. There is a great deal of evidence that suggests that genetic and environmental influences play an important role in both the pathogenesis and progression of prostate cancer. Although the incidence of latent or clinically insignificant prostate cancer is relatively similar in both Asia and the United States, the rate of clinically significant prostate cancer is much higher in the United States.[35,36] In addition, Asian men who migrate to this country, after one generation, have higher incidences of prostate cancer at a level that approaches the average U.S. incidence.[37] Furthermore, the incidence of prostate cancer in Japan has been increasing in conjunction with the increased influence of Western diet and lifestyle.[38] These observations support the belief that environmental factors are important in tumor progression, and diet has been implicated as one important environmental factor in both the progression and initiation of prostate cancer.

One dietary agent that has been suspected as a causative agent is fat, in particular animal fat. The mechanism of action is speculative, but some investigators have shown that dietary fat can influence androgen metabolism.[39] Other potential mechanisms include alterations in eicosanoid synthesis (prostaglandin and leukotrienes), membrane phospholipid composition, and free radical formation from fatty acid oxidation.[40,41]

Armstrong and Doll have reported that prostate cancer mortality rates for different countries are highly correlated with estimates of total fat consumption.[42] In a separate study of 28 countries, a correlation of 0.704 was found between dietary fat and prostate cancer risk.[43] Rose and Connolly confirmed these findings and additionally demonstrated a strong correlation between animal fat consumption (expressed as percent of total calories) and prostate cancer mortality.[44] No relationship was observed when only vegetable fats were examined.[44] Case-control studies in general support the relationship between prostate cancer and dietary fat intake.[45–49] Several studies show a positive relationship with increasing estimates of fat intake and increased risk[46–48]; however, most studies do not show a dose-response relationship. Interestingly, no clear relationship between obesity and prostate cancer risk has been demonstrated.[44]

A recent case-control study of U.S. male physicians has reported that certain plasma fatty acids (α-linolenic acid) are associated with increased risk of prostate cancer.[50] The relative risks (RRs) of prostate cancer for men in the three highest quartiles of plasma α-linolenic acid level were 3.0 (95% confidence interval [CI], 1.2 to 7.3), 3.4 (95% CI, 1.6 to 7.5), and 2.1 (95% CI, 0.9 to 4.9). Although a true dose-response effect was not seen, α-linolenic levels were positively correlated with meat and dairy food intake. The relative risk for red meat consumption at least five times per week versus less than once per week was 2.5 (95% CI, 0.9 to 6.7). Adjustment for plasma α-linolenic acid did not appreciably change this estimate. Dairy consumption was not associated with prostate cancer in this analysis. In addition, no relationship was seen for other fatty acids examined: oleic acid, linoleic acid, eicosapentaenoic acid (an omega-3 fatty acid), and palmitic and stearic acid.

These results are supported by another earlier prospective report, the Health Professionals Follow-up Study.[51] Using dietary histories, the investigators reported that α-linolenic acid intake was positively associated with prostate cancer and also with advanced prostate cancer. Intake of red meat was also positively and independently associated with advanced prostate cancer. Again, no relationship was seen with dairy intake.

Diet and Bladder Cancer

The effect of diet and behavior on bladder cancer has also been found to be the strongest risk factor for the development of bladder cancer. Cigarette smoking has been estimated to account for about 40 to 50% of all bladder cancers. Another major potential etiologic factor is diet; currently major areas of interest include total energy intake, fat intake, protein intake, vitamin intake, and even water intake. The use of artificial sweeteners, coffee, and alcohol have been investigated with equivocal results.[52–55]

A cross-national investigation of bladder cancer mortality and diet has shown significant variability in mortality in different countries and a positive correlation with dietary total fat, animal fat, animal protein, meat, and alcohol.[56] In this study, tobacco consumption was only weakly correlated with mortality from bladder cancer. Riboli and associates also reported a significantly increased risk of bladder cancer with high intake of saturated fat.[57] In a case-control study of 432 cases, the highest quartile of saturated fat intake had a significantly increased risk of bladder cancer (RR, 2.25; 95% CI, 1.42 to 3.55). No significant association was found for retinol, carotene, or vitamin E. Risch and coworkers, in a case-control study, reported that increased cholesterol intake was associated with a mild but significant increase in risk; in addition, intake of vitamin A, retinol, β-carotene, or vitamin C had no effect on the incidence of bladder cancer.[52]

A case-control study of 351 bladder cancer patients using detailed questionnaires and interviews reported a significant effect of diet on bladder cancer.[58] An increased risk of bladder cancer was associated with higher kilocalorie intake, but only in patients under 65 years of age. Increased total fat and protein intake were each associated with increased risk. However, when adjusted for total kilocalorie intake, only total fat intake showed a positive trend (highest quartile odds ratio [OR], 1.59; 95% CI, 0.93 to 2.17); total protein intake showed a negative association. Vitamin intake was only significant for carotenoid consumption, which was associated with decreased risk in patients under 65 years of age.

A case-control study from Sweden also suggested a role of dietary fat in the incidence of bladder cancer.[59] High intake of fried foods was associated with a relative risk of 1.7 (95% CI, 1.4 to 4.2). In addition, high fat intake was correlated with a positive trend (RR, 1.7; 95% CI, 1.0 to 2.8). A cohort study of Seventh-Day Adventists[55] reported that high consumption of meat, poultry, and fish was associated with significantly increased risk for bladder cancer. Alcohol and coffee consumption was not associated with increased risk in multivariate analysis. The data also suggested decreased risk with frequent consumption of fruit juices and green vegetables.

In contrast, a prospective study of Japanese-American men in Hawaii showed no relationship between calorie intake, protein intake, or fat intake and incidence of bladder cancer.[53] In this study, only low consumption of fruit was significantly associated with risk of bladder cancer.

Many epidemiologic studies have also focused on vitamin consumption as well. Data on the consumption of vitamin A, carotenes, or green, yellow, or leafy vegetables have been equivocal, with some studies showing no effect[52,54,57,58] and others showing a modest protective effect.[59] Steineck et al. reported some protective effect with vitamin A supplement usage.[59] Information on the effect of vitamin C is limited. Nomura et al.[54] reported decreased risk with increased consumption of vitamin C in women only; Risch et al.[52] and Riboli et al.[57] reported no effect. Chyou and associates[53] and Mills and coworkers[55] have reported decreased risk with fruit and fruit juice consumption, respectively.

Diet and Renal Cell Carcinoma

Limited data are available on the effect of diet on renal cell carcinoma (RCC). Other than cigarette smoking and excess body weight, risk factors for RCC are poorly understood.[60] Much emphasis has been placed on the possible roles of occupational exposures, use of diuretics, history of renal disease, and other factors; however, the effect of diet has not been studied extensively.

Chow and colleagues, in a case-control study of 690 patients and 707 controls, reported significantly increased risks of RCC with increasing consumption of red meat, high-protein foods, and staple foods (grains, breads, and potatoes).[60] The relative risk for the highest quartile of protein intake was 1.9 (95% CI, 1.0 to 3.6) after adjustment for total caloric intake. No alteration in risk was seen for total fat, saturated fat, or vitamin intake (vitamin C, vitamin E, β-carotene) with adjustment for total caloric intake. The authors suggested that, although no independent effect of protein on RCC has been established, the consumption of high amounts of protein may be related to the development of other chronic renal conditions that may be associated with RCC.

Similarly, McLaughlin et al. reported a significant increase in risk for RCC in Shanghai, China, with increasing meat consumption, especially in the highest quartile (OR, 4.0; 95% CI, 1.4 to 11.4).[61] Decreased risk was observed with increasing fruit and vegetable consumption. No significant effect was seen for tea, coffee, or alcohol consumption. A separate case-control study in Minnesota also by McLaughlin et al. reported a positive association of increased meat consumption with risk for RCC.[62] Maclure and Willett reported, in a case-control study, a significantly increased risk for RCC with increased beef consumption (RR, 3.4; 95% CI, 1.6 to 7.2) without adjustment for smoking.[63] Increased risk was seen for soft drinks, colas, and diet sodas.

Other studies, however, have not confirmed these findings.[64–66] Krieger and associates, in a case-control study, noted a nonsignificantly increased risk for RCC with increased meat consumption.[64] No alteration in risk was seen with alcohol, coffee, or tea consumption. McCredie and colleagues also found no association of RCC with increased red meat intake.[66]

MODES OF THERAPY

Various forms of nutritional therapy are available to the clinician today. The best way to decide on the most appropriate form of therapy is to have a nutritional support plan. Several points must be considered in formulating a nutritional support plan: (1) category and extent of malnutrition (nutritional assessment), (2) extent of hypermetabolism (total urinary nitrogen), (3) individual protein and calorie requirements, (4) goal of nutritional therapy, (5) presence of functioning gastrointestinal tract, (6) appetite, (7) route of delivery of nutrients (central vs. peripheral vein vs. gastrointestinal tract), and (8) presence of specific organ dysfunction.

Nutritional Support with Chemotherapy, Radiotherapy, or Surgical Therapy in Cancer Patients

In order to establish the efficacy of nutritional supplementation therapy on the cancer patient, end-points or goals should be established. These goals may include improvement in quality of life, decreased morbidity (i.e., improved resistance to infection, less hospitalization), improved functional status, or simply improved nutritional status. Initially, it was hoped that nutritional therapy with total parenteral nutrition could improve patient tolerance for chemotherapy or radiation therapy and even prolong survival; unfortunately, there is currently no convincing evidence to support this belief. However, in patients with severe malnutrition, perioperative nutritional support, if given for at least 10 days preoperatively, can reduce morbidity and mortality.

Chemotherapy

When patients undergo intensive chemotherapy, oral intake is often decreased, adequate caloric intake becomes suboptimal, and nutrition status often worsens. Total parenteral nutrition (TPN) has been given in conjunction with chemotherapy in the hope that maintenance or improvement of the nutritional status would improve patient outcome. The use of nutritional support for chemotherapy showed favorable results initially in animal studies. Nutritional supplementation improved nutritional status, reduced toxicity of chemotherapy, and enhanced survival in experimental animals.[15] These results have not been reproduced in randomized human studies, and many studies have demonstrated a worse outcome with TPN.[67,68] A review by Koretz[69] of 17 trials showed no beneficial effect of TPN on survival, with some studies showing decreased survival. Hematologic factors and gastrointestinal side effects were not necessarily improved with TPN. However, rates of infection were in general significantly higher in the TPN-treated groups. Additionally, lean body mass, albumin level, and CHI have not been shown to improve with TPN in these patients.

A meta-analysis of 12 controlled randomized trials by the American College of Physicians further examined the role of TPN and chemotherapy.[70] Overall, patients receiving TPN were only 81% as likely to survive as control patients. Likelihood of complete or partial response was only 68% versus controls. Furthermore, risk of significant infection was increased fourfold with the use of TPN ($p <$ 0.0001). The effect of TPN on hematologic and gastrointestinal toxicity was small and not considered clinically significant. Therefore, the American College of Surgeons has recommended that the routine use of parenteral nutrition for patients undergoing chemotherapy should be strongly discouraged, that therapy should be reserved for those patients whose malnutrition is regarded as life threatening, and that consideration be given to the potential complications associated with therapy. Many of the studies reviewed included patients who were not severely malnourished; because complications associated with TPN may be reduced in severely malnourished patients,[71] further studies will be needed to assess the role of TPN with chemotherapy in this select group.

In contrast, one select group of patients, bone marrow transplant recipients, may exhibit improved clinical outcome with TPN. Weisdorf and coworkers, in a randomized study of 137 patients, showed significant improvement in overall survival, time to relapse, and disease-free survival in patients treated starting 7 days prior to transplant.[72] However, Szeluga and associates, in a separate randomized trial in 65 leukemia patients, reported no difference in survival, hematopoietic recovery, or length of hospitalization.[73] Patients in this study were randomized to receive either 4 weeks of TPN or enteral feeding consisting of dietary counseling or tube feeding.

Radiation Therapy

Limited data are available on the use of nutritional support with radiotherapy. Patients undergoing radiotherapy are at additional risk for radiation enteritis, which may exacerbate any existing malnutrition. The use of TPN in patients undergoing radiotherapy has been evaluated in several randomized prospective trials.[74,75] These studies fail to show any significant benefit in terms of response to therapy, survival, or decreased complications.[15,74] Some studies do show increased weight gain with TPN, but it is unclear if these benefits are sustained. The use of oral supplementation or oral elemental diets has also been shown to have no appreciable effect on the response to chemotherapy, but there may be some decrease in bowel toxicity. In the absence of significant benefit, the routine use of nutritional supplementation in patients undergoing radiotherapy is not recommended. Further studies are necessary to evaluate whether severely malnourished patients undergoing radiotherapy may benefit from supportive nutritional therapy.

Perioperative Nutritional Therapy

The use of preoperative TPN in cancer patients has received considerable attention. Cancer patients have a high incidence of protein-calorie malnutrition; more than 30% of cancer patients undergoing major upper gastrointestinal procedures have significant malnutrition.[76] It has been clearly established that those patients with severe malnutrition have higher rates of morbidity and mortality following surgery. The goal of perioperative nutritional support has been to reduce the risk of perioperative morbidity and mortality in malnourished patients. Although improved nutritional status may be considered an end-point of therapy, the risk and expense of the use of TPN precludes its use unless there is some clinical benefit to the patient.

Initial studies of perioperative TPN and the effect on morbidity and mortality have suggested that there may be a slight benefit. Mullen et al., in a nonrandomized study, compared the effects of 7 days of preoperative TPN versus a standard oral diet in 145 patients scheduled for major intra-abdominal or intrathoracic surgery.[77] Patients were entered into the TPN group (n = 50) based on clinical assessment. Significant reductions in morbidity (18% TPN vs. 39% controls) and mortality (4% TPN vs. 29% for controls) were seen in the TPN-treated group. Stratification of results in risk groups revealed that the benefit of TPN was significant only in the high-risk group.

In a nonrandomized study by Starker and colleagues,[7] 59 patients with malnutrition preoperatively were given 1 week of TPN. Malnutrition was defined as weight loss greater than 10% and serum albumin level less than 3.5 mg/dl. Subgroup analysis revealed that those patients who failed to demonstrate a rise in serum albumin level following one week of TPN had a significantly higher incidence of postoperative complications (45% vs. 4.3%). In a second phase of the study, those patients who failed to show a rise in serum albumin level within 1 week were continued on TPN for 4 to 6 weeks. This group did show a rise in serum albumin level after 4 to 6 weeks of TPN, and their incidence of postoperative complications was significantly reduced (12.5 vs. 45%). These data suggest that malnourished patients who receive TPN for 1 week preoperatively may benefit from additional TPN if they fail to respond to initial treatment.

Randomized studies have in general not reproduced the beneficial effects of TPN seen in uncontrolled studies. Most of these studies have shown no improvement in morbidity or mortality in patients treated with TPN perioperatively.[78] One of the earliest prospective randomized trials to show a significant reduction in morbidity and mortality in TPN-treated patients was reported by Muller and coworkers.[79] In this study, 59 patients with gastrointestinal carcinoma were randomized to receive either 10 days of preoperative TPN or a regular diet; significant reductions in major complications and mortality postoperatively were demonstrated in the TPN group. This study has been criticized because of the subsequent reporting of a third group treated with TPN and intralipid that had a significantly higher mortality compared to controls.[80] A meta-analysis by Detsky et al. of 11 controlled trials suggested that TPN may reduce the risk for complications from major surgery and fatalities.[71] The analysis showed a 20% reduction in complications and a 32% reduction in fatalities, although neither reduction was statistically significant. Many of the studies examined suffered from design flaws, including the use of well-nourished patients, small sample size, inadequate treatment regimen, and the use of enteral nutrition in control patients. Detsky et al. state that the design flaws may have limited the ability of these trials to show the effectiveness of TPN. Nevertheless, the authors concluded that perioperative nutritional support will most likely benefit those patients who are severely malnourished preoperatively or those patients who are expected to have adequate nutritional intake for prolonged periods postoperatively (at least 10 to 14 days).[71]

In 1991, a well-controlled prospective study on the use of TPN perioperatively was reported.[81,82] A total of 395 malnourished patients who required laparotomy or noncardiac thoracotomy were randomly assigned to receive either TPN for 7 to 15 days preoperatively and 3 days postoperatively or no TPN at all.

Patients were selected from a pool of 3259 candidates; patients with a history of recent surgery, recent TPN, or expected death within 90 days were excluded from the pool. Patients were excluded if a delay in surgery (>7 days) was contraindicated or TPN was contraindicated. Patients with major concurrent organ system disease were also excluded, based on the belief that their concurrent disease may significantly affect their overall outcome independently of their nutritional status. A small group of patients (3.0%) were excluded because TPN was considered essential (pancreatitis, partial bowel or gastric outlet obstruction). Following exclusions, 2448 patients (75%) remained; of these, 951 patients were malnourished. Of the malnourished group, 169 patients were discharged without surgery and of the 459 patients who consented to participate in the study, 395 patients (86%) underwent surgery. Nutritional status was assessed by both the SGA and the nutritional risk index.

Rates of major complications during the first 30 postoperative days were similar in the two groups (25.5% TPN, 24.5% control). Major infectious complications occurred more commonly in the TPN-treated group (14.1 vs. 6.4% in controls; p = 0.01). An increase in the number of episodes of pneumonia, fascitis, and bacteremia was observed in the TPN group. Noninfectious complications were slightly but not significantly reduced in the TPN group (22.2 vs. 16.7% for controls; p = 0.20). The increase in complications seen in the control group were primarily anastomotic leaks, bronchopleural fistulas, and other gastrointestinal complications (bleeding, obstruction, perforation, and ischemia).

When patients were subdivided into groups based on nutritional status, subgroup analysis showed that, in patients with severe malnutrition, the frequency of noninfectious complications was significantly lower than in control patients (42.9 vs. 5.3% for controls; $p = 0.03$). This significant difference was observed when stratification was based on the nutrition risk index (which relies on serum albumin and weight loss). When stratification was based on the SGA, a decrease in noninfectious complications in the severely malnourished patients was also seen (22.6 vs. 42.1% for controls) but the difference was not significant ($p = 0.21$). Furthermore, the frequency of infectious complications was not increased in these patients compared to controls (15.8 vs. 21.4% for controls; $p = 1.00$). Use of TPN in patients with mild or borderline malnutrition provided no benefit but resulted instead in a higher incidence of postoperative infections.

These results suggest that there is little or no benefit of TPN in patients who are mildly or moderately malnourished and that use of TPN is associated with increased incidence of infectious complications in these patients. Conversely, the use of TPN in severely malnourished patients is probably efficacious; in this group, the incidence of noninfectious complications is reduced and the incidence of infectious complications is not increased.

Postoperative Nutritional Support

The efficacy of parenteral nutrition in the postoperative period is less well established. This is particularly true in previously well-nourished patients undergoing elective surgery in whom a return to oral intake is expected within 5 to 7 days. Abel et al.[83] studied the effect of immediate postoperative parenteral hyperalimentation and found no improvement of the course of malnourished patients undergoing cardiac surgery. However, the nutritional regimen that they used supplied a daily caloric intake of only 1000 to 1400 kcal. Holter and Fischer[84] demonstrated that a combined preoperative (3-day) and postoperative (10-day) period of nutritional support reduced complication rates in malnourished patients with gastrointestinal carcinoma and weight loss.

It has been shown that immediate postoperative parenteral nutrition results in a reduction in hospitalization time in a group of bladder cancer patients undergoing radical cystectomy and diversion.[85,86] This occurred in patients with no significant degree of preoperative malnutrition. There was a markedly shorter length of hospitalization for patients receiving TPN (median stay 17 days) in the postoperative period as compared to those receiving 5% dextrose (median stay 24 days). This difference was found to be highly significant ($p < 0.002$). It should be noted that this study was randomized but not double blind and was a retrospective review of data not collected during the actual performance of the study. The initial goal of the study was to examine the metabolic effects of nutritional supplementation and not duration of hospitalization. Further studies are necessary to document the application of this finding to patients undergoing other major surgical procedures. The cost saving of a major disease in duration of hospitalization following elective surgery warrants that the effect of nutrient support following injury be seriously examined, particularly as the age of the population increases. However, it seems clear that the routine use of 5% dextrose solution for postoperative nutrition should be re-evaluated.

CONCLUSIONS

Nutritional support of the malnourished hospitalized patient must be viewed as a primary form of therapy today. Severe malnutrition is ominous for all hospitalized patients, especially those facing major surgery. If urologists ignore the starving patient's nutritional needs, they cannot hope to have great success with their other therapeutic modalities. Careful and judicious use of nutritional therapy is essential in treating patients with cancer to decrease morbidity from cancer therapy and also from nutritional therapy itself.

REFERENCES

1. Kaminski MV, Fitzgerald MJ, Murphy RJ, et al: Correlation of mortality with serum transferrin and energy. JPEN J Parenter Enteral Nutr 1977; 1:27.
2. Pietsch JB, Meakins JL, MacLean LD: The delayed hypersensitivity response: applications in clinical surgery. Surgery 1977; 82:349.
3. Seltzer MH, Cooper DN, Ingler P, et al: Instant nutritional assessment. JPEN J Parenter Enteral Nutr 1979; 3:157.
4. Nirgiotis JG, Andrassy RJ: Preserving the gut and enhancing the immune response: the role of enteral nutrition in decreasing sepsis. Contemp Surg 1992; 41:17.
5. Bistrian BR, Blackburn GL, Sherman M, et al: Therapeutic index of nutritional depletion in hospitalized patients. Surg Gynecol Obstet 1975; 141:512.
6. Blackburn GL, Bristrian BR, Maini BS, et al: Nutritional and metabolic assessment of the hospitalized patient. JPEN J Parenter Enteral Nutr 1977; 1:11.
7. Starker PM, LaSala PA, Askanazi J, et al: The influence of preoperative total parenteral nutrition upon morbidity and mortality. Surg Gynecol Obstet 1986; 162:569.
8. Blackburn GL, Harvey KB: Nutritional assessment as a routine in clinical medicine. Postgrad Med 1982; 71:46.
9. Hensle TW: Nutritional support of the surgical patient. Urol Clin North Am 1983; 10:109.
10. Bistrian BR, Blackburn GL, Scrimshaw NS, et al: Cellular immunity in semi-starved state in hospitalized adults. Am J Clin Nutr 1975; 28:1148.
11. Herrmann VM: Nutritional assessment. *In* Torosian MH (ed): Nutrition for the Hospitalized Patient, p 233. New York, Marcel Dekker, 1995.
12. McClave SA, Mitoraj TE, Theilmeier KA, et al: Differentiating subtypes (hypoalbuminemic vs marasmic) of protein-calorie malnutrition: incidence and clinical significance in a university hospital setting. JPEN J Parenter Enteral Nutr 1992; 16:337–342.
13. Bistrian BR: Assessment of hospital protein-calorie malnutrition. *In* Hill G (ed): Nutrition and the Surgical Patient, pp 39–54. Edinburgh, Churchill Livingstone, 1981.

14. Rutten P, Blackburn GL, Flatt HP, et al: Determination of optimal hyperalimentation infusion rate. J Surg Res 1975; 18:477.
15. Heys SD, Park GM, Garlick PJ, et al: Nutrition and malignant disease: implications for surgical practice. Br J Surg 1992; 79:614–623.
16. Clark RG, Karatzas T: Pre-operative nutritional status. Br J Clin Pract 1988; 63(Suppl):2–7.
17. Hill GL: Malnutrition and surgical risk: guidelines for nutritional therapy. Ann R Coll Surg 1987; 69:263–265.
18. Detsky AS, Baker JP, Mendelson RA, et al: Evaluating the accuracy of nutritional assessment techniques applied to hospitalized patients: methodology and comparisons. JPEN J Parenter Enteral Nutr 1984; 8:153–159.
19. Pettigrew RA, Hill GL: Indicators of surgical risk and clinical judgment. Br J Surg 1986; 73:47–51.
20. Detsky AS, McLaughlin JR, Baker JP, et al: What is subjective global assessment of nutritional status? JPEN J Parenter Enteral Nutr 1987; 11:8–13.
21. Parnes HL, Aisner J: Protein calorie malnutrition and cancer therapy. Drug Safety 1992; 7:404–416.
22. Langstein HN, Norton JA: Mechanisms of cancer cachexia. Hematol Oncol Clin North Am 1991; 5:103–123.
23. Morrison SD: Control of food intake in cancer cachexia: a challenge and a tool. Physiol Behav 1976; 17:98–107.
24. Young VR: Energy metabolism and requirements in the cancer patient. Cancer Res 1977; 37:2336–2347.
25. Knox LS, Crosby LO, Feurer ID, et al: Energy expenditure in malnourished cancer patients. Ann Surg 1983; 197:152–162.
26. Lundholm K, Hom G, Scherstein T: Insulin resistance in patients with cancer. Cancer Res 1978; 38:4665.
27. Holroyde CP, Reichard A: Carbohydrate metabolism in cancer cachexia. Cancer Treat Rep 1981; 65(Suppl):67–78.
28. Eden E, Edstrom S, Bennegard K, et al: Glucose flux in relation to energy expenditure in malnourished patients with and without cancer during periods of fasting and feeding. Cancer Res 1984; 44:1718–1724.
29. Heber D, Byerly LO, Chlebowski RT, et al: Medical abnormalities in glucose and protein metabolism in noncachectic lung cancer patients. Cancer Res 1982; 42:4815.
30. Jeevanandam M, Lowry SF, Horowitz GD, Brennan MF: Cancer cachexia and protein metabolism. Lancet 1984; 2: 1423.
31. Norton JA, Stein TP, Brennan MF: Whole body protein synthesis and turnover in normal man and malnourished patients with and without known cancer. Ann Surg 1981; 194: 123.
32. Heber D, Tchekmedyian NS: Pathophysiology of cancer: hormonal and metabolic abnormalities. Oncology 1992; 29(Suppl 2):28–31.
33. Lowry SF, Muldawer LL: Tumor necrosis factor and other cytokines in the pathogenesis of cancer cachexia. Principles Pract Oncol 1990; 4:1–12.
34. Torti F, Dieckmann B, Beutler G, et al: A macrophage factor inhibits adipose gene expression: an in vitro model of cachexia. Science 1985; 229:867–869.
35. Wingo PA, Tong T, Bolden S: Cancer statistics, 1995. CA Cancer J Clin 1995; 45:8–30.
36. Yatani R, Chigusa I, Akazaki K, et al: Geographic pathology of latent prostatic carcinoma. Int J Cancer 1982; 29: 611–616.
37. Mandel JS, Schuman LM: Epidemiology of cancer of the prostate. Rev Cancer Epidemiol 1980; 1:1–65.
38. Boyle P, Kevi R, Lucchini F, et al: Trends in diet-related cancers in Japan: a conundrum. Lancet 1993; 342:752.
39. Hamalainen E, Adlercreutz H, Pusk P, et al: Diet and serum sex hormones in healthy men. J Steroid Biochem 1984; 20:459–464.
40. Cave WT: Dietary n-3 polyunsaturated fatty acid effects on animal tumorigenesis. FASEB J 1991; 5:1571–1579.
41. Marshall L, Szczeniewski A, Johnston PV: Dietary alphalinolenic acid and prostaglandin synthesis: a time course study. Am J Clin Nutr 1983; 38:895–900.
42. Armstrong B, Doll R: Environmental factors and cancer incidence and mortality in different countries, with special reference to dietary practices. Int J Cancer 1975; 15:617–631.
43. Knekt P, Reunanen A, Aromaa A, et al: Serum cholesterol and risk of cancer in a cohort of 39,000 men and women. J Clin Epidemiol 1988; 41:519–530.
44. Rose DP, Connolly JM: Dietary fat, fatty acids and prostate cancer. Lipids 1992; 27:798–803.
45. Rotkin ID: Studies in the epidemiology of prostatic cancer: expanded sampling. Cancer Treat Rep 1977; 61:173–180.
46. Graham S, Haughey B, Marshall J, et al: Diet in the epidemiology of carcinoma of the prostate gland. J Natl Cancer Inst 1983; 70:687–692.
47. Kolonel LN, Nomura AM, Hinds NW, et al: Role of diet in cancer incidence in Hawaii. Cancer Res 1983; 43:2397s–2402s.
48. Ross RK, Shimizu J, Paganini-Hill A, et al: Case-control studies of prostate cancer in Blacks and Whites in Southern California. J Natl Cancer Inst 1987; 78:869–874.
49. West DW, Slattery ML, Robison LM, et al: Adult dietary intake and prostate cancer risk in Utah: a case-control study with special emphasis on aggressive tumors. Cancer Causes Control 1991; 2:85–94.
50. Gann PH, Hennekens CH, Sacks FM, et al: Prospective study of plasma fatty acids and risk of prostate cancer. J Natl Cancer Inst 1994; 86:281–286.
51. Giovannucci EJ, Rimm EB, Colditz GA, et al: A prospective study of dietary fat and risk of prostate cancer. J Natl Cancer Inst 1993; 85:1571–1579.
52. Risch HA, Burch JK, Miller AB, et al: Dietary factors and the incidence of cancer of the urinary bladder. Am J Epidemiol 1988; 127:1179–1191.
53. Chyou PH, Nomura AM, Stemmermann GN: A prospective study of diet, smoking, and lower urinary tract cancer. Ann Epidemiol 1993; 3:211–216.
54. Nomura AM, Kolonel LN, Hankin JH, et al: Dietary factors in cancer of the lower urinary tract. Int J Cancer 1991; 48: 199–205.
55. Mills PK, Beeson WL, Phillips RL, et al: Bladder cancer in a low risk population: results from the Adventist Health Study. Am J Epidemiol 1991; 133:230–239.
56. Hebert JR, Miller DR: A cross-national investigation of diet and bladder cancer. Eur J Cancer 1994; 30A:778–784.
57. Riboli E, Gonzalez CA, Gonzalo LA, et al: Diet and bladder cancer in Spain: a multi-centre case-control study. Int J Cancer 1991; 49:214–219.
58. Vena JE, Graham S, Freudenheim J, et al: Diet in the epidemiology of bladder cancer in western New York. Nutr Cancer 1992; 18:255–264.
59. Steineck G, Hagman U, Gerhardsson M, et al: Vitamin A supplements, fried foods, fat and urothelial cancer: a case-referent study in Stockholm in 1985–1987. Int J Cancer 1990; 45:1006–1011.
60. Chow WH, Gridley G, McLaughlin JK, et al: Protein intake and risk of renal cancer. J Natl Cancer Inst 1994; 86:1131–1139.
61. McLaughlin JK, Gao YT, Gau RN, et al: Risk factors for renal-cell cancer in Shanghai, China. Int J Cancer 1992; 52: 562–565.
62. McLaughlin JK, Mandel JS, Blot WJ, et al: A population-based case-control study of renal cell carcinoma. J Natl Cancer Inst 1984; 72:275–284.
63. Maclure M, Willett W: A case-control study of diet and risk of renal adenocarcinoma. Epidemiology 1990; 1:430–440.
64. Krieger N, Marrett LD, Dodds L, et al: Risk factors for renal cell carcinoma: results of a population-based case-control study. Cancer Causes Control 1993; 4:101–110.
65. Talmani R, Baron AE, Barra S, et al: A case-control study of risk factor for renal cell cancer in northern Italy. Cancer Causes Control 1990; 1:125–131.
66. McCredie M, Ford JM, Stewart HJ: Risk factors for cancer of the renal parenchyma. Int J Cancer 1988; 42:13–16.
67. Pearlstone DB, Pisters PW, Brennan MF: Nutrition and

cancer. *In* Torosian MH (ed): Nutrition for the Hospitalized Patient, p 393. New York, Marcel Dekker, 1995.
68. Brennan MF: Total parenteral nutrition in the cancer patient. N Engl J Med 1981; 305:375–382.
69. Koretz RL: Nutritional support: how much for how much? Gut 1986; 27(S1):85–95.
70. McGeer AJ, Detsky AS, O'Rourke K: Parenteral nutrition in patients receiving cancer chemotherapy. Ann Intern Med 1989; 110:734–736.
71. Detsky AS, Baker JP, O'Rourke K, et al: Perioperative parenteral nutrition: a meta-analysis. Ann Intern Med 1987; 107:195–203.
72. Weisdorf SA, Lysne J, Wind D, et al: Positive effect of prophylactic total parenteral nutrition on long term outcome of bone marrow transplantation. Transplantation 1987; 43: 833–838.
73. Szeluga DJ, Stuart RK, Brookmeyer R, et al: Nutritional support of bone marrow transplant recipients: a prospective randomized clinical trial comparing total parenteral nutrition to an enteral feeding program. Cancer Res 1987; 47:3309.
74. Donaldson SS: Nutritional support as an adjunct to radiation therapy. JPEN J Parenter Enteral Nutr 1984; 8:302–310.
75. Pezner R, Archambeau JO: Critical evaluation of the role of nutritional support for radiation therapy patients. Cancer 1985; 55:263–267.
76. Daly JM, Redmond HP, Gallagher H: Perioperative nutrition in cancer patients. JPEN J Parenter Enteral Nutr 1992; 16(6 Suppl):100s–105s.
77. Mullen JL, Buzby GP, Matthews DC, et al: Reduction of operative morbidity and mortality by combined preoperative and postoperative nutritional support. Ann Surg 1979; 192:604–613.
78. Buzby GP: Overview of randomized clinical trials of total parenteral nutrition for malnourished surgical patients. World J Surg 1993; 17:173–177.
79. Muller JM, Brenner U, Dienst C, et al: Preoperative parenteral feeding in patients with gastrointestinal carcinoma. Lancet 1982; 1:68–71.
80. Muller JM, Keller HW, Brenner U, et al: Indications and effects of preoperative parenteral nutrition. World J Surg 1986; 10:53–63.
81. Buzby GP, Blouin G, Colling CL, et al: Perioperative total parenteral nutrition in surgical patients. N Engl J Med 1991; 325:525–532.
82. Buzby GP, Williford WO, Petson OL, et al: A randomized clinical trial of total parenteral nutrition in malnourished surgical patients: the rationale and impact of previous clinical trials and pilot study on protocol design. Am J Clin Nutr 1988; 47:357–365.
83. Abel RM, Fischer JE, Buckley MJ, et al: Malnutrition in cardiac surgical patients: results of a prospective, randomized evaluation of early postoperative parenteral nutrition. Arch Surg 1976; 111:45.
84. Holter AR, Fischer JE: The effects of perioperative hyperalimentation on complications in patients with carcinoma and weight loss. J Surg Res 1977; 23:31.
85. Askanazi J, Hensle TW, Starker PM, et al: Effect of immediate postoperative nutritional support on length of hospitalization. Ann Surg 1986; 23:236.
86. Hensle TW, Askanazi J, Rosenbaum LH, et al: Metabolic changes associated with radical cystectomy. J Urol 1985; 134:1032.

52

ANESTHESIA FOR MAJOR CANCER SURGERY

PEMA DORJE, M.D. *and* KEVIN K. TREMPER, M.D., PH.D.

General anesthesia is a combination of amnesia, analgesia, and muscle relaxation. This state can be achieved by the inhalation of a variety of vapors to produce each of these conditions in proportion to the concentration achieved in the central nervous system. It can also be achieved through the use of three different pharmacologic agents targeted to produce each affect to the degrees desired: amnesics, analgesics, and neuromuscular blocking agents. As the concentration of inhalation anesthetics increases, there is also a progressive depression of cardiovascular function and respiratory function. Because of the requirements of the surgical procedures or the patient's pre-existing cardiac disease, the concentration of the inhalation agent required to produce sufficient muscle relaxation may produce a relative overdose with respect to its affect on the cardiovascular system. For this reason, modern general anesthesia usually requires titration of the three classes of agents described above to optimize the conditions for surgery while maintaining cardiovascular stability. The goals of modern anesthesia are (1) to achieve this state quickly and safely by choosing the appropriate techniques and agents, taking into consideration the patient's medical condition; (2) to maintain this state throughout the surgical procedure while compensating for the effects of varying degrees of painful stimuli and blood and fluid loss; and (3) to reverse the muscle relaxation and amnesia, bringing patients back to their own physiologic control while maintaining sufficient analgesia to minimize postoperative pain and the associated adrenergic response.

This anesthetic state may also be accomplished by placing local anesthetics directly on or around the spinal cord or peripheral nerves. These local anesthetics block nerve conduction by blocking sodium channels to a degree that is proportional to their concentration. For procedures that are conducted below the diaphragm, it is possible to provide analgesia and muscle relaxation with either spinally or epidurally administered local anesthetics and narcotics. The narcotics block specific receptors and therefore diminish the sensation of pain without affecting nerve conduction that controls motor and sympathetic function. All local anesthetics will block sympathetic sensory and motor function in that order. As the desmatomal level rises, it is usually found that the level of the motor blockade will be two dermatomes below the sensory level and the sympathetic blockade will be two dermatones above the sensory level. There is great variability in this effect, but the sympathetic blockade is always greater than the motor or sensory blockade. Because the sympathetic chain is thoracolumbar in origin, a high spinal or epidural sympathectomy level has the potential of producing a total sympathectomy, resulting in maximal peripheral vasodilatation. If the sympathectomy level rises to the T1–T4 level, the cardiac sympathetic enervation is also blocked. The combination of complete peripheral vasodilatation and lack of cardiac sympathetic enervation produces profound hypotension and bradycardia. For this reason spinal and epidural anesthetic levels are usually maintained below the T1–T4 level. Because the diaphragm is enervated by the phrenic nerve (C3–5), as the sympathetic level rises there would be significant hemodynamic effects as a result of the sympathetic blockade prior to motor effects blocking diaphragmatic function at the cervical level. The duration of anesthetic action is related to the perfusion of the tissue and the metabolism of the anesthetic. The local perfusion can be reduced by the addition of epinephrine, producing local vasoconstriction. Regional anesthetic techniques have the benefit of blocking pain conduction and the associated autonomic response to pain, lasting not only throughout the procedure but in recovery. They have the disadvantage of producing a peripheral sympathectomy and can only be used in procedures in the lower half of the body. Over the past decade, regional and general anesthetics have been used in combination to take advantage of both techniques in improving not only the anesthetic course but the postoperative recovery.

Anesthetic administrations are accomplished with a high degree of safety 30 to 40 million times per year in the United States in spite of the serious potential complications that may be associated with errors in technique or judgment. The high degree of success of both surgical and anesthetic outcomes is due to the efforts of thousands of surgeons and anesthesiologists advancing the art and science of each of these fields. It obviously was not always this way. Patients in the early 1800s approached a surgical procedure as though they were facing an execution. There was the unavoidable pain and most certainly hemorrhage, possibly shock, and very likely postoperative infection. Most patients would put their estates and personal affairs in order in anticipation of the worst outcome. There were obvious limitations on what procedures surgeons could attempt, and pain was unavoidable. Because there was very little that could be done to alleviate pain, the ability to withstand pain was considered one of man's most noble virtues. This opinion lingers today, in that one who complains of pain is often considered weak or of lesser character than one who endures pain silently. Even though the development of modern techniques and analgesics have provided us with the ability to nearly eliminate all perioperative pain, there still remain judgmental feelings about patients who complain of pain. Pain is not only unpleasant but it has significant adverse physiologic effects; therefore, it should be obvious that physicians should encourage patients to alert health care personnel when pain is felt.

This chapter reviews anesthetic principles as they relate to patients undergoing major urologic surgical procedures. It reviews preoperative assessment of these patients with malignancies and common coexisting diseases and how that may affect the perioperative management. It also examines intraoperative management with respect to hemodynamic monitoring, coagulation assessment, and the rationale for blood and blood component transfusions. Specific anesthetic techniques are reviewed for the most common urologic oncologic procedures. Finally, common problems in the postoperative period are examined, including nausea, vomiting, and pain management. For a more comprehensive review of anesthetic principles, the reader is referred to *Anesthesia* by R. Miller and *Anesthesia and Co-Existing Disease* by R. Stoelting.[1,2]

PREOPERATIVE WORK-UP

The aim of the preoperative anesthetic assessment is to evaluate the patient's medical condition, form an anesthetic and postoperative care plan, and discuss the plan with the patient. During the preoperative work-up, the impact of the cancer and its attendant chemotherapy and radiation therapy and the associated medical conditions of the patient are carefully evaluated to ensure their preoperative optimization to the extent achievable. Preoperative work-up consists of a careful, unhurried review of history, physical examination, chart, and laboratory results, paying particular attention to the effects of the disease's process on the functional status of the heart, lung, brain, kidney, liver, and bone marrow. The patient's physical status is described by the time-honored American Society of Anesthesiologists (ASA) stratification of physical status (Table 52–1).[3]

TABLE 52–1. PHYSICAL STATUS CLASSIFICATION OF THE AMERICAN SOCIETY OF ANESTHESIOLOGISTS*

Class	Physical Status
1	Patient has no organic, physiologic, biochemical, or psychiatric disturbances.
2	Patient has mild to moderate systemic disturbances that may or may not be related to the disorder requiring surgery (e.g., essential hypertension, diabetes mellitus).
3	Patient has severe systemic disturbance that may or may not be related to the disorder requiring surgery (e.g., heart disease that limits activity, poorly controlled essential hypertension).
4	Patient has severe systemic disturbance that is life-threatening with or without surgery (e.g., congestive heart failure, persistent angina pectoris).
5	Patient is moribund and has little chance for survival, but surgery is to be performed as a last resort.

*Adapted from Dripps R, Lamont A, Eckenhoff J: The role of anesthesia in surgical mortality. JAMA 1961; 178:261, with permission. Copyright 1961, American Medical Association.

Cardiovascular System

The most common major perioperative complications can be attributed to cardiac causes: myocardial infarction (MI), dysrhythmias, or cardiac failure. The preoperative cardiac evaluation of cancer patients is composed of two components: (1) routine evaluation of the heart for major surgery, and (2) evaluation of the cardiac effect of malignancy and its treatment.

Routine Cardiovascular Evaluation

Hypertension and coronary artery disease (CAD) are the most common cardiovascular diseases in adult patients presenting for surgery. Hypertensive patients should be investigated and treated to render them normotensive prior to elective surgery. The incidence of hypotension and myocardial ischemia is higher in untreated than adequately treated hypertensive patients.[4,5] Their medications should be continued throughout the perioperative period. However, diuretics may be better omitted on the day of surgery to minimize circulatory and electrolyte disturbances. There is, however, no evidence in an otherwise healthy patient of increased postoperative complications unless the patient's preoperative diastolic pressure is 110 mm Hg or greater. Hypertensive patients with significant left ventricular hypertrophy may be at increased risk of perioperative cardiac events.

CAD is the leading cause of death in the United States and continues to be a major cause of postoperative morbidity and mortality. In patients known to have CAD, the major risk factors for perioperative cardiac events are cardiac failure, unstable angina, and recent infarction. Congestive cardiac failure is the single most important factor predicting postoperative cardiac morbidity. Cardiac failure must be under optimal medical control before elective surgical procedures, and aggressive hemodynamic monitoring in the perioperative period is essential in most cases.

Much of the anesthetic preoperative evaluation is directed toward detecting the presence and degree of ischemic heart disease. Establishing risk factors for perioperative cardiac events in patients with CAD continues to be a challenge and is an evolving science. Since Detsky's[6] modification of Goldman et al.'s multivariate cardiac risk indicators,[7] new approaches to cardiac evaluation for noncardiac surgery have been described.[8,9] The main feature of the new approach[8] is a *combination* of a simplified, validated, and easy to use *clinical risk indicator, functional cardiac reserve* assessed from the patient's daily activity, and the *degree of surgical risk*.[10–13] The combination approach has been shown to be a cost-effective way of screening and categorizing surgical patients into those who need and those who do not need further cardiac work-up.[10,12] In those patients whose functional cardiac reserve cannot be assessed because of respiratory, vascular, or orthopedic diseases, the cardiac reserve is assessed by stressing the heart pharmacologically.

Paul and Eagle[8] proposed a simplified and easy to use set of clinical risk factors (Table 52–2) that help to place an individual patient into one of three groups. Patients with unstable angina or more than two clinical markers have a very high risk of CAD and should be considered for cardiac catheterization and coronary revascularization before the surgical procedure, if feasible. Patients with no clinical risk factors fall in the low-risk group and need no further cardiac work-up.

Patients who fall in the intermediate-risk group are then assessed in light of their functional capacity by history and the degree of risk depending on the type of surgery (see Fig. 52–1). Functional capacity is assessed from the history obtained during the preoperative clinical evaluation. Emergency, intrathoracic, aortic, peripheral vascular, intra-abdominal, and major orthopedic surgery are all procedures associated with high perioperative cardiac complications. Head and neck, ophthalmologic, peripheral limb, and prostate surgery are associated with low cardiac risk.

TABLE 52–2. EAGLE INDEX*

- Age greater than 70 years
- Angina
- Prior myocardial infarction
  - by history
  - by ECG-Q wave
- Diabetes mellitus
- Congestive heart failure

*From Paul SD, Eagle K: A stepwise strategy for coronary risk assessment for noncardiac surgery. Med Clin North Am 1995; 79:1241, with permission.

A history of a prior MI is obviously important information to take into consideration. Large retrospective studies have found that the incidence of reinfarction is related to the time elapsed since the previous MI.[14–16] Mortality from reinfarction has been reported to be between 20 and 50% and occurs within the first 48 hours after surgery. In the era of angioplasty and thrombolytic therapy, the time interval may be less applicable and the risk assessment must be more individualized.[9] Patients with recent MI are not a homogeneous group, but rather have variable extent of myocardial damage and functional impairment and varying degrees of risk for further myocardia ischemia. Silent ischemia on ambulatory electrocardiography or poor symptom-limited exercise tolerance may indicate increased risk of ischemic cardiac events.[17–19] A patient with non–Q wave MI who has exercise limitation should have a cardiac evaluation because the probability of significant coronary artery stenosis is very high. If a patient with non–Q wave MI has returned to full exercise capacity, then the risk for perioperative cardiac events is small. Aggressive hemodynamic monitoring and intervention may reduce the risk of perioperative reinfarction.[15] The risk cannot be completely eliminated by optimizing hemodynamic status alone because local coronary vasoconstriction and/or thromboembolic events precipitated by the stress response and coagulation disturbances can cause infarction.[20] Prior coronary revascularization substantially reduces the risk of reinfarction. Anesthetic technique has not been shown to change the incidence of reinfarction, although regional anesthetic/analgesic techniques appear to minimize the stress response and catecholamine surge in the perioperative period.[21,22]

Among the valvular diseases, aortic stenosis and mitral valvular disease can cause major intraoperative hemodynamic disturbances. Symptomatic aortic stenosis must be evaluated using two-dimensional echocardiography by a cardiologist. The cardiac output and the valve area obtained from the echocardiogram can be used to calculate the valvular pressure gradient. In severe stenosis, preoperative transarterial valvuloplasty should be considered.

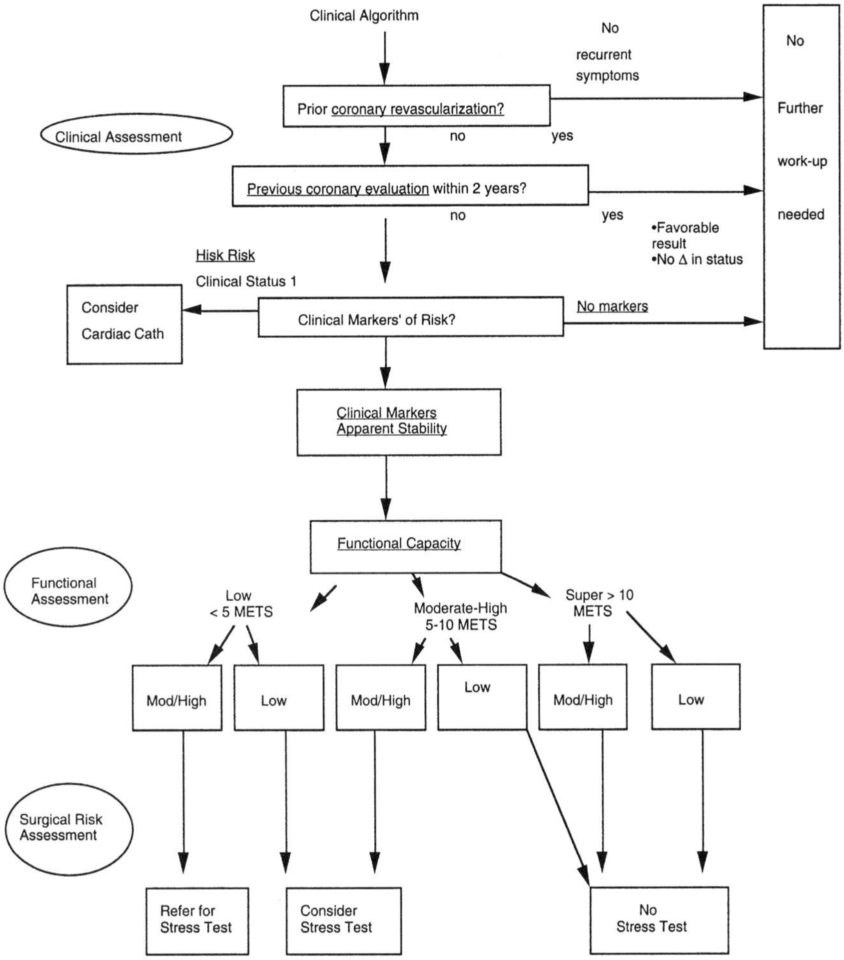
Clinical Algorithm
Clinical Assessment
Prior coronary revascularization?
no
yes
No recurrent symptoms
No Further work-up needed
Previous coronary evaluation within 2 years?
no
yes
•Favorable result
•No Δ in status
Hisk Risk
Clinical Status 1
Consider Cardiac Cath
Clinical Markers' of Risk?
No markers
Clinical Markers Apparent Stability
Functional Capacity
Functional Assessment
Low < 5 METS
Moderate-High 5-10 METS
Super > 10 METS
Mod/High
Low
Mod/High
Low
Mod/High
Low
Surgical Risk Assessment
Refer for Stress Test
Consider Stress Test
No Stress Test

FIGURE 52–1. Strategy for preoperative risk assessment for patients undergoing noncardiac surgery. +, Angina, MI by history or electrocardiogram (Q waves), congestive heart failure (CHF) (or ventricular tachycardia), diabetes mellitus; †, controlled angina, uncontrolled CHF, angina or CHF after recent MI; °, moderate- or high-risk surgery—vascular, thoracic, major abdominal, orthopedic; ++, low-risk surgery—head and neck, eye, prostate, hernia, breast.

Effects of Malignancy and Its Treatment on the Heart

Cardiac toxicity of the anthracyclines (daunomycin, doxorubicin) may be in the form of non–dose-related acute toxicity and dose-related cardiomyopathy.[23] The acute form occurs during the treatment and manifests mainly in the form of a variety of arrhythmias. The manifestation of acute toxicity is no indication of subsequent development of cardiomyopathy.

Cardiac toxicity is believed to result from free radical damage. The myocardial tissue is deficient in catalase,[24] and anthracycline therapy reduces glutathione peroxidase activity,[24] thus making the heart vulnerable to free radical damage. The peak plasma drug level may be very important in the pathogenesis of cardiomyopathy.[25] The known risk factors are shown in Table 52–3.[26]

Cardiac toxicity can be minimized by giving the anthracycline over a longer period of time without affecting its antitumor activity.[25] Dexrazoxane, by chelating intracellular iron, a cofactor in the free radical process, has marked cardioprotective effect without compromising antitumor effect.[27] This drug may allow larger doses of anthracyclines to be used without cardiotoxicity.

The cardiomyopathy persists after discontinuation of the anthracycline and may present from the subclinical to frank congestive cardiac failure. Radionucleotide angiography and M-mode echocar-

TABLE 52–3. RISK FACTORS ASSOCIATED WITH ANTHRACYCLINE CARDIAC TOXICITY*

- Peak plasma drug level
- Total cumulative dose over 550 mg/m^2 (daunomycin)
- Concomitant cyclophosphamide therapy
- Prior mediastinal irradiation
- Age over 65 years

*Adapted from Von Hoff D, Layard M, Basa P, et al: Risk factors for doxorubicin-induced congestive heart failure. Ann Intern Med 1979; 91: 710, with permission.

diography are used to assess cardiac dysfunction, but cardiac biopsy via right heart catheter is required to confirm the diagnosis. The signs, symptoms, and treatment are those of any congestive cardiac failure. If the cardiomyopathy is refractory to digoxin and diuretics, then a β-adrenergic agonist or a phosphodiesterase inhibitor must be tried.

Other therapies associated with cardiac complications include cyclophosphamide, 5-fluorouracil, and chest radiation therapy.[28] Symptoms and electrocardiographic changes suggestive of cardiac ischemia caused by 5-fluorouracil have been reported.[29] Cyclophosphamide may cause pericarditis and pericardial effusion. Cardiac radiation may cause pericardial disease, myocardial fibrosis, conduction defects, and valvular dysfunction.[30]

Assessment of the Respiratory System

The preoperative respiratory evaluation is divided into three sections: (1) upper airway evaluation; (2) routine pulmonary evaluation; and (3) effects of malignancy and its treatment on the pulmonary function.

Evaluation of the Upper Airway

In a closed claims study of 1541 anesthesia-related injuries to the patient, respiratory events constituted 34% of the cases, the majority of which led to death or brain damage.[31] These statistics put emphasis on the importance of careful preoperative evaluation of the upper airway and of developing a well-thought-out plan for management of those patients who have a clinically difficult airway and of those who may present with an unanticipated difficult airway.

The signs of a difficult airway may be clinically obvious or may be so subtle that a trained physician's careful evaluation is required to recognize it. During the evaluation of the upper airway for anesthesia, one must ensure that the lungs can be ventilated and the trachea can be intubated after the induction of anesthesia. The anatomic variations that would suggest difficulty in mask ventilation and/or intubation are thick beard, protruding upper jaw, receding lower jaw, and thyromental distance less than three fingerbreadths. A thick neck in an obese patient is also a warning sign, particularly if it is associated with history of snoring at night and somnolence during daytime. Pathologic changes in the oral cavity, temporomandibular joint, or upper cervical spine joints, significant abscess, and hematoma in the neck could contribute to difficult airway.

Radiation therapy in the neck area can cause extensive fibrosis, making airway manipulation more difficult. A mass in the mediastinum could compress on the trachea. After induction of anesthesia, the compressed trachea could collapse, making it impossible to ventilate by face mask or to pass the endotracheal tube past the obstruction. This potential problem must be kept in mind when evaluating the chest x-ray. Vincristine may cause laryngeal nerve palsy,[32] and, if the patient has hoarseness, the vocal cord must be evaluated by an otolaryngologist by indirect laryngoscopy. Autonomic neuropathy as a paraneoplastic effect[33] of many tumors or as side effect of prolonged vincristine therapy, longstanding diabetes, and alcoholism may cause delayed gastric emptying and increase the risk of regurgitation of gastric contents during induction of and emergence from anesthesia.

The basic principle to remember while dealing with a patient with a difficult airway is that the airway must be secured before the general anesthesia is administered. The patient's wakefulness should not be given away lightly. Awake tracheal intubation with fiberoptic scope after topical application of local anesthesia to the upper airway and awake tracheostomy under local anesthesia are some of the ways by which the airway may be secured.

Routine Pulmonary Evaluation

A careful history and clinical examination are usually sufficient to assess the respiratory status. If the patient has significant respiratory disease, then chest x-ray, clinical spirometry, and blood gases on room air are usually recommended. The results of the preoperative evaluation must be seen in light of the known risk factors[34] (Table 52–4).

Arterial P_{CO_2} greater than 45 mm Hg in a patient with advanced chronic lung disease is indicative of difficulty in weaning the patient from the mechanical ventilator, particularly if the surgery is extensive and close to the diaphragm.

Upper abdominal procedures produce marked diaphragmatic dysfunction[35] that persists even when the surgical pain is controlled by epidural analgesia or other means. The pattern of respiration shifts from predominantly abdominal to rib cage breathing. Reduced excursion of the diaphragm leads to atelectasis in the basal region, resulting in hypoxemia. The diaphragm regains its normal function by 24 hours. An increased number of risk factors present in any individual is likely to in-

TABLE 52–4. RISK FACTORS FOR POSTOPERATIVE PNEUMONIA*

- Chest and abdominal surgery
- Chronic respiratory disease
- P_{CO_2} greater than 45 mm Hg on room air
- Obesity
- Old age (greater than 70 years)
- Severe malnutrition
- History of cigarette smoking
- A variety of neurologic and muscle conditions related to cancer and its treatment

*Adapted from Windsor J, Hill G: Risk factors for postoperative pneumonia. Ann Surg 1988; 208:209, with permission.

crease the chance of developing postoperative pulmonary complications by a high margin.

Effects of Malignancy and Its Therapy on the Lung

Cancer and its treatment are associated with a variety of neurologic and muscular disorders.[33] These disorders frequently involve muscles of respiration and can have a major influence on the choice and use of muscle relaxant and the way the postoperative respiratory care is planned. The neurologic evaluation is briefly discussed later in this chapter. Cancer and its treatment may be associated with inflammatory, acute necrotizing, cachectic, carcinoid, and steroid myopathies. The presence of myopathy and its involvement of respiratory muscle must be looked for when evaluating a cancer patient for surgery.

Pulmonary damage caused by anticancer treatments is typified by bleomycin pulmonary toxicity (BPT). Bleomycin is primarily used for the treatment of testicular cancers, lymphomas, and squamous cell carcinomas. In the tissues it forms a complex with iron and catalyzes reduction of molecular oxygen to superoxide or hydroxyl radicals, which in turn cause DNA cleavage.[36] In the cells it is degraded by bleomycin hydrolase, which makes it incapable of binding to metal cofactors. The bleomycin hydrolase level is low in lung and skin, making these organs particularly susceptible to its toxicity. Genetic variations in the activity of this enzyme may explain why some patients are more susceptible than others to BPT.[37–39] It has minimal myelotoxicity because of the high hydrolase activity in the bone marrow. Bleomycin is eliminated by renal excretion, 45 to 70% in the first 24 hours.

Preoperative evidence of BPT has been suggested as one of the risks for perioperative acute respiratory failure (see Table 52–5). Animal studies show that pulmonary injury is exacerbated by high concentration of inspired oxygen.[40,41] Limited clinical data, albeit sometimes conflicting, suggest that the oxygen administered during anesthesia may play a role in the development of perioperative acute respiratory failure.[40,41] Surgery within a short period from the last dose of bleomycin has also been suggested as a risk factor, but no safe period has been determined. Large volumes of crystalloid have also been mentioned,[49] but the evidence for this is weak. Use of large tidal volumes during one-lung ventilation is suspected to play a role in the pathogenesis of postpneumonectomy pulmonary edema.[50] Patients with BPT have reduced lung volume, and therefore it is prudent to use reduced tidal volumes.

TABLE 52–5. RISK FACTORS FOR THE DEVELOPMENT OF BPT

- Age greater than 70 years[36]
- History of cigarette smoking[42,43]
- Chest radiation therapy[44–46]
- Renal insufficiency
- Total dose greater than 450 mg[47]
- Single dosing instead of divided or continuous infusion
- Concurrent cyclophosphamide or cisplatin[48]
- Hyperoxia exposure[40,41]
- Genetic predisposition[37–39]

History of dyspnea, tachypnea, or dry cough and bibasilar rales on auscultation are the most common symptoms and signs of BPT. A pulmonary function test, chest x-ray, and baseline arterial blood gas measurement have been recommended in the presence of any of the clinical signs, but history and physical examination are more important indicators of the severity of disease than pulmonary function studies.[51] No matter what the test results are, patients with a history of bleomycin therapy undergoing general anesthesia should be ventilated on ambient air and minimal oxygen added, when required, to keep the arterial oxygen saturation at 90%. This can be achieved with a good measure of safety in the era of pulse oximetry. Intraoperative fluid restriction may not be advisable, but fluid overload must be avoided. There are isolated case reports of dramatic improvement resulting from the early administration of corticosteroid in acute respiratory failure.[41,52] Prophylactic use of corticosteroid may be justified if the patient requires high concentrations of oxygen. Mitomycin-C–treated patients may develop acute postoperative respiratory failure that also appears to improve with steroid therapy.[53]

Other agents associated with pulmonary fibrosis include busulfan, carmustine, methotrexate, cyclophosphamide, and thoracic radiation. If the patient receives a transfusion before the onset of respiratory failure, then transfusion-related acute lung injury must be considered in the differential diagnosis.

Effects of Malignancy and Its Therapy on the Nervous System

A variety of motor neuron diseases, stiff muscles with myoclonus, plexopathies, and myopathies have been described to be associated with malignancy and its treatment.[33] Autonomic neuropathy also can occur from the effect of malignancy or vincristine. The neurologic deficit may be due to direct compression or infiltration, or a paraneoplastic effect of cancer, or to chemotherapy and radiation. Intracranial metastasis and raised pressure or spinal bony metastasis may contraindicate placement of an epidural catheter for pain relief. Baseline motor and sensory function levels must be established, particularly if any regional or peripheral nerve blocks are being considered for pain relief.

Autonomic neuropathy may increase the risk of regurgitation during induction of anesthesia because of poor gastric emptying and/or produce intraoperative hemodynamic instability because of lack of normal autonomic function. The diagnosis of postoperative myocardial ischemia may also be difficult to assess because angina may be absent in these patients.

Succinylcholine used to facilitate tracheal intubation may precipitate massive hyperkalemia in many of these neurologic conditions. The neuromuscular blockers must be chosen and used with greater caution because unexpected sensitivity and resistance may be encountered. Also, monitoring the neuromuscular blockade may be misleading in the presence of unrecognized neuropathies. The perioperative implications of involvement of the muscles of respiration was alluded to under the respiratory section.

Hematologic and Hemostatic Disorders

The incidence of hemostatic disorder is high in malignant diseases.[54] Deep venous thrombosis is frequently the first or the presenting symptom of malignancy of the pancreas, lung, or female reproductive tract. Severe bleeding disorders may be associated with widespread metastasis of cancer of the prostate, lung, colon, breast, and ovary and malignant melanoma. Chemotherapy and radiation can cause severe bone marrow suppression, resulting in leukopenia, thrombocytopenia, and anemia. L-Asparaginase causes liver damage and factor deficiencies. Wilms' tumor can cause von Willibrand's syndrome. Vitamin K deficiency may be present from malnutrition, broad-spectrum antibiotic therapy, or obstructive biliary disease. Vitamin K is required for the post-translational gamma-carboxylation of vitamin K–dependent factors. Because of multiple coagulopathies such as disseminated intravascular coagulation, hepatic insufficiency, and vitamin deficiency, vitamin K should be tried when the prothrombin time is prolonged in cancer patients. Intraoperative coagulopathies may also result from hypothermia. In a small proportion of patients undergoing transurethral resection of the prostate, urokinase from the prostatic tissue may cause fibrinolysis.

Veno-oclusive disease of the liver associated with hepatic radiation and as a complication of a variety of chemotherapeutic agents is clinically indistinguishable from Budd-Chiari syndrome. The obstruction results from endothelial thickening of terminal hepatic venules. Thrombosis is common, and the incidence of deep venous thrombosis is high in cancer patients with malignancy.

Thrombocytopenia is common in patients with malignancy. A syndrome akin to idiopathic thrombocytic purpura is associated with Hodgkin's and other lymphoma. Thrombocytosis is common with a variety of malignancies and may predispose to thrombotic complication if there are other risk factors. Mithramycin is associated with bleeding disorders that may persist up to 2 weeks after therapy.

Malignancy and Endocrinopathy

Malignant tumors can secret a variety of hormones clinically presenting as paraneoplastic syndromes. Adrenocorticotrophic hormone, antidiuretic hormone, and parathormone are commonly involved. Neck radiation may cause thyroid or parathormone deficiency. Suramin, aminoglutethimide, ketoconazole, and high-dose corticosteroid therapy as a part of an antiemetic regimen during chemotherapy could produce adrenal insufficiency under increased stress and may need coverage with hydrocortisone.

Laboratory Tests

The combination of carefully obtained history and physical examination is the optimal way of evaluating the patient preoperatively for disease processes and of selecting the appropriate laboratory investigations. Current practice of laboratory investigation must be viewed critically because the majority of the test results do not benefit the patient. Laboratory tests in general are poor screening devices for diseases.[55] Marginally abnormal tests may lead to additional tests, leading to increased cost and inefficiency. Such test results may expose the patient to the risks of additional invasive evaluation. The medicolegal risk to the physician may be increased if the busy physician ordering the barrage of tests has failed to follow up the results.

Korvin and colleagues[56] reviewed the biochemical and hematologic tests performed on 1000 patients on admission to the hospital and found many abnormal results, none of which unequivocally benefited the patient. In a review of 5003 preoperative screening tests performed on 2570 healthy patients undergoing cholecystectomy,[57] abnormal results were obtained in 225. Action resulting from these abnormalities occurred in 17 cases. In only four patients could a conceivable benefit have arisen from a preoperative screening test. When compared with the results of the history and physical examination, routine preoperative investigations provided little further information that altered management. Similar studies have looked at the value of preoperative chest x-rays and electrocardiography. The extent of preoperative laboratory investigation in cancer patients must be based on the results of thorough history and physical examination.

Malignancy's association with a variety of paraneoplastic effects and thrombotic and hemorrhagic disorders, and the effect of chemotherapy on coagulation and organ function, may prompt the clinician to order a wider range of investigations.

PREOPERATIVE FASTING

Pulmonary aspiration of gastric contents is a devastating anesthetic complication, but its incidence is low and its risk and clinical importance may be overrated. Many of the patients who aspirate have a known risk factor, and aspiration could have been prevented by better risk assessment and alterations in the anesthetic management. The routine, healthy, elective surgical patient without known risk factors appears to be relatively safe from this feared complication, and acid aspiration prophylaxis is not indicated.

To reduce gastric volume, patients are fasted preoperatively (NPO) for 6 to 8 hours. Gastric transit time for food is variable and unpredictable, whereas water and clear liquid have a 50% emptying time of less than 30 minutes. Therefore, it is illogical to have the same protocol for solid and liquid ingestion. In light of recent publications on this subject[58] many centers have relaxed their liquid ingestion guidelines in ASA 1 and 2 patients.[20,59] Clear liquid is allowed up to 4 hours before the surgery in adults and 2 hours in children. If the patient has hiatal hernia, preoperative opioid medication, autonomic neuropathy from diabetes, alcoholism, certain cancer and its medications, pregnancy, trauma, bowel obstruction, prior esophageal surgery, anticipated difficult airway, or the like, then the NPO time is not relaxed for clear liquids. The commonly used clear liquids include water, apple juice, and carbonated drinks, although some centers allow black coffee and tea. The relaxed preoperative fasting guideline can cause confusion about the protocol among health care personnel and for the patient. In high-risk patients, medications such as metoclopramide, famotidine, and sodium bicitra may be given preoperatively to reduce gastric volume and increase its pH to >2.5.

INTRAOPERATIVE MONITORING

There has been a steady decline in anesthesia-related deaths in spite of increasing number of seriously ill patients presenting for surgery.[60] This improvement coincides with widespread application of monitors of anesthesia delivery system and patient parameters. At Harvard Medical School, the major accident rate of 1:75,700 and associated death rate of 1:150,400 before (1976–1985) compares well with the corresponding rates of 1:392,000 and 0 after (1985–1990) the adoption of improved monitoring methods.[61] Improved safety in anesthesia is presumed to be the result of, at least in part, improvements in monitoring.

Patients undergoing major cancer surgery usually have reduced physiologic reserve because of age-related diseases and the effect of cancer and chemotherapy. In addition, the surgery may be associated with massive blood loss and fluid shifts. Therefore, adequate means of monitoring their hemodynamics, electrolytes, and acid-base and coagulation status are required.

Systolic Pressure Variation

An intra-arterial catheter is normally used for continuous display of blood pressure and access for repeated arterial blood sampling that is required during and after major surgery. In addition, the difference in the systolic blood pressure caused by the phases of mechanical ventilation is a good indicator of intravascular volume. This pressure difference is called the systolic pressure variation (SPV). The reduction in the venous return during the inspiratory phase of the mechanical ventilation reduces the left ventricular stroke volume and the systolic blood pressure (Fig. 52–2). This is the physiologic basis of the variation. The positive pressure during inspiratory phase may be viewed as a negative or a reversed but recurring form of fluid challenge. The SPV is normally around 6 mm Hg, and it increases with increasing intravascular volume deficit. An SPV of 12 mm Hg is associated with significant hypovolemia, and the variation can exceed 25 mm Hg in severe hypovolemia.

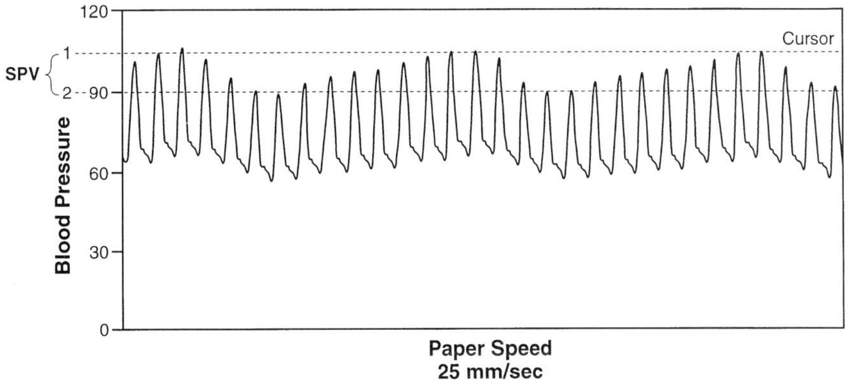

120
Cursor
SPV
1
2
90
60
30
0
Blood Pressure
Paper Speed
25 mm/sec

FIGURE 52–2. Radial arterial pressure tracing during posterior spinal fusion showing the effect of mechanical ventilation. The low-pressure tracings (cursor 2) correspond to mechanical inspiration and the high-pressure tracings (cursor 1) to expiration. The difference between the two cursors is the systolic pressure variation (SPV). The SPV in this tracing is about 15 mm Hg, suggesting hypovolemia.

Animal[62] and clinical studies[63–65] have shown SPV to be a reliable indicator of intravascular volume. SPV, pulmonary artery occlusion pressure (PAOP), and left ventricular end-diastolic area index (EDA) by echocardiographic estimate have been compared in patients after aortic surgery.[64] In this study there was a good correlation between the EDA and the SPV (r=0.8). Each volume loading caused a significant increase in the EDA and cardiac index and a simultaneous reduction in the SPV. Results of this clinical study suggest that SPV may be superior to PAOP as a volume monitor in mechanically ventilated patients. In the authors' experience, the SPV disappears during hypervolemia and cardiac failure. The SPV thus becomes a simple, effective, and continuous hemodynamic monitor in patients being mechanically ventilated. The SPV may not be valid if the chest is open or if the pulmonary compliance is altered.

Pulmonary Artery Catheterization

Pulmonary artery catheterization (PAC) has been in clinical use for 25 years, and over 2 million catheters are used in this country annually, resulting in estimated associated cost in the vicinity of $2 billion. It is an example of a technological advancement achieving wide acceptance without being subjected to vigorous evaluation. There is a lack of properly designed prospective studies showing favorable outcome with its use. The information obtained from PAC certainly alters the clinical management of the patient, but it is difficult to prove that it alters the outcome. A recent multicenter survey[66] found an unacceptable level of knowledge of the technical limitations and principles of pulmonary artery monitoring among users in academic environments. The ASA Task Force[67] examined the evidence for benefits and risks from pulmonary artery catheters used in settings encountered by anesthesiologists. They concluded that it is difficult to draw meaningful conclusions about the effectiveness and safety of PAC because of deficiencies in the currently available data.

Intracardiac pressures, cardiac output, and mixed venous saturation are the main data obtained from PAC, from which other hemodynamic and respiratory indices can be derived. Preload assessment, as indicated by ventricular end-diastolic filling pressure, is one of the most important indications for the use of PAC, but the pressure-volume correlation of the ventricles can be poor in the population in whom they are most needed. Studies of patients with cardiac disease and sepsis,[68] burns,[69] and trauma[70] show poor correlation in ventricular pressure-volume relation, presumably because of compliance changes of the ventricle and of the vascular bed in which the catheter tip is placed.

Physicians supervising trainees must be aware of the reviews and recommendations of the anesthesia and critical task forces in the United States and Europe and ensure that the trainees under them have the knowledge levels necessary. Achieving clinical competency in the use of PAC and understanding its limitations are essential to improve the risk-benefit ratio of its use. Measured pressures by themselves can be misleading, but relating their trends to the clinical condition of the patient may be more meaningful. In difficult cases, data from alternative sources such as SPV and echocardiography must be used when available.

A central venous catheter may be used during major surgery as access for fluid and medication and for monitoring the adequacy of venous filling. One must appreciate that the correlation between the right ventricular pressure and volume can be poor in situations of right ventricular dysfunction secondary to burns, sepsis, or ischemia. This poor correlation may be secondary to altered compliance of the right ventricle, presence of certain valvular diseases, and changing venous tone, which may affect the ventricular pressure more than the volume. Head-down lithotomy positioning can make interpretation of filling pressures difficult. However, careful monitoring and study of the central venous pressure waveforms can give much diagnostic insight into valvular diseases, dysrhythmias, and cardiac tamponade.[71] Prominent c-v waves of tricuspid regurgitation, marked elevation of the right atrial pressure in tricuspid stenosis, and absence of y-descent of the atrial pressure wave form of cardiac tamponade are some of the examples.

Coagulation Monitoring

Malignancy is associated with a variety of thrombotic and hemorrhagic complications. The diagnosis and management of intraoperative and postoperative hemorrhagic disorder must be guided by coagulation tests. The clinical utility of the test results provided by an institutional laboratory is limited by delays in obtaining results. On-site portable hematologic assays for whole blood activated partial thromboplastin time, prothrombin time, and platelet count have become available.[72–74] These tests use disposable plastic reagent cartridges and are technically easy to perform, and the results are ready in only a few minutes. With the availability of this point-of-service laboratory support, the management of intraoperative bleeding disorder is not hampered by delays in necessary test results. The undelayed test results eliminate the guess work in blood component therapy to correct coagulation defects, and this may result in better patient outcome and reduce inappropriate use of blood products.

Other devices available for on-site use are the thromboelastograph and Sonoclot Analyzer. Both of these devices are viscoelastometers of whole blood that give a qualitative measure of the kinetics of clot formation and dissolution and of clot quality. The graphic output of these instruments can sometimes suggest the presence of heparin-like substances in the blood as the cause of coagulopathy, as can happen during liver transplant and rarely in metastatic bladder carcinoma. If a heparin-like substance is suspected, its presence can be confirmed by the effect of heparinase on a sample of blood. If the thromboelastogram returns to normal, then the patient's coagulopathy may respond to protamine.

BLOOD COMPONENT THERAPY

As patients with malignancy live longer because of improvements in therapy, the demand for blood component therapy has increased markedly. Stored blood is cold and contains high levels of potassium, hydrogen ion, and citrate and no calcium. Blood transfusion at fast rates and in large volumes during surgery can be a major biochemical and hemodynamic challenge to patients with organ disease and reduced physiologic reserve. Because of the likelihood of polytransfusion of blood products, and altered immune status in cancer patients, an increase in the number of serious, and many times unexpected, complications can occur.[75] The contaminating leukocytes in the blood products appear to be responsible for many of these complications (Table 52–6).[76]

Physicians involved in the care of cancer patients must work closely with the blood bank for effective management with a strong emphasis on prevention of complications. Some of the complications of blood component therapy that are particularly relevant to patients with malignancy are briefly discussed here.

Transfusion-Associated Graft-Versus-Host Disease

Donor lymphocytes in cellular blood products engraft and mount an immunologic reaction against the recipient when the recipient fails to mount a rejection response against the donor lymphocytes.[77,78] Three factors may influence the occurrence of transfusion-associated graft-versus-host disease (TA-GVHD): (1) the immune status of the patient, (2) the human lymphocyte antigen (HLA) match between the host and the donor,[79,80] and (3) the dose and viability of injected leukocytes.[75,78] TA-GVHD has a mortality of around 90% and the risk factors are not completely defined. Immunodeficiency, high-dose chemoradiotherapy, Hodgkin's disease, and blood transfusions from relatives[79–81] are some of the main risk factors. Onset of symptoms is marked by a high fever within 3 to 30 days of the transfusion, followed by maculopapular rash within 1 to 2 days. Severe constitutional changes, abnormal liver function tests, and sepsis and bleeding secondary to bone marrow hypoplasia and pancytopenia are other features of TA-GVHD. Currently gamma irradiation of the cellular blood products is the only effective method of preventing TA-GVHD.[82,83] The request for irradiated blood must be initiated by the physician caring for the patient.

TABLE 52–6. POTENTIAL ADVERSE EFFECTS OF LEUKOCYTES*

Immunologically mediated effects
Alloimmunization to human leukocyte antigens
Febrile nonhemolytic transfusion reactions
Platelet refractoriness
Transplant rejection
Graft-versus-host disease
Immunosuppression
Viral disease reactivation
Infectious disease transmission
Viruses (e.g., cytomegalovirus, human T-cell lymphotropic virus I/II, Epstein-Barr virus)
Bacteria (e.g., *Yersinia enterocolitica*)
Reperfusion injury

*From Miller J, Mintz P: The use of leukocyte-reduced blood components. Hematol Oncol Clin North Am 1995; 9:69, with permission.

Transfusion-Transmitted Viral Diseases

Cytomegalovirus (CMV) is a leukocyte-associated virus that can be transmitted by cellular blood products and causes disease in immunosuppressed patients. Serologic testing can identify previously infected individuals, if recent intravenous immunoglobulin or unscreened blood products have not been given. In seropositive individuals, CMV disease is caused either by the reactivation of the dormant virus or from the new CMV strain transmitted by transfusion. It therefore appears that both seronegative and seropositive recipients are at risk of transfusion-associated CMV infection and disease.[84] Antiviral therapy for CMV disease is associated with significant morbidity and cost, and therefore the importance of prevention cannot be overemphasized. Use of seronegative blood products or leukocyte reduction of cellular blood products are effective means of preventing the transmission of the infection.

Patients with malignancy are likely to have underlying immunodeficiency or are likely to be immunosuppressed because of the disease and its therapy. They are also likely to be recipients of multiple transfusions, so preventive measures must be initiated early in management. Cryoprecipitate and fresh frozen plasma are acellular and do not pose a risk. The result of the latest study of the risk of viral infection following transfusion of 1 unit of blood is shown in Table 52–7.

Although the probability of contracting acquired immunodeficiency syndrome (AIDS) from a transfusion is very small, the concern among the public is substantial. The previous statistics confirm that

TABLE 52–7. RISK OF TRANSFUSION-TRANSMITTED VIRAL INFECTION*

HIV	1:493,000
HTLV	1:641,000
Hepatitis C	1:103,000
Hepatitis B	1:63,000

Risk of blood among units whose units passed all screening tests. New screening tests should reduce the risk even further.

*Adapted from Schreiber GB, Busch MP, Kleinman SH, et al: The risk of transfusion-transmitted viral infections. N Engl J Med 1996; 334, 1685, with permission.

the blood supply is safer today than it has ever been. These impressive results have been the result of a comprehensive program of donor screening and blood testing. The current incidence of HIV-infected bank blood is not due to false-negative testing but due to the fact that the test is for the antibody to the virus and not the virus itself, therefore leaving a 6-week window period where the virus is present but the test is negative. This results in an estimated 20 to 25 contaminated units per year from the 12,000,000-unit supply collected nationally. In 1996, a new P-24 antigen test was introduced that will reduce the number of infected units of blood by an estimated 25% (i.e., approximately six additional contaminated units will be detected per year at an estimated cost of $10 million per detected unit). Given the age and the disease process that face the urologic oncologic patient, the concern regarding contracting AIDS from a blood transfusion should be extremely small. Its risk (approximately 1:500,000) should be discussed with patients relative to all the other risks associated with their cancer, the surgical procedure, and their concurrent chronic medical problems. In general, for any patient with severe cardiac or pulmonary disease, the risk of not receiving a red cell transfusion would appear to dramatically outweigh the risk of HIV infection. A study has found that, in patients who are at high risk for cardiac disease who are undergoing vascular surgery, there was a substantial increase in cardiac morbidity when the hematocrit was allowed to decrease below 28%.[86] Consequently, it is suggested that, in elderly patients with significant cardiopulmonary disease, the hematocrit be maintained in the range of 30%.

Alloimmunization and Platelet Refractoriness

Alloimmunization to a class 1 antigen on the platelet is the leading cause of platelet refractoriness, with an incidence reported to be between 30 and 70% in multiply transfused patients.[75] A poor 1-hour post-transfusion platelet increment, corrected for number of platelets transfused and the estimated blood volume of the recipient, is suggestive of alloimmunization. Other causes of platelet refractoriness, such as sepsis, hypersplenism, and disseminated intravascular coagulation, must be ruled out. Diagnosis is confirmed by detecting lymphocytotoxic antibodies. Serial measurements of this antibody are a useful monitor because the condition can sometimes regress. Alloimmunization is managed by transfusing HLA-matched or cross-matched platelets. Limited efficacy and increased pressure on the supply of compatible platelets puts the patients at increased risk of thrombocytopenic bleeding. Use of preventive measures for patients at risk is the preferred approach. Effective means of prevention include ultraviolet irradiation and leukoreduction of cellular blood products.[75]

Transfusion-Associated Acute Lung Injury

Leukoagglutinating and lymphocytotoxic antibodies in donor blood products cause a rare but underrecognized serious reaction manifested by noncardiogenic pulmonary edema within 2 to 6 hours of transfusion.[75] The agglutinated leukocytes lodge in the pulmonary vasculature and cause capillary leak syndrome and exudation of fluid into the pulmonary interstitium. This condition should be suspected in all cases of unexplained pulmonary edema after transfusion. Treatment is mainly supportive. The donor blood should be identified and further donation from that donor should be restricted to non–plasma-containing products. Multiparous donors are frequently responsible for the reaction.

Immunomodulation and Allogenic Blood Transfusion

Animals receiving allogenic blood transfusion (ABT) and tumor cell infusion or tumor inoculation have a significantly higher rate of pulmonary metastasis than do control animals.[87] These studies also show that this effect has an immunologic mechanism involving the donor leukocytes in the allogenic blood. Concern about the effect of ABT in patients undergoing cancer surgery has stimulated over 70 studies, the majority of which were done retrospectively in colorectal cancer and have yielded conflicting results.[87] Several meta-analyses of these studies, however, have concluded that ABT has a deleterious effect on the prognosis of patients. Two randomized prospective studies of patients with colorectal cancer have concluded that ABT is associated with higher cancer recurrence rate. Several other prospective nonrandomized studies have shown no adverse effect of ABT.[88,89] A randomized prospective study of the influence of ABT for prostate cancer has shown no deleterious effect,[90] although three other retrospective studies[91–93] showed increased recurrence rate. Retrospective studies on kidney tumors show adverse effect in three studies,[94–96] and no effect in other studies.[97,98]

Lander et al. concluded that the available data support the concept that allogenic blood products increase cancer recurrence rate after potentially curative surgical resection.[99]

The effect of ABT on the incidence of bacterial infection in the postoperative period has been studied in trauma, burn, and cancer patients. The retrospective, prospective nonrandomized, and prospective randomized studies all showed a significantly increased risk of bacterial infectious complication associated with ABT. In a prospective randomized study of colorectal cancer, Heiss and colleagues[100] showed that the odds ratio for developing bacterial infectious complication in patients receiving ABT versus syngeneic blood transfusion was 2.84, while there was no difference in the noninfectious complication rates. Patients who received larger volume ABT seem to have higher infectious complication rates. In a prospective randomized study of cancer patients, nonleukodepleted ABT was associated with a significantly higher postoperative bacterial infection rate compared to leukodepleted ABT.[101] The association between ABT and bacterial infection must be validated with properly controlled prospective randomized clinical studies.

Intraoperative Autotransfusion during Cancer Surgery

Increasing demand on a limited supply of homologous blood, increasing cost of transfusion, the risk of transfusion reactions, the risk of transmission of infections, and the possible impact of the immunomodulatory effect of transfusion have led to increased interest in the use of intraoperative autotransfusion during major cancer surgery. There is continued but unsubstantiated concern about the transfusion of blood that is potentially contaminated by malignant cells. The stress of surgery, homologous blood transfusion, and high-dose opioid treatment all contribute to make immunosuppression inevitable in the perioperative period. However, the role of the host immune factors in the prevention of dissemination of malignancy has not been established.

Intraoperative autotransfusion has been studied in hepatic resection,[102,103] urologic malignant neoplasm,[104] and bladder cancer.[105] These studies could not show increased dissemination of cancer caused by autotransfusion. Studies have failed to show a correlation between the circulating tumor cells and subsequent development of metastasis,[105] which suggests that the presence of circulating tumor cells has no prognostic significance. Patients with renal cell carcinoma with caval extension already have circulating tumor cells, and intraoperative autotransfusion is routinely used.

The filters in the cell savers routinely used in clinical practice are extremely efficient in removing white blood cells and cancer cells.[106,107] Although some may view the routine use of filters as a solution to an unestablished problem, their use may lead to better acceptance of intraoperative autotransfusion by clinicians who continue to have concerns about the possibility and consequences of transfusion of malignant cells.

FLUID THERAPY, ELECTROLYTES, AND ACID-BASE DISTURBANCES

Cancer and its chemotherapy can cause a variety of electrolytes and acid-base disorders. Major fluid shifts during surgery can compound the problem. Hypercalcemia is usually a late manifestation of cancer with poor prognosis, and therefore not likely to be encountered in patients presenting for major surgery. Hypocalcemia may be caused by radiation therapy to the neck and mediastinum or cisplatin-based chemotherapy, or may occur as a part of the tumor lysis syndrome.

Cisplatin is potentially nephrotoxic and causes hypomagnesemia, hypokalemia, hypophosphatemia, and hypocalcemia. Refractory hypocalcemia and hypokalemia will respond to replacement therapy once hypomagnesemia is corrected. In most cases these electrolyte disturbances disappear once cisplatin is stopped, but in a minority of cases they can persist for long periods of time. Hypomagnesemia makes the patient more prone to torsades de pointes–type ventricular fibrillation.

A variety of tumors and anticancer drugs such as vincristine, cyclophosphamide, and cisplatin show up on the long differential diagnosis for the syndrome of inappropriate antidiuretic hormone secretion. The syndrome is characterized by hypotonic hyponatremia and a urinary osmolality greater than 100 mmol/kg.

Large volumes of normal saline causes a metabolic acidosis that may be dilutional or may result from hyperchloremia caused by normal saline. How or why hyperchloremia causes metabolic acidosis is not obvious when analyzed by the conventional Henderson-Hasselbalch approach to acid-base balance. A revolutionary approach to acid-base analysis proposed by Stewart[108] makes it more easy to explain hypochloremic metabolic alkalosis and hyperchloremic metabolic acidosis. Instead of the conventional H^+ and HCO_3^- as the important determinants of acid-base status, the new approach makes distinction between *independent* variables (P_{CO_2}, net strong ion charge, and total weak acids) and *dependent* variables (HCO_3^-, HA, A, CO_3^{2-}, OH^-, and H^+). Only changes in independent variables can affect H^+. Interested readers are referred to the review by Stewart for a full description and implication.[108]

When large quantities of fluid therapy are required, Normosol or Plasmalyte may be better choices because they have less chloride and therefore are less prone to cause metabolic acidosis. In addition, the magnesium content of the fluid may be very desirable in patients who have recently received cisplatin therapy. The magnesium in Normosol may cause hypotension if this solution is given at very fast rates.

ANESTHESIA FOR UROLOGIC CANCER SURGERY

Anesthesia for Transurethral Resection of the Prostate

Literature on the advantages of regional anesthesia over general anesthesia for transurethral resection of the prostate (TURP) shows conflicting results. The regional anesthesia may cause less hemodynamic instability, reduced blood loss, no immunosuppression, earlier recognition of TURP syndrome and bladder perforation, and reduced postoperative pain because of pre-emptive analgesias.

Bowman and coauthors compared low spinal and general anesthesia for prostate surgery and found no difference in blood transfusion requirements or dysrhythmia rate in the two groups.[109] However, the general anesthesia group was associated with a greater incidence of intraoperative hypotension and postoperative hypertension. A series of studies have looked at postoperative cognitive function and found temporary impairments, but there was no difference between general and regional anesthesia groups. There is disagreement in the literature concerning intraoperative blood loss and the method of anesthesia during TURP. A large mass of resected tissue, long resection time, infection from an indwelling catheter, and general anesthesia are associated with increased blood loss.[110] Other studies show no association between the method of anesthesia and intraoperative blood loss.[111,112]

A significant fall in lymphocyte count and a decrease in lymphocyte response to certain mutagens is associated with general anesthesia.[113] These authors suggested that this transient immunosuppression associated with general anesthesia should be avoided during TURP for cancer of the prostate. Perhaps the real advantage of regional anesthesia for TURP is reduced postoperative pain.[109,114] There was significantly less postoperative pain and analgesic requirements in patients who had regional anesthesia,[109] presumably because of the pre-emptive analgesic effect of regional anesthesia. Addition of 0.1 mg morphine to the intrathecal local anesthesia produces longer pain relief without significant increase in itching or nausea.[114] Spinal anesthesia is associated with a significant incidence of transient hearing disturbances and a small incidence of post-dural puncture headache. Failure of the return of TURP irrigating fluid in a normal way may suggest bladder perforation. Extraperitoneal perforation may cause periumbilical or lower abdominal pain, but this may be absent when the spinal anesthesia is above T10. Peritoneal perforation causes abdominal and shoulder pain.

TURP Syndrome

The irrigating fluids used in TURP are chosen for their optical and electrical properties. Glycine and Cytal (a mixture of sorbitol and mannitol) are the most commonly used irrigating fluids. The prostate glands are rich in venous sinuses, and absorption of the irrigating fluid is inevitable. Depending on the volume absorbed and the duration of resection, the absorbed fluid produces volume and biochemical disturbances whose symptoms and signs are manifested in the central nervous system (CNS) and the cardiovascular system. The CNS effects range from confusion to coma. The main cause of CNS effects is dilutional hyponatremia. A serum sodium level of 120 mEq/L or less is associated with TURP syndrome. In addition, glycine and resultant hyperammonemia may have CNS effects. Glycine is believed to be a neurotransmitter at many inhibitory nerve terminals, but the role of glycine in CNS effects is currently speculative. Oxidative biotransformation of the excess glycine may lead to the buildup of ammonia (a known neurotoxin) in the body as the urea cycle is overwhelmed. Arginine is an essential amino acid and a major ingredient in the urea cycle. It is tempting to hypothesize that adding arginine in the irrigating fluid may prevent hyperammonemia. Distilled water used as irrigating fluid can cause water intoxication in addition to dilutional hyponatremia. The hypo-osmolar effect of distilled water can lead to hemolysis and cerebral and cardiac edema. For this reason an isotonic solutions is preferable to distilled water for resection of the prostate.

The cardiovascular effects of absorbed irrigating fluid result from volume overload and hyponatremia. Initial hypertension and bradycardia may be followed by hypotension and pulmonary edema. Dilutional hyponatremia is likely to be associated with dilutional hypocalcemia and hypomagnesemia, but their physiologic effect in this setting is unknown. Severe hyponatremia may explain the widened QRS complex and ventricular ectopy.

Treatment consists of cardiorespiratory support, fluid restriction, and loop diuretics. Mechanical ventilation and invasive hemodynamic monitoring may be required. Fluid overload may manifest in the recovery room as the spinal anesthesia and its vasodilatory effect wears off. Hypertonic saline may be given if the serum sodium level is below 120 mEq/L. Hypertonic saline (3 to 5%) should be given at a rate no faster than 100 ml/hour. Faster rates of infusion can cause pontine myelinolysis.

Use of irrigating fluids at room temperature causes a significant decrease in body temperature, leading to shivering and stress. Prewarmed irrigating fluid has been effective in preventing the hypothermia without leading to increased blood loss.[115] Septicemia must be considered in the differential diagnosis of unexplained hypotension and tachycardia in the perioperative period in patients who had a preoperative indwelling urinary catheter.

Radical Prostatectomy

Improvements in the surgical technique[116] and intensive scrutiny of the cost effectiveness of the perioperative care[117–120] of patients undergoing radical retropubic prostatectomy (RRP) have resulted in major changes in their perioperative management. There has been substantial reduction in the duration of surgery, blood loss, transfusion rates, and length of hospital stay. Because of these improvements, invasive hemodynamic monitoring is rarely indicated in these patients. Studies have shown no difference in postoperative morbidity or complication rates between patients receiving general or epidural anesthesia for RRP.[121] However, the type of anesthesia may influence intraoperative blood loss. In a randomized study of 100 patients undergoing RRP, it has been shown that patients who received epidural anesthesia alone had significantly less intraoperative blood loss when compared to general anesthesia alone or combined general and epidural anesthesia.[122] This suggests that general anesthesia is an independent predictor of increased intraoperative blood loss. This may be due to increased venous pressure secondary to positive pressure ventilation or to the vasodilatory effect of isoflurane. Epidural anesthesia is associated with significantly reduced postoperative analgesic requirements.[123]

Perineal prostatectomy with or without laparoscopic lymphadenectomy requires general anesthesia because of the positioning and the gas insufflation in the peritoneal cavity. Preoperative autologous blood collection can reduce perioperative homologous transfusion, but this impact is tempered by its cost and preoperative anemia despite a reasonable interval between collection and surgery.[124] In good hands, the frequency of transfusion requirement is so small that autologous blood collection is not cost effective.

Radical Nephrectomy

Anesthetic management for the radical nephrectomy presents special challenges to the anesthesiologist. Renal cell carcinoma has the propensity to extend along the renal veins and the inferior vena cava (IVC) sometimes all the way to the right atrium.[125,126] The majority of the tumor mass in the IVC arises from tumors of the right kidney. Intraoperative tumor embolization leading to acute right heart failure is a feared complication. The anesthetic plan depends on the surgical approach. When the tumor involves the suprahepatic IVC with or without right atrium extension, deep hypothermic circulatory arrest provides excellent operating conditions.[125] Its disadvantages are substantial increase in cost and technical complexity. When the right atrium is not involved, the hepatic IVC thrombus may be managed with venous bypass.[127] Attwood et al. used femoral and right atrial cannulation for this purpose,[128] but a more peripheral venous access can be used for the bypass. We have used Biomedicus 15-French cannulas placed percutaneously in the femoral and internal jugular veins by the anesthesiologist at the time of induction. This approach is used routinely for the venous bypass for liver transplant recipients at our institution. The savings in surgical time is substantial.

Invasive monitoring is not routinely necessary for a simple radical nephrectomy. When the IVC is involved by the thrombus, a pulmonary artery catheter and an arterial line should be considered because of the possibility of acute pulmonary embolism and increased bleeding. Blood loss from partial nephrectomy is substantially more than from radical nephrectomy. Perioperative blood transfusion does not seem to affect survival after operation for renal cell cancer.[97]

Retroperitoneal Lymph Node Dissection

Retroperitoneal lymph node dissection for nonseminomatous germ cell testicular tumor stage I and II is usually indicated in young healthy patients. Patients in stage III will have received a course of chemotherapy usually consisting of cisplatin, vinblastine, and bleomycin. The surgery is conducted after chemotherapy has rendered the tumor markers normal, and therefore the surgery is not urgent. Patients should be allowed to recover from the side effects of chemotherapy. The surgery is time consuming and there is a risk of damage to renal vessels and the ureters. The major side effects of the chemotherapy include myelosuppression, pulmonary toxicity, nausea and vomiting, paralytic ileus, weight loss, anemia, nephrotoxicity, hypomagnesemia, and peripheral neuropathy. Coagulation screening and baseline neurologic examination are essential, especially when the postoperative pain plan includes epidural analgesia. The management of BPT has already been discussed. Invasive arterial pressure monitoring is required to monitor intraoperative volume status (see previous discussion of SPV).

POSTOPERATIVE PAIN MANAGEMENT

Postoperative pain management traditionally relied on intermittent intramuscular injection of opioids on an as-needed basis. This method of pain relief resulted in large fluctuations in the blood lev-

TABLE 52–8. INTRAVENOUS PCA DOSAGE SCHEDULE

Drug	Loading Dose (mg/kg)	PCA Dose (mg)	Lockout (min)	Infusion/hr (mg)
Morphine	0.05–0.1	0.5–3.0	6–10	0.5–3.0
Meperidine	0.5–1.0	5–30	6–10	5–20
Hydromorphine	0.01–0.02	0.1–0.3	6–10	0.1–0.3

els of the analgesic, and the pain relief was deploringly inadequate. Patient-controlled analgesia (PCA) developed from the recognition of this inadequacy. PCA has received widespread acceptance by patients, nursing staff, and physicians because it provides more prompt and nonfluctuating analgesia that more closely matches the patient's need over time. In PCA the patient administers opioid intravenously or opioid or local anesthesia epidurally. Thus PCA can adjust to the individual variability in pain tolerance, and in the pharmacokinetics and pharmacodynamics. It is very important that the patient understands the PCA well and has a chance to ask questions about its use. Some of the concerns patients usually have are reduced contact with the nursing staff, inadvertent overdose, inadequate analgesia, and opioid addiction. The factors that must be considered when initiating PCA are the loading dose, a constant infusion rate, demand dose, the lockout interval, the maximum dose, and the monitoring protocol. The lockout interval for morphine and meperidine is 6 to 10 minutes. The maximums or restrictions are safeguards in the PCA units that can be changed after careful consideration. Demand dosing and constant rate infusion plus demand dosing are the most commonly used modes. The dosage schedule of morphine, meperidine, and hydromorphine used in intravenous PCA in our institution is given in Table 52–8. In epidural PCA, usually a mixture of dilute local anesthetic and opioid is used.

The use of transdermal narcotic delivery is now receiving attention and may become available for postoperative pain. The method is practical and inexpensive and aims to maintain continuous delivery and constant blood levels. Fentanyl has been the drug of choice and in chronic pain has been well received by patients. Side effects must be carefully managed as they occur.

Pain Assessment and Measurement

Pain is a highly subjective and multidimensional experience encompassing many sensory and affective components. A multitude of factors influence the manner in which patients experience pain and appreciate the effectiveness of therapy provided for its relief. Objective measurement of pain is difficult but important. Observer pain scores based on behavioral and autonomic signs of pain intensity are unreliable. Currently the visual analogue scale is the most widely used pain assessment tool. It is a simple, sensitive, and reproducible instrument.

Uncontrolled postoperative pain has other morbidity in addition to the suffering of pain and immobility. The metabolic effects of the stress response to surgical trauma have a neuroendocrine mechanism. If afferent input to the CNS is attenuated by epidural local anesthesia, the stress response can be minimized but may not be completely abolished. The reasons may be that the epidural blockade may not be high enough or dense enough to prevent complete inhibition of noxious afferent input. In addition, local release of chemical mediators such as interleukin may be playing a part. The increased metabolic demand and the high catabolic state of the skeletal muscle may contribute to the postoperative fatigue syndrome. PCA does not reduce postoperative fatigue syndrome, presumably because of incomplete suppression of the stress response. The neuroendocrine response to surgical stress may affect the incidence of postoperative cardiac ischemia. Postoperative epidural analgesia with local anesthesia and opioids is associated with a decrease in sympathetic nervous activity, improved cardiac hemodynamics, and coronary vasodilatory effect. This may account in part for the improved outcome in high-risk surgical patients managed with epidural analgesia.[31,129–131]

Hyperalgesia is an altered state of sensibility in which the pain response to a noxious stimulus is greatly increased.[132] Bradykinin released at the site of injury initiates and maintains the state of hyperalgesia. Bradykinin also stimulates the phospholipase–cyclo-oxygenase cascade and the resulting synthesis of prostaglandins that are responsible for the release of substance P at the nerve terminals. Bradykinin, prostaglandin, and substance P reinforce each other via a vicious cycle and maintain the state of hyperalgesia. Allodynia is a condition in which even light pressure and touch is perceived as intensely painful. Primary hyperalgesia occurs at the site of injury and becomes evident within minutes of the injury. Secondary hyperalgesia occurs in response to thermal stimuli and has a delayed onset. Both peripheral and CNS sensitization is involved in the pathogenesis of secondary hyperalgesia. Administration of opioids, local anesthetic, and nonsteroidal anti-inflammatory agents (NSAIDs) before the surgical trauma may prevent or minimize the peripheral and central sensitization and reduce both the intensity and the duration of postoperative pain.

Postoperative epidural analgesia is associated with reduced pulmonary complications after thoracic and upper abdominal procedures. The ability to cough and take deep breaths is better with adequate pain control, and this can reduce postoperative pneumonia.

The immunosuppression associated with surgical trauma may increase the risk of postoperative in-

TABLE 52–9. KETOROLAC DOSAGE*

Dose	Patients <65 years old	Patients >65 years old and/or <50 kg
Single dose—intramuscular	60 mg × 1 dose only	30 mg × 1 dose only
Single dose—intravenous	30 mg × 1 dose only	15 mg × 1 dose only
Multiple dose, intramuscular or intravenous	30 mg every 6 hr, not more than 120 mg/day	15 mg every 6 hr, not more than 60 mg/day
Oral (10-mg tablets)	2 tabs followed by 1 tab every 4–6 hr, not more than 40 mg/24 hr	1 tab every 4–6 hr, not more than 40 mg/24 hr

*Adapted from Package insert: Toradol. Palo Alto, CA, Syntex Laboratories, 1995, with permission.

fection. Further immunoalteration may be induced by the administration of opioids[133–137] and blood transfusions. The use of epidural local anesthesia and analgesia may help to reduce opioid use and preserve immune function. There are no clinical studies looking at the effect of opioid-induced perioperative immunosuppression on the distant seeding of cancer cells.

Nonsteroidal Anti-inflammatory Drugs

Ketorolac is the only parenteral NSAID for short-term analgesia available in the United States. It has a fast onset of action, and the analgesic effect lasts about 4 to 6 hours. It is highly bound to plasma proteins and metabolized to inactive forms in the liver. No dosage adjustment is necessary in patients with cirrhosis. Clearance is significantly reduced in the elderly and in patients with renal disease. Its analgesic potency compares well with that of opioids (2 mg intramuscular ketorolac equals 3 to 5 mg intramuscular morphine).

Ketorolac is contraindicated in patients with active peptic ulcer disease and recent gastrointestinal bleeding or perforation. Advanced renal impairment and hypovolemia are also contraindications for its use. In mild renal impairment the dose should be reduced. It should not be used in patients with cerebrovascular bleeding, bleeding diathesis, and incomplete hemostasis. It should not be used as a prophylactic analgesic preoperatively and intraoperatively if hemostasis is critical.[138]

The combined duration of parenteral and oral use should not exceed 5 days (Table 52–9).[139] Exceeding the recommended dose or shortening the dosing interval may lead to increased frequency and severity of adverse reactions.

MANAGEMENT OF POSTOPERATIVE NAUSEA AND VOMITING

Postoperative nausea and vomiting (PONV) is one of the most common and unpleasant complications of surgery for both inpatients and day surgical patients. The reported incidence of PONV varies between 25 to 43% for inpatients and 8 to 45% for ambulatory surgical patients.[140,141] In a climate where total cost of an illness is becoming increasingly important, PONV is a major contributor to direct and indirect costs for both the hospital and patient.[141] PONV is perceived by patients to account for equal or more debilitation than surgery itself and may cause them to lose wages as a result of absence from work.[142] Many patients place nausea and vomiting as the most unpleasant consequence of surgery. Reducing the incidence of PONV and its associated problems in targeted high-risk groups[143] (Table 52–10) can improve care and reduce costs. Recent trends in more effective and aggressive postoperative pain management have shifted the focus onto PONV. The goal of effective prevention and management of PONV is more achievable with the availability of a more effective antiemetic drug with fewer side effects: ondansetron.

There is no literature about the incidence of PONV in cancer patients. Patients who have experienced significant chemotherapy-induced nausea and vomiting are known to experience nausea from the mere anticipation of chemotherapy. This may suggest that this group of patients has an altered sensitivity of the reflexes governing nausea and vomiting. Furthermore, the chemotherapy-induced nausea and vomiting usually requires a much higher dose of ondansetron for control, so these patients may be at high risk for PONV and may need higher doses of antiemetic.

Ondansetron, a selective 5-HT_3 antagonist,[144] is more effective than metoclopramide and droperidol

TABLE 52–10. RISK FACTORS FOR POSTOPERATIVE NAUSEA AND VOMITING*

- Intravenous anesthetics except Propofol
- Inhalational anesthetic agents
- Opioids
- Previous history of postoperative nausea and vomiting or motion sickness
- Obesity
- Female
- Children
- Abdominal and gynecological surgery

*From Kenny G: Risk factors for postoperative nausea and vomiting. Anaesthesia 1994; 49(suppl):6, with permission.

in controlling chemotherapy-induced nausea and vomiting. Large multicenter studies have demonstrated that ondansetron (4 mg) administered intravenously is effective in preventing and treating PONV.[145-147] Another large multicenter study has shown that ondansetron 16 mg given orally 1 hour before the surgery, is effective in preventing PONV.[148] A small pilot study has shown that prophylactic ondansetron was superior to both droperidol and metoclopramide in the prevention of emetic sequela in females undergoing minor gynecologic procedures.[146] Large multicenter studies comparing ondansetron with other antiemetics in the management of PONV are underway.[149] In all the studies conducted to date, the use of ondansetron was associated with very few side effects.

CONCLUSION

This chapter has attempted to review some of the most pertinent aspects of anesthetic care and perioperative management for patients undergoing major urologic procedures. It has stressed the importance of the preoperative work-up to allow optimization of the patient's medical condition prior to undergoing the stress of the surgical procedure. It has also reviewed the various modalities available in postoperative pain management not only to improve patient comfort and satisfaction but also morbidity. For a more in-depth review of specific anesthetic theory and techniques, the reader is referred to comprehensive textbooks (e.g., refs. 1 and 2).

REFERENCES

1. Miller R: Anesthesia, 4th edition. New York, Churchill Livingstone, 1994.
2. Stoelting R, Dierdorf SF (eds): Anesthesia and Co-Existing Disease. New York, Churchill Livingstone, 1993.
3. Dripps R, Lamont A, Eckenhoff J: The role of anesthesia in surgical mortality. JAMA 1961; 178:261.
4. Ryhanen P, Hollman A, Horttonen L: Blood pressure changes during and after anesthesia in treated and untreated hypertensive patients. Ann Chir Gynaecol 1978; 67:180.
5. Prys-Roberts C: Hypertension and anesthesia—fifty years on. Anesthesiology 1979; 50:281.
6. Detsky A: Predicting cardiac complications in patients undergoing non-cardiac surgery. J Gen Intern Med 1986; 1:211.
7. Goldman L, Caldera D, Nussbaum S, et al: Multifactorial index of cardiac risk in noncardiac surgical procedures. N Engl J Med 1977; 297:845.
8. Paul SD, Eagle K: A stepwise strategy for coronary risk assessment for noncardiac surgery. Med Clin North Am 1995; 79:1241.
9. Fleisher L: Preoperative cardiac evaluation for noncardiac surgery: a functional approach. Anesth Analg 1992; 74: 586.
10. Coley CM: Usefulness of dipyridamole-thallium scanning for preoperative evaluation of cardiac risk for nonvascular surgery. Am J Cardiol 1992; 69:1280.
11. Eagle KA: Dipyridamole-thallium scanning in patients undergoing vascular surgery. JAMA 1987; 257:2185.
12. Eagle K: Combining clinical and thallium data optimizes preoperative assessment of cardiac risk before major vascular surgery. Ann Intern Med 1989; 110:859.
13. Lette J: Preoperative and long-term cardiac risk assessment. Ann Surg 1992; 216:192.
14. Shah KB, Kleinman BS, Sami H, et al: Reevaluation of perioperative myocardial infarction in patients with prior myocardial infarction undergoing noncardiac operations. Anesth Analg 1990; 71:231.
15. Rao TK, Jacobs KH, El-Etr A, et al: Reinfarction following anesthesia in patients with myocardial infarction. Anesthesiology 1983; 59:499.
16. Tarhan S, Moffitt EA, Taylor W, et al: Myocardial infarction after general anesthesia. JAMA 1972; 220:1451.
17. Jereczek M, Andersen D, Schroeder J, et al: Prognostic value of ischemia during Holter monitoring and exercise testing after acute myocardial infarction. Am J Cardiol 1993; 72:8.
18. Currie P, Ashby D, Saltissi S: Prognostic significance of transient myocardial ischemia on ambulatory monitoring after myocardial infarction. Am J Cardiol 1993; 71:773.
19. Gill JB, Cains J, Roberts R, et al: Prognostic importance of myocardial ischemia detected by ambulatory monitoring early after acute myocardial infarction. N Engl J Med 1996; 334:65.
20. Kamat S, Kleiman N: Platelets and platelet inhibitors in acute myocardial infarction. Cardiol Clin 1995; 133:435.
21. de Leon-Casasola OA, Parker B, Lema M, et al: Postoperative epidural bupivacaine-morphine therapy: experience with 4,227 surgical cancer patients. Anesthesiology 1994; 81:368.
22. Bode RJ, Lewis KP, Zarich S, et al: Cardiac outcome after peripheral vascular surgery: comparison after general and regional anesthesia. Anesthesiology 1996; 84:3.
23. Myers C: Anthracyclines and DNA intercalators. *In* Holland J, Frei EI, Bast RJ, et al (eds): Cancer Medicine, Vol 1, p 764. Philadelphia, Lea & Febiger, 1993.
24. Doroshow J, Locker G, Myers C: The enzymatic defenses of the mouse heart against reactive metabolites. J Clin Invest 1980; 65:128.
25. Legha SS, Benjamin RS, Mackay B, et al: Reduction of doxorubicin cardiotoxicity by prolonged continuous intravenous infusion. Ann Intern Med 1982; 96:133.
26. Von Hoff D, Layard M, Basa P, et al: Risk factors for doxorubicin-induced congestive heart failure. Ann Intern Med 1979; 91:710.
27. Seifert CF, Nesser M, Thompson D: Dexrazoxane in the prevention of doxorubicin-induced cardiotoxicity. Ann Pharmacother 1994; 28:1063.
28. Van Hoff DD, Rozencweig M, Piccart M: The cardiotoxicity of anticancer agents. Semin Oncol 1982; 9:23.
29. Soukop M, McVie J, Calman K: Fluorouracil cardiotoxicity. Br Med J 1978; 1:547.
30. Harrigan P, Otis D, Recht A, et al: The effect of adjuvant radiation therapy (RT) on cardiac events in breast cancer patients treated with doxorubicin (Dox) [Meeting abstract]. Proc Annu Meet Am Soc Clin Oncol 1995; 14: A109.
31. Caplan R, Posner K, Ward R, et al: Adverse respiratory events in anesthesia: a closed claims analysis. Anesthesiology 1990; 72:828.
32. Delaney P: Vincristine-induced laryngeal nerve paralysis. Neurology 1982; 32:1285.
33. Stubgen J: Neuromuscular disorder in systemic malignancy and its treatment. Muscle Nerve 1995; 18:636.
34. Windsor J, Hill G: Risk factors for postoperative pneumonia. Ann Surg 1988; 208:209.
35. Ford GT, Whitelaw W, Rosenal T, et al: Diaphragm function after upper abdominal surgery in humans. Am Rev Respir Dis 1983; 127:431.
36. Mathes D: Bleomycin and hyperoxia exposure in the operating room. Anesth Analg 1995; 81:624.
37. Schrier D: The role of strain variation in murine bleomycin-induced pulmonary fibrosis. Am Rev Respir Dis 1983; 127:63

38. Chandler D: Possible mechanisms of bleomycin-induced fibrosis. Clin Chest Med 1990; 11:21.
39. Comis R: Bleomycin pulmonary toxicity: current status and future directions. Semin Oncol 1992; 19:64.
40. Hulbert JC: Risk factors of anesthesia and surgery in bleomycin-treated patients. J Urol 1983; 130:163.
41. Ingrassia T, Ryu J, Trastek V, et al: Oxygen exacerbated bleomycin pulmonary toxicity. Mayo Clin Proc 1991; 66: 173.
42. Hansen S: Enhanced pulmonary toxicity in smokers with germ-cell cancer treated with cis-platinum, vinblastine and bleomycin: a long-term follow-up. Eur J Cancer Clin Oncol 1989; 25:733.
43. Lower E: Bleomycin causes alveolar macrophages from cigarette smokers to release hydrogen peroxide. Am J Med Sci 1988; 295:193.
44. Einhorn L: Enhanced pulmonary toxicity with bleomycin and radiotherapy in oat cell lung cancer. Cancer 1976; 37: 2414.
45. Samuels M: Large-dose bleomycin therapy and pulmonary toxicity. JAMA 1976; 235:1117.
46. Catane R, Schwade JG, Turrisi A, et al: Pulmonary toxicity after radiation and bleomycin: a review. Int J Radiat Oncol Biol Phys 1979; 5:1531.
47. Blum RH, Carter SK, Agre K: A clinical review of bleomycin, a new antineoplastic agent. Cancer 1973; 31:903.
48. Yee G: Cisplatin-induced changes in bleomycin elimination. Cancer Treat Rep 1983; 67:587.
49. Goldiner P: Factors influencing postoperative morbidity and mortality in patients treated with bleomycin. Br Med J 1978; 1:1664.
50. Slinger P: Perioperative fluid management for thoracic surgery: the puzzle of postpneumonectomy pulmonary edema. J Cardiothorac Vasc Anesth 1995; 9:442.
51. Selvin BL: Cancer chemotherapy: implications for the anesthesiologist. Anesth Analg 1981; 60:425.
52. Gilson A: Reactivation of bleomycin lung toxicity following oxygen administration. Chest 1985; 88:304.
53. Thompson CC, Bailey MK, Conroy J, et al: Postoperative pulmonary toxicity associated with mitomycin-C therapy. South Med J 1992; 85:1257.
54. Nand S, Messmore H: Hemostasis in malignancy. Am J Hematol 1990; 35:45.
55. Roizen M: Preoperative evaluation. *In* Miller RD (ed): Anesthesia, Vol 1, p. 827. New York, Churchill Livingstone, 1994.
56. Korvin C, Pearce RH, Stanley J: Admissions screening: clinical benefits. Ann Intern Med 1975; 83:197.
57. Turnbull J, Buck C: The value of preoperative screening investigations in otherwise healthy individuals. Arch Intern Med 1987; 147:1101.
58. Kallar SK, Everett LL: Potential risks and preventive measures for pulmonary aspiration: new concepts in preoperative fasting guidelines. Anesth Analg 1993; 77:171.
59. Green C, Pundit S, Schork A: Preoperative fasting time: is the traditional policy changing? Results of a national survey. Anesth Analg 1996; 83:123.
60. Rosenberg J, Wahr J: Cardiac arrest during anesthesia. *In* Paradis N, Halperin H, Nowak R (eds): Cardiac Arrest, p. 783. Baltimore, Williams & Wilkins, 1996.
61. Eichhorn J: Effect of monitoring standards on anesthesia outcome. Int Anesth Clin 1993; 31:181.
62. Pizov R, Ya'ari Y, Perel A: Systolic pressure variation is greater during hemorrhage than during sodium nitroprusside-induced hypotension in ventilated dogs. Anesth Analg 1988; 67:170.
63. Pizov R, Segal E, Kaplan L, et al: The use of systolic pressure variation in hemodynamic monitoring during deliberate hypotension in spine surgery. J Clin Anesth 1990; 2: 96.
64. Coriat P, Vrillon M, Perel A, et al: A comparison of systolic blood pressure variations and echocardiographic estimates of end-diastolic left ventricular size in patients after aortic surgery. Anesth Analg 1994; 78:46.
65. Rooke GA, Schwid HA, Shapira Y: The effect of graded hemorrhage and intravascular volume replacement on systolic pressure variation in humans during mechanical and spontaneous ventilation. Anesth Analg 1995; 80:925.
66. Iberti T, Fischer EP, Leibowitz A, et al: A multicenter study of physicians' knowledge of the pulmonary artery catheter. JAMA 1990; 264:2928.
67. ASA Task Force: Practice guidelines for pulmonary artery catheterization. Anesthesiology 1993; 78:380.
68. Calvin J, Dridger A, Subbald W: Does the pulmonary wedge pressure predict the left ventricular preload in critically ill patients? Crit Care Med 1981; 9:437.
69. Martyn J, Snider MT, Szyfelbein S, et al: Right ventricular dysfunction in acute thermal injury. Ann Surg 1980; 191: 330.
70. Shah D, Broner B, Dutton R, et al: Cardiac output and pulmonary wedge pressure: use for evaluation of fluid replacement in trauma patients. Arch Surg 1977; 112:1161.
71. Mark J: Central venous pressure monitoring: clinical insights beyond the numbers. J Cardiothorac Vasc Anesth 1991; 5:163.
72. Despotis G, Santoro S, Spitznagel E, et al: Prospective evaluation and clinical utility of on-site monitoring of coagulation in patients undergoing cardiac operation. J Thorac Cardiovasc Surg 1994; 107:271.
73. Despotis G, Santoro S, Spitznagel E, et al: On-site prothrombin time, activated partial thromboplastin time, and platelet count. Anesthesiology 1994; 80:338.
74. Despotis G, Hogue CW J, Santoro S, et al: Effect of heparin on whole blood activated partial thromboplastin time using a portable, whole blood coagulation monitor. Crit Care Med 1995; 23:1674.
75. Friedberg R: Issues in transfusion therapy in the patient with malignancy. Hematol Oncol Clin North Am 1994; 8: 1223.
76. Miller J, Mintz P: The use of leukocyte-reduced blood components. Hematol Oncol Clin North Am 1995; 9:69.
77. Anderson KC, Weinstein HJ: Transfusion associated graft versus host disease. N Engl J Med 1990; 323:315.
78. Greenbaum B: Transfusion-associated graft-versus-host disease: historical perspectives, incidence, and current use of irradiated blood products. J Clin Oncol 1991; 9: 1889.
79. Petz L, Yam CP, Cecka M, et al: Transfusion-associated graft-versus-host disease in immunocompetent patients: report of a fatal case associated with transfusion of blood from a second degree relative, and a survey of predisposing factors. Transfusion 1993; 33:742.
80. Kanter M: Transfusion-associated graft-versus-host disease: do transfusions from second degree relatives pose a greater risk than those from first degree relatives? Transfusion 1992; 32:323.
81. Thaler M, Shamiss A, Orgad S, et al: The role of blood from HLA-homozygous donors in fatal transfusion associated graft-versus-host disease after open heart surgery. N Engl J Med 1989; 321:25.
82. Pelszynski M, Moroff G, Luban N, et al: Effect of irradiation of red blood cells units on T-cell inactivation as assessed by limiting dilution analysis: implications for preventing transfusion-associated graft-versus-host disease. Blood 1994; 83:1683.
83. Jeter EK, Spivey MA: Non-infectious complications of blood transfusion. Hematol Oncol Clin North Am 1995; 9:187.
84. Bowden R: Transfusion-transmitted cytomegalovirus infection. Hematol Oncol Clin North Am 1995; 9:155.
85. Schreiber GB, Busch MP, Kleinman SH, et al: The risk of transfusion-transmitted viral infections. N Engl J Med 1996; 334:1685.
86. Nelson AH, Fleisher LA, Rosenbaum SH: Relationship between postoperative anemia and cardiac morbidity in high-risk vascular patients in the intensive care unit. Crit Care Med 1993; 21:860.
87. Bordin J, Blajchman M: Immunosuppressive effects of allogenic blood transfusion: implications for the patient

with malignancy. Hematol Oncol Clin North Am 1995; 9: 205.
88. Heiss M, Juach K, Delanoff C, et al: Blood transfusion modulated tumor recurrence—a randomized study of autologous versus homologous blood transfusion in colorectal cancer. J Clin Oncol 1994; 12:1859.
89. Busch O, Hop W, van Papendrecht M: Blood transfusions and prognosis in colorectal cancer. N Engl J Med 1993; 328:1372.
90. Ness P, Walsh P, Zahurak M, et al: Prostate cancer recurrence in radical surgery patients receiving autologous or homologous transfusion. Transfusion 1992; 32:31.
91. Heal J, Chuang C, Blumberg N: Perioperative blood transfusions and prostate cancer recurrence and survival. Am J Surg 1988; 156:374.
92. McClinton S, Moffat L, Scott S, et al: Blood transfusion and survival following surgery for prostate carcinoma. Br J Surg 1990; 77:140.
93. Eickoff J, Gote H, Baek J: Perioperative blood transfusion in relation to tumor recurrence and death after surgery for prostatic cancer. Br J Urol 1991; 68:608.
94. Mikulin T, Powel C, Urwin G, et al: Relation between blood transfusion and survival in renal adenocarcinoma. Br J Surg 1986; 73:1036.
95. Manyonda I, Shaw D, Foulkes A, et al: Renal cell carcinoma: blood transfusion and survival. Br Med J 1986; 293: 537.
96. Edna T, Vada K, Hesselberg F, et al: Blood transfusion and survival following surgery for renal carcinoma. Br J Urol 1992; 70:135.
97. Jakobsen E, Eickhoff JH, Andersen J, et al: Perioperative blood transfusion does not affect survival after operation for renal cell cancer. Eur Urol 1994; 26:145.
98. Moffat L, Sunderland G, Lamont D, et al: Blood transfusion and survival following nephrectomy for carcinoma of kidney. Br J Urol 1987; 60:316.
99. Lander D, Hill G, Wong K, et al: Blood transfusion-induced immunomodulation. Anesth Analg 1996; 82:187.
100. Heiss M, Mempel W, Juach K, et al: Beneficial effect of autologous blood transfusion on infectious complications after colorectal cancer surgery. Lancet 1993; 342:1328.
101. Jensen L, Anderson A, Christiansen P, et al: Postoperative infection and natural killer cell function following blood transfusion in patients undergoing elective colorectal cancer surgery. Br J Surg 1992; 79:513.
102. Zulim R, Rocco M, Goodnight J, et al: Intraoperative autotransfusion in hepatic resection for malignancy. Arch Surg 1993; 128:206.
103. Fujimoto J, Okamoto E, Yamanaka N, et al: Efficacy of autotransfusion in hepatectomy for hepatocellular carcinoma. Arch Surg 1993; 128:1065.
104. Klimberg I, Sirois R, Wajsman Z, et al: Intraoperative autotransfusion in urologic oncology. Arch Surg 1986; 121: 1326.
105. Hart O, Klimberg IW, Wajsman Z, et al: Intraoperative autotransfusion in radical cystectomy for carcinoma of the bladder. Surg Gynecol Obstet 1989; 168:302.
106. Dale R, Kipling RM, Smith M, et al: Separation of malignant cells during autotransfusion. Br J Surg 1988; 75: 581.
107. Torre G, Ferrari M, Favre A, et al: A new technique for intraoperative blood recovery in cancer. Eur J Surg Oncol 1994; 20:565.
108. Stewart P: Modern quantitative acid-base chemistry. Can J Physiol Pharmacol 1983; 61:1444.
109. Bowman G, Hoerth J, McHlothlen J, et al: Anesthesia for transurethral resection of the prostate: spinal or general? J Am Assoc Nurse Anesth 1981; 49:63.
110. Mackenzie A: Influence of anesthesia on blood loss in transurethral prostatectomy. Scott Med J 1990; 35:14.
111. McGowan S, Smith G: Anesthesia for transurethral prostatectomy. Anaesthesia 1980; 35:847.
112. Nielsen K, Andersen K, Asbjorn J, et al: Blood loss in transurethral prostatectomy: epidural versus general anesthesia. Int Urol Nephrol 1987; 19:287.
113. Whelan P, Morris P: Immunologic responsiveness after transurethral resection of the prostate: general versus spinal anesthesia. Clin Exp Immunol 1982; 48:611.
114. Kirson L, Goldman J, Slover R: Low dose intrathecal morphine for postoperative pain control in patients undergoing transurethral resection of the prostate. Anesthesiology 1989; 71:192.
115. Heathcote P, Dyer P: The effect of warm irrigation on blood loss during transurethral prostatectomy under spinal anesthesia. Br J Urol 1986; 58:669.
116. Walsh P: Radical prostatectomy: a procedure in evolution. Semin Oncol 1994; 21:662.
117. Klein EA, Licht MR: Reducing length of stay after radical prostatectomy. Semin Urol 1995; 13:137.
118. Koch MO, Smith JA Jr, Hodge EM, et al: Prospective development of a cost-efficient program for radical retropubic prostatectomy. Urology 1994; 44:311.
119. Kramolowsky EV, Wood NL, Rollins K, et al: The role of the physician in effecting change in hospital charge for radical prostatectomy. J Am Coll Surg 1995; 180:513.
120. Kramolowsky EV, Wood NL, Rollins K, et al: Impact of physician awareness on hospital charges for radical retropubic prostatectomy [see comments]. J Urol 1995; 154: 139.
121. Shir Y, Frank SM, Brendler CB, et al: Postoperative morbidity is similar in patients anesthetized with epidural and general anesthesia for radical prostatectomy. Urology 1994; 44:232.
122. Shir Y, Raja SN, Frank SM, et al: Intraoperative blood loss during radical retropubic prostatectomy: epidural versus general anesthesia. Urology 1995; 45:993.
123. Shir Y, Raja SN, Frank SM: The effect of epidural versus general anesthesia on postoperative pain and analgesic requirements in patients undergoing radical prostatectomy. Anesthesiology 1994; 80:49.
124. Yamada AH, Lieskovsky G, Skinner D: Impact of autologous blood transfusions on patients undergoing radical prostatectomy using hypotensive anesthesia. J Urol 1993; 149:73.
125. Montie J, el Ammar R, Pontes J, et al: Renal cell carcinoma with inferior vena cava tumor thrombi. Surg Gynecol Obstet 1991; 173:107.
126. Casanova GA, Zingg EJ: Inferior vena caval tumor extension in renal cell carcinoma. Urol Int 1991; 47:216.
127. Couillard DR, deVere White RW: Surgery of renal cell carcinoma. Urol Clin North Am 1993; 20:263.
128. Attwood S, Lang DM, Goiti J, et al: Venous bypass for surgical resection of renal carcinoma invading the vena cava: a new approach. Br J Urol 1988; 61:402.
129. Yeager M, Glass DD, Neff R, et al: Epidural anesthesia and analgesia in high risk surgical patients. Anesthesiology 1987; 66:729.
130. Christensen T, Kehlet H: Postoperative fatigue. World J Surg 1993; 17:220.
131. Tuman K, McCarthy RJ, March RJ, et al: Effects of anesthesia and analgesia on coagulation and outcome after major vascular surgery. Anesth Analg 1991; 73:696.
132. Walters E: Injury related behavior and neuronal plasticity: an evolutionary perspective on sensitization, hyperalgesia, and analgesia. Int Rev Neurobiol 1994; 36:325.
133. Guan L, Townsend R, Eisenstein T, et al: Both T cells and macrophages are targets of kappa-opioid-induced immunosuppression. Brain Behav Immun 1994; 8:229.
134. Guan L, Townsend R, Eisenstein T, et al: The cellular basis for opioid-induced immunosuppression. Adv Exp Med Biol 1995; 373:57.
135. Hoffman KE, Maslonek KA, Dykstra L, et al: Effects of central administration of morphine on immune status in Lewis and Wistar rats. Adv Exp Med Biol 1995; 373:155.
136. Hernandez MC, Flores LR, Bayer BM: Immunosuppression by morphine is mediated by central pathways. J Pharmacol Exp Ther 1993; 267:1336.
137. Heath D: The treatment of hypercalcaemia of malignancy. Clin Endocrinol 1991; 34:155.

138. Read J, Bainton R: Operative hemorrhage in association with ketorolac. Anaesthesia 1994; 49:73.
139. Package insert: Toradol. Palo Alto, CA, Syntex Laboratories, 1995.
140. Watcha M, White P: Postoperative nausea and vomiting. Anesthesiology 1992; 77:162.
141. Hirsch J: Impact of postoperative nausea and vomiting in the surgical setting. Anaesthesia 1994; 49(Suppl):30.
142. Rosen M, Camu F: Foreword. Anaesthesia 1994; 49(Suppl):1.
143. Kenny G: Risk factors for postoperative nausea and vomiting. Anaesthesia 1994; 49(Suppl):6.
144. Markham A, Saurian EM: Ondansetron: an update of its therapeutic use in chemotherapy-induced and postoperative nausea and vomiting. Drugs 1993; 45:931. [Published erratum appears in Drugs 1993; 46:268]
145. Claybon L: Single dose intravenous ondansetron for the 24 hour treatment of postoperative nausea and vomiting. Anaesthesia 1994; 49:24.
146. McKenzie R, Kovac A, O'Connor T, et al: Comparison of ondansetron versus placebo to prevent postoperative nausea and vomiting in women undergoing ambulatory gynecologic surgery [see comments]. Anesthesiology 1993; 78:21.
147. Scuderi P, Wetchler B, Sung Y, et al: Treatment of postoperative nausea and vomiting after outpatient surgery with the 5-HT3 antagonist ondansetron [see comments]. Anesthesiology 1993; 78:15.
148. Rust M, Cohen L: Single oral dose ondansetron in the prevention of postoperative nausea and emesis. Anaesthesia 1994; 49:16.
149. Joslyn A: Ondansetron, clinical development for postoperative nausea and vomiting: current studies and future directions. Anaesthesia 1994; 49(Suppl):34.

53

ACUTE AND CHRONIC RENAL DISEASE IN UROLOGIC ONCOLOGY

GLENN M. CHERTOW, M.D. *and* BARRY M. BRENNER, M.D.

ASSESSMENT OF RENAL FUNCTION

The most common measure used to estimate renal function in humans is the serum creatinine concentration. Creatinine is freely filtered, is secreted in only small amounts in states of normal or near-normal function, and is not reabsorbed. Unlike creatinine, blood urea nitrogen, although commonly used to evaluate renal function, is a relatively poor surrogate. A number of clinical factors, including dietary protein intake, gastrointestinal bleeding, drugs that promote catabolism (e.g., glucocorticoids, tetracyclines), and states of impaired renal perfusion (e.g., volume depletion, congestive heart failure, hepatic cirrhosis), can alter the blood urea nitrogen concentration independently of renal function.

The creatinine clearance can be determined using the following formula:

$$\text{CrCl (ml/min)} = \frac{\text{urine concentration of creatinine (mg/dl)} \times \text{urine volume (ml/min)}}{\text{plasma concentration of creatinine (mg/dl)}}$$

The creatinine clearance closely approximates the glomerular filtration rate when the glomerular filtration rate exceeds 50 to 60 ml/min. However, as renal function deteriorates, the creatinine clearance tends to overestimate glomerular filtration, because of the relative contribution of secreted creatinine, which rises as renal function declines. In contrast, the urea nitrogen clearance (calculated as above but using urine and serum urea nitrogen concentrations) tends to underestimate glomerular filtration because of proximal tubular urea reabsorption. Taking the average of the creatinine and urea clearances is a reasonably accurate method of estimating renal function when the glomerular filtration rate reaches 20 ml/min or below.

When using urine collections to estimate renal function, it is important to recall that the urine creatinine content can be used to confirm whether the collection is complete. For men of average body size, the daily creatinine excretion in steady state should be between 16 and 24 mg of creatinine per kilogram of body weight; for women the value is 12 to 20 mg/kg body weight, depending on body build and the presence or absence of edema. Other urinary constituents, including urea nitrogen and sodium, vary substantially day to day as a result of dietary variability and should not be used to evaluate completeness of the sample.

If obtaining a timed collection of urine is not feasible, an approximation of creatinine clearance can be obtained using the Cockcroft-Gault formula[1]:

$$\text{CrCl (ml/min)} = \frac{(140-\text{age}) \times \text{weight} (\times 0.85 \text{ if female})}{\text{serum creatinine} \times 72}$$

This formula takes into account the age-related loss of glomerular filtration as well as the contribution of creatinine generation (using body weight as a surrogate for muscle mass) toward the steady state serum creatinine concentration, and is a better measure of renal function than the serum creatinine concentration alone. Of course, the Cockcroft-Gault equation may overestimate creatinine clearance in the obese or markedly edematous patient. For this reason, the use of ideal body weight may result in a more accurate estimate.

If a more precise estimate of renal function is required, as for a patient in whom a prolonged course of cisplatin chemotherapy is anticipated, a radiolabeled tracer, such as ^{125}I-iothalamate, can be used. This method is reliable, precise, and valid (compared with inulin clearance, the gold standard) and widely available at major medical centers.

The urinalysis is an important diagnostic tool that is rapid, inexpensive, and relatively easy to perform. Urine dipsticks can detect modest degrees of hematuria, pyuria, and proteinuria, and are often the first clue to the presence of acute or chronic renal disease. A microscopic analysis may provide insight into the severity and/or duration of renal disease (see later).

Radiographic studies, widely used in urologic diseases, are rarely useful in assessing renal function. Nuclear medicine studies can be used to determine glomerular filtration rate, but this information can be more easily estimated with other techniques. Renal ultrasound can be used to help determine the chronicity of disease (e.g., reduced kidney size with longstanding disease) as well as the presence or absence of urinary tract obstruction (see later).

ACUTE RENAL FAILURE

Acute renal failure, an abrupt decline in glomerular filtration rate accompanied by the accumulation of nitrogenous waste products, is variably defined by clinical criteria. A conservative designation is a 25 to 50% increase in the serum creatinine concentration from baseline. Some investigators use alternative definitions, including a doubling of the baseline serum creatinine or an increase in the serum creatinine concentration above an arbitrary ceiling, such as 2.0 or 2.5 mg/dl. Oliguria, usually defined as a urine output less than 400 ml/day, occurs in 20 to 40% of cases,[2-4] depending on the clinical setting, and generally carries a less favorable prognosis.[5] Acute renal failure requiring dialysis is associated with in-hospital mortality rates exceeding 40% in most published studies.[6-9] The most common causes of acute renal failure in the urologic oncology setting are outlined in Table 53–1.

Regardless of the definition employed, acute renal failure occurring in the setting of genitourinary malignancy, related either to surgical or medical therapy, is a serious complication. We begin our discussion of acute renal failure with a section on the general diagnostic and therapeutic approach to the patient with acute renal failure. This is followed by a detailed discussion of perioperative acute renal failure and drug-induced nephrotoxic syndromes, with a special focus on chemotherapeutic agents commonly used in the management of urologic malignancy. Bilateral nephrectomy and its complications, including the need for long-term renal replacement therapy, is deferred to subsequent sections of the chapter.

TABLE 53–1. CAUSES OF ACUTE RENAL FAILURE IN UROLOGIC ONCOLOGY

Acute tubular necrosis
Prolonged hypotension
Sepsis syndrome
Pigment nephropathy (hemoglobin or myoglobin)
Multiple myeloma
Radiocontrast
Structural
Ureteral, bladder neck, or urethral obstruction
Partial nephrectomy
Drug induced
Chemotherapeutic agents
Cisplatin
Carboplatin
Ifosfamide
Interleukins
Other agents
Amphotericin B
Gentamicin and other aminoglycosides
Ciprofloxacin
Trimethoprim-sulfamethoxazole

General Approach to Diagnosis of Acute Renal Failure

For the purposes of diagnosis and management, the approach toward a patient with acute renal failure should focus on three areas: (1) diseases characterized by renal hypoperfusion, without frank necrosis or other parenchymal damage ("prerenal azotemia"); (2) diseases characterized by urinary tract obstruction ("postrenal acute renal failure"); and (3) diseases characterized by inflammation, infiltration, or ischemic or toxic injury to the renal parenchyma ("intrinsic" acute renal failure).

The history and physical examination virtually always provide insight into the cause(s) of acute renal failure in the patient with urologic malignancy. Along with a few relatively inexpensive laboratory studies, information from the history and physical examination can determine the cause(s) of acute renal failure in a large majority of cases. Important historical information to seek should include nausea, vomiting, diminished oral intake, and subjective assessment of reduced urine output, which can be associated with volume depletion; polyuria, which can be associated with a variety of metabolic disturbances (e.g., hypercalcemia, hypokalemia) as well as with urinary tract obstruction; and drug exposures, including the use of over-the-counter analgesic agents. Other unusual signs or symptoms should be elicited, such as fever, dysuria, and hematuria, but these rarely account for the decline in glomerular filtration.

The physical examination should focus first on the assessment of volume status. Volume depletion, with prerenal azotemia, is the most common etiology of acute renal failure in most published reports.[3,10] Prerenal azotemia is especially prevalent among patients with active malignancy, particularly those who are elderly, or recent recipients of chemotherapy. Vital signs may show tachycardia and hypotension, with orthostatic changes (fall in diastolic blood pressure greater than 10 mm Hg, heart rate increase more than 10 beats/minute). Relative hypotension, without frank orthostasis, may be seen in less severe instances. When the patient is volume depleted, jugular venous pressure is often less than 5 cm H_2O and undetectable on routine physical examination. Dry mucous membranes and poor skin turgor support the diagnosis of prerenal azotemia but are nonspecific.

In contrast, patients with volume overload, as might accompany subacute renal insufficiency with sufficient time for sodium retention, often manifest jugular venous distention (jugular venous pressure exceeding 8 cm H_2O), pulmonary rales, and peripheral edema. These findings are critical to recognize because the administration of intravenous crystalloid or colloid (the usual empirical treatment for presumed prerenal azotemia) to patients with acute renal failure who are volume replete can be hazardous. Other physical examination findings characteristic of more chronic or acute advanced renal disease should be sought, including pallor (resulting from anemia), a pericardial friction rub (caused by uremic pericarditis); asterixis, myoclonus, or stupor (nonspecific findings but characteristic of uremic neurologic disease); excoriations (caused by severe pruritus); and/or the nitrogenous "uremic" fetor.

Laboratory studies are often helpful in differentiating various etiologies of acute renal failure (Table 53–2). The ratio of the blood urea nitrogen and serum creatinine concentrations is often used to differentiate prerenal azotemia from other causes of acute renal failure, with a ratio exceeding 20:1 characteristic of the former. Unfortunately, the ratio can be misleading, particularly in otherwise ill persons, such as those with malignant disease, who may have markedly reduced protein intake as a result of anorexia, and/or muscle wasting resulting from tumor-associated catabolism or longstanding malnutrition. A more useful tool to differentiate prerenal azotemia from other causes of acute renal failure is the fractional excretion of sodium.[11,12] The fractional excretion of sodium $[(U_{Na}/P_{Na})/(U_{Cr}/P_{Cr})]$ tends to be substantially less than 1% in persons with acute renal failure and prerenal azotemia. Exceptions are relatively common, as in persons with acute tubular necrosis secondary to radiocontrast agents, aminoglycosides, or sepsis syndrome, whose fractional excretions of sodium are often low despite ischemia or toxic injury sufficient to result in tubular damage.[13–15] In contrast, persons with acute renal failure caused by drug-induced acute tubular necrosis or acute interstitial nephritis, or urinary tract obstruction, other common causes of acute renal failure in the urologic oncology population, tend to exhibit fractional excretions of sodium in excess of 1%.[11,12,16]

TABLE 53–2. USEFUL LABORATORY STUDIES IN THE DIAGNOSIS OF ACUTE RENAL FAILURE IN THE PATIENT WITH UROLOGIC MALIGNANCY

Blood chemistries
Creatinine
Urea nitrogen
Sodium
Potassium
Bicarbonate
Calcium
Phosphate
Uric acid
Magnesium
Creatine kinase
Leukocyte count
Eosinophil count
Urine chemistries
Sodium
Creatinine
Urine sediment
Muddy brown casts
Leukocyte casts
Red blood cell casts
Eosinophils

Other, more subtle laboratory abnormalities, although not in themselves diagnostic, can aid in the differential diagnosis of acute renal failure in the urologic oncology setting. Mild degrees of hypernatremia (in the range of 142 to 145 mEq/L), hyperkalemia (in the range of 5 to 6 mEq/L), and metabolic acidosis (serum bicarbonate concentration in the range of 18 to 21 mEq/L) can be seen with disorders of distal tubular function, including those related to interstitial nephritis,[17] or papillary necrosis; the hyperkalemia and hyperchloremic metabolic acidosis (so-called type IV renal tubular acidosis) is particularly common in urinary tract obstruction.[18–20] Pyuria, rash, eosinophiluria, and eosinophilia in excess of 3 to 5% are occasionally observed in cases of interstitial nephritis.[21] Relative wasting of potassium and magnesium can be seen in some cases of acute renal failure, particularly those associated with the use of cisplatin, ifosfamide, and/or aminoglycoside antibiotics; these syndromes are addressed in more detail later. Relative hypophosphatemia and hypouricemia may indicate a Fanconi's syndrome, also seen in association with the administration of these same drugs.[22] Finally, elevations of the serum uric acid, phosphate, and potassium concentrations, although evident in most cases of severe acute or chronic renal failure, may be most striking in cases of tumor lysis syndrome, usually associated with treatment of hematopoietic malignancies.[23]

The microscopic urinalysis provides a vital piece of the diagnostic puzzle in many cases of acute renal failure. The urinalysis is usually bland in cases of prerenal azotemia, except for the presence of hyaline casts. Certain microscopic findings point toward specific intrinsic renal diseases. Acute tubular necrosis is characterized by the presence of abundant granular "muddy brown" casts. Interstitial nephritis and pyelonephritis are characterized by abundant white and red blood cells and occasional leukocyte casts. Inflammatory diseases of the glomerulus, relatively rare in the setting of urologic malignancy, are characterized by abundant red blood cells and, in a fraction of cases, red blood cell casts, a finding rather specific for the presence of inflammatory glomerular disease.

Imaging studies are frequently used in the differential diagnosis of acute renal failure. As noted earlier, ultrasonography is the diagnostic modality of choice in identifying urinary tract obstruction, with a sensitivity and specificity of approximately 90%.[24,25] Rarely, urinary tract obstruction can be present without dilatation of the urinary collecting system, including in cases of retroperitoneal fibrosis,[26] with concomitant volume depletion, and with a variety of tumors (adenocarcinoma of the cervix or colon, or lymphoma) encasing or infiltrating the renal pelvis or ureter(s).[27] Computed tomography can be used to follow up cases of hydronephrosis detected by ultrasound, and to determine the specific etiology responsible for the obstruction to flow.[28] Magnetic resonance imaging has improved resolution of intrarenal structure compared with computed tomography, particularly with regard to the differentiation of soft tissue densities (tumor vs. hematoma), but is rarely required in the work-up of acute renal failure.

Estimating the Risk of Acute Renal Failure

Hospital-acquired acute renal failure develops in approximately 5% of hospitalized patients, although various baseline factors and in-hospital exposures modify that risk. In the urologic oncology population, drug exposures, particularly to chemotherapeutic agents and nephrotoxic antimicrobials, are the most important risk factors for the development of acute renal failure. However, demographic factors and comorbidities should be taken into account when considering a patient's "renal risk profile." It is worth noting the demographics of the urologic oncology population specific to each malignancy because these factors may strongly influence susceptibility to acute renal failure, as well as predict ultimate renal recovery. Persons with carcinoma of the bladder and prostate tend to be from older age groups, compared with those with renal cell carcinoma or testicular or other germ cell neoplasms. Several studies have suggested that advanced age is an important risk factor for the development of acute renal failure in a variety of clinical settings.[29] In fact, age-associated nephrosclerosis and renal dysfunction, rather than age per se, is the more likely culprit.[30] Therefore, an elder person with preserved renal function may be at reduced risk compared with a younger individual with evidence of renal dysfunction. Important comorbidities that might also increase acute renal failure risk include hepatic dysfunction, especially hyperbilirubinemia, pancreatitis, sepsis syndrome, diabetes with renal involvement, congestive heart failure and other states of renal hypoperfusion, and atherosclerotic vascular disease (often with "silent" renovascular involvement). Efforts to maintain optimal renal perfusion with volume expansion should be enforced at all times, if the risk of pulmonary edema or other complications is thought to be low. There is probably no role for the prophylactic use of loop or osmotic diuretics or low-dose dopamine, although these interventions remain controversial and widely used (see later).[31]

Specific Acute Renal Failure Etiologies in Urologic Oncology

Perioperative Complications

Adverse perioperative events can occasionally lead to acute renal failure in the patient with urologic malignancy. The most important of these complications is prolonged intraoperative hypotension, resulting in ischemic renal injury, or acute tubular necrosis. Prerenal azotemia and acute tubular necrosis can be thought of as two points along a spectrum of hypoperfusion; if the severity and/or duration of hypoperfusion are severe and prolonged, acute tubular necrosis can ensue. In contrast to states of prerenal azotemia, in which restoration of perfusion rapidly returns function toward normal, renal function can be impaired for up to 8 weeks or more in severe cases of acute tubular necrosis. In addition to prolonged hypotension, sepsis, rhabdomyolysis, hemolysis (including transfusion reaction and hematomata), exposure to intravenous contrast, and nephrotoxic antibiotics (including the intraperitoneal administration of polymixin and aminoglycosides, including kanamycin or neomycin) are other important causes of perioperative acute tubular necrosis.

Management of acute tubular necrosis depends largely on restoring adequate perfusion and abrogating any toxic or otherwise unnecessary exposures. Various pharmacologic agents have been examined prophylactically or in the early stages of established acute tubular necrosis, including mannitol,[32] loop diuretics,[33] low-dose dopamine,[34,35] other vasodilators,[36–38] free radical scavengers,[39] growth factors,[40] and monoclonal antibodies.[41] Unfortunately, none has proved beneficial in prospective, placebo-controlled trials in humans.[31] Nevertheless, a short trial of diuretics is reasonable (e.g., furosemide, 40- to 200-mg intravenous bolus or 10 to 40 mg/hour by continuous infusion) because subsequent management, including blood product support and the timing of dialysis if required, will be greatly influenced depending on urine output and fluid balance.

Dialysis may be required if renal recovery is delayed for more than several days, especially if the patient is catabolic or in markedly positive fluid balance. Conventional, or intermittent, hemodialysis, performed three or more times per week, is the treatment of choice for most patients with acute renal failure requiring dialysis; peritoneal dialysis or continuous hemofiltration or hemodiafiltration can be used for patients who are hemodynamically unstable.[42] The optimal timing or intensity of dialysis for acute renal failure is unknown.[43,44] Access to the circulation is usually achieved with a temporary percutaneous Silastic catheter rather than a permanent arteriovenous fistula or graft, as might be used in a patient with chronic renal failure, in the hope that residual renal function might recover. Potential sites for this catheter include the internal jugular, subclavian, and femoral veins. A cuffed internal jugular catheter is the preferred route under most circumstances.

The duration of functional impairment is highly variable, ranging from days to several weeks. An increase in urine output and blunting of the intradialytic rate of rise of serum creatinine are two nonspecific but encouraging signs of renal recovery. If either of these findings is observed, a quantitative estimate of glomerular filtration should be obtained. If the creatinine clearance exceeds 5 to 10 ml/min and the patient is otherwise stable, a trial off dialysis can be attempted.

The other important perioperative complication relates to acute urinary tract obstruction, usually as a result of bleeding with retroperitoneal hematoma formation. True surgical errors, such as the inadvertent suturing of the ureters, can rarely result in perioperative acute renal failure as a result of urinary tract obstruction, if the obstruction is bilateral or if the patient has a solitary functioning kidney. Such errors are rare but can be detected by maintaining a high level of suspicion, and with early use of abdominal ultrasonography. If identified promptly, perioperative acute renal failure caused by obstruction rarely results in sufficient injury to require dialysis support. All patients with progressive renal failure in the perioperative setting should undergo ultrasonography before other invasive diagnostic or therapeutic maneuvers are initiated.

Management of acute renal failure associated with urinary tract obstruction is dictated by (1) the level of obstruction (upper vs. lower tract); (2) the acuity of the obstruction and its clinical consequences, including renal dysfunction and infection; and (3) the performance status and overall level of care elected by the patient. Benign causes of urinary tract obstruction, including bladder outlet obstruction and nephrolithiasis, should be ruled out because conservative management, including Foley catheter placement and intravenous fluids, respectively, will usually relieve the obstruction in most cases. Among patients with urologic malignancies, ureteral obstruction resulting from tumor is the most common and concerning cause of urinary tract obstruction. If technically feasible, ureteral obstruction resulting from tumor is best managed by cystoscopic placement of a ureteral stent. Otherwise, the placement of nephrostomy tubes with external drainage may be required. Intravenous antibiotics should also be given if there are signs of pyelonephritis or urosepsis. Fluid and electrolyte status should be carefully monitored after obstruction is relieved.

Renal Complications of Cancer Chemotherapy for Urologic Neoplasms

Cisplatin. Cisplatin is one of the most important chemotherapeutic agents available in urologic oncology. Its inclusion in regimens for testicular carcinoma has markedly improved short-term response rates and long-term survival, such that the large majority of patients with testicular carcinoma can be cured of their disease. It also is active in advanced bladder carcinoma, often in combination with methotrexate and other agents (see later). Its toxicities include myelosuppression, nausea, and high-frequency hearing loss, but its major side effect is nephrotoxicity, with various manifestations seen in up to 50% or more of patients exposed to the drug, the proportion of patients affected being dose dependent.[45–47]

The characteristic pattern of nephrotoxicity is a progressive nonoliguric renal failure, with associated electrolyte abnormalities. Magnesium wasting can be severe, with associated hypokalemia and hypocalcemia largely as secondary phenomena,[48,49] and can be exacerbated by the concomitant use of aminoglycosides, amphotericin B, and/or loop diuretic agents.[49,50] Now frequently used in combination with ifosfamide, cisplatin can enhance the toxicity of that drug, presumably as a result of its proximal tubular toxicity.

Because of cisplatin's potent antitumor activity, and the lack of satisfactory alternative agents, there has been tremendous interest in strategies aimed at ameliorating cisplatin-associated nephrotoxicity. In addition to careful dosing, volume expansion is a reliable means of reducing the odds of complications.[51] Many practitioners, including those at our hospital, advise that a brisk urine output be maintained for at least 12 hours before and 12 hours after cisplatin administration. The use of hypertonic saline as the infusion medium (to enhance volume expansion), and other nephroprotective agents, such as probenecid, sodium thiosulfate, and ethiofos, have been or are currently under study.[52,53]

Carboplatin. Carboplatin, a cisplatin analog, has a similar range of activity against multiple tumors, including testicular carcinoma. However, its primary dose-limiting side effect is myelosuppression rather than renal insufficiency. In phase I and II trials, little if any nephrotoxicity was attributed to the drug.[54] More recently, nephrotoxicity has been described, usually after repeated courses at doses in excess of 800 mg/m^2, after previous cisplatin chemotherapy, in combination with other potential nephrotoxic agents (e.g., ifosfamide),[55] or in patients with baseline renal insufficiency. Reversible renal dysfunction and hypomagnesemia are the abnormalities most commonly reported.[56,57] Based on limited anecdotal evidence,[58] and extrapolation from our experience with cisplatin, pre- and post-administration volume expansion would be advisable, if tolerated, in patients treated with this drug.

Ifosfamide. Ifosfamide is an alkylating agent structurally related to cyclophosphamide that has been used with increasing frequency over the past several years for the treatment of "high-risk" testicular carcinoma and other aggressive malignancies. It is associated with perhaps the most interesting of the antineoplastic drug-related nephrotoxic syndromes. Ifosfamide, or a toxic metabolite, causes tubulointerstitial injury, resulting in impairment of glomerular filtration and proximal tubular dysfunction, characterized by the overexcretion of glucose, amino acids, phosphate, bicarbonate, potassium, and uric acid (Fanconi's syndrome). Fanconi's syndrome is clinically evident in approximately 5% of patients, but subclinical or isolated abnormalities (e.g., aminoaciduria, phosphaturia) are present in up to two thirds of patients.[59,60] Those with pre-existing renal dysfunction, a history of nephrectomy, prior high-dose therapy or high cumulative dose, or coadministration of cisplatin or carboplatin are at highest risk of nephrotoxicity.[61,62] Young children may be at the highest risk.[63] Furthermore, approximately 10% of children with Wilms' tumor treated with ifosfamide have developed rickets as a result of phosphate wasting and inadequate enzymatic conversion to 1,25-OH vitamin D.[64]

Although commonly employed, the use of Mesna does not appear to abrogate the direct nephrotoxicity of ifosfamide. To our knowledge, there are no proven prophylactic or therapeutic strategies for ifosfamide-induced nephrotoxicity. Extra caution should be given toward patients treated with platinum-based antineoplastic agents, amphotericin B, and aminoglycosides because of their overlapping nephrotoxic profiles.

Methotrexate. Methotrexate is a commonly used antimetabolite, in clinical use for several decades, with selected utility in urologic oncology—specifically, in the treatment of choriocarcinoma and in some systemic chemotherapeutic regimens for advanced carcinoma of the bladder and urothelium. At standard doses, as would typically be used for choriocarcinoma, there is relatively little nephrotoxicity. At higher doses (e.g., 12 g/m^2), however, nephrotoxic effects are seen in approximately 10% of treated patients, characterized by a nonoliguric acute renal failure.[65] Volume expansion and urinary alkalinization can reduce the risk of significant complications.[66]

More important perhaps than the effect of the drug on the kidney is the effect of renal insufficiency on disposition of the drug.[67] Particularly when methotrexate is used in combination chemotherapy with other potentially nephrotoxic agents (e.g., regimens with cisplatin and vinblastine with or without doxorubicin for advanced urothelial carcinoma[68]), patients with acute or chronic renal insufficiency may develop marked elevations in their plasma concentrations of methotrexate and its metabolites, if the dose is not properly adjusted.

Agents without Direct Nephrotoxicity. For a more detailed discussion of the disposition of various antineoplastic agents without direct nephrotoxicity (e.g., bleomycin, melphalan), the reader is referred to the excellent review by Shuler et al.[69]

Other Conventional Agents. Drugs less commonly used for urologic malignancies that have important but rarely reported nephrotoxicities include doxorubicin (nephrotic syndrome), mitomycin C (hemolytic-uremic syndrome),[70] suramin (acute renal failure),[71] intravesicular thiotepa (ureteral obstruction and acute renal failure),[72] and intravesicular bacillus Calmette-Guérin (rhabdomyolysis and acute renal failure).[73]

Interleukins. Interleukin-2 is a potent cytokine released by a subset of activated T-lymphocytes. Interleukin-2, alone or in combination with lymphokine-activated killer cells, has been shown to possess antineoplastic activity and has been used with some success in metastatic malignancies, including renal cell carcinoma, a tumor otherwise resistant to conventional chemotherapeutic agents.[74–76]

Toxicities with interleukin-2 therapy are severe but usually self-limited, including chills, nausea, vomiting, hypotension, weight gain, and disorientation in more than 50% of patients in all series, despite the use of various agents to ameliorate these effects. Renal dysfunction develops in 80 to 100% of patients.[74–80] Clinically, the syndrome is characterized by marked sodium avidity, edema formation, and mild to moderate elevations of the serum creatinine and urea nitrogen concentrations. In the series reported by Rosenberg et al.,[75] 13% of patients developed advanced renal failure, defined as a serum creatinine greater than 6.0 mg/dl. Fractional excretion of sodium is typically reduced; the urine sediment is usually bland. Most investigators postulate that the renal lesion associated with interleukin-2 administration is caused by the marked capillary leak syndrome induced by the drug, with a reduction in renal perfusion and plasma oncotic pressures. These findings are confounded in most studies by the concurrent use of indomethacin, a potent cyclo-oxygenase inhibitor, known to impair renal perfusion via its effect on vasodilatory prostaglandin synthesis. No defects in renal electrolyte excretion, glycosuria, or aminoaciduria have been demonstrated.[79] Hypophosphatemia has been commonly observed, most likely resulting from respiratory alkalosis induced directly by interleukin-2 or from pulmonary interstitial edema, as a result of the capillary leak syndrome.

Prior nephrectomy and pre-existing renal dysfunction are factors that increase the risk and severity of nephrotoxicity.[80,81] Little is known regarding potential means of preventing interleukin-2–induced renal failure. Modifications of the timing of drug administration have not yielded any important differences. It would be advisable to avoid the use of indomethacin, if possible, although this agent may be essential to allow systemic tolerability of the drug itself. Preliminary studies with few patients have shown some benefit of pentoxifylline[82] or low-dose dopamine[83] at reducing the severity of renal dysfunction and edema formation in this syndrome.

Although largely unpublished to date, there appears to be a similar spectrum of nephrotoxicity associated with the use of interleukin-12.

Renal Syndromes Associated with Primary Diseases and Supportive Therapies

In addition to acute and chronic renal failure, there are several renal syndromes associated with urologic malignancy that merit brief discussion. These include renal infiltration by genitourinary lymphoma, electrolyte abnormalities associated with renal cell carcinoma or surgical procedures of the prostate or bladder, and membranous nephropathy, a form of nephrotic syndrome, perhaps paraneoplastic, observed concurrently with several renal neoplasms. It is worth noting that tumor lysis syndrome, an important cause of acute renal failure in patients with hematologic malignancy, is extremely rare in nonhematopoietic neoplasms,[84,85] even among those tumors large in size that are sensitive to chemotherapy or radiation therapy, such as choriocarcinoma or other nonseminomatous germ cell tumors. Although of theoretical interest, tumor lysis syndrome therefore is not discussed in detail.

Infiltrative Genitourinary Lymphoma. Lymphoma only rarely originates in the genitourinary tract.[86,87] However, extrarenal malignant lymphoma infiltrates the kidneys in more than one third of cases, sometimes resulting in nephromegaly, hypertension, and occasionally acute renal failure.[88–92] Richmond et al.[90] described a large and well-detailed case series of patients with lymphoma confirmed by postmortem examination. The renal parenchyma was infiltrated in 40% of patients overall. Involvement was usually bilateral, in the form of multiple nodules, and was more common among younger lymphoma patients compared with older, and women compared with men. Renal insufficiency and hypertension were attributed to lymphomatous infiltration in 12% and 9% of patients, respectively. Subsequent studies have confirmed the widespread histologic involvement but have suggested that clinically significant disease develops in less than 5% of patients.

Clearly the most important adverse renal manifestation of lymphoma relates to ureteral obstruction (see earlier). However, in cases of acute renal failure, particularly when associated with nephromegaly (kidney size greater than 12 to 15 cm, depending on body size) and a bland urine sediment, lymphomatous infiltrative disease should be considered. The differential diagnosis of renal failure with nephromegaly includes diabetic nephropathy, human immunodeficiency virus–associated nephropathy, hypokalemic nephropathy, and other infiltrative diseases, such as amyloidosis.

Electrolyte Abnormalities. Hypo- or hypernatremia, hypo- or hyperkalemia, and a variety of acid-base disturbances can be seen in chronically ill patients with advanced urologic malignancy because of anorexia, nausea, vomiting, or diarrhea. Generally, these conditions can be readily managed with the thoughtful use of replacement intravenous solutions. However, particularly in cases of disordered osmoregulation (hypo- and hypernatremia), the clinician should carefully investigate for more subtle causes of electrolyte imbalance, including adrenal insufficiency resulting from metastatic tumor or infection, or the syndrome of inappropriate antidiuretic hormone secretion. Postoperative bladder irrigation is an important special situation to consider. Patients with carcinoma of the bladder or prostate whose genitourinary tracts are irrigated with saline or glycine-containing solutions may develop severe degrees of hyponatremia related to free water absorption via the bladder wall, especially in the presence of ongoing pain or narcotic therapy (potent stimuli for antidiuretic hormone secretion). Urine output should be carefully monitored during bladder irrigation; if urine output declines without other cause, the irrigant should be temporarily stopped and the serum sodium concentration should be checked. Likewise, inappropriately large urinary volumes, particularly in a patient at risk for urinary tract obstruction, should prompt an investigation into the possibility of nephrogenic diabetes insipidus, including renal ultrasonography and serum electrolytes. A careful drug exposure history is critical in these cases; electrolyte abnormalities associated with remote amphotericin or cisplatin exposure may persist long after the accompanying renal insufficiency has resolved.

Hypercalcemia accompanies renal cell carcinoma in approximately 5% of cases.[93] Hypercalcemia can exert numerous deleterious effects on the kidneys. At the vascular level, hypercalcemia promotes renal vasoconstriction, thereby limiting renal perfusion.[94] If hypercalcemia is severe and protracted, the tubules and interstitium can be affected by calcium precipitation, fibrosis, and scarring.[95] This may in turn lead to disorders of tubular function, including mild to moderate degrees of hypernatremia, hyperkalemia, and non–anion gap metabolic acidosis. Furthermore, hypercalcemia inhibits the action of antidiuretic hormone, thereby promoting polyuria and hemoconcentration.

Hypercalcemia associated with renal cell carcinoma, as with other malignancies, can be effectively managed with a stepwise approach. The intravascular volume compartment should be expanded, with or without concomitant use of loop diuretics to augment sodium delivery and sodium and calcium excretion. Thiazide diuretic agents should not be used because they tend to reduce, rather than increase, calcium excretion. Hypotonic intravenous fluids (e.g., 0.45% saline) may be preferred to saline or other isotonic solutions, depending on the initial serum sodium concentration. The addition of a biphosphanate (e.g., pamidronate) or calcitonin is often required for long-term control of hypercalcemia. Other potential hypocalcemic agents, generally less effective and/or potentially more toxic, include corticosteroids, nonsteroidal anti-inflammatory drugs, and mithramycin.

Renal Complications of Urinary Diversion. The initial method of urinary diversion for patients who required bladder resection was anastomosis of the ureter(s) to a segment of large bowel (i.e., ureterocolic anastomosis), until it was discovered that serious electrolyte and acid-base disturbances frequently occurred as a result of the efficient absorption of urinary constituents by the colonic mucosa.[96,97] As a result, diversion of the ureters to a segment of small bowel—the "ileal conduit"—has become the standard method of urinary diversion for patients with bladder carcinoma.

The most common metabolic complication of ileal diversion (to a lesser extent than in ureterocolic diversion) is a hyperchloremic metabolic acidosis caused by the loss of urinary bicarbonate with concomitant ileal reabsorption of ammonium, chloride, and hydrogen ions.[98,99] The degree of acid-base disturbance correlates directly with the length of the ileal segment, postoperative urinary leakage, and the presence of underlying renal dysfunction.[100]

Several factors in play after urinary diversion conspire to promote nephrolithiasis, usually of the struvite type.[101,102] Metabolic acidosis leads to hypocitraturia. Citrate is a potent inhibitor of calcium oxalate stone formation because it competes with oxalate for the binding of free calcium in the urine; with hypocitraturia, calcium oxalate or uric acid crystals can then serve as a nidus for struvite stone formation. Hypercalciuria is also promoted after urinary diversion via several mechanisms, including bone demineralization (related to metabolic acidosis) and changes in renal calcium excretion associated with an increase in intestinal ammonium and sulfate reabsorption. Finally, the anatomic connection to the bowel and its flora, particularly *Proteus* species and to a lesser extent *Providencia, Klebsiella, Morganella,* and *Citrobacter* species, makes the formation and maintenance of struvite stones a particular problem for this group of patients. Urinary tract obstruction, nephrocalcinosis, and repeated bouts of pyelonephritis are important complications associated with ileal conduits that can adversely affect renal function over time.

The management of patients with struvite or other kidney stones following urinary diversion is straightforward. A large fluid intake (greater than 2 to 3 L/day) is essential. Suppressive antibiotics (e.g., trimethoprim-sulfamethoxazole) can limit morbidity associated with chronic struvite calculi but rarely sterilize; occasionally extracorporeal shock-wave lithotripsy (followed by antibiotic therapy) or percutaneous nephrolithostomy is required. Oral base replacement with sodium bicarbonate or potassium, calcium, or magnesium citrate may be helpful in selected cases.

Nephrotic Syndrome. The occurrence of nephrotic syndrome in association with malignancy is widely recognized, with membranous nephropathy being the most common histopathologic correlate, at least among carcinomas and other solid tumors.[103,104] Nephrotic syndrome resulting from membranous nephropathy,[105,106] minimal change disease,[107] and amyloidosis[108] has been reported in association with renal cell carcinoma; the initial two entities are also seen in Hodgkin's and non-Hodgkin's lymphomas. Likewise, minimal change disease has been reported in association with benign renal neoplasms, including oncocytoma[109] and angiomyolipoma,[110] in both cases being sensitive to corticosteroid therapy.

In affected patients with renal cell carcinoma, empirical corticosteroid therapy would be ill advised, given the potential adverse consequences of therapy and the relative likelihood of membranous nephropathy in this group. Rather, pathology should be obtained at the time of partial or total nephrectomy. Treatment with an angiotensin-converting enzyme inhibitor will reduce (although not eliminate) the level of proteinuria in approximately 40% of patients with membranous nephropathy.[111] Although dietary protein restriction may reduce proteinuria, it should be prescribed with caution in the setting of malignancy because of the strong potential for protein-energy malnutrition in patients with cancer.

Patients whose biopsies are consistent with minimal change disease should be treated with corticosteroids (e.g., prednisone, 1 mg/kg per day or 2 mg/kg every other day) if there are no contraindications; the response is usually complete and brisk. In contrast, patients with malignancy-associated membranous nephropathy are unlikely to respond to corticosteroid therapy alone. The risk of cytotoxic therapies (i.e., cyclophosphamide, chlorambucil) or plasmapheresis, as have been used for idiopathic membranous nephropathy, is probably prohibitive, particularly because these agents exert little or no effect on the underlying malignancy.

Antibiotics Used for Infections of the Genitourinary Tract and with Neutropenia. Supportive therapies for urologic malignancy, including antibiotics, are important causes of acute and chronic renal failure. Antibiotics are frequently used periprocedure, but the short duration of therapy and the specific agents used (usually first- or second-generation cephalosporins) have infrequent nephrotoxicity. In contrast, three drugs commonly used in the treatment of fever and neutropenia (as often induced with chemotherapy) warrant brief discussion: gentamicin (and other aminoglycosides), ciprofloxacin (and other quinolones), and amphotericin B.

Aminoglycosides have been widely used in critically ill patients for nearly three decades, and still today are included in most multidrug antibiotic regimens for their rapid bactericidal activity against most gram-negative bacilli, including *Pseudomonas* and *Enterobacter* species. Nephrotoxicity develops in up to 40% of patients, depending in part on several factors, including dose and duration of drug administration, advanced age, obesity, baseline renal insufficiency, and other underlying diseases.[112,113] The characteristic clinical course is that of a nonoliguric acute tubular necrosis, developing 7 to 10 days after initiation of therapy. Relative wasting of potassium and magnesium may accompany the renal dysfunction.[114,115] Coadministration of vancomycin,[116] first-generation cephalosporins, and diuretic agents[117] has been reported to increase the risk of aminoglycoside-induced nephrotoxicity, but these reports are controversial because it is difficult to distinguish drug-specific from underlying disease-related effects.

A current controversy exists regarding the most safe and effective means of administering aminoglycoside antibiotics for fever and neutropenia. The current standard regimen is 3 to 5 mg/kg per day of gentamicin in three divided doses, although several experimental studies in animals and small studies in humans have suggested that less frequent dosing (e.g., once daily) may result in significantly less nephrotoxicity without a reduction in efficacy.[118,119] Larger clinical trials in humans will be required to settle this controversy.

Ciprofloxacin, also active against gram-negative bacilli, is being used increasingly in empirical antibiotic regimens, particularly as an aminoglycoside substitute in patients at high risk for aminoglycoside toxicity, because of their similar spectra of activity. Although initially thought to be free of significant nephrotoxicity, numerous reports of acute interstitial nephritis associated with the use of ciprofloxacin and related drugs have been published in recent years, and have been reviewed.[120]

Amphotericin B is a broad-spectrum antifungal agent, commonly used in empirical antibiotic regimens for fever unresponsive to antibacterial drugs, and prescribed for the treatment of systemic fungal infections in immunocompromised hosts. In urologic oncology, these infections would most commonly be seen in men with testicular or bladder carcinoma, who have been rendered neutropenic for prolonged periods of time, related to high-dose combination chemotherapy. Amphotericin B causes several nephrotoxic syndromes. First, progressive renal insufficiency can develop in some cases, particularly with prolonged exposure, as a result at least in part of amphotericin B–induced vasoconstriction and ischemia.[121] Volume depletion and other states of hypoperfusion increase the risk of amphotericin B–induced acute renal failure; volume loading prior to infusion can ameliorate toxicity.[122,123] Second, amphotericin B frequently causes a syndrome of potassium and magnesium wasting, occasionally to such a degree that parenteral replacement of electrolytes through a central venous catheter is required.[50] Third, nephrogenic diabetes insipidus and a hyperchloremic metabolic acidosis can develop as an additional tubular toxicity.[50] It is important to recall that the fluid and electrolyte abnormalities seen in a majority of patients whose cumulative dose has exceeded 2 to 3 g often persist after the renal function normalizes. In addition to vigilant oral replacement of potassium and magnesium, the distal diuretic amiloride (2.5 to 10 mg/day) can be a useful adjunctive potassium- and magnesium-sparing therapy.

CHRONIC RENAL FAILURE IN UROLOGIC ONCOLOGY

Nephron Mass Reduction

On the basis of several experimental models of renal disease, Brenner and colleagues have determined that the loss of functional renal mass is associated with a compensatory increase in intraglomerular pressure and single-nephron glomerular filtration rate.[124] These hemodynamic changes are ultimately maladaptive because they appear to accelerate the progression of renal disease, regardless of the experimental model or clinical scenario. Patients with renal cell carcinoma who undergo partial or subtotal nephrectomies are the human clinical analogs to experimental models of renal ablation (e.g., five-sixths nephrectomy).[125]

The short-term renal consequence of uncomplicated uninephrectomy is hyperfiltration; that is, total glomerular filtration rate exceeds 50% of prenephrectomy values, despite a 50% reduction in renal mass. Although initially beneficial, hyperfiltration can result in the development of systemic hypertension, proteinuria, and progressive renal dysfunction, depending on several factors. Although the ill effects of uninephrectomy in healthy kidney transplant donors are modest, at least over the first 10 to 20 years after surgery,[126] the renal complication rate increases in the setting of advanced age (with underlying age-related glomerulosclerosis), more extreme degrees of renal ablative surgery (two-thirds, three-fourths, or five-sixths nephrectomy), and the presence of underlying renal dysfunction or systemic hypertension. Several studies have formally examined the development and extent of renal injury in patients with more than

50% reduction in renal mass as a result of surgery for carcinoma.[127–130] Novick and colleagues showed that the extent of proteinuria was directly correlated with the time since surgery, and inversely correlated with the estimated volume of remnant renal tissue.[131] Furthermore, in four of five patients who were biopsied for moderate to severe proteinuria, the pathologic lesion found was focal and segmental glomerulosclerosis, the characteristic histologic finding associated with hemodynamic renal injury.[124,131]

Although acute renal failure complicates nephron-sparing surgery in up to 18% of cases (11% in the largest study of 259 patients, 3% requiring dialysis), few studies have followed patients for enough time to accurately estimate the risk of end-stage renal disease. In a recent report, Polascik and coworkers[132] suggested that improved surgical technique, including renovascular occlusion with regional hypothermia, intraoperative sonography, and injection of the collecting system with methylene blue (to verify anastomoses), may reduce the risk of perioperative (and ultimately, chronic) renal failure; prospective validation of these observations is needed.

Therefore, on the basis of extensive experimental and some clinical evidence, it would be advisable to treat survivors of nephron-sparing surgery with angiotensin-converting enzyme inhibitors, even in the absence of frank systemic hypertension, in an effort to abrogate hyperfiltration. An angiotensin receptor antagonist (e.g., losartan) is an acceptable alternative. A modest reduction in dietary protein intake to approximately 0.6 to 0.8 g/kg per day may provide additional therapeutic benefit, and could be considered after the perioperative period when protein requirements may exceed these values.

Radiation Nephritis

Germ cell tumors, particularly those exclusively or largely of seminomatous type, are the urologic malignancies most commonly treated with primary radiation therapy. Renal radiation exposure will occur in those patients with para-aortic and retroperitoneal lymph node involvement, some of the common sites of metastatic disease.

Although initially described in the early part of the century,[133,134] radiation nephritis was not recognized as an important clinical entity until the 1950s. Among several series reported in the early 1950s, Kunkler et al.[135] described 137 adult men with seminomas who received abdominal x-irradiation. Renal failure and/or hypertension developed in 27 (20%). Renal failure developed only in patients who had received at least 2300 cGy over a course of several weeks. These authors noted that nephrotoxic effects were delayed for several months, and occasionally up to 1 year after exposure. At that time renal failure developed, often in association with proteinuria, hypertension, and edema. One third of their patients died with uremia.

Subsequent experience has shown the clinical consequences of renal irradiation to be varied.[136,137] Acute radiation nephritis occurs in up to 40% of exposed patients, after a latency period of approximately 6 to 12 months.[138] Its clinical course is roughly analogous to a rapidly progressive glomerulonephritis, with the abrupt onset of hypertension, proteinuria, hematuria, and progressive renal failure. Churchill et al.[139] reported a shortened latency period of acute radiation nephritis with combined radiation and bleomycin-vinblastine therapy in a patient treated for testicular carcinoma, suggesting the possibility of a radiation-sensitizing or other synergistic effect within the kidney.

A more indolent form of radiation nephritis is insidious in onset, with a latency period ranging from 18 months to 14 years following exposure, but with similar symptomatology.[136] More rarely, proteinuria without renal dysfunction, and variable degrees of hypertension, including malignant hypertension, have been reported.[136]

Bone marrow transplantation–associated hemolytic-uremic syndrome, an entity reminiscent of acute radiation nephritis, has been ascribed to the use of cyclosporine for graft-versus-host disease prophylaxis. However, the initiating or potentiating effects of total body irradiation on this syndrome are unknown. It has been distinguished clinically from radiation nephritis by its earlier onset, usually within 100 days of transplantation.[140,141]

The adverse effects of radiation can be limited by techniques that shield at least part of the renal volume from radiation exposure, and by limiting the dose and duration of exposure, particularly in individuals with pre-existing functional impairment.[142] Hypertension should be aggressively controlled; angiotensin-converting enzyme inhibitors may be the antihypertensive drugs of choice based on several experimental studies and anecdotal clinical experience.[143–145] Indeed, radiation nephritis has been associated with hypertension and marked elevations of plasma renin activity in humans.[146] Rarely, uninephrectomy has been required to control hypertension.

End-Stage Renal Disease

The treatment of urologic malignancy only rarely results in end-stage renal disease. Some of the special treatment considerations of bilateral nephrectomy or nephrectomy of a solitary functional kidney are addressed later. Chronic renal failure develops in two other distinct settings; abruptly, in the setting of acute renal failure resulting from severe ischemic acute tubular necrosis and/or nephrotoxin exposure without renal recovery, or more insidiously, as a result of progressive loss of function, often after subtotal nephrectomy for bilateral renal cell carcinoma.

Acute renal failure usually results in a self-limited injury of moderate severity. More severe or sequential injuries (e.g., complicated surgery followed by sepsis and radiocontrast exposure) will sometimes lead to sufficient injury that a prolonged course of dialysis is required. Renal function will fortunately recover in most cases, although "progression" to end-stage disease can occur in up to one third of cases requiring dialysis.[147]

If prolonged renal replacement therapy is required, the options are threefold: hemodialysis, peritoneal dialysis, or transplantation. Hemodialysis is most often used in the United States, on a schedule of three times weekly for 3 to 4 hours each time. It is the most efficient form of dialysis, and can be employed in virtually all subjects as long as access to the circulation can be achieved and maintained. Continuous ambulatory peritoneal dialysis is an alternative dialytic modality that may be preferred by persons who wish to play a more active role in their dialysis care. This form of therapy requires the by-hand instillation of relatively large volumes of fluid (dialysate) into the abdomen through a catheter four to five times daily, or with an automated device at night. A history of previous abdominal surgery and/or radiation therapy makes this option less attractive and sometimes not viable, given the disruption and diminished transport capacity of the peritoneum (the dialysis "membrane," in this case).

Although most patients with urologic cancer and end-stage renal disease would fare best on hemodialysis, some characteristics that might allow the institution of peritoneal dialysis include prostate cancer rather than renal cell carcinoma or bladder cancer, assistance at home, adequate vision and dexterity, and, most importantly, substantial residual renal function (more than 2 ml/min) given the relative inefficiency of peritoneal compared with hemodialysis.

Transplantation can be considered in a select group of patients with urologic cancer. Advanced age would disqualify some individuals with prostate or bladder cancer. However, survivors of testicular cancer or renal cell carcinoma who develop end-stage renal disease related to cisplatin nephrotoxicity and/or surgical resection, respectively, for example, might be reasonable candidates for transplantation, assuming eradication of their malignant disease. It would be advisable for potential transplant recipients to remain free of disease for at least 2 to 5 years, depending on the underlying malignancy, because the immunosuppressive therapy required to prevent graft rejection can be deleterious and may enhance tumor growth in some instances.[148,149]

Finally, not all patients with end-stage renal disease are appropriate candidates for long-term renal replacement therapy. For example, an individual with metastatic prostate cancer, widespread retroperitoneal disease, and failed nephrostomies might elect not to undergo long-term dialysis because of discomfort, inconvenience, or other personal reasons. This decision would seem reasonable to most physicians. These and other difficult decisions regarding provision of care are best made together by the patient, the family, and the principal care providers (e.g., primary care physician, urologist, and oncologist). However, it is important to note that the provision of dialysis for acute renal failure and long-term dialysis for end-stage renal failure are not inexorably linked. For any given individual, a short-term trial of dialysis for therapy-related acute renal failure might be requested, and reasonable, whereas long-term dialysis might be refused.

SPECIAL ISSUES IN UROLOGIC ONCOLOGY AND NEPHROLOGY

Toxic Nephropathy and Transitional Cell Carcinoma

Although not a renal complication of urologic malignancy per se, it is worth noting the association between urothelial malignancy and a variety of causes of toxic nephropathy. This association was first reported in 1965 by Hultengren et al.[150] in six patients with papillary necrosis and tumors of the renal pelvis, five of whom were known to abuse phenacetin-containing analgesic drugs. Several subsequent epidemiologic studies confirmed this finding in larger patient groups.[151,152] Gonwa et al.[152] reported that 5% of cases of transitional cell carcinoma were associated with analgesic abuse; conversely, Bengtsson et al.[153] reported that 8% of patients with suspected analgesic nephropathy developed carcinoma of the renal pelvis over an average 5-year follow-up period. The relative risk of urothelial malignancy associated with other analgesic agents, including nonsteroidal anti-inflammatory drugs, aspirin, and acetaminophen, is unknown.

Other forms of toxic nephropathy, including "Balkan nephropathy,"[154] and a recently described nephropathy seen in association with the consumption of Chinese herbs,[155,156] are similarly associated with an increased risk of transitional cell carcinoma. These and related nephrotoxic syndromes are characterized by a chronic interstitial nephritis, with accompanying fluid and electrolyte disturbances (see earlier). Inquiry into the use of all prescription and nonprescription drugs and dietary supplements should be included in the initial work-up of the patient with known or suspected transitional cell carcinoma of the renal pelvis or collecting system.

Nephroendocrinopathy of Bilateral Nephrectomy

The bilateral nephrectomy survivor, in addition to requiring renal replacement therapy, requires close attention to the manifestations of "nephroendocrinopathy," with total or near-total loss of the kidney-derived hormones renin and erythropoietin and the lack of enzymatic conversion of 25-OH vitamin D.

In past years, bilateral nephrectomy was occasionally performed for severe and potentially disabling hypertension in persons with end-stage renal disease who were refractory to medical therapy. This practice has fallen out of favor, largely because of improved efficacy and tolerability of antihypertensive agents, and the accompanying metabolic derangements discussed later. In these cases, the absence of renin, and the resultant loss of the potent vasoconstrictor angiotensin II, was thought to be the primary mechanism responsible for the improvement in blood pressure control. However, the patient rendered anephric by surgery for malignancy may suffer ill consequences from the absence of renin. A fraction of patients may develop hypotension that is difficult to remedy. A number of therapies have been tried in these cases, usually without success, including high-sodium diets, compressive leg stockings, and various sympathomimetic agents (e.g., pseudoephedrine).

Bilateral nephrectomy will almost universally result in anemia because of the loss of erythropoietin. Although blood transfusion may still be necessary in the perioperative setting, the anemia can usually be corrected by starting erythropoietin replacement soon after surgery. Most patients will respond to 2000 to 4000 units two to three times per week, via either the subcutaneous or intravenous route. Although several of the causes of erythropoietin unresponsiveness, including severe hyperparathyroidism[157] and aluminum toxicity,[158] would probably not be relevant in the patient abruptly rendered anephric, iron deficiency,[159] and generalized inflammation,[160] as might accompany chronic infection or metastatic malignancy, should be carefully looked for if the patient does not respond to erythropoietin within several weeks.

Finally, the kidney is responsible for 1-hydroxylation of 25-OH vitamin D, the final step in the pathway of vitamin D activation. Without 1-hydroxylation at the kidney, functional vitamin D deficiency ensues. Functional vitamin D deficiency can be problematic for all patients with end-stage renal disease, but is particularly hazardous to the anephric patient because the combination of hyperphosphatemia, resulting from absent renal phosphate clearance, and the lack of 1,25-OH vitamin D, independently promoting parathyroid hormone production, can lead quickly to secondary hyperparathyroidism and raging osteitis fibrosa cystica (so-called renal osteodystrophy). Virtually all patients will have abnormalities in calcium and phosphate metabolism following bilateral nephrectomy. These can be best managed by a multimodality approach: (1) dietary phosphate restriction to less than 1 g/day, (2) administration of calcium carbonate or acetate with or just after meals as a dietary phosphate binder, and (3) administration of 1,25-OH vitamin D (calcitriol).

REFERENCES

1. Cockcroft DW, Gault MH: Prediction of creatinine clearance from serum creatinine. Nephron 1976; 16:31–36.
2. Swan R, Merrill J: Clinical course of acute renal failure. Medicine 1953; 32:215–228.
3. Hou SH, Bushinsky DA, Wish JB, et al: Hospital-acquired renal insufficiency: a prospective study. Am J Med 1983; 74:243–248.
4. Shusterman N, Strom BL, Murray TG, et al: Risk factors and outcome of hospital-acquired acute renal failure. Am J Med 1987; 83:65–71.
5. Anderson RJ, Linas SL, Berns AS, et al: Nonoliguric acute renal failure. N Engl J Med 1977; 296:1134–1138.
6. McMurray SD, Luft FC, Maxwell DR, et al: Prevailing patterns and predictor variables in patients with acute tubular necrosis. Arch Intern Med 1978; 138:950–955.
7. Maher ER, Robinson KN, Scoble JE, et al: Prognosis of critically-ill patients with acute renal failure: APACHE II score and other predictive factors. Q J Med 1989; 72: 857–866.
8. Lien J, Chan V: Risk factors influencing survival in acute renal failure treated by hemodialysis. Arch Intern Med 1985; 145:2067–2069.
9. Abreo K, Moorthy V, Osborne M: Changing patterns and outcome of acute renal failure requiring hemodialysis. Arch Intern Med 1986; 146:1338–1341.
10. Baslov JT, Jorgensen HE: A survey of 499 patients with acute anuric renal insufficiency: causes, treatment, complications and mortality. Am J Med 1963; 34:753–765.
11. Espinel CH: The FENa test: use in the differential diagnosis of acute renal failure. JAMA 1976; 236:579–581.
12. Miller TR, Anderson RJ, Linas SL, et al: Urinary diagnostic indices in acute renal failure: a prospective study. Ann Intern Med 1978; 89:47–50.
13. Fang LST, Sirota RA, Ebert TH, Lichenstein NS: Low fractional excretion of sodium with contrast media-induced acute renal failure. Arch Intern Med 1980; 140:531–533.
14. Vaz AJ: Low fractional excretion of urine sodium in acute renal failure due to sepsis. Arch Intern Med 1983; 143: 738–739.
15. Zarich S, Fang LST, Diamond JR: Fractional excretion of sodium: exceptions to its diagnostic value. Arch Intern Med 1985; 145:108–112.
16. Lins RL, Verpooten GA, DeClerck DS, DeBroe ME: Urinary indices in acute interstitial nephritis. Clin Nephrol 1986; 26:131–133.
17. Kristjansson K, Laxdal T, Ragnarsson J: Type 4 renal tubular acidosis (sub-type 2) associated with idiopathic interstitial nephritis. Acta Paediatr Scand 1986; 75:1051–1054.
18. Early LE: Extreme polyuria in obstructive uropathy: report of a case of "water-losing nephritis" in an infant, with a discussion of polyuria. N Engl J Med 1956; 255: 600–605.
19. Pelleya R, Oster JR, Perez GO: Hyporeninemic hypoaldosteronism, sodium wasting and mineralocorticoid-resistant hyperkalemia in two patients with obstructive uropathy. Am J Nephrol 1983; 3:223–227.
20. Battle DC, Arruda JAL, Kurtzman NA: Hyperkalemic distal renal tubular acidosis associated with obstructive uropathy. N Engl J Med 1981; 304:373–380.
21. Ditlove J, Werdmann P, Bernstein M, Massry SG: Methicillin nephritis. Medicine (Baltimore) 1977; 56:483–491.
22. Bergeron M, Gougoux A, Vinay P: The renal Fanconi syndrome. *In* Scriver CR, Beaudet AL, Sly WS, Valle D (eds): The Metabolic and Molecular Bases of Inherited Disease, 7th edition, pp 3691–3704. New York, McGraw-Hill, 1995.

23. Zusman J, Brown DM, Nesbit ME: Hyperphosphatemia, hyperphosphaturia and hypocalcemia in acute lymphoblastic leukemia. N Engl J Med 1973; 289:1335–1340.
24. Rao KG, Hackler RH, Woodlief RM, et al: Real-time renal ultasonography in spinal cord injury patients: prospective comparison with excretory urography. J Urol 1986; 135: 72–77.
25. Talner LB, Scheible W, Ellenbogen PH, et al: How accurate is ultrasonography in detecting hydronephrosis in azotemic patients? Urol Radiol 1981; 3:1–6.
26. Lalli AF: Retroperitoneal fibrosis and inapparent obstructive uropathy. Radiology 1977; 122:339–342.
27. Curry ND, Gobien RP, Schabel SI: Minimal-dilatation obstructive uropathy. Radiology 1982; 143:531–534.
28. Kaye AD, Pollack HM: Diagnostic imaging approach to the patient with obstructive uropathy. Semin Nephrol 1982; 2:55–73.
29. Bullock ML, Umen AJ, Finkelstein M, Keane WF: The assessment of risk factors in 462 patients with acute renal failure. Am J Kidney Dis 1985; 5:97–103.
30. Chertow GM, Lazarus JM, Christiansen CL, et al: Preoperative renal risk stratification. Circulation 1996 (in press).
31. Denton MD, Chertow GM, Brady HR: Renal-dose dopamine for the treatment of acute renal failure: a review of the rationale and results of experimental and human studies. Kidney Int 1996; 49:4–14.
32. Flores J, DiBona DR, Beck CH, Leaf A: The role of cell swelling in ischemic renal damage and the protective effect of hypertonic solute. J Clin Invest 1972; 51:118–126.
33. Bailey RR, Natale R, Turnbull DI, Linton AL: Protective effect of furosemide in acute tubular necrosis and acute renal failure. Clin Sci 1973; 45:1–17.
34. Goldberg LI: Cardiovascular and renal implications of dopamine: potential clinical applications. Pharmacol Rev 1972; 24:1–29.
35. Parker S, Carlon GC, Isaacs M, et al: Dopamine administration in oliguric and non-oliguric renal failure. Crit Care Med 1981; 9:630–632.
36. Wagner K, Schultze G, Molzahn M, Neumayer HH: The influence of long-term infusion of the calcium antagonist diltiazem on postischemic acute renal failure in conscious dogs. Klin Wochenschr 1986; 64:135–140.
37. Conger JD, Falk SA, Hammond WS: Atrial natriuretic peptide and dopamine in a rat model of ischemic acute renal failure in the rat. Kidney Int 1991; 40:21–28.
38. Marbury TC, Rahman SN, Sweet RM, et al: A randomized, double-blind, placebo-controlled multi-center clinical trial of anaritide atrial natriuretic peptide in the treatment of ATN. J Am Soc Nephrol 1995; 6:470.
39. Zager RA, Gmur DJ: Effect of xanthine oxidase inhibition on ischemic acute renal failure in the rat. Am J Physiol 1989; 257:F953-F958.
40. Miller SB, Martin DR, Kissane J, Hammerman MR: Insulin-like growth factor I accelerates recovery from ischemic acute tubular necrosis in the rat. Proc Natl Acad Sci USA 1992; 89:11876–11880.
41. Kelly KJ, Williams WW, Colvin RB, Bonventre JV: Antibody to intercellular adhesion molecule-1 protects the kidney against ischemic injury. Proc Natl Acad Sci USA 1994; 91:812–816.
42. Chertow GM, Owen WF Jr, Lazarus JM: Conventional hemodialysis in the treatment of acute renal failure. *In* Bellomo R, Ronco C (eds): Acute Renal Failure in the Critically Ill, pp 265–297. Berlin, Springer-Verlig, 1995.
43. Conger J: A controlled evaluation of prophylactic dialysis in post-traumatic acute renal failure. J Trauma 1975; 15: 1056–1063.
44. Gillum D, Dixon B, Yanover M, et al: The role of intensive dialysis in acute renal failure. Clin Nephrol 1986; 25: 249–255.
45. Higby DJ, Wallace HJ Jr, Holland JF: Cis-diamminedichloroplatinum (NSC-119875). A phase I study. Cancer Chemother Rep 1973; 57:459–463.
46. Gonzalez-Vitale JC, Hayes DM, Cvitkovic E, Sternberg SS: The renal pathology in clinical trials of cis-platinum (II) diamminedichloride. Cancer 1977; 39:1362–1371.
47. Rossof AH, Slayton RE, Perlia CP: Preliminary clinical experience with cis-diamminedichloroplatinum (II) (NSC 119875, CACP). Cancer 1972; 30:1451–1456.
48. Schilsky RL, Barlock A, Ozols RF: Persistent hypomagnesemia following cisplatin chemotherapy for testicular cancer. Cancer Treat Rep 1982; 66:1767–1769.
49. Buckley JE, Clark VL, Meyer TJ, Pearlman NW: Hypomagnesemia after cisplatin combination chemotherapy. Arch Intern Med 1984; 144:2347–2348.
50. Douglas JB, Healy JK: Nephrotoxic effects of amphotericin B, including renal tubular acidosis. Am J Med 1969; 46:154–162.
51. Vogelzang NJ, Torkelson JL, Kennedy BJ: Hypomagnesemia, renal dysfunction and Raynaud's phenomenon in patients treated with cisplatin, vinblastine and bleomycin. Cancer 1985; 56:2765–2770.
52. Ozols RF, Corden BJ, Jacob J: High-dose cisplatin in hypertonic saline. Arch Intern Med 1984; 100:19–24.
53. Gandara DR, Perez EA, Wiebe V, DeGregorio MW: Cisplatin chemoprotection and rescue: pharmacologic modulation of therapy. Semin Oncol 1991; 18:49–55.
54. Koeller JM, Trump DL, Tutsch KD, et al: Phase I clinical trial and pharmacokinetics of carboplatin (NSC 24 241240) by single monthly 30 minute infusion. Cancer 1986; 57:222–225.
55. Wright JE, Elias A, Tretyakov O, et al: High-dose ifosfamide, carboplatin, and etoposide pharmacokinetics: correlation of plasma drug levels with renal toxicity. Cancer Chemother Pharmacol 1995; 36:345–351.
56. Deray G, Ben-Othman T, Brillet G, et al: Carboplatin-induced acute renal failure. Am J Nephrol 1990; 10:431–432.
57. Vogelzang NJ: Nephrotoxicity from chemotherapy: prevention and management. Oncology 1991; 5:97–102.
58. Reed E, Jacob J: Carboplatin and renal dysfunction. Ann Intern Med 1989; 110:409.
59. Rossi R, Godde A, Kleinebrand A, et al: Unilateral nephrectomy and cisplatin as risk factors of ifosfamide-induced nephrotoxicity: analysis of 120 patients. J Clin Oncol 1994; 12:159–165.
60. Elias AD, Eder JP, Shea T: High dose ifosfamide with mesna uroprotection: a phase I study. J Clin Oncol 1990; 8:170–178.
61. Pratt CB, Meyer WH, Jenkins JJ, et al: Ifosfamide, Fanconi's syndrome, and rickets. J Clin Oncol 1991; 9:1495–1499.
62. Rossi R, Danzebrink S, Hillebrand D, et al: Ifosfamide-induced subclinical nephrotoxicity and its potentiation by cisplatinum. Med Pediatr Oncol 1994; 22:27–32.
63. Suarez A, McDowell H, Niaudet P, et al: Long-term follow-up of ifosfamide renal toxicity in children treated for malignant mesenchymal tumors: an International Society of Pediatric Oncology report. J Clin Oncol 1991; 9:2177–2182.
64. Burk CD, Restano I, Kaplan B: Ifosfamide-induced renal tubular dysfunction and rickets in children with Wilm's tumor. J Pediatr 1990; 117:331–335.
65. Ackland SP, Schilsky RL: High-dose methotrexate: a critical reappraisal. J Clin Oncol 1987; 5:2017–2031.
66. Pitman SW, Frei E III: Weekly methotrexate-calcium leukovorin rescue: effect of alkalinization on nephrotoxicity; pharmacokinetics in the CNS; and use in CNS non-Hodgkin's lymphoma. Cancer Treat Rep 1977; 61:695–701.
67. Jolivet J, Cowan KH, Curt GA: The pharmacology and clinical use of methotrexate. N Engl J Med 1983; 309: 1094–1104.
68. Sternberg CN, Yagoda A, Scher HI, et al: M-VAC (methotrexate, vinblastine, doxorubicin and cisplatin) for advanced transitional cell carcinoma of the urothelium. J Urol 1988; 139:461–468.
69. Shuler C, Golper TA, Bennett WM: Prescribing drugs in renal disease. *In* Brenner BM (ed): The Kidney, 5th edi-

tion, Vol 2, pp 2653–2702. Philadelphia, WB Saunders Co, 1995.
70. Lesesne JB, Rothchild N, Erickson B, et al: Cancer associated hemolytic-uremic syndrome: analysis of 85 cases from a national registry. J Clin Oncol 1989; 8:170–178.
71. Figg WD, Cooper MR, Thibault A, et al: Acute renal toxicity associated with suramin in the treatment of prostate cancer. Cancer 1994; 74:1612–1614.
72. Schellhammer PF: Renal failure associated with the use of thio-tepa. J Urol 1973; 110:498–501.
73. Armstrong RW: Complications after intravesical instillation of bacillus Calmette-Guerin: rhabdomyolysis and metastatic infection. J Urol 1991; 145:1264–1266.
74. Rosenberg SA, Lotze MT, Muul LM, et al: Observations on the systemic administration of autologous lymphokine-activated killer cells and recombinant interleukin-2 to patients with metastatic cancer. N Engl J Med 1985; 313:1485–1491.
75. Rosenberg SA, Lotze MT, Muul LM, et al: A progress report on the treatment of 157 patients with advanced cancer using lymphokine-activated killer cells and interleukin-2 or high-dose interleukin-2 alone. N Engl J Med 1987; 316:889–897.
76. Fisher RI, Coltman CA, Doroshow JH, et al: Metastatic renal cancer treated with interleukin-2 and lymphokine-activated killer cells. Ann Intern Med 1988; 108:518–523.
77. Shalmi CL, Dutcher JP, Feinfeld DA, et al: Acute renal dysfunction during interleukin-2 treatment: suggestion of an intrinsic renal lesion. J Clin Oncol 1990; 8:1839–1846.
78. Belldegrun A, Webb DE, Austin HA III, et al: Effects of interleukin-2 on renal function in patients receiving immunotherapy for advanced cancer. Ann Intern Med 1987; 106:817–822.
79. Kozeny GA, Nicolas JD, Creekmore S, et al: Effects of interleukin-2 immunotherapy on renal function. J Clin Oncol 1988; 6:1170–1176.
80. Guleria AS, Yang JC, Topalian SL, et al: Renal dysfunction associated with the administration of high-dose interleukin-2 in 199 patients with metastatic melanoma or renal carcinoma. J Clin Oncol 1994; 12:2714–2722.
81. Belldegrun A, Webb DE, Austin HA III, et al: Renal toxicity of interleukin-2 administration in patients with metastatic renal cell cancer: effect of pre-therapy nephrectomy. J Urol 1989; 141:499–503.
82. Thompson JA, Benyunes MC, Bianco JA, Fefer A: Treatment with pentoxifylline and ciprofloxacin reduces the toxicity of high-dose interleukin-2 and lymphokine-activated killer cells. Semin Oncol 1993; 20:46–51.
83. Memoli B, DeNicola L, Libetta C, et al: Interleukin-2-induced renal dysfunction in cancer patients is reversed by low-dose dopamine infusion. Am J Kidney Dis 1995; 26: 27–33.
84. Barton JC: Tumor lysis syndrome in nonhematopoietic neoplasms. Cancer 1989; 64:738–740.
85. Drakos P, Bar-Ziv J, Catane R: Tumor lysis syndrome in nonhematologic malignancies. Am J Clin Oncol 1994; 17: 502–505.
86. Ferry JA, Harris NL, Papanicalaou N, Young RH: Lymphoma of the kidney. A report of 11 cases. Am J Surg Pathol 1995; 19:134–144.
87. Bhatia S, Randive NU, Soman CS, Naresh KN: Primary bilateral renal lymphoma. Am J Surg Pathol 1996; 20:257.
88. Armstrong D, Myers WPL: Renal failure incident to reticulum cell sarcoma of the kidneys. Ann Intern Med 1966; 65:109–117.
89. Tsokos GC, Balow JE, Spiegel RJ, Magrath IT: Renal and metabolic complications of undifferentiated and lymphoblastic lymphomas. Medicine (Baltimore) 1981; 60: 218–229.
90. Richmond J, Sherman RS, Diamond HD, Craver LF: Renal lesions associated with malignant lymphoma. Am J Med 1962; 32:184–207.
91. Truong LD, Soroka S, Sheth AV, et al: Primary renal lymphoma presenting as acute renal failure. Am J Kidney Dis 1987; 9:502–506.
92. Martinez-Maldonado M, Ramirez-Arellano GA: Renal involvement in malignant lymphoma: a survey of 49 cases. J Urol 1966; 95:485–488.
93. Chisholm GD, Roy RR: The systemic effects of malignant renal tumours. Br J Urol 1971; 43:687–700.
94. Humes HD, Ichikawa I, Troy JL, Brenner BM: Evidence for a parathyroid hormone-dependent influence of calcium on the glomerular filtration. J Clin Invest 1978; 61: 32–40.
95. Lins LE: Reversible renal failure caused by hypercalcemia: a retrospective study. Acta Med Scand 1978; 203: 309–314.
96. Ferris DO, Odel HM: Electrolyte pattern of the blood after bilateral ureterosigmoidostomy. JAMA 1905; 136:634–640.
97. Annis D, Alexander MK: Differential absorption of electrolytes from large bowel in relation to ureterosigmoid anastomosis. Lancet 1952; 2:603–606.
98. McDougal WS: Metabolic complications of urinary intestinal diversion. J Urol 1992; 147:1199–2002.
99. McDougal WS, Koch MO: Effect of sulfate on calcium and magnesium homeostasis following urinary diversion. Kidney Int 1989; 35:105–108.
100. Castro JE, Ram MD: Electrolyte imbalance following ileal urinary diversion. Br J Urol 1970; 42:29–32.
101. Terai A, Arai Y, Kawakita M, et al: Effect of urinary intestinal diversion on urinary risk factors for urolithiasis. J Urol 1995; 153:37–41.
102. Assimos DG: Nephrolithiasis in patients with urinary diversion. J Urol 1996; 155:69–70.
103. Lee JC, Yamauchi H, Hopper J Jr: The association of cancer and the nephrotic syndrome. Ann Intern Med 1966; 64:41–51.
104. Row PG, Cameron JS, Turner DR, et al: Membranous nephropathy: long term follow-up and association with neoplasia. Q J Med 1975; 44:207–239.
105. Couser WC: Renal mass and the nephrotic syndrome in a 71 year old man. N Engl J Med 1980; 303:985–995.
106. Alpers CE, Contran RS: Neoplasia and glomerular injury. Kidney Int 1986; 30:465–473.
107. Abouchacra S, Duguid WP, Somerville PJ: Renal cell carcinoma presenting as nephrotic syndrome complicated by acute renal failure. Clin Nephrol 1993; 39:340–342.
108. Tang AL, Davies DR, Wing AJ: Remission of nephrotic syndrome in amyloidosis associated with a hypernephroma. Clin Nephrol 1989; 32:225–228.
109. Forland M, Bannayan GA: Minimal-change lesion nephrotic syndrome with renal oncocytoma. Am J Med 1983; 75:715–720.
110. Borras M, Panades MJ, Ramos J, Montoliu J: Minimal-change nephrotic syndrome associated with renal angiomyolipoma. Nephron 1994; 68:138–139.
111. Thomas DM, Hillis AN, Coles GA: Enalapril can treat the proteinuria of membranous nephropathy without detriment to systemic or renal hemodynamics. Am J Kidney Dis 1991; 18:38–43.
112. Leehey DJ, Braun BI, Tholl DA, et al: Can pharmacokinetic dosing decrease nephrotoxicity associated with aminoglycoside therapy? J Am Soc Nephrol 1993; 4:81–90.
113. Cronin RE, Henrich WL: Toxic nephropathy. *In* Brenner BM (ed): The Kidney, 5th edition, Vol 2, pp 1680–1711. Philadelphia, WB Saunders Co, 1995.
114. Patel R, Savage A: Symptomatic hypomagnesemia associated with gentamicin therapy. Nephron 1979; 23:50–52.
115. Bar RJ, Wilson HE, Mazzaferri EL: Hypomagnesemic hypocalcemia secondary to renal magnesium wasting: a possible consequence of high dose gentamicin therapy. Ann Intern Med 1975; 82:646–649.
116. Rybak MJ, Albrecht LM, Burke SC, Chandrasekar PH: Nephrotoxicity of vancomycin alone and with an aminoglycoside. J Antimicrob Chemother 1990; 25:679–687.
117. Moore RD, Smith CR, Lipsky JJ, et al: Risk factors for nephrotoxicity in patients treated with aminoglycosides. Ann Intern Med 1984; 100:352–357.

118. Gilbert DN: Once-daily aminoglycoside therapy. Antimicrob Agents Chemother 1991; 35:399–405.
119. Prins JM, Buller HR, Kuijper EJ, et al: Once versus thrice daily gentamicin in patients with serious infections. Lancet 1993; 341:335–339.
120. Lo WK, Rolston KVI, Rubenstein EB, Bodey GP: Ciprofloxacin-induced nephrotoxicity in patients with cancer. Arch Intern Med 1993; 153:1258–1262.
121. Cheng JT, Witty RT, Robinson RR, Yarger WE: Amphotericin B nephrotoxicity: increased renal resistance and tubule permeability. Kidney Int 1982; 22:626–633.
122. Fisher MA, Talbot GH, Maislin G, et al: Risk factors for amphotericin B-associated nephrotoxicity. Am J Med 1989; 87:547–552.
123. Heidemann HTH, Gerkens JF, Spickard WA, et al: Amphotericin B nephrotoxicity in humans decreased by salt repletion. Am J Med 1983; 75:476–481.
124. Brenner BM, Meyer TW, Hostetter TH: Dietary protein intake and the progressive nature of renal disease: the role of hemodynamically mediated glomerular injury in the pathogenesis of progressive glomerular sclerosis in aging, renal ablation, and intrinsic renal disease. N Engl J Med 1982; 307:652–659.
125. Neuringer JR, Brenner BM: Hemodynamic theory of progressive renal disease: a 10-year update in brief review. Am J Kidney Dis 1993; 22:98–104.
126. Hakim R, Goldszer RC, Brenner BM: Hypertension and proteinuria: long-term sequelae of uninephrectomy in humans. Kidney Int 1984; 29:1072–1076.
127. Novick AC, Streem S, Montie JE, et al: Conservative surgery for renal cell carcinoma: a single-center experience with 100 patients. J Urol 1989; 141:835–839.
128. Solomon LR, Mallick NP, Lawler W: Progressive renal failure in a remnant kidney. BMJ 1985; 291:1610–1611.
129. Rutsky EA, Dubovsky EV, Kirk K: Long-term follow-up of a human subject with a remnant kidney. Am J Kidney Dis 1991; 18:509–513.
130. Campbell SC, Novick AC, Streem SB, et al: Complications of nephron sparing surgery for renal tumors. J Urol 1994; 151:1177–1180.
131. Novick AC, Gephardt G, Guz B, et al: Long-term follow-up after partial removal of a solitary kidney. N Engl J Med 1991; 325:1058–1062.
132. Polascik TJ, Pound CR, Meng MV, et al: Partial nephrectomy: technique, complications and pathologic findings. J Urol 1995; 154:1312–1318.
133. Baerman G, Linser P: Uber die lokale und allgemeine wirkung der rontgenstahlen. Munch Med Wochenschr 1904; 51:1996–2000.
134. Warthin AS: Changes produced in kidneys by roentgen irradiation. Am J Med Sci 1907; 113:736–741.
135. Kunkler PB, Farr RF, Luxton RW: The limit of renal tolerance to X-rays. Br J Radiol 1952; 25:190–197.
136. Luxton RW: Radiation nephritis: a long-term study of fifty-four patients. Lancet 1961; 1:580–581.
137. Madrazo A, Schwartz G, Churg J: Radiation nephritis: a review. J Urol 1975; 114:822–827.
138. Jennette JC, Ordonez NG: Radiation nephritis causing nephrotic syndrome. Urology 1983; 22:631–634.
139. Churchill DN, Hong K, Gault MH: Radiation nephritis following combined abdominal radiation and chemotherapy (bleomycin-vinblastine). Cancer 1978; 41:2162–2164.
140. Shulman H, Striker G, Deeg HJ, et al: Nephrotoxicity of cyclosporin A after allogeneic marrow transplantation. N Engl J Med 1981; 305:1392–1395.
141. Atkinson K, Biggs JC, Hayes J, et al: Cyclosporin A associated nephrotoxicity in the first 100 days after allogeneic bone marrow transplantation: three distinct syndromes. Br J Haematol 1983; 54:59–67.
142. Keane WF, Crosson JT, Staley NA, et al: Radiation-induced renal disease: a clinicopathologic study. Am J Med 1976; 60:127–137.
143. Moulder JE, Fish BL, Cohen EP: Treatment of radiation nephropathy with ACE inhibitors. Int J Radiat Biol Phys 1993; 27:93–99.
144. Juncos LI, Carrasco-Duenas S, Cornejo JC, et al: Long-term enalapril and hydrochlorothiazide in radiation nephritis. Nephron 1993; 64:249–255.
145. Cohen EP, Lawton CA, Moulder JE: Bone marrow transplant nephropathy: radiation nephritis revisited. Nephron 1995; 70:217–222.
146. Shapiro AP, Cavallo T, Cooper W, et al: Hypertension in radiation nephritis: report of a patient with unilateral disease, elevated renin activity levels, and reversal after unilateral nephrectomy. Arch Intern Med 1977; 137:848–851.
147. Chertow GM, Christiansen CL, Cleary PD, et al: Prognostic stratification in critically ill patients with acute renal failure requiring dialysis. Arch Intern Med 1995; 155: 1505–1511.
148. Penn I: Renal transplantation for Wilm's tumor: report of 20 cases. J Urol 1979; 122:793–794.
149. Penn I: The effect of immunosuppression on pre-existing cancers. Transplantation 1993; 55:742–747.
150. Hultengren N, Lagergren L, Ljunqvist A: Carcinoma of the renal pelvis in renal papillary necrosis. Acta Chir Scand 1965; 130:314–320.
151. Piper JM, Tonascia PHJ, Matanoski GM: Heavy phenacetin use and bladder cancer in women aged 20 to 49 years. N Engl J Med 1985; 313:292–295.
152. Gonwa TA, Corbett WT, Schey HM, Buckalew VM: Analgesic-associated nephropathy and transitional cell carcinoma of the urinary tract. Ann Intern Med 1980; 93: 249–252.
153. Bengtsson U, Angervall L, Ekman H, Lehmann L: Transitional cell tumors of the renal pelvis in analgesic abusers. Scand J Urol Nephrol 1968; 2:145–150.
154. Cukuranovic R, Ignjatoivc M, Stefanovic V: Urinary tract tumors and Balkan nephropathy in the South Morava river basin. Kidney Int Suppl 1991; 40:S80-S84.
155. Cosyns JP, Jadoul M, Squifflet JP, et al: Urothelial malignancy in nephropathy due to Chinese herbs. Lancet 1994; 344:188.
156. Cosyns JP, Jadoul M, Squifflet JP, et al: Chinese herbs nephropathy: a clue to Balkan endemic nephropathy. Kidney Int 1994; 45:1680–1688.
157. Massry SG: Pathogenesis of the anemia of uremia: role of secondary hyperparathyroidism. Kidney Int 1983; 24: S204–S212.
158. Kaiser L, Schwartz KA: Aluminum-induced anemia. Am J Kidney Dis 1985; 6:348–352.
159. Macdougall IC, Hutton RD, Cavill I, et al: Poor response to treatment of renal anaemia with erythropoetin corrected by iron given intravenously. BMJ 1989; 299:157–158.
160. Lazarus JM, Denker BM, Owen WF Jr: Management of the patient with renal failure. *In* Brenner BM (ed): The Kidney, 5th edition, Vol 2, pp 2424–2506. Philadelphia, WB Saunders Co, 1995.

54

PAIN CONTROL AND SUPPORTIVE CARE OF THE TERMINAL PATIENT

GILBERT Y. WONG, M.D. *and* PETER R. WILSON, PH.D.

Pain can be defined as "an unpleasant sensory and emotional experience associated with actual or potential tissue damage, or described in terms of such damage."[1] Cancer pain, in particular, may have a severe impact on multiple levels affecting the functioning of both patient and family. Unfortunately, pain accompanying cancer is often inadequately treated, although it is the major fear and concern of many patients.[2,3]

We are only beginning to understand the effects of pain and stress on the human organism. There is accumulating evidence that pain and stress can inhibit immune function with involvement of natural killer cells, resulting in enhanced tumor growth or metastases.[4–7] In humans, there are also supportive findings that the alleviation of pain and stress may improve the survival of cancer patients.[8,9] Thus the pressing need for adequate management of cancer-related pain may be more important than previously realized.[10]

The multidisciplinary approach to the management of cancer and cancer pain is likely to be the most effective and successful means of treatment. This team of specialists might include internists, oncologists, surgeons, anesthesiologists, neurologists, physiatrists, psychiatrists, nurses, and social workers. The different members of the team could then contribute expertise to the management of the patient in pain with urologic cancer.

PAIN ASSESSMENT

There are multiple causes and mechanisms of cancer-related pain that may coexist. Therefore, a thorough, detailed history and physical are essential to assist in the diagnosis of the potential mechanisms involved in the pain of cancer. A complete review of the patient's record in conjunction with a careful patient history may reveal important clues to determining the source(s) of the pain. Important elements of the patient's history include the pain history, oncologic history, medical history, and psychosocial history, which will aid the eventual diagnosis and guide the treatment.

A detailed pain history will consider the location, distribution, quality, intensity, and temporal characteristics related to the patient's pain experience. Associated sensory phenomena may include paresthesias, dysesthesias, and numbness. Subjective muscle weakness is also important to note. Presently, patient self-report is the most valuable means to assess the subjectively influenced feeling of pain. There are a number of pain measurements developed to assess cancer pain, including a 0 to 10 numerical pain intensity scale, a 100-mm visual analogue scale, the McGill Pain Questionnaire, and the Memorial Pain Card. No one instrument has been shown to be superior to others. Measurements of pain intensity, function, and pain relief should be made at appropriate intervals to evaluate adequacy of pain therapies.

Also, it is important not to underestimate the potential effect of psychological modulation of existing nociceptive pain mechanisms. A general psychological and behavioral assessment, which might include psychometric testing, may be essential to thorough evaluation. As the physician-patient relationship develops, a sense of the patient's feelings of anger, frustration, depression, and anxiety, if present, may be revealed. These emotions may all potentially exacerbate the subjective feelings of pain that the cancer patient could be experiencing, and must be addressed.

Every patient should receive a comprehensive physical examination. Assessment should include thorough inspection of the site of pain, related adjacent sites (referred pain patterns), sites of known tumor invasion, and a musculoskeletal and neurologic examination. The careful neurologic examination is important to be able to identify any neuropathic pain process(es) that may occur from infiltrating tumor or peripheral nerve(s) or possible spinal cord involvement.

Various diagnostic studies may be helpful to confirm and define a clinical diagnosis of a particular pain syndrome. Plain radiologic studies may be useful as a screening procedure. Imaging studies such as computed tomography (CT) scanning and magnetic resonance imaging (MRI) may provide detailed visualization of bony and soft tissues and extent of tumor infiltration. Electromyelography may assist in the interpretation of neurologic dysfunction. Nuclear medicine procedures such as bone scan or gallium scan may offer additional information in regard to bony or soft tissue involvement.

Frequent reassessment cannot be overemphasized in the treatment of cancer pain. Cancer pain is a dynamic and progressive process that can continue to evolve with time until death. Consistent follow-up will allow the opportunity to re-evaluate existing pain problems and to identify acute processes that occur in response to the disease or therapy.

CARE OF THE TERMINAL PATIENT

Because of the previous lack of attention paid to the needs of dying patients and their families within existing medical systems, the hospice movement evolved in the 1960s. The needs and concerns of the family became the focus, with the family included as part of the care team. The needs of the terminal cancer patient differ significantly from those of cancer pain patients at an earlier stage of disease. The psychological and social implications of a short prognosis are considerable, and the need for pain and symptom relief is even more pressing.

Collectively, the various end-points may be to optimize the one common theme, the so-called quality of life.[11] The essential character of life is difficult to define, but there may be identifiable physical, emotional, and social elements that apply to terminally ill patients.[11] The major goals of care of the terminally ill are to provide the patient with a support system to help the patient live as actively as possible in the face of impending death, to provide relief from pain and other symptoms, and to provide psychological care for the patient and family.[2]

Supportive Care

Hospice care has been called "a blend of clinical pharmacology and applied compassionate psychology."[12] It is a philosophy of providing intensive symptom control combined with psychosocial and spiritual support to dying patients and their families. For hospice purposes, the definition of the terminal period is less than 6 months of life.[13] Hospice can be a program of supportive services for terminally ill patients and their families, provided either at home or in designated inpatient settings. Presently, most hospice care, however, is home based. In many cases, the patient, "primary care giver" (caring family member or close friend), nurse, social worker, and physician constitute the "care team." Periodic nurse home visits by a health care nurse with physician guidance are essential to home terminal care.

In terminal illness, the primary aim is no longer to prolong life but to make the life that remains as comfortable and meaningful as possible. The question of "what is appropriate treatment?" given a patient's circumstances and prospects must be addressed. Comfort-oriented care focuses on alleviating symptoms, including pain, and usually is not directly aimed at the underlying causes. There is often a compromise between prolonging life and maximizing comfort. In early stages of cancer, the priority is prolongation of life. This might involve painful and destructive procedures. However, in terminal stages, comfort is the overriding aim, and "curative" procedures are abandoned.

Symptom Control

Symptom control is the hallmark of terminal care, with common symptoms including pain, dysphagia, anorexia, fecal incontinence, vomiting, constipation, diarrhea, pain, and nausea. A variety of drugs can be used to treat such symptoms (Table 54–1).

TABLE 54–1. DOSAGES FOR MEDICATIONS TREATING COMMONLY ACQUIRED SYMPTOMS

Drug	Dosing Schedule
Antiemetics	
Promethazine hydrochloride (Phenergan)	12.5–25 mg PO q 4 h
Metoclopramide (Reglan)	10 mg PO before each meal and q HS
Scopolamine (Transderm Scōp)	1 patch (0.5 mg) behind each ear; lasts up to 3 days
Antidiarrheals	
Diphenoxylate/atropine (Lomotil)	15–20 mg/day in 3–4 divided doses PRN
Loperamide (Imodium)	4 mg PO, may repeat 2 mg PRN up to 16 mg/day
Laxatives	
Psyllium (Metamucil)	1 tsp up to t.i.d.
Docusate (Peri-Colace)	100 mg PO
Bisacodyl (Dulcolax)	5 mg PO

The issue of pain control is discussed throughout the chapter. However, an important issue to pain control, in the context of supportive care of the cancer patient, is the compromise between analgesia with medications and increased sedation with altered sensorium. This complex issue, with significant implications, is preferably discussed with the patient and family in the earlier stages of treatment to attempt to meet their desires. In certain cases, however, the confusional state resulting from the metabolic changes associated with the disease process may be difficult to improve.

Psychological Care of the Patient and Family

The caregiver treating the cancer patient with pain can be faced with complex diagnostic and therapeutic challenges. Patients with cancer pain face many complex emotional problems such as anxiety, depression, anger, and denial. For these cases, psychiatric involvement in the management of the cancer pain patient and family can be integral. Patients with severe cancer pain and associated emotional problems may require more aggressive psychotherapy in addition to adjunctive psychotropic drugs.[2]

Especially true in cancer or terminal patients is the lowered threshold toward feeling abandoned or believing that needs are ignored. The care team should be continually involved in an active manner, not with passive, uninterested dialogue. This interaction may be achieved by simple and direct communication with the patient and family. Team members should avoid giving patients and family conflicting or contradictory information, which can generate anxiety and loss of confidence. The diagnosis of cancer is accompanied by a sense of helplessness and loss of control, resulting in anxiety and fear. Thus the cancer patient should be continually encouraged to be active and participate in self-care whenever possible. The primary goal is to assist the patient to accept, in a positive manner, the reality of the terminal illness. Unfortunately, some patients continue in the denial stage throughout the illness. In such cases it is particularly important to maintain dialogue with the family and significant others.

Psychosocial interventions, if necessary, are optimally introduced early in the course of disease. These should be regarded as part of a multidisciplinary approach to management of the pain, not a substitute for analgesic therapy. Psychosocial interventions may involve both cognitive and behavioral techniques. Cognitive techniques are designed to influence how one interprets events and bodily sensations.[14] Behavioral techniques are directed to helping patients cope with pain and helping them to modify their reactions to pain.[14]

Support of the family of the cancer patients is an essential part in the care of the dying. Communication between the care team and patient's family should be open and maintained throughout the process. Integrating the family in the case of the patient can be beneficial for all. A family that is content and at ease will have a positive impact on the patient. Peer support groups are one type of vehicle that can be especially helpful to both patient and family in regard to providing a social outlet, emotional support, and access to education and information. Another route is pastoral care that can provide access to spiritual care and support of the patient and family.

ETIOLOGY OF PAIN

There are multiple causes of cancer-related pain that may coexist: tumor pain, pain resulting from cancer treatment, cancer-related biochemical or physiologic alterations, pain unrelated to the cancer, or a combination of these categories.

Tumor Pain

Bone

Tumor invasion of the bone, from either primary or metastatic cancer, is the most common cause of pain in cancer patients.[2,15] Prostate cancer is a frequent cause of bony metastases. Primary tumors of metastases can cause pain by various mechanisms. Bony metastatic deposits are believed to cause pain by stretching or invading periosteum or by direct bony involvement. There is some evidence that prostaglandins, prostacyclins, or both are involved. There may be local pain at tumor sites or distant referred pain—for example, knee pain from hip deposits. Pathologic fractures are an obvious source of pain. Decisions to debulk painful tumors by surgery, radiotherapy, or chemotherapy and immobilize pathologic fractures in order to reduce pain must be made. Because of the complex innervation of the periosteum of long bones, neural blockade is rarely indicated.[16] Involvement of vertebral bodies by tumor usually causes localized pain. However, extension of the mass may involve neurologic structures and result in syndromes ranging from isolated peripheral neural irritation and deficits to paraplegia or quadriplegia. CT, MRI, or myelography is used to delineate tumor invasion of anatomic structures that may produce signs and symptoms. Urgent decompression may be necessary to prevent or minimize damage to the spinal cord, nerve roots, or cauda equina.

Nerves

Tumor compression or infiltration of peripheral nerves is the second most frequent cause of pain in cancer patients.[2,17] Primary or metastatic tumors may infiltrate nerve roots, nerve trunks, and plexuses. Mechanisms of pain production in such cases are not clear, but they may involve direct mechanical (pressure) irritation, chemical (prostaglandin) irritation, local inflammatory reactions, and impairment of neural blood supply. Involvement of neural structures may produce motor, sensory, or autonomic disturbances. Pain can be localized or diffuse, sharp or dull, and constant or intermittent, with or without causalgic (burning) characteristics. Careful neurologic assessment is essential to define any functional impairment.

Tumor compression of the neuraxis may be debilitating and is considered a medical emergency. The tumor typically enters the epidural space by direct spread of vertebral metastases.[18] Epidural spread may also occur by direct invasion of retroperitoneal tumor or blood-borne seeding of the epidural space.

Pathologic fractures, particularly of vertebral bodies in prostate cancer, may produce localized neurologic lesions, with radiculopathy, plexopathy, or neuropathy. Neck or back pain may result from vertebral body involvement of radicular compression. Pain from either source may be unilateral or bilateral. Neurologic symptoms vary with site and extent of compression and include motor and sensory deficits. Progression to paraplegia, with loss of bladder and bowel sphincter control, may occur. Confirmation of extent and severity of involvement may require myelography, CT, or MRI. Careful documentation is required before diagnostic or therapeutic maneuvers involving epidural or intrathecal spaces are attempted. Extension of neural involvement after such a procedure might result from tumor swelling, hematoma or bleeding, or nerve damage from mechanical or chemical trauma. Decisions whether to debulk an infiltrating mass by surgery, radiotherapy, or chemotherapy must be made.

Pain Associated with Cancer Therapy

Pain may be associated with surgical therapy. Wound pain occurs during healing and may increase total discomfort in the acute postoperative period. Direct nerve trauma or entrapment of nerves in scar tissue may lead to delayed neuralgic pain, with pain and sensory loss, dysesthesia, and hyperesthesia. Pain may increase with movement, and symptoms of causalgia may occur.

Although chemotherapy often relieves cancer pain by decreasing the tumor mass, pain syndromes may be related to the use of these drugs. Certain chemotherapeutic agents, such as vinca alkaloid drugs, may produce a peripheral neuropathy characterized by burning pain exacerbated by minor stimuli in one or more extremities.[19]

Radiotherapy is often used to decrease the tumor size with the hope that symptoms (including pain) are reduced even if a cure is not possible. However, radiotherapy itself can cause direct neurologic damage, resulting in pain. Neuralgic pain associated with motor and sensory deficits can occur soon after radiation involving peripheral nerves or plexuses. Radiation may also cause a fibrotic reaction around peripheral nerves or plexuses, which may appear within a few months or may be delayed for many years. There may be motor, sensory, and autonomic changes and associated skin changes with lymphedema.

Pain Related to Cancer-Associated Biochemical or Physiologic Alterations

Paraneoplastic syndromes may be a concomitant problem with cancer, and may be a potential cause of pain.[2] These syndromes may not be necessarily related to the malignancy but are promoted and supported by the cancer.

Pain Unrelated to Cancer or Cancer Therapy

Pain that is unrelated to cancer or cancer therapy may occur in patients with cancer. For example, pain may arise from pre-existing osteoarthritis, fibromyalgia, headaches, or irritable bowel syndrome. Therefore, it is essential to define the precise mechanisms of pain in patients with cancer so that they can receive appropriate treatment.

TREATMENT OF CANCER PAIN

Many cancer patients can achieve satisfactory pain relief with simple conservative treatment involving systemic analgesics and rehabilitative interventions. However, in some cases more invasive treatments—for example, nerve blocks or spinal delivery systems—may be indicated concurrently. Management of cancer pain will likely be most successful with the assistance of a multidisciplinary pain clinic, which can offer a multimodal treatment approach ranging from systemic analgesic therapy to interventional therapy, with appropriate psychosocial support.

Systemic Analgesic Therapy

Nonopioid, opioid, and adjuvant analgesic drugs are the mainstay of treatment for many patients with cancer pain.[39] A key concept is the individualization of the analgesic regimens and therapy for each cancer patient. Frequent reassessment of the patient's response to treatment is essential in determining the accuracy of the pain diagnosis and efficacy of the selected therapy. Worsening of previously controlled pain or new pain must prompt a thorough re-evaluation to rule out the possibility of a new tumor growth or spread. Also, patients must

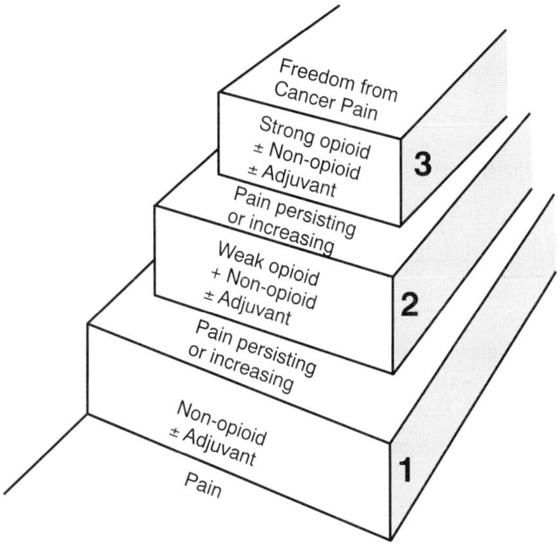
Freedom from Cancer Pain
Strong opioid
± Non-opioid
± Adjuvant
3
Pain persisting or increasing
Weak opioid
+ Non-opioid
± Adjuvant
2
Pain persisting or increasing
Non-opioid
± Adjuvant
1
Pain

FIGURE 54–1. World Health Organization three-step analgesic ladder. (From World Health Organization: Cancer Pain Relief and Palliative Care: Report of a WHO Expert Committee [World Health Organization Technical Report Series, No 804]. Geneva, World Health Organization, 1990, with permission.)

TABLE 54–2. DOSAGES FOR ACETAMINOPHEN AND NSAIDs IN ADULTS*

Drug	Dosing Schedule
Acetaminophen and over-the-counter NSAIDs	
Acetaminophen	650 mg PO q 4 h
Aspirin	650 mg PO q 4 h
Ibuprofen	400–600 mg PO q 6 h
Prescription NSAIDs	
Choline magnesium trisalicylate (Trilisate)	1000–1500 mg PO t.i.d.
Diflunisal (Dolobid)	500 mg PO q 12 h
Etodolac (Lodine)	200–400 mg PO q 6–8 h
Ketoprofen (Orudis)	25–60 mg PO q 6–8 h
Naproxen (Naprosyn)	250–275 mg PO q 6–8 h
Parenteral NSAIDs	
Ketorolac tromethamine (Toradol)	15–30 mg IV or IM q 6 h

*Adapted from Jacox A, Carr DB, Payne R, et al: Management of Cancer Pain: Clinical Practice Guideline No. 9 (AHCPR Publication No. 94-0592). Rockville, MD, Agency for Health Care Policy and Research, 1994.

be closely followed, particularly when beginning or changing analgesic requirements. In general, intramuscular administration of drugs should not be considered because of local pain and unreliable absorption by this route. Also, there is no place for "placebo" treatment in patients with proven terminal cancer; no useful information is gained from this practice.

The World Health Organization has developed a three-step analgesic ladder for management of cancer pain (Fig. 54–1).[20,42] In the first step, patients with mild to moderate cancer-related pain should be treated with a nonopioid analgesic, which should be combined with adjuvant drugs if a specific indication for one exists. In the second step, patients who have limited opioid exposure and present with moderate to severe pain or who fail to achieve adequate relief after a trial of a nonopioid analgesic should be treated with an opioid typically used for moderate pain, such as codeine, hydrocodone, oxycodone, or propoxyphene. This opioid drug is typically combined with a nonopioid and may be coadministered with an adjuvant analgesic. There is no place for meperidine in long-term pain therapy because of the accumulation of toxic metabolites. In the third step, patients who present with severe pain or fail the second step of the analgesic ladder should receive an opioid conventionally used for severe pain. The drugs placed in this category may include morphine, oxycodone, hydromorphone, methadone, fentanyl, and levorphanol.

Nonopioids (Table 54–2)

These first-step agents are useful alone for mild to moderate pain and provide additive analgesia when used in combination with opioid drugs in the treatment of more severe pain.[40] These drugs may potentiate the effects of opioid analgesics with less side effects.[21,22] In contrast to opioid drugs, nonopioid analgesic agents such as aspirin (ASA), nonsteroidal anti-inflammatory drugs (NSAIDs), and acetaminophen, do not cause tolerance or physical dependence. However, they do have a ceiling effect and should not be used in doses higher than recommended for nonmalignant pain.

NSAIDs may have a unique role in the management of pain from bone metastases.[23] Reports suggest that both ASA and indomethacin relieve bone pain possibly through inhibition of prostaglandin synthesis, which may be important in development of bone metastases.

Although relatively safe, ASA and NSAIDs must be used with caution in patients with disturbances of the gastrointestinal tract, decreased renal function, and blood clotting disorders.[24] Acetaminophen hepatic toxicity is rare unless large doses (above 4 g/day) are ingested, or in patients with compromised liver function.

Almost all the nonopioid medications at this first step of the analgesic ladder are administered by the oral route. Presently, ketorolac is the only NSAID that is available for parenteral administration. However, it must not be used for more than 5 days.

Opioids (Table 54–3)

Patients who do not achieve adequate symptom relief with the first step of the analgesic ladder need to progress to the second step, which includes "mild" opioids. Opioids are defined as a structurally related class of natural or synthetic agents that have morphine-like properties and range in chemical nature from alkaloid derivatives to peptides that bind to different opiate receptors.[25]

TABLE 54–3. DOSAGES FOR OPIOID ANALGESICS IN OPIOID-NAIVE ADULTS OF 50 KG BODY WEIGHT OR MORE*

Drug	Dosing Schedule
Opioid agonists	
Morphine	30 mg PO q 3–4 h 10 mg IV q 3–4 h
Morphine, controlled-release (MS Contin, Oramorph)	90–120 mg PO q 12 h
Hydromorphone (Dilaudid)	7.5 mg PO q 3–4 h 1.5 mg IV q 3–4 h
Levorphanol (Levo-Dromoran)	4 mg PO q 6–8 h 2 mg IV q 6–8 h
Methadone	20 mg PO q 6–8 h 10 mg IV q 6–8 h
Oxymorphone (Numorphan)	1 mg IV q 3–4 h
Fentanyl (Duragesic patch)	25–100 μg/hour transdermally (replace every 3 days)
Combination opioid-NSAID preparations	
Codeine (with aspirin or acetaminophen)	180–200 mg PO q 3–4 h
Hydrocodone (Lorcet, Lortab, Vicodin, others)	30 mg PO q 3–4 h
Oxycodone (Roxicodone, Percocet, Percodan, Tylox, others)	30 mg PO q 3–4 h
Propoxyphene (Darvocet-N 100)	1–2 tabs PO q 4 h

*Adapted from Jacox A, Carr DB, Payne R, et al: Management of Cancer Pain: Clinical Practice Guideline No. 9 (AHCPR Publication No. 94-0592). Rockville, MD, Agency for Health Care Policy and Research, 1994.

If the pain is continuous, analgesics should be given on a scheduled basis (around-the-clock), with additional "rescue" doses as required, so that there will be continuous serum levels of the analgesic medication. Opioids should be administered by the most convenient route capable of providing adequate analgesia. In most cases, the oral route is the most appropriate because of convenience and cost effectiveness. There are a number of other routes available for drug administration, including sublingual, rectal, subcutaneous, intravenous, intranasal, and transdermal. The persistence of inadequate pain relief must be addressed by stepwise escalation of the opioid dose until adequate analgesia is achieved or unmanageable side effects occur. In most cases, the development of side effects can be alleviated by medical management.

Studies of the patterns of chronic opioid drug use in patients with cancer and in those with other medical illnesses have demonstrated that tolerance and physical dependence occur, but that psychological dependence (addiction) is rare.[26] Tolerance occurs with long-term administration of opioids, but increasing doses of the drugs continue to produce analgesia. Because of the evolving nature of cancer pain, the development of tolerance must be closely monitoried by frequent reassessments. The use of a combination of drugs such as nonopioids or adjuvants and opioid drugs may improve analgesia without escalation of the narcotic dose.[22]

Lack of knowledge of the equianalgesic doses of opioid drugs, when switching one medication to another, is the most common cause of ineffective treatment of the cancer pain.[19] Also, lack of attention to the pharmacokinetic profile has also limited the effective use of certain drugs. Therefore, cancer-related pain should be managed with physician supervision, and a thorough understanding of the pharmacology and pharmacokinetics of the analgesic medications.

All patients receiving opioids should be closely monitored for side effects and complications. The most common adverse effects of opioids are constipation, nausea and vomiting, somnolence or cognitive impairment, and respiratory depression. In fact, all patients taking opioids should be managed with a bowel stimulant program unless contraindicated (e.g., diarrhea). Many of the other symptoms may be treatable with medical management and medications. Overall, side effects are not usually a limiting factor in the use of oral opioids.[27]

There are specific considerations to certain medications within the opioid class. Meperidine should not be used because of accumulation of its metabolite normeperidine, which can cause toxic effects, including seizures. Typically, mixed agonist-antagonist drugs are not ideal drugs for cancer pain because of limited efficacy at higher doses. Also, mixed agonist-antagonist drugs (such as buprenorphine and pentazocine) have the potential to precipitate withdrawal symptoms and increased pain if long-term opioid medications have been administered.

Adjuvant Drugs (Table 54–4)

Adjuvant drugs, which alter neural processing, may be useful when combined with opioid or nonopioid analgesics. In some neuropathic pain states, they may be drugs of choice.[28]

Corticosteroids, such as dexamethasone and prednisone, are commonly used adjuvant analgesics.[29] These drugs may produce analgesia by preventing release of prostaglandins, leading to a reduction of local inflammation and swelling, and may also elevate mood and increase appetite.

Antidepressants such as tricyclic antidepressants and selective serotonin reuptake inhibitors may be effective adjuvants to nonopioid and opioid analgesics by elevating mood, and may exert an independent nonopioid analgesic action.[41]

Amphetamines may potentiate the analgesic action of narcotics and also antagonize their sedative effects, elevate mood, and increase activity of the patient.[30] These drugs, however, are not commonly prescribed because of bureaucratic considerations.

Benzodiazepines such as diazepam may be helpful in the management of acute anxiety and panic attacks that occur in certain cancer patients. Furthermore, there is some evidence that benzodiaze-

TABLE 54–4. DOSAGES FOR ADJUVANT ANALGESIC DRUGS FOR CANCER PAIN*

Drug	Dosing Schedule
Corticosteroids	
Dexamethasone	16–96 mg PO, IV
Prednisone	40–100 mg PO
Anticonvulsants	
Carbamazepine	200–600 mg PO b.i.d.
Phenytoin	300–500 mg PO
Antidepressants/selective serotonin reuptake inhibitors	
Amitriptyline	10–50 mg PO q HS
Nortriptyline	10–75 mg PO q HS
Doxepin	25–150 mg PO q HS
Trazodone	75–225 mg PO q HS
Tramadol (Ultram)†	50–400 mg PO total q D
Psychostimulants	
Dextroamphetamine	5–10 mg PO
Benzodiazepines	
Valium	2–10 mg b.i.d.–q.i.d.
Clonazepam	0.5 mg PO t.i.d. (starting dose) to 5–6 mg PO t.i.d.

*Adapted from Jacox A, Carr DB, Payne R, et al: Management of Cancer Pain: Clinical Practice Guideline No. 9 (AHCPR Publication No. 94-0592). Rockville, MD, Agency for Health Care Policy and Research, 1994.
†Not an antidepressant.

pines may exert some mild analgesic action.[31] This class of medications should not be used as the sole medication to control pain in cancer.

Diagnostic Neural Blockade

Accurately placed nerve blocks can provide specific information on particular involvement of nervous structures and pathways of pain transmission. Also, these nerve blocks can be performed diagnostically or prognostically to predict the potential desirable or undesirable outcome of a permanent (neurolytic) nerve block.

Therapeutic Neural Blockade

Peripheral nerves and the central neuraxis can be blocked for variable periods by a number of different agents: for hours by injection of local anesthetics, days by freezing (cryoanalgesia), and weeks to months by thermocoagulation (radiofrequency) or injection of alcohol, phenol, or other chemicals (e.g., ammonium sulfate).[32] However, prior to any permanent neurolytic procedures, temporary (diagnostic) blocks are performed to assess the potential permanent intended or unintended effects, such as sensory, motor, or autonomic changes. Also, the decision to perform a neurolytic procedure must consider the potential for neuroma formation and deafferentation pain syndromes. In many cancer patients, the limited survival of the patient negates the issues of many of these potential problems. In all cases, therapeutic nerve blocks must be incorporated into the overall management, including systemic analgesic therapy.

The results of peripheral neurolysis have been disappointing, with numbness and pain relief persisting for a few weeks only. Furthermore, as axonal regeneration occurs, a neuroma can form at the site of damage, potentially resulting in painful allodynia and hyperesthesia. However, this process may take 3 to 6 months to occur.

Central neuraxis blockade, such as subarachnoid neurolysis with alcohol or phenol, while assuming some risk, can be beneficial in certain cancer patients. In certain pain syndromes that are localized to a limited number of dermatomes, pain can be controlled by blockade of dorsal roots as they traverse the cerebrospinal fluid within the spinal cord, resulting in a chemical dorsal rhizotomy. Although complications are usually slight, there is a theoretical possibility of cord damage, ranging from minor sensory deficit to quadriplegia.

Spinal Opioids (Epidural and Intrathecal)

The delivery of opioids directly to the spinal cord is highly effective in providing analgesia in many patients.[33,34,43] Compared to neurolytic procedures, spinal opioids have the distinct advantage of preserving sensory, motor, and some autonomic neural function, although bladder control might be impaired. The spinal route of administration of opioids is typically considered only after simpler routes have been demonstrated to provide inadequate pain relief or intolerable adverse effects. The continuous administration of the opioids occurs through a reservoir or pump to a catheter placed in either the epidural or intrathecal space. This reservoir or pump may allow the patient to remain at home and receive subsequent refillings by a hospice nurse or trained family member.

Superior Hypogastric Block

The sympathetic nervous system may be blocked at various levels in the body to interrupt pain transmission of visceral pain states. The superior hypogastric plexus is a sympathetic nervous system structure located in the retroperitoneum that transmits nociceptive information from the pelvic viscera via the hypogastric nerves. Neural blockade of the superior hypogastric plexus that interrupts pain transmission has been claimed to be a successful therapeutic technique for pelvic pain of neoplastic origin.[35,36]

Neurosurgical Treatment

A neurosurgical approach to the treatment of pain involves ablation of neural structures. The neural connection between the periphery and the brain is disrupted to alleviate the pain. Peripheral neurectomy itself is rarely an effective intervention because peripheral nerve fibers will regenerate in time. Neuroma formation or deafferentation pain may then develop, with worsening of the pain syndrome. Other neurosurgical techniques include section of spinal nerve roots, dorsal root entry zone (DREZ) lesioning, and spinothalamic tractotomy.

Anterolateral cordotomy is performed on the side opposite the pain, and cephalad enough to produce adequate pain and temperature relief. The most appropriate patient is the individual with pain in a unilateral limb distribution. If cordotomy is made at higher levels (e.g., C2 vertebral level), ventral gray matter of the spinal cord may be sectioned along with the spinothalamic tract. As a result, motor deficit of an extremity will result. This procedure may be carried out either by open surgery or by a percutaneous radiofrequency lesion.

Dorsal rootlets corresponding to the distribution of pain can be lesioned by heat. The DREZ (dorsal root entry zone) lesions are produced by a radiofrequency current or laser in the superficial layers of the dorsal horn.[37,38] Potential complications may include limb weakness, numbness, paresthesias, and proprioceptive loss.

In recent years, neurosurgical ablative procedures have perhaps been considered less often with refinement of stepwise systemic analgesic therapies, availability of specialists trained to perform neurolytic blocks, and the technological advances of spinal drug delivery systems.

CONCLUSION

Cancer pain can be complicated both to understand and to treat. As evidence, cancer pain is often inadequately managed, although it is the major fear and concern of many patients. Furthermore, studies have shown that, with proper care, many of these cancer patients can have adequate pain control. Thus, with accumulating evidence suggestive of possible effects of pain and stress affecting immune functioning and influencing survival, there is an even more pressing need for optimal pain control. The expertise of a pain specialist or multidisciplinary pain clinic may be invaluable in guiding the management of these cancer patients with often complicated pain-related symptomatology.

REFERENCES

1. Merskey H, Bogduk N: Classification of Chronic Pain, 2nd edition. Seattle, IASP Press, 1994.
2. Bonica JJ, Ventafridda V, Twycross RG: Cancer pain. *In* Bonica JJ (ed): The Management of Pain, 2nd edition, Vol 1, pp 400–446. Philadelphia, Lea & Febiger, 1990.
3. Cleeland C: Research in cancer pain: what we know and what we need to know. Cancer 1991; 67(Suppl):823–827.
4. Keller SE, Weiss JM, Schleifer SJ, et al: Suppression of immunity by stress: effect of a graded series of stressors on lymphocyte stimulation in the rat. Science 1981; 213: 1397–1400.
5. Laudenslager ML, Ryan SM, Drugan RC, et al: Coping and immunosuppression: inescapable but not escapable shock suppresses lymphocyte proliferation. Science 1983; 221: 568–570.
6. Sklar LS, Anisman H: Stress and coping factors influence tumor growth. Science 1979; 205:513–515.
7. Visintainer MA, Volpicelli JR, Seligman MEP: Tumor rejection in rats after inescapable or escapable shock. Science 1982; 216:437–439.
8. Lillemoe KD, Cameron JL, Kaufman HS, et al: Chemical splanchnicectomy in patients with unresectable pancreatic cancer. Ann Surg 1993; 217:447–457.
9. Spiegel D, Bloom JR, Kraemer HC, Gettheil E: Lancet 1989; 2:888–891.
10. Liebeskind JC: Pain can kill. Pain 1991; 44:3–4.
11. Morris JN, Suissa S, Sherwood S, et al: J Chronic Dis 1986; 1:47–62.
12. Reuben DB, Mor V, Hiris J: Clinical symptoms and length of survival in patients with terminal cancer. Arch Intern Med 1988; 148:1586–1591.
13. Smith JL: Care of People Who Are Dying: The Hospice Approach. *In* Patt RB (ed): Cancer Pain, pp 543–552. Philadelphia, JB Lippincott, 1993.
14. Jacox A, Carr DB, Payne R, et al: Management of Cancer Pain: Clinical Practice Guideline No. 9 (AHCPR Publication No. 94-0592). Rockville, MD, Agency for Health Care Policy and Research, 1994.
15. Twycross RG, Fairfield S: Pain in far-advanced cancer. Pain 1982; 14:303–310.
16. Carter RL, et al: Patterns and mechanisms of bone metastases. J R Soc Med 1985; 78(Suppl 9):2–6.
17. Daut RL, Cleeland CA: The prevalence and severity of pain in cancer. Cancer 1982; 50:1913.
18. Rodriguez M, Dinapoli RP: Spinal cord compression: with special reference to metastatic epidural tumors. Mayo Clin Proc 1980; 55:442–448.
19. Foley KM: The treatment of cancer pain. N Engl J Med 1985; 313:84–95.
20. World Health Organization: Cancer Pain Relief. Geneva, World Health Organization, 1986.
21. Hodsman NB, Burns J, Blyth A, et al: The morphine sparing effects of diclofenac sodium following abdominal surgery. Anaesthesia 1987; 42:1005–1008.
22. Weingart WA, Sorkness CA, Earhart RH: Analgesia with oral narcotics and added ibuprofen in cancer patients. Clin Pharmacol 1985; 4:53–58.
23. Brodic GN: Indomethacin and bone pain. Lancet 1974; 2: 1160.
24. Insel PA: Analgesic-antipyretics and antiinflammatory agents: drugs employed in the treatment of rheumatoid arthritis and gout. *In* Gillman AG, Rall TW, Nies AS, Taylor P (eds): Goodman and Gillman's The Pharmacological Basis of Therapeutics, 8th edition, pp 638–681. New York, Pergamon Press, 1990.
25. Martin WR: Pharmacology of opioids. Pharmacol Rev 1984; 35:4.
26. Porter J, Jick JH: Addiction rare in patients treated with narcotics. N Engl J Med 1980; 302:123.
27. Ventafridda V, Tamburini M, Caraceni A, De Conno F, et al: A validation study of the WHO method for cancer pain relief. Cancer 1987; 59:850–856.
28. Swerdlow M: Anticonvulsant drugs and chronic pain. Clin Neuropharmacol 1984; 7:51–82.
29. Bruera E, Roca E, Cedaro L, et al: Action of oral methylprednisolone in terminal cancer patients: a prospective randomized double blind study. Cancer Treat Rep 1985; 69: 751–754.

30. Joshi JH, de Jongh CA, Schnaper N, et al: Amphetamine therapy for enhancing the comfort of terminally ill patients (PTS) with cancer. Proc Am Soc Clin Oncol 1982; 1:C-213.
31. King SA, Strain JJ: Benzodiazepines and chronic pain. Pain 1990; 41:3–4.
32. Wilson PR, Wedel DJ: Role of pain clinic in bone cancer pain. *In* Sim FH (ed): Diagnosis and Management of Metastatic Bone Disease, p 109–117. New York, Raven Press, 1988.
33. Wang JK, Nauss LA, Thomas JE: Pain relief by intrathecally applied morphine in man. Anesthesiology 1979; 50:149.
34. Behar M, Magora F, Olshwang D, Davidson J: Epidural morphine in treatment of pain. Lancet 1979; 1:527–529.
35. Plancarte R, Amescua C, Patt RB, Aldrete JA: Superior hypogastric block for pelvic cancer pain. Anesthesiology 1990; 73:236–239.
36. de Leon-Casasola OA, Kent E, Lema MJ: Neurolytic superior hypogastric plexus block for chronic pelvic pain associated with cancer. Pain 1993; 54:145–151.
37. Nashold BS, Ostdahl RH: Dorsal root entry zone lesions for pain relief. J Neurosurg 1979; 51:59–69.
38. Nashold BS, Bullitt, X: Dorsal root entry zone lesions to control central pain in paraplegics. J Neurosurg 1981; 55: 414–419.
39. American Pain Society: Principles of Analgesic Use in the Treatment of Acute and Cancer Pain, 3rd edition, 1993.
40. Beaver WT: Nonsteroidal antiinflammatory analgesics in cancer pain. *In* Foley KM, Bonica JJ, Ventafridda V (eds): Advances in Pain Research and Therapy, Vol 16, pp 109–131. New York, Raven Press, 1990.
41. Charney DS, Menkes DB, Heninger GR: Receptor sensitivity and the mechanism of action of antidepressant treatment. Arch Gen Psychiatry 1981; 38:1160–1180.
42. Portenoy RK: 3-step analgesic ladder for management of cancer pain. Pharmacy Prac News 1991 (August).
43. Yaksh TL: Spinal opiate analgesia: characteristics and principles of action. Pain 1981; 11:293.

55

THE RANDOMIZED CLINICAL TRIAL

BRENT A. BLUMENSTEIN, PH.D.

A randomized clinical trial (RCT) is a clinical study comparing interventions in which the interventions are assigned to participating patients or subjects using a random process. RCTs have the greatest potential for yielding a valid comparison of interventions because randomization implements explicit control over extraneous factors that might otherwise interfere with comparison of the interventions. However, RCTs are complex undertakings and have many pitfalls where missteps in the design, execution, and analysis can threaten the potential for validity. This chapter reviews selected aspects of the RCT principles, focusing on those aspects of RCTs that illustrate why they are superior to other means of comparing interventions. There are a number of other works that provide coverage of other details of RCTs.[1–6] Also, of special note to readers seeking additional details on the topic of clinical trials management is the entire supplemental issue (volume 16, number 2S, 1995) of the journal *Controlled Clinical Trials*, in which there are six articles and a glossary addressing the issues of the management of multicenter studies.

This chapter focuses primarily on RCTs of interventions designed to mitigate or cure a disease or condition in cancer patients, with examples from urologic cancer. However, many of the principles discussed also apply to RCTs of interventions designed to prevent disease in individuals who are unafflicted with that disease, and also to diseases other than urologic cancers. Unless otherwise indicated, the reader may assume that all principles discussed in this chapter apply equally to all types of RCTs.

INTERVENTION AND ARM

The term "intervention" is used to refer to the clinical maneuvers being studied. The term "arm" is used in preference to the more restrictive term "treatment" because the maneuvers studied are often quite complex and more precisely defined as an algorithm of intended actions, including contingencies. For example, the term "intervention" can refer to not only application of a treatment but also specific instructions about how to respond to adverse effects of the treatment, or what to do when an initial treatment fails. As another example of the restrictiveness of the term "treatment" in the context of a RCT is in studies of disease prevention where the object of the study may be a vitamin, and those under study are individuals not afflicted with the disease or condition that is to be prevented; the study subjects are therefore not being "treated." Also, the term "treatment" is very much stretched when one of the arms is "no treatment."

A RCT is said to have arms, usually two but sometimes more. Participants are randomly assigned to the arms of a RCT. Associated with each arm is an intervention, and the intent is that each participant assigned to an arm is to receive the intervention associated with that arm. Thus, the term "arm" refers to a group of patients for whom the intent is that each is to receive the intervention associated with that arm.

RCTs are designed to compare outcomes between the arms. The outcome comparison statistic, whether it is a difference in means, a difference in proportions, a hazard ratio, or some other statistic, provides a measure of between-arm differences with respect to the outcome. Therefore, when data from a RCT are presented, it is most correct to state the results as a between-arm comparison. The conclusion that the RCT provides evidence that there is or is not a difference with respect to the interventions is a conclusion based on having the between-arm comparison. Conclusions stated in terms of comparisons of interventions require a careful inspection of the RCT results in order to assess the degree to which the results in each arm reflect the outcome for the intervention associated with that arm. Therefore, the results section of articles reporting the results of a RCT should present between-arm comparisons and data demonstrating the degree to which each arm reflects an outcome related to the associated intervention; conclusions about between-interventions differences and other speculations should appear in the discussion.

PATIENTS, PARTICIPANTS, AND INVESTIGATORS

The individuals enrolled in studies of disease prevention are usually referred to as participants rather than patients. Unfortunately, the term "participant" is also used to refer to the clinicians or other type of individuals who enroll patients or other individuals to a RCT. The term "investigator" is preferred for those enrolling participants to a RCT regardless of the type of trial.[7]

THE PROTOCOL

A RCT must have a detailed protocol. As an example, the top-level subject headings for protocols in the Southwest Oncology Group are listed in Table 55–1. There are other possibilities for these subject headings,[1] and in some RCTs there may not exist a document explicitly identified as a protocol, but there is an alternative implementation of the functions of the protocol in document(s) with names such as the Manual of Operations.[7]

One of the most important aspects of the protocol is the explicit and clear identification of the primary and secondary objectives and identification of the outcome measures (end-points) associated with each objective. The primary objective should be simple and have an associated outcome that is unambiguous and readily assessable for all patients randomized. The trial size is computed based on the primary objective and outcome measure. The primary objective, the associated primary outcome, and the criteria used to compute the trial size constitute a criterion for success, although this criterion for success is often not explicitly stated as such.

TABLE 55–1. FIRST-LEVEL HEADINGS FOR A SOUTHWEST ONCOLOGY GROUP PROTOCOL

Schema
Objectives
Background
Drug Information
Staging Criteria
Eligibility Criteria
Stratification
Treatment Plan
Toxicities To Be Monitored and Dosage Modifications
Study Calendars
Criteria for Evaluation and End-point Definitions
Statistical Considerations
Discipline Review
Registration Guidelines
Data Submission Schedule
Special Instructions
Ethical and Regulatory Considerations
Bibliography
Master Forms Set
Appendix

Often it seems desirable to have a primary objective that is a composite of both an efficacy outcome and a safety outcome, and perhaps other outcomes. One approach is to use as the primary outcome a score that is a combination of efficacy and adverse event outcomes. The problem with this approach is that there must be a prospectively identified weighting of these two types of outcome, such as the prolongation of x deaths by y or more years is worth z deaths from adverse effects of the intervention. It is very difficult to specify such weighting a priori, however, and it is likely an exercise in fantasy to formulate an approach to the computation of a trial size based on such a score. Another approach is shift the focus to defining the criterion for success by identifying two or more objectives, perhaps based on efficacy, adverse effects, quality of life, cost of care, or the like, and then to explicitly state the criterion for each of these identified objectives. Overall success is then defined as meeting the criteria for success associated with all objectives. Conditional successes based on meeting subsets of criteria could also be defined, or definitions of success for subsets of objectives could be deferred for consensus development following completion of the RCT. The sample size is computed to be the larger of the independently computed trial sizes for each separate objective. In this approach the problem of assigning the a priori weighting is avoided by transferring the consideration to the definition of a type of composite success, but an implicit weighting scheme is still present in the criteria used to compute the trial sizes associated with each objective. Also, this method does not allow for a composite success to be defined conditionally on the magnitudes of the outcome; for example, more adverse effects may be acceptable for larger magnitudes of outcome benefit. The problem of basing the criterion for success on a mixture of outcomes does not have a generally satisfactory solution.

ELIGIBILITY CONSIDERATIONS

The types of patients to be enrolled into a RCT are identified in the protocol using eligibility criteria, which may be highly restrictive or more open.[8] If restrictive, then the RCT results will be less like general clinical practice and therefore less generalizable, but may have the advantage of protecting some types of patients from harm or providing information on aspects of the interventions that might be observed if the eligibility criteria were more open.

As a RCT is conducted, patient elegibility issues are inevitable and criteria for defining eligibility with respect to the analysis of the RCT should be clearly stated in the protocol. The guiding principle is to include all "eligible patients randomized" in the primary analyses of any RCT because including all eligible patients preserves the randomization. Invariably some patients not meeting the eligibility criteria will be randomized, however, usually as a result of incomplete review of prerandomization materials or lack of rigor by investigators. The definition of "eligible patients randomized" is a key step in the design and analysis of RCTs. There are two possibilities regarding the discovery of randomized patients not meeting eligibility criteria: (1) the discovery is based on subsequent review of data or materials collected prior to randomization, and the discovery of such cases is equally likely in each arm of the RCT; or (2) that discovery is based on data or material that becomes available following randomization or data or material collected prior to randomization, and subsequent discovery is not equally likely in each arm. The declaration of a patient as ineligible for the purposes of exclusion from the analyses can only be based on condition 1 because the data or materials used to discover the ineligibility are equally applicable to both arms and are not influenced by any differences in intervention. In condition 2 there is a possibility of a difference between arms with respect to the ease of declaring patients ineligible because behaviors following randomization are likely influenced by differences between the arms in what is done to the patient. Therefore, the definition of "eligible patients randomized" as used in this chapter refers to all patients randomized except those found to be ineligible under condition 1. All other patients randomized, including those discovered under condition 2, are regarded as eligible for the purposes of analysis.

INTERIM ANALYSES

The protocol should also include specification of a formal analysis plan.[1,9] The analysis plan lays out the schedule of all formal analyses, including the formal final analysis. A formal analysis is one that potentially could change the course of the trial or that is used to represent the final results of the trial. These formal analyses should be planned with adjusted significance levels so that there is protection against erroneous conclusions resulting from multiple looks at the data. In addition, a formal analysis plan minimizes the temptation to engage in "data-directed analyses" and maximizes validity of the final result. The protocol should also specify a plan for monitoring the trial's progress and following the formal analysis plan, including the possibility of a data and safety monitoring committee that is at least to some degree independent of the investigators.[10] The monitoring plan should specify that trial results will not be revealed before either the data are mature or a criterion for early presentation for results is met (as specified in the analysis plan) in order to avoid the possibility of publication of results that have insufficient statistical power[11] or have an adverse effect on accrual.[12]

The difference in the duration of survival as measured from the date of randomization is often a preferred primary outcome in cancer trials. The date of death is generally easy to obtain and there is no subjectivity in its ascertainment, and a prolongation of survival usually represents a direct benefit to the patient, for example. However, in diseases in which survival is long, such as early-stage prostate cancer, the trials may have to be quite large and take a long time to complete; therefore, there are strong temptations to use an alternative primary outcome, such as progression-free survival, response to therapy, or local control. The justification for using an alternative to survival as the primary outcome usually takes one or both of two forms: the alternative primary outcomes is claimed to be a surrogate outcome for survival, or the alternative primary outcome may be argued to represent a direct patient benefit. The use of putative surrogate outcomes for survival can often give erroneous results, however, and there will likely be other excellent examples of the failure of surrogate outcomes in the future.[13,14]

An example of a current surrogate outcome issue in early-stage prostate cancer is that of neoadjuvant hormonal therapy (NHT). The report of an RCT of NHT based on looking at pathologic stage as the primary outcome showed a significant difference,[15] but a subsequent report failed to show that this difference in pathologic findings translated to a difference in progression based on prostate-specific antigen (PSA) findings at 1 year of follow-up.[16] Thus there remain many questions, including questions about the meaning of the pathologic outcome, whether there was sufficient statistical power to claim there is no difference in PSA progression, and whether there would ultimately be a difference in survival. Unfortunately, this trial was not sized for a survival difference because only 303 patients were randomized.[15] In contrast, the Southwest Oncology Group recently initiated a NHT trial in which survival is the primary outcome, and this trial requires the randomization of 1740 patients.

Whenever the use of survival as the primary outcome appears not to be feasible, because of either trial size or duration, there should be decisive and exhaustive efforts devoted to pursuing administrative solutions, such as trial simplification and expansion to include investigators, that would assure very rapid accrual, rather than the dangerous and potentially wasteful use of an alternative or surrogate primary outcome.

RANDOMIZATION

Randomization is a fundamental design principle throughout scientific research because it provides an explicit mechanism for controlling extraneous factors. In the RCT (as well as in other types of scientific study designs that use randomization) the effects of extraneous factors are controlled because the assignment of the interventions is probabilistically independent of extraneous factors. Preintervention patient characteristics that are potentially related to the outcome in a RCT are called extraneous factors (relative to the primary objective of the RCT) because they are not the objective of the trial. The probabilistic independence between arm and extraneous factors is the basis of the potential for validity of RCT results because the comparisons of the outcomes between arms are independent of the extraneous factors. Within a given trial, the probabilistic independence between arms and extraneous factors means that there is a high likelihood that the patients assigned to each arm of the trial will be similar with respect to extraneous factors. Therefore, it is unlikely that an observed between-arm difference in outcome is confounded by differences between the arms with respect to extraneous factors.

The probabilistic independence between arm and extraneous factors applies to *all* extraneous factors, those measured as well as those not measured. Thus it is likely the patients assigned to each arm will be similar with respect to previously identified extraneous factors and also those that are not currently known.

Suppose two interventions for early stage prostate cancer are to be compared—for example, radical prostatectomy versus watchful waiting—with respect to a difference on overall survival. Some preintervention patient characteristics, such as Gleason score, PSA, patient age, and general health, have a putative prognostic relationship to overall survival in early-stage prostate cancer patients, and these are referred to as extraneous factors. In a RCT, patients with high Gleason scores are not more likely to receive one intervention over another because the intervention assignment is probabilistically independent of Gleason score. Similarly, the patients assigned to each arm will also likely be similar with respect to unmeasured extraneous factors. Thus the comparison of the arms will likely not be confounded by uneven distribution of extraneous factors between the arms.

The probabilistic independence between intervention assignment and extraneous factors implemented by randomization means there is a very high likelihood that the groups of patients assigned to each intervention will have similar characteristics, but randomization does not guarantee that the groups will be similar in all respects. In this context, "similar" means that extraneous factors have approximately the same distribution in each of the arms; that is, there are no glaring imbalances in the distribution of patient characteristics across the arms. The possibility of imbalances exists because randomization is a probabilistic process, not a deterministic process. The existence of between-arm differences does not mean that the random assignment process was executed improperly. In fact, it is likely that the arms will have at least one characteristic on which there will be a statistically significant difference. The random process of playing card shuffling and distribution has some elements of similarity and contrasting dissimilarities to randomization in clinical trials. Playing cards are shuffled and then distributed (a random process) in order to form hands (analogous to the patients groups in an RCT), but in card games the players use their skills in order to exploit the small differences between hands. Thus, although there is a similarity of intent and outcome with respect to the use of randomization, there is also a big difference between the RCT and playing cards: In a RCT there does not exist an analogy for the player, who in card games acts as an agent to selectively manipulate the outcome for the assigned hand using an assessment of small imbalances and the knowledge gained by observing the actions of the other players. Thus in a RCT there will likely be small between-arm patient differences, but these small differences are not being actively exploited by an agent acting with at least some knowledge of the differences and intent to exploit them.

Consider the alternative of simply collecting data on groups of patients treated using the interventions to be compared where the choice of intervention is a patient/physician choice—that is, randomization is not used to assign interventions. When randomization is not used, extraneous factors are not probabilistically independent of intervention assignment, and this leads to a high likelihood of an imbalance with respect to extraneous factors. For example, patients who are not surgical candidates would not likely receive a surgical treatment. Now there are statistical methods that can provide limited adjustments for the effect of extraneous factor imbalances between intervention groups. The most common are regression models, including logistic regression for dichotomous outcomes and proportional hazard regression (Cox regression) for time-to-event outcomes. In these statistical models, the known extraneous factors are entered into the model as covariates. These regression model methods have gross limitations, however, including limitations in the types of imbalances that can be effectively adjusted for, the inability to completely adjust for even simple imbalances when there are strong correlations between two or more extraneous factors, and the inability to control for imbalances in extraneous factors that are not known about and therefore unmeasured (this is called the missing covariate problem). Therefore, when interventions are to be compared using data in which the intervention has not been randomly assigned, it is not possible to feel confident that the effect of imbalances in extraneous factors can be adjusted for completely using advanced statistical methods.

Because of the possibility of randomization imbalances, the presentation of any RCT should always include analyses assessing the degree to which the patient groups are similar. This assessment can also serve to demonstrate to the reader that the randomization was done correctly. The objective is to discover the presence of gross randomization imbalances. This is done by using statistical tests for imbalances in the distribution of preintervention patient characteristics across the arms. The statistical tests usually done are univariate tests; that is, they test for the existence of an imbalance for one characteristic at a time. However, a collection of K univariate tests must be interpreted with care because even if the randomization process is executed properly, the probability that at least one test will be significant at the 0.05 level is $1 - (1 - 0.015)^K$. Thus, for five statistical tests this probability is 0.23, and therefore there exists a high probability (0.23) of finding a significant difference by chance alone. It follows that, when a series of univariate tests with a 0.05 level of significance are used to assess the quality of a randomization, there is a high probability of making a type I error—that is, concluding that there is a flaw in the randomization when there is not one. If a series of univariate tests are used to assess the quality of the randomization, then there should be an adjustment in the significance level used in the individual tests, or the presentation of the results from such testing should include a strong cautionary statement about the high probability of a type I error.

Multivariate statistical tests provide an alternative to assessing randomization quality, but are seldom used. Multivariate tests test for distributional differences using more than one patient characteristic and are particularly accurate (i.e., avoid type I errors) when there exist strong correlations between characteristics. For example, the T^2 test is a generalization of the univariate t test and can be used for a collection of continuous measurements. However, multivariate testing is much more difficult to do, especially when there are mixed data types, such as both continuous and discrete measurements. When there are mixed data types, the T^2 test cannot be used and advanced regression methods must be used; for example, logistic regression with arm as the outcome variable can be used to test for the dependence of the probability of assignment to a specific arm on the extraneous factors (covariates).

It should be noted that the potential for randomization imbalances to invalidate the results from a RCT is relatively a much smaller potential problem than the potential for incomplete adjustment for between-group differences in nonrandomized intervention comparisons. In the RCT, the test assessing for randomization flaws is a test for an unlikely event (assuming that randomization was done properly), whereas in nonrandomized intervention comparisons, the between-intervention-group differences in extraneous factors are relatively easy to identify when measured but are difficult to adjust for using statistical models, and unmeasured extraneous factors are not adjusted for in any way. Therefore, two articles comparing the same interventions, one presenting the results from a RCT and the other presenting a nonrandomized comparison (e.g., case series data), may look somewhat similar in that the same kinds of tables and statistical models are used, but the RCT results have a much greater potential for validity. The reader will only know that this huge difference in potential for validity exists if the reader has a thorough understanding of the principles underlying the RCT and the limitations of making intervention comparisons from data in which randomization is not used.

ANALYSIS BY INTENT-TO-TREAT (ANALYSIS BY ARM)

One of the most difficult concepts and bothersome aspects of RCTs analysis for those who do not understand the reasons is the principle of analysis by intent-to-treat. Analysis by intent-to-treat is another term for analysis by arm. In an analysis by arm, the outcomes for all eligible patients randomized to each arm are compared to those for other arms regardless of the intervention actually received. Recall that an arm in a RCT is the name for a group of randomly assigned patients where the intent is that each patient in that arm receive the intervention associated with that arm. The bothersome aspect of analysis by arm is that not all patients in a given arm *will* receive the intervention associated with that arm, and in fact some may receive an intervention associated with another arm of the RCT. The term "intent-to-treat" is used in order to emphasize boldly that the analysis is based on intent rather than the intervention actually received. To those who have not considered carefully the principles underlying the design of RCTs, the comparison of outcomes for groups of patients when not every patient in each group received the same intervention seems like heresy. To make matters worse, the analyses by arm are (should be) featured as the primary analysis presenting the definitive results of the trial, and other analyses, such as those analyzing patients according to the treatment actually received, are (should be) presented as secondary analyses with strong warnings about the potential for bias in these types of secondary analyses.

For example, at the end of the Prostate Cancer Intervention Versus Observation Trial (PIVOT),[17] the primary analysis will feature a comparison of the survival between the eligible patients randomized to the arm where the intent is to treat surgically to those randomized to the arm where the intent is to use an intervention based on expectant management. Because of refusals or postrandomization discovery of comorbid conditions precluding the initiation of the intended intervention, however, there will be patients in both arms who do not receive the intended intervention. Thus the primary analysis will include patients in the surgery arm who did not receive surgery, and patients in the expectant management arm who refused expectant management and got surgery almost immediately, and patients in both arms who received other forms of initial therapy (such as external beam radiation therapy or brachytherapy).

The underlying and dominant principle on which analysis by arm is based is the preservation of the between-arm (patient group) comparability created through the random assignment of patients to the arms. Recall that the purpose of randomization is to assign interventions in a way that is probabilistically independent of extraneous factors, with the effect of creating groups of patients (the arms) who are likely to be comparable in all regards, even those not measured. When patients are removed from the analysis because of not receiving the intended intervention, or are reassigned to another arm because of receiving the intervention associated with that arm, then there is a high likelihood of eroding the between-group comparability. Furthermore, there is a high likelihood that intervention deviations will occur for reasons that are not independent of the intended intervention and the outcome, leading to an even greater potential for biased results.

For example, in the PIVOT[17] it will be likely that at least some of the patients randomized to the surgical intervention arm will be discovered after randomization to have a condition that precludes surgery. However, conditions that preclude surgery are also likely indicators of a reduced potential for survival. Therefore, an estimate of survival for surgery based on removing patients who did not receive surgery from the analysis will lead to an estimate of survival that is biased upward relative to that which would be estimated using all patients who received surgery. An even more serious bias would be present in a comparison of survival in patients who received surgery and those who received expectant management wherein some of the patients randomized to the surgery arm who did not receive surgery received expectant management instead.

Actually the concept of analysis by intent-to-treat may be more reflective of clinical practice in settings outside of the RCT. The literature is permeated with outcome estimates from clinical series of patients treated in a specific fashion. Consider two kinds of estimates: (1) those based only on patients who received the intervention, and (2) those based on patients who were identified as being candidates for and committing to the specific intervention. Both types of estimates would seem to be useful (provided the population could be adequately characterized), but the second type of estimate would seem to be more relevant.

There is a cost to the preservation of between-arm comparability provided by analysis by arm. For example, whenever an intervention has some degree of efficacy, the estimated outcome using all patients assigned to the associated arm will be attenuated because of the patients who do not receive the intervention (as described for the PIVOT example). The greater the percentage of intervention deviations, the larger will be the effect on the attenuation. Therefore, if many intervention deviations are expected, then the trial size must be adjusted upward based on an estimate of the amount of attenuation expected. If a large percentage of patients are expected to not receive the intended intervention, then it might be useful to redefine the description of the intervention to be less treatment specific.

Thus the analysis by arm leads to the following presentation style for the result of a RCT. The analytic results should be stated in terms of arms (not interventions)—for example, arm A is (not) significantly different than arm B. All statements regarding specific interventions should be clearly labeled as conclusions based on assuming that the results from the arms are representative of outcomes for the applicable interventions. Analyses by intervention received (as compared to analyses by arm) should be clearly labeled as secondary analyses, with clearly worded applicable cautionary statements about the potential for lack of comparability between intervention patient groups. Appropriate methods for attempting a statistical adjustment for differences between the characteristics of the patients in the intervention groups should be part of any such secondary analyses.

REPRESENTATIVES AND RANDOMIZATION

In statistics textbooks, the most common paradigm underlying the validity of the statistical methods described is that of obtaining a statistical estimate of or testing a hypothesis about a feature of a population using a random sample of data from that population. Specifically, the sample is the observational unit on which data have been collected, and the population is the conceptual framework of units that could have been members of the sample. The simplest method of sampling is called simple random sampling, whereby each unit in the population has an equal chance of becoming a member of the sample. Thus the concept of random sampling forms the basis for arguing that a statistical procedure—for example, the estimation of a mean or a median or the test of a hypothesis—is unbiased or valid for the population of interest. If the sample is not randomly selected, then it is difficult to argue that it is representative, and therefore estimates will be biased and hypothesis tests are not valid. In the usual textbook presentation, statistical validity and representativeness are therefore tied together under the paradigm of a random sampling from a population.

The act of obtaining a random sample from a population is not an explicit concern when planning and executing a RCT, however. In fact, it would be very difficult to argue that the participants included in a RCT (the sample) are representative of a meaningful population. First, RCTs are only done by investigators who have a clinical research interest, and the potential patients available to that investigator for recruitment to a RCT are not likely representative of the general population of potentially eligible patients. Second, not all potentially eligible patients are approached for participation in a RCT, often because of circumstances of availability, or of perceptions of the likelihood of refusal to participate. Finally, not all potentially eligible patients offered the opportunity to participate in a RCT will do so. These processes interfere with representativeness of the patients enrolled into a RCT, and are complex and undefinable. Therefore, it is futile to argue that the patients enrolled in a RCT are representative of anything other than themselves. (*Note*: It is difficult to argue that statistical estimates reported for a clinical series, or even a collection of clinical series, are representative of a usefully definable population for the same reasons cited for RCTs, even though the erosion of representativeness from selections and refusals are somewhat diminished. It could be claimed that the patients included in clinical series therefore are somewhat more representative of a usefully definable population, but in neither case is the ideal of a random sample from a population even approached.)

The basis for the statistical validity of the results from a RCT cannot therefore be based on the "random sample from a population" paradigm. Instead, statistical validity is based on the act of randomization. (It is important to note that intervention assignment based on randomization is conceptionally and operationally distinct from random sampling.) The validity of tests of hypotheses in randomized clinical trials is based on referring the statistic computed from the data obtained (e.g., a difference in proportions) under the randomization used in the trial to the distribution of such possible statistics computed using the data observed and all possible random assignments that could have been made. This procedure is called a randomization testing and is conditional on the data values obtained from the trial.[18] If there is no intervention effect, then the statistic observed will likely be a value indicating no effect and therefore be in the middle of the distribution of statistical values generated from all permutations of random assignments on the observed data. If the observed statistical value is not in the middle of the distribution of all possible assignments, however, then it is concluded that either there is no effect and the random assignment "chosen" for the RCT produced an unusual outcome, or there is evidence that assumption of no effect is incorrect. Randomization testing is loosely analogous to assessing the fairness of dealing in a poker game. If a player is dealt four aces, then either the dealing is fair and a highly unusual event has occurred, or there is evidence of unfair dealing. In applications of the randomization test, a P value quantifies the probability of the observed outcome under the assumption of no effect.

When statistical inference is based on the paradigm of randomization (as compared to the paradigm of a random sample from a population), then the argument for generalizability of the results must be based on an assessment of the similarity of the characteristics of the patients included in the RCT to those to whom the results might be applied. Therefore, it is important that the patients included in a RCT be carefully characterized in any report of the results so that the reader can make this assessment.

The explicit computation of a randomization test for a RCT is not often done because the number of all possible random assignments is usually quite large, and therefore the computations would be prodigious even using today's computers.[19] An exception is the use of Fisher's exact test for comparing proportions. It can be shown mathematically that Fisher's exact test is in fact a randomization test and although the computations are burdensome, they are not prodigious. When the computations are prodigious, approximations to randomization tests are used. For example, it has been shown that traditional statistical tests (t test, log rank test, χ-square test, etc.) provide good approximations to randomization test P values for sufficiently large sample sizes.[18] In this case the use of traditional statistical tests does not mean that there has been a shift to a "random sample from a population" paradigm; instead, the P value from the traditional test is regarded as an approximation to the randomization test P value. Most applications of traditional statistical tests to RCTs are not identified as approximations to randomizations tests, however, and in fact there is seldom any discussion of the issue of random sampling versus randomization tests in the presentation of RCTs.

DISCUSSION

This chapter has attempted to discuss some of the fundamental principles in the design, conduct, and analysis of RCTs. Specifically, definitions of the concepts and terminology of the RCT has been defined, the need for a protocol and some of its elements have been identified, the principle of randomization and its applicability to RCTs has been described, the important principle of the analysis by intent-to-treat and its rationale have been detailed, and some of the principles underlying the generalizability of RCTs have been defined. Many more principles and issues have not been covered, however, mainly because of space limitations. These include trial management, data quality, surrogate outcomes, large simple trials, crossover designs, neoadjuvant studies, double or single blinding, factorial designs, intervention-by-intervention interactions (in factorial designs), stratification, interventions-by-stratification interactions, quality-of-life outcomes, economic outcomes, prerandomization, and ethical issues, among others. The reader no doubt realizes that the subject of the RCT is a deep one.

The main theme of the RCT topics chosen to be included in this article has been to convince the reader of the superiority of the RCT for intervention comparisons as contrasted to the use of comparisons based on clinical series data. This approach to topic selections was motivated by the author's observation that, although many clinicians are able to articulate that RCT methodology is superior, it is rare that a clinician is able to articulate adequately the reasons why.

RCTs are not simply superior to the use of clinical series data for the comparison of interventions; RCTs are vastly superior for all the reasons given in this article, and many reasons that are not described because of space restrictions. The author's personal observation is that there is a general lack of appreciation for this quantification of the superiority of RCTs, and too often evidence from RCTs and clinical series data are almost equally weighted when critically appraising the relative merits of two or more interventions.

There are two additional relevant observations. First, often those who are able to articulate that the RCT is the superior methodology for addressing interventional issues continue to spend inordinate efforts promoting clearly inferior approaches, such as registries or other forms of gathering clinical series data, instead of addressing the difficult administrative and consensus development issues involved in promoting meaningful RCTs. Second, there are too few RCTs addressing truly important issues and too many clinical series articles.

As a result of the paucity of RCT data addressing issues in early-stage prostate cancer patients, for example, clinicians have only clinical series data on which to base important treatment decisions. This sad state of affairs is evident in recently published treatment guidelines for early-stage prostate cancer, wherein it was found that there are no acceptable RCT data on which to base recommendations for treatment decisions.[20] Because the trials that need to be done in order to provide the needed data have yet to be opened (PIVOT is one exception,[17] adjuvant radiation therapy in pathologic stage C prostate cancer is another[21]), it could be a decade or more before definitive answers can be known concerning some of these important questions (a little less time for the exceptions cited).

RCTs are not completely absent from urologic cancer research literature. For example, there have been over 20 RCTs addressing the scientific hypothesis concerning the potential benefit from the use of antiandrogens in metastatic prostate cancer, including a meta-analysis of these RCTs.[11,22,23] The difference between the situation in early-stage versus late-stage prostate cancer appears to be related to the ease with which the trial can be done, especially how easy it is to convince the patient to allow the treatment selection to be chosen randomly and how quickly the final results become available. Also, there are a number of factors that make surgical RCTs more difficult,[24] and many of the urologic oncology trials that need to be done are trials that would include surgical or surgical-type interventions, such as brachytherapy versus prostatectomy or brachytherapy versus external beam radiotherapy. Thus it is possible to do RCTs in urologic cancers, but it appears that the will to do RCTs evaporates when the trials to be done are difficult. There are also important and difficult issues in other urologic cancers that remain to be addressed adequately, such as a comparison of nephrectomy to partial nephrectomy.

PIVOT is an example of a really difficult and important RCT in early-stage prostate cancer.[17] PIVOT has accrued over 200 patients in 1.5 years, although whether PIVOT will be successful ultimately remains to be seen. PIVOT provides an example that it is not impossible to initiate and have some success with a very difficult RCT. Fortunately, many of the RCTs that need to be done would not be as difficult as PIVOT.

What is needed today in urologic cancer clinical research are leaders who are willing to undertake the difficult role of advocating the necessary RCTs. The role as a leader means a commitment to the time necessary to implement such RCTs through consensus development, rigorous protocol creation, recruitment of sufficient numbers and types of investigators to enable the trial to be done, insistence on high standards for data collection and monitoring, and continued education of investigators and sponsors regarding the importance of participation. Although such activities can be frustrating, the potential for a meaningful contribution to clinical science is great.

REFERENCES

1. Simon RM: Design and conduct of clinical trials. *In* De Vita VT, Hellman S, Rosenberg SA (eds): Principles and Practice of Oncology, 4th edition, pp 418–440. Philadelphia, JB Lippincott Co, 1993.
2. Simon R: A decade of progress in statistical methodology for clinical trials. Stat Med 1991; 10:1789–1817.

3. Meinert CL: Clinical Trials. New York, Oxford University Press, 1986.
4. Buyse ME, Staquet MJ, Sylvester RJ: Cancer Clinical Trials: Methods and Practice. Oxford, England, Oxford University Press, 1984.
5. Pocock SJ: Clinical Trials. Chichester, England, John Wiley & Sons, 1983.
6. Friedman LM, Furberg CD, DeMets DL: Fundamentals of Clinical Trials. Boston, Wright, 1981.
7. Blumenstein BA, James KE, Lind KL, Mitchell HE: Functions and organization of coordinating centers for multicenter clinical trials. Controlled Clin Trials 1995; 16(2S): 4S–29S.
8. George SL: Reducing patient eligibility criteria in cancer clinical trials. J Clin Oncol 1996; 14:1364–1370.
9. Green SJ, Fleming TR: Guidelines for the reporting of clinical trials. Semin Oncol 1988; 15:455–461.
10. Harrington D, Crowley J, George SL, et al: The case against independent data monitoring committees. Stat Med 1994; 13:1411–1414.
11. Blumenstein BA: Some statistical considerations for the interpretation of trials of combined androgen therapy. Cancer 1993; 72(Suppl):3834–3840.
12. Crowley J, Green S, Liu PY, Wolf M: Data monitoring committees and early stopping guidelines: the Southwest Oncology Group experience. Stat Med 1994; 13:1391–1399.
13. Fleming TR: Surrogate markers in AIDS and cancer trials. Stat Med 1994; 13:1423–1435.
14. Fleming TR: Evaluating therapeutic interventions: some issues and experiences. Stat Sci 1992; 7:428–456.
15. Soloway MS, Sharifi R, Wajsman Z, et al: Randomized prospective study comparing radical prostatectomy alone versus radical prostatectomy preceded by androgen blockade in clinical stage B2 (T2bNxM0) prostate cancer. J Urol 1995; 154:424–428.
16. Soloway MS, Sharifi R, Wajsman Z, et al: Randomized prospective study—radical prostatectomy alone vs radical prostatectomy preceded by androgen blockade in cT2b prostate cancer—initial results [Abstract]. J Urol 1996; 155(suppl):555A.
17. Wilt TJ, Brawer MK: The Prostate Cancer Intervention Versus Observation Trial: a randomized trial comparing radical prostatectomy versus expectant management for the treatment of clinical localized prostate cancer. J Urol 1994; 152:1910.
18. Kempthorne O: The randomization theory of experimental inference. J Am Stat Assoc 1955; 50:946–967.
19. Edgington ES: Randomization Tests. New York, Marcel Dekker, 1980.
20. Middleton RG, Thompson IM, Austinfeld MS, et al: Prostate Cancer Clinical Guidelines Panel summary report on the management of clinically localized prostate cancer. J Urol 1995; 154:2144–2148.
21. Thompson IM, Paradelo JC, Crawford ED, et al: An opportunity to determine optimal treatment of pT3 prostate cancer: the window may be closing. Urology 1994; 44: 804–811.
22. Prostate Cancer Trialists' Group: Maximum androgen blockade in advanced prostate cancer: an overview of 23 randomised trials with 3238 deaths in 5710 patients. Lancet 1995; 346:265–269.
23. Blumenstein BA: Overview analysis issues using combined androgen deprivation overview analysis as an example. Urol Oncol 1995; 1:95–100.
24. McLeon RS, Wright JG, Soloman MJ, et al: Randomized controlled trials in surgery: issues and problems. Surgery 1996; 119:483–486.

INDEX

Note: Page numbers in *italics* refer to illustrations; page numbers followed by "t" refer to tables.